Revised as per the CBME curri

Mudaliar and Men

Clinical Obstetrics

THIRTEENTH EDITION

Revised as per the CBME curriculum

Mudaliar and Menon's
Clinical Obstetrics

THIRTEENTH EDITION

A L Mudaliar
MD, LLD, DSc, DCL (Oxon), FRCOG, FACS, FRCF Ed (Hon)

M K Krishna Menon
BA, MD, FRCOG, FAMS

Edited by

T Radha Bai Prabhu
MD, DGO, MNAMS, FRCOG, FRCS, PhD, DSc

Professor and HOD, Department of Obstetrics and Gynaecology,
Sri Muthu Kumaran Medical College Hospital and Research Institute, Chennai

Former Director and Superintendent, Institute of Obstetrics and Gynaecology and
Government Hospital for Women and Children, Chennai

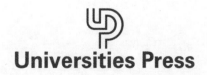

Universities Press

MUDALIAR AND MENON'S CLINICAL OBSTETRICS, THIRTEENTH EDITION

UNIVERSITIES PRESS (INDIA) PRIVATE LIMITED

Registered Office
3-6-747/1/A & 3-6-754/1, Himayatnagar, Hyderabad 500 029, Telangana, India
info@universitiespress.com; www.universitiespress.com

Distributed by
Orient Blackswan Private Limited

Registered Office
3-6-752, Himayatnagar, Hyderabad 500 029, Telangana, India

Other Offices
Bengaluru, Chennai, Guwahati, Hyderabad, Kolkata, Mumbai, New Delhi, Noida, Patna, Visakhapatnam

© Universities Press (India) Private Limited 2011, 2015, 2023
First edition published in Great Britain by Oliver and Boyd, SW Edinburgh 1938
Fifth edition published in India 1962
Seventh edition 1972: Reprinted 1974, 1975
Eighth edition 1978
Ninth edition 1990: Reprinted 1991, 1992, 1994, 1995 (Twice), 1997, 1998, 1999 (Twice), 2000, 2001, 2002, 2003 (Twice), 2005
Tenth edition 2005: Reprinted 2006 (Twice), 2007, 2008
First Universities Press Impression 2008: Reprinted 2009, 2010 (Twice), 2011
Eleventh edition 2011: Reprinted 2012 (Three times), 2013, 2014
Twelfth edition 2015: Reprinted 2016, 2017, 2018, 2019, 2020
Thirteenth edition 2023

ISBN 978-93-93330-36-9

501879

Cover and book design
© Universities Press (India) Private Limited 2023

All product and company names are trademarks™ or registered® trademarks of their respective holders. Use of them does not imply any affiliation with or endorsement by them.

Typeset in Life BT 10.5/12.5 pt *by*
e-Leaf Technologies, Chennai

Printed in India at
SS Colour Impression Pvt Ltd, Chennai 600 106

Published by
Universities Press (India) Private Limited
3-6-747/1/A & 3-6-754/1, Himayatnagar, Hyderabad 500 029, Telangana, India

Table of Contents

Preface to the Thirteenth Edition

It has been nearly seven years since the twelfth edition of *Mudaliar and Menon's Clinical Obstetrics* was published. In the last few years, there have been numerous advances and developments in the fields of obstetrics and gynecology. In 2019, the National Medical Council (NMC) introduced the Competency-Based Medical Education (CBME) curriculum for undergraduate students, which focusses on imparting knowledge, clinical expertise, communication skills and ethics in medical practice to students of medicine. Keeping these developments in mind, in this 13th edition, we have endeavoured to meet the recommendations made by the NMC to help students optimally benefit from the book.

To keep up with the recent advances in the subject, we have made a sincere effort to revise all the chapters and to update them with the most current information available at the time of publication. While topics such as prenatal diagnosis, abnormal labour, hypertensive disorders and MTP have been thoroughly updated in keeping with the most recent international guidelines, this edition also features new topics such as Zika and COVID infections. Epilepsy and asthma, shoulder dystocia and bronchial asthma have been covered in newly added chapters. A new chapter has also been added on medical ethics and medicolegal issues, as these are important aspects of medicine that should be taught to students of the subject so that they may learn to ethically practice medicine.

Each chapter opens with a mention of the CMBE competencies covered therein as well as a list of learning objectives that outline the knowledge and skills a student would acquire from that chapter. Evidence-based information is provided in accordance with the latest guidelines recommended by national and international bodies. Examination is the most difficult challenge faced by a medical student. Keeping this in mind, essential points are presented in boxes, tables and algorithms for better comprehension and ease of memorisation. A number of clinical photographs and USG images have been added to aid in the visualisation of concepts. In most chapters, discussions on clinical scenarios have been added to help students to understand the clinical aspects and problem-based approach to various ailments. To encourage students to self-learn, the essay questions, short answer questions and MCQs at the end of each chapter have been extensively updated.

The list of people I would like to thank for their invaluable contributions to this edition is too long to include here. In particular, however, I would like to acknowledge Dr K Jayashree Srinivasan for contributing the chapter on ethics and medicolegal issues and Dr Arasar Seeralan for meticulously editing the section on newborn and neonatal problems. Thanks are also due to Dr Sampathkumari, Dr Karthiga Prabhu, Dr Sravani Chitra, Dr Bharathy Dhala, Dr B H Parameshwar Keerthi and Professor M P Kanchana for their help.

I am deeply indebted to Professor Colleen Srinivasan for the tutelage and guidance I received from her. A former student of Professor Krishna Menon, she recalled him often in her lectures. It is largely the knowledge and skills imparted to me by this great teacher, clinician, academician and surgeon par excellence that gave me the strength and confidence to take on the daunting task of editing this prestigious book.

I consider myself privileged to have had the opportunity to edit this thirteenth edition. It is my hope that undergraduate and postgraduate students as well as teachers will benefit from it, and that it will help students not only to pass their exams, but also to apply the knowledge so acquired to clinical practice in the future.

T Radha Bai Prabhu

Email: radhaprabhu54@ymail.com

Acknowledgements

- I take this opportunity to thank all those whose invaluable contributions, efforts and time went into the revision of this classic textbook.
- Special thanks are owed to Dr Jayashree Srinivasan, my friend and Professor of Obstetrics and Gynaecology, Saveetha Medical College, Chennai, for writing the chapter on 'Ethics and Medicolegal Issues in Obstetrics' and for her final round of checks to ensure that everything was in order.
- I am extremely thankful to Dr Arasar Seeralan, Professor of Paediatrics, ACS Medical College Hospital and Research Institute, Chennai, for diligently updating the neonatology section.
- Thanks are due to Dr Sampathkumari, Professor of Obstetrics and Gynaecology, Sri Muthukumaran Medical College Hospital, Chennai, for updating the MCQs.
- I thank Dr Karthiga Prabhu, my niece and Professor of Obstetrics and Gynaecology, SRM Medical College Hospital and Research Institute, Chennai, for going through the manuscript and sharing with me her valuable inputs and suggestions. She also significantly helped with the editing of this book and prepared insightful case-based scenarios, which I am sure will be very useful to students.
- I am grateful to Dr Sravani Chithra, Assistant Professor of Obstetrics and Gynaecology, Sri Muthukumaran Medical College Hospital and Research Institute, Chennai, for preparing PowerPoint Presentations for this book. She also provided me with a number of interesting clinical photographs.
- My heartfelt thanks to Dr Bharathy Y Dhala, Consultant Radiologist, Athena Diagnostics, Chennai, and Dr B H Parameshwar Keerthi, Consultant Radiologist, BM Scans, Kancheepuram, for the excellent and valuable USG images they contributed to the book. I would also like to thank Dr M P Kanchana, Professor of Pathology, Institute of Obstetrics and Gynaecology, for her excellent HPE photographs.
- I must thank the team at Universities Press, especially Mr Madhu Reddy and Dr Sudha Ganesan for entrusting this prestigious book to me, and to Mr Ravi Vishwakarma for putting me in touch with Universities Press. I thank Dr Alpa Agrawal for her inputs, suggestions and immense cooperation during this revision and Ms Malini Gopalakrishnan for her efforts in meticulously copy editing the book. I also thank the rest of the team for the untiring work that went into bringing out this edition.
- I would like to acknowledge my postgraduate students and department faculty for collecting numerous clinical photographs that have been included in this book.
- I thank all my teachers and also my students, who have always been a source of inspiration and are the reason I became a teacher.
- I must mention my mother, who was always my pillar of strength; though she is no longer with me, it is from her memory that I drew the strength and confidence to take on this project.
- Finally, I thank God for his blessings and for giving me this opportunity and the time and wherewithal to complete the revision of this book to the best of my abilities.

T Radha Bai Prabhu

Preface to the Fifth Edition

The delay in bringing out this 5th edition of the book has been great. I regret the delay, but it has, however, been of benefit in several respects.

It is with pleasure that I record here that Dr M K Krishna Menon, BA, MD, Director, Institute of Obstetrics and Gynaecology, Government Hospital for Women and Children, Madras, and Professor of Obstetrics and Gynaecology, Madras Medical College, has found it possible to associate himself with me in the preparation of this edition. Dr Krishna Menon collaborated with me when the first book was brought out in 1938 and gave much valuable help in the 4th edition of this book. In this edition, all the statistics collected in the recent years have been made available by him and in many respects, he has been responsible for the revision of certain chapters. The book is, therefore, being issued in the joint names of both of us. I am thankful to the Government of Madras for giving him permission to associate himself with the publication of this edition. This book, however, is not an official publication.

I am also thankful to Dr A Venugopal Mudaliar, MS, FACS, Honorary Surgeon, General Hospital, Madras, for having once more helped me in regard to some of the chapters.

I am thankful to Dr V Rajagopalan, FFARCS, for his help and advice in the preparation of the chapter on Anaesthesia and Analgesia in Labour.

This edition is being published by Orient Longmans Ltd., to whom I am deeply indebted. They have spared no pains in the production of the book in a proper manner.

I trust this book with be useful for undergraduates, for candidates appearing for post-graduate qualifications in Obstetrics and for junior practitioners. Our intention has always been to emphasise the clinical and practical aspects in the practice of Obstetrics, and we hope the book will be found suitable as a text-book of clinical obstetrics.

A L Mudaliar

'Kensington'

Kilpauk, Madras

South India

1st July 1962

Preface to the First Edition

An apology is needed for adding still another volume to the many text-books and treatises on Obstetrics. I resisted the temptation to play the role of author for long, but because of the constant persuasion of my students and colleagues and the encouragement I received at their hands, I have ventured on this publication. For over twenty-five years, it has been my privilege to work in one of the largest of the maternity institutions of the East, and to have been in contact with students and post-graduates from all over India and the Near East. The Government Hospital for Women and Children, Madras, has for long been the centre of clinical instruction for students from the Universities of Madras, Andhra, Lahore, and Lucknow, and for some time, from Rangoon and other parts of India. As a post-graduate centre of training, it attracts graduates from all the Universities in India, as well as from Hong-Kong, Burma, Federated Malaya States, Ceylon, and French and Portuguese India.

It is this contact with a large and varied student population and with postgraduates from different schools that has enabled me to realise more clearly the needs of students and practitioners and to appreciate their difficulties. This book is an attempt to put in print the teaching and practice of the clinic. To students, the subject requires to be presented in a manner that will interest them in it and at the same time enable them to appreciate the rationale of the methods of treatment adopted. The need of the practitioner is for a clear-cut presentation of diagnosis and treatment, so that when confronted by a case he is in a position to select a suitable line of treatment. The specialist does not require such detailed guidance. Experience has taught him what to choose and what to discard, what to rely on and what not to attempt. The beginner, however, needs a guiding hand. I have ventured therefore to lay down definite lines of treatment for each case. This has been based upon my experience and a study of the results of such treatment at the clinic. Honest differences of opinion as to the best line of treatment of some obstetric complications still exist, although the field is gradually being reduced. Fortunately, the efficacy of conservative measures is becoming better appreciated.

Statistics are useful, but anyone who has approached obstetric problems from this point of view realises its limitations. Nowhere is this so evident as in the Tropics. Many of the patients who come with obstetric complications, such as placenta previa, eclampsia or contracted pelvis, also suffer from anaemia, malaria, or nutritional deficiency, diseases which have their own adverse effects on the prognosis of the case. A writer on clinical obstetrics in the Tropics cannot but lay emphasis on tropical diseases complicating pregnancy and parturition. Unfortunately, to date, this subject has not received the attention it deserves, and only of late has there been any proper consideration of the problem. I have stressed this subject, so that the practitioner in the Tropics may better understand these complications as they occur in pregnancy and the methods of dealing with them. Much work yet remains to be done in this field.

In describing obstetric operations, I have tried to indicate their limitations. It should be remembered that nature frequently plays a role better than any obstetrician. When, however, the need for interference does arise, meticulous care is required at every step of the operation, and it is my hope that the technical details given in this section will be of value.

It is a pleasure to acknowledge the invaluable assistance given by my junior colleagues in the hospital—Drs R K K Tampan, P V Venkataswami and M K Krishna Menon. Dr R K K Tampan assisted me in the preparation of the greater part of the book before he left to undertake post-graduate studies at Edinburgh. His presence there was most valuable, as he saw the book through the press. Drs Ventakaswami and Krishna Menon helped me during the preparation of the latter half of the work and with the revision of the proofs as they came from the press. I also acknowledge the assistance given by the steno-typist, Mr A Ranganathan, whose careful and accurate transcription of the work is beyond all praise. I thank Mr P M Ratnasabapathi, the artist, for his skill and patience in drawing the illustrations, and Miss M P Russell, M.A., who compiled the Index.

My thanks are specially due to Dr John Sturrock of Edinburgh who perused the manuscript and offered many valuable suggestions. To the publishers, Messrs Oliver and Boyd, I am indebted. The task of publishing the work of an author so far away from Edinburgh is not an easy one, and I realise that many difficulties have had to be overcome. Their unfailing courtesy and ready co-operation and the promptness with which they undertook and published this work has placed me under a deep debt of gratitude to them. I thank them most sincerely for their kindness.

A L Mudaliar

Egmore, Madras

South India

September 1938

Competency Mapping

Mapping of *Mudaliar and Menon's Clinical Obstetrics*, 13th edition, to the Competency-Based Medical Education (CBME) curriculum

Chapter	Core competencies	Integrations
Chapter 1	OG 14.1	AN 53.2, AN 53.3
Chapter 2	OG 2.1	AN 49.2
Chapter 3	OG 3.1	AN 77.1, AN 77.2, AN 77.3
Chapter 4	OG 3.1, OG 4.1	AN 77.4, AN 79.4, AN 79.5, AN 80.3, AN 80.6
Chapter 5	OG 7.1	PY 9.8
Chapter 6	OG 6.1	AN 79.6, PY 9.10
Chapter 7	OG 14.1	
Chapter 8	OG 5.1, OG 5.2, OG 8.1–8.8	
Chapter 9	OG 4.1, OG 5.2, OG 8.7	AN 77.6, AN 79.5, AN 79.6
Chapter 10	OG 8.8, OG 9.4, OG 15.1, OG 16.3	
Chapter 11	OG 8.3, OG 8.8, OG 16.3	
Chapter 12	OG 13.1	PY 9.8, AN 80.5
Chapter 13	OG 13.1	
Chapter 14	OG 13.1, OG 13.5	PE 18.4, PY 18.5
Chapter 15	OG 5.1, OG 13.1, OG 15.1, OG 15.2	AN 49.5, PY 9.8, PH 1.41, PE 18.4, PE 18.5
Chapter 16	OG 13.1	
Chapter 17	OG 17.1, OG 17.3, OG 19.1	PY 9.8, CM 10.3, PE 7.8, PE 7.7
Chapter 18	OG 9.5	
Chapter 19	OG 1.3, OG 6.1, OG 9.1, OG 37.7	AN 78.5
Chapter 20	OG 9.3	AN 78.3
Chapter 21	OG 4.3, OG 9.4	PA 30.5
Chapter 22	OG 10.1	
Chapter 23	OG 10.1	
Chapter 24	OG 13.2	
Chapter 25	OG 4.1, OG 8.3, OG 8.4, OG 16.3	
Chapter 26	OG 13.2	
Chapter 27	OG 4.1, OG 11.1	
Chapter 28	OG 12.8	
Chapter 29	OG 12.2	
Chapter 30	OG 12.1	

Chapter	Core competencies	Integrations
Chapter 31	OG 12.3	
Chapter 32	OG 12.4	
Chapter 33	OG 12.6	
Chapter 34	OG 7.1	
Chapter 35	OG 12.7, OG 35.11, OG 8.7	
Chapter 36	OG 12.5	
Chapter 37	–	
Chapter 38	OG 29.1	
Chapter 39	OG 9.3	
Chapter 40	OG 15.1, OG 15.2, OG 14.4	
Chapter 41	OG 14.2, OG 14.3	
Chapter 42	OG 15.1, OG 15.2	
Chapter 43	OG 14.3	
Chapter 44	OG 13.1, OG 14.4	
Chapter 45	OG 8.5, OG 14.1, OG 14.2	
Chapter 46	OG 2.1	
Chapter 47	OG 16.1, OG 16.2	
Chapter 48	OG 14.2, OG 14.3	
Chapter 49	OG 17.3, OG 19.1	
Chapter 50	OG 18.1, OG 18.2, OG 18.4	PE 20.3
Chapter 51	OG 17.1, OG 17.2, OG 36.2	PE 20.16
Chapter 52	OG 18.1	PE 20.8, PE 20.16
Chapter 53	OG 18.1	PE 20.19
Chapter 54	OG 18.3, OG 18.4	PE 27.24, PE 27.25
Chapter 55	OG 15.1, OG 15.2	
Chapter 56	OG 15.1	
Chapter 57	OG 15.1	
Chapter 58	OG 1.1, CM 10.1	FM 3.28
Chapter 59	OG 1.2, OG 1.3	CM 9.2
Chapter 60	OG 10.2	
Chapter 61	OG 10.2	
Chapter 62	OG 8.8, OG 20.3	AN 81.1, AN 81.2, AN 81.3, RD 1.13, FM 3.21
Chapter 63	OG 9.2, OG 20.1, OG 20.3	FM 3.21, FM 3.27
Chapter 64	OG 19.1, OG 19.2, OG 19.4, OG 21.1, OG 21.2	AN 77.5, PH 1.39, FM 3.24, PY 9.6, CM 9.5
Chapter 65	–	FM 3.19
Chapter 66	–	PE 18.1, PE 18.2, CM 10.1, CM 10.4, FM 3.21, FM 3.25

The Pelvis

Learning Objectives

» To describe the pelvic bones and muscle attachments
» To discuss the different types of pelvises and pelvic diameters
» To describe and demonstrate pelvic assessment in a model
» To demonstrate pelvic adequacy

BOUNDARIES OF A TRUE PELVIS

- The pelvis is an important structure from the obstetric point of view as it forms the canal through which the fetus has to pass. The pelvis is divided by the linea terminalis into two parts:
  i. An upper part, known as the **pelvis major** or **false pelvis**, which has no obstetric significance
  ii. A lower part called the **pelvis minor** or **true pelvis**
- The **linea terminalis** is formed by the upper border of the sacral vertebra, the arcuate line of the ilium and the pectineal line of the pubis.
- The **true pelvis** (Table 1.1) lies below and behind the linea terminalis and is important in childbearing.

Table 1.1 The boundaries of the true pelvis

Above	Promontory and alae of the sacrum, linea terminalis and the upper margin of the pubic bones
Below	The pelvic outlet

STRUCTURE OF THE PELVIS

The **pelvic cavity** is cylindrical and extends from the brim or inlet above to the outlet below. The cavity of the true pelvis is shaped like a bent cylinder, with the posterior wall deeper than the anterior wall. The depth of the posterior wall is 10 cm (12 cm when measured along the curvature of the sacrum) and that of the anterior wall is 5 cm.

AXIS OF THE BIRTH CANAL

In an erect posture, the upper part of the pelvic cavity is directed downward and backward, while the lower part curves downward and forward. This is the axis of the birth canal and is called the **curve of Carus** (Fig. 1.1).

The axis of the birth canal is the direction in which the fetus progresses as it descends through the birth canal.

It is an imaginary line joining the midpoints of the AP diameters of the inlet, cavity and outlet. This line runs downward and backward in the upper half of pelvis, then turns downward and forward in the lower half of the pelvis. The descent of the fetal head follows the curve of Carus, downward and backward until it reaches the ischial spines. At this level, the contraction of the pelvic floor muscles directs the fetal head downward and forward until delivery.

In an erect posture, the upper part of the pelvic cavity is directed downward and backward and the lower part curves downward and forward. This is the axis of the birth canal and is called the **curve of Carus.**

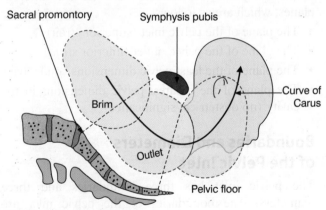

Fig. 1.1 Curve of Carus

WALLS OF THE PELVIS

The walls of the true pelvis are partly bony and partly ligamentous. Its boundaries are presented in Table 1.2.

Table 1.2   Walls of the true pelvis

Posterior	The anterior surface of the sacrum
Lateral	The inner surface of the ischial bones and the sacrosciatic notches and ligaments
Anterior	The pubic bones, the ascending superior rami of the ischial bones and the obturator foramina

■ MUSCLES OF THE TRUE PELVIS

A series of broad and thick muscles and their investing fasciae cover the bones and ligaments of the true pelvis (Table 1.3).

Table 1.3   Muscles of the true pelvis

Location	Muscles forming the walls
Sides	The pyriformis
Posteriorly	The coccygeus muscles
Laterally	The obturator internus
Inferiorly	The levator ani

The pelvic diaphragm is a musculo-aponeurotic part separating the pelvis above from the perineum and vulva below. This is formed by the levator ani and the coccygei muscles. Three orifices—the urinary meatus, the vulval outlet and the anus—pierce this diaphragm.

■ PLANES AND DIAMETERS OF THE PELVIS

In the true pelvis, the diameters are taken in different planes, which are as follows:

- The plane of the pelvic inlet (superior strait)
- The plane of the pelvic outlet (inferior strait)
- The plane of the least pelvic dimensions (midpelvis)
- The plane of the greatest pelvic dimensions in the cavity (no obstetrical significance)

Boundaries and Diameters of the Pelvic Inlet

The pelvic inlet has three boundaries and three diameters. The boundaries of the pelvic inlet are described in Table 1.4.

Table 1.4   The three boundaries of the pelvic inlet

Posterior	Sacral promontory and alae of the sacrum
Lateral	Linea terminalis
Anterior	Horizontal rami of the pubic bones and symphysis pubis

The three diameters at the brim are as follows (Fig. 1.2):

1. Anteroposterior
2. Transverse
3. Right and left oblique

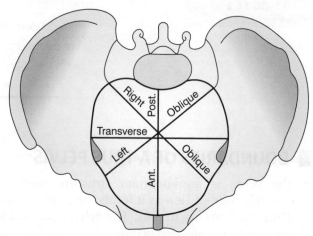

Fig. 1.2   Diameters of the pelvic inlet

Anteroposterior Diameters

There are three **anteroposterior diameters** (Fig. 1.3), which are as follows:

1. The obstetric conjugate
2. The diagonal conjugate
3. The anatomical conjugate (conjugate vera)

Obstetric conjugate

- The **obstetric conjugate** is the most important one, since it is the shortest AP diameter through which the presenting part of the fetus must pass at the time of delivery.
- This diameter is the distance between the sacral promontory and the nearest point on the posterior surface of the symphysis pubis. It generally measures 10 cm or more but may be considerably shortened in an abnormal pelvis.
- This conjugate cannot be measured clinically but can be estimated indirectly by measuring the diagonal conjugate.

Diagonal conjugate

- The **diagonal conjugate** is the distance from the promontory of the sacrum to the apex of the pubic arch. It is about 1.5–2 cm greater than the obstetric conjugate.
- Since the diagonal conjugate can be clinically measured, the obstetric conjugate is calculated by subtracting 1.5–2 cm from the diagonal conjugate, depending on the thickness of the pubic arch.

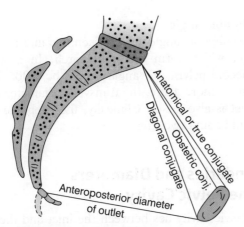

Fig. 1.3 AP diameters of the pelvis

How to measure the diagonal conjugate

- In an adequately spacious pelvis, the sacral promontory is not felt.
- The measurement is taken by inserting the middle and index fingers of the right hand into the vagina until the middle finger touches the sacral promontory.
- Then, the hand is lifted to touch the undersurface of the pubic bone and is marked by the other hand. The distance between the two points is the diagonal conjugate. If this measurement is >12 cm, it is adequate for the normal fetal head to enter the pelvic brim.

> The obstetric conjugate is the shortest AP diameter at the inlet and is obtained by subtracting 1.5–2 cm from the diagonal conjugate.

Anatomical conjugate

- The **anatomical conjugate** or the **true conjugate** is the distance between the sacral promontory and the upper portion of the inner surface of the symphysis pubis.
- It generally measures 11 cm.

Transverse Diameter of the Inlet

This is the greatest distance between the linea terminalis on either side (Fig. 1.2). It measures about 13.5 cm and usually intersects the diagonal conjugate at a point, 4 cm in front of the promontory.

Oblique Diameters

When the head enters the pelvic brim, the engaging diameter of the fetal head occupies one of the oblique diameters (Fig. 1.2) or the transverse diameter of the pelvic brim. The right oblique diameter extends from the right sacroiliac joint to the iliopectineal eminence on the opposite side and is occupied by the suboccipitobregmatic diameter of the fetal head in the occipitoanterior position. The left oblique diameter extends from the left sacroiliac

joint to the opposite iliopectineal eminence. The right and left oblique diameters measure about 13 cm each.

Sacrocotyloid diameter

This is the distance from the midpoint of the sacral promontory to the iliopectineal eminence on the same side (Fig. 1.4).

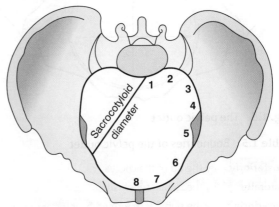

Fig. 1.4 The sacrocotyloid diameter

Clinical significance of the sacrocotyloid diameter

This diameter has clinical significance in the occipitoposterior position. When the head enters the pelvic brim, the biparietal diameter (9.4 cm) occupies the sacrocotyloid diameter. Since the sacrocotyloid diameter is only 9 cm long, the biparietal diameter cannot descend directly; instead, the head enters by lateral tilting (asynclitism) movements and also gets deflexed.

Posterior sagittal diameter

It is the part of the AP diameter that lies posterior to the transverse diameter. This diameter increases from the pelvic brim to the outlet. At the brim, the posterior sagittal diameter measures 5 cm.

> **Clinical importance of the pelvic brim**
> - The cardinal movement of engagement occurs at the pelvic brim.
> - Engagement is said to have occurred when the widest transverse diameter of the fetal skull namely, the biparietal diameter, has passed through the brim of the pelvis.

Boundaries and Diameters of the Pelvic Outlet

The outlet (Fig. 1.5 and Table 1.5), though irregular in outline, roughly resembles two triangles in different planes with their bases meeting at the line of the interischial spine.

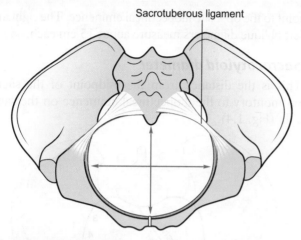

Sacrotuberous ligament

Fig. 1.5 The pelvic outlet

Table 1.5 Boundaries of the pelvic outlet

Posteriorly	By the tip of the coccyx
Laterally	By the ischial tuberosities
Anteriorly	By the pubic arch formed by inferior rami of the ischium and the pubis as they converge towards the symphysis pubis

The outlet has three diameters—the anteroposterior diameter, the transverse diameter and the posterior sagittal diameter.

Anteroposterior diameter

This is the distance from the inferior border of the symphysis pubis to the posterior aspect of the tip of the sacrum. It measures 12 cm.

Transverse diameter

The transverse diameter is the distance between the inner edges of the ischial tuberosities and usually measures 10.5–11 cm.

Posterior sagittal diameter

It extends from the middle of the transverse diameter to the tip of the sacrum. The posterior sagittal diameter of the outlet usually exceeds 7 cm.

Waste space of Morris

Normally, the width of the pubic arch is such that a disk of 9.4 cm (diameter of a well-flexed head) can pass through the pubic arch at a distance of 1 cm from the inferior border of the symphysis pubis. This distance is known as the waste space of Morris. When the subpubic angle is narrow, as in an android pelvis, the head delivers more posteriorly, increasing the space between the subpubic angle and the fetal head. This is compensated if the posterior sagittal diameter is adequate. In these cases, a liberal episiotomy is required to prevent perineal lacerations.

Subpubic angle

The subpubic angle lies between two inferior pubic rami, which form the pubic arch. In a normal gynecoid pelvis, this angle should be >90°. If this angle is more acute, the transverse diameter of the outlet is also lesser. Clinically, the subpubic angle should admit two fingers.

Boundaries and Diameters of the Pelvic Cavity

The pelvic cavity lies between the inlet and the outlet. The anterior wall of the cavity is formed by the pubic bone and is shallow. The posterior wall is deep, concave and is formed by the sacrum. There are two planes in the cavity—the plane of greater pelvic dimension and the plane of least pelvic dimension.

Plane of the greatest pelvic dimension

This plane has no obstetrical significance. It passes through the junction of the second and third sacral vertebrae, and laterally through the ischial bones over the middle of the acetabulum and posterior surface of the symphysis pubis. It is nearly circular. Its anteroposterior diameter measures 12.5 cm and its transverse diameter measures 12.75 cm.

Plane of the least pelvic dimension (midpelvis)

The **midpelvis** is otherwise known as the **plane of the least pelvic dimension**. At this plane, there are three diameters, which are presented in Table 1.6.

Table 1.6 Diameters of the midpelvis

Transverse diameter or interspinous diameter	This is the **distance between the two ischial spines** and is the smallest diameter of the pelvis; it measures 10 cm
Anteroposterior diameter	It extends from the lower border of the symphysis pubis to the junction of the 4th and 5th sacral vertebrae; this distance should be a minimum of 11.5 cm
Posterior sagittal diameter	It extends from the midpoint of the inter ischial diameter to the junction of the 4th and 5th sacral vertebrae; this measures 6 cm

Mid-cavity assessment

In a mid-cavity contraction, the ischial spines are prominent, the sacrum is flat and not curved, the pelvic side walls are converging, the sacrosciatic notch does not allow two fingers and the subpubic arch is narrow and does not admit two fingers.

The ischial spine is an important landmark in the cavity for the following reasons:

- Interspinous diameter is the smallest diameter in the pelvis
- Internal rotation occurs when the occiput is in this plane
- Marks the beginning of the forward curve of the pelvis
- Most cases of deep transverse arrest occur here
- Ischial spines represent zero station in the pelvis
- The head is considered engaged when the vault is felt vaginally at or below this level
- External os of the cervix lies at this level
- Corresponds to the origin of the levator ani muscle; the levator ani muscles are situated at this level and their ischiococcygeous part is attached to the ischial spines
- It is the landmark used for administering a pudendal block—the pudendal nerve curves around the ischial spines

THE JOINTS OF THE PELVIS

Sacroiliac Joints

The sacroiliac joints are synovial joints between the articular surfaces of the sacrum and the ilium. A large number of short but strong bundles of fibres enter the sacroiliac ligaments, resulting in minimal rotatory movement. After puberty, the range of movement is much greater and is increased temporarily in the later months of pregnancy.

Pubic Symphysis

The pubic bones are united by the superior pubic ligament, inferior pubic ligament (**arcuate ligament**) and an inter-pubic disc of fibrocartilage. The symphysis pubis has a certain degree of mobility, which increases during pregnancy.

Sacrococcygeal Joint

It is a synovial hinge joint between S5 and the first coccygeal vertebra. It has a weak capsule reinforced by sacrococcygeal ligaments. It allows both flexion and extension.

Clinical Significance of the Pelvic Joints

- There is relaxation of the sacroiliac joints during pregnancy due to hormonal changes. Marked mobility of the pelvis has been observed at term due to the upward gliding movement of the sacroiliac joint.

- Relaxation of the symphysis pubis may start in early pregnancy but increases during the last three months. This regresses after delivery.
- When vaginal delivery is conducted in the dorsal lithotomy position, displacement of the sacroiliac joint is greatest, and the diameter of the outlet increases by 1.5–2 cm.
- McRoberts manoeuvre, which is performed in cases of shoulder dystocia, is based on the mobility of the sacroiliac joint.

CLASSIFICATION OF PELVIC SHAPES

Caldwell and Moloy's Classification

Caldwell and Moloy have, on the basis of X-ray studies, attempted a **morphological classification of the pelvis**. This takes into consideration the anatomical varieties in pelvic architecture presumably caused by racial, sexual or other complex inherited influences rather than by any pathological bony changes. Four parent types of pelvic shapes have been recognised in this system (Fig. 1.6).

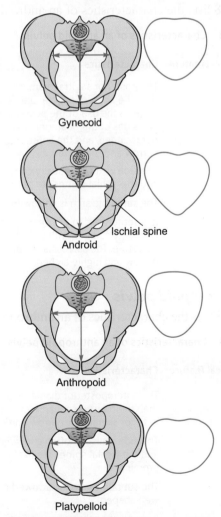

Gynecoid

Ischial spine

Android

Anthropoid

Platypelloid

Fig. 1.6 Caldwell–Moloy's classification of pelvises

1.   Gynecoid pelvis

Table 1.7 lists the characteristics of a gynecoid pelvis.

Table 1.7   Characteristics of a gynecoid pelvis

Anatomical feature	Characteristics
Inlet	Since the transverse diameter is only slightly greater than or equal to the anteroposterior diameter, the inlet is slightly oval or round. The posterior sagittal diameter at the inlet is slightly less than the anterior sagittal diameter. The sides of the posterior segment are rounded and wide.
Midpelvis	In the midpelvis, the side walls of the pelvis are straight, and the spines are not prominent. The transverse diameter at the ischial spines is 10 cm or more.
Outlet	At the outlet, the pubic arch is wide.
Sacrum	The sacrum is inclined neither anteriorly nor posteriorly, and the sacrosciatic arch is well-rounded.

2.   Android pelvis

Table 1.8 lists the characteristics of an android pelvis.

Table 1.8   Characteristics of an android pelvis

Anatomical feature	Characteristics
Inlet	The posterior sagittal diameter is less than the anterior sagittal diameter. This restricts the use of the posterior space. The sides of the posterior segment are not rounded, and the anterior pelvis is narrow and triangular.
Midpelvis	The side walls are usually convergent, and the ischial spines are prominent.
Outlet	The subpubic arch is narrowed.
Sacrum	It is set forward in the pelvis and is usually straight, with little or no curvature. The sacrosciatic notch is narrow and highly arched.

3.   Anthropoid pelvis

Table 1.9 lists the characteristics of an anthropoid pelvis.

Table 1.9   Characteristics of an anthropoid pelvis

Anatomical feature	Characteristics
Inlet	The anteroposterior diameter is greater than the transverse diameter. The anterior segment is narrow and pointed.
Midpelvis	The side walls are often convergent, and the ischial spines are likely to be prominent.
Outlet	The subpubic arch is narrowed but well-shaped.
Sacrum	It usually has six segments and is straight. The sacrosciatic notch is large.

4.   Platypelloid pelvis

This pelvis is the rarest of the pure varieties and is found in less than 3% of women. The characteristics of the platypelloid pelvis are as follows:

- Transverse oval inlet
- Very wide, rounded subpubic angle
- Very wide, flat posterior segment
- Narrow sacrosciatic notch
- Average sacral inclination
- Very wide subpubic arch
- Straight side walls
- Very wide interspinous and intertuberous diameters

Intermediate or mixed types of pelvises

Most pelvises are of the intermediate or mixed type. In such cases, the type of pelvis is determined by the posterior segment, and its tendency is determined based on the anterior segment. For example, in a pelvis with a gynecoid posterior segment and android anterior segment, the pelvis is designated as a **gynecoid pelvis with android tendency**. Pelvises with the parent types of Caldwell and Moloy's classification are considered abnormal when any of the diameters are substantially reduced.

Gynecoid pelvis is seen in nearly 50% of cases, android in 25%, anthropoid in 20% and platypelloid in 5% of cases.

Clinical significance

Small, gynecoid pelvis

In this type, though the shape is normal, the diameters are proportionately reduced. Hence, there is a **delay at every stage of labour** due to the lack of space. Powerful uterine contractions are required to push the presenting part downward. This type can cause cephalopelvic disproportion (CPD).

Android pelvis

With this type of pelvis, the **occipitoposterior position** is common. Due to the funnel-like shape of the pelvis, progressive difficulty is faced, rotation fails to occur, and transverse arrest is common.

Android pelvis → Occipitoposteriors → Incomplete rotation and deep transverse arrest
Anthropoid pelvis → POP (persistent occipitoposterior)

Anthropoid pelvis

In this type of pelvis, persistent occipitoposterior position is common.

Platypelloid pelvis

In this type of pelvis, there is asynclitic engagement. Face presentation can occur.

■ ABNORMALITIES OF THE PELVIS

Certain diseases may affect the pelvic bones and alter the development of the normal pelvis. Some of the variations are described here.

Rachitic Flat Pelvis

This occurs in a child who suffers from rickets and is not treated. It is uncommon nowadays since vitamin D supplementation is universally and routinely given to all children.

Naegele's Pelvis

This occurs due to arrested development of one ala of the sacrum.

Robert's Pelvis

This occurs due to the arrested development of both alae of the sacrum (Fig. 1.7).

Obliquely Contracted Pelvis

An obliquely contracted pelvis can occur due to various reasons.

1. **Kyphoscoliosis** is defined as a deviation of the normal curvature of the spine in the sagittal and coronal planes and can include a rotation of the spinal axis.

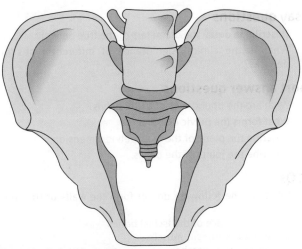

Fig. 1.7   Robert's pelvis

There may be a congenital deformity of the spine or the condition may develop secondary to diseases such as tuberculosis or rickets. Kyphoscoliosis affecting the lower thoracolumbar region can affect the pelvic diameters. Pelvic diameters can also be affected following tuberculosis of the pelvic joints and rickets. These conditions may result in an obliquely contracted pelvis.

2. An obliquely contracted pelvis may occur following the shortening of the lower limbs due to **poliomyelitis or accidents**. In these situations, the pelvic diameters are reduced on the side where the leg is normal. This is due to the woman putting her weight on her normal leg, which results in the acetabulum getting pushed inside the pelvis.

KEY POINTS

✓ *The pelvis forms a canal through which the fetus passes during delivery.*

✓ *The diameters of the pelvis are taken in different planes, namely the plane of the pelvic inlet, plane of the pelvic outlet, plane of least pelvic dimension and plane of greatest dimension.*

✓ *The smallest diameter of the true pelvis is the interspinous diameter.*

✓ *The transverse diameter is the widest at the brim. Therefore, the head engages in the transverse diameter.*

✓ *At the outlet, the AP diameter is greater, and therefore, the head has to rotate by 90°.*

✓ *The interspinous diameter is the smallest. Therefore, arrest of descent and non-rotation occurs at this level. The most important plane in obstructed labour is the plane of least pelvic dimension.*

✓ *In a small gynecoid pelvis, all measurements are lesser than normal. This can lead to CPD.*

✓ *The fetal head descends along the axis of the pelvis. Therefore, the same axis should be followed at the time of instrumental delivery.*

✓ *If the subpubic angle is narrow, the head is pushed backwards. This may result in a perineal tear.*

✓ *Relaxation of the sacroiliac joints and symphysis pubis occurs during pregnancy and is maximum at term due to hormones.*

✓ *In shoulder dystocia, the McRoberts manoeuvre is successful due to the mobility of the sacroiliac joint, which increases the diameter of the pelvis.*

✓ *Backache and suprapubic pain are caused by the relaxation of the pelvic joints.*

✓ *Gynecoid pelvis is the most favourable for childbirth and android is the least favourable.*

✓ *Anthropoid pelvis favours direct OP presentation and face-to-pubis delivery.*

✓ *Platypelloid pelvis is associated with face presentation.*

Essay questions

1. Describe in detail the diameters of the true pelvis.
2. What is the clinical significance of different types of pelvises?

Short answer questions

1. What are the boundaries of a true pelvis?
2. What forms the pelvic diaphragm?
3. Describe the plane of the least pelvic dimension.
4. Describe the joints of the pelvis.

MCQs

1. Which of the following do not form the walls of the true pelvis?
   a) Inner surface of the ischial bones
   b) Ischiocavernosus muscle
   c) Sacrosciatic notches
   d) Sacrosciatic ligaments
2. Which of the following is the most important diameter for the delivery of the fetus?
   a) The obstetrical conjugate
   b) The diagonal conjugate
   c) The anatomical conjugate
   d) The anteroposterior diameter of the outlet
3. Occipitoposterior position and deep transverse arrest are common in which of the following pelvises?
   a) Gynecoid pelvis
   b) Android pelvis
   c) Anthropoid pelvis
   d) Platypelloid pelvis
4. Which of the following describes the diagonal conjugate?
   a) It measures less than the obstetrical conjugate.
   b) It is the distance from the sacral promontory to the apex of the pubic arch.
   c) It is the distance between the sacral promontory to the nearest point on the posterior surface of the symphysis pubis.
   d) It is the distance between the sacral promontory and the upper portion of the inner surface of the symphysis pubis.
5. Which of the following is the shortest anteroposterior diameter at the brim?
   a) Diagonal conjugate
   b) Obstetrical conjugate
   c) Anatomical conjugate
   d) True conjugate
6. What is the diameter between the sacroiliac joint of one side and the iliopectineal eminence of the opposite side called?
   a) Anteroposterior diameter
   b) Transverse diameter
   c) Depth of pelvis
   d) Oblique diameter
7. In which of the following types of pelvises is a persistent occipitoposterior position common?
   a) Android pelvis
   b) Platypelloid pelvis
   c) Gynecoid pelvis
   d) Anthropoid pelvis

Answers

1. (b), 2. (a), 3. (b), 4. (b), 5. (b), 6. (d), 7. (d)

Fill in the blanks

1. The linea terminalis is formed by _____.
2. The diagonal conjugate is the distance from the _____ to the _____.
3. The smallest diameter of the pelvis is the _____.
4. The transverse diameter of the pelvic inlet measures _____ cm.

Answers

1. the upper border of the sacral vertebra, the arcuate line of the ilium and the pectineal line of the pubis, 2. sacral promontory, the apex of the pubic arch, 3. interspinous diameter, 4. 13.5

Anatomy of the Female Genital Organs

Learning Objectives

» To know the structure of the uterus, the parts of the uterus and its importance in labour

» To understand the blood supply to the uterus and its clinical significance

» To discuss the innervation of the uterus and explain how the sensory fibres from the pelvis are transmitted

» To describe the perineal body and the anatomical basis of episiotomy and perineal tears

» To describe the appearance of the cervix through a speculum

» To describe the structures that are palpable during vaginal and rectal examinations

■ EXTERNAL GENITAL ORGANS

The **external female genital organs** (Fig. 2.1) comprise the following:

- The mons pubis
- The labia majora
- The labia minora
- The clitoris
- The vestibule
- The hymen and the vaginal orifice, the external urethral meatus and the perineum

All these organs constitute the **vulva**.

Mons Pubis or Mons Veneris

The mons pubis is a rounded fold of skin covering a pad of fat that lies over the symphysis pubis. The outer surface is covered with hair after puberty. In women, pubic hair is distributed in a triangular area, the base of which is formed by the upper margin of the symphysis. A few hairs are distributed downward, over the outer surface of the labia majora.

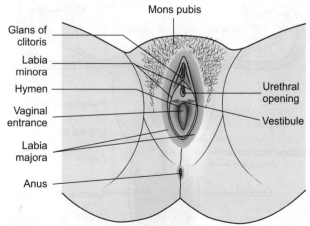

Fig. 2.1 The external female genitalia

Labia Majora

The labia majora are two elongated folds of adipose tissue that are covered with skin and extend downward and backward from the mons veneris. They meet anteriorly in the anterior commissure and posteriorly in the posterior commissure in front of the anus. The labia majora are richly supplied with sebaceous glands.

Beneath the skin, there is a layer of dense connective tissue that is rich in elastic fibres and adipose tissue; no muscular element is found.

There are venous plexuses in the adipose tissue, which get enlarged in pregnancy. The slightest trauma can result in a hematoma.

Labia Minora

The labia minora are two thin, reddish folds of tissue, one on each side. These folds are exposed only when the labia majora are separated. The lower portion of the labia minora fuses along the middle to form a fold known as the **fourchette**, which is usually lacerated during childbirth. Between the fourchette and the vaginal orifice is a boat-like depression—the **fossa navicularis**.

The labia minora are highly sensitive for the following reasons:

- They are richly supplied with nerve endings
- There are no hair follicles in the skin covering this area
- The labia minora has sweat glands and sebaceous glands which keep the area moist
- The sweat glands, known as apocrine glands, are under the influence of the sex hormones

Clitoris

The clitoris is situated in the anterior-most part of the vulva and projects between the two folds of the labia minora. It corresponds to the penis in the male.

The clitoris has a glans, a body and two crura. The glans is supplied with nerve endings and corpuscles and hence is highly sensitive. It has a rich supply of blood and hence a tear involving the clitoris causes heavy bleeding.

Vestibule

The vestibule is an area that extends from the clitoris above to the anterior margin of the hymen below, and laterally to the labia minora. The **urethral orifice** is situated in the centre of the vestibule.

The **vestibule** is not usually visible since it is covered by the labia. The aggregation of veins in this area is known as a vestibular bulb. These veins are situated close to the ischiopubic rami and under the vestibular mucus membrane.

Though they are generally pushed behind the pubic rami during childbirth, the posterior end of these veins, which encircle the vagina, can be injured during childbirth and could result in hemorrhage or hematoma.

Hymen and Vaginal Orifice

The hymen is composed of elastic and collagenous connective tissue and is an incomplete septum covering the vaginal orifice. Generally, the hymen is circular or somewhat crescentic and is usually ruptured at the first coitus.

At childbirth, the hymen is extensively lacerated and is later represented by a large number of cicatrized nodules of varying sizes called **carunculae myrtiformes**.

Perineum

The perineum is a wedge-shaped area extending from the posterior wall of the vagina to the anterior wall of the anus. It is supported by the pelvic and urogenital diaphragms.

Posteriorly, the **pelvic diaphragm** comprises the following:

1. Levator ani muscle
2. Coccygeus muscle
3. The fascia covering these muscles

The **urogenital diaphragm** consists of the following:

1. The deep transverse perineal muscles
2. The constrictor of the urethra
3. The internal and external fascial coverings

Blood supply to the perineum

The major blood supply to the perineum is via the internal pudendal artery which is a branch of the internal iliac artery and its branches. The internal pudendal artery has **three** branches supplying the vulvar region namely:

1. **Clitoral artery** – supplies the clitoris
2. **Perineal artery** – supplies the skin, subcutaneous tissue and muscles of the vulva

3. **Inferior rectal artery** – supplies the skin and musculature

The internal pudendal artery also anastomoses with superficial and deep pudendal vessels which are branches of the femoral artery.

Nerve supply to the perineum

The **pudendal nerve**, which originates from the S2, S3 and S4 levels of the spinal cord along with its branches, primarily supplies the perineum. This is the main reason for the use of a **pudendal block** during operative vaginal deliveries.

Bartholin's Glands

Bartholin's glands are a pair of small, globular structures, 0.5–1 cm in diameter. They are also called the greater vestibular glands. These glands are situated on either side of the vaginal orifice and are covered by the posterior end of the bulb of the vestibule. They are compound racemose glands and lead into a narrow duct that opens below the hymen on the inner surface of the labia minora near its posterior end.

These glands can get infected (bartholinitis) and form a **Bartholin's abscess**. Their rich vascularity and proximity to vascular vestibular erectile tissue could be a source of excessive bleeding when the removal of these glands is attempted.

■ THE INTERNAL GENITAL ORGANS

The **internal female genital organs** (Fig. 2.2) comprise the following:

- Vagina
- Uterus
- Fallopian tubes
- Ovaries

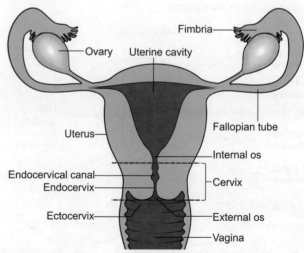

Fig. 2.2 The internal genital organs in the female

Vagina

Position

This is a musculo-membranous tube extending from the vulva outside to the uterus inside.

- It is situated between the bladder in front and the rectum behind.
- Further, it is directed upward and backward and is slightly curved posteriorly.
- The **vaginal canal** is a transverse or H-shaped slit with the lower end narrower than the upper end. The lengths of the anterior and posterior **vaginal walls** vary.
- The anterior wall measures 6–8 cm and the posterior wall measures 7–10 cm in length.
- The cervix dips into the vaginal canal.
- The **vault of the vagina,** which surrounds the cervix, consists of four pouches or fornices. The **anterior fornix** is in close relation with the bladder, the **posterior fornix** with the pouch of Douglas and the rectum, and the **right** and **left lateral fornices** are in close relation with the ureter and the uterine artery on the side.

Relations

The anterior, lateral and posterior relations are described below.

Anterior

The vagina is in contact with the bladder and urethra, from which it is separated by connective tissue referred to as the **vesicovaginal septum**.

Lateral

The vagina is supported by the free edges of the levator ani muscles.

Posterior

In its upper third, the vagina is related to the pouch of Douglas and is therefore in close contact with the peritoneal cavity. A thin septum formed by the vaginal wall and the peritoneum separates the two. The lower portion of the vagina is in relation with the rectum and the perineal body. The connective tissue between the rectum and the vagina forms the **rectovaginal septum**.

Histology

The **vaginal mucosa** consists of non-cornified, stratified squamous epithelium. Beneath the epithelium, there is a thin, fibromuscular coat, usually consisting of an inner circular layer and an outer longitudinal layer of smooth muscle. Normally, no glands are present in the vagina. **Vaginal epithelial cells** exfoliate into the vagina; the vaginal smear study of these exfoliated cells

explains the hormonal pattern. The **vaginal epithelium** is rich in glycogen, which is broken down by the commensal lactobacilli present in the vagina. This helps in maintaining the acidic pH of the vagina, thereby protecting it from infections, particularly during the sexually active and reproductive periods.

Blood supply

There is an abundant supply of blood to the vagina. The upper third of the vagina is supplied by the cervicovaginal branches of the uterine arteries, the middle third by the inferior vesical arteries, and the lower third by the middle rectal and pudendal arteries. The vaginal artery may branch directly from the internal iliac artery.

Venous drainage

There is extensive venous plexus immediately surrounding the vagina. Vessels follow the course of the arteries. Eventually, these veins drain into the internal iliac veins.

Lymphatic drainage

The lymphatics from the lower third of the vagina along with those of the vulva drain into the inguinal lymph nodes. Lymphatics from the mid-vaginal area drain into the internal iliac nodes and those from the upper third of the vagina drain into the iliac nodes.

Nerve supply

The nerve supply to the vagina is from S2, S3 and S4 sacral nerves and the sympathetic supply is from the hypogastric plexus of nerves. In addition, the lower end of the vagina has a sensory supply from the pudendal nerve.

Perineal Body

The perineal body is a fibromuscular wedge filling the angle between the lower one-third of the vagina and the anal canal. It is the median raphe of the levator ani and is reinforced by the central tendon of the perineum, on which the bulbocavernosus muscles, superficial transverse perineal muscles and the external anal sphincter converge. These structures, which contribute to the perineal body, provide much support to the perineum (Fig. 2.3).

Muscular attachments of the perineal body
- External anal sphincter
- Bulbospongiosus
- Superficial transverse perineal muscle
- Deep transverse perineal muscle
- Anterior fibres of levator ani
- Few fibres from the external urinary sphincter

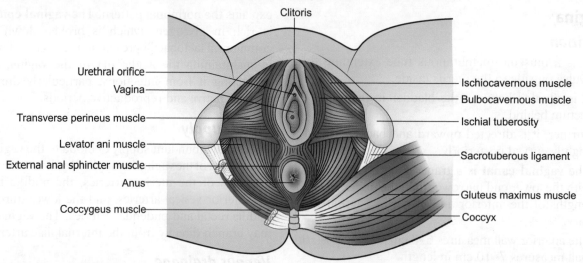

Fig. 2.3 Muscles of the pelvis

Clinical significance

The perineal body is an important structure that welds the pelvis and perineum together.

- Injury to this body due to prolonged pressure and stretching during delivery or by obstetric trauma weakens the support to the pelvic organs, leading to prolapse.
- The anatomic structures involved in a mediolateral episiotomy include the vaginal epithelium, transverse perineal muscles, bulbocavernosus muscle and perineal skin. A deep or large mediolateral episiotomy may expose the ischiorectal fossa. It may also involve the levator ani fibres.

Uterus

Appearance

The uterus is a pear-shaped muscular organ situated in the pelvis between the bladder anteriorly, and the rectum posteriorly.

Size

The uterus varies in size and shape, these parameters being influenced by age and parity (Table 2.1). Before puberty, the organ ranges in length from 2.5–3.5 cm. The uterus of an adult nulliparous woman is 6–8 cm in length, whereas that of a multiparous woman is 9–10 cm in length.

Table 2.1 Length of the uterus at different ages

Age group	Length of the uterus (cm)
Pre-pubertal female	2.5–3.5
Adult nulliparous	6–8
Adult multiparous	9–10

In adults, the uterus weighs about 50–70 g. The length of the cavity is 3–5 cm. The cavity is triangular, with its base above and its apex at the junction between the body and the cervix. The anterior and posterior walls are almost in contact and hence the cavity has the appearance of a narrow slit. The capacity of the undistended uterus is only 4 mL.

Parts of the uterus

The uterus consists of **two unequal parts**:

1. The upper triangular portion, known as the **uterine body** or the **corpus**
2. The lower cylindrical or fusiform portion, which projects into the vagina; this is known as the **cervix**

   The **isthmus** is the portion of the uterine cavity between the internal cervical os and the endometrial cavity. It has a special obstetrical significance because it forms the **lower uterine segment** during pregnancy. In adults, the uterine body is larger than the cervix. The cervix is 1/3rd to 1/4th of the size of the uterine body. The part of the uterus that lies above the insertion of the fallopian tubes is known as the fundus of the uterus.

Uterine body or the corpus

The wall of the uterine body is composed of **three layers**, which are as follows:

1. Serous
2. Muscular
3. Mucous

The **serous layer** is formed by the peritoneum, which covers the anterior two-thirds and the whole of the posterior surface of the uterus. The **myometrium or the muscular layer** forms the greater part of the uterus and consists of non-striated muscles bound by connective tissue with elastic fibres. The muscle fibres are arranged in **three layers**:

1. The outer longitudinal layer runs anteroposteriorly over the fundus, which is continuous with the fallopian tube and ligaments.
2. The inner circular fibres are prominent near the orifices, that is, near the tubal ostia and internal os.
3. Between the two are the interlacing muscle fibres, which form a characteristic 'figure of eight' around the blood vessels. These muscles help in contracting the blood vessels, functioning like '**living ligatures**' to control hemorrhage. The muscle fibres diminish progressively from the fundus to the cervix. The muscle content of the cervix is only 10%.

When the uterus does not contract and instead, remains atonic, this ligature effect is not active. As a result, the vessels remain open, increasing blood loss, particularly following delivery. This condition is known as postpartum hemorrhage (PPH) and could even be life-threatening if not diagnosed and managed immediately.

The **endometrium** is the **mucosal layer** that lines the uterine cavity. Due to the cyclical hormonal changes during the reproductive years, the endometrium normally ranges in thickness from 0.5 mm to as much as 15 mm. The endometrium is made up of surface epithelium, glands and interglandular mesenchymal tissue, in which there are numerous blood vessels.

Uterine cervix

The uterine cervix is the portion of the uterus that lies below the isthmus. Anteriorly, the upper boundary of the cervix, that is, the internal os, corresponds to the level at which the peritoneum is reflected upon the bladder.

The cervix comprises **two parts**:

1. The supravaginal portion
2. The infravaginal portion

The **supravaginal portion of the cervix** is covered on its posterior surface by the peritoneum and laterally, is attached to the cardinal ligaments. Anteriorly, it is separated from the overlying bladder by loose connective tissue.

The external os is located at the lower extremity of the **infravaginal portion** of the cervix. The external os is nearly circular in nulliparous women, but after delivery, the orifice may become a transverse slit. The length of the cervical canal is about 2.5–3.5 cm from the internal os to the external os.

Structure

The cervix is composed of connective tissue, collagen, muscle fibres and blood vessels. The physical properties of the cervix depend on the collagen and connective tissue. The cervical change associated with the onset of labour is collagen breakdown, which results in the softening of the cervix.

The cervical canal is lined with mucosa composed of a single layer of very high, columnar epithelium that rests upon a thin basement membrane. Near the external os, the columnar epithelium of the cervical canal and the squamous epithelium of the ectocervix meet at the squamocolumnar junction.

Ligaments of the uterus

The following ligaments keep the uterus in position:

- Broad ligaments
- Round ligaments
- Uterosacral ligaments
- Mackenrodt's ligaments

Broad ligaments

The broad ligament on each side of the uterus is a double layer of peritoneum directed from the lateral margin of the uterus to the lateral wall of the pelvis. It serves to divide the pelvic cavity into an anterior and a posterior compartment. While superiorly there is a free border, the inferior border merges with the pelvic floor. The lateral (outer) third of the upper free margin forms the infundibulopelvic ligament and the medial (inner) two-thirds form the mesosalpinx enclosing the fallopian tube and the round and ovarian ligaments. Below and medially, the uterine artery is enclosed by the broad ligament. The broad ligament also encloses the extraperitoneal connective tissue, the true ligament of the ovary, the paroophoron and epoophoron, and certain blood vessels, nerves and lymphatics.

Round ligaments

The round ligaments extend on either side from the anterolateral angle of the uterus just below and in front of the insertion of the fallopian tubes. They are enclosed between the serous layers of the broad ligaments and pass laterally through the internal abdominal rings into the inguinal canals, and finally merge in the labia majora. In non-pregnant women, the round ligament could be 3–5 mm in diameter. During pregnancy, the round ligaments undergo considerable hypertrophy and increase appreciably in both length and diameter. These ligaments correspond to the gubernaculum testis in men.

Uterosacral ligaments

The two uterosacral ligaments are condensations of the visceral pelvic fascia. Anteriorly, they extend from the posterolateral aspect of the supravaginal portion of the cervix and upper vagina to encircle the rectum;

posteriorly, they are attached to the fascia over the second and third sacral vertebrae.

Mackenrodt's ligaments

Also known as **cardinal ligaments**, these are thickened bands of fibromuscular tissue stretching across the pelvis. They run along the base of the broad ligaments, attaching medially to the side of the cervix uteri and vaginal vault and laterally to the wall of the pelvis.

Blood supply to the uterus

The uterus derives its blood supply principally from the uterine and the ovarian arteries (Fig. 2.4). The **uterine artery** arises from the anterior branch of the internal iliac artery. It runs downward, forward and medially in the base of the broad ligament, crosses above the ureter and passes to the side of the uterus. Just before the main branch turns abruptly upward, a small branch separates; this is the **cervicovaginal artery**, which supplies the lower portion of the cervix and the upper portion of the vagina.

> In a subtotal obstetric hysterectomy, it is important to identify the cervicovaginal artery and ligate it before removing the uterus.

The main artery, which proceeds upward in the broad ligament along the lateral border of the uterus, has a number of branches. One branch extends to anastomose with the ovarian artery, a second passes into the mesosalpinx, supplying the fallopian tube and a third passes into the fundus.

The main uterine artery, which proceeds upwards along the lateral border of the uterus, branches into the myometrium—these branches are called the **arcuate arteries**. These arteries enter the myometrium obliquely and run parallel to the surface of the uterus to meet the arcuate artery of the opposite side, thus encircling the uterine body.

From the arcuate arteries, radial arteries branch off at right angles and run towards the endometrium, dividing into short **basal arteries** and long coiled **spiral arteries**. The basal arteries supply the basal endometrium. The coiled spiral arteries supply the middle and superficial parts of the endometrium. The spiral arteries respond to hormones, while the basal arteries do not.

Clinical importance of blood supply of the uterus

- The pelvis has extensive collateral circulation with the internal iliac artery, anastomosing with the aorta, external iliac and femoral artery. This is an important point to note since ligation of the internal iliac artery can be performed in cases of obstetrical hemorrhage without compromising blood supply to other pelvic structures.
- In normal pregnancies, the cytotrophoblast cells of the developing placenta migrate through the decidua and part of the myometrium to invade both the endothelium and the highly muscular tunica media of

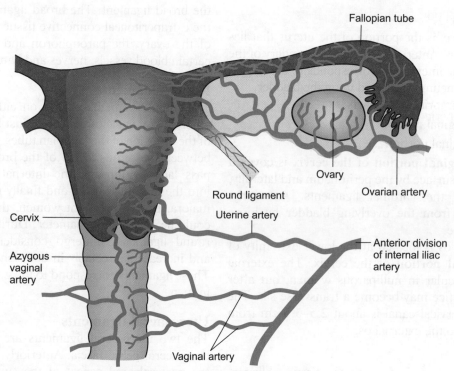

Fig. 2.4 Arterial supply of the internal genital organs

Labels: Fallopian tube, Ovary, Ovarian artery, Round ligament, Uterine artery, Anterior division of internal iliac artery, Cervix, Azygous vaginal artery, Vaginal artery

the maternal spiral arteries. As a result, these vessels transform from small muscular arterioles to large-capacity vessels of low resistance, thereby greatly facilitating blood flow to the placenta as compared to other areas of the uterus.

- This can be observed by Doppler studies of uterine arteries which show low-resistance blood flow from 11 weeks onwards. High-resistance flow can predict the development of pre-eclampsia and growth restriction at a later date.

> Ligation of the uterine artery helps in reducing blood loss when there is excessive postpartum hemorrhage.

Venous drainage

The veins that emerge from the uterine fundus, fallopian tube and ovary form the **pampiniform plexus**. From this, two ovarian veins emerge and later fuse to form a single ovarian vein, which on the left side, joins the renal vein and on the right side, joins the inferior vena cava. The uterine veins accompany the uterine arteries and terminate in the corresponding internal iliac vein.

Lymphatic drainage

Though the endometrium is abundantly supplied with lymphatics, true lymphatic vessels are confined largely to the basal layer. The lymphatics from the various segments of the uterus drain into several sets of lymph nodes. Those from the cervix terminate mainly in the internal iliac nodes, which are situated near the bifurcation of the common iliac vessels.

The lymphatics from the body of the uterus are distributed to two groups of lymph nodes. One set of vessels drains into the internal iliac nodes; the other set, after joining certain lymphatics from the ovarian region, terminates in the periaortic lymph nodes (Fig. 2.5).

Innervation

The nerve supply of the uterus is derived principally from the sympathetic nervous system and partly from the parasympathetic system.

The **parasympathetic system** is represented on either side by the pelvic nerve, which consists of fibres from the second, third and fourth sacral nerves and ends in the ganglion of Frankenhauser. The **sympathetic system** enters the pelvis through the hypogastric plexus, which arises from the aortic plexus just below the promontory of the sacrum. After descending on either side, it also enters the uterovaginal plexus of Frankenhauser, which consists of ganglia of varying sizes situated on either side of the cervix, just above the posterior fornix and in front of the rectum.

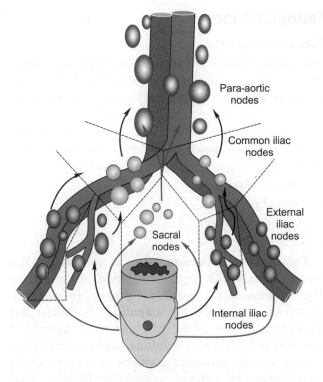

Fig. 2.5 Lymphatic drainage of the internal genital organs

Branches from these plexuses supply the uterus, bladder and the upper part of the vagina and comprise both myelinated and non-myelinated fibres.

Functions

The sympathetic fibres cause muscular contraction and vasoconstriction, whereas the parasympathetic fibres inhibit contraction and lead to vasodilatation. Since the Frankenhauser plexus is derived from both sources, it has certain functions of both components of the autonomic nervous system.

The eleventh and twelfth thoracic nerve roots carry sensory fibres from the uterus, transmitting the pain of the uterine contractions to the central nervous system.

The sensory nerves from the cervix and upper part of the birth canal pass primarily through the pudendal nerve. The nerves from the lower portion of the vagina pass through the ilioinguinal and pudendal nerves. The motor fibres to the uterus leave the spinal cord at the level of the seventh and eighth thoracic vertebrae.

> Knowledge of the innervation of the uterus is important to provide epidural and labour analgesia and also for epidural or spinal anesthesia during cesarean section.
>
> In epidural analgesia, the sensory fibres travelling through T11, 12 and L1 from the body of the uterus and the pain sensation from the cervix, vagina and perineum, which pass via S2, 3 and 4, are blocked.

Fallopian Tubes

Position and size

The fallopian tubes are situated on either side of the uterus and lie in the medial four-fifths of the upper border of the broad ligament. They are attached to the uterine cornua and measure 8–14 cm in length. They are convoluted, and their free ends are near the ovaries.

Each fallopian tube is divided into four parts, which are as follows:

1. Interstitial portion
2. Isthmal portion
3. Ampullary portion
4. Infundibular portion

The **interstitial portion** refers to the part of the tube that fuses with the muscular part of the uterus. The **isthmus** is the narrowest portion immediately adjacent to the uterus. The **ampulla** is the widest and the outermost part of the tube and has a fimbriated end; this is known as the **infundibulum**. This opens directly into the peritoneal cavity by an ostium, which is surrounded by a number of radiating fimbriae. One of the fimbrial projections, known as fimbria ovarica, is longer than the others and reaches the ovary. This is believed to facilitate the picking up of the ovum.

The wall of each tube consists of two layers of muscles—the inner circular and the outer longitudinal layers. The fallopian tube is not uniform in thickness. While the narrowest isthmus measures 2–3 mm in diameter, the widest ampullary portion measures 5–8 mm.

Tubal sterilisation procedures are preferably done in the isthmus so that recanalisation techniques, if performed later, have a higher success rate. This is based on the uniform thickness of the muscle layer in this segment.

The lumen of the tube is lined by a single layer of columnar cells, some of them ciliated and others secretory. The fallopian tube is covered by the peritoneum.

Ovaries

The ovaries are two almond-shaped bodies that are situated near the fimbriated extremity of the fallopian tubes and are attached to the posterior surface of the broad ligament by the **mesovarium** and to the lateral pelvic wall by the **infundibulopelvic ligament**.

The **ovarian ligament** extends from the upper end of the lateral wall of the uterus just below and behind the insertion of the fallopian tube, to the inner pole of the ovary.

The **ovary** is divided into **three** regions, which are as follows:

1. Hilum
2. Medulla
3. Cortex

The **hilum** is the small area composed of connective tissue and non-striated muscle fibres through which the ovarian vessels, lymphatics and nerves pass into the ovary from the broad ligament.

The **cortex** of the ovary is the outer layer in which the Graafian follicles are situated. Its surface is lined by a single layer of cells called the germinal epithelium, continuous at the hilum with the peritoneum of the broad ligament.

The **medullary portion** is the central portion of the ovary, composed of connective tissue and a large number of blood vessels. The ovary has no peritoneal covering.

Blood supply

Ovarian arteries branch directly from the aorta. The ovarian artery on each side reaches the hilum of the ovary through the infundibulopelvic ligament. At the hilum, it branches off into many smaller arteries which enter the ovary. The main stem passes along the mesosalpinx and reaches the uterine cornua, where it anastomoses with the ovarian branches of the uterine artery.

KEY POINTS

✓ *The uterus is situated in the pelvis between the bladder anteriorly and the rectum posteriorly. It is divided into the body and the cervix.*

✓ *The cervix dips into the vagina. The vault of the vagina which surrounds the cervix consists of four pouches called the fornices.*

✓ *The wall of the uterine body is composed of three layers, namely the serosa, muscular and mucosal layers.*

✓ *The uterus is supported by ligaments. These are the uterosacral ligaments and Mackenrodt's ligaments.*

✓ *The pain of uterine contractions is felt at the T12–L2 level.*

✓ *Pain from the lower vagina, perineum and labia is transmitted to the S2–S4 level.*

✓ *The ovarian arteries, which are direct branches from the abdominal aorta, supply the ovary.*

✓ *The isthmus is the narrowest portion of the fallopian tube.*

Essay questions

1. What are the different anatomical relations of the vagina? Describe the blood supply and venous and lymphatic drainage of the vagina.
2. Describe the structure, supports, anatomical relationship and blood and nerve supply of the uterus.

Short answer questions

1. Describe the pelvic and urogenital diaphragms.
2. Describe the blood supply to the uterus.
3. Describe the innervations of the uterus.
4. What are the Bartholin's glands?
5. What is the perineal body?
6. Describe the ligaments supporting the uterus.

MCQs

1. Which of the following is not a branch of the internal pudendal?
   a) Clitoral artery
   b) Perineal artery
   c) Inferior rectal artery
   d) Superior vesical artery
2. Which of the following forms the fallopian tube from the medial to the lateral side?
   a) Interstitial portion, isthmal portion, ampullary portion and infundibular portion
   b) Interstitial portion, ampullary portion, isthmal portion and infundibular portion
   c) Interstitial portion, isthmal portion infundibular portion and ampullary portion
   d) Isthmal portion, interstitial portion, ampullary portion and infundibular portion
3. Which of the following does not support the vagina?
   a) Perineal body
   b) Levator ani muscle
   c) Broad ligament
   d) Cardinal ligament

4. Which of the following ligaments corresponds to the gubernaculum of the testis in males?
   a) Broad ligament
   b) Round ligament
   c) Uterosacral ligaments
   d) Mackenrodt's ligaments
5. Which of the following corresponds to the penis in males?
   a) Clitoris
   b) Vestibule
   c) Mons pubis
   d) Labia minora
6. Which of the following is highly sensitive and richly supplied by nerve endings?
   a) Mons pubis
   b) Labia minora
   c) Glans of clitoris
   d) Labia majora
7. Which of the following arteries supplies blood to the uterus?
   a) Uterine artery
   b) Ovarian artery
   c) Uterine and ovarian arteries
   d) External iliac artery

Answers

1. (d), 2. (a), 3. (c), 4. (b), 5. (a), 6. (c), 7. (c)

Fill in the blanks

1. The main blood supply to the perineum is from the _____.
2. The lower uterine segment is formed by the _____ of the uterus.
3. The round ligament corresponds to the _____ in men.
4. The lower one-third of the vagina drains into the _____ lymph nodes.
5. Ovarian artery is a branch of the _____.

Answers

1. internal pudendal artery, 2. isthmus, 3. gubernaculum testis, 4. inguinal, 5. aorta

Physiology of Ovulation and Menstruation

Learning Objectives

» To know the physiology of ovulation and menstruation
» To understand the hormonal control of ovulation
» To understand the synchronisation between ovulation and menstruation

■ PHYSIOLOGY OF OVULATION

Before delving into the complex gynecological abnormalities and aberrations, it is essential to have a clear understanding of the basic biological processes necessary for a successful conception.

The organs of generation do not mature till the second decade of life. After a certain period, which varies from individual to individual, some of the functions of these organs cease. The essential organ of reproduction in the female is the ovary as ova are produced in it.

The **accessory organs** include the following:

• The oviducts or fallopian tubes—in which fertilisation occurs
• The uterus—in which the fertilised ovum is implanted and in which the fetus develops and grows
• The vagina—the passage through which the spermatozoa ascend
• The mammary glands—which undergo changes during pregnancy, may also be considered as accessory organs as they aid in providing nourishment to the infant during the initial period of its extrauterine life

Menstruation is defined as a periodic physiologic discharge of blood, mucus and other cellular debris from the uterine endometrium, which occurs at more or less regular intervals (except during pregnancy and lactation), from the time of puberty to menopause.

Menarche indicates the onset of the first menstruation. The average age of menarche is between 12 and 14 years. It may start as early as 10 years or as late as 16 years and still be within normal limits.

Menopause is defined as the final cessation of menstruation due to the loss of ovarian function. This occurs, on average, at about 51 years, but there are wide variations. With menopause, there is exhaustion of the ovarian follicles in the ovary, resulting in hormonal changes and estrogen deficiency.

In a **normal menstrual cycle**, there is cyclical hormone production from the hypothalamus and pituitary, which act on the ovary and stimulate the growth of the ovarian follicle with the parallel proliferation of the uterine endometrium in preparation for the implantation of the embryo. A normal menstrual cycle lasts 21–35 days with 2–6 days of flow and an average blood loss of 20–60 mL.

■ OVARIAN FOLLICULAR DEVELOPMENT

The formation of primary oocytes is an intrauterine event. At 20 weeks of gestation, there are as many as 6–7 million oocytes. However, these oocytes undergo atresia continuously; at birth, only 1–2 million oocytes remain. By puberty, this number of oocytes is reduced to 300,000, and by the time of menopause, the ovary has only rare, interspersed oocytes in a dense stroma.

Follicular Changes

Follicular development (Fig. 3.1) is a dynamic process that continues from menarche until menopause. Initially, there is gonadotropin-independent recruitment of primordial follicles, after which, the follicle-stimulating hormone (FSH) assumes control of follicular differentiation and growth and allows a cohort of follicles to continue differentiating.

The epithelioid cells that are derived from the germinal epithelium surround the oocyte as a single layer of cells, forming the **primary follicle**. These follicular cells proliferate to form multilayered **granulosa cells** surrounding the oocytes, forming a **preantral follicle.**

As the follicle grows, the ovarian stroma organises itself into a fibrous **outer theca externa** and an **inner theca interna**. These two layers are separated by a highly polymerised membrane. At the time of ovulation, the luteinising hormone (LH) acts on this membrane to depolymerise it and allow vascularisation of granulosa cells.

With the collection of follicular fluids, the granulosa cells divide into a cumulus oophorus containing the ovum in the centre and the membrana granulosa lining the cavity forming the antral follicle (**Graafian follicle; Fig. 3.2**).

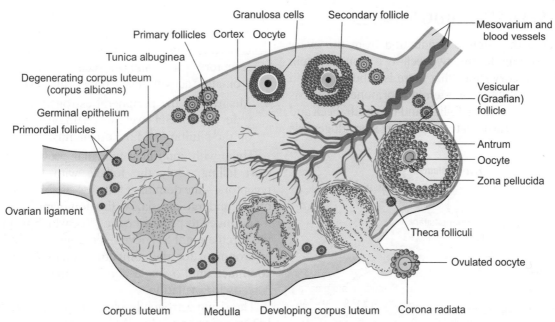

Fig. 3.1 Sequential development of the follicle, formation of corpus luteum and follicular atrophy in the ovary

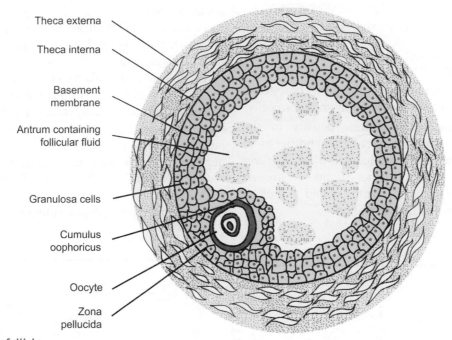

Fig. 3.2 Graafian follicle

The maturing follicle shows an increased rate of growth during the last few days of the **proliferative phase.** This is associated with the increased production of estrogens, which cause characteristic changes in the endometrium, the vaginal mucosa and the cervical mucus. This phase is also associated with increased LH secretion with the rupture of the Graafian follicle, ovulation, and later, the development of the **corpus luteum**. Ovulation is the process by which the mature ovum is released from the ovary.

The corpus luteum produces considerable quantities of progesterone and also some estrogen. These hormones prepare the endometrium for implantation, render the cervical mucus hostile to sperm penetration, and alter the vaginal mucosa. Unless the corpus luteum is exposed to massive stimulation from the products of conception, its functional life is limited. Fourteen days after ovulation, steroid secretion decreases so markedly that the endometrium is desquamated and shed in the form of menstrual bleeding.

■ OVARIAN STEROIDOGENESIS

It is believed that steroid production from the ovary occurs according to the two cell–two gonadotropin theory. This theory states that there is subdivision and compartmentalisation of steroid hormone synthesis activity in the developing follicle and that both theca and granulosa cells participate in ovarian steroidogenesis (Fig. 3.3).

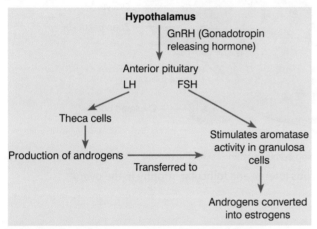

Fig. 3.3 Algorithm for ovarian steroidogenesis

1. Theca cells possess LH receptors. The LH stimulates the theca cells to produce androgens—androstenedione and testosterone from cholesterol. These androgens are transferred to granulosa cells.

2. The FSH stimulates aromatase activity in the granulosa cells, which convert these androgens to estrogens. These locally produced estrogens, along with the FSH, serve to further stimulate estrogen production, FSH receptor synthesis and granulosa cell proliferation and differentiation.

3. At low concentrations, androgens stimulate estrogen aromatase activity in granulosa cells. At high concentrations, they inhibit the expression of FSH receptors on granulosa cells, thereby inhibiting aromatase activity and leading to atresia of the follicle.

4. Meanwhile, the peripheral estrogen level rises and reduces the FSH level by exerting negative feedback on the pituitary and hypothalamus.

Thus, with continued follicular growth, FSH levels start falling. Only the follicle with the most FSH receptors—the dominant follicle—is able to survive; the others undergo atresia. As the dominant follicle grows, it continues to produce estrogens, which further lower the circulating FSH levels, creating an unfavourable environment for the competing follicles. This process continues until a single dominant follicle remains and is ready for ovulation.

The rising estrogen levels exert positive feedback on LH secretion and induce LH receptors on the granulosa cells. This leads to the luteinisation of the granulosa cells, production of progesterone and initiation of ovulation that occurs 10–12 hours after the LH peak.

The **midcycle LH surge** increases the concentration of prostaglandins and proteolytic enzymes in the follicular wall (Fig. 3.4).

The follicle wall weakens, and the oocyte is extruded, leading to ovulation. After ovulation, the remaining follicular granulosa cells take up lipids and yellow lutein pigment and form the corpus luteum. Corpus luteum steroids (estradiol and progesterone) provide negative feedback and cause a decrease in FSH and LH secretion, inhibiting subsequent follicular recruitment.

Progesterone from the corpus luteum supports the endometrium. Corpus luteum function depends

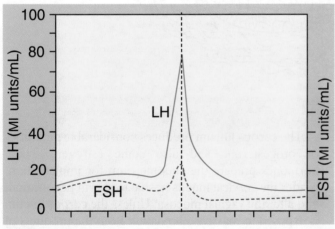

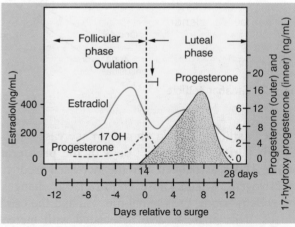

Fig. 3.4 Plasma hormone levels during the ovarian cycle (note that the cycle is divided into follicular and luteal phases based on both histological and endocrine criteria)

on continued LH production. In the absence of pregnancy, the corpus luteum regresses after 12–16 days to form the corpus albicans. The estrogen and progesterone levels wane, the negative feedback is removed and FSH and LH levels rise again and recruit another set of follicles.

If pregnancy occurs, the placental hormone, chorionic gonadotropin (hCG), mimics LH action and continually stimulates the corpus luteum to secrete progesterone. Continued luteal function is essential for pregnancy until the placental hormones take over.

CHANGES THAT OCCUR DURING THE MENSTRUAL CYCLE

Cyclical Changes in the Endometrium

The endometrial histology changes cyclically in accordance with ovarian hormone production. Broadly, the endometrium proliferates and is ultimately shed with each cycle if pregnancy does not occur.

These changes are seen in the superficial two-thirds of the endometrium, which is known as the **decidua functionalis**. The deeper one-third of the endometrium, known as the **decidua basalis**, does not undergo these changes and acts as a source of endometrial regeneration after each menses.

The **proliferative phase** that begins after the menses is characterised by progressive mitotic growth of the endometrium in response to rising levels of estrogen. The straight, narrow and short endometrial glands with low columnar epithelium transform into long, tortuous structures with a pseudostratified pattern. The stroma is dense and compact, and vascular structures are infrequently seen (Fig. 3.5).

The **secretory phase,** which begins after ovulation, is brought about by the effect of progesterone. There is evidence of glandular secretions in the form of glycogen-containing vacuoles in the endometrial cells. The stroma becomes edematous, and the spiral arteries lengthen and coil.

In the absence of implantation, the **menstrual phase** begins. It is brought about by the regression of the corpus luteum and the withdrawal of estrogen and progesterone, leading to spiral artery spasms and endometrial ischemia. This results in an irregular breakdown and shedding of the endometrium.

The endometrium begins to shrink, and bleeding occurs from the spiral arteries exposed by the shedding of the functional layer of the endometrium. After several days, the basal epithelium regenerates and proliferative changes appear in the endometrium as a result of estrogen stimulation from the new ripening follicles.

Changes in the Vagina

The vaginal epithelium also undergoes cyclical hormonal changes, which can be demonstrated in vaginal smears.

Changes in the Cervix

The changes that take place in the cervix either assist or prevent the transport of sperm.

Cervical secretion is closely related to the phases of the menstrual cycle. Just after menstrual bleeding, the cervical canal appears to be closed, and the cervical secretion is not very copious. Just before ovulation, copious amounts of thin cervical secretions are seen. This increased amount of thin mucus favours the ascent of spermatozoa into the upper genital tract. The 'spinnbarkeit' or 'threadability' of the mucus is particularly noticeable at this time and is considered a presumptive sign of ovulation. A few days after ovulation, the amount of cervical mucus decreases again, as does its spinnbarkeit.

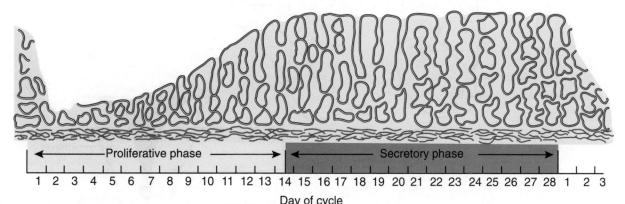

Fig. 3.5   Changes in the endometrium during the menstrual cycle

Alterations in the mucus may also be seen in a dried smear. Before ovulation, cervical mucus crystallises, producing a 'fern pattern'. If ovulation has occurred, the fern pattern is not seen. These changes are of clinical diagnostic importance as they help in determining the fertile period.

The specific biochemical characteristics of the alkaline cervical mucus at the time of ovulation also facilitate sperm migration into the upper genital tract. In contrast, sperm penetrability is reduced or absent during the luteal phase of the menstrual cycle.

NEUROHORMONAL CONTROL OF OVARIAN FUNCTION

The **hypothalamu**s is situated at the base of the brain, above the optic chiasma and below the third ventricle. It is connected directly to the pituitary gland. The hypothalamus secretes **gonadotropin-releasing hormone** (GnRH), also called luteinising

hormone-releasing hormone (LHRH), which is a deca-peptide. LHRH is released in a pulsatile fashion. It controls the secretion of **luteinising hormone** (LH) and **follicle-stimulating hormone** (FSH) from the anterior pituitary, which in turn regulates steroidogenesis in the ovary. Estrogen and progesterone from the ovary regulate the hypothalamus and pituitary by feedback mechanism (Fig. 3.6).

Premenstrual decrease in the concentration of estrogen and progesterone due to the regression of corpus luteum function exerts a positive feedback effect on the hypothalamus, increasing FSH release and stimulating follicular estrogen synthesis.

Rising 17β-estradiol has a dual effect on the hypothalamo–pituitary axis. It inhibits gonadotropin release from the pituitary (negative feedback) and stimulates LHRH secretion by the hypothalamus, which results in increased pituitary LH secretion.

With a further rise in the estradiol level in the preovulatory phase, the negative feedback control

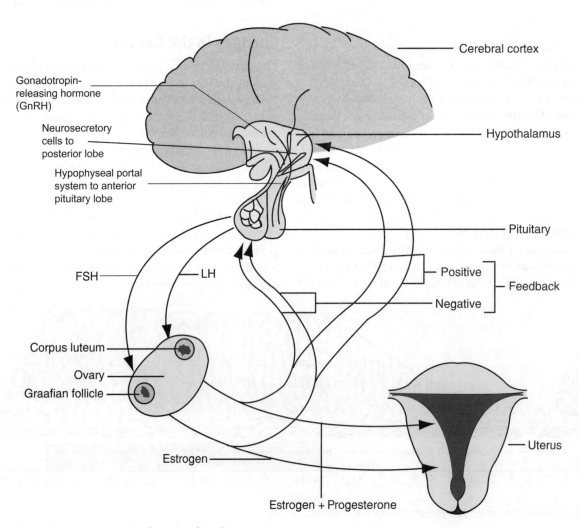

Fig. 3.6 Neurohormonal control of ovarian function

is disturbed, resulting in a preovulatory rise in LH release. The initial rise of LH induces the luteinisation of the theca interna cells with the resulting preovulatory release of progesterone (1 mg/L). This causes the 'LH surge' 12–24 hours prior to ovulation.

The FSH levels remain relatively constant throughout the follicular phase, with a slight rise just prior to ovulation, a return to the base level at the time of ovulation, and again rising a little premenstrually.

The estradiol level rises gradually with the growth of the follicle under the influence of the FSH, reaches its peak level at or just before the LH surge and returns to the follicular level in two days. A second peak is seen in the midluteal phase.

The LH surge induces ovulation followed by corpus luteum formation and increasing progesterone synthesis. A level of progesterone of more than 2 mg/mL suppresses the LHRH. As a result, the pulsatile release of the LH in the luteal phase is less frequent.

The corpus luteum regresses after its fixed lifespan. This leads to a drop in estradiol and progesterone levels, and thereafter, menstruation.

17β-estradiol increases gradually in the follicular phase (the range is 50–100 pg/mL) and reaches its peak (300–400 pg/mL) at or around the time of the LH surge. This level drops after ovulation and shows a second peak in the midluteal phase (100–200 pg/mL) before dropping again to reach its minimum value before menstruation. There are numerous metabolites of estrogen; 17β-estradiol is the most potent, estriol is the least potent, and estrone is midway between the two.

Progesterone has a negligible concentration in the blood during the follicular phase. Just prior to the LH surge, it increases to 1.5 ng/mL; after ovulation, the values rise to reach the midluteal level of 5–10 ng/mL. During the midluteal phase, serum progesterone levels are usually higher than 7 ng/mL. The concentration of progesterone decreases a few days before the onset of menstruation.

KEY POINTS

✓ Menstruation is defined as a periodic discharge of blood, mucus and other cellular debris from the uterine mucosa.

✓ Menarche refers to the onset of menstruation. Menopause is defined as the cessation of the menses.

✓ The hypothalamus secretes, in a pulsatile fashion, GnRH, which controls the secretion of luteinising hormone and follicle-stimulating hormone from the anterior pituitary. These, in turn, regulate steroidogenesis in the ovary.

✓ Both theca and granulosa cells participate in the synthesis of ovarian steroid hormones—estrogen and progesterone.

✓ The endometrium changes in an orderly fashion in response to cyclic hormone production by the ovary. The vaginal epithelium and the cervix also undergo cyclic changes.

Essay questions

1. Describe the changes in the cervical mucus during the different phases of the menstrual cycle.
2. Describe the changes in the endometrium during the different phases of the menstrual cycle.
3. What do you understand of the 'two cell–two gonadotropin' theory of ovarian steroidogenesis?

Short answer questions

1. Define menarche and menopause.
2. Describe the hormonal changes that take place during the menstrual cycle

MCQs

1. What is the average blood loss in a normal menstrual cycle?
   a) 20–60 mL
   b) <20 mL
   c) 60–80 mL
   d) >80 mL

2. If pregnancy does not occur, how long does the corpus luteum take to regress?
   a) After 12–16 days
   b) After <7 days
   c) After 16 days
   d) After 7–12 days

3. How many oocytes are present at the time of puberty?
   a) 3,000
   b) 30,000
   c) 300,000
   d) 300

4. When does the ovary contain the maximum number of oocytes?
   a) 20 weeks of gestation
   b) At birth
   c) At puberty
   d) At 20 years of age

5. When does the LH surge occur?
   a) 12–24 hours before ovulation
   b) At the time of ovulation
   c) 12–24 hours after ovulation
   d) 3 days after ovulation

6. Which of the following is not characteristic of the proliferative phase in the endometrium?
   a) Mitotic growth of the endometrium
   b) The endometrial glands become long and tortuous with a pseudostratified pattern
   c) The stroma is dense and compact
   d) Glycogen-containing vacuoles appear in the endometrial cells

Answers
1. (a), 2. (a), 3. (c), 4. (a), 5. (a), 6. (d)

Fill in the blanks

1. Natural estrogen with the greatest potency is _____.
2. The duration of a normal menstrual cycle is _____.
3. The onset of menstruation at puberty is known as _____.
4. The final cessation of menstruation is known as _____.

Answers
1. 17 β-estradiol, 2. 21–35 days, 3. menarche, 4. menopause

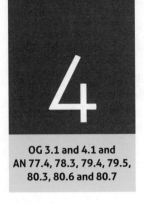
Fertilisation of the Ovum and Development of the Placenta, Embryo and Fetus

---

Learning Objectives

» To describe male and female gametogenesis
» To describe the process of fertilisation and implantation
» To discuss the embryology of the fetus
» To describe the formation and functions of the placenta
» To describe the development of the umbilical cord and the types of attachment
» To describe normal fetomaternal circulation

■ FERTILISATION

Spermatogenesis and Oogenesis

Gametogenesis (Fig. 4.1), the production of sperm and eggs, takes place through the process of meiosis. During meiosis, two cell divisions separate the paired chromosomes (diploid), resulting in gametes. Each one of these gametes contains half the number of chromosomes as the parent (haploid). The production of sperm is called spermatogenesis and the production of eggs is called oogenesis.

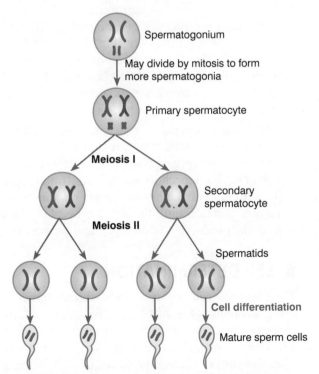

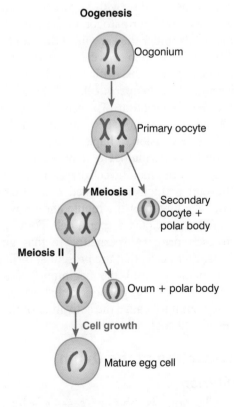

Fig. 4.1 Flowcharts for spermatogenesis and oogenesis

Oogenesis

Oogenesis occurs in the outermost layers of the ovaries. The process starts with a germ cell, called an oogonium, which undergoes mitosis to replicate and increase in number; oogenesis results in the production of up to one to two million cells in the embryo. The first cell that undergoes meiosis is called a primary oocyte. This cell begins the first meiotic division but is arrested in the first prophase stage. At the time of birth, all the cells are in the prophase stage. At adolescence, anterior pituitary hormones facilitate the development of a number of follicles in the ovary. This results in the primary oocyte completing its first meiotic division. The cell divides unequally, with most of the cellular material and organelles going to one cell, called a secondary oocyte, and only one set of chromosomes and a small amount of cytoplasm going to the other cell. This second cell, which is called a polar body, usually dies. A secondary meiotic arrest occurs at the metaphase stage. At ovulation, this secondary oocyte is released, following which, it travels towards the uterus through the fallopian tube. If the secondary oocyte is fertilised, the meiosis II is completed, producing a second polar body and a fertilised egg containing all 46 chromosomes, half of which are from the sperm.

Spermatogenesis

Spermatogenesis occurs in the walls of the seminiferous tubules, with stem cells at the periphery of the tube and spermatozoa in the lumen of the tube. Immediately under the capsule of the tubule are diploid, undifferentiated stem cells called spermatogonia. These cells undergo mitosis, with one offspring going on to differentiate into a sperm cell and the other giving rise to the next generation of sperm. Meiosis begins with a cell called a primary spermatocyte. At the end of the first meiotic division, a haploid cell is produced, called a secondary spermatocyte. This haploid cell must go through another meiotic cell division. The cell produced at the end of meiosis is called a spermatid. When it reaches the lumen of the tubule and grows a flagellum (or 'tail'), it is called a sperm cell. Four sperms result from each primary spermatocyte that goes through meiosis. Stem cells that are present at birth are inactive and remain so until the beginning of adolescence. During adolescence, gonadotropic hormones from the anterior pituitary cause the activation of these cells and the production of viable sperm.

Fertilisation of the Ovum

Definition

• Fertilisation is the process of fusion of the spermatozoa and the ovum. It usually occurs in the ampullary region of the fallopian tube. After the ejaculation of the seminal fluid into the posterior fornix, the spermatozoa ascend through the cervical mucous plug and the uterine cavity to reach the fallopian tube. If an ovum is present in the outer end of the tube, fertilisation occurs here, ten to twelve hours after the intercourse.

• The fertilised ovum then moves down the fallopian tube by tubal peristalsis and enters the uterine cavity at the end of about three days, having reached the blastocyst stage during transit (Fig. 4.2).

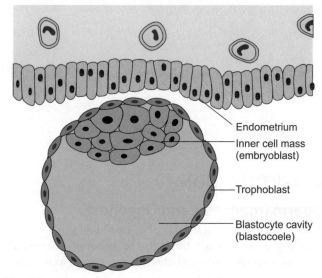

Fig. 4.2 Blastocyst

• The chorionic cells surrounding the blastocyst now begin the process of embedding the fertilised ovum in the uterine cavity (Fig. 4.3). This is chiefly achieved by the direct erosion of the uterine mucosa in the progestational phase. The embedding of the fertilised ovum in the uterine cavity is also aided by the cytolytic property of the cells.

• The invasive chorionic cells promote implantation and the establishment of circulation for the rapidly growing conceptus. They also start secreting the hormone human chorionic gonadotrophin (hCG). This hormone of embryonic origin maintains corpus luteum function until the developing placenta takes over the production of estrogen and progesterone.

■ SEX DETERMINATION

The human cell contains 46 chromosomes. The ovum contains 44 somatic chromosomes and two X chromosomes, whereas the spermatozoon contains 44 chromosomes and one X and one Y chromosome. After maturation, these are reduced to 22 X in the ovum and 22 X or 22 Y in the spermatozoon. After the union of the gametes, the zygote will contain either 44 XX

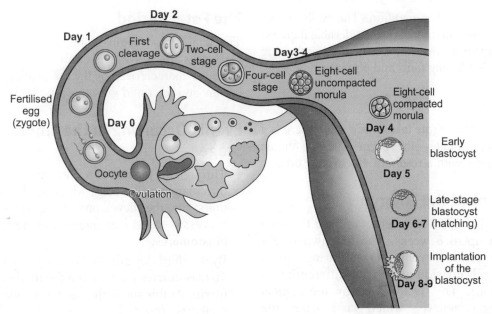

Fig. 4.3 Ovulation, fertilisation and implantation

chromosomes or 44 XY chromosomes. The presence of an X and a Y chromosome results in a male child, whereas the presence of two X chromosomes results in a female child.

Important aspects of sex determination during development
- A zygote containing 46 (2X) chromosomes will result in a female child and one containing 46 (XY) chromosomes will result in a male child.
- The Y chromosome is essential for the transformation of a gonad into a testis. The absence of the Y chromosome leads to ovarian development.
- Two X chromosomes are required for ovarian formation. The presence of only one X chromosome may lead to ovarian dysgenesis.
- Once the gonad has differentiated into a testis, it secretes testosterone and the anti-Müllerian hormone. The anti-Müllerian hormone inhibits the development of the Müllerian system or the female reproductive organs.
- Testosterone stimulates the development of the Wolffian system in the male.

Importance of the Y Chromosome

The female sex is considered neutral; it is the Y chromosome that directs gonadal differentiation towards forming the testes. In the absence of the Y chromosome, the gonad develops into an ovary. For proper ovarian formation, both the X chromosomes are required (XX). If only one X chromosome is present (XO), ovarian dysgenesis results.

Development of the Testes

The development of the testes is regulated by the sex determining region (*SRY*)—a gene located on the short arm of the Y chromosome. For up to eight weeks, the urogenital tracts are indistinguishable in the two sexes. Thereafter, differentiation of the internal and external genitalia to the male phenotype is dependent upon testicular function.

Hormonal secretions from the testes

Once the gonad has differentiated into a testis, it secretes two substances—testosterone, the male hormone, and the anti-Müllerian hormone (AMH). The anti-Müllerian hormone inhibits the development of the Müllerian system in the fetus. In the external genitalia, the testosterone is converted to dihydrotestosterone (DHT) in the presence of 5α-reductase, which is essential for the development of the external genitalia in the male. Testosterone stimulates the development of the Wolffian system in the male.

Genetic sex is established at fertilisation, **gonadal sex** is determined by the *SRY* gene on the Y chromosome, and **phenotypic sex** is dependent on the secretion of testosterone and anti-Müllerian hormone from the fetal testes.

▌ EARLY DEVELOPMENT OF THE EMBRYO

With the arrival of the fertilised ovum in the uterus, extensive changes begin in the uterus and the neighbouring organs of generation. The walls of the uterus hypertrophy, and there is a considerable increase in the blood supply to meet the needs of the enlarging uterus and the developing fetus and placenta (Fig. 4.4).

Zygotic Stage

The formation of the zygote takes place when there is a fusion of the male gamete—the sperm—and the female gamete—the egg—with a resultant 46 chromosomes.

Development of the Embryo

The conceptus is known as an embryo from the time of fertilisation up to 8 weeks. The first two weeks constitute the pre-embryonic stage, during which there is rapid cell division and initial differentiation (cell maturation). This is followed by the critical period of organogenesis, which lasts from the third to the eighth week of development following fertilisation.

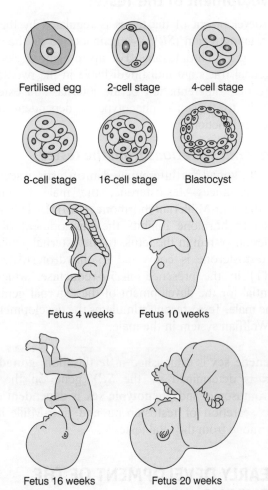

Fertilised egg   2-cell stage   4-cell stage

8-cell stage   16-cell stage   Blastocyst

Fetus 4 weeks   Fetus 10 weeks

Fetus 16 weeks   Fetus 20 weeks

Fig. 4.4   Stages of embryonic and fetal development

The Fetal Period

The fetal period begins eight weeks after fertilisation (10 weeks after LMP) and continues until delivery. This period is characterised by the maturation of tissues and organs and the rapid growth of the body.

Events Occurring in the Embryonic Stage

- Through the process of mitosis, the zygote subdivides into many smaller cells, which are the early building units for the development of the embryo. This process is called cleavage and the resulting cells are **blastomeres.**
- By the third day after fertilisation, a cluster of about 16 blastomeres passes from the uterine tube into the uterus. At this stage, the cluster is called a morula or mulberry.
- By the time some 30 blastomeres have been produced, pools of clear fluid accumulate between some of the internal cells. These spaces soon coalesce into a common subcentral cavity. The resulting hollow cellular ball is a blastula and is called a **blastocyst.**
- While it is within the uterine cavity, the blastocyst loses its gelatinous capsule, imbibes fluid, and expands to a diameter of 0.2 mm. Six to nine days after fertilisation, the naked and sticky blastocyst comes into contact with the uterine lining and adheres to it. The endometrium is most receptive between day 20–24 of the menstrual cycle for implantation.

Trophoblast formation

The compact mass of cells at one pole of the blastocyst is called the **inner cell mass.** This forms the embryo, while the outer mass of cells forms the **trophoblast**. The cells of the trophoblast differentiate further into an inner cellular layer, which is termed the **cytotrophoblast or Langhans' layer**, and an outer syncytial layer termed the **syncytiotrophoblast**.

Implantation process

The syncytiotrophoblast throws out a large number of irregular villous processes, which exert a histolytic action on the uterine mucosa. This not only facilitates the embedding of the ovum in the maternal tissues but also, a little later, provides channels by which the developing embryo can draw nourishment from maternal blood. This process is called **implantation** (Fig. 4.5) and occurs 6–9 days after fertilisation or on day 19–20 of the menstrual cycle.

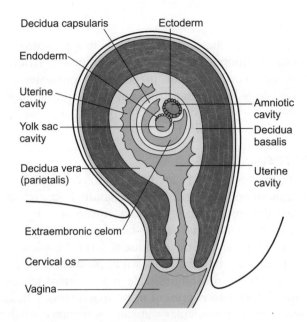

Fig. 4.5 Early stage of implantation

Formation of the yolk sac in the embryo

While these changes are occurring in the trophoblast, the inner mass undergoes differentiation, which results in the formation of two hollow vesicles. Of the two vesicles so formed, one remains in close contact with the trophoblast and constitutes the **amnio-embryonic vesicle**; the other is placed more centrally and is usually referred to as the **yolk sac.** By six weeks of pregnancy, the embryo is 4–5 mm long, cardiac development is complete and cardiac activity is seen. The partitioning of the **primitive heart** is completed by eight weeks; then, the limb buds are formed. Development of the CNS takes place three weeks after fertilisation.

Events Occurring in the Fetal Period

- At 10 weeks of pregnancy, the embryo is called a **fetus** and is nearly 4 cm long.
- Respiratory system development is seen at 11 weeks of gestation with the appearance of bronchioles. However, alveoli appear later. The development of the lungs is complete by 25 weeks of gestation.
- By the end of 12 weeks, centres of ossification appear in most of the fetal bones and the external genitalia begin to show signs of differentiation.
- By 14 weeks, it is possible to assign the sex of the fetus based on the appearance of the external genitalia.
- By 28 weeks, the fetus weighs about 1 Kg. At the end of 32 weeks, the fetus weighs about 1.8 Kg. The skin is still wrinkled.

- By 36 weeks, the fetal body becomes more rounded because of the deposition of subcutaneous fat.

FETAL MEMBRANES AND THE PLACENTA

Amnion

Structure

The amnion is a double-layered, translucent membrane that encloses the amniotic fluid. Its outer layer is mesodermal connective tissue and its inner layer is the ectoderm. Although it generally consists of a few layers of stratified squamous cells, patches of low cuboidal cells are also seen. It is avascular and provides major tensile strength to the fetal membranes.

Function

The amnion is metabolically active. It maintains amniotic fluid homeostasis and produces many bioactive compounds like growth factors and cytokines. The chorion and amnion arise from the placenta at its margin to envelop the fetus. They strip easily from the fetal surface of the placenta and can be separated from one another by careful dissection.

Chorion

Structure

The chorion consists of two layers—an outer **trophoblast** and an inner primary **mesenchyme**. The mucous membrane that covers the ovum is called the **decidua capsularis**, the portion on which the ovum rests is termed the **decidua basalis** and the rest of the lining of the uterus is called the **decidua vera**. With the growth of the embryo and the expansion of the amniotic cavity, the decidua capsularis is compressed and becomes thinner; the circulation through it is gradually cut off, and the villi of the corresponding part of the chorion atrophy and disappear. This portion of the chorion becomes smooth and, as it takes no share in the formation of the placenta, it is sometimes termed the non-placental part of the chorion or **chorion laeve**. On the other hand, the villi on the part of the chorion that is in contact with the decidua basalis increase greatly in size and complexity. Hence, the chorion is named chorion **frondosum** (Fig. 4.6).

Liquor Amnii

The fluid that collects within the amniotic cavity surrounding the embryo is called amniotic fluid or **liquor amnii**.

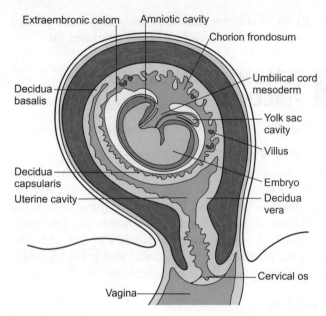

Fig. 4.6 Relationship of the chorion to the placenta

Source

In early pregnancy, amniotic fluid is an ultrafiltrate of maternal plasma. By the beginning of the second trimester, the amniotic fluid becomes an extension of the fetal extracellular fluid space which diffuses through the fetal skin and is similar to fetal plasma. After 20 weeks, increasing stratification and cornification of the skin prevents diffusion. The fetal urine then becomes the major contributor to the amniotic fluid and fetal swallowing is probably the major route of fluid removal. The fetal kidneys start producing urine at 12 weeks of gestation. Towards term, saliva and lung fluid may also contribute to the composition of the fluid.

Composition

In the later part of pregnancy, the amniotic fluid is slightly alkaline (pH is about 7.2) and hypotonic. The concentration of electrolytes is essentially the same as that of maternal blood. As pregnancy advances, there is a decrease in the concentration of both sodium and chloride. This is due to the addition of the highly hypotonic fetal urine to the existing amniotic fluid. The concentration of urea, uric acid and creatinine gradually increases in the amniotic fluid as pregnancy reaches term. The average values near term are presented in Table 4.1.

Table 4.1 Composition of amniotic fluid near term

Component	Content
Protein	0.5 g
Non-protein	24 mg
Nitrogen/Uric acid	4–5 mg
Sugar	19 mg
Calcium	5.5 mg
Creatinine	2.2 mg per 100 mL of amniotic fluid

Hormones

Recent studies have demonstrated the presence of various hormones in the liquor amnii—cortisone, 17-hydroxy corticosteroids, pregnanediol, progesterone, 17-ketosteroids, pregnanetriol and estriol. In addition, human chorionic gonadotropin (hCG) and human placental lactogen (hPL) are also present.

Other substances

Prostaglandin E_1 and E_2 are found in the amniotic fluid throughout pregnancy; only prostaglandin F seems to be present during labour. A high concentration of $F_{2\alpha}$ has been found in maternal venous blood samples obtained during labour and in the decidua at term. Infusions of both E_2 and $F_{2\alpha}$ have been shown to produce rhythmic uterine activity indistinguishable from normal labour. Although bilirubin is present in normal amniotic fluid, it has acquired particular clinical significance in the prenatal assessment of rhesus hemolytic disease of the newborn.

Volume

It has been shown that amniotic fluid volume increases steadily throughout pregnancy to a maximum of 800–1,200 mL at 34–38 weeks. It averages at about 50 mL at 12 weeks of pregnancy, 400 mL at 20 weeks, and 1 litre at 36 weeks. After 38 weeks, fluid volume declines by approximately 125 mL/week, to an average volume of 800 mL at 40 weeks. There is further decrease in amniotic fluid approaching 100–600 mL at 43 weeks (Table 4.2). The presence of an excessive amount of liquor amnii is called **hydramnios**. Diminution in the volume of amniotic fluid is called **oligohydramnios**.

Table 4.2 Amniotic fluid volume at various stages of pregnancy

Period of gestation (in weeks)	Volume of liquor amnii (in mL)
12	50
20	400
35	1,000
43	100–600

Causes of hydramnios

Pregnancy-related
- Multiple pregnancy
- Maternal diabetes
- Hydrops fetalis

Fetal malformations
- Anencephaly, hydrocephalus
- Spina bifida
- Esophageal atresia

Idiopathic

Causes of oligohydramnios
Pregnancy-related
- Placental insufficiency during pregnancy like severe pregnancy-induced hypertension (PIH)

Complications
- Rupture of the membrane

Fetal malformations
- Fetal bilateral renal agenesis

Appearance

The colour of the amniotic fluid changes during the normal course of pregnancy. Prior to 20 weeks, it usually ranges from a pale straw colour to deep yellow, depending upon the amount of **bilirubin** present. At this stage of pregnancy, bilirubin is a normal constituent of amniotic fluid and does not necessarily indicate rhesus hemolytic disease in the fetus.

After mid-pregnancy, the concentration of bilirubin decreases, and by 36 weeks, the normal amniotic fluid is virtually colourless. White floccules may sometimes appear in the fluid during the last four to five weeks. These are clumps of desquamated fetal skin cells and free lipid material, the **vernix caseosa**, which may be found on the skin of the infant at birth. Abnormal colouring usually results from contamination with blood or meconium, but it may also be due to bilirubin. High bilirubin levels after 30 weeks must be regarded as abnormal. Golden-coloured amniotic fluid is seen in cases of Rh-isoimmunisation, bloodstained amniotic fluid in abruption, tobacco juice-like or dark brown amniotic fluid in cases if intrauterine death, and greenish amniotic fluid when there is meconium-stained liquor.

Functions of amniotic fluid

The amniotic fluid serves several important functions, which are as follows:
- It provides a medium in which the fetus can move.
- It allows musculoskeletal development of the fetus.
- It protects the fetus from trauma.
- It maintains the temperature of the fetus.
- It promotes growth and development of the lungs and gastrointestinal tracts.
- It promotes surfactant synthesis.

Clinical importance

Amniotic fluid analysis has clinical importance in various situations, which are as follows:
- For the study of sex-linked disease, chromosomal abnormalities and metabolic disorders
- In the evaluation of Rh-isoimmunisation
- In the evaluation of intrauterine fetal infections
- In the estimation of fetal lung maturity

Amniotic fluid measurement is important in the evaluation of the well-being of the fetus. The amount of amniotic fluid can be measured by ultrasound. **Amniotic fluid index (AFI)** is defined as the sum of vertical depths of the largest amniotic fluid pocket in each of the four uterine quadrants. The normal range is 5–24 cm.

Interpretation of AFI

- <5 cm is considered oligohydramnios
- 5–8 cm is considered low normal
- 8–18 cm is normal
- 18–24 cm is high normal
- >24 cm is indicative of polyhydramnios

■ THE UMBILICAL CORD

The umbilical cord extends from the fetal umbilicus to the placenta and conveys fetal blood to and from the placenta. It usually begins at or near the centre of the fetal surface of the placenta. The umbilical cord is formed by an outer covering of amniotic ectoderm containing the vitello-intestinal duct and the yolk sac or umbilical vesicle. The umbilical cord incorporates within itself the body stalk and its contained umbilical vessels (two umbilical arteries and one umbilical vein) and the allantois (Fig. 4.7a and b).

The umbilical cord is spirally twisted and increases in length as pregnancy progresses so that at the end of pregnancy, it is about 50 cm long. On cross-section, the cord shows a covering of amniotic epithelium, generally two arteries and one vein and the remains of the allantois with Wharton's jelly, which holds everything together (Fig. 4.7a and b).

Abnormalities

Length

- A short umbilical cord is one that is <30–35 cm in length. It may be associated with congenital malformations, fetal growth restriction and intrapartum distress of abruptio placenta.
- A long umbilical cord is >80 cm in length. An excessively long cord could lead to cord entanglement, cord prolapse and fetal distress, increasing fetal morbidity.

Single umbilical artery

Single umbilical artery is associated with an increased risk of chromosomal aberrations and congenital malformations in the fetus. Neonates with isolated single umbilical artery have increased rates of prematurity, growth restriction and adverse neonatal outcomes.

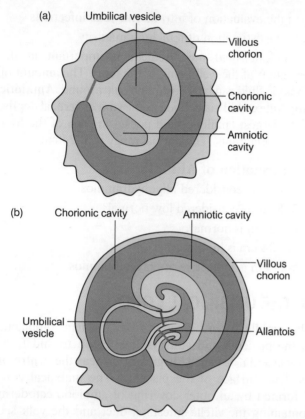

(a)
- Umbilical vesicle
- Villous chorion
- Chorionic cavity
- Amniotic cavity

(b)
- Chorionic cavity
- Amniotic cavity
- Villous chorion
- Umbilical vesicle
- Allantois

Fig. 4.7 Development of umbilical cord: (a) the amniotic cavity, chorionic cavity and the yolk sac and (b) the development of umbilical cord from the stalk of the yolk sac and the connecting stalk

Types of Cord Insertion

Marginal insertion

Cord insertion at the placental margin is also known as **Battledore placenta** (Fig. 4.8). This does not cause any increase in the risk to the mother or fetus.

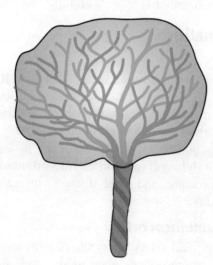

Fig. 4.8 Battledore placenta

Velamentous insertion

The umbilical vessels separate in the membranes at a distance from the placental margin (Fig. 4.9). This occurs more frequently with twins than in singleton pregnancies.

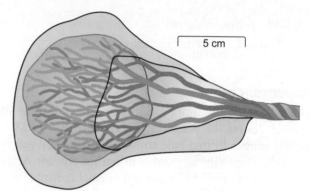

5 cm

Fig. 4.9 Velamentous insertion

Vasa previa

This is usually associated with velamentous insertion when some of the fetal vessels in the membranes cross the region of the cervical os or below the presenting part (Fig. 4.10). Sometimes, this can also occur with a succenturiate-lobed placenta or with marginal insertion of the cord. When the membranes rupture, it presents as antepartum hemorrhage due to the tearing of a fetal vessel, which results in fetal bleeding, and leads to fetal distress and fetal death if not delivered immediately.

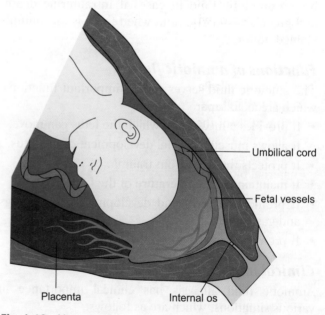

- Umbilical cord
- Fetal vessels
- Placenta
- Internal os

Fig. 4.10 Vasa previa

■ PLACENTA

Development

- After the embedding of the fertilised ovum, a mass of syncytiotrophoblast (**the trophoblastic shell**) develops around the periphery. At first, these cells simply digest the endometrial and stromal cells. But with the growth of the embryo, in order to supply oxygen and nutrition, the maternal vessels open up, bathing the fertilised ovum in a 'lake' of maternal blood. This ensures a supply of oxygen and food to the developing embryo. The **chorionic villi** attach the fetus to the uterus.
- At first, the cells are composed of the syncytiotrophoblasts. Later, there appears a core of discrete, pale cells called the cytotrophoblast or **Langhans' layer**.
- About the same time, the mesoderm is growing into the villus and the afferent and efferent vessels are being developed in situ. The villus is now mature. Most of the chorionic villi, which branch and rebranch in a complicated manner, float freely in the maternal blood 'lake' and expose a very large area to the blood circulating there; these are called **nutritive villi**. The vessels in the villi join each other until they converge in the body stalk to form the umbilical vessels. Other villi are attached directly to the decidua, particularly in the region of the decidua basalis. Their main function is to ensure anatomical fixation of the growing ovum. The trophoblast from these anchoring villi spreads over the surface of the decidua basalis so that the entire maternal blood space is lined with trophoblastic cells. The villus surface of the syncytiotrophoblast is bathed directly by maternal blood, but fetal blood is contained within fetal capillaries in the villi of the placenta. This type of placenta is called a **hemochorioendothelial placenta**.
- Fetal blood is separated from the syncytiotrophoblasts by the walls of the fetal capillaries, the mesenchyme in the villous space and the cytotrophoblasts. Fetal blood does not come into direct contact with maternal blood.

Structure of Chorionic Villi

- Villi can be seen in the human placenta as early as 12 days after fertilisation. The trophoblast undergoes rapid proliferation and forms numerous processes known as the **primary chorionic villi** on the surface of the chorion. These increase in size and ramify, and the chorionic mesenchyme invades the solid trophoblastic column, forming **secondary villi**. Branches of the umbilical vessels grow into these villi, and in this way, are converted into **tertiary chorionic villi**. The young villus is a delicate structure covered with a layer of **syncytiotrophoblast.** It is sometimes condensed into deeply staining knots at its free tip. Beneath this is the **cytotrophoblast** composed of discrete cubical cells (Fig. 4.11). First, this is two layers thick, then a single layer thick, and in the mature villus, it disappears entirely.
- The mesodermal core of the young villus is comparatively thick, whereas that in the mature organ is very thin. The capillaries of the villus are thin-walled structures with no special features. Metabolites must pass through these several layers on their way to and from the fetal bloodstream.
- In the mature or ageing villus, certain stigmata of age are apparent. The syncytium may be represented by an extremely thin film, and in a few places, may be replaced by little clots of fibrin—the fibrin nodes. The Langhans' layer disappears, and the mesodermal core is greatly attenuated.

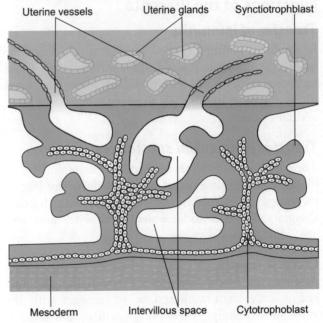

Uterine vessels   Uterine glands   Synctiotrophblast

Mesoderm   Intervillous space   Cytotrophoblast

Fig. 4.11 Structure of the chorionic villus

Placenta at Term

The placenta anchors the fetus to the uterine wall and is important for the nutritive, respiratory and excretory functions of the fetus.

Structure

At term, the human placenta is a discoid organ measuring 15–20 cm in diameter and 2–3 cm in thickness and weighing about 500 g. Usually, it is implanted on the posterior or anterior surface of the uterine cavity, well towards the fundus. There are two circulations—the fetal and maternal circulation. On examination of the maternal surface of the expelled placenta, one can see that it is divided by depressed areas of varying depths into irregularly shaped lobes known as cotyledons. The cotyledons are filled with loose villi attached only to the major villous stalks. The number of cotyledons varies from 10 to 38. The depressed areas are the bases of the placental septa, which are mostly made up of fibrous tissue. The septa, which are maternal in origin, extend only to about three quarters of the way to the chorionic plate; very few functional vessels are seen in it at term. The increase in the weight of the fetus is proportional to that of the placenta from 12–30 weeks of pregnancy. Thereafter, there is very little increase in the weight of the placenta; there is no further rise in the post-term period. At term, around 150 mL of blood may be transferred from the placenta to the newborn if there is a delay of ten minutes before the cord is tied.

Functions of the Placenta

Transfer of immunity

In humans, immune bodies are transferred from the mother to the fetus through the chorionic villi. These protect the newborn at birth. This forms the basis for maternal immunisation to protect newborns from certain diseases.

Transfer of essential substances

The supply of substances required for maintaining fetal life and the elimination of waste products are largely facilitated by diffusion across the placental barrier. Oxygen, carbon dioxide, water, electrolytes and urea are included in this group.

Oxygen supply

At first, the blood that flows through the placental site is only slightly altered by its contact with the villi. Subsequently, when the growth of the fetus is accelerated, marked changes take place. Due to the continuous passage of oxygen from the maternal blood in the intervillous space to the fetus, the oxygen saturation of this blood resembles that in the maternal capillaries and is less than that of the mother's arterial blood. The average oxygen saturation of the intervillous space blood is estimated to be 65–75%, with a partial pressure of oxygen of about 30–40 mmHg. The oxygen saturation of the umbilical vein blood is approximately 60%, with a partial pressure of oxygen of about 20 mmHg. Despite the relatively low partial pressure of oxygen, the fetus normally does not suffer from a lack of oxygen. The cardiac output in a human fetus in late pregnancy is considerably greater (per unit of weight) than in an adult. This, along with the increased oxygen-carrying capacity of the fetal blood due to its higher hemoglobin concentration, compensates effectively for the low oxygen tension.

Supply of nutrition

Many nutritional substances such as glucose, amino acids, calcium, phosphorus, iron and probably some of the vitamins cross the placental barrier.

Glucose transfer

In the early months of pregnancy, glycogen is stored in the placenta until the fetal liver and pancreas are sufficiently developed to take over the function of storing and utilising this carbohydrate. As it contains glycolytic enzymes, the placenta too is able to convert its store of glycogen into absorbable glucose. Most of the fetal carbohydrate is absorbed from the mother's blood in the form of glucose, which passes readily through the placenta.

Vitamins

The water-soluble vitamins, B1 and C, pass through the placenta readily and the latter is retained in excess in fetal blood. Riboflavin is transmitted by the absorption and degradation of its dinucleotide precursor. The fat-soluble vitamins A, E and K are also probably transmitted through the placenta, but definite evidence concerning the permeability of the placenta to vitamin D is lacking.

Hormones

The placenta produces many steroid and protein hormones. It produces large amounts of estrogens, progesterone, chorionic gonadotropin (hCG) and human placental lactogen (hPL). It also produces chorionic adrenocorticotropin (ACTH), growth hormone, chorionic thyrotrophin, parathyroid-related protein (PTHrP), calcitonin and relaxin.

Abnormalities of the Placenta

Circumvallate placenta

The fetal surface of the placenta presents a central depression surrounded by a thickened greyish-white ring. The ring is composed of a double fold of amnion and chorion, with degenerated decidua and fibrin in-between. Large vessels terminate abruptly at the margin of the ring (Fig. 4.12).

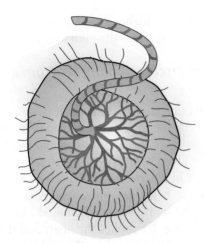

Fig. 4.12 Circumvallate placenta

Clinical significance

There is an increased risk of antepartum hemorrhage, both from placental abruption and fetal hemorrhage, increasing fetal morbidity.

Succenturiate lobes

One or more small accessory lobes may develop in the membranes at a distance from the periphery of the main placenta (Fig. 4.13).

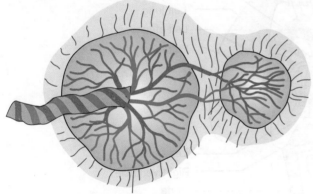

Fig. 4.13 Succenturiate placenta

Multiple placentae with a single fetus

Occasionally, the placenta is separated into lobes. When the division is incomplete, the vessels extend from one lobe to the other before uniting to form the umbilical cord, it is called **placenta bipartite**. If the lobes are separated entirely and the vessels remain distinct, the condition is known as **placenta duplex** (two lobes; Fig. 4.14) or **placenta triplex** (three lobes).

Membranaceous placenta

In this condition, the placenta develops as a thin membranous structure occupying the entire periphery of the chorion and all the fetal membranes are covered with functioning villi.

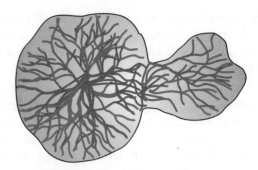

Fig. 4.14 Placenta duplex

Maternal Circulation in the Placenta

Blood leaves the maternal circulation and flows into a 'lake' lined by the fetal syncytium, not the maternal endothelium. This blood then drains back into the maternal veins. There is normally no gross intermingling of the maternal and fetal blood. There is still no clear understanding of the supply and drainage of the intervillous space. It has been stated that arterial blood enters at the base of the cotyledons and flows upward to the subchorial lake and laterally to the marginal sinus, where all of the venous drainage of the placenta takes place.

It has been shown that the spiral arteries lie more or less perpendicular to the uterine wall, while the veins generally run parallel to it, thus facilitating the closure of the veins during uterine contractions and preventing the squeezing of vital maternal blood from the intervillous space. The spiral arteries pour their blood into the intervillous space. The arterial blood then filters in all directions, gradually draining downward to pass out through the basally distributed veins. See Chapter 5 for the description of uteroplacental blood flow.

■ PHYSIOLOGY OF THE FETUS

- During the **early period** of its development, the fertilised ovum is dependent on the remains of the cells of the discus proligerus adhering to it or on the fluid of the fallopian tube into which it is immersed for its nourishment.

- From the **second week** onwards, blood vessels traverse the chorionic villi and come into close contact with the maternal blood. From this period, the growth of the fetus is maintained by the fetomaternal circulation.

- In the **fully formed fetus**, blood passes from the fetus to the placenta through the umbilical arteries and returns through the umbilical vein. There is no communication between fetal and maternal circulations.

- The placenta represents the fetal organ of respiration, nutrition and excretion. Thus, the umbilical arteries carry dark venous blood to the placenta. This blood loses its carbonic acid and takes up oxygen.

- The oxygen requirement of the fetus is small as it is protected from the loss of heat, its movements are sluggish, and only the oxidative processes that are required for the building up of the developing tissues are needed. However, the fetus requires a rich supply of nutrition for its growth.

Fetal Circulation

The fetal blood flows to and from the placenta at the attachment of the umbilical cord (Fig. 4.15).

Deoxygenated fetal blood flows to the placenta through the two umbilical arteries. The vessels course through the chorionic plate and into the larger stem villi. They festoon into small, free-floating, finely branched villi. The vessels follow the branching villi, which become smaller and smaller and end in smaller terminal villi containing only capillary networks. Blood

with significantly higher oxygen content returns from the placenta to the fetus through a single umbilical vein.

How fetal circulation differs from adult circulation

Fetal circulation differs from adult circulation in some respects. Fetal blood is not oxygenated in the lungs, so a major portion of the right ventricular output bypasses the lungs. The chambers of the fetal heart work in parallel, not in a series as in the adult. As a result, the brain and the heart get more oxygenated blood than the rest of the body. Well-oxygenated blood enters the left ventricle which supplies the heart and the brain and less oxygenated blood enters the right ventricle which supplies the rest of the body.

The blood flow in the fetus

- The blood vessels traverse the umbilical cord and enter the umbilicus of the fetus. Here the umbilical vein, which carries oxygenated blood from the placenta, passes directly into the liver. Before

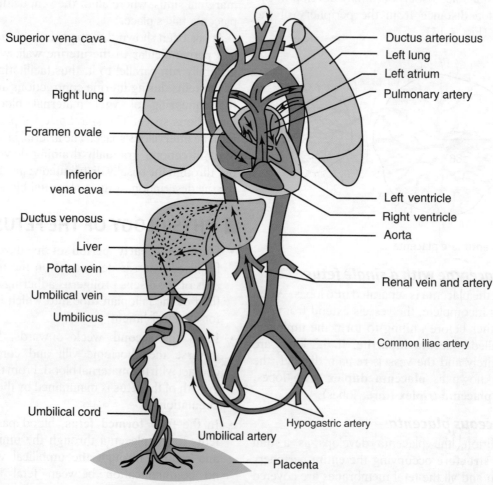

Fig. 4.15 Fetal circulation (Adapted from Parer JJ. Fetal circulation. Sciarra JJ (ed). *Obstetrics and Gynecology*, Vol. 3. Maternal and Fetal Medicine. Maryland: Harper & Row. 1984.)

doing so, however, it gives off a branch, **the ductus venosus,** which carries the greater part of the blood directly into the inferior vena cava and then to the right atrium. Here, the bloodstream impinges on the eustachian valve and is directed through the foramen ovale into the left atrium, from where it passes into the left ventricle, to be driven into the aorta.

- As this arterial blood passes into the inferior vena cava through the ductus venosus, it is mixed with the venous blood returning from the lower limbs and the lower part of the trunk. The well-oxygenated blood courses along the medial aspect of the inferior vena cava, and the less oxygenated blood along the lateral aspect. Once this blood enters the right atrium, the well-oxygenated blood is preferentially shunted through the foramen ovale into the left heart and then into the brain.

- After these tissues have extracted oxygen, the less oxygenated blood returns to the right ventricle through the superior vena cava. The less oxygenated blood coursing through the lateral aspect of the inferior vena cava also enters the right ventricle from the right atrium. Only a small part of the blood passes through the lungs, while the greater part traverses through the ductus arteriosus, which communicates with the aortic arch (Fig. 4.16 and 4.17).

- The aorta divides into the common iliacs, which further divide into the internal and external iliacs. From the internal iliacs, the hypogastric arteries leave, and ascending alongside the bladder to the umbilical vein as the umbilical arteries in the cord,

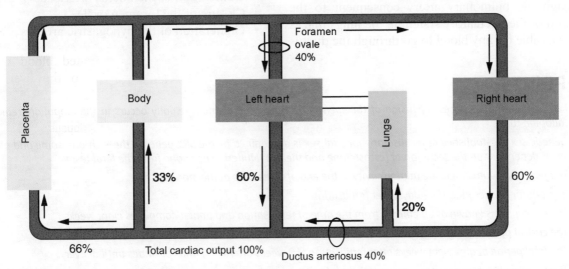

Fig. 4.16 Diagram representing the fetal circulatory system and the approximate proportions of blood flowing through its various elements

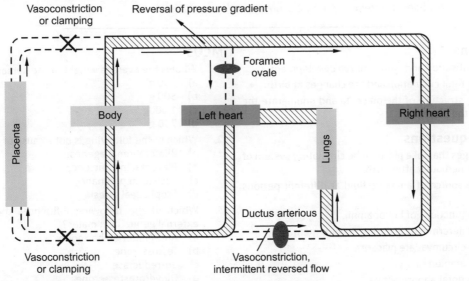

Fig. 4.17 Diagram showing the transition from fetal to adult-type circulation

they reach the placenta. Here, they split up into arterioles and capillaries in the villi.

CHANGES IN CIRCULATION AFTER BIRTH

After the birth of the child, when the first inspiration takes place, the circulation of the newborn undergoes the following changes:

- The resistance to the blood flow through the lungs is diminished, and the blood passes from the pulmonary arteries through the lungs into the left atrium.
- The pressure in the left atrium increases, whereas that in the right atrium decreases, so that the foramen ovale closes and remains closed.
- The increased rush of blood from the right ventricle through the pulmonary artery consequent to the suction of the circulatory system in the lungs makes it impossible for any blood to go through the ductus arteriosus, which therefore collapses, becomes obliterated and shrinks.
- Consequent to the ligature applied on the umbilical cord, the supply of blood from the vein is cut off, the walls of the umbilical vein agglutinate, and the vein is reduced to a cord-like ligament passing to the liver, the **ligamentum teres**.
- The ductus venosus also collapses and shrinks and becomes a vestigial structure. The hypogastric arteries contract and thrombose and form the obliterated hypogastric arteries of the adult.

Circulatory changes at birth
- Obliteration of the umbilical vein
- Obliteration of the ductus venosus
- Obliteration of the ductus arteriosus
- Closure of the foramen ovale
- Obliteration of the hypogastric arteries

KEY POINTS

✓ *Fertilisation is the process of fusion of the spermatozoa and the ovum. It usually occurs in the ampullary region of the fallopian tube.*

✓ *Genetic sex is established at fertilisaton, gonadal sex is determined by the* **SRY** *gene on the Y chromosome and phenotypic sex is dependent on the secretion of testosterone and the anti-Müllerian hormone from the fetal testes.*

✓ *The fertilised ovum enters the uterine cavity at the end of three days at the morula stage.*

✓ *Implantation takes place 6–9 days after fertilisation.*

✓ *The conceptus is known as an embryo from the time of fertilisation and until it completes eight weeks.*

✓ *The critical period of organogenesis lasts from the third to the eighth week of development.*

✓ *The fetal period begins eight weeks after fertilisation (10 weeks after LMP) and continues until delivery.*

✓ *The human placenta is hemochorioendothelial. At term, the placenta measures 15–20 cm in diameter, 2–3 cm in thickness and weighs about 500 g.*

✓ *The changes that occur in the fetal circulation at birth include the obliteration of the umbilical vein, ductus venosus, ductus arteriosus and hypogastric arteries, and the closure of the foramen ovale.*

Essay questions

1. Describe fertilisation and early embryo development.
2. Describe the fetal circulation and the changes at birth.
3. Describe the structure of the placenta and enumerate the functions of the placenta.

Short answer questions

1. List the changes that take place in the circulatory system of the infant immediately after birth.
2. Describe the source of amniotic fluid at different periods of gestation.
3. Describe the functions of liquor amnii.
4. Describe sex determination during development.
5. Describe the circumvallate placenta.
6. Describe the amnion.
7. Describe placental abnormalities.

MCQs

1. What is the average weight of the human placenta at term?
   a) 250 g
   b) 500 g
   c) 1,000 g
   d) 750 g

2. Which of the following is not a cause of oligohydramnios?
   a) Bilateral renal agenesis
   b) Placental insufficiency
   c) Post-term pregnancy
   d) Esophageal atresia

3. Which of the following influences the development of external genitalia in males?
   a) Anti-Müllerian hormone
   b) Testosterone
   c) 5α-reductase
   d) Dihydrotestosterone

4. Which of the following is true regarding sex determination of the fetus?
   a) The presence of only one X chromosome is adequate for normal ovarian formation.
   b) Dihydrotestosterone (DHT) stimulates the development of the Wolffian system in the male.
   c) The sex determining region is located on the short arm of the Y chromosome.
   d) Testosterone inhibits the development of the Müllerian system in the fetus.

5. At which stage does the fertilised ovum enter the uterine cavity?
   a) Four-cell stage
   b) Eight-cell stage
   c) Morula stage
   d) Blastocyst stage

6. At which stage is the volume of amniotic fluid maximum?
   a) 25 weeks
   b) 30 weeks
   c) 36 weeks
   d) 40 weeks

7. Where is the *SRY* gene located?
   a) Short arm of Y
   b) Long arm of Y
   c) Short arm of X
   d) Long arm of X

8. Which of the following stimulate the development of the Wolfian system in the male?
   a) AMH
   b) Testosterone
   c) Estrogen
   d) Progesterone

9. Which of the following makes up the umbilical cord?
   a) 2 umbilical arteries and 1 umbilical vein
   b) 1 umbilical artery and 2 umbilical veins
   c) 2 umbilical arteries and 2 umbilical veins
   d) 1 umbilical artery and 1 umbilical vein

Answers
1. (b), 2. (d), 3. (d), 4. (c), 5. (c), 6. (c), 7. (a), 8. (b), 9. (a)

Fill in the blanks

1. The embryonic period lasts for _____ from the time of fertilisation.
2. The sex of the fetus may be assigned based upon the appearance of the external genitalia by _____.
3. The presence of an excessive amount of liquor amnii is known as _____.
4. Testosterone is converted into dihydrotestosterone in the presence of the enzyme _____.

Answers
1. 8 weeks, 2. 14 weeks, 3. polyhydramnios, 4. 5α-reductase

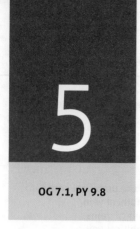

5

OG 7.1, PY 9.8

Maternal Changes During Pregnancy

Learning Objectives

» To know the anatomical changes associated with pregnancy
» To understand the physiological changes in the various systems of the body during pregnancy
» To describe the symptoms produced by these changes during pregnancy
» To interpret the hematological and biochemical changes in pregnant women
» To describe the hormonal changes in pregnancy

■ INTRODUCTION

During pregnancy, to meet the demands of the growing embryo and the fetus, the maternal body undergoes various changes. These include anatomical changes (Fig. 5.1) in various organs of the body to increase space and blood supply to the uterus for the development of the fetus and physiological changes in the various systems of the body for its nourishment. These changes are facilitated by the adaptations of various organ systems and by the increase in the general metabolism. These changes are only temporary, and in a normal pregnancy produce no deleterious effects on the mother.

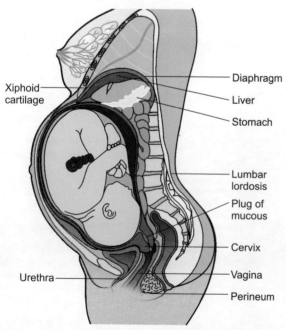

Xiphoid cartilage
Diaphragm
Liver
Stomach
Lumbar lordosis
Plug of mucous
Cervix
Vagina
Urethra
Perineum

Fig. 5.1 The abdominal cavity of a pregnant woman; there is increased lumbar lordosis and displacement of the abdominal viscera

■ CHANGES IN THE GENITAL TRACT

Uterus

Size

In a nulliparous woman, the uterus is a pear-shaped organ, about 6.5 cm long and weighing 70 g. It is located within the pelvis. At term, the uterus fills up the greater part of the abdominal cavity and undergoes considerable hypertrophy. At this stage, the uterus is about 32 cm long, 24 cm wide and 22 cm deep and weighs about 1 Kg.

Shape

In the first few weeks of pregnancy, the body of the uterus assumes a globular form and later becomes almost spherical. Then, it grows rapidly, more in length than in breadth, and assumes an oval form by the end of pregnancy.

Uterine wall

At the beginning of pregnancy, the uterine wall becomes thicker, and then it gradually thins. At term, the uterine wall is only 1.5 cm thick and is soft and easily indentable. Uterine enlargement is most marked at the fundus.

Enlargement of the uterus

This occurs due to the interplay of hypertrophy and hyperplasia.

- **Hypertrophy** is the increase in the volume of an organ or tissue due to the enlargement of its component cells.
- **Hyperplasia** is a condition in which the size of the cells remains approximately the same but the number of cells increases.

Uterine enlargement in pregnancy is largely the result of **hypertrophy** of the existing muscle fibres, which are stimulated chiefly by the action of estrogen and perhaps, progesterone. **Hyperplasia** of the formation of new muscle fibres occurs to a lesser extent.

Mechanical distension, which generally occurs after 12 weeks of pregnancy, is a result of the effect of expanding products of conception. The uterus grows out of the pelvis by about 12 weeks of pregnancy. The growth of the uterus is usually proportionate to the period of pregnancy, but under certain conditions, it may be smaller or larger than the period of pregnancy would warrant.

Arrangement of muscle fibres

The uterine muscle fibres are arranged in **three** layers (Fig. 5.2).

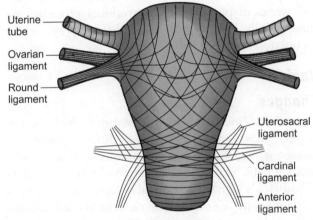

Fig. 5.2 Arrangement of muscle fibres

1. The **outer layer** arches over the fundus.
2. The **middle layer** is made up of an interlacing network of fibres perforated by blood vessels. The muscle fibres are doubly curved, forming a figure of eight around the perforating vessels. After delivery, the fibres contract and constrict the perforating vessels, leading to a stoppage of bleeding, and hence are known as the **living ligatures of the uterus.**
3. The **inner layer** consists of sphincteric fibres around the opening of the fallopian tube and the internal os.

During pregnancy, there is an increase in uterine connective tissue, which makes it softer. The isthmic portion also softens like the other parts of the uterus, but this happens much earlier than in the fundal region.

Hegar's sign

This is the softening of the lower uterine segment just above the cervix. When the uterine segment is compressed between examining fingers, its walls feel very thin. Hegar's sign is noted by the **sixth to eighth week of pregnancy.** While the fundal region dilates and relaxes to hold the growing fetus, the isthmic region closes like a sphincter to hold the conceptus inside.

Position

In the standing position, the long axis of the uterus corresponds to the axis of the pelvic inlet. In the supine position, the uterus rests upon the spine, the aorta and the inferior vena cava. As an abdominal organ, the uterus is rotated to the right due to the presence of the rectosigmoid on the left. This is known as **dextrorotation**. This dextrorotation should be corrected before clinically assessing the height of the fundus or at the time of cesarean section.

Uterine blood vessels

Blood supply

To keep pace with the growth of the uterus as well as the growing fetus, the blood supply to the uterus increases manyfold. The arteries hypertrophy, the veins increase in size, and the lymphatics of the uterus enlarge and multiply during pregnancy so that the full-term uterus is richly supplied with blood and lymph.

Uteroplacental blood flow

An increase in the blood supply to the placental bed is brought about by the **spiral arterioles** (Fig. 5.3), which undergo characteristic changes whereby they are converted to thin-walled dilated sinuses. The invasion of the trophoblast destroys the muscle walls and the elastic layer of the spiral arterioles so that they become non-sensitive to the pressor reagents.

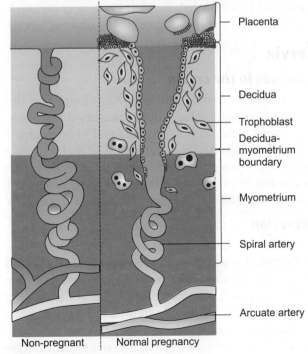

Fig. 5.3 Uteroplacental blood flow

Trophoblast invasion

The trophoblastic invasion occurs in **three** stages, which are as follows:

1. Pre-invasive stage
2. Intraluminal stage
3. Wall replacement

During the **pre-invasive phase** (up to 12 weeks), trophoblasts invade the endothelium of the spiral arterioles of the decidua. During the **intraluminal stage** (12–20 weeks), the **myometrial spiral arteriolar wall is invaded by the trophoblast, which is subsequently replaced** by fibrinoid material. Unlike the systemic veins, the pelvic veins do not possess a surrounding supporting sheath; hence, they dilate enormously during pregnancy and act as a reservoir when blood is pumped out of the placenta during contractions. The uterine blood flow is increased to 500–700 mL/minute at term.

Uterine contractility

From early pregnancy, uterine contractions known as Braxton Hicks contractions occur, which are painless, irregular and intermittent. They occur at long intervals, last for a shorter period and are not associated with dilatation of the cervix or descent of the presenting part. The contractions do not show any coordination or diminishing gradient. In the later stages of pregnancy, these contractions may cause some discomfort, leading to **false labour**. As pregnancy advances, there is a gradual increase in muscle tone and sensitivity. Close to term, these contractions become more frequent, regular and coordinated; they last longer and eventually transition into true labour pains at the onset of labour.

Cervix

Changes in the cervix

The cervix becomes soft and blue from the first trimester onwards. This is due to increased vascularity and edema along with hyperplasia and hypertrophy of the cervical glands. The latter results in an eversion of the endocervical columnar epithelium, which appears as **erosion** in pregnancy. This area is soft, velvety and red and may bleed at the time of taking a Pap smear.

Secretion

Cervical secretion increases in pregnancy. The endocervical mucosal cells produce copious amounts of tenacious mucus which plugs the cervical canal soon after conception. The plug is dislodged at the onset of labour resulting in a **bloody show.** The basal cells near the squamocolumnar junction undergo changes due to the effect of hormones. They become slightly bigger with prominent deep-stained nuclei. The cervical

stroma also shows changes. It loosens, the collagen and hydroxyproline content decreases and there is an increase in water content. These changes lead to softening and ripening near term.

Fallopian Tube

The fallopian tube on either side is generally stretched out in pregnancy and is more vascular.

Round Ligaments

These are thickened and hypertrophied.

Ovaries

There is no ovulation during pregnancy. The ovaries become enlarged, especially the one containing the corpus luteum. The corpus luteum functions for the first 6–7 weeks of pregnancy and produces progesterone; subsequently, it contributes little to progesterone production and regresses.

Vagina

Changes

The vagina increases in vascularity, which is one of the most marked changes during pregnancy. Consequently, there is more copious secretion and a characteristic violet discolouration during pregnancy (**Chadwick's sign**). The vaginal mucosa thickens; there is hypertrophy of smooth muscle cells and a loosening of the connective tissue.

Secretion

The vaginal secretion, derived partly from the cervix and partly from the transudation from the vaginal epithelium, is acidic. During normal pregnancy, its pH varies between 3.8 and 4.4. This acidic pH is due to the production of lactic acid by *Lactobacillus acidophilus* from glycogen in the vaginal walls. The increased vascularity at the time of pregnancy is not confined to the genitalia, but also extends to other adjacent organs.

■ CHANGES IN THE BREASTS

Marked changes take place in the breasts during pregnancy. These changes are more obvious in primigravidae than in multiparas. The majority of changes occur particularly at two different periods of pregnancy—around the second month and at the fifth month. In the second month of pregnancy, the breasts increase in size and sensitivity, and a bluish discolouration appears in the form of streaks (due to distended veins), especially at the periphery. The nipple becomes more erectile and the areola becomes more deeply pigmented (Fig. 5.4).

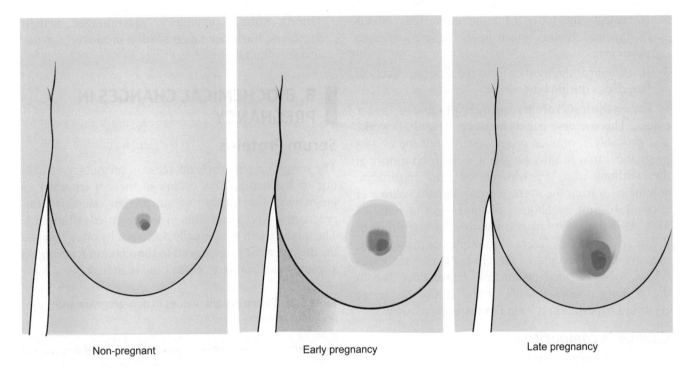

| Non-pregnant | Early pregnancy | Late pregnancy |

Fig. 5.4   Changes in the breasts during pregnancy

Prominent tubercles, called **Montgomery's follicles**, are seen in the primary areola. These are hypertrophic sebaceous glands. Around the fifth month, a less deeply pigmented area forms around the primary areola. This is known as the secondary areola, and on this too, some tubercles, **secondary Montgomery's follicles**, may appear (Fig. 5.5).

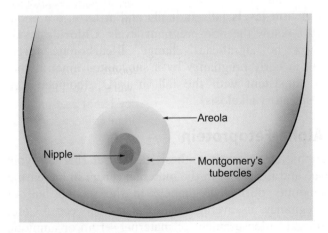

Fig. 5.5   Montgomery's follicles

Secretion

After the first few months, some clear, sticky fluid may be expressed from the nipples, which later becomes yellowish in colour. This is known as **colostrum**.

PHYSIOLOGICAL CHANGES IN PREGNANCY

A. HEMATOLOGICAL CHANGES IN PREGNANCY

Volume and Composition of Blood

Increase in volume

During pregnancy, the **total blood volume** increases by 30%, the **plasma volume** increases by about 50% and red **cell volume** increases by about 20%. This accounts for the **hemodilution** in pregnancy. This is also described as '**physiological anemia of pregnancy**'. The maternal blood volume starts increasing during the first trimester (at around 6 weeks), increases most rapidly during the second trimester, and plateaus during the last weeks of pregnancy. The maximum volume increase is reached at 32–34 weeks of gestation. In multiple pregnancy, there is a much greater increase in blood volume than the average. The presence of a fetus is not essential for this hypervolemia as this is also seen in a hydatidiform mole. **Pregnancy-induced hypervolemia** serves **three** purposes, which are as follows:

1. It meets the demands of the enlarged uterus and its hypertrophied vascular system.

2. It protects the fetus from the deleterious effects of impaired venous return in the supine and erect positions.

3. It safeguards the mother from the adverse effects of blood loss during parturition.

The **erythrocyte volume** also increases, but to a lesser extent. This increase begins between 10 and 20 weeks and probably continues progressively until the end of pregnancy. In a healthy pregnant woman on a normal diet without iron supplementation, the erythrocyte volume rises from the average non-pregnant volume of about 1,400 mL to about 1,650 mL—an increase of 18%. As in the case of plasma volume, the magnitude of the increase is much larger in multiple pregnancy. The increase in the volume of the circulating erythrocytes is due to accelerated production rather than due to the prolongation of the life of the RBCs. Moderate erythroid hyperplasia is found in the bone marrow.

Change in composition

- The **erythrocyte count** falls from an average non-pregnant value of about 4.5 million/mm^3 to a minimum of about 3.7 million/mm^3 at about 30 weeks.
- The **hemoglobin concentration** falls from an average of 13–14 g/L whole blood in the healthy, non-pregnant woman to an average minimum of 11–12 g/L.
- The **hematocrit** level drops from an average non-pregnant value of about 40% to a minimum of 33–34% in the last ten weeks of pregnancy. Most studies suggest that there is no change in the hemoglobin concentration of erythrocytes from the average value of 320–330 g/L.
- There is a marked increase in the **leukocyte count**— from a non-pregnant level of 7,000–10,000/mm^3 to more than 12,000/mm^3 in the postpartum period. The activity of alkaline phosphatase in the WBCs is increased, and an occasional myelocyte may be seen.

Coagulation Factors in Pregnancy

Fibrinogen level in normal pregnancy

- **Blood fibrinogen** is said to increase in pregnancy, especially as term approaches. Fibrinogen level in normal pregnancy increases by about 50%—the fibrinogen level in the non-pregnant woman is, on an average, 260 mg/dL, whereas at term, it ranges from 288–576 mg/dL.
- All **clotting factors** except XI and XIII increase during pregnancy.
- In about 5–7% of pregnant women, **platelet levels** decrease.
- **Clotting time** and **bleeding time** are unchanged in normal pregnancy.

- During normal pregnancy, **plasminogen activity** increases; **fibrinogen degradation products** increase, usually after labour.

B. BIOCHEMICAL CHANGES IN PREGNANCY

Serum Proteins

The serum protein levels decrease in pregnancy, usually due to **hydremia**. This occurs in the last trimester of pregnancy. The average serum protein values in non-pregnant and pregnant women are presented in Table 5.1. The total protein level usually decreases by one gram and the drop is most pronounced in the albumin fraction. As a result, the albumin:globulin ratio is altered.

Table 5.1 Serum protein values in non-pregnant and pregnant women

Protein	Non-pregnant state	Pregnant state
Total protein (g/dL)	7.19	6.46
Albumin (g/dL)	3.78	2.44
Globulin (g/dL)	3.41	4.02

Serum Electrolytes

In normal pregnancy, there is a small but consistent decline in the concentration of most serum electrolytes. **Sodium levels** fall in early pregnancy by 2–3 mEq/L to a relatively constant level. **Potassium levels** also fall in early pregnancy by 0.2–0.3 mEq/L but may rise again to non-pregnant levels in late pregnancy. **Calcium levels** fall gradually and at term, are about 10% below the non-pregnant levels. **Chloride levels** show no significant change. **Bicarbonate levels** fall in early pregnancy by a substantial amount that is consistent with the fall in pCO$_2$ (compensated respiratory alkalosis).

Alpha-Fetoprotein

Alpha-fetoprotein is synthesised in the fetal liver and yolk sac and is present in the maternal serum in increasing amounts during pregnancy. In the second half of pregnancy, its average value ranges between 53 and 55 g/L. Measurement of maternal serum or amniotic fluid alpha-fetoprotein (AFP) is advocated for the diagnosis of conditions like neural tube defects and omphalocele.

Lipids

The total serum lipids, triglycerides (neutral fats), cholesterol and phospholipids rise during pregnancy.

■ C. METABOLIC CHANGES

Weight Changes During Pregnancy

One of the most noticeable alterations in pregnancy is the gain in weight. The enlarging uterus, the growing fetus, the placenta and liquor amnii, the acquisition of fat and water retention, all contribute to this increase in weight (Table 5.2).

Table 5.2 Analysis of weight gain during pregnancy

Tissues and fluids	Weight gain (g)
Fetus	3,400
Placenta	650
Amniotic fluid	800
Uterus	970
Breasts	405
Blood	1,450
Extravascular fluid	1,480
Total	12,500

The increase in weight varies from person to person. The total weight gain over the course of pregnancy in a healthy primigravida is approximately 12.5 Kg.

Rate of increase

The rate of weight gain varies according to the stage of pregnancy. In the first three months, there may be no substantial gain, especially if the woman has severe vomiting and anorexia. The rate of weight gain between 20 weeks and delivery is about 0.5 Kg per week. A woman gains 5 Kg in the second trimester and another 5 Kg in the third trimester. Weight gain in pregnancy is directly related to the birth weight of the fetus. **Low weight gain** has been found to be associated with preterm or low-birth-weight infants. The woman's weight before pregnancy also influences the net weight gain. Heavier women are likely to gain more weight than thin women. Extreme eating habits influence weight gain. Excessive weight gain may be associated with pre-eclampsia and gestational diabetes mellitus.

Water Metabolism

Water retention is a normal physiological change of pregnancy. The minimum amount of extra water an average woman retains during pregnancy is about 6.5 L. Of this, 3.5 L is the water content of the fetus, placenta and the amniotic fluid and 3.0 L is accumulated due to an increase in maternal blood volume and uterine size (Table 5.3). There is an increase in venous pressure below the level of the uterus due to the partial occlusion of the vena cava. This leads to the accumulation of about a litre of water, which leads to pitting edema of the ankles and legs in a substantial proportion of pregnant women, especially at the end of the day.

Table 5.3 Water retained during pregnancy

Source of water	Amount (in litres)
Fetus, placenta and amniotic fluid	3.5
Increase in maternal blood volume and uterine size	3
Increase in venous pressure due to partial occlusion of the inferior vena cava	1

Carbohydrate Metabolism

Carbohydrate, protein and fat metabolism is altered so as to supply the fetus with nutrients, glucose and free fatty acids. Maternal carbohydrate metabolism is altered in pregnancy in favour of a hyperglycemic state that is induced by the placental hormones. This metabolic change is required to supply glucose and glycogenic precursors for the fetus as well as to provide an additional fuel substrate to the mother. The fetus continuously consumes glucose from the maternal circulation.

There are two metabolic phases in pregnancy, which are as follows:

1. **Anabolic phase of pregnancy (early pregnancy):** In early pregnancy, energy is stored. This store serves as an important calorie reserve to meet the maternal energy needs in cases where the fetal energy and glucose requirements exceed those supplied by the maternal diet.

2. **Catabolic phase of pregnancy (late pregnancy):** The fetus competes with the mother for circulating glucose and there is an increased nutrient flow across the placenta to the fetus. The insulin resistance in late pregnancy serves to maintain adequate maternal glucose concentration so as to supply glucose to the fetus.

The **fasting blood sugar value** is lower in pregnancy than it is in the non-pregnant state. Lower fasting blood glucose levels and the higher concentration of plasma-free fatty acids in normal pregnant women represent an **accelerated starvation stage. Placental lactogen** promotes lipolysis and increases free fatty acid concentration in maternal plasma. It also antagonises insulin action in the periphery, thereby allowing glucose to be available to the fetus.

- Other hormones—estrogen, progesterone and cortisol—also induce a diabetogenic state in pregnancy.
- Besides these, the placental enzyme, insulinase, accelerates the degradation of insulin, thus contributing to the **diabetogenic state** of pregnancy. To compensate for the anti-insulin state, the endogenous insulin secretion and insulin response to glucose load are increased in pregnancy.
- After an oral glucose load, the rise in the blood glucose level slows down due to decreased gastric emptying and delayed absorption in pregnancy. Due to the peripheral resistance to insulin, blood sugar does not return to the fasting level after two hours, as it does in the non-pregnant state.
- The basal concentration of insulin is normal in the first and second trimesters, but it is elevated by as much as 50–80% in the third trimester. This results in the lowering of fasting blood sugar.
- There is also significant peripheral antagonism to insulin due to increased progesterone, cortisol levels, growth hormone and human placental lactogen (hPL) levels. Moreover, there is accelerated degradation of insulin by insulinase from the placenta.

Fat Metabolism

In pregnancy, the storage of fat increases from early gestation and reaches a maximum during the second trimester. This level decreases slightly in the third trimester due to fetal consumption. The levels of cholesterol, phospholipids and free fatty acids are high in pregnancy and decrease in the puerperium with breastfeeding. All these changes help in meeting the fetal need for fatty acids. As a pregnant woman is already in a state of accelerated starvation, with increased levels of fatty acid as fuel usage, **ketonuria** and **ketonemia** develop faster during pregnancy in pathological conditions like hyperemesis gravidarum, starvation or uncontrolled diabetes mellitus.

Protein Metabolism

In early pregnancy, amino acids are actively transported across the placenta to fetal circulation. During the second half of pregnancy, the amino acid requirement by the fetus is further increased.

The total protein content increases in pregnancy. The fetus and placenta contain approximately 500 g of protein; 500 g of protein is added to the uterus as contractile protein and to the maternal blood as hemoglobin and plasma proteins. The albumin concentration decreases due to hemodilution.

Mineral Metabolism

Copper and ceruloplasmin levels increase in the plasma, while the levels of calcium and magnesium reduce slightly. A small but significant increase in the free calcium concentration occurs in late pregnancy. Even though the concentration of zinc in plasma is decreased in pregnancy, the total amount of zinc is increased due to the increased plasma volume induced by pregnancy.

Iron Metabolism

Investigations reveal that in pregnancy, there is a tendency for serum iron levels to be lowered, especially after the 24th week after an increase in the total iron binding capacity of the serum. Serum folate and vitamin B levels fall in normal pregnancy. Vitamin B6 and ascorbic acid levels also show a drop in normal pregnancy. The amount of iron absorbed from the diet, together with the mobilised iron stores, is usually insufficient to meet the demands of pregnancy.

SYSTEMIC CHANGES IN PREGNANCY

■ CARDIOVASCULAR SYSTEM

Heart

As the diaphragm is elevated by the enlarging uterus, the heart is displaced upward. It rotates on its anteroposterior axis, which results in the displacement of the apex beat to the fourth intercostal space and outwards to the left by 3 cm in the third trimester. These changes may give a false impression of cardiac enlargement. Sometimes, there is an increase in the cardiothoracic diameter.

The extent of these changes is influenced by the size and position of the uterus, the strength of the abdominal muscles and the configuration of the abdomen and thorax (Fig. 5.6). The cardiac volume increases by 75 mL. With the slight hypertrophy of the left ventricle due to the cardiac overload by increased blood volume in late pregnancy, the left ventricular mass and end diastolic pressures are increased.

Heart sounds

Heart sounds may be altered in pregnancy. The **first sound** is loud at the apex with a split, owing to the early closure of the mitral valve. There is no change in the aortic and pulmonary components of the **second sound**. The **third heart sound** is heard in 75% of normal pregnant women and is due to rapid ventricular filling during early diastole. **Systolic ejection murmurs**, which occur due to the increased blood flow through the great vessels, are heard at the base of the heart.

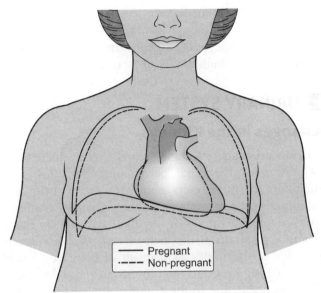

Fig. 5.6 Anatomical changes in the position of the heart and lungs

These murmurs increase in intensity during inspiration. The **ECG** shows a prominent S wave in lead I and conspicuous Q wave and an inverted P wave in lead III.

Pulse rate

The resting pulse rate increases by about 10 beats/minute.

Cardiac output

The cardiac output rises early in pregnancy from a mean of about 4.5 L/minute at pre-pregnancy to about 5.5 L/minute by about the twelfth or sixteenth week (Table 5.4). Nearly 2/3rd of this increase is achieved in the first trimester. It increases to 6.0 L/minute by mid-pregnancy and remains at that level until about the last eight weeks, after which, there is a steady decline to about 5–5.5 L/minute at term. The increased output is brought about by a slight increase in the heart rate and stroke volume. Whether this increased output necessarily leads to hypertrophy of the heart is debatable. It is possible that the reserve power of the heart is able to cope with the increased needs of pregnancy, as the strain on the heart is not sudden but gradual. At the time of labour, the cardiac output further increases to 15% in the first stage of labour and 50% in the second stage of labour due to uterine contraction. Further increase is seen soon after delivery due to the emptying of the uterine blood into the general circulation as well as by the shifting of blood from the lower limbs as the pressure on the IVC is relieved. The cardiac output returns to normal two weeks after delivery.

Table 5.4 Cardiac output in pregnancy

Period of gestation	Mean cardiac output (in L/min)
Pre-pregnancy	4.5
12–16 weeks	5.5
Mid-pregnancy to 32 weeks	6
After 32 weeks	5–5.5

Blood pressure

Blood pressure normally ranges from 110–120 mmHg systolic and from 75–85 mmHg diastolic. The arterial blood pressure decreases to a nadir in mid-pregnancy and rises thereafter. Variations in blood pressure are of great significance during pregnancy, and any rise up to or above 140 mmHg systolic or 90 mmHg diastolic should alert the obstetrician.

Other Changes

Varicose veins

During pregnancy, there is an increased tendency **of veins** to become **varicosed**. While venous pressure in the veins of the arm is unaltered, the pressure in the femoral and other leg veins is high. This high pressure in the femoral veins drops immediately after delivery. Varicose veins in the lower half of the body tend to develop in pregnant women. The usual sites are the legs, vulva, rectum, anus and vagina, in that order.

The causes of varicose veins are as follows:

- Increased venous congestion below the diaphragm caused by the greater intra-abdominal pressure of pregnancy
- Obstruction of the common iliac veins owing to the rush of blood from the enlarged hypogastric veins
- Disturbed vasomotor conditions
- Increase in the total amount of blood and consequent enlargement of the veins to accommodate this increase
- Hereditary factors play an important role in the development of varicose veins

Supine hypotension syndrome

When the pregnant woman is in the supine position, the enlarged gravid uterus presses on the inferior vena cava, which reduces the venous return to the heart, and in turn, decreases cardiac output. This causes significant hypotension and is referred to as the **supine hypotension syndrome**. This can be avoided by asking the woman to lie on her left side.

■ RESPIRATORY SYSTEM

The lower ribs flare out in pregnancy. The subcostal angle increases from 68° in early pregnancy to 103° at term. The level of the diaphragm is raised by about 4 cm, and the transverse diameter of the chest increases by about 2 cm. In pregnancy, respiration is more diaphragmatic than costal. There is little change in the respiration rate during pregnancy. Maternal oxygen consumption increases by 20–40% during pregnancy The vital capacity is not altered. The tidal volume is increased by 200 mL, and the residual volume is reduced by 200 mL. Increased volume of air, together with reduced residual volume, improves gaseous exchange.

There is an increased awareness of a desire to breathe even early in pregnancy. This **physiological dyspnea** is due to increased tidal volume and decreased blood pCO_2, which paradoxically causes dyspnea. Hyperventilation decreases pCO and increases pO_2, thus favouring gas transfer across the placenta. These changes occur because of the central effect of progesterone, which exerts a direct action on the respiratory centre. Pulmonary arterial pressure is not increased in pregnancy and, therefore, to accommodate the augmented blood flow, there is vasodilatation. This causes increased vascular markings in the lung fields in the skiagram.

■ GASTROINTESTINAL SYSTEM

Many pregnant women experience symptoms like nausea, indigestion and constipation. There is evidence of motor sluggishness, reduced intestinal secretion and altered liver function. The stomach and the intestines are displaced by the enlarging uterus. The appendix is displaced upwards and laterally and the physical findings in appendicitis are altered.

- **Heartburn** is common in pregnancy due to the reflux of acidic secretions into the lower esophagus. This is because intra-esophageal pressure is lower and intragastric pressure is higher than normal during pregnancy. Also, the position of the stomach is altered, and the lower esophageal sphincter tone is decreased.
- During labour, the **gastric emptying time** is prolonged appreciably and is a risk factor for aspiration during general anesthesia.
- **Hemorrhoids** are common due to increased pressure on the veins below the level of the uterus.
- **Gallbladder contractions** are reduced, leading to stasis. This is because progesterone inhibits

cholecystokinin-mediated smooth muscle contraction of the gallbladder. This, along with increased cholesterol, explains the increased risk of gallstones in multiparous women.

■ URINARY SYSTEM

Changes in the Kidneys

During pregnancy, kidney size is slightly increased. Dilatation of the renal pelvis and elongation and dilatation of the ureters above the pelvic brim are commonly seen in pregnancy. These changes are more marked on the right side. In the early weeks, these changes result from the lack of tone of the smooth muscles of the ureter as a result of increased levels of circulating progesterone. In the later months, these changes occur due to the compression of the ureters by the enlarging uterus.

Changes in the Ureters

The right ureter shows greater alterations than the left, which is protected to a certain extent by the sigmoid. Further, the dextrorotation of the uterus and a hugely dilated right ovarian vein complex in pregnancy may increase the compression on the right ureter. Urinary stasis in the dilated ureters can predispose to urinary tract infection.

Renal Function

The glomerular filtration rate (GFR) increases by 50% and renal plasma flow increases by 75% during pregnancy. Late in pregnancy, urinary flow and sodium excretion are grossly affected by posture, averaging at less than half the rate of excretion when supine as compared to the lateral recumbent position. Several tests of renal function used clinically may be altered by normal pregnancy. Creatinine clearance is a useful test to estimate renal function during pregnancy.

Amino acids and water-soluble vitamins are lost in the urine of pregnant women in much greater amounts than in non-pregnant women. As a consequence of increased **GFR**, the serum concentration of creatinine and urea decrease. Urine concentration tests may yield misleading results.

Glycosuria is common during pregnancy but is not necessarily pathologic. It is a result of the increase in GFR without an increase in the tubular reabsorption of filtered glucose. However, the possibility of diabetes mellitus should be considered and evaluated further in the presence of persistent glycosuria. Proteinuria does not normally occur during pregnancy.

Changes in the Bladder

From the fourth month onwards, the bladder shows hyperplasia of its muscle and connective tissue. The trigone is elevated and there is a marked widening and deepening of the trigone by the end of pregnancy. Due to the early engagement of the head in a primigravida, the base of the bladder is pushed upward and forward. This results in the base of the bladder becoming more concave, a change from its original convexity. A pregnant woman may complain of increased frequency of micturition in the early weeks of pregnancy due to the pressure exerted by the enlarging uterus on the bladder and nearing term, when the fetal head enters the pelvis.

■ NERVOUS SYSTEM

The nervous system is in a more excitable condition in the pregnant woman. **Temperamental changes** are not infrequent. **Melancholia** and **real psychosis** may develop, especially in those with a family history. From 12 weeks of pregnancy, women experience frequent awakening and lack of sleep. The maximal sleep disturbances occur postpartum and may contribute to 'postpartum blues' or depression.

■ ENDOCRINE SYSTEM

During pregnancy, the endocrine system shows tremendous changes.

- **The placenta, the new organ, secretes a variety of hormones.**
- **There are changes in the pre-existing endocrine system.**

Placental Hormones

Human chorionic gonadotropin

It is a glycoprotein with the highest carbohydrate content of any hormone in the human body. Like all glycoproteins, it consists of **two subunits**: an α (92 amino acids) and a β (145 amino acids) subunit. Of these, the α subunit is structurally and immunologically similar in hCG, LH, FSH and TSH. Human chorionic gonadotropin is synthesised by the syncytiotrophoblast cells of the placenta even before implantation and can be detected in the peripheral blood by radioimmunoassay soon after implantation and well before the first missed period. The **titres** are increased in twin pregnancy, hydatidiform mole and choriocarcinoma. The titres are also high if the fetus has Down syndrome. Low titres are recorded in ectopic pregnancy and threatened abortion (Table 5.5).

Table 5.5   hCG titres

Increased hCG titres	Decreased hCG titres
Multiple pregnancy	Ectopic pregnancy
Hydatidiform mole	Threatened abortion
Down syndrome	

Functions

hCG is mainly luteotrophic and helps to maintain the corpus luteum of pregnancy till about the sixty-eighth day, when the placenta takes over and the corpus luteum is no longer necessary. It also stimulates fetal testicular testosterone secretion to promote male sexual differentiation. hCG stimulates the maternal thyroid gland—in women who have a hydatidiform mole or choriocarcinoma, biochemical or clinical hyperthyroidism may develop.

Estrogen

During pregnancy, the placenta is the major site of the production of estrogen. However, this production depends on the presence of a normal fetoplacental unit. Pregnancy is a **hyperestrogenic state** which lasts till delivery. The enzyme systems necessary for estrogen production are distributed between the fetal tissues (the fetal adrenals and liver) and the placenta and hence, both need to function optimally (Fig. 5.7). To produce estriol, the steroids must shuttle back and forth between the fetus and the placenta for successive steps in biosynthesis. In the non-pregnant woman, estradiol is the most important estrogen secreted when compared to the pregnant state where estriol is quantitively more.

Estriol is largely derived from the fetal precursors—dehydroepiandrosterone (DHEA) sulphate secreted by the adrenals and hydroxylated in the fetal liver to 16-hydroxy dehydroepiandrosterone sulphate (as the placenta lacks 16-hydroxylase) is desulphated and aromatised in the placenta to give estriol. Near term, the fetus is the source of 90% of the placental estriol precursor. There is also a minor contribution from the placenta, where estriol is metabolised from estradiol and estrone. The maternal pituitary has little or no influence on estrogen synthesis in pregnancy. The rate of formation of placental estrogen is severely limited in anencephaly and reduces strikingly after fetal demise.

Progesterone

This is the chief hormone of the corpus luteum and the syncytiotrophoblast of the placenta. It has been traditionally regarded as **the hormone that sustains pregnancy**. During the early weeks of pregnancy, the luteal source is vital for the sustenance of the conceptus, after which the placental source takes over, although the

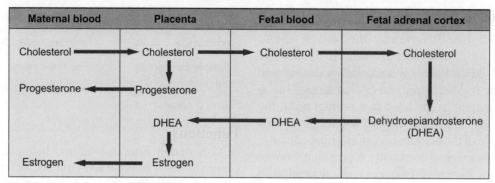

Fig. 5.7 Biosynthesis of hormones in pregnancy

corpus luteum continues to contribute insignificantly throughout pregnancy. This probably takes place around the 60th day. The biosynthesis of progesterone by the placenta is complex and is dependent on the mother and the fetus for the precursors, namely, cholesterol and pregnenolone. The highest level of progesterone in the blood is found in the umbilical vein, with a substantial arteriovenous difference.

Progesterone is excreted in the maternal urine as pregnanediol. During the first six to eight weeks, the pregnanediol excretion remains at the level of the luteal phase of the normal menstrual cycle. Thereafter, the excretion rises steadily, reaching its highest value at 36 weeks of gestation.

Functions

Progesterone causes secretory changes in the endometrium and prepares it for the implantation of the blastocyst. After implantation, progesterone is necessary for sustaining the viability of the blastocyst; it also reduces the excitability of the uterine musculature, thus preventing early fetal expulsion. Besides these actions, progesterone causes smooth muscle relaxation and there is evidence that it stimulates the respiratory centre, resulting in the lowering of alveolar and arterial pCO_2, normally seen in pregnancy. The growth of the breasts during pregnancy is largely under the influence of both estrogen and progesterone. While estrogen stimulates the proliferation of the duct system, growth and pigmentation of the nipples and areola, the development of the alveoli and lobules is influenced by progesterone. For progesterone to be effective, the breast must be previously primed by estrogen.

Functions of progesterone in pregnancy
- Prepares the endometrium for the implantation of the blastocyst
- Sustains the viability of the blastocyst
- Reduces the excitability of the uterine musculature
- Causes smooth muscle relaxation
- Helps in the development of the alveoli and the lobules of the breast

---

Androgens

Both testosterone and androstenedione are found in greater quantities in women in late pregnancy than in non-pregnant women. However, the free circulating androgens in pregnant women are less than those in non-pregnant women as the binding proteins are increased. There is no correlation between these levels and the sex of the fetus. Maternal plasma testosterone and androstenedione are converted to estradiol in the placenta.

Human placental lactogen (HPL)

It was also known as **human chorionic somatomammotropin (hCS)**. Human placental lactogen is produced by the syncytiotrophoblast, and unlike the human chorionic gonadotropin, there is a close correlation between its production and the placental weight throughout pregnancy. From a very low level in early pregnancy, it rises to peak levels of 5–15 µg/mL at term. Although negligible quantities are found in the fetal serum, amniotic fluid levels increase concomitantly with those in maternal blood. The production rate at term is greater than any other human hormone. It is a polypeptide with structural similarity to human growth hormone and human prolactin.

Functions

Human placental lactogen causes lipolysis and inhibits gluconeogenesis. It also leads to an increase in the maternal levels of insulin, which may contribute to some anabolic effect on the mother and fetus. It also has a potent angiogenic action.

Prostaglandins

A prostaglandin is a 20-carbon, unsaturated fatty acid containing a cyclopentane ring formed from the essential fatty acid, arachidonic acid. Prostaglandins are divided into **three groups** according to their configuration—**PGA_2, PGE** and **PGF_2**—of which the latter two are important in reproductive physiology. Prostaglandins are widely distributed in the body, including in the endometrium, decidua and amniotic fluid. The highest concentrations of PGF_2 and PGF are found in the decidua and myometrium during labour, and there is reason to believe that this is the mechanism by which the product of conception is expelled.

Changes in the endocrine glands during pregnancy

Pituitary hormones

- *Gonadotropins:* Both maternal FSH and LH are reduced in pregnancy, and when pregnancy occurs, the rhythmicity of gonadotropin secretion is interrupted, and no further ovulation occurs. LH is suppressed to a greater extent than FSH.
- *Adrenocorticotropic hormone (ACTH):* Increased production of ACTH is reflected by the rising levels of corticosteroids.
- *Melanocyte stimulating hormone (MSH):* MSH, a polypeptide, is chemically similar to ACTH. It serves no purpose in pregnancy and is responsible for the changes in skin pigmentation which are characteristic of pregnancy, e.g., increased pigmentation of the areola of the nipple, darkening of the linea alba and the occasional mask-like pigmentation of the face (chloasma).
- *Hormones of the posterior pituitary:* These are oxytocin and vasopressin (an anti-diuretic hormone). Oxytocin induces uterine contractions and is responsible for the ejection of milk during lactation. During pregnancy, the uterus is less sensitive, but at term, it responds strongly to oxytocin injections. The most important action of **vasopressin** is its antidiuretic activity. There is an increase in the level of the antidiuretic hormone during pregnancy.

Adrenal hormones

- *Corticosteroids:* The fetus produces corticosteroids in pregnancy and is capable of converting some amount of the progesterone it receives from the placenta to corticosteroids. However, the maternal adrenal cortex is the chief source of corticosteroid secretion. There is no evidence that the placenta produces the adrenocorticoid. The urinary excretion of glucocorticoids increases considerably with advancing pregnancy, reaching a peak during the last trimester. Two to four days after delivery, the excretion returns to normal.
- *Aldosterone:* The increased secretion of aldosterone is reflected in its increased urinary excretion. The stimulus for its increased secretion is probably the increased activity of the renin–angiotensin system, which itself is due to the reduced mean blood pressure in the kidneys during pregnancy. However, the primary stimulus is thought to be progesterone, as the aldosterone level rises to combat the suggested sodium-losing effect of progesterone.

Thyroid hormones

In pregnancy, there is a slight increase in the size of the thyroid gland due to hyperplasia and increased vascularity. There is an increase in the levels of thyroxine-binding globulin, and the placenta produces a number of thyroid-stimulating factors. One of the important functions of the thyroid hormone is to increase the rate of oxygenation of tissue cells. There is a progressive increase in oxygen consumption in pregnancy as indicated by rising values of BMR up to 25%.

Insulin

Pregnancy is associated throughout with an altered response to glucose loading. In late pregnancy, a detectable rise in plasma insulin level is not associated with a proportional drop in maternal blood glucose, indicating an insulin-resistant state. Human placental lactogen and raised levels of corticosteroids are responsible for the insulin-resistant state.

Renin

The activity in the plasma of the enzyme, renin, is considerably raised in pregnancy. The extra renin is derived from the maternal kidneys and is produced in response to reduced mean blood pressure in the kidneys, ureteral obstruction by the gravid uterus and reduced concentration of body sodium.

■ SKELETAL SYSTEM

Pelvis

During pregnancy, the pelvis shows increased vascularity, and the pelvic ligaments become lax due to the effect of hormones. As a result, the pelvic joints become tender. Mobility also increases at the sacrococcygeal, sacroiliac and pubic joints. In some cases, the pregnant woman has severe pain over the joint, difficulty in walking and discomfort in the lower portion of the back. With the increasing protuberance of the abdomen, the centre of gravity falls anteriorly and, as a result, there is compensatory **lordosis**, and rotation of the pelvis on the femur (Fig. 5.8). This lordosis leads to anterior neck flexion and slumping of the shoulder girdle, producing traction on the ulnar and median nerves and leading to numbness and weakness in the upper extremity.

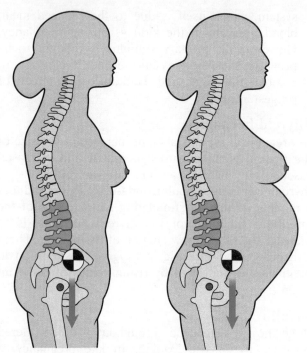

Fig. 5.8   Postural changes in pregnancy—with the enlargement of the gravid uterus, there is increased lumbar lordosis and a tendency, to some degree, for kyphosis

■ SKIN

Abdominal Wall

The abdominal wall distends as the pregnancy advances, and grows thinner, especially around the umbilicus. The rectus muscles may separate in the midline, creating a **diastasis recti**. The skin over the abdomen shows depressed lines, which are pinkish or bluish in appearance. These lines are called the **striae gravidarum** or **stretch marks**. They are curved, irregular, arranged more or less concentrically, sometimes radially, around and over the thighs on the anterior aspect, sometimes on the posterior aspect as far as the knees, as well as under the breasts. These lines are caused by the rupture of the subcuticular elastic fibres. After delivery, they heal, leaving pearly white or silvery bright lines, now known as **linea albicans**.

Pigmentation

Occasionally, brownish patches appear on the face, giving rise to **chloasma** otherwise called the **melasma gravidarum** or the **mask of pregnancy**. The midline of abdominal skin becomes brownish black and is called **linea nigra**. There is also increased hyperemia, sweating and sebaceous secretion. Vascular **angiomata, spider naevi** and **palmar erythema are commonly seen in pregnancy due to the** hyper-estrogenic state associated with pregnancy.

KEY POINTS

✓   *The maternal system undergoes many adaptations in normal pregnancy to enable the rapid growth of the embryo and the fetus.*

✓   *The uterus grows proportionate to the period of pregnancy and its blood supply increases tremendously.*

✓   *The uterine blood flow increases to 500–700 mL/minute at term.*

✓   *The **spiral arterioles** undergo characteristic changes, whereby they are converted to thin-walled dilated sinuses.*

✓   *The blood volume starts to increase by six weeks of pregnancy and reaches its peak at 32–34 weeks.*

✓   *Increase in plasma volume is more (50%) than the red cell volume (20%) resulting in physiological anemia.*

✓   *There is a marked increase in the **leukocyte count** from a non-pregnant level of 7,000–10,000/mm³ to more than 12,000/mm³ in the postpartum period.*

✓   *The total weight gain in healthy primigravidas is approximately 12.5 Kg. The weight increases by 0.5 Kg per week from the second trimester onwards.*

✓   *Cardiac output increases by 40% from 6 weeks to peak at mid-pregnancy around 25–30 weeks.*

✓   *There is a drop in blood pressure in the second trimester.*

✓   *Maternal oxygen consumption increases by 20–40% during pregnancy.*

✓   *The glomerular filtration rate (GFR) increases by 50% and renal plasma flow increases by 75% during pregnancy.*

Essay questions

1.   Describe the changes that occur in the genital tract during pregnancy.
2.   Describe uterine and breast changes that occur during normal pregnancy.
3.   Describe the physiological changes occurring in various systems of the body during pregnancy.

Short answer questions

1.   Write a short note on supine hypotension syndrome.
2.   Write a short note on human chorionic gonadotropin.
3.   What are Braxton Hicks contractions?
4.   Write a short note on weight gain in pregnancy.

MCQs

1. Softening of the lower uterine segment just above the cervix is called:
   a) Hegar's sign
   b) Chadwick's sign
   c) Osiander's sign
   d) Palmer's sign

2. At what period of gestation is the Hegar's sign noted?
   a) 6–8 weeks
   b) 8–10 weeks
   c) 10–12 weeks
   d) 12–14 weeks

3. What is the characteristic violet discolouration of the vagina during pregnancy called?
   a) Hegar's sign
   b) Chadwick's sign
   c) Osiander's sign
   d) Palmar's sign

4. At what period of gestation does the uterus grow out of the pelvis?
   a) 8 weeks
   b) 10 weeks
   c) <8 weeks
   d) 12 weeks

5. What is the total weight gain during pregnancy?
   a) 5 Kg
   b) 8 Kg
   c) 10 Kg
   d) 12.5 Kg

6. In which of the following conditions is hCG increased?
   a) Twins
   b) Molar pregnancy
   c) Down syndrome
   d) All of the above

Answers

1. (a), 2. (a), 3. (b), 4. (d), 5. (d), 6. (d)

Fill in the blanks

1. The irregular, pink, depressed lines seen over the lower abdomen and thighs during pregnancy are known as _____.

2. The brownish-black midline of the abdominal wall during pregnancy is known as _____.

3. Brownish patches over the face during pregnancy are known as _____.

4. The clear fluid that can be expressed from the breast during the latter part of pregnancy is called _____.

5. The irregular, intermittent, painless uterine contractions that occur during pregnancy are known as _____.

6. The increase in the volume of an organ or tissue due to the enlargement of its component cells is known as _____.

7. The acidic pH of the vagina is due to the production of lactic acid by _____.

8. Human chorionic gonadotropin is synthesised by the _____.

Answers

1. striae gravidarum, 2. linea nigra, 3. melasma gravidarum, 4. colostrum, 5. Braxton Hicks contractions, 6. hypertrophy, 7. *Lactobacillus acidophilus*, 8. syncytiotrophoblast of the placenta

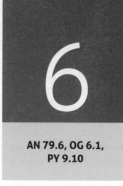

6

AN 79.6, OG 6.1, PY 9.10

Diagnosis of Pregnancy

Learning Objectives

» To know the signs and symptoms of pregnancy

» To discuss the investigations to diagnose pregnancy

» To understand the basis of urine and serum pregnancy tests and their interpretations

» To know the applications of serum β-hCG assay

» To discuss the USG diagnosis of pregnancy

■ INTRODUCTION

Though the history and examination findings may suggest a pregnancy, laboratory investigations and USG assessment are essential to confirm the diagnosis of pregnancy.

SIGNS AND SYMPTOMS OF PREGNANCY

The duration of pregnancy is 280 days, calculated from the first day of the last menstrual period. This period is divided into three trimesters; the signs and symptoms of pregnancy vary in different trimesters.

■ FIRST TRIMESTER

Subjective Symptoms

Amenorrhea

- In a woman who is in her reproductive years and is sexually active, amenorrhea is highly suggestive of pregnancy unless proven otherwise.

- However, amenorrhea can also occur due to various other reasons such as anovulation, premature ovarian failure, severe illness or emotional disturbances.

- On the other hand, in a woman who is pregnant, a history of amenorrhea may be absent due to various reasons such as the following:

  — **There could be cyclical bleeding** in the first 8–12 weeks of pregnancy, either from a bicornuate uterus or uterus didelphys.

  — There could be bleeding at the time of implantation.

  — Intermittent bleeding may occur from a normal uterus prior to the fusion of the decidua vera and decidua capsularis.

  — Pathological lesions in the genital tract can also give rise to bleeding during pregnancy.

Morning sickness

In the early weeks of pregnancy, nausea and vomiting are common. Morning sickness starts at around 4–6 weeks of pregnancy and continues till about 16 weeks. Usually, it is present in the early hours of the morning and reduces as the day progresses. In some cases, however, sickness may continue throughout the day. Women with multiple pregnancy or molar pregnancy experience higher degrees of vomiting. Though the cause of this symptom is unknown, it usually coincides with the rising levels of hCG in early pregnancy. Nausea and vomiting can also be caused by other conditions such as gastric acidity and GI tract upset.

These symptoms can be minimised by eating small meals at more frequent intervals and avoiding spicy and oily foods, which precipitate these symptoms. Occasionally, vomiting may be severe enough to cause weight loss, dehydration, acidosis and hypokalemia. This condition is termed **hyperemesis gravidarum**. Intravenous fluid replacement, correction of electrolytes and dextrose replacement are required to correct ketosis (further details in Chapter 18, *Hyperemesis gravidarum*).

Excessive salivation and pica

Excessive salivation is an early symptom of pregnancy. The woman's palate may change during pregnancy, and she may crave certain foods. This is called **pica of pregnancy.** Excessive salivation and pica are not diagnostic of pregnancy as they are purely subjective and may occur in various neurotic conditions as well.

Irritability of the bladder

Frequency of micturition is a common symptom of pregnancy. It occurs due to the pressure exerted on the bladder by the growing uterus. As the uterus increases in size and becomes an abdominal organ, this pressure is relieved, and the symptom gradually disappears.

Fatigue
Easy fatigability is very frequent in early pregnancy.

Headache
Some women complain of excessive headaches due to vasodilatation. However, when the headache is intense and associated with other symptoms, it is important to rule out neurological conditions.

Signs of Pregnancy

Changes in the breasts
Changes in the breasts are marked, particularly in primigravidae. There is a general enlargement, with a prominence of the veins, increased pigmentation and characteristic primary and secondary areolae. The nipples become more prominent, erectile and turgescent. **Montgomery's follicles** appear first on the primary areolae, and later, on the secondary areolae.

The **secondary areolae** develop from the twentieth week onwards, while the other changes generally take place during the first trimester, from the fourth to the twelfth week of pregnancy. The presence of a little fluid in the breast can usually be detected from week 12 onwards by gently squeezing the breast in the direction of the nipple. The fluid is clear and contains some colostrum corpuscles.

Occasionally, changes in the breast similar to those caused by pregnancy are found in women with prolactin-secreting pituitary tumours or in women on certain drugs. In multiparas, the changes in the breasts are not of much diagnostic value because pregnancy may take place in a lactating woman. Pigmentation of the areola and the production of a milky secretion from the breasts may be remnants of a prior pregnancy.

Bluish discolouration of the vagina
Due to the increased blood flow to the pelvic organs, a number of changes are seen in the cervix and vagina. A bluish discolouration of the vagina is detected between the fourth and eighth weeks of pregnancy. The vulva and vaginal mucous membranes, because of the congestion of the blood vessels, present a violet or light blue tint, and later, a purplish or deep blue tint. The discolouration increases in intensity up to the sixteenth week to reach its maximum and then persists throughout pregnancy. This sign was first described by Jacquemier and later emphasised by Chadwick and hence, is known as **Jacquemier's sign or Chadwick's sign.**

Besides discolouration, there may be a sensation of increased warmth in the genitalia due to the increased blood supply to these parts. At a later stage, increased vaginal pulsations may be felt, which are referred to as **Osiander's sign**. This sign, however, may be produced by any condition that causes congestion of the pelvic organs.

Uterine changes
The uterus undergoes remarkable changes in pregnancy. In the early weeks, there are changes in the size, shape and position of the uterus. These can be detected by bimanual abdomino-vaginal examination.

Appearance
The **virgin uterus** is pyriform or pear-shaped and is usually anteflexed. During the first 8–10 weeks of gestation, the uterus gradually becomes rounded or globular and more anteflexed.

Position
Occasionally, a retroverted uterus does not become anteverted during pregnancy; instead, it grows in the retroverted position. This condition is called a **retroverted gravid uterus.** The retroverted pregnant uterus may become incarcerated in the hollow of the sacrum or sacculated.

Size
The uterus in the early weeks of pregnancy lies within the pelvic cavity. By the twelfth week, it gradually rises upwards towards the abdomen.

Other changes
The uterus becomes much softer during pregnancy. The softening is particularly noticeable in the cervix and in the lower uterine segment. This softening of the cervix is an important sign and can be recognised from the fourth week onwards.

Hegar's sign
The softening and compressibility of the isthmus or lower uterine segment are collectively called **Hegar's sign**. This is observed from about the sixth or eighth week to the twelfth week of pregnancy. This sign is more difficult to recognise in multiparas than in primiparas. It is, however, not positively diagnostic of pregnancy since softening can sometimes occur due to other reasons also.

Elicitation of Hegar's sign
Hegar's sign can be elicited in several ways.
- In women with a lax abdominal wall and a roomy vagina, two fingers are introduced into the vagina,

behind the cervix, while the fingers of the other hand are pressed down into the abdomen from above the symphysis pubis. The fingers of the two hands will almost meet as if there is no resisting tissue in between, and the cervix and body of the uterus will appear as two independent masses.

- Alternatively, two fingers are passed into the anterior fornix. The fingers of the other hand are placed above the symphysis, behind the body of the anteflexed uterus, and pressed downward to meet the vaginal fingers. Because of the danger of causing an interruption of pregnancy, these manipulations must be gentle, and pressure over the body of the uterus must be avoided (Fig. 6.1). Since the advent of USG imaging, these signs are no longer elicited on a routine basis.

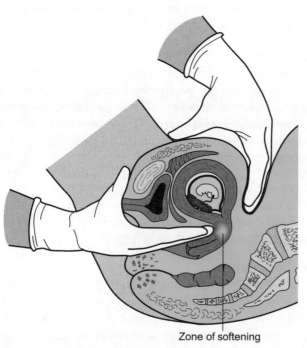

Zone of softening

Fig. 6.1   Eliciting Hegar's sign

Changes in the cervix

- In a nulliparous woman, the external os is circular, the mucous membrane is smooth and intact, and the orifice is closed. In a parous woman, on the other hand, the orifice is a transverse, patulous slit, which may admit the tip of the finger (Fig. 6.2a and b). In women who have a history of premature labour or abortion, the cervix may not show the characteristic signs. On the other hand, the cervix of a nullipara may be torn and may resemble a multiparous cervix as a result of operative manipulations.

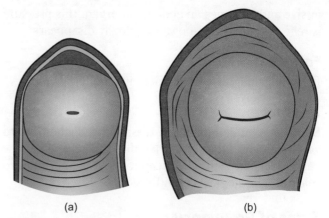

Fig. 6.2   (a) Nulliparous cervix and (b) cervix in a parous woman (note the transverse slit and the irregular cicatrices)

- The cervix softens by 6–8 weeks of pregnancy. The cervix in the non-pregnant state feels like the nasal cartilage, whereas during pregnancy, it becomes soft like the lips of the mouth. Softening of the cervix is otherwise called **Goodell's sign**.

Changes in the cervical mucus

A slide made of cervical mucus collected from a pregnant woman and observed under the microscope after drying shows a beaded pattern characteristic of the effect of progesterone.

■ SECOND TRIMESTER

Subjective Symptoms

During this period, some of the signs and symptoms that were present in the first trimester of pregnancy gradually disappear and other signs and symptoms become apparent. Morning sickness, increased salivation and frequency of micturition generally disappear by this time.

Fetal movement

An important symptom that may be felt during the second trimester is **quickening,** which is the first perception of fetal movement by the mother. The mother may feel the active fetal movements at the end of week 16—initially as a flutter and later as vigorous movements. In a primigravida, this may be delayed to 18–20 weeks of gestation. Based on the date of quickening, an approximate gestational age of the fetus may be arrived at. However, this is not accurate as it is patient-dependent. Peristaltic movements of the intestines may sometimes be mistaken for fetal movements.

Objective Signs

Changes in the skin

- **Pigmentation** is one of the characteristic changes that take place in pregnancy. This is more marked on the forehead and cheeks in the form of dark brown patches and more noticeable in those who are fair. This is called **chloasma**. Pigmentation and **striae** may also be seen on the breasts and over the abdominal wall (see Chapter 5, *Maternal changes in pregnancy*).
- Due to the stretching of the skin and disruption of the underlying collagen, linear stretch marks appear; these are known as **striae gravidarum. Linea nigra** is a linear pigmented line extending from the umbilicus to the symphysis pubis. These skin changes occur due to the stimulation of melanocytes by hormones.
- These changes may occasionally be absent during pregnancy. On the other hand, the use of steroidal contraceptives may be associated with these findings in non-pregnant women.
- There may also be reddening of the palms called **palmar erythema**. Due to the increasing levels of estrogen, **spider nevi** may develop, characterised by a central arteriole with thin radiating vessels.

Changes in the breasts

In the second trimester, there is further enlargement of the breasts, with the appearance of secondary areolae, striae, Montgomery follicles and secretions.

Changes in the shape and size of the uterus

The uterus, being a progressively growing organ in pregnancy, gradually increases in size and becomes ovoid in shape. It can be felt at different levels of the abdomen at different periods of pregnancy.

Intermittent uterine contractions

This is known as the **Braxton Hicks sign** and is found irrespective of whether the fetus is alive or dead. It may be detected by palpation as early as week 16. These contractions, as a rule, occur throughout pregnancy at fairly long intervals and last for a few seconds. They may be easily elicited by keeping the hand in full contact with the abdominal wall over the uterus, upon which the gradual relaxation and contraction of the uterus can be felt. These contractions are painless and not associated with cervical changes.

Active fetal movements

When felt or seen, fetal movements are evidence of continuing pregnancy and a live child. They may be noticed after the sixteenth or eighteenth week of pregnancy. Fetal movements may be elicited by external manipulations that produce passive movement of the fetus in utero.

Palpation of the fetal parts

By about the middle of pregnancy, the fetus generally grows to a size that allows it to be recognised by abdominal palpation. As pregnancy progresses, this sign is of great value, not only in detecting pregnancy but also in ascertaining the position of the fetus in utero nearing term.

External ballottement

In the second trimester, the amount of liquor is relatively greater than the size of the baby. Therefore, when the uterus is externally tapped with one hand, the fetus moves; this fetal movement can be felt with the other hand (Fig. 6.3). External ballottement can be elicited from 20–24 weeks of gestation. It depends upon the amount of liquor amnii present in the uterine cavity and is difficult to elicit when the abdominal wall is thick, in the presence of abdominal obesity, and in cases where the liquor amnii is very much diminished in quantity.

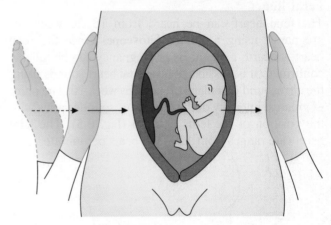

Fig. 6.3   External ballottement

Internal ballottement

Internal ballottement can be elicited between 16 and 18 weeks of gestation. With two fingers in the vagina, upward pressure is applied at the fornix. This results in the fetus moving up and then settling on the fingers again (Fig. 6.4). Before week 18, the fetus is too small to respond to the digital impulse; after week 28, the fetus is relatively too large, filling so much of the uterine cavity that it cannot move about as freely as before. This sign may not be elicited in conditions associated with a deficiency of the liquor amnii and in cases where the fetus is not presenting by the cephalic pole.

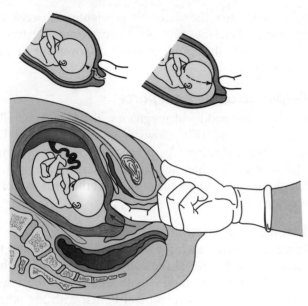

Fig. 6.4 Internal ballottement

Auscultatory signs

On auscultation over the abdomen, besides the fetal heart, various other sounds may be heard. The fetal heart should be differentiated from these sounds.

Fetal heart

The fetal heart can be heard from 18–20 weeks of pregnancy using a **Pinard fetoscope**. Once the fetal heart is heard, a diagnosis of pregnancy can be reliably confirmed. It is possible to hear fetal heart sounds using the ultrasound Doppler technique by week 10. The point of greatest intensity of the fetal heart sounds varies with the position of the fetus in utero (Fig. 6.5). The fetal heart rate ranges from 120–160 beats per minute.

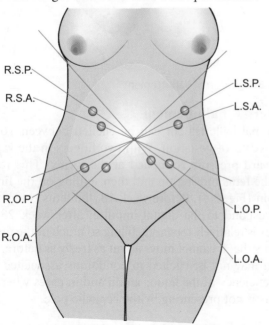

Fig. 6.5 Position of the fetal heart in several positions of vertex and breech presentations

Funic souffle

This is a sharp, whizzing sound synchronous with the fetal heartbeat, which is heard rarely due to the rush of blood through the umbilical arteries.

Other sounds that may be heard are due to the movements of the fetus, intestinal movements and maternal aortic pulsation. The **uterine souffle** is a soft, blowing sound that is synchronous with the maternal pulse and is produced by the passage of blood through the dilated uterine arteries.

■ THIRD TRIMESTER

During this period of pregnancy, painless uterine contractions persist, fetal movements are more easily felt and seen, fetal parts are easily palpable, and the fetal heart is heard clearly if the fetus is alive; ballottement is generally not elicitable. The uterus enlarges progressively until, at term, it occupies almost the entire abdomen.

INVESTIGATIONS FOR THE CONFIRMATION OF PREGNANCY

In early pregnancy, none of the physical signs and symptoms can entirely confirm the presence of pregnancy. Therefore, pregnancy should be confirmed by laboratory investigations.

■ DETECTION OF hCG IN BLOOD OR URINE

The diagnosis of pregnancy is based on the detection of serum β-hCG (Table 6.1) either in the woman's urine or her serum. The techniques that are used to detect β-hCG are bioassays and immunological tests. Of these, the bioassay techniques have become obsolete and are not used anymore.

Immunoassay

Human chorionic gonadotrophin has both α and β hCG subunits. Antigen–antibody reactions are used to detect the presence of these subunits in serum or urine. The tests to detect hCG antibodies to alpha subunits are not specific because they cross-react with LH, which has an identical alpha subunit. However, antibodies against the beta subunit of hCG are highly specific and do not cross-react with LH. This specificity is the basis of the detection of hCG in urine or blood.

Different immunoassays use different combinations of antibodies. A positive test indicates the presence

Table 6.1 Characteristics of tests to detect hCG to establish a diagnosis of pregnancy

Characteristics	Radioimmunoassay	Immuno-radiometric assay	ELISA (more sensitive)	ELISA (less sensitive)
Sensitivity (mIU/mL of hCG)	5	150	25	<50
Turnaround time (minutes)	240	30	80	5–15
Post-conception age when first positive (days)	10–18	18–22	14–17	18–22
Gestational age when first positive (weeks)	3–4	4	3–5	4

(Adapted from Shields AD. Pregnancy Diagnosis. *Medscape Drugs & Diseases.* Updated March 28, 2014. http://emedicine.medscape.com/article)/262591-overview)

of hCG from any source. It could be from a normal intrauterine pregnancy, ectopic pregnancy, non-viable intrauterine pregnancy, gestational trophoblastic disease or hCG-secreting ovarian tumours.

ELISA Technique

The enzyme-linked immunosorbent assay uses a monoclonal antibody that binds to the hCG in the test sample. A second antibody, which is tagged with an enzyme, is added to sandwich the test sample of hCG. When the substrate for this enzyme is added, colour develops. The development of colour signals that the test is positive and its absence signals a negative test. The sensitivity of ELISA for hCG in serum is 50 mIU/mL.

Home Pregnancy Tests

A number of relatively inexpensive pregnancy test kits are available, which can be used for home testing. Most of these are based on the enzyme-linked immunological assay.

Urine pregnancy test

Urine pregnancy test is the commonest method of diagnosing pregnancy in the clinic or at home. The test is usually done one week after a missed period. It is more sensitive if performed after 45 days of amenorrhea. The first morning specimen is usually recommended for testing because the hCG level is highest in such a sample. However, the test can be performed with a random sample also. The urine pregnancy test employs the enzyme-linked immunosorbent assay. It can detect hCG at a threshold of 25–50 mIU/mL.

Serum pregnancy test

This is the most sensitive method to detect hCG in serum. It is available as a qualitative test and a quantitative test. It can detect serum hCG levels as low as 5–20 mIU/mL. Serum tests are useful when pregnancy following

ART techniques needs to be confirmed, when ectopic pregnancy is suspected and in the follow-up of molar pregnancy.

Applications of serum β-hCG assays

- Serum β-hCG assays are most often used to confirm pregnancy. More than 95% of women show detectable levels of serum β-hCG 8–10 days after fertilisation. Therefore, a serum pregnancy test may be positive even before missing a period and is useful in confirming pregnancy following IVF.
- The levels of hCG peak at 12–14 weeks of gestation and then gradually decline. Early high levels may indicate the presence of multiple or molar pregnancy.
- The normal doubling time of β-hCG is 48 hours. In women with missed miscarriage or ectopic pregnancy, this doubling does not occur. Therefore, it is useful in the evaluation of a missed abortion and ectopic pregnancy.
- Quantitative hCG assays are important in the follow-up of trophoblastic diseases.
- A false-negative result can occur if the test is performed too early or in those with irregular cycles. In these individuals, the pregnancy test should be repeated.
- A false-positive result can also occur in cases where exogenous hCG was administered during infertility treatment or in the presence of β-hCG-secreting tumours.

ULTRASOUND DIAGNOSIS OF PREGNANCY

Currently, ultrasound is the most widely used tool to diagnose pregnancy. The following are the characteristic USG features on transvaginal ultrasound examination:

- The gestational sac is detected as a well-defined white ring by the fourth to fifth week (Fig. 6.6).

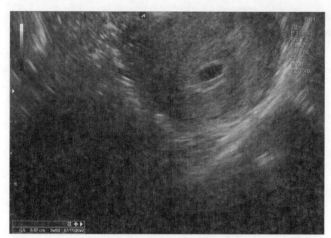

Fig. 6.6 Early pregnancy: Intrauterine gestation sac with a small yolk sac (*Image courtesy*: Dr Parameshwar Keerthi, Kancheepuram)

- The yolk sac appears at five weeks.
- The fetal pole appears at 5.5 weeks.
- The fetal cardiac activity is detectable at 6 weeks of gestation.
- At 8–14 weeks, the crown–rump length of the embryo allows the accurate estimation of gestational age (Fig. 6.7).

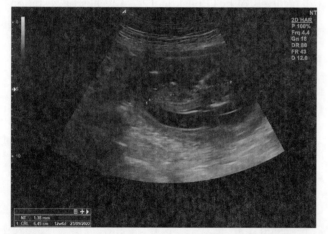

Fig. 6.7 Measurement of crown–rump length (*Image courtesy*: Dr Parameshwar Keerthi, Kancheepuram)

It takes another 4–7 days to visualise all these structures by transabdominal USG.

CALCULATION OF ESTIMATED DATE OF DELIVERY

Precise knowledge of the age of the fetus is important in order to assess the growth of the fetus, to interpret the various investigations performed during pregnancy and to determine the time of delivery. The estimated date of delivery (EDD) can be determined based on accurate knowledge of the date of onset of the **last menstrual period (LMP)**, clinical examination and USG assessment.

CALCULATING EDD FROM LMP

- The average duration of pregnancy is 266 days from conception and 280 days from the date of the last menstrual period in women with 28-day cycles. If the cycle is longer or shorter, an adjustment should be made in calculating the EDD.
- In a woman who has had regular menstrual cycles in the past, once in 28–30 days, the EDD is calculated by using Naegele's rule.

Naegele's rule: Add seven days to the first day of the LMP and either go back three months or go forward nine months. For example, if the first day of the LMP was October 1, the EDD will be July 8.

- For women who have always had a 40-day cycle, after calculating the EDD using Naegele's rule, another 10 days should be added to arrive at the correct EDD. However, this EDD should be confirmed using USG.
- If the pregnancy falls in a leap year, six days should be added to arrive at the correct EDD.
- In women with irregular cycles and those who have conceived despite the use of contraceptive methods or conceived during lactational amenorrhea, the determination of EDD is challenging.

CALCULATING EDD BY CLINICAL ASSESSMENT

- Under normal conditions, the uterus enlarges uniformly, and its height is proportionate to the period of pregnancy (Fig. 6.8; Table 6.2). The anteverted fundus of the pregnant uterus is just palpable at the symphysis after 12 weeks of gestation. The fundus is at the level of the umbilicus at 22–24 weeks and at 36 weeks of gestation, the fundus is at the level of the xiphisternum. At 40 weeks, the fundal height drops to a lower level corresponding to 32 weeks and there is a falling forward of the uterus.
- The duration of pregnancy cannot be accurately determined by this method because of the inconsistency of the location of the umbilicus, the thickness of the abdominal wall and the aberrations produced by obesity, multiple pregnancy, hydramnios and oligohydramnios.

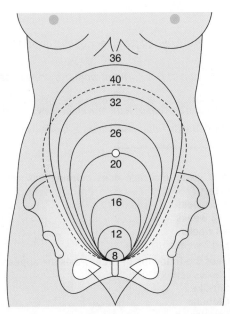

Fig. 6.8 Assessment of the height of uterus by palpation

Table 6.2 Conditions with variation in the height of the uterus

Height more than the period of amenorrhea	Height less than the period of amenorrhea
Vesicular mole	Ectopic pregnancy
Hydramnios	Retroverted gravid uterus
Multiple pregnancy	Intrauterine fetal demise
Concealed, accidental hemorrhage	Oligohydramnios
Uterine tumour associated with pregnancy	Missed abortion

- It has been shown that between 18 and 34 weeks, the fundal height in centimetres equals the gestational age in weeks. These measurements are taken after emptying the bladder (discussed in detail in the chapter on antenatal care).

USG ASSESSMENT OF GESTATIONAL AGE

- Crown–rump length (CRL) measurement gives an accurate estimate of gestational age in the first trimester. With this, the EDD can be calculated accurately to within 3–5 days. The crown–rump length measurement is taken along the length of the fetus in a straight line from the top of the head to the bottom of the buttocks (without correction for body curvature). This measurement is usually taken at 7–14 weeks of gestation.
- Biparietal measurement between 15 and 24 weeks of gestation predicts gestational age with an error of 7–10 days.
- After 26 weeks of gestation, the error increases to 14–21 days and hence, this feature is not used to assess the gestational age after such time.
- Femur length (FL) and humerus length correlate strongly with gestational age with an error of 7–11 days up to 26 weeks of gestation, after which the error increases to 14–21 days.
- A combination of measurements is better than a single measurement for the assessment of gestational age.

DIFFERENTIAL DIAGNOSES

The differential diagnosis for pregnancy includes the following:
- Distended bladder
- Fibroid uterus
- Cystic ovarian tumours

PSEUDOCYESIS (PHANTOM PREGNANCY)

This condition may occur in women who have an intense desire to become pregnant. A deposit of fat is seen in the anterior abdominal wall and omentum, and the intestines become distended with flatus. In such cases, signs of pregnancy may be present— menstruation may cease, the mammary signs of gestation may appear, and the abdomen may become progressively prominent. The woman may imagine that she feels fetal movements; striae may appear both on the abdomen and breasts. In extreme cases, these signs may continue to progress, and eventually, spurious labour may set in. The diagnosis of this condition is not difficult. Ultrasound is useful in such cases; needless to say, the pregnancy tests will invariably be negative.

KEY POINTS

✓ The presumptive symptoms of pregnancy are amenorrhea, nausea, vomiting, increased frequency of micturition, fatigue and perception of fetal movements by the woman.

✓ A definite diagnosis of pregnancy is made in the first trimester by the detection of β-hCG in the woman's urine or serum and by USG assessment.

✓ Definitive signs of pregnancy are the detection of fetal heart sounds and the perception of fetal movements by the examiner.

✓ Gestational age is assessed based on the LMP and by clinical examination; the definite assessment is made by USG.

Essay questions

1. Describe and discuss the signs and symptoms of pregnancy.
2. What are the investigations employed to diagnose pregnancy?
3. Describe the objective signs of pregnancy in the first and second trimesters.
4. Describe the methods of calculating the expected date of delivery.

Short answer questions

1. At six weeks of gestation, what are the structures visualised by TVS?
2. Write a short note on the various pregnancy tests available.
3. What are the differential diagnoses for pregnancy?
4. When the uterus is larger than the period of gestation, what conditions would you suspect?
5. What is uterine souffle?

MCQs

1. Which of the following is used to make the earliest diagnosis of pregnancy?
   a) History
   b) Examination
   c) Ultrasound
   d) Assessment of hCG
2. By what gestational age can the fetal heartbeat be detected by ultrasound?
   a) Fourth week
   b) Sixth week
   c) Eighth week
   d) Tenth week
3. Which of the following is NOT a cause of amenorrhea in a normally menstruating woman?
   a) Pregnancy
   b) Anovulation
   c) Mullerian agenesis
   d) Premature ovarian failure
4. What is the minimum hCG concentration that can be detected by the ELISA test?
   a) 50 mIU/mL
   b) 100 mIU/mL
   c) 150 mIU/mL
   d) 200 mIU/mL
5. Which of the following is the most accurate parameter for the assessment of gestational age by ultrasound?
   a) Crown–rump length
   b) Biparietal diameter
   c) Abdominal circumference
   d) Femur length
6. By what gestational age does morning sickness begin in pregnancy?
   a) 4–6 weeks
   b) 6–8 weeks
   c) >8 weeks
   d) 8–12 weeks
7. Which of the following best describes the appearance of a nulliparous cervix?
   a) Slit-like
   b) Globular
   c) Circular
   d) Transverse
8. At what gestational age is quickening felt?
   a) 6 weeks
   b) 8 weeks
   c) 10 weeks
   d) Second trimester
9. When is the uterus palpable above the symphysis pubis?
   a) 6th week
   b) 8th week
   c) 10th week
   d) 12th week
10. What is a pulsation in vagina in pregnancy called?
    a) Chadwick's sign
    b) Jacquemier's sign
    c) Osiander's sign
    d) Hegar's sign

Answers
1. (d), 2. (b), 3. (c), 4. (a), 5. (a), 6. (a), 7. (c), 8. (d), 9. (d), 10. (c)

Fill in the blanks

1. The first perception of fetal movements by the pregnant woman is termed as _____.
2. Quickening is first felt in the _____ trimester.
3. The average duration of pregnancy is _____ days from conception.
4. Irregular, intermittent and painless uterine contractions are known as _____ contractions.
5. Excessive vomiting during the first trimester of pregnancy, which may be associated with dehydration and acidosis, is known as _____.
6. A sharp whizzing sound synchronous with the fetal heartbeat heard due to the rush of blood through the umbilical arteries is known as _____.

Answers
1. quickening, 2. second, 3. 266, 4. Braxton Hicks, 5. hyperemesis gravidarum, 6. funic souffle

Case scenario-based discussion

1. A 28-year-old woman who has been married for 6 months visits the clinic with a history of two months' amenorrhea. She wants to know whether she is pregnant.
   a) What history should be taken in this case? What are the early symptoms of pregnancy?
   b) How will you confirm this woman's pregnancy?
   c) What is the most sensitive pregnancy test and what are the indications?
   d) How would you confirm pregnancy by USG assessment?

Answers

a) It is important to ask about the woman's last menstrual period as well as the regularity of her menstrual cycles in the past. It is also important to ask about subjective symptoms such as nausea, vomiting, increased frequency of micturition, giddiness and early fatiguability.

b) A urine pregnancy test should be performed, preferably with the first morning sample. This test is an immunological test that detects the presence of hCG in the urine.

c) The most sensitive pregnancy test is the serum β-hCG assay, which can detect 2–20 mIU/mL of hCG in the serum. It is useful for confirming pregnancy and very useful following ART techniques and in the follow-up of molar pregnancy and ectopic gestations, where serial measurements can be made.

d) On USG, the gestational sac is detected as a well-defined white ring by the fourth to fifth week. The yolk sac appears at five weeks, The fetal pole is seen at 5.5 weeks and fetal cardiac activity is detected at 6 weeks of gestation. At 8–14 weeks, the crown-rump length of the embryo can be measured.

7

OG 14.1

The Fetus in Normal Pregnancy

Learning Objectives

» To know the various diameters of the fetal skull
» To know the engaging diameters in various presentations
» To describe the lie, attitude, presentation and position of the fetus
» To describe the moulding of the fetal skull
» To discuss the clinical significance of sutures and fontanelles of the fetal skull

■ INTRODUCTION

In the process of labour, the fetus is a passenger who travels through a passage—the pelvis. Therefore, it is important to understand the fetus and its relationship with the pelvis. From the obstetric point of view, the fetal head is the most important part of the fetus because the head is in the lower part of the uterus in >95% of cases and is the first part of the fetus to enter the pelvis at the time of labour. Moreover, because of its bony structure, the fetal head is the most difficult part of the fetus to pass through the pelvis. This chapter will discuss the anatomy of the fetal skull and its relation to the maternal pelvis so as to elucidate the positional changes of the fetal head in the pelvis and the difficulties that may arise in the course of labour.

■ THE FETAL SKULL

• The fetal skull (Fig. 7.1) consists of the vault, the base and the face. The vault of the skull is subject to some degree of compression. The bones that form the vault of the skull are the two frontal bones, the two parietal bones, the occipital bone, the two temporal bones and the wings of the sphenoid.

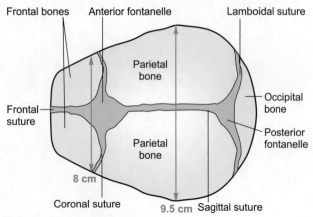

Fig. 7.1 The fetal skull (top view)

• These bones are not firmly united by bony union. In between the two bones, there is a thin piece of membrane, which is called a suture.
• Where two or more sutures meet, there is a wider expanse of membrane termed the fontanelle (Fig. 7.1). The bones at the base of the skull and the facial bones are firmly united, and therefore, are not compressible.

Sutures of the Fetal Skull

The following are the sutures of the fetal skull (Fig. 7.2):
• The frontal suture, situated between the two frontal bones
• The sagittal suture, situated between the two parietal bones
• The coronal suture, situated between the frontal and parietal bones
• The lambdoidal suture, situated between the posterior margins of the parietal bones and the occipital bone
• The temporal suture, situated on either side, between the inferior margin of the parietal bone and the upper margin of the temporal bone of the corresponding side

In labour, when the cephalic pole of the fetus is the presenting part, all the sutures except the temporal suture can be felt.

Fontanelle

The fontanelle is an area covered by membranes in which the suture lines meet (Fig. 7.2; Table 7.1).
• The anterior fontanelle is otherwise called bregma. It is the meeting point of the sagittal, coronal and frontal sutures. It is diamond-shaped, measures 2–3 cm and gets ossified by 1–1½ years of age.
• The posterior fontanelle is a Y-shaped triangular area and the meeting point of the sagittal and lambdoid sutures. It closes by 2–3 months of age.

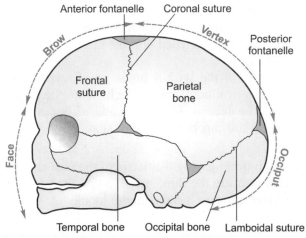

Fig. 7.2 The fetal skull: Sutures and fontanelles

Table 7.1 Fontanelles in the fetal skull: Shape, location, boundaries and sutures

Fontanelle	Shape and location	Bones forming it	Sutures felt
Anterior	Lozenge- or diamond-shaped

Junction of the sagittal and coronal sutures | Two parietal bones on either side posteriorly and two frontal bones in front | Sagittal, coronal and frontal |
| Posterior | Small, triangular area

Junction of the sagittal and lambdoidal sutures | Two parietal bones and the occipital bone | Lambdoidal |
| Temporal | Junction of the temporal and lambdoidal sutures | Inferior margin of the parietal bone and the upper margin of the temporal bone | |

Diameters of the Fetal Skull

The diameters of the fetal skull (Table 7.2; Fig. 7.3 and 7.4) are important as the skull is the first to enter the pelvic brim in various types of cephalic presentations. These diameters also indicate the shape and size of the fetal skull and the approximate measure of the head circumference. It is important to know the engaging diameter for each type of cephalic presentation and the engagement of the fetal head.

The engaging diameters

When the fetal head enters the pelvic brim, one of the anteroposterior (AP) diameters of the fetal skull occupies the transverse or oblique diameters of the pelvic brim—this is called the engaging diameter. The engaging diameter varies with the different types of cephalic presentations such as vertex (occipitoanterior and posterior positions), face and brow presentations.

Table 7.2 Diameters of the skull

Diameter	Measurement (in cm)
Bitemporal	8
Biparietal	9.5
Suboccipito-bregmatic	9.5
Submento-bregmatic	9.5
Occipitofrontal	11.5
Verticomental	13.5

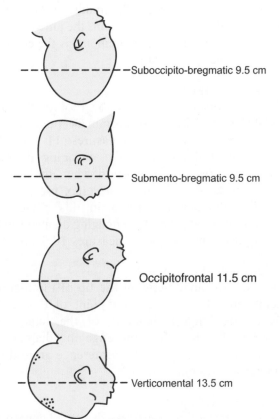

Fig. 7.3 Diameters of the fetal skull

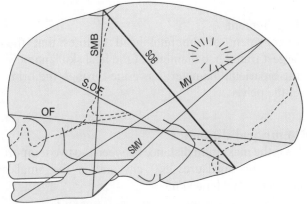

Fig. 7.4 Engaging diameters of the fetal skull
SOB: Suboccipito-bregmatic diameter in occipitoanterior position
SMB: Submento-bregmatic in face presentation
OF: Occipitofrontal in occipitoposterior position
SOF: Suboccipitofrontal in occipitoposterior position
MV: Mentovertical (also called verticomental) in brow presentation

Suboccipito-bregmatic diameter

This measures 9.5 cm and is the distance between the middle of the anterior fontanelle and a point just below the occipital protuberance. This is the engaging diameter in the occipitoanterior position (vertex presentation). The circumference of the fetal head at this point is 27.5 cm.

Submento-bregmatic diameter

This is the distance between the middle of the anterior fontanelle and a point that represents the junction of the chin and neck. It measures 9.5 cm and is the engaging diameter in face presentation.

Occipitofrontal diameter

This is the distance between the root of the nose or glabella and the most prominent point on the occipital protuberance. It measures 11 cm. The occipitofrontal diameter is the engaging diameter in the occipitoposterior position when the head is in an attitude of deflexion in a vertex presentation. The circumference is 34 cm in this plane. The suboccipitofrontal is another engaging diameter in the occipitoposterior position; it measures 10.5 cm.

Verticomental diameter

This is the distance between the tip of the mentum or chin and the most distant point of the vertex. This is the longest diameter of the fetal skull, measuring 13 cm and is the engaging diameter in a brow presentation. The circumference around this diameter is 37.5 cm.

Biparietal diameter

This is the maximum transverse distance between the two parietal eminences. It measures 9.5 cm.

Engagement

Engagement of the fetal head denotes that the largest transverse diameter of the fetal skull, namely the biparietal diameter, has gone through the brim of the pelvis.

Bitemporal diameter

This is the maximum distance between the two temporal bones. This measures 8.0 cm and is the smallest diameter of the fetal skull.

Moulding of the Fetal Skull

As the fetal skull bones are united only by fibrous tissue, they can slide and override each other to adjust to the shape and size of the maternal pelvis. This process occurs during labour and is known as moulding. Because of moulding, the diameters of the fetal skull become slightly shortened and the circumference also reduces.

The base of the skull is made up of several bones united by a firm bony union which cannot be reduced in size. The face is, likewise, made of bones united firmly and is incapable of compression.

Though the engaging diameters of the face and the vertex measure the same, i.e., 9.5 cm, the vertex is preferred because it can undergo moulding.

Table 7.3 presents the various terms used to describe the fetal skull.

Table 7.3 Various terms used to describe the fetal skull

Term	Description
Occiput	It is the most prominent part of the occipital bone; it is located just behind the posterior fontanelle
Sinciput	It is the area between the orbital ridges anteriorly and the bregma and the coronal sutures above
Vertex	It is a diamond-shaped area bound on either side by the parietal eminences, anteriorly by the anterior fontanelle and posteriorly by the posterior fontanelle (Fig. 7.5)
Face	It is the area between the chin and the root of the nose (glabella)
Glabella	It is the root of the nose/area between the two orbital ridges
Cephalic prominence	On abdominal palpation, while performing the second pelvic grip, it is the most prominent bony part of the skull that is felt first; it could be either the occiput or the sinciput
	The significance of this will be discussed in detail in the chapter on obstetric examination of the patient
Denominator	This term refers to an arbitrary point chosen for each fetal presenting part to describe its position with reference to the different quadrants of the maternal pelvis, e.g., for vertex presentation, it is the occiput, and for face presentation, it is the chin
Engagement	Engagement is said to have occurred when the widest transverse diameter of the fetus has passed through the brim of the pelvis
	In a cephalic presentation, this is the biparietal diameter and in breech presentation, it is the bitrochanteric diameter

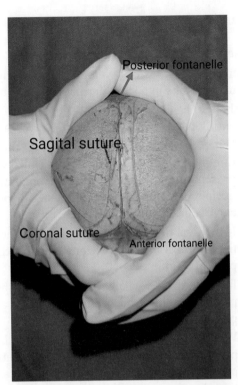

Fig. 7.5 The boundaries of vertex (*Image courtesy*: Dr Jayashree Srinivasan, Professor, Saveetha Medical College)

CLINICAL SIGNIFICANCE OF SUTURES AND FONTANELLES OF THE FETAL SKULL

- As the head descends into the pelvis, the direction of the sagittal suture of the fetal skull and the fontanelle, which is felt easily and low down, help in identifying the type of presentation—whether occipitoanterior (OA)/occipitoposterior (OP) or brow presentation.
  — In a well-flexed head in the OA position, the posterior fontanelle is low down and is easily palpable, whereas the anterior fontanelle is not palpable.
  — In the OP position with a deflexed head, the anterior fontanelle is easily palpable; one may also be able to palpate the posterior fontanelle at a higher level.
  — In the brow presentation, only the anterior fontanelle is palpable along with the forehead up to the orbital ridges.
  — In the face presentation, the fontanelle is not palpable.
- In hydrocephalus, the sutures and the fontanelles are widely separated due to the excessive collection of CSF within the ventricles. If the fetus cannot be

saved due to excessive destruction of the brain tissue, in order to facilitate vaginal delivery, the head can be decompressed by passing a needle or craniotomy scissors through the wide fontanelles to drain the fluid.

- As the sutures between the bones are membranous, the vault of the skull is compressible, thereby reducing the diameter of the fetal skull. This is called moulding of the fetal skull. The degree of moulding is graded as follows:

Grade 1: Sutures opposed
Grade 2: Sutures overlapped, but reducible
Grade 3: Sutures overlapped, but irreducible

Grades 2 and 3 moulding indicate that there is excessive compression of the fetal head, indicating obstructed labour and the risk of the fetus developing hypoxia.

▮ FETAL ATTITUDE

The attitude of the fetus refers to the relation of the different parts of the fetus to one another. Normally, the fetal attitude is one of universal flexion. In the occipitoposterior position, there could be a deflexed attitude.

Universal Flexion

In this attitude, the spinal column is bent forward, the head is flexed, the chin rests against the sternum, the arms are flexed and folded across the chest, the lower extremities are flexed so that the thighs are against the abdomen and the legs are bent (at the knee joint), resting on the thighs with the feet crossed in an attitude of dorsiflexion. In this position, the fetus forms an ovoid mass corresponding roughly to the shape of the uterine ovoid. This allows the space occupied by the fetus to be reduced to the minimum. Thus, this attitude of universal flexion has an important bearing on the mechanism of delivery. When the fetal ovoid (in this attitude of universal flexion) lies longitudinally in the uterine ovoid, the uterus is subjected to very little stretching. In such a position, the fetus may have either the head or the breech at the lower pole of the uterus.

Significance of Fetal Attitude

- An attitude of universal flexion allows the smaller diameters of fetal parts to enter the pelvis as seen in the occipitoanterior position.
- In the occipitoposterior position, the fetus maintains an extended attitude. In the OP position, the fetal

spine is posterior, and is splint against the maternal spine, and therefore, unable to flex. As a result, the spine gets straightened out and the fetus attains a military attitude, and its head gets deflexed.

FETAL LIE

- Fetal lie is the relation between the longitudinal axis of the fetal ovoid and the longitudinal axis of the uterine ovoid.
- When the longitudinal axis of the fetus corresponds to the longitudinal axis of the uterine ovoid, it is called a longitudinal lie and the presentation is either cephalic or breech (podalic presentation). In labour, nearly 99% of fetuses present in a longitudinal lie (Fig. 7.6a and b).

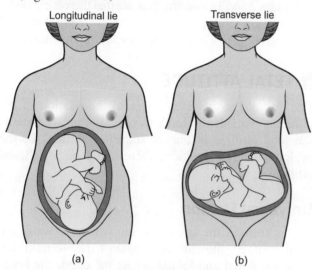

Fig. 7.6 (a) Longitudinal and (b) transverse lie

When the longitudinal axis of the fetus is either oblique or transverse to that of the uterine ovoid, the lie is said to be an oblique or transverse lie. Multiparity, placenta previa, hydramnios and uterine anomalies are some of the factors contributing to transverse lie.

FETAL PRESENTATION

- Fetal presentation refers to the portion of the fetal ovoid that is in relation to the lower pole of the uterus and is the first to engage in the pelvis when labour starts.
- The presenting part is the portion of the fetus that lies lowest and is the first to be felt by vaginal examination.
- When the fetus presents by the head, it is known as cephalic presentation. In this presentation, the part of the cephalic pole lying lowest may vary—it may be vertex/face/brow presentation.

- When the fetus presents by breech in the lower pole (podalic pole), it is known as a podalic presentation.
- When the fetus lies transverse and obliquely in the uterus, it results in a shoulder presentation.
- In the cephalic presentation, depending on the presenting part, various presentations can occur:
  — When the head is well flexed so that the chin is in contact with the thorax, it is called a vertex presentation. In the vertex presentation, both occipitoanterior and occipitoposterior positions can occur.
  — If the fetal neck is fully extended and the face is the foremost in the birth canal, it is called a face presentation.
  — If the fetus is partially extended with the brow presenting lowermost, it is called a brow presentation.
  — When more than one part of the fetus is in the presenting position, it is called a compound presentation.

DENOMINATOR

The denominator is an arbitrary point chosen for each fetal presenting part to describe its position with reference to the different quadrants of the maternal pelvis (Table 7.4). It is generally a bony landmark.

Table 7.4 Presentations and denominators

Presentation	Presenting part	Denominator
Cephalic	Vertex	Occiput
Cephalic	Face	Mentum or chin
Cephalic	Brow	Frontal eminence
Breech	Pelvis	Sacrum
Shoulder	Shoulder	Acromion

The four quadrants in any plane of the pelvis may be divided into two right quadrants and two left quadrants:
1. Right anterior
2. Right posterior
3. Left anterior
4. Left posterior

FETAL POSITION

Depending upon the position of the denominator with reference to the four quadrants of the pelvic cavity, the position of the fetus (Fig. 7.7a–d) in utero is determined.

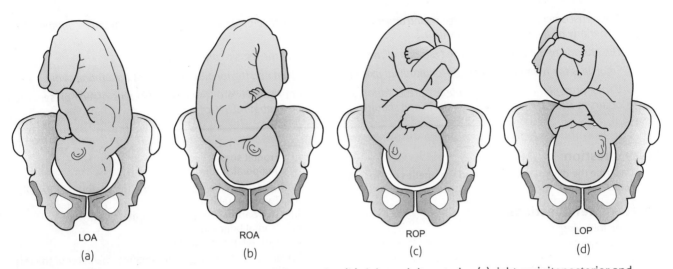

LOA	ROA	ROP	LOP
(a)	(b)	(c)	(d)

Fig. 7.7 Various vertex presentations: a) Left occipitoanterior, (b) right occipitoanterior, (c) right occipitoposterior and (d) left occipitoposterior

FREQUENCY OF PRESENTATIONS AND POSITIONS

- Vertex presentation is the commonest presentation, occurring in nearly 96% of the cases, whereas breech presentation occurs in 3%, face presentation in 0.5% and shoulder presentation in about 0.5% of cases.
- Among the vertex presentations, the position most adopted by fetuses is the left occipitoanterior, which occurs in nearly 70% of cases.
- Right occipitoposterior position occurs in over 25% of cases. The rest are either left occipitoposterior or right occipitoanterior.

Factors that Influence the Increased Frequency of Cephalic Presentations

The cephalic presentations, in particular the vertex presentations, are the most common type of presentation. This can be explained by the following theories:

- Due to the effect of gravity, the head, which is the heaviest part of the fetus, occupies the lower pole.
- The entire podalic pole of the fetus, the breech and its flexed extremities are bulkier than the cephalic pole and therefore move to the upper pole where more space is available.

- Until about the thirty-second week, the amniotic cavity is large in relation to the fetal mass, and there is no crowding of the fetus by the uterine walls. After 32 weeks of gestation, the ratio of the amniotic contents to the fetal mass alters by relative diminution of the amniotic fluid. As a result, the uterine walls are more closely apposed to the fetal parts, and the pyriform shape of the uterus exerts its effect. At this stage, the fetus, if presenting by breech, changes its polarity to make use of the roomier fundus for its bulkier and more motile podalic pole.
- The high incidence of breech presentation in hydrocephalic fetuses is in accord with this theory, which says that the cephalic pole. which is larger, tends to occupy the upper pole.
- In the presence of a uterine septum, due to the decrease in the space available in the fundus, the breech occupies the lower pole.
- By altering the natural adjustment of the fetal ovoid to the uterine cavity, conditions such as prematurity, placenta previa, hydramnios, uterine malformations, contracted pelvis and tumours of the lower segment can predispose to malpresentations. Grand multiparity with a lax abdominal wall can also result in malpresentations.

KEY POINTS

✓ *The diameters of the fetal skull are important because these are the first diameters to enter into the pelvic brim in various types of cephalic presentations.*

✓ *When the fetal head enters the pelvic brim, one of the AP diameters of the fetal skull occupies the transverse or oblique diameters of the pelvic brim. This is called the engaging diameter.*

✓ *Engagement of the fetal head denotes that the largest transverse diameter of the fetal skull, namely the biparietal diameter (9.4 cm), has gone through the brim of the pelvis.*

✓ The vertex is a diamond-shaped area bound on either side by the parietal eminences, anteriorly by the anterior fontanelle and posteriorly by the posterior fontanelle.

✓ The attitude of the fetus refers to the relation of the different parts of the fetus to one another.

✓ Fetal lie is the relation between the longitudinal axis of the fetal ovoid and the longitudinal axis of the uterine ovoid.

✓ Vertex presentation is the commonest presentation, occurring in nearly 96% of the cases, whereas breech presentation occurs in 3%, face presentation in 0.5% and shoulder presentation in about 0.5% of cases.

Essay question

1. Describe the diameters, sutures and fontanelles of the fetal skull.

Short answer questions

Define the following:

1. Fetal attitude
2. Fetal lie
3. Fetal presentation
4. Fetal position
5. Anterior fontanelle
6. Moulding of the fetal skull

MCQs

1. What is the suture between the parietal bone and the occipital bone called?
   a) Frontal suture
   b) Sagittal suture
   c) Coronal suture
   d) Lambdoidal suture

2. Which is the engaging diameter of a face presentation?
   a) Suboccipito-bregmatic
   b) Submento-bregmatic
   c) Occipitofrontal
   d) Verticomental

3. Which of the following sutures is used to identify the position of the fetal skull?
   a) The frontal suture
   b) The sagittal suture
   c) The coronal suture
   d) The lambdoidal suture

4. What is the incidence of vertex presentation at term?
   a) 80%
   b) 86%
   c) 90%
   d) 96%

5. In what type of presentation is the engaging diameter occipitofrontal?
   a) Face
   b) Brow
   c) Occipitoposterior
   d) Occipitoanterior

6. Which of the following is the longest diameter of the fetal head?
   a) Biparietal
   b) Verticomental
   c) Occipitofrontal
   d) Submento-bregmatic

7. Which of the following is the suture between the frontal and parietal bones?
   a) Coronal suture
   b) Sagittal suture

c) Frontal suture
   d) Temporal suture

8. Which of the following bones form the posterior fontanelle?
   a) Two parietal bones
   b) Two parietal bones and occipital bone
   c) Frontal bones in front
   d) Parietal and frontal bones

9. Which of the following is the smallest diameter of the fetal skull?
   a) Biparietal diameter
   b) Bitemporal diameter
   c) Occipitofrontal diameter
   d) Verticomental diameter

10. Which is the engaging diameter in a brow presentation?
    a) Biparietal diameter
    b) Bitemporal diameter
    c) Suboccipito-frontal diameter
    d) Verticomental diameter

11. How much does the biparietal diameter measure?
    a) 9.5 cm
    b) 13.5 cm
    c) 11 cm
    d) 8 cm

12. What is the relation between the longitudinal axis of the fetal ovoid and the longitudinal axis of the uterine ovoid called?
    a) Fetal attitude
    b) Fetal lie
    c) Fetal position
    d) Fetal presentation

13. What is the commonly adopted vertex presentation?
    a) Left occipitoanterior
    b) Right occipitoposterior
    c) Left occipitoposterior
    d) Right occipitoanterior

Answers
1. (d), 2. (b), 3. (b), 4. (d), 5. (c), 6. (b), 7. (a), 8. (b), 9. (b), 10. (d), 11. (a), 12. (b), 13. (a)

Fill in the blanks

1. The parts of the fetal skull are _____.
2. The anterior fontanelle is otherwise called _____.
3. The bones that meet in the posterior fontanelle are _____.
4. The maximum transverse diameter of the fetal skull is the _____.
5. When more than one part of the fetus presents it is called a _____.
6. When the longitudinal axis of the fetus is oblique to that of the uterine ovoid, the lie is said to be _____.

Answers
1. vault, base and face, 2. bregma, 3. two parietal bones and the occiput, 4. biparietal diameter, 5. compound presentation, 6. an oblique lie

Preconceptional and Antenatal Care

Learning Objectives

» To know the importance of preconceptional counselling

» To describe and discuss the objectives of antenatal care

» To be able to assess the period of gestation, elicit obstetric history, past medical and surgical history, family history and medication history

» To plan the number of antenatal visits and management at each antenatal visit

» To know the investigations in each trimester of pregnancy

» To know the indications for USG in the first and second trimesters of pregnancy

» To identify high-risk maternal problems and if necessary, refer high-risk mothers to higher centres

» To discuss the planning of antenatal care for low-risk and high-risk mothers

» To discuss prophylactic medications, nutrition advice and vaccines in pregnancy

■ PRECONCEPTIONAL CARE

Preconceptional care involves measures and interventions that are undertaken before the woman becomes pregnant in order to improve the maternal and neonatal outcomes. The objective of such care is to identify and correct potential risk factors that may have adverse effects on a pregnancy.

General Measures

- A detailed medical, obstetric and family history should be taken to identify potential risk factors.
- A detailed general examination including weight, BP, testing for anemia and assessment of the cardiovascular system should be carried out.
- The presence of anemia and malnutrition should be identified and corrected.
- Women should be advised on ideal body weight prior to conception as both underweight and obesity can have an adverse effect on the mother and fetus.
- All women planning pregnancy should be started on 0.4 mg of folic acid to prevent neural tube defects in the fetus. Those who are at an increased risk because of a previously affected child and those who are epileptic and on antiepileptic medications should be given 4 mg of folic acid daily.
- The woman should be advised against smoking, alcohol consumption and substance abuse.
- Vaccination history against rubella, chickenpox and hepatitis B should be verified. The rubella status of the woman's partner should also be checked.

If the woman is seronegative, the fetus may be vulnerable to anomalies if exposed to rubella during the period of organogenesis. Such women should therefore be offered rubella vaccination and be advised not to become pregnant within one month of immunisation. Similarly, vaccination against chickenpox and hepatitis B can also be given prior to initiating infertility treatment.

- Pre-existing medical conditions such as diabetes, obesity, hypothyroidism, seizure disorders and HIV should be managed appropriately before attempting conception. The woman's current medications should be evaluated in detail to avoid the use of teratogenic drugs and to switch her to safer drugs. Women who have cardiac diseases, autoimmune disorders, chronic renal disease and those who have had renal transplant should seek the obstetrician's opinion as well as that of the respective specialist to check whether pregnancy is a feasible option (Table 8.1).

Screening for Diseases

- In women with a history of recurrent pregnancy loss, genetic studies and other investigations are required.
- Genetic risk factors in the family should be identified.
- Women who have a history of early-onset pre-eclampsia/eclampsia require APLA screening.
- Screening for sexually transmitted diseases and UTI and treatment prior to pregnancy are important to prevent preterm labour and intrapartum infections.

Table 8.1 Evaluation of medical conditions

Medical condition	Recommendations
Pre-existing diabetes	• Should be aimed at good glycemic control • Should be aimed at HbA1C <7 before conception • Evaluate for retinopathy, nephropathy, cardiac status, etc.
Epilepsy	• Use monotherapy, less teratogenic drugs, increase the dose of folic acid
Heart disease	• Look for absolute contraindication to pregnancy • Assess the functional state of the heart • Avoid warfarin in those on valve replacement
Hypertension	• Avoid ACE inhibitors • Evaluate the cardiac status, look for retinopathy and nephropathy
Hematological disorders	• In areas where hemophilia and thalassemia are prevalent, women should be counselled on the risk of inheritance and the need for prenatal diagnostic tests during pregnancy

Prevention of Unintended Pregnancies

Preconception care also entails counselling regarding the prevention of unintended pregnancies and spacing of children.

■ ANTENATAL CARE

Aims of Antenatal Care

- To confirm pregnancy, assess gestational age, identify pre-existing medical illness, identify high-risk factors, order investigations and provide prophylactic mediations
- To monitor the well-being of the mother and baby
- To manage the 'minor ailments' of pregnancy
- To prevent, identify and manage conditions that may adversely affect the mother and the baby
- To provide advice, reassurance, education and support to the woman and her family
- To determine the timing and mode of delivery
- To achieve safe delivery of the baby
- To ensure that the infant is born under optimum conditions

Frequency of Antenatal Visits

- The WHO proposed a minimum of four antenatal visits during the antenatal period; these should be focused visits—the first visit in the first trimester to conduct a thorough assessment of the woman; the second visit between 20 and 22 weeks to order an anomaly scan as well as other screening investigations and to start the woman on suitable prophylactic medication; the third visit at 30–34 weeks to identify evolving high-risk factors and to assess fetal growth and the fourth visit at 38 weeks of gestation to plan the timing and mode of delivery. The current WHO guidelines recommend at least eight contacts between the pregnant woman and the healthcare professional.
- Most women, especially those with high-risk pregnancies, should have antenatal care through more than four antenatal visits.
  — The booking visit should be before 10 weeks of pregnancy
  — The second-trimester visit at 20–22 weeks
  — Four weekly appointments from 20–32 weeks
  — Fortnightly visits from 32–36 weeks and weekly visits thereafter

■ THE FIRST TRIMESTER VISIT

The booking visit should ideally be planned at 10 weeks of gestation. It is usually scheduled as soon as pregnancy is suspected. The following are the objectives of the booking visit:

- To confirm pregnancy
- To assess gestational age
- To rule out abnormal pregnancies
- To diagnose multiple pregnancy
- To review the woman's medical history
- To identify high-risk pregnancies
- To assess the woman's general condition
- To order investigations
- To provide prophylactic medication

Confirmation of Pregnancy

Based on symptoms

A history of amenorrhea and the presence of characteristic symptoms such as nausea, vomiting, giddiness, breast tenderness and increased urinary frequency are suggestive of pregnancy.

Biochemical test

A positive urine or serum pregnancy test indicates the presence of serum β-hCG, which confirms pregnancy.

Ultrasonography (USG)

- The earliest evidence of pregnancy is the appearance of the gestational sac, which is visualised by transvaginal USG (TVS) as early as 4 weeks after conception. It is clearly made out between 4.5 and 5 weeks of gestation. The mean sac diameter is 2–3 mm at 4 weeks of gestation.
- The gestational age can be calculated from the mean sac diameter. Adding 30 to the mean sac diameter will give the gestational age in days. For example, if the mean gestational sac diameter is 10 mm, the gestational age is 10 + 30 = 40 days (6 weeks).
- The gestational sac should be evaluated for the presence of a yolk sac and the fetal pole (Fig. 8.1). The yolk sac appears at 5 weeks, when the sac diameter is 10 mm. Normally, the size of the yolk sac is 6 mm; it normally disappears at 12–14 weeks. In the presence of large yolk sacs, an abnormal pregnancy should be suspected (Fig. 8.1).
- By 5.5 weeks, the fetal pole appears as a 1–2 mm large structure.
- Cardiac activity appears at 6 weeks of gestation, when the embryo is >5 mm in size.

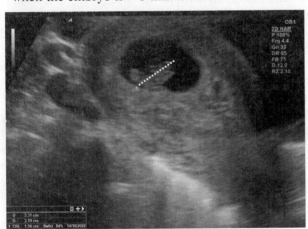

Fig. 8.1 USG showing gestational sac with the fetal pole (*Image courtesy*: Dr Parameshwar Keerthi, BM Scans, Kancheepuram)

Dating of Pregnancy (Assessment of Gestational Age) and Calculating Expected Date of Delivery

History

- The woman should be asked about the first day of her last menstrual period (LMP).
- She should be asked about the regularity of her previous menstrual cycles and the use of contraception prior to missing the period.
- In a woman who has had regular menstrual cycles in the past, once in 28–30 days, the expected date of delivery (EDD) is calculated using Naegele's rule—add 7 days to the first day of LMP and either go back 3 months or go forward 9 months.
- In women who have always had 40-day cycles, after calculating the EDD, another 10 days are added to arrive at the actual EDD.
- EDD based on LMP should be confirmed by USG dates.
- In women who have had very irregular cycles, Naegele's rule is not dependable. In such cases, USG parameters should be used to calculate EDD.
- Only 4–5% of women deliver on their due date.

USG to assess the gestational age

USG assessment of gestational age is discussed in detail in Chapters 6 and 10.

- Crown–rump length (CRL) measurement gives an accurate estimate of the gestational age in the first trimester. With this, the EDD can be calculated accurately to within 3–5 days.
- The CRL is measured along the length of the fetus in a straight line from the top of the head to the bottom of the buttocks.
- Usually, this measurement is recorded between 7 and 14 weeks of gestation.
- If, for some reason, the EDD is not calculated in the first trimester, then in the second trimester of pregnancy, the biparietal diameter (BPD) is measured to assess the gestational age. It is the widest transverse diameter of the fetal head, recorded between 14 and 20 weeks of gestation.
- With the BPD measurement, the EDD can be accurately calculated to ±7 days.
- The margin of error in calculating the EDD increases with increasing gestational age. For this reason, gestational age should be assigned before 20 weeks of gestation. If a woman visits the obstetrician for the

first time late in her second trimester or in her third trimester, femur length and transcerebellar diameters can also be used to assess the gestational age.

Accurate estimation of gestational age in first trimester is important for the following reasons:
- To accurately calculate the EDD
- To monitor the fetal growth
- To avoid iatrogenic prematurity
- To plan induction for post-term pregnancy
- To interpret screening investigations such as Down screen

Booking History

1. Demographic details

Age
Pregnant women at the extremes of age are vulnerable to more complications than those in their twenties and early thirties. Pregnancy in the teenaged mother can result in the development of anemia, pre-eclampsia, cephalopelvic disproportion (CPD) and more operative deliveries. Fetal growth restriction (FGR), preterm birth and miscarriages are also more common in teen pregnancies. Women who are above 35 years of age are predisposed to diabetes, hypertension, malpresentations, macrosomic babies and genetic abnormalities in the fetus, especially Down syndrome. A macrosomic baby could result in CPD and obstructed labour.

Occupation
It is important to enquire whether the pregnant woman is working and about the nature of her work. Women who work or commute for long hours are vulnerable to preterm births and IUGR. The working status may negatively affect the woman's nutritional needs, resulting in anemia. Women working in laboratories and radiology departments are vulnerable to infection and radiation exposure.

Residence
It is advisable for pregnant women to receive obstetric care at a healthcare centre that is not too far from their place of residence. This is especially true for women who are diagnosed with hypertension, placenta previa, multiple pregnancy and malpresentations and those nearing term.

Socioeconomic status
Socioeconomic status has a bearing upon the nutritional status of the individual. Women from low socioeconomic groups are more likely to be anemic and underweight and are at a higher risk of going into preterm labour and delivering growth-restricted and low-birth-weight babies. On the other hand, obesity and diabetes are more common among women from higher socioeconomic strata.

2. Marital history
The number of years of marriage and history of consanguinity should be elicited. Consanguineous marriages may be associated with congenital anomalies of the fetus such autosomal recessive disorders and single gene defects. It is important to enquire whether the woman has had infertility treatment. In women who have had such treatment, it must be ascertained whether the pregnancy was spontaneous or induced.

3. Menstrual history
A detailed menstrual history is important with regards to the regularity of the cycles, duration of flow and the first day of last menstrual period. In women who have irregular cycles, those who do not remember their LMP and those who conceived during lactational amenorrhea, the gestational age should be calculated based on the USG parameters. Besides the date of the last menstrual period, the amount of bleeding in the last menstrual cycle is also important. Scanty bleeding may be associated with ectopic pregnancy or implantation bleeding may be wrongly taken as LMP.

4. Medical history
History of past and current medical illnesses (hypertension, diabetes, renal disease, epilepsy, bronchial asthma, cardiac disease, thyroid disorders and autoimmune diseases) and past and current medications should be elicited. Medications may need to be changed or their dose adjusted in pregnancy.

Surgical history
Appendicectomy, ovarian cystectomy (for adhesions), any surgical treatment on the cervix such as cone biopsy and large loop excision of transformation zone (LLETZ) for cervical intraepithelial neoplasia (CIN) lesions can predispose the woman to preterm labour.

5. Obstetric history
The woman's obstetric score should be calculated at the time of the booking visit. Obstetric score is defined in terms of gravidity, para, abortions, ectopic pregnancy, living children, etc.

- **Gravidity** is the number of times the woman has conceived including the current pregnancy (all pregnancy events should be included—abortions, ectopic, medical termination of pregnancy [MTP], preterm birth, intrauterine death, etc.). The following terms are used to describe gravidity:
  — Gravida: A woman who is pregnant
  — Primigravida: A woman who is pregnant for the first time
  — Multigravida: A woman who has conceived more than once
  — Elderly primi: A woman who is pregnant for the first time at the age of 35 or more (in western countries, such terminology is no longer used as most women get pregnant after 30 years of age)
  — Nulligravida: A woman who has never been pregnant
- **Parity** is the number of times the woman has had a viable birth (as it involves delivery, the current pregnancy should not be included).
- The **period of viability** is defined as the gestational age at which >50% of the newborns are able to survive outside the uterus. The period of viability in India varies from 24–28 weeks of gestation depending on the available neonatal facility.
- In women who have delivered twins, the labour process is one, therefore, they are called para 1 and live 2.
- For each conception, the following history should be elicited:
  — Period of gestation and outcome of each pregnancy (such as spontaneous abortion, termination of pregnancy, ectopic, hydatidiform mole, preterm delivery, term delivery)
  — Any antenatal complications, e.g., anemia, pre-eclampsia and GDM; the treatment given for the same should be noted
  — Details of labour onset—spontaneous onset or induced (and indication for induction)
  — Gestational age at delivery—preterm, term, post-term—and mode of delivery

  — Mode of delivery—spontaneous vaginal delivery, instrumental delivery such as forceps and ventouse, cesarean section (elective or induced); indication for cesarean section; place and year of delivery
  — Intrapartum complications, the birth weight of the baby, baby's condition at birth, neonatal complications and neonatal admission
  — Postpartum complications such as PPH, maternal morbidity and whether blood transfusion was given should be noted

Table 8.2 presents an example of how obstetric history is recorded.

Gynecological history
- History of heavy periods can predispose to anemia in pregnancy.
- Previous surgery on the cervix can predispose to cervical incompetence.

Contraception history
A history of using any contraceptive method prior to the current pregnancy should be elicited. After using oral contraceptive pills or the use of injectable contraceptives such as DMPA, the EDD may not be accurate as some cycles may be anovulatory after stopping the contraceptive. Occasionally, a woman may become pregnant due to contraceptive failure.

6. *Family history*
- Consanguinity
- Hypertension, diabetes, pre-eclampsia, eclampsia
- Multiple pregnancy
- Congenital malformations, mental retardation, recurrent abortions, unexplained neonatal death
- Hereditary disorders
- Blood transfusion in family members may indicate hereditary hematological disorders
- History of keeping pets such as cats at home (they may predispose to toxoplasmosis)

Table 8.2 Record of obstetric history

S. no.	Year	Period of gestation	Outcome of pregnancy	Antenatal complications	Labour onset	Mode of delivery	Sex/birth weight/ neonatal complications	Postnatal complications
1		14 weeks	Spontaneous abortion	-	-	-	-	-
2		38 weeks	Term delivery	GDM	Induced	LSCS on indication	M/3.9 Kg/hypoglycemia	NIL

7.   Social history

*   Family support—nuclear or joint family, socioeconomic status
*   Dietary history
*   Smoking, drug abuse, alcoholism

8.   History of current pregnancy

*   The woman should be asked whether the pregnancy is a planned or unplanned.
*   In the current pregnancy, the LMP, previous investigations and medications including folic acid intake and any complaints in the current pregnancy, any minor ailments such as nausea, heartburn, vomiting, constipation, shortness of breath, dizziness, swelling, backache, frequency of micturition, abdominal discomfort and headaches should be enquired about.
*   **Warning signs** such as bleeding and pain should also be enquired about. It is also important to enquire about history of exposure to possible viral infections, fever, intake of medications in the first trimester as well as inadvertent exposure to radiation such as X-rays or CT scan, which can predispose to congenital anomalies of the fetus. There may be excessive vomiting, which should not be ignored.

Booking Examination

General examination

*   Short stature may be associated with a small gynecoid pelvis, which can predispose to CPD.
*   Low BMI is associated with fetal growth restriction, preterm labour and low-birth-weight babies. High BMI is associated with pre-eclampsia, GDM, operative interventions and anesthesia complications.
*   Evidence of anemia should be looked for.
*   Jaundice may be present in active viral infections or in hemolytic anemia complicating pregnancy.
*   Cardiovascular and respiratory system examinations should be carried out.
*   BP should be measured in the recumbent/sitting position, and Korotkoff sounds should be taken to define diastolic BP.
*   Thyroid enlargement should be looked for.
*   The breasts should be examined to look for retracted nipples and lumps.
*   Abdominal and obstetrical examinations should be carried out.
*   Pelvic examination may be carried out if required.
*   The woman's gait should be observed—shortening of the limb may occur following polio, injury, tuberculosis of the hip joint or it may be congenital.

*   The spine should be examined to look for kyphosis and scoliosis. Spinal deformities and shortening of the limbs can affect the pelvic diameters.

Abdominal examination

Both abdominal and vaginal examinations should be performed only after asking the woman to empty her bladder.

*   Until 12 weeks of gestation, the uterus is a pelvic organ, and therefore, is not palpable per abdomen. If the uterus feels larger than the period of amenorrhea, the possibility of multiple gestation, molar pregnancy, concurrent adnexal masses or incorrect EDD calculation should be suspected and confirmed by USG.
*   Undiagnosed abdominal pathology, liver and splenic enlargement should be looked for.
*   Any scars from previous surgery/presence of hernia should be recorded.
*   First-trimester vaginal examination is mandatory when a woman presents with amenorrhea, pain and bleeding for the diagnosis of ectopic pregnancy and various types of miscarriages. With the availability of USG, bimanual pelvic examination is not usually carried out for the assessment of gestational age. However, vaginal examination and examination of external genitalia are important for the diagnosis of vulval ulcers, warts, labial adhesions, discharge and undiagnosed vaginal septum, prolapse and other vaginal and vulvar pathologies. In women who have never had a Pap test in the past, it can be carried out.

Booking investigations

1. **Complete hemogram:** This yields hemoglobin levels and hematocrit value which will indicate the presence and severity of anemia (Hb levels should be more than 11 g%).
2. **Blood group and RhD status:** If the woman is Rh-negative, her partner's Rh type should be checked. If the partner is Rh-positive, the pregnancy should be monitored for the development of Rh-isoimmunisation, and prophylactic measures should be undertaken where necessary. Indirect Coomb's test should be carried out in the first trimester itself in those who have had previous pregnancy events or blood transfusions to identify whether Rh-isoimmunisation has already occurred or not.
3. **Urine examination:** Urine is tested for glucose and protein during every visit. If urine is nitrite-positive or if there are >6 pus cells per high power field (hpf), the midstream specimen should be sent for

culture and sensitivity to diagnose asymptomatic bacteriuria, which may predispose to pregnancy loss, preterm labour, pyelonephritis and pre-eclampsia.

4. **Screening for infections:** Hepatitis B and C screening should be carried out for all pregnant women to prevent perinatal transmission to the newborn.

   - **Syphilis:** In order to prevent congenital syphilis, all women should be screened for syphilis using the Venereal Disease Research Laboratory (VDRL) or rapid plasma reagin (RPR) test.

   - **Human immunodeficiency virus:** All women should be offered HIV testing using enzyme-linked immunosorbent assay (ELISA) and Western blot test. Universal screening is recommended for all pregnant women to prevent transmission to the newborn and the uninfected partner. If a woman is HIV-positive, early treatment can be initiated.

   - **Rubella:** Testing for rubella IgG antibodies is ideally discussed and performed in the prenatal period. If found to be not immune to rubella (i.e., if IgG antibodies are absent), the woman is advised vaccination against rubella before attempting pregnancy. If identified for the first time in pregnancy, vaccination is carried out in the postnatal period to protect future pregnancies.

   - **TORCH (toxoplasmosis, rubella, cytomegalovirus and Herpes simplex) screen:** This is not routinely carried out in all pregnancies. Screening for toxoplasmosis may be required if the individual has pets at home. TORCH may be indicated while investigating pregnancy losses, congenital anomalies and calcifications in the brain.

5. **Screening for diabetes:** All pregnant women should be screened for gestational diabetes mellitus (GDM). An oral glucose challenge test (OGCT) is carried out by giving the woman a 75 g glucose load, irrespective of the last meal. A single blood sample is taken after two hours (discussed in detail in Chapter 31, *Diabetes complicating pregnancy*). In women who are unable to tolerate a glucose load because of vomiting, a fasting and postprandial blood sugar test or a random blood sugar test is performed along with HbA1C levels.

6. **Screening for thyroid disorders:** If there are signs and symptoms indicating a thyroid disorder, a thyroid function test is carried out. In known cases of hypothyroidism, TSH levels are checked to determine whether the condition is under control.

7. **Screening for aneuploidy:** Screening for trisomy 21 (Down syndrome), trisomy 18 and trisomy 13 should be carried out. Universal screening of all pregnant women should be performed based on NT thickness.

Selective screening by first-trimester screening (FTS) is recommended for high-risk women—those over 35 years of age, those who already have an affected child, those with a positive family history of aneuploidy and those who are diabetic.

   - **First-trimester USG screening for increased nuchal thickness:** The accumulation of fluid behind the fetal neck is referred to as nuchal thickness (NT). It is measured by USG between the 11th and 14th week of pregnancy (between the 1st day of the 11th week and the last day of the 13th week).

   - **First-trimester screening (FTS) with USG and biochemical screening:** First-trimester screening involves measuring the NT thickness by USG and measuring human chorionic gonadotrophin and pregnancy-associated plasma protein (PAPP)-A levels. When the fetus has Down syndrome, the PAPP-A level is low and serum β-hCG is raised.

8. **USG assessment in the first trimester:** USG in the first trimester of pregnancy yields the following information:

   - Confirmation of intrauterine pregnancy
   - Diagnosis of abnormal pregnancy such as ectopic pregnancy and molar pregnancy
   - Presence of heterotrophic pregnancy (presence of both intrauterine and extrauterine pregnancy)

   In intrauterine pregnancies, USG yields the following information:

   - Whether single or multiple pregnancy
   - Viability of the fetus
   - Gestational age of the fetus
   - In multiple pregnancy, the type of chorionicity—dizygotic/monozygotic pregnancy
   - Pregnancy complications such as miscarriages
   - NT thickness to identify Down syndrome in fetus
   - Congenital anomalies such as anencephaly (anomaly scan is carried out at 18–20 weeks of gestation)
   - Congenital anomalies of the uterus
   - Associated benign tumours of the uterus such as fibroids
   - Adnexal pathology such as ovarian tumours (corpus luteal cyst is the physiological cyst of pregnancy and disappears after 12 weeks of gestation)

By the end of the first trimester, high-risk pregnancies should be identified as such. However, it should be borne in mind that even women with low-risk pregnancies may subsequently develop complications that put them in the high-risk category. Table 8.3 lists the findings that are categorised as high-risk.

Table 8.3 Features of high-risk pregnant women

Feature	Findings
Age	<18 years and >35 years
Gravida	Primigravida and grand multipara
Previous obstetric history	History of cesarean section, preterm labour, premature rupture of membranes, termination of pregnancy >2 occasions, stillbirth, neonatal death, intrauterine growth restriction, macrosomia, pre-eclampsia/eclampsia, GDM, fetal abnormality, PPH, genetic disease in the family
Current pregnancy	Pre-eclampsia, GDM, anemia, other medical illness, smoking, Rh incompatibility, bleeding in early and late pregnancy, poor weight gain, pregnancy following ART techniques
Examination	Short stature <145 cm, BP >140/90, pre-pregnancy weight >85 Kg/<45 Kg, uterus large/small for gestational age, multiple pregnancy, malpresentations, polyhydramnios

SECOND AND THIRD TRIMESTERS OF PREGNANCY

Subsequent Antenatal Visits

At each subsequent antenatal visit, the following information are obtained.

History

- General questions regarding maternal well-being
- Any specific complaints such as pain, bleeding, headache, diminished urine output, reduced/loss of fetal movements, sudden increase in weight, generalised edema, breathlessness and vomiting
- Enquiry regarding fetal movements—these are usually felt by 18 weeks in a primigravida and by 16 weeks in a multigravida; the perception of the first fetal movement by the mother is called quickening and depends on the observation of the individual
- Any other specific complaints or concerns

Examination

The examination of a pregnant woman in her second or third trimester should be done to look for the following:

- Anemia and pedal edema
- Blood pressure
- Maternal weight (the average weight gain from the second trimester onwards is 0.5 Kg per week)

- Abdominal palpation for fundal height; this is done as follows:
  - There are three landmarks on the abdomen—the symphysis pubis, umbilicus and xiphisternum.
  - Between the symphysis pubis and the umbilicus, two equidistant lines are drawn.
  - At 12 weeks of gestation, the uterus is palpable per abdomen just above the symphysis pubis, especially in thin individuals.
  - The first line corresponds to 16 weeks and the second line corresponds to 20 weeks of gestation; if the fundus is felt at the level of the umbilicus, it corresponds to 24 weeks of gestation.
  - Another two lines are drawn between the umbilicus and xiphisternum at equal distance. The third line corresponds to 28 weeks of gestation and the fourth line corresponds to 32 weeks of gestation; fundal height at the xiphisternum corresponds to 36 weeks of gestation.
  - The uterus cannot grow upwards beyond the xiphisternum because of the presence of diaphragm; therefore, the uterus enlarges in the transverse direction.
  - There is also descent of the presenting part (cephalic/breech) into the pelvis; as a result, the fundal height decreases, and at 38 weeks, corresponds to 34 weeks and at 40 weeks, corresponds to 32 weeks of gestation.
  - At every visit, the fundal height should be checked by palpation to see whether it corresponds to the EDD.
  - If the height of the uterus is more than the period of gestation, the possibility of multiple pregnancy, hydramnios, incorrect dates, a large-for-gestational age baby and uterine/adnexal tumours should be considered.
  - If the height of the uterus is lower than that corresponding to the period of gestation, the possibility of incorrect dates, oligohydramnios and IUGR should be considered.
- Abdominal palpation for fetal parts: Also called external ballottement, this is done by placing the hands on either side of the uterus, tapping the abdomen with one hand and feeling for the movement of the fetus with the other hand; fetal movement can be elicited up to 24 weeks of gestation.
- Checking the fetal heart: From 16 weeks onwards, the fetal heart can be heard using a handheld Doppler; a fetoscope can be used after 24 weeks of gestation.

Differentiating between 32 and 40 weeks of gestation

- At 40 weeks, as the height of the fundus decreases and the pressure on the abdominal organs and the discomfort due to the elevated diaphragm are reduced. Consequently, the patient feels relieved. This is called '**lightening**'.
- Due to the transverse enlargement of the uterus, the flanks will be full.
- The woman is asked to sit at the edge of the bed with her legs hanging. At 40 weeks of gestation, the uterus will fall forward in this position, especially in multigravid women.
- Because the uterus is falling forward, it may be possible to keep a hand behind the fundus. This is called **shelving** (Fig. 8.2).

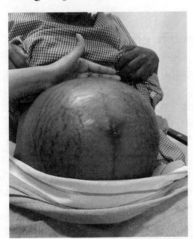

Fig. 8.2 Falling forward of the uterus and shelving

Clinical assessment of fetal growth

- With a flexible inch tape, the distance between the symphysis pubis and the fundus is measured (symphysio-fundal height [SFH]; Fig. 8.3).
- From 20–34 weeks of gestation, this measurement in centimetres equals the gestational age in weeks.
- If the SFH is less than 4 cm for the period of gestation, IUGR, isolated oligohydramnios and incorrect dates should be suspected, and appropriate investigations carried out. Serial measurement is taken and plotted on a graph (gravidogram). This is a very simple and inexpensive method to pick up IUGR in low-resource settings. This measurement is not applicable when there is an oblique or transverse lie.
- If the SFH is more than the expected measurement, macrosomia, multiple pregnancy and incorrect dates should be considered.

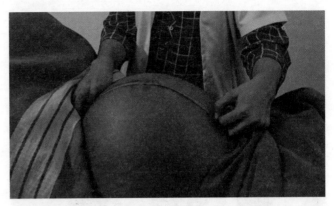

Fig. 8.3 Measurement of symphysio-fundal height

Investigations at each visit

- Full blood count
- Urinalysis for protein, blood, glucose and pus cells
- Screening for GDM at 24–26 weeks and at 34 weeks
- In Rh-negative mothers, indirect Coombs test
- Indications for USG in the second and third trimesters of pregnancy (Table 8.4)

Table 8.4 USG assessment in the second and third trimesters of pregnancy

Gestational age	Investigations
18–22 weeks	• Anomaly scan • Doppler study in high-risk cases for pre-eclampsia and FGR
After 24 weeks	• Fetal echo in type I diabetes, GDM, family history/mother suffering from heart disease, mother suffering from autoimmune diseases, especially SLE
32–34 weeks	• In cases of placenta previa, adherent placenta (MRI may be indicated) is looked for
Serial scans from 28 weeks every 3–4 weeks	• In FGR, diabetes, pre-eclampsia

Assessment at 36 Weeks of Gestation

- The general condition of the woman is assessed.
- The woman should be educated on the symptoms of labour pains.
- Complications should be looked for.

Abdominal examination

- The uterus should be examined for longitudinal or transverse enlargement.
- The uterus should be examined for overdistension.
- The presence of scars and hernia should be noted.

• From 36 weeks onwards, the lie of the fetus (longitudinal, transverse or oblique), its presentation (cephalic or breech) and the degree of engagement of the presenting part should be assessed and recorded. 95% of fetuses at term present by the vertex in labour; hence this is called normal presentation.

• The height of the uterus should be assessed with the ulnar border of the left hand (Fig. 8.4).

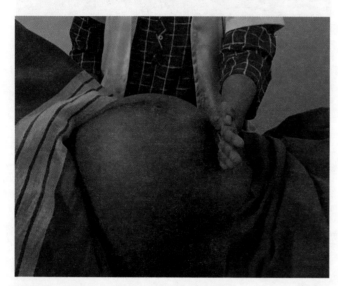

Fig. 8.4 Demonstration of fundal height

• Abdominal palpation involves four manoeuvres (Leopold's manoeuvre)—the fundal grip, the lateral grip, the first pelvic grip (Pawlik's grip) and the second pelvic grip.

Before palpating the abdomen, the clinician should explain the procedure to the woman. In order to achieve good relaxation, she should be asked to lie on her back with her thighs and knees flexed. The clinician stands on the woman's right side, facing her head.

Fundal grip (Fig. 8.5a)
— The clinician places the palms of her hands on either side of the fundus and palpates the abdomen to see which part of the fetus is occupying the fundus.

— If the breech is occupying the fundus, it will be broad, soft and not independently ballotable from the body. When the breech is moved, the body of the fetus moves as well.

— If the head is occupying the fundus, it is rounded, hard and independently ballotable.

— In transverse lie, the uterus is enlarged transversely, and the head will be palpated in one of the loins.

Umbilical grip (Fig. 8.5b)
— The palms of the hands are closely applied to the uterus and the abdomen is palpated from the fundus to the lower part of the uterus to identify the side of the spine and the limbs.

— On the side of the spine, there is uniform resistance that feels curved on palpation. On the side of the limbs, it feels nodular and irregular. The fingers can be dipped between the nodules.

— The fetal spine is felt more easily. It is anterior in the occipitoanterior position and is felt towards the flank in the occipitoposterior position.

— The limbs will be more anterior and can be felt easily in certain presentations such as the direct occipitoposterior position, when the dorsum is posterior in transverse lie and in multiple pregnancy.

The first pelvic grip (Fig. 8.5c)
— The first pelvic grip or the Pawlik's grip helps in identifying the presenting part, i.e., the part of the fetus that occupies the lower pole of the uterus. The right hand of the examiner is held wide open and applied to the lower abdomen, above the symphysis pubis (the woman should be asked to empty her bladder before performing this manoeuvre). The presenting part is grasped between the fingers and palpated to see whether the head or the breech is occupying the lower pole.

— The head will feel hard and rounded, whereas the breech will feel soft, broad and irregular.

— In a transverse lie, the lower pole will be empty.

— The presenting part is moved to see whether it is possible to move it from side to side. If it is possible to move it easily, the presenting part is said to be mobile/floating. If it is not movable, then it indicates that the presenting part has entered the pelvic brim, where it may be just fixed or engaged.

The second pelvic grip (Fig. 8.5d)
— The second pelvic grip helps in reconfirming the presenting part as well as in identifying the attitude of the fetus. It also helps to determine whether the head is engaged or not.

— In carrying out the second pelvic grip, the clinician faces the patient's feet and places her hands on either side of the woman's abdomen. Palpating in this manner confirms the presenting part of the fetus.

— To identify the attitude of the fetus, the side of the spine is palpated. The first bony prominence felt

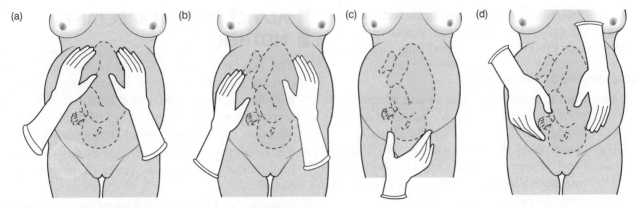

Fig. 8.5 (a) Fundal grip, (b) lateral (umbilical grip), (c) first pelvic grip (Pawlik's grip) and (d) second pelvic grip

on the side of the spine is the occiput and the bony prominence felt on the opposite side is the sinciput. Whether the head is flexed, extended or deflexed is made out by identifying the relation between the occiput and the sinciput.

— When the head is well-flexed, the occiput is at a lower level than the sinciput.
— When the head is extended, as in brow and face presentations, the occiput is at a higher level than the sinciput and one can feel a groove between the fetal spine and the occiput.
— When the head is deflexed, as in the occipitoposterior position, both the occiput and sinciput are at the same level.

Engagement

Engagement indicates that the greatest transverse diameter of the fetal head—the biparietal diameter—has gone through the brim of the pelvis. When the head is engaged, only the sinciput or none of the parts of the fetal head are palpable per abdomen and the hand will be diverging.

Cephalic prominence

It is the part of the fetal head that is felt first and is prominent on palpation.

• In a well-flexed head, the cephalic prominence is the sinciput.
• In the extended head, the cephalic prominence is the occiput.

Abdominal palpation also yields the following information:

• CPD (discussed in Chapter 45, *Cephalopelvic disproportion and obstructed labour*)
• The amount of liquor
• The gestational age and estimated weight of the fetus can be calculated by clinical examination

using the symphysio-fundal height (SFH); serial measurements are necessary to do this as accurately as possible

---

Assessment of fetal weight by Johnson's rule

• Approximate fetal weight in grams = Symphysio-fundal height in cm − N × K (constant 155) (N = 12 if the fetal head is above the ischial spines and 11 if the fetal head is below the ischial spines.)

Assessment of gestational age by MacDonald's rule

• Duration of gestation in weeks = Fundal height × 8/7

Auscultation

The fetal heart is located using either a fetoscope or a handheld Doppler. The fetal heart is always heard on the side of the back. In cephalic presentations, it is heard below the level of the umbilicus and in breech presentation, above the level of the umbilicus.

Vaginal examination

• After explaining the procedure to the woman and obtaining her consent, a vaginal examination should be performed. After cleaning the vulval area with an antiseptic solution, two fingers of a gloved hand are inserted gently into the vagina to examine it. The bladder should be emptied prior to examination.
• In all primigravid women and multigravidae in whom there is a history of an obstetric mishap, the vaginal examination is carried out after 38 weeks of gestation to check the adequacy of the pelvis.
• It is done prior to the induction of labour to assess the favourability of the cervix (discussed in Chapter 16, *Induction of labour*).

- Vaginal examination is contraindicated in cases of suspected or confirmed placenta previa or in the presence of PROM to avoid introducing infection.

Assessment of the pelvis

It is important to assess the capacity and adequacy of the pelvis prior to delivery. Though a definite diagnosis of CPD is made after delivery, in certain situations—a small, gynecoid pelvis in a short woman, an obliquely contracted pelvis due to polio, kyphoscoliosis and injury or infection affecting the joints—CPD can be diagnosed before delivery.

While assessing the pelvis, the following findings should be noted:

- Whether sacral promontory is reached or not
- Curvature of the sacrum from above, downwards and laterally
- Whether the walls of the sides of the pelvis are parallel or converging
- Whether the sacro-sciatic notch admits two fingers
- Whether the ischial spines are prominent or not
- Whether both spines are reached with the stretched index and middle fingers
- Whether the subpubic angle is acute or obtuse and whether it admits the backs of two fingers
- The intertuberous diameter—the distance between the two ischial tuberosities—should admit approximately four knuckles
- In addition to assessing the pelvis, it is important to assess for CPD (discussed in Chapter 45, *Cephalopelvic disproportion and obstructed labour*)

Mode of delivery

It is often at the 36 weeks' appointment that a decision is made regarding the mode of delivery (i.e., whether vaginal delivery or planned cesarean section).

Assessment at 40 Weeks of Gestation

The well-being of the mother and the fetus should be assessed. If fetal well-being is satisfactory, and there are no maternal contraindications, a decision can be made to await spontaneous delivery for another 7 days with a kick chart and careful fetal surveillance. Membrane sweeping can be done at 40 weeks.

Assessment at 41 Weeks of Gestation

If undelivered at 41 weeks, labour can be induced, or a cesarean section can be performed.

ADVICE TO THE EXPECTANT MOTHER

- The expectant mother should be instructed about diet, relaxation and sleep, bowel habits, exercise, bathing, clothing, avoidance of hard and tiring work, recreation and follow-up visits. The need for regular attendance at the clinic should be emphasised.
- The restriction of sexual intercourse and its avoidance in the first and last few weeks of pregnancy are beneficial.
- Women should be informed about the warning signs in pregnancy and be instructed to report immediately in case of any of the following:
  - Bleeding per vaginum
  - Abdominal or pelvic pain
  - Swelling of the face or limbs
  - Generalised edema
  - Blurring or dimness of vision
  - Persistent headache, frontal headache and vomiting
  - Reduced urine output
  - Leakage of fluid
  - Fever
  - Persistent vomiting
  - Breathlessness
  - Dizziness
  - Dysuria
  - Diminished fetal movements/excessive fetal movements

Nutrition and Diet During Pregnancy

- In a country like India where malnutrition is rampant, affecting both maternal and fetal well-being, it is essential that the pregnant mother be suitably advised regarding her diet. Nutritional advice should take into account the foods available locally, the beliefs regarding them, cooking facilities, patterns of meals, and whether the pregnant woman is a working woman and the type of work she is doing.
- In general, the pregnant woman should be advised to eat whatever she likes in the amounts she desires and salted to taste, as long as the diet contains calories, proteins and various nutrients in recommended amounts (Table 8.5).
- She should be advised to consume food rich in proteins, iron, calcium and fibre. She should also be advised to consume adequate quantities of milk,

Table 8.5 Recommended daily nutritional allowance during pregnancy

Nutrient	Non-pregnant women	Pregnant women	Lactating women
Energy (Kcal)	2,200	2,500	2,600
Protein (g)	45–50 (1 g/Kg)	60–75 (1.5 g/Kg)	70–75
Calcium (g)	0.8	1.2	1.2
Iron (mg)	15	60	30
Folate (µg)	180	400	280
Vitamin D (µg)	5	10	12

fruits and vegetables. Water consumption should be adequate to prevent constipation and urinary tract infection in pregnancy. As pregnancy advances, the woman should be advised to eat frequently and in small quantities so as to avoid gastric regurgitation.

- With regard to **dietary supplements**, according to the Government of India, 100 mg of elemental iron and 500 µg of folic acid should be taken daily for 100 days during pregnancy. Calcium supplementation is also advised in doses of 1,000 mg/day. IFA (iron-folic acid) tablets are also prescribed during the lactation period.
- Besides iron supplementation, deworming with one tablet of albendazole is also done to prevent anemia.

Weight Gain in Pregnancy

Depending on the pre-pregnancy weight, different levels of weight gain are recommended for pregnant women (Table 8.6).

Table 8.6 Recommended weight gain in pregnancy

BMI	Recommended weight gain in pregnancy
Low BMI (<20)	12.5–18 Kg
Normal BMI (20–25)	11.5–16 Kg
High BMI (26–30)	7–11.5 Kg
Obese (>30)	Not more than 6 Kg

Immunisation

- Vaccination in pregnancy protects not only the mother but also her baby for six months postpartum. The Federation of Obstetric and Gynecological Societies of India recommends immunisation against tetanus, diphtheria, pertussis and influenza during pregnancy.
- It is important that all pregnant women be immunised against **tetanus**, as neonatal tetanus is one of the most common causes of high perinatal mortality.

- Tetanus toxoid can be given in two doses separated by eight weeks—the first at 16–20 weeks and the second at 20–24 weeks. For those who have already been immunised, one booster dose of tetanus toxoid should be given in a subsequent pregnancy, preferably four weeks before the expected date of delivery.
- If the subsequent pregnancy occurs within 5 years, only one booster is given.
- Tetanus, diphtheria and acellular pertussis (T-dap) vaccination can be considered instead of the second dose of tetanus toxoid to offer protection against diphtheria and pertussis in addition to tetanus.
- Pregnant women should be advised to take a flu vaccine during the flu season.
- During epidemics and pandemics such as swine flu and COVID-19, necessary vaccines should be advised.

Care of the Breasts

- The objectives are cleanliness and improvement of **circulation** to keep the lacteal sinuses and ducts open to allow colostrum and milk to escape freely under the pressure of secretion.
- The woman should wash her breasts twice daily and avoid wearing tight brassieres.
- Washing with lukewarm water after each act of breastfeeding is recommended.
- Retracted nipples should be identified during pregnancy. The syringe method can be attempted after 36 weeks of gestation (earlier attempts may induce preterm labour due to nipple stimulation) to rectify this.

▋ COMMON CONCERNS DURING PREGNANCY

Exercise

Pregnant women may exercise provided they do not get excessively fatigued. Women who are accustomed to aerobic exercises before pregnancy may continue this during pregnancy. However, they should not intensify the exercise. Women who had a more sedentary lifestyle should be advised against activity more strenuous than walking. Women who have hypertensive disorders, multiple pregnancy, a growth-restricted fetus or heart disease should avoid high-impact exercise; minimal walking can be allowed.

Work

Women can continue with their employment until they go into labour if the pregnancy is uncomplicated. When there is a history of preterm labour or complications such as FGR and pre-eclampsia, women should be advised to take adequate rest.

Travel

Travel by car and train is safe for pregnant women. Driving two-wheelers should be avoided. Four-wheeler driving can be undertaken with care until the early third trimester of pregnancy. Long-distance air travel should be avoided as it may be associated with venous thrombosis.

Nausea and Morning Sickness

Nausea and vomiting are very common symptoms in the early weeks of pregnancy and usually disappear by 14 weeks of gestation. The severity of the symptoms can be reduced by simple dietary measures such as eating dry food like bread and biscuit, low-fat food, carbohydrate-rich food such as rice and mashed potatoes and drinks such as lemonade. Deep fried, greasy and spicy food should be avoided. Instead of large meals, small quantities of food should be taken every 2–3 hours. Adequate fluid intake should be advised.

Bowel Habits

Constipation is common in pregnancy because of the prolonged transit time caused by the relaxing effect of progesterone and compression of the large bowel by the uterus. Women should be encouraged to drink at least 8–12 glasses of fluid every day in the form of water, milk, juice or soup. Fibre intake should be increased in the form of whole grain breads and cereals, vegetables, fruits and legumes. Regular exercises such as walking and swimming should be advised. Laxatives should be avoided as far as possible.

Coitus

If there is a history of previous abortion, intercourse should be avoided in the second and third months. Intercourse does not affect the fetus but is best avoided from week 36 of pregnancy until six weeks after delivery.

Drugs

It is advisable to avoid using drugs, if possible, particularly in the early weeks, when embryogenesis is taking place. Most drugs cross the placenta to reach the embryo or the fetus. If a drug is required and administered during pregnancy, the benefit must clearly outweigh any inherent risks.

Heartburn

Heartburn is caused by **gastroesophageal reflux** due to the relaxation of the lower esophageal sphincter. Eating small and frequent meals, avoiding lying supine or prone, and using antacids whenever necessary may help relieve symptoms. Oily and spicy food, coffee and alcohol should be avoided as these may aggravate the problem.

Increased Vaginal Discharge

Increased vaginal discharge is common during pregnancy and unless associated with itching/irritation, it is usually non-pathological and may be due to increased mucus production by the cervical glands.

Increased Frequency of Micturition

Increased urinary frequency and urinary incontinence can occur during pregnancy. The enlarging uterus in early pregnancy and the presenting part in the latter part of pregnancy exert pressure on the bladder to cause these symptoms. Women should be reassured and advised not to restrict fluids. Regular pelvic floor exercises during and after pregnancy should be advised. UTI may be associated with similar symptoms and may have to be evaluated.

Backache

Back pain is very common in pregnancy due to the relaxation of the pelvic joints and ligaments caused by progesterone. Faulty posture can also predispose to backache. It can be minimised by having women squat rather than bend over to reach down, using back support while sitting and avoiding high-heeled shoes. Women should be advised to rest on a hard, firm bed and to avoid lifting heavy weights and standing for long hours. They should be advised to sleep on one side with a pillow between their legs. Massaging of the back muscles and hot or cold compression on the back help in relieving the pain.

Leg Cramps

During pregnancy, muscle cramps can occur due to calcium and potassium deficiency and due to weight gain. Women should be advised to maintain a well-balanced diet that contains calcium and potassium. Remaining well-hydrated, regularly walking and rotating the ankles and toes while resting will encourage circulation and prevent cramps. Women should be advised to rest with their legs elevated and wear supportive stockings. At the time of cramps, the application of local heat, warm baths and massaging the calves and feet would help.

Carpal Tunnel Syndrome

Tingling and numbness (**paresthesia**) over the thumb and the lateral two and half fingers are common complaints. This is due to the compression of the median nerve and peri-neural edema. Splinting of the wrists and small doses of diuretics are advised in severe cases (Fig. 8.6).

Varicosities

These are exaggerated by pregnancy and prolonged standing. Treatment is usually limited to periodic rest with elevation of legs and use of elastic stockings.

Hemorrhoids

These are exaggerated during pregnancy due to increased pressure on the rectal veins caused by the obstruction of venous return by the large uterus and

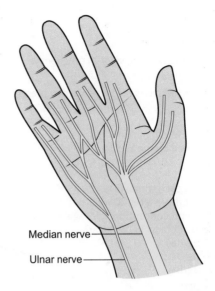

Median nerve

Ulnar nerve

Fig. 8.6 Carpal tunnel syndrome is a complication of pregnancy

the tendency to develop constipation during pregnancy. Treatment consists of topically applied anesthetics, warm soaks and stool softeners.

KEY POINTS

✓ *The main objectives of prenatal care are to ensure the good health of the mother and safe delivery of a healthy child. It should ideally start at the preconception stage.*

✓ *Women should be examined at regular intervals to identify risk factors for the pregnancy. High-risk pregnancies should be followed-up more frequently.*

✓ *Maternal weight gain, blood pressure, presence of pallor, height of the uterine fundus, amount of amniotic fluid and the presenting part should be recorded at each visit.*

✓ *The presence of warning signs should be enquired about and managed accordingly.*

✓ *Preconceptional care involves measures and interventions that are undertaken before the woman becomes pregnant with the aim to improve maternal and neonatal health.*

✓ *The WHO proposes a minimum of four antenatal visits during the antenatal period; these should be focused visits.*

✓ *The first visit should be at less than 10 weeks of gestation; at this visit, a detailed history should be taken and a thorough examination carried out.*

✓ *The booking visit should ideally be at or before 10 weeks of gestation.*

✓ *Booking investigations include a complete hemogram, blood group and Rh status, urine analysis along with culture and sensitivity if necessary and screening for diabetes and sexually transmitted infections such as hepatitis B, C, syphilis and HIV infection.*

✓ *Fetal growth should be assessed by clinical methods and if necessary, by USG.*

✓ *Women should be educated on the warning signs in pregnancy.*

✓ *They should be advised about the ideal diet and nutrition supplements during pregnancy.*

✓ *Necessary vaccination should be administered during pregnancy.*

Essay questions

1. What is the antenatal care given to a woman presenting at 10 weeks of gestation?
2. Discuss the nutritional advice to be given to a pregnant woman.
3. Discuss the minor ailments experienced by pregnant women and how they are managed.

Short answer questions

1. What is the ideal time for the first prenatal visit and what are its goals?
2. Define the following terms:
   a) Parity
   b) Nullipara
   c) Primipara

d) Gravida
e) Nulligravida
f) Multigravida

3. Enumerate the warning signs in pregnancy.
4. What is Naegle's rule?
5. What immunisation is recommended in pregnancy?

MCQs

1. What is the minimum number of antenatal visits recommended by the WHO?
   a) Four
   b) Five
   c) Once in each trimester
   d) At least three after 20 weeks
2. What is the preconceptional dosage of folic acid to prevent neural tube defects in the baby?
   a) 100 µg/day
   b) 200 µg/day
   c) 300 µg/day
   d) 400 µg/day
3. During the first pelvic grip, if the sinciput is at a lower level than the occiput, what does it imply?
   a) The fetal head is engaged
   b) The fetal head is deflexed or extended
   c) The fetal head is fixed
   d) The fetal head is free
4. Which of the following is the goal of preconception care?
   a) To reduce maternal and child mortality
   b) To prevent unintended pregnancies
   c) To prevent complications during pregnancy and delivery
   d) All of the above
5. What is the recommended schedule for antenatal visits?
   a) Once in 4 weeks up to 28 weeks
   b) Once in 15 days from 28–36 weeks
   c) Weekly after 36 weeks
   d) All of the above
6. How often should hemoglobin be estimated in pregnant women?
   a) Once in every trimester
   b) Once at the first visit
   c) Once at 20 weeks
   d) Once at the time of labour
7. What is Johnson's formula used to calculate?
   a) Fetal height
   b) EDD
   c) Fetal weight
   d) Gestation age

8. Which grip determines whether the head has entered the pelvis or not?
   a) Fundal grip
   b) Umbilical grip
   c) First pelvic grip
   d) Second pelvic grip
9. Where is the fetal heart heard in the cephalic presentation?
   a) Above the umbilicus
   b) Below the umbilicus
   c) At the level of the umbilicus
   d) None of these

Answers
1. (a), 2. (d), 3. (b), 4. (d), 5. (d), 6. (a), 7. (c), 8. (d), 9. (b)

Fill in the blank

1. In a diabetic woman, during the preconception visit, the _____ should be measured to assess the adequacy of control.

Answers
HbAiC

Case scenario-based discussion

1. A 22-year-old IT professional who has been married for 3 months comes to the clinic for preconceptional advice.
   a) What is the goal of preconceptional care?
   b) Discuss in detail the history to be elicited and examinations to be carried out.
   c) What investigations would you carry out?
   d) What medications and vaccination would you advice?

Answers
a) The goal of preconceptional care is to identify and correct the potential risk factors that may have an adverse effect on pregnancy so as to achieve a healthy pregnancy and a healthy neonate.
b) A detailed medical and family history should be taken to identify potential risk factors. A detailed general examination should be carried out to check the woman's weight and BP and assess her cardiovascular system. The presence of anemia and malnutrition should be identified and corrected. Pre-existing medical conditions such as diabetes, obesity, hypothyroidism, seizure disorders and HIV should be managed appropriately before attempting conception. The current medications should be evaluated in detail to avoid using teratogenic drugs and to switch to safer drugs. The woman should be advised on the cessation of smoking, alcohol and substance abuse and to maintain the ideal body weight. Temporary contraception may also be discussed.
c) General investigations such as complete hemogram, urine analysis, blood sugar levels and serology are recommended as part of preconception care. In obese individuals, a thyroid function test should also be carried out.
d) All women planning pregnancy should be started on 0.4 mg of folic acid to prevent neural tube defects in the fetus. The woman's vaccination history against rubella, chickenpox and hepatitis B should be verified. If seronegative, she should be given these vaccinations.

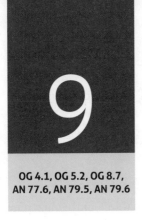

9

**OG 4.1, OG 5.2, OG 8.7,
AN 77.6, AN 79.5, AN 79.6**

Drugs in Pregnancy

Learning Objectives

» To know about the development of the embryo, fetus and the period of organogenesis
» To know the Food and Drug Administration (FDA) classification for drug use in pregnancy
» To know the effects of various drugs on fetal development
» To know what drugs are contraindicated in pregnancy
» To discuss the various mandatory vaccinations during pregnancy

INTRODUCTION

- A teratogen is a substance, organism or physical agent capable of causing the abnormal development of the embryo or fetus.
- A teratogen can cause abnormalities of structure (congenital anomalies), abnormalities of function or growth restriction.
- Every pregnancy carries a risk of major and minor congenital anomalies of the fetus.
- Drug exposure has been associated with 2–3% of all birth defects. The effect of a drug on the fetus could be any of the following:
  — No effect
  — Pregnancy loss
  — Fetal malformations
  — Growth restriction
  — Functional disorder
- Drugs used in pregnancy may have a temporary or a permanent teratogenic effect on the fetus.

THE EFFECT OF TERATOGENS ON FETAL DEVELOPMENT

The susceptibility of the conceptus to teratogenic agents varies with the developmental stage at the time of exposure as well as the dose and the duration of drug exposure.

- The result of exposure to a teratogen is determined by the **timing of the exposure.**
- Exposure to a teratogen prior to 31 days (from the LMP) produces all or none of the effects. The insult either results in an abortion or the survival of the fetus without any congenital anomalies.
- While exposure during the critical period of embryogenesis may lead to malformations, the same

exposure in the fetal period may lead to growth restriction or functional disorders. By 10 weeks after the last menstrual period, all the organ systems have formed and continue to develop and grow. Exposure to drugs and medications in the second and third trimesters of pregnancy can affect the growth and function of the organs.

- The **dose and the duration** of exposure to the drug are also important.
- A drug must cross the placenta to have an effect on the fetus. Most drugs are transferred across the placenta by passive diffusion.

DEVELOPMENT OF THE EMBRYO AND THE PERIOD OF ORGANOGENESIS

- The conceptus is known as an embryo from the time of fertilisation up to 8 weeks.
- The first two weeks are referred to as the **stage of blastogenesis**. This is also known as the segmental period/the presomite period, which extends from the date of ovulation to 14 days. During this period, there is rapid cell division, and the blastocyst is vulnerable to exogenous factors. If exposed to a teratogen during this period, either the embryo dies or, if the injury is slight, the cells overcome the harmful effect as each cell is a totipotent cell. In the latter scenario, normal embryonal growth occurs. This is also known as the **'all or none' law**.
- This is followed by the **period of organogenesis** (the classic teratogenic period), which extends from 31–71 days after the last menstrual period in a normal 28-day menstrual cycle (17–57 days from fertilisation, i.e., third to the eighth week of development following fertilisation).

- The **fetal period** begins 8 weeks after fertilisation (10 weeks following LMP) and continues until delivery. This period is characterised by the maturation of tissues and organs and rapid growth of the body.

Period of Organogenesis

- The stage of organogenesis extends from the beginning of the 3rd week to the 8th week and is the most critical period with regard to structural malformations.
- Exposure to teratogenic drugs during this critical period is more likely to be associated with a structural defect than exposure in the third trimester.
- Malformation patterns noted at birth are also related to the gestational age at exposure.
- Drug exposure early in the period of organogenesis—as early as 31 days—leads to neural tube and cardiac defects which develop early. On the other hand, exposure later in the period—as late as 71 days—leads to palate and ear defects. Closure of the neural tube occurs between 22–28 days after conception.

FOOD AND DRUG ADMINISTRATION (FDA) CLASSIFICATION FOR DRUG USE IN PREGNANCY

The Food and Drug Administration (FDA) has developed a rating system for the use of drugs in pregnancy to provide therapeutic guidance based on the potential benefits and maternal and fetal risks. The drugs have been classified as follows:

- Category A:
  — Controlled studies on women show no risk to the fetus
  — Examples are multivitamins
- Category B:
  — Animal studies show no fetal risk; however, there are no controlled studies on pregnant women
  — Adverse effects seen in animal studies, but no evidence of risk in humans in well-controlled studies
  — Examples include penicillin, ampicillin, paracetamol and ranitidine
- Category C:
  — Risk cannot be ruled out
  — Either animal or human studies are unavailable, or animal studies show adverse effects but no human studies available

- — The potential benefits may outweigh the potential risks
  — Examples include acyclovir, aspirin and zidovudine
- Category D:
  — Positive evidence of risk
  — Examples include phenytoin, carbamazepine and warfarin
- Category X:
  — Animal and human studies show fetal abnormalities and they are contraindicated in pregnancy
  — An example is isotretinoin

Some Category X Drugs

- Androgens—danazol
- Folic acid antagonists—methotrexate
- Lithium
- Streptomycin
- Tetracycline
- Thalidomide
- Retinoids above the recommended levels

DRUGS USED IN MEDICAL DISORDERS AND PREGNANCY

Certain medical disorders in pregnancy may require to be treated with suitable drugs. Hence it is necessary for the obstetrician to be aware of the possible teratogenic effects of drugs and how to administer them with caution.

Anticonvulsants

- In women on anticonvulsant medications for epilepsy during pregnancy, the risk of fetal malformations is 2–3 times that in the general population. The risk of malformation is increased when multiple drugs and higher doses are used. Women on multiple drugs may be shifted to monotherapy.
- Valproate, carbamazepine and phenytoin are category D drugs; lamotrigine is a category C drug.
- Valproic acid and carbamazepine carry a risk of approximately 1% for neural tube defects. Sodium valproate is associated with brachycephaly with a high forehead and small nose and lips.
- Carbamazepine, phenytoin and phenobarbital are folic acid antagonists. They cause neural tube defects, cleft lip and cardiac defects. It is recommended that women on anticonvulsants be prescribed 4–5 mg of folic acid daily.

- Phenytoin use in pregnancy has been associated with fetal hydantoin syndrome (also known as the fetal anticonvulsant syndrome) with the newborn presenting with microcephaly, developmental delay, mental retardation, growth deficiency, hypoplasia of the nail, nasal bone hypoplasia and hypertelorism.
- Lamotrigine is an inhibitor of dihydrofolate reductase and the incidence of congenital anomalies is similar to that among the general population.
- In women on anticonvulsant therapy who have been seizure-free for more than two years and for whom the electroencephalogram is reported normal, withdrawing the drug before pregnancy may be beneficial.
- Maternal vitamin K supplementation in the last month of pregnancy and neonatal administration may be required to prevent neonatal bleeding.

Antibiotics

Table 9.1 lists some of the commonly used antimicrobial agents and their effects on the fetus.

Table 9.1 Antimicrobial medicines and their effects on the fetus

Drug	Effects
Penicillin, metronidazole, nitrofurantoin, cephalosporins	Category B
Erythromycin	Category B, but erythromycin estolate is contraindicated in pregnancy because of hepatotoxicity—erythromycin can be given
Aminoglycosides	Category C—nephrotoxicity or ototoxicity have been reported in preterm newborns—to be used in divided doses and with caution
Tetracyclines	Category D—maternal hepatotoxicity—used in the second half of pregnancy, interferes with tooth development and may cause permanent yellow/grey/brown discolouration of the teeth and enamel hypoplasia

- Antibiotics are commonly used to prevent or treat infection in pregnancy.
- Penicillin and its derivatives are safe in pregnancy. No increase in birth defects has been noted with the use of erythromycin and metronidazole in early or late pregnancy.
- Cephalosporins are safe in pregnancy. No increase in birth defects has been shown with nitrofurantoin use in pregnancy.

- Sulfonamides used in the third trimester of pregnancy can lead to hyperbilirubinemia in the neonate and should be avoided in women with glucose-6-phosphatase deficiency.
- Tetracycline is contraindicated in pregnancy as it inhibits bone growth, interferes with tooth development and causes enamel hypoplasia and discolouration of teeth.
- Antituberculous drugs—except streptomycin, isoniazid, rifampicin, ethambutol and pyrazinamide are safe to use in pregnancy.
- Antiviral acyclovir is safe in pregnancy.
- Primaquine is contraindicated in pregnancy.
- Fluoroquinolones (ciprofloxacin, norfloxacin, levofloxacin) have an affinity for bone and cartilaginous tissue, and therefore should be avoided in pregnancy.
- The aminoglycosides—gentamycin and tobramycin used in the first trimester for pyelonephritis can result in ototoxicity.

Antifungal Agents

- Nystatin is safe to use in pregnancy.
- Fluconazole is a category C drug.

Antiretrovirals

- Zidovudine is a category C drug and is safe and effective to use in pregnancy.
- Efavirenz is a category D drug and not recommended during the first 8 weeks of pregnancy due to the increased risk of malformations.

Analgesics

- Aspirin taken in the first trimester of pregnancy has not been shown to be associated with teratogenic effects.
- No teratogenicity has been reported with non-steroidal anti-inflammatory agents (NSAIDs), but chronic use can lead to oligohydramnios, constriction of the fetal ductus arteriosus and pulmonary hypertension.
- Acetaminophen and codeine have not been shown to be associated with congenital malformation. But, narcotics are associated with addiction and withdrawal symptoms in the neonatal period.

Anticoagulants

- Common indications for anticoagulants in pregnancy are antiphospholipid syndrome, prosthetic valves, treatment of deep vein thrombosis and pulmonary embolism.

- Warfarin is an oral anticoagulant which crosses the placenta. Warfarin embryopathy occurs in 5% of patients exposed to the medication between 6–9 weeks of gestation. Warfarin embryopathy presents with nasal hypoplasia, bilateral optic atrophy, mental retardation and stippling of the bone, especially the vertebra and femoral epiphysis, which can be seen on radiological examination. There may be fetal intracranial hemorrhage if warfarin is used in the second and third trimesters. It can present with agenesis of the corpus callosum and Dandy–Walker syndrome.
- Both unfractionated heparin (UFH) and low-molecular-weight heparin (LMWH) are used in pregnancy. Because of their large molecular weight, they do not cross the placenta to cause adverse effects on the fetus. They are category B drugs.

Cardiovascular Drugs

- Antihypertensives are commonly used in pregnancy to treat chronic hypertension and pre-eclampsia.
- Alpha-methyl dopa and beta-blockers have not been shown to be associated with teratogenicity.
- However, with the use of beta-blockers, there may be an increased risk of intrauterine growth restriction.
- Labetalol and nifedipine are safely used in pregnancy.
- Increased risk of congenital malformations has been reported with angiotensin-converting enzyme inhibitors (ACE inhibitors) with craniofacial deformities, fetal limb contractures, hypoplastic lungs, renal tubular dysplasia and oligohydramnios. It is a category D drug and contraindicated in pregnancy.

Thyroid Medications

- Antithyroid medications propylthiouracil and methimazole cross the placenta and can cause fetal goitre.
- Methimazole has been associated with scalp defects and esophageal atresia.
- Therefore, the drug of choice for hyperthyroidism in pregnancy is propylthiouracil.

Antipsychotic Drugs

- Lithium exposure in early pregnancy has been shown to be associated with cardiovascular defects, especially Ebstein's anomaly. It has been recommended that in women on lithium, the drug therapy be changed. However, withdrawal of lithium may exacerbate the condition. Therefore, the decision to change the drug depends on the maternal and fetal benefits.

- Drugs used in the treatment of depression such as imipramine, amitriptyline and selective serotonin-re-uptake inhibitors are associated with neonatal withdrawal effects. Cardiovascular defects have also been observed.

Drugs Used for Respiratory Ailments

- Antihistamine chlorpheniramine is safe in pregnancy. Cetirizine and loratadine are used as second-line therapy.
- The cough suppressant codeine is safe to use in pregnancy.
- Asthmatics are treated with terbutaline inhalers. Inhaled corticosteroids can also be used.

Drugs for Nausea and Vomiting of Pregnancy

- Promethazine antihistamine has antiemetic and sedative effects and can be given safely for nausea and vomiting in pregnancy.
- Metoclopramide is an effective antiemetic and prevents reflux esophagitis.
- Antiemetic doxylamine can be combined with pyridoxine.
- Ondansetron is also used in pregnancy.
- Antacids are safe for use in pregnancy.
- Histamine-receptor antagonists such as cimetidine and ranitidine are also safely used.

Vitamins and Minerals

- Folic acid, iron and calcium are safely used in pregnancy.
- Vitamin A in high doses is a teratogen and therefore, contraindicated in pregnancy.

Retinoids

- Retinoids are known to be teratogenic in humans.
- **Isotretinoin** is widely used for treating cystic acne. It is shown to be associated with retinoic acid embryopathy with craniofacial and cardiac defects, optic nerve anomalies, blindness, cleft palate and mental retardation.

Hormones

- Androgens: Exposure to exogenous sex hormones before 7 weeks does not affect the genitalia. Between 7 and 12 weeks, the female genitalia can masculinise if exposed to androgens. Exposure at 12–20 weeks can lead to genital ambiguity.

- Oral contraceptives: These have not been shown to be associated with congenital anomalies.
- Diethylstilbestrol exposure: The drug is associated with structural abnormalities of the Müllerian ducts, the most common being hypoplastic T-shaped uterine cavity, cervical collars, hoods, septa and withered fallopian tubes. The drug is also associated with the development of clear cell adenocarcinoma of the cervix and/or vagina.

Habit-Forming Drugs

Alcohol

The consumption of alcohol during pregnancy may lead to the birth of a hyperactive child who is mentally retarded and has characteristic facial features like a broad upper lip, midfacial hypoplasia, low-set ears and epicanthic folds, micrognathia, microphthalmia, flattened nasal bridge and short nose. Congenital heart and joint defects are common. These features constitute the fetal alcohol syndrome. There may be microcephaly, mental retardation and behavioural problems. A newborn may present with withdrawal symptoms.

Cocaine

Cocaine addiction can cause abruptio placenta, preterm labour, FGR, intrauterine death and miscarriages. Other anomalies that are noted are microcephaly, limb defects and genitourinary malformations. The newborn may also present with withdrawal symptoms.

Use of Vaccines in Pregnancy

- Vaccination in pregnancy protects not only the mother but also the baby for 6 months postpartum. The FOGSI recommends immunisation against tetanus, diphtheria, pertussis and influenza during pregnancy.
- Two doses of tetanus toxoid injection at least 28 days apart should be given to all pregnant mothers commencing from the second trimester. If the subsequent pregnancy occurs within 5 years, only one booster is given.
- Tetanus, diphtheria and acellular pertussis (T-dap) vaccination can be considered instead of the second dose of tetanus toxoid to offer protection against diphtheria and pertussis in addition to tetanus.
- Influenza vaccination is recommended for mothers from 26 weeks onwards. In the case of a pandemic, the influenza vaccine can be given earlier to protect the mother.

- According to the CDC recommendations, tetanus, diphtheria, influenza, hepatitis, meningococcal and rabies vaccines are considered safe, if indicated.
- The vaccines that are contraindicated or whose safety is not established are BCG, varicella, measles, mumps and rubella. Following MMR and varicella vaccines, women should be counselled to avoid pregnancy for 4 weeks.
- Certain vaccines need special considerations. Yellow fever vaccine is a live-attenuated vaccine, and therefore, is best avoided during pregnancy. However, if the woman is travelling to an endemic area, it may have to be given. Anthrax, Japanese encephalitis, pneumococcal, polio and typhoid vaccines should be considered under special situations.
- Swine flu and COVID vaccines are safe to use in pregnancy during epidemics and pandemics.
- Women can be safely vaccinated in the postnatal period with influenza and rubella vaccines (rubella vaccine is given along with postnatal contraception).

Chemotherapeutic Drugs

- Methotrexate is a folic acid antagonist. Its use in the first trimester of pregnancy, exposure between 6–8 weeks of gestation and a dose greater than 10 mg/week have been shown to be associated with CNS abnormalities, limb defects and craniofacial abnormalities.
- The use of cyclophosphamide is associated with missing and hypoplastic digits on the hands and feet, cleft palate, imperforate anus and microcephaly.

Thalidomide

It is absolutely contraindicated in pregnancy. It causes abnormalities in the limbs, ears and the cardiovascular system.

Women of the reproductive age should use medications only under medical supervision. Necessary precautions should be taken to rule out pregnancy prior to the use of drugs.

While administering any drug during pregnancy, the obstetrician/physician should be aware of its effects on the fetus, especially during the first trimester. However, if the maternal benefits are greater than the risks or if the drug is life-saving, then the drug should not be withheld.

RADIATION EXPOSURE IN PREGNANCY

A pregnant woman may either require imaging studies or she may be inadvertently exposed to radiation before the pregnancy is diagnosed. It has been shown that a threshold dose of 5 rads is required to cause adverse effects on the fetus. There is an increased risk of congenital anomalies, growth restriction, mental retardation and childhood leukemia above this level. The doses of radiation from dental X-rays and chest X-rays are very low, and hence they can be undertaken if absolutely necessary.

- Radiation exposure with chest X-ray: <0.01 mGy (10 mGy = 1 rad)
- Abdomen and pelvic X-rays: 1.1 to 1.4 mGy
- CT scan and fluoroscopic studies can be associated with an exposure of 10 rads; therefore, they should be avoided during pregnancy
- There is no ionizing radiation with MRI, and thus it can be used if absolutely necessary

KEY POINTS

✓ A teratogen is a substance, organism or physical agent capable of causing abnormal fetal development.

✓ The susceptibility of the conceptus to teratogenic agents varies with the developmental stage at the time of exposure as well as the dose and duration of drug exposure.

✓ The classic teratogenic period is from 31–71 days after the last menstrual period in a normal 28-day menstrual cycle (17–57 days from fertilisation).

✓ Major congenital anomalies occur in 2–3% of all pregnancies due to drug exposure.

✓ The use of anticonvulsant drugs in pregnancy increases the risk of fetal malformations by 2–3 times. Phenytoin use in pregnancy has been associated with fetal hydantoin syndrome, also known as fetal anticonvulsant syndrome.

✓ Penicillin and cephalosporins are safe to use in pregnancy.

✓ Warfarin embryopathy occurs in 5% of patients exposed to the medication at 6–9 weeks of gestation.

✓ Female genitalia can masculinise if exposed to androgens between 7 and 12 weeks of gestation.

✓ Women in the reproductive age group should restrict the use of drugs unless pregnancy is ruled out.

Essay questions

1. Describe the Food and Drug Administration (FDA) classification for drugs used during pregnancy.
2. Define 'teratogen'. What is the teratogenic period? What are the effects of teratogens on the development of the embryo and fetus?

Short answer questions

Write short notes on the following:

1. Warfarin embryopathy
2. Fetal hydantoin syndrome
3. Antibiotics safe to use in pregnancy
4. Use of antiepileptic drugs in pregnancy
5. Vaccines that can be safely used in pregnancy
6. Vaccines that are contraindicated in pregnancy

MCQs

1. What is the most crucial time when structural malformations can occur in the fetus?
   a) Just before implantation
   b) Between fertilisation and implantation
   c) Embryonic period
   d) Fetal period
2. According to the FDA, the drugs for which animal studies indicate no fetal risk but for which there are no human studies are categorised into which of the following groups?
   a) Category A
   b) Category B
   c) Category C
   d) Category D
3. Which of the following vaccines can be used in pregnancy?
   a) Rubella vaccine
   b) Varicella vaccine
   c) Mumps vaccine
   d) Influenza vaccine
4. Which of the following drugs causes the discolouration of teeth in the fetus?
   a) Ampicillin
   b) Gentamycin
   c) Tetracycline
   d) Azithromycin
5. Which of the following categories of drugs is not associated with any fetal risks?
   a) Category A
   b) Category B
   c) Category C
   d) Category D
6. What cardiac drugs should be avoided in pregnancy?
   a) ACE inhibitors
   b) Beta-blockers
   c) Methyl-dopa
   d) Digoxin
7. Which of the following is a characteristic of warfarin embryopathy?
   a) Nasal hypoplasia
   b) Stippling of the bone
   c) Bilateral optic atrophy
   d) All of the above

8. The prolonged use of which of the following drugs reduces the amniotic fluid levels?
   a) Warfarin
   b) Tetracyclin
   c) Indomethacin
   d) Labetalol
9. Which of the following medications causes structural abnormalities of the Müllerian ducts?
   a) Methyl-dopa
   b) Calcium blockers
   c) Diethyl stilbestrol
   d) Morphine

Answers
1. (c), 2. (b), 3. (d), 4. (c), 5. (a), 6. (a), 7. (d), 8. (c), 9. (c)

Fill in the blanks

1. Tetracycline given in late pregnancy causes _____.
2. The administration of indomethacin during pregnancy may lead to _____.

Answers
1. discolouration of teeth, 2. the constriction of fetal ductus arteriosus

Case scenario-based discussion

1. A 28-year-old gravida 2, para 1, alive 1, visits the clinic with history of 2 months of amenorrhea and complaints of nausea and vomiting that is not manageable. While detailing her history, she reveals that she had a respiratory infection one week prior to missing her period, and that an X-ray chest was taken and antibiotics were prescribed.
   a) What is the effect of antibiotics on the embryo at this stage?
   b) At what threshold level is radiation harmful to the fetus?
   c) How much is the radiation exposure in a chest X-ray?
   d) Which imaging modality does not emit radiation?
   e) How would you manage her nausea and vomiting?

Answers
a) The first two weeks following ovulation are known as the stage of blastogenesis. If exposed to a teratogen during this period, the embryo either dies or, if the injury is slight, overcomes the harmful effects of the drug entirely. This is called the `all or none' effect.
b) It has been shown that a threshold dose of 5 rads is required to cause adverse effects on the fetus.
c) The radiation exposure with chest X-ray is <0.01 mGy.
d) There is no ionising radiation with MRI.
e) Nausea and vomiting can be treated with doxylamine, pyridoxine and promethazine, which are effective antiemetics. Metoclopramide prevents reflux esophagitis. Antacids are also safe in pregnancy.

10

OG 8.8, OG 9.4, OG 15.1, OG 16.3

Imaging Techniques

Learning Objectives

» To know the indications for USG in the first trimester of pregnancy
» To know how to perform USG evaluation of the fetus in the second and third trimesters of pregnancy
» To know how to assess the cervix by USG for cervical insufficiency

■ ULTRASONOGRAPHY (USG)

Principles of Ultrasound

The use of ultrasound in medicine was developed from **SONAR (sound navigation and ranging) systems** used to detect submarines. Ultrasound uses the principle of inverse piezoelectric effect—when mechanical pressure is applied to the surface of piezoelectric crystals, these materials produce an electric current. Inversely, when an electric pulse is applied to a piezoelectric material, a mechanical wave is produced, which is the ultrasound beam. An **ultrasound scanner** is made up of transducers containing piezoelectric crystals. When excited by an electric pulse, the crystals generate ultrasonographic waves that pass from the ultrasound transducer into the tissues in their path. When these waves meet a tissue interface, they are reflected to the transducer and converted into an electric signal, which is processed and digitalised as an ultrasound image on the monitor.

> **Sound is the orderly transmission of mechanical vibrations through a medium.** The number of vibrations that occur per second is known as the frequency of sound and is measured in hertz (Hz).
>
> 1 Hz = 1 cycle/second
>
> The human ear can detect frequencies in the range of 20–20,000 Hz (20 kilohertz). Any sound above this range is known as ultrasound. Most types of medical diagnostic equipment have a range of 1–15 megahertz (MHz).
>
> 1 MHz = 1,000,000 cycles/second

Obstetric ultrasound uses a frequency of 2–12 MHz. The higher the frequency, the better the resolution; however, tissue penetration is limited. For this reason, high-frequency probes are used to examine structures closer to the surface and lower frequency probes are used to study deeper tissues.

A **transvaginal transducer** uses a frequency of 5–10 MHz, and is useful in early pregnancy, in assessing the length of the cervix and for localising the placenta in placenta previa. **Abdominal transducers** use a frequency of 2–6.5 MHz and are commonly used in obstetrics. A dense structure like bone appears white on the screen (echogenic), while fluid appears black (anechoic)—this happens when an entire wave is transmitted and nothing is reflected back. Structures made up of a few echoes are referred to as echo-poor or hypoechoic.

■ TIMING OF USG EXAMINATION IN OBSTETRICS

- The first USG is carried out at 11–13 weeks +6 days.
- The second scan is carried out at 18–20 weeks of gestation to identify anomalies of the fetus.
- A third-trimester scan is indicated to assess fetal growth and well-being, to diagnose evolving anomalies and to evaluate the placenta in cases of placenta previa and to diagnose adherent placenta.

> **Safety of ultrasound**
> Ultrasound waves at very high intensity can cause human tissue damage from heat and cavitation. However, the low intensity at which real-time imaging is done is devoid of any fetal risks. The ionising radiation from X-ray causes fetal damage. In contrast, diagnostic ultrasound has been shown to be harmless. Even though **duplex Doppler imaging** uses higher energy intensities than ultrasound, no adverse effects have been noted.

USES OF ULTRASOUND IN THE FIRST TRIMESTER

The first-trimester scan is usually carried out at 11–13 weeks +6 days of gestation. However, in the presence of pain or bleeding or when there is a need to confirm pregnancy and the viability of the fetus, USG can be performed at any time. Either a transabdominal or transvaginal scan can be carried out, but a transvaginal scan is more useful in the first trimester. In order to perform an effective transabdominal scan (TAS), the woman's bladder should be full.

▍ INDICATIONS FOR FIRST-TRIMESTER SCANS

1. USG Examination for Confirmation of Intrauterine Pregnancy

- The earliest evidence of pregnancy is the appearance of the gestational sac, which is identified by transvaginal USG (TVS) as early as 4 weeks inside the uterine cavity and is clearly made out between 4.5 and 5 weeks of gestation. The mean sac diameter at 4 weeks of gestation is 2–3 mm.
- The gestational sac should be evaluated for the presence of a yolk sac and the fetal pole. The yolk sac appears at 5 weeks, when the sac diameter is 10 mm by TVS (Fig. 10.1).

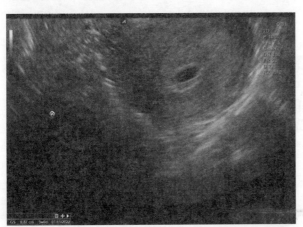

Fig. 10.1 Intrauterine gestational sac with a small yolk sac (*Image courtesy:* Dr B H Parameshwar Keerthi, BM Scans, Kancheepuram)

- The normal yolk sac measures 6 mm in diameter and disappears at 12–14 weeks. In the presence of large yolk sacs, abnormal pregnancy should be suspected.

- By 5.5 weeks, the fetal pole appears as a 1–2 mm wide structure. Cardiac activity appears at 6 weeks of gestation, when the embryo is >5 mm in size (Fig. 10.2).

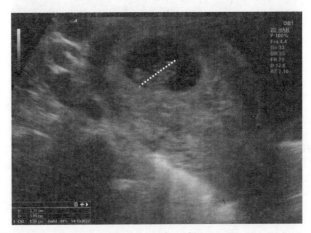

Fig. 10.2 Fetal pole within the sac (*Image courtesy:* Dr Parameshwar Keerthi, Kancheepuram)

Confirmation of intrauterine pregnancy by TVS	
Gestational sac:	4.5–5 weeks
Yolk sac:	5 weeks
Fetal pole:	5.5 weeks
Fetal cardiac activity:	6 weeks
(It takes another 4–7 days to visualise all these structures by transabdominal scan.)	

2. Assessment of Gestational Age (Dating of Pregnancy) by USG

- Gestational age can be calculated from the mean sac diameter. Adding 30 to the mean sac diameter will give the gestational age in days. For example, if the mean sac diameter is 10 mm, the gestational age will be 10 + 30 = 40 days (6 weeks).
- The crown–rump length (CRL) measurement gives an accurate estimate of the gestational age in the first trimester, with which the EDD can be calculated accurately to within 3–5 days. This measurement is taken along the length of the fetus in a straight line from the top of the head to the bottom of the buttocks (without correction for body curvature; Fig. 10.3). Usually, the measurement is taken at 7–14 weeks of gestation. At a lower gestational age (7–10 weeks), the accuracy in calculating the gestational age is ±3 days; at 11–14 weeks, the accuracy is ±5 days.

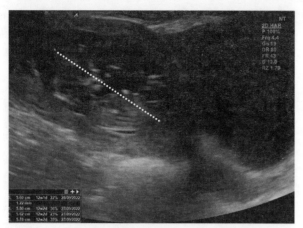
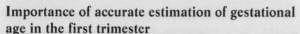

Fig. 10.3 Measurement of crown–rump length (*Image courtesy:* Dr Parameshwar Keerthi, Kancheepuram)

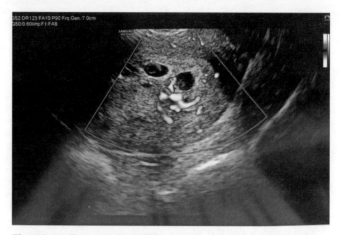

Fig. 10.4 Transvaginal USG showing two gestational sacs with yolk sacs

> **Importance of accurate estimation of gestational age in the first trimester**
> - To accurately calculate the EDD
> - To monitor fetal growth
> - To avoid iatrogenic prematurity
> - To plan induction for post-term pregnancy
> - To interpret screening investigations such as Down screen

3. Viability of Pregnancy

A pregnancy is said to be viable when fetal heart pulsations are demonstrated within the gestation sac. These are visualised by week 6 using the vaginal method and by week 7 using the abdominal method.

4. USG Diagnosis of Multiple Pregnancy

In multiple pregnancies, multiple gestational sacs can be identified. The diagnosis of an ongoing multiple pregnancy is made when the fetal viability is confirmed in all the sacs. In a first-trimester scan for multiple gestation, chorionicity should always be assessed. In dichorionic twins, each fetus is in a separate gestational sac (Fig. 10.4). The presence of the lambda sign and a thick separating membrane confirms dichorionicity. In monochorionic twins, two fetuses are seen in a single gestational sac. The presence of a T sign and a thin separating membrane confirms monochorionicity.

5. USG in the Evaluation of Miscarriages

- Threatened miscarriage: Cardiac activity is present; subchorionic hemorrhage may be present.
- Inevitable miscarriage: The cervix is open and the sac lies low in the uterus or in the cervical canal.

- Incomplete miscarriage: A smaller amount of the products of conception are seen in the uterine cavity than in the previously confirmed pregnancy.
- Complete miscarriage: The uterine cavity is empty.
- Missed miscarriage: It may present as blighted ovum (anembryonic pregnancy) or early fetal death.

> **Minimal criteria for diagnosing miscarriage by USG**
> - The mean sac diameter is ≥ 25 mm and no embryo is seen by TVS (30 mm if TAS is used [anembryonic pregnancy]).
> - The CRL is ≥ 7 mm and fetal heart tones are absent (with TAS, CRL is >10 mm and fetal heart is absent).
> - No fetal cardiac activity is present. This is especially definitive in cases where it was previously seen.

Additional guidelines suggested by the Society of Radiologists in Ultrasound, USA

- The absence of an embryo with a heartbeat at least two weeks after an ultrasound scan that showed a gestational sac **without a yolk sac** indicates a miscarriage.
- The absence of an embryo with a heartbeat at least 11 days after an ultrasound scan that showed a gestational sac **with a yolk** sac is also diagnostic.

6. USG in the Diagnosis of Ectopic Pregnancy

- A gestational sac may be evident as early as when the serum β-hCG level is 300 IU/mL, but should always be evident by the time it reaches 1,000 mIU/mL (discriminatory level).

- Failure to visualise a gestational sac at the discriminatory level of serum β-hCG indicates either a failed intrauterine pregnancy or an ectopic pregnancy or pregnancy of unknown location.
- In the presence of a gestational sac with a yolk sac or embryo within the uterine cavity, a diagnosis of an intrauterine pregnancy is confirmed. However, it is important to remember that heterotopic pregnancy may rarely occur, especially in those women who conceived through in vitro fertilisation.

USG features of ectopic pregnancy

- On USG, ectopic pregnancy appears as an intact, well-defined tubal ring (the 'bagel sign') in which the yolk sac and/or the embryonic pole with or without cardiac activity is seen within a completely sonolucent sac in the adnexal region (Fig. 10.5). Colour Doppler may show a 'ring of fire' appearance.
- An empty uterine cavity and the presence of an adnexal mass and/or fluid in the POD confirms ectopic pregnancy.

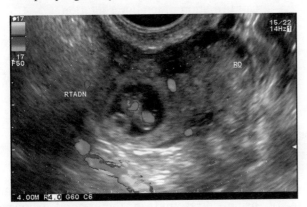

Fig. 10.5 Fetal pole with yolk sac within the sonolucent sac in the adnexal region (*Image courtesy*: Mediscan Systems, Chennai)

7. USG in the Diagnosis of Hydatidiform Mole

The ultrasound diagnosis of a hydatidiform mole is based on the presence of numerous cystic spaces of varying sizes with intervening echogenic areas in the uterine cavity—classically known as a **snowstorm appearance** (Fig. 10.6). Internal and peripheral vascularity is noted.

8. Screening for Down Syndrome by Nuchal Translucency (NT)

Nuchal translucency is a sonographic finding of a collection of fluid under the nuchal skin (Fig. 10.7). The subcutaneous translucent area between the skin and the soft tissue over the fetal spine in the sagittal

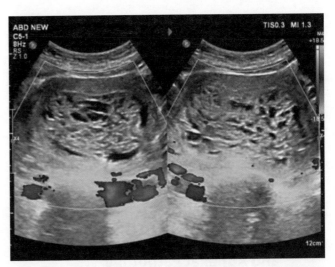

Fig. 10.6 A complete hydatidiform mole (*Image courtesy*: Dr Parameshwar Keerthi, Kancheepuram)

plane is measured at 11–13 weeks +6 days of gestation. Accurate gestational age is important in interpreting the measurements. Between 10 and 12 weeks, nuchal translucency is less than 2 mm and at 13 weeks, it is 2–3 mm. Increased value suggests trisomy 13, trisomy 18, trisomy 21, Turner syndrome, Klinefelter syndrome or triploidy. Other markers of aneuploidy in the first trimester are unossified nasal bone and absence or reversal of flow in the ductus venosus.

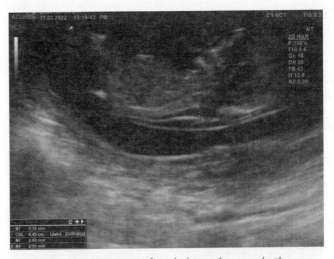

Fig. 10.7 Measurement of nuchal translucency in the sagittal plane (*Image courtesy*: Dr Parameshwar Keerthi, Kancheepuram)

9. USG Diagnosis of Incompetent Cervix (Cervical Insufficiency)

The normal cervix has a length of 2.5 cm or more. The width of the cervical canal at the level of the internal os is less than 4 mm. At 16–28 weeks of gestation, if the length of the cervix is less than 2 cm in a woman with no previous history of preterm delivery and <2.5 cm in a woman with previous history of preterm delivery, a diagnosis of incompetent cervix is made. In cervical insufficiency, there may also be widening of the internal os of more than 8 mm presenting with funneling. Funneling can be demonstrated by applying suprapubic pressure. A cervical length of <25 mm at 16–28 weeks of gestation by transvaginal USG is associated with an increased risk of spontaneous preterm delivery.

10. Use of USG in Prenatal Diagnostic Procedures

USG is useful for interventions such as chorion villus sampling, amniocentesis, embryo transfer and so on.

11. USG in the Evaluation of Uterine and Adnexal Pathology

USG is also helpful in evaluating uterine and adnexal pathologies such as fibroids and adnexal masses complicating pregnancy. Uterine anomalies such as bicornuate uterus can also be diagnosed in the first trimester.

12. USG in Early Identification of C-section Scar Pregnancy

The first-trimester scan is also useful in diagnosing cesarean section scar pregnancy.

USG IN THE DIAGNOSIS OF CONGENITAL MALFORMATIONS OF THE FETUS

1. Anencephaly

Some anomalies like anencephaly and encephalocele may be diagnosed at as early as 9–10 weeks and are easily diagnosed by 11 weeks of gestation. The absence of a cranial vault gives a 'frog's eye' appearance to the fetus (Fig. 10.8).

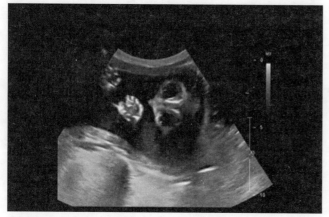

Fig. 10.8   Frog's eye appearance in anencephaly (*Image courtesy:* Dr Parameshwar Keerthi. Kancheepuram)

2. Other Anomalies

Anomalies such as omphalocele and holoprosencephaly can also be diagnosed in the first trimester of pregnancy.

ROLE OF ULTRASOUND IN THE SECOND AND THIRD TRIMESTERS

Ultrasound is carried out in the second or third trimester of pregnancy for the indications listed in the box below.

> **Indications for USG in the second and third trimesters**
> - Screening for fetal anomalies (usually done in the second trimester)
> - Assessment of the fetus
>   — Evaluation of fetal growth
>   — Estimation of fetal weight
>   — Confirmation/calculation of gestational age
>   — Fetal well-being—biophysical profile
>   — Follow-up of fetal anomaly
>   — Confirmation of fetal presentation
>   — Confirmation of fetal demise
> - Placental localisation and abnormalities such as separation
> - For interventions such as amniocentesis, fetal blood sampling, and so on

USE OF ULTRASOUND IN THE SECOND TRIMESTER

Systematic screening for fetal anomalies is the main aim of using ultrasound in the second trimester of pregnancy. This is also known as **targeted fetal examination (TAFE).**

Timing of the Scan

The second-trimester scan is performed at 18–20 weeks of gestation to diagnose congenital anomalies of the fetus and to assess the gestational age. As per the recent amendment of the MTP Act, in cases where anomalies are diagnosed before 24 weeks of gestation, the pregnancy can be terminated. From 26–28 weeks onwards, USG is used to assess fetal growth.

The components of the second-trimester scan are as follows:

- A general survey to assess the fetal number, viability and placental location
- Fetal biometry to assess the gestational age in the early second trimester and to assess the fetal growth from the late second trimester onwards

- Fetal environment to study the placenta, umbilical cord and amniotic fluid
- Associated uterine and adnexal pathology and to assess the cervical length
- Diagnosis of structural anomalies of the fetus

Fetal Biometry

Fetal biometry involves the measurement of the following:

- Biparietal diameter (BPD)
- Femur length (FL)
- Abdominal circumference (AC)
- Head circumference (HC)

These measurements are used to assess the gestational age in the early second trimester and to measure the fetal growth from the late second trimester onwards.

Assessment of gestational age

- Biparietal diameter (BPD) measured between 15 and 24 weeks of gestation predicts gestational age with an error margin of 7–10 days.
- BPD is measured at the level of the thalamus, falx and cavum septum pellucidum in the transverse section (Fig. 10.9).

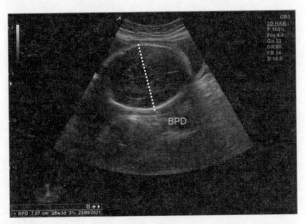

Fig. 10.9 USG picture showing the measurement of the biparietal diameter (*Image courtesy*: Dr Parameshwar Keerthi, Kancheepuram)

- After 26 weeks of gestation, the error increases to 14–21 days. Hence, this method is not used to assess the gestational age after 26 weeks.
- BPD measurement also becomes unreliable when there is a change in the shape of the head as in a dolichocephalic head. In these circumstances, head circumference (HC) is taken (Fig. 10.10).
- Femur length (FL) and humerus length correlate strongly with gestational age with an error margin of

7–11 days up to 26 weeks of gestation, after which the margin increases to 14–21 days (Fig. 10.11).

- A combination of measurements is better than a single measurement for the assessment of gestational age. Table 10.1 presents the accuracy of the various USG parameters in predicting the EDD.
- The measurement of the transverse diameter of the cerebellum between 14 and 24 weeks is also useful in assessing the gestational age.

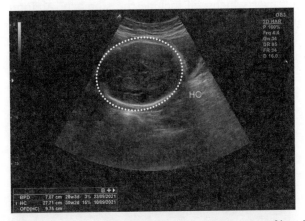

Fig. 10.10 USG picture showing the measurement of head circumference (*Image courtesy*: Dr Parameshwar Keerthi, Kancheepuram)

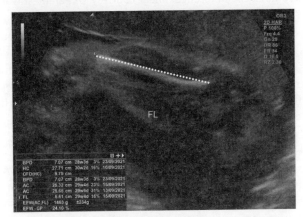

Fig. 10.11 USG picture showing the measurement of femur length (*Image courtesy*: Dr Parameshwar Keerthi, Kancheepuram)

Table 10.1 Accuracy of gestational age estimation using USG parameters

Measurement used	Gestational age at assessment	Accuracy
Mean gestational sac diameter	5 weeks	±5–7 days
CRL	7–10 weeks	±3 days
CRL	11–14 weeks	±5 days
BPD, HC, AC, FL	14–24 weeks	±7–10 days
BPD, HC, AC, FL	After 26 weeks	14–21 days

Estimation of fetal growth

In order to assess fetal growth, the gestational age of the fetus must be accurately established before 24 weeks of gestation. Fetal growth is assessed by serially measuring the abdominal circumference (AC) of the fetus, which is a measure of hepatic size and the amount of abdominal adipose tissue. This measurement is taken in the transverse section of the fetal abdomen at the level of the intrahepatic portion of the umbilical vein of the fetal liver which will include the stomach. Abdominal circumference can also be taken (Fig. 10.12).

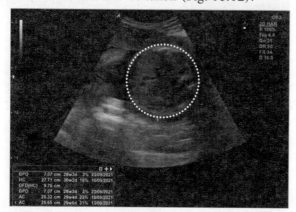

Fig. 10.12 USG picture showing the measurement of abdominal circumference (*Image courtesy:* Dr Parameshwar Keerthi, Kancheepuram)

The serial measurement of biparietal diameter alone is not sufficient to accurately measure fetal growth as it is associated with high false-negative rates. This is due to the **brain-sparing effect**, wherein the brain is less affected by growth retardation than organs such as the liver and spleen. The growth rates of the fetal head and abdomen are studied together to assess **fetal growth** in IUGR.

In women at risk of **small-for-gestational age (SGA) babies**, both HC and AC are measured, and their ratio (HC:AC) is calculated. A large head–trunk ratio is seen in an asymmetrically growth-retarded fetus. A symmetrically small fetus shows a normal head–trunk ratio, suggesting either **fetal abnormality** or a normal but genetically small fetus.

The finding of a large abdominal circumference (on or above the 90th percentile) or a fetus with accelerated growth should suggest the possibility of **maternal diabetes mellitus**. Excessive fetal growth is associated with polyhydramnios (amniotic column of more than 8 cm) and a large placenta (more than 4 cm thick) suggests poor control of **maternal diabetes**.

Estimation of fetal weight

Fetal weight is usually obtained by measuring **BPD** and **AC**. In late pregnancy, if the fetal head is engaged or in breech presentation or if the shape of the head is dolicocephalic, then the measurement of BPD becomes unreliable. In these situations, **HC**, **AC** and **FL** are used to estimate fetal weight.

Assessment of fetal well-being

Fetal well-being is assessed by performing a **biophysical profile as discussed in Chapter 11**, *Antepartum fetal surveillance: Tests of fetal well-being.*

Assessment of Fetal Environment

The fetal environment is assessed by evaluating the placenta, amniotic fluid and the umbilical cord.

Evaluation of the placenta

The placenta (Fig. 10.13) is easily recognised by a stronger echo pattern compared to that of the underlying myometrium. By week 8, the placental site is easily recognised. Placental localisation is an integral part of an obstetric examination and is reasonably accurate in skilled hands. The texture and pattern of the placenta have been graded by ultrasound according to **Grannum's grading system**. In pregnancies complicated by hypertensive disease and intrauterine growth retardation, a mature placenta may be seen in earlier gestational periods.

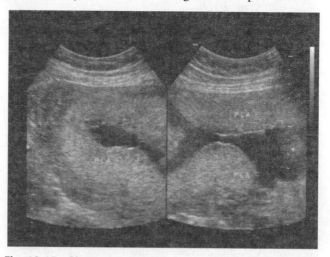

Fig. 10.13 Placenta on USG

- USG is useful in localising the placenta.
- In cases with placenta previa, the distance between the placental margin and the internal os can be measured.
- USG also helps in the diagnosis of adherent placenta.
- Other placental abnormalities such as infarctions and calcifications can be diagnosed.

Estimation of amniotic fluid volume (AFI)

The amniotic fluid volume can be assessed either **subjectively** or by measuring the maximum vertical pocket or the amniotic fluid index. A **maximum vertical pocket** of 2–8 cm is considered normal. **Amniotic fluid index** (Fig. 10.14) is calculated by adding the vertical depths of the largest pocket in each of the four uterine quadrants. The normal value is between 5 and 24 cm. When the AFI is <5 cm, a diagnosis of oligohydramnios is made.

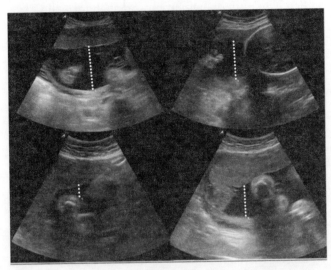

Fig. 10.14 Measurement of AFI by USG—measurements taken from four quadrants of the uterus (*Image courtesy:* Dr Parameshwar Keerthi, Kancheepuram)

- Causes of polyhydramnios include multiple pregnancy, fetal abnormalities such as anencephaly, duodenal atresia, hydrops fetalis and maternal diabetes mellitus.
- Causes of oligohydramnios include rupture of membranes, intrauterine growth restriction, anomalies of the urinary tract such as renal agenesis and urethral stenosis and postdated pregnancy.

Evaluation of the umbilical cord

USG is very useful in diagnosing umbilical cord abnormalities such as single umbilical artery and nuchal cord. Umbilical vessels have two arteries and one vein (Fig. 10.15). With the use of Doppler, abnormal insertions of the umbilical cord such as marginal insertion (battledore placenta) can be diagnosed. Umbilical cord entry into the fetal abdomen should be evaluated as this helps in the diagnosis of anterior abdominal wall defects such as omphalocele.

Diagnosis of Structural Defects by USG (Targeted Anomaly Scan)

A targeted anomaly scan at 18–20 weeks of gestation identifies more than 70% of major anomalies and nearly 50% of minor anomalies. A number of anomalies can be detected, some of which are detailed below.

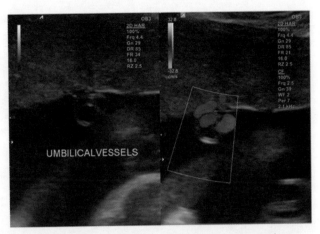

Fig. 10.15 Normal umbilical vessels with two arteries and one vein (*Image courtesy:* Dr Parameshwar Keerthi, Kancheepuram)

Anencephaly

The absence of a cranial vault gives a 'frog's eye' appearance to the fetus. This anomaly is readily detected from 10–11 weeks onwards (Fig. 10.8).

Hydrocephalus

It is defined as the presence of excessive cerebrospinal fluid and is diagnosed by the enlargement of the ventricles, i.e., ventriculomegaly (Fig 10.16).

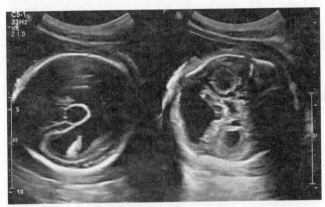

Fig. 10.16 Hydrocephalus—the first image shows a dilated lateral ventricle with a dangling choroid plexus and the second image shows a dilated fourth ventricle (*Image courtesy:* Dr Parameshwar Keerthi, Kancheepuram)

Duodenal atresia

Duodenal atresia has a characteristic 'double-bubble' appearance of the stomach on ultrasound (Fig. 10.17).

Jejunal atresia

It presents with dilated loops of the bowel on USG. The triple-bubble sign is the classic radiographic appearance of jejunal atresia. The third bubble is seen due to the proximal obstruction caused by the atretic jejunum.

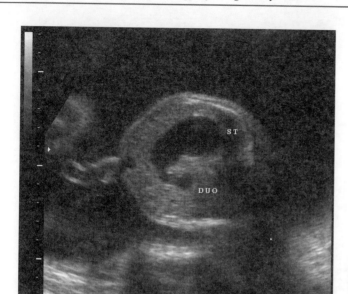

Fig. 10.17 Double-bubble appearance on USG in duodenal atresia

Diaphragmatic hernia

This is suspected when cystic structures are seen within the chest. Parts of the bowel may be seen passing through the diaphragm.

Clubfoot

This is diagnosed when the length of the entire foot can be seen in the same section as the tibia and fibula.

Single umbilical artery (Fig. 10.18)

The umbilical cord should normally contain two arteries and one vein. Eighty per cent of fetuses with a single umbilical artery are normal; others may be associated with abnormalities of the urinary tract, heart and gastrointestinal tract.

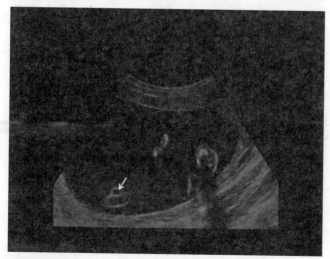

Fig. 10.18 Single umbilical artery (*Image courtesy:* Dr Parameshwar Keerthi, Kancheepuram)

Hydrops fetalis

In this condition, there is either fetal ascites or plural and pericardial effusion with skin edema. It may be due to Rh-isoimmunisation or other non-immune causes.

Markers of chromosomal abnormalities

Some of the abnormalities detected on USG may indicate an underlying chromosomal abnormality.

Cystic hygroma:	Turner syndrome or trisomy 21
Duodenal atresia:	Trisomy 21
Omphalocele:	Trisomy 13 or 18
Hyperechogenic bowel:	Fetal aneuploidy and cystic fibrosis

USES OF USG IN THE THIRD TRIMESTER OF PREGNANCY

Assessment of Fetal Growth

- Fetal growth assessment is carried out by measuring the abdominal circumference. Serial measurements are taken and plotted on a graph. AC value of less than the 10th percentile is diagnostic of growth restriction.
- Similarly, fetal weight is calculated using BPD, FL and AC and plotting these values on a graph. Values less than the 10th percentile indicate either growth restriction or a small-for-gestational age fetus.

Assessment of Fetal Well-Being

Fetal well-being is assessed using biophysical profile and Doppler velocimetry (discussed in detail in Chapter 11, *Antepartum fetal surveillance: Tests of fetal well-being*).

Other uses of third-trimester USG are as follows:

- Evaluation of antepartum hemorrhage
- In PPROM, for serial evaluation of liquor volume
- Evolving anomalies such as cardiac anomalies and hydrocephalus
- Confirmation of fetal death
- Confirmation of fetal presentation in obese patients
- Monitoring during external cephalic version
- Guidance during fetoscopy and cordocentesis
- Guidance during fetal therapy such as intrauterine fetal transfusion and twin-to-twin transfusion
- Fetal growth, fetal well-being, multiple gestation and estimation of fetal weight

DOPPLER VELOCIMETRY

The **Doppler shift** is a principle of physics. When sound waves strike a moving target, their frequency changes in proportion to the velocity and direction of the moving target. This principle is used to determine the rate and volume of blood flow through various maternal and fetal vessels.

The **waveforms** of different vessels are studied and based on the systolic and diastolic blood flow, various indices are calculated. The vessels commonly studied are maternal uterine arteries, middle cerebral arteries and fetal umbilical arteries.

Doppler ultrasound is useful in the evaluation of high-risk pregnancies such as pre-eclampsia, GDM, fetal growth restriction and fetal anemia. It is also useful in diagnosing umbilical cord abnormalities. Doppler studies measure the blood flow in the placental unit and in the fetal blood vessels. They are useful in differentiating healthy fetuses from hypoxic fetuses, especially in IUGR. They are also helpful in deciding the timing of delivery. Arterial Doppler includes uterine artery Doppler, umbilical artery Doppler and middle cerebral artery Doppler. Venous Doppler measures blood flow in the ductus venosus.

Doppler ultrasonography of the umbilical artery assesses the blood flow to the fetus via the umbilical artery. With normal placental function, in order to maintain the blood flow to the fetus, there is low-resistance flow so that even during diastole. there is good flow to the fetus (Fig. 10.19).

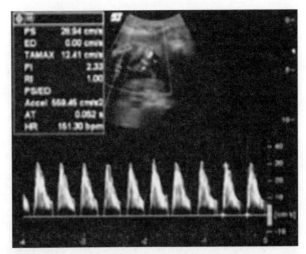

Fig. 10.20b Umbilical artery Doppler assessment

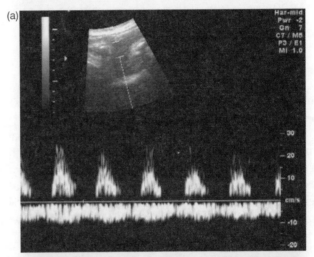

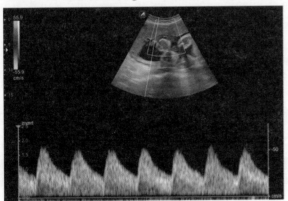

Fig. 10.19 Normal umbilical artery velocimetry with good diastolic blood flow (*Image courtesy:* Dr Parameshwar Keerthi, Kancheepuram)

When the placental resistance increases, the diastolic flow is either absent (Fig. 10.20a and b) or reversed (Fig. 10.21a and b). Reversed diastolic flow warrants immediate termination of pregnancy irrespective of the period of gestation.

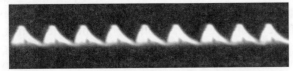

Fig. 10.20a Umbilical artery velocimetry with absent diastolic blood flow

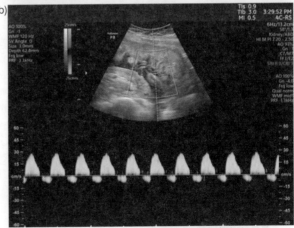

Fig. 10.21a and b Umbilical artery velocimetry with reversed diastolic blood flow

Various indices are calculated to confirm adequate blood flow to the fetus.

- **Systolic/diastolic ratio (S/D ratio)** is the ratio of the maximum systolic to the minimum diastolic blood flow.

- **Resistance index or RI** is calculated by the formula:

$$\frac{\text{(Peak systolic velocity} - \text{end diastolic velocity)}}{\text{Systolic velocity}}$$

OR

$$(S - D)/S$$

- **Pulsatility index (PI)** is calculated by the formula:

$$\frac{\text{(Peak systolic velocity} - \text{end diastolic velocity)}}{\text{Mean velocity}}$$

OR

$$(S - D)/\text{mean}$$

The systolic–diastolic ratio (S/D) is the most commonly used index to assess the blood flow to the fetus. S/D ratio mean value decreases with fetal age as follows:

- At 20 weeks, the 50th percentile for the S/D ratio is 4
- At 30 weeks, the 50th percentile is 2.83
- At 40 weeks, the 50th percentile is 2.18

If there is an increase in the resistance to blood flow through the umbilical artery, this is seen as an increase in systolic/diastolic (S/D) flow ratio.

Umbilical artery Doppler is considered abnormal when the S/D ratio is more than the ninety-fifth percentile for the gestational age or if the diastolic flow is either absent or reversed. It has been reported that perinatal mortality for reversed end diastolic flow is approximately 33% and that for absent diastolic flow, it is about 10%.

Middle Cerebral Artery (MCA) Blood Flow (Fig. 10.22)

In normal pregnancies, the diastolic flow in the cerebral arteries is lower than that in the umbilical arteries (UA) at any gestational age. Therefore, the cerebrovascular resistance remains higher than the placental resistance and the pulsatility index of the MCA and umbilical artery (MCA/UA ratio; otherwise called cerebroplacental ratio or CPR)

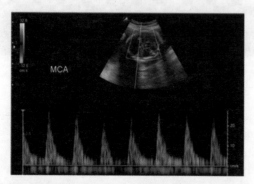

Fig. 10.22 Middle cerebral artery Doppler (*Image courtesy:* Dr Parameshwar Keerthi, Kancheepuram)

is greater than 1. The index drops to less than 1 if the flow distribution is in favour of the brain in pathological pregnancies. In the presence of fetal hypoxia, to spare the vital organ—the brain—blood is shunted to the cerebral arteries. This is known as the **brain-sparing effect**. An increased diastolic flow in the middle cerebral arteries is an early sign of fetal hypoxia.

Indications for Doppler Velocimetry

Screening for fetal anomalies
- Markers for congenital heart disease and cardiac anomalies
- Evaluation of vascular malformations in the fetus
- Diaphragmatic hernia, renal anomalies

Clinical indications
- Screening for pre-eclampsia in first and second trimesters
- Diagnosing fetal anemia (in Rh-isoimmunised pregnancies)
- Evaluation of the growth-restricted fetus
- Assessment of fetal hypoxia in high-risk pregnancies as a method of fetal surveillance

Other imaging modalities that use ultrasound are as follows:

- 3D ultrasound: It is useful in evaluating facial defects and provides a 3D image of the fetus.
- 4D ultrasound: 3D images are viewed in real time. It is useful in evaluating cardiac activity.
- Fetal echocardiography: This is used to diagnose structural and functional defects.

X-RAYS

With the advent of USG, the use of X-ray in obstetrics is restricted to maternal indications such as X-ray chest for a medical condition in the mother. If an X-ray is definitely indicated, the abdomen is shielded to minimise the effect of radiation on the fetus. The effect of X-ray radiation on the fetus depends on the gestational age at exposure and the amount of radiation received by the fetus. If inadvertent exposure occurs in the preimplantation stage, it is lethal to the fertilised ova and the embryo, and miscarriage occurs. Exposure during the period of organogenesis has a teratogenic effect. Exposure during the fetal period can also result in growth restriction and can have central nervous system effects like microcephaly and mental retardation. The amount of radiation received by the fetus in most diagnostic procedures is less than

2 rads. The possibility of adverse effects on the fetus at this radiation dose is minimal.

MAGNETIC RESONANCE IMAGING (MRI)

MRI has the ability to acquire images in any plane with a high soft tissue contrast. This technique uses powerful **magnets** to produce **radiofrequencies; it does not produce ionising radiation.** This is an advantage over computed tomography. No harmful human effects from MRI have been noted so far. Therefore, MRI may be performed without any fetal risks, provided there is a very definite indication for the same. However, MRI is not recommended for use in the first trimester.

The **indications for MRI during pregnancy** are as follows:

- **Evaluation of intraabdominal malignancies** like lymphoma and renal cell carcinoma
- **Evaluation of retroperitoneal space**, for example, detection of adrenal tumours like pheochromocytoma
- Characterisation of **uterine and ovarian masses**
- **To assess fetal anatomy** when ultrasound is equivocal due to reduced liquor and fetal movements
- **Following road traffic accidents**

During pregnancy, imaging procedures that are not associated with ionising radiation such as ultrasound and MRI should be considered instead of X-rays and computed tomography wherever possible.

KEY POINTS

✓ *Ultrasound is the use of high-frequency sound waves to visualise internal structures. Most types of medical diagnostic ultrasound equipment use a range of 1–10 megahertz (MHz).*

✓ *In the first trimester, ultrasound is used to diagnose pregnancy, confirm fetal viability, detect multiple pregnancy and diagnose pregnancy complications like missed abortion, ectopic pregnancy and hydatidiform mole.*

✓ *In the second and third trimesters, it is used to detect fetal anomalies, estimate gestational age, fetal growth and fetal weight and assess fetal well-being.*

✓ *Ultrasound is devoid of any known fetal risks and is safe in pregnancy.*

✓ *The imaging modalities used during pregnancy include ultrasound, Doppler, and occasionally, magnetic resonance imaging.*

✓ *X-rays and computed tomography produce ionising radiation, which may have potential biological hazards in high doses. However, in routine diagnostic doses, they are safe and are used for maternal indications.*

✓ *Ultrasound and MRI are safe in pregnancy and are the imaging techniques of choice.*

Essay questions

1. Discuss the indications for first-trimester USG.
2. What are the uses of second-trimester USG?

Short answer questions

1. How does ultrasound help in the estimation of gestational age?
2. What are the diagnostic criteria for missed miscarriage?
3. Describe the role of magnetic resonance imaging (MRI) during pregnancy.
4. Write short note on nuchal translucency.

MCQs

1. At what period of gestation is the crown–rump measurement taken to estimate the gestational age?
   a) 4–6 weeks
   b) 6–12 weeks
   c) 14–16 weeks
   d) 18–20 weeks
2. At how many weeks of gestation is fetal cardiac activity seen by abdominal ultrasonography?
   a) 4 weeks
   b) 5 weeks
   c) 6 weeks
   d) 7 weeks
3. What is the earliest gestational age at which a diagnosis of anencephaly can be made by USG?
   a) 6 weeks
   b) 7 weeks
   c) 8 weeks
   d) 9 weeks
4. Which is the best parameter to assess gestational age in the first trimester?
   a) BPD
   b) Head circumference
   c) Abdominal circumference
   d) Crown–rump length
5. In which of the following is a snowstorm appearance seen on USG?
   a) Hydatidiform mole
   b) Ectopic pregnancy
   c) Missed abortion
   d) None of these
6. At what level is abdominal circumference measured?
   a) Kidney
   b) Intrahepatic portion of umbilical vein
   c) Liver
   d) Bladder

7. At what gestational age is nuchal translucency best measured?
   a) 15 weeks
   b) 7 weeks
   c) 10 weeks
   d) 11–13+6 weeks

8. Which of the following cervical length is indicative of cervical insufficiency with previous history of preterm labour?
   a) <3 cm
   b) <2.5 cm
   c) <4 cm
   d) <2 cm

9. Ultrasound in the first trimester is used to identify all except:
   a) Intrauterine pregnancy
   b) Confirm cardiac activity\viability
   c) To measure nuchal translucency for Down syndrome
   d) For fetal anomaly

10. Which of the following is used to assess fetal well-being?
    a) Biophysical profile
    b) Measuring BPD
    c) Measuring AC
    d) Measuring FL

11. In which of the following conditions is polyhydramnios seen?
    a) Renal agenesis
    b) Maternal DM
    c) Urethral stenosis
    d) IUGR

Answers
1. (b), 2. (d), 3. (d), 4. (d), 5. (a), 6. (b), 7. (d), 8. (b), 9. (d), 10. (a), 11. (b)

Fill in the blanks

1. Systematic screening for fetal anomalies in the second trimester is done between _____ weeks of gestation.
2. The earliest ultrasound confirmation of intrauterine pregnancy is the demonstration of the _____.
3. The normal value for amniotic fluid index is _____.
4. The double bubble sign is seen in _____.

Answers
1. 18–20 weeks, 2. intrauterine gestational sac, 3. 5–24, 4. duodenal atresia

Case-scenario based discussion

1. A 28-year-old gravida 2, para 1, live 1 presents at 10 weeks of gestation for antenatal booking. While taking her obstetric history, she reveals that she had a spontaneous preterm birth at 32 weeks of gestation and that there were no known risk factors.
   a) This woman is at high risk for what complication?
   b) What information should one look for in the first-trimester USG?
   c) What screening method should be adopted to predict preterm labour in this woman?
   d) If a bicornuate uterus was diagnosed in the first trimester of pregnancy, what measure should be taken?

Answers
a) The risk of recurrent preterm delivery is very high in this woman.
b) One should look for Müllerian anomalies such as bicornuate uterus.
c) She should be screened by transvaginal USG for cervical length at 16–24 weeks of gestation. A cervical length of <25 mm is indicative of a short cervix.
d) As a bicornuate uterus may be associated with cervical incompetence, this woman may need cervical encirclage.

11

OG 8.3, OG 8.8, OG 16.3

Antepartum Fetal Surveillance: Tests of Fetal Well-Being

Learning Objectives

» To describe the indications for antepartum surveillance
» To describe the methods to assess the well-being of the fetus in utero

---

DEFINITION AND GOAL

Antenatal fetal assessment is the assessment of fetal well-being in utero before the onset of labour. The goal of antenatal fetal surveillance is to identify fetuses at risk of intrauterine hypoxia and acidosis early, so that timely intervention and delivery can be undertaken to prevent fetal death. At the same time, antenatal assessment helps in identifying normal fetuses so that unnecessary interventions can be avoided.

Certain maternal factors, fetal factors and some complications of pregnancy have been shown to increase the risk of fetal hypoxia. Early detection of antenatal fetal hypoxia is helpful for timely intervention and prevention of fetal loss. Usually, antepartum fetal surveillance is performed in pregnancies with a high risk of antepartum fetal death. These tests depend upon fetal activities like breathing movement, fetal movement, amniotic fluid production and fetal heart rate.

Indications for fetal surveillance

Maternal indications:
- Hypertension
- Type I diabetes, GDM
- Chronic renal disease
- Febrile illness
- Rh isoimmunisation
- Antepartum hemorrhage and placental abnormalities
- APLA, sickle cell disease
- Postdated pregnancy
- PROM

Fetal indications:
- IUGR
- Oligohydramnios and polyhydramnios
- Decreased fetal movement in high-risk and normal pregnancy
- Multiple pregnancy
- Previous stillbirth, neonatal deaths

TIMING OF ANTENATAL FETAL ASSESSMENT

- Antenatal fetal assessment should be initiated only when the estimated fetal maturity is sufficient to expect a reasonable chance of survival in case delivery becomes necessary. The timing also varies depending on the underlying risk factor and indication. The frequency of investigations varies depending on the indication.
- In women presenting with reduced or absent fetal movements, immediate assessment is mandatory.
- In women with multiple pregnancy (dizygotic twins), Rh-incompatibility or medical disorders such as pre-eclampsia/GDM, the assessment should start at 28–32 weeks of gestation. Monozygotic twins are monitored from the period of viability.
- In those with previous stillbirths, the evaluation should start 2–3 weeks prior to the time of occurrence of the previous adverse event.
- PPROM and FGR fetuses are evaluated at the time of diagnosis.
- In women who have crossed the EDD, the surveillance starts at 40 weeks.

TESTS FOR FETAL WELL-BEING

- Fetal movement counting
- Non-stress test
- Fetal breathing
- Amniotic fluid volume

FETAL MOVEMENT COUNTING (KICK CHART)

Normal Fetal Movements

Normally, fetuses move about 10 times per hour, more so in the evening. They may have rest cycles lasting for 40 minutes each. In the event of fetal hypoxia, due to placental insufficiency, the fetus reduces its activity to conserve oxygen consumption. This is perceived as reduced or absent fetal movement by the mother. Cessation of fetal movement is the last event, and it occurs 24–48 hours before fetal demise. If 10 movements are not felt by the mother in a 12-hour period, investigations should be initiated. Fetal movements can be either counted by the pregnant woman or they can be visualised with real-time ultrasound.

Methods of Counting Fetal Movements

Cardiff count-to-ten

The pregnant woman is asked to count fetal movements starting at a fixed time every day. The time at which she perceives the 10th movement every day is noted. There should be at least 10 movements in 12 hours. If there are <10 movements in a 12-hour period, the woman should be advised to report immediately. The perception of less than four movements in a 24-hour period is called a 'fetal alarm signal' and indicates that fetal demise is imminent. The appropriate intervention should be performed in such cases.

Counting in four blocks

Alternatively, a 12-hour period can be divided into four blocks. Fetal movement is counted for the first one hour during each block. The number of fetal movements counted is multiplied by four to arrive at the movements in 12 hours.

Counting fetal movements for one hour every day

A pregnant woman may find it cumbersome to count fetal movements for a prolonged period or repeatedly. As an alternative, she may be asked to count the movements for one hour every day. The perception of 3–4 fetal movements in a 1-hour period is reassuring.

Advantages

- It is a non-invasive, inexpensive test in which the woman can monitor her own fetus.
- Even low-risk women are advised to monitor their babies using a kick chart nearing delivery.

Limitations

- Maternal obesity, hydramnios, placental localisation (anterior placenta) and the use of medications by the woman may modify the perception of fetal movements.
- It also depends on the woman's focused attention. Therefore, women should be given clear instructions on how to count fetal movements.

Evaluation of reduced fetal movement

- When a woman presents with reduced fetal movement, the well-being of the fetus should be evaluated.
- This is done by using cardiotocography to assess fetal heart rate and its reactivity to fetal movements and USG to demonstrate fetal movement and assess the amniotic fluid volume.

■ NON-STRESS TEST (NST)

The non-stress test is a non-invasive way of assessing the well-being of the fetus in utero. The fetus is evaluated by cardiotocography (CTG) for fetal heart rate and its reactivity to fetal movements.

Cardiotocography (CTG)

Continuous electronic recording of fetal heart rate is called CTG. The cardiac function of the fetus is controlled by the parasympathetic and sympathetic systems. Normal physiological events such as fetal movements, uterine contractions and stimulation as well as adverse events such as fetal hypoxia alter the sympathetic and parasympathetic activity, which manifests as fetal heart rate changes. The fetal heart rate changes are recorded using an abdominal transducer; this is called external cardiotocography. CTG also records uterine contractions in labour. The machine also has a button (event marker) that the woman can press whenever she feels a fetal movement (Fig. 11.1).

Technique

- A transabdominal Doppler ultrasonic transducer is used to record the fetal heart rate while a tocodynamometer is applied to detect uterine contractions at the same time.
- The non-stress test is carried out for 20–40 minutes.
- The pregnant woman is given an event marker to mark every time the fetus moves.

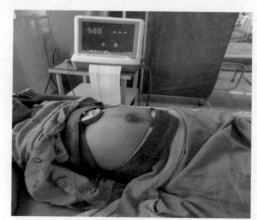

Fig. 11.1 CTG machine in use

- The response of the fetal heart rate (FHR) to fetal movement forms the basis of the NST.

The components of CTG

Baseline heart rate

The normal baseline heart rate is 110–160 beats/minute (bpm) depending on the gestational age. The baseline heart rate indicates the balance between the sympathetic and parasympathetic systems controlling the fetal heart. In mature fetuses, the heart beats at lower rates—usually <130–140 bpm—indicating the maturity of the parasympathetic system; in preterm fetuses, the control of the sympathetic system predominates, resulting in a heart rate >140 bpm.

- When the baseline heart rate is <110 bpm, it is called **bradycardia**. During the antenatal period, bradycardia is rare. It may be seen in a case of a congenital heart block or when there is an abruption.
- When the baseline heart rate is >160 bpm, it is called fetal **tachycardia**. During the antenatal period, it is seen in association with maternal fever, hyperthyroidism, fetal anemia or arrhythmia.

Variability

The fetal heart rate is not fixed and keeps fluctuating above and below the baseline for 5–25 beats. This is called variability. A number of conditions such as fetal hypoxia, CNS depressants, fetal sleep cycles, congenital anomalies, prematurity or fetal tachycardia can reduce this variability. If the variability is between 6–10, it is reduced, and if it is <5, it is silent. Variability of >25 beats is also abnormal as may be seen in acute hypoxia. Baseline variability rather than baseline rate is the best indicator of fetal well-being.

Accelerations

Acceleration is an abrupt increase in the FHR from the baseline. The heart rate increases >15 bpm above baseline for >15 seconds and then comes back to the baseline rates.

- In response to a fetal movement or a stimulus such as acoustic stimulation, a healthy fetus shows at least two accelerations within a period of 20 minutes; this is called a reactive CTG (Fig. 11.2).
- If accelerations are not noted over 20 minutes, the test can be extended for 40 minutes (Fig. 11.3).
- When there are no fetal movements or FHR accelerations in response to fetal movements for a period of 40 minutes, it is called a non-reactive CTG.

Decelerations

- Decelerations are abrupt falls in the FHR from the baseline (Fig. 11.4).

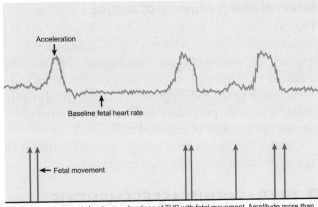

Reactive non-stress test showing accelerations of FHR with fetal movement. Amplitude more than 15 beats per minute, duration longer than 15 seconds.

Fig. 11.2 Reactive NST showing accelerations of FHR with fetal movement—an amplitude of >15 bpm for >15 seconds

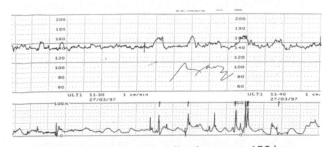

Fig. 11.3 Reactive CTG—baseline heart rate 130 bpm, variability >10 with accelerations with fetal movements and no decelerations

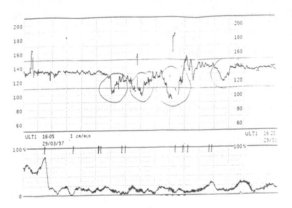

Fig. 11.4 Decelerations with fetal movements

Interpretation of NST

- *Reactive:* A reactive test is the presence of two or more accelerations that peak at 15 bpm or more, each lasting 15 seconds or more, in response to fetal movement. A reactive test indicates that the fetus, at that particular period of testing, is not compromised. In other words, it is a good sign.
- *Non-reactive:* The NST is considered non-reactive if there are no fetal movements or fetal heart accelerations with fetal movements over a period of 40 minutes.

Interval and frequency of testing

The frequency of performing NST depends on the presence/absence of obstetric complications. As a routine, in uncomplicated pregnancies, it may be repeated at an interval of seven days or twice weekly. In women with post-term pregnancy, diabetes, fetal growth restriction and pregnancy-induced hypertension, a non-stress test may be required daily.

Contraction stress tests using oxytocin infusion or nipple stimulation are not used commonly.

ULTRASOUND ASSESSMENT OF FETAL WELL-BEING

Fetal Breathing Movement

This is assessed by USG. Two types of fetal breathing movements have been described, which are as follows:

1. **Gasps**: These occur at a frequency of 1–4 per minute.
2. **Irregular bursts**: These occur at a frequency of 240 per minute.

Fetal breathing movements show a diurnal variation and are reduced at night. These movements are increased after maternal meals.

Fetal hypoxia leads to the diminution or absence of breathing movements. In addition, labour, hypoglycemia, sound stimuli and cigarette smoking also affect these movements. Because of the multiplicity of factors that affect fetal breathing, its role as a marker of fetal health is not clear. It is therefore used in conjunction with other variables as a component of the biophysical profile.

Amniotic Fluid Volume

Decreased uteroplacental perfusion leads to decreased fetal renal blood flow, decreased urine output, and thereby, oligohydramnios. Thus, the assessment of amniotic fluid by USG has become an integral part of antepartum fetal surveillance. The methods to measure amniotic fluid volume (Fig. 11.5) include measurement of the largest vertical pocket and amniotic fluid index (the sum of the largest vertical pockets in the four quadrants).

Oligohydramnios is defined as an amniotic fluid index (AFI) of less than 5.0 cm. If AFI is 5–8 cm, oligohydramnios should be suspected. AFI of 8–24 cm is normal, and AFI of >25 cm indicates **polyhydramnios.**

BIOPHYSICAL PROFILE

A combination of five fetal biophysical variables to assess fetal health was found to be better than any of them used alone. This combination was designated as the biophysical profile by Manning et al.

The following are the variables of the biophysical profile:

1. Fetal heart rate acceleration
2. Fetal breathing
3. Fetal movements
4. Fetal tone
5. Amniotic fluid volume

A normal variable is assigned a score of 2 and an abnormal variable a score of 0. Thus, the highest score possible for a normal fetus is 10. The scores for the various components of the biophysical profile are presented in Table 11.1. The presence of oligohydramnios (largest vertical pocket <2 cm) warrants further evaluation, regardless of the composite score.

The possibility of antepartum death in a structurally normal fetus with a normal biophysical profile is 1 in 1,000. The most common causes of fetal death after a normal biophysical profile are fetal/maternal hemorrhage, umbilical cord accidents and abruptio placentae. The interpretation and management of a pregnancy after arriving at a biophysical profile are as presented in Table 11.2.

MODIFIED BIOPHYSICAL PROFILE

It takes about 30–60 minutes to perform a biophysical profile. A modified biophysical profile, which includes non-stress test and amniotic fluid volume, has been used as the first-line antepartum screening test. This test can be performed in 10 minutes, is associated with good neonatal outcome and is accepted as a means of antepartum fetal surveillance.

DOPPLER STUDY

Doppler studies measure the blood flow in the placental unit and in the fetal blood vessels. They are useful in

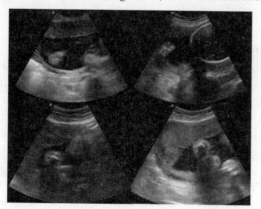

Fig. 11.5 Measurement of AFI (*Image courtesy:* Dr B H Parameshwar Keerthi, BM Scans, Kancheepuram)

Table 11.1 Components and their scores for the biophysical profile

Component	Score 2	Score 0
Non-stress test	>2 accelerations of >15 seconds in 20–40 minutes	0 or 1 acceleration in 20–40 minutes
Fetal breathing	>1 episode if rhythmic breathing lasting >30 seconds within 30 minutes	<30 seconds of breathing in 30 minutes
Fetal movement	>3 discrete body or limb movements within 30 minutes	<2 movements in 30 minutes
Fetal tone	>1 episode of extension of a fetal extremity with return to flexion or opening or closing of hand	No movement or extension/flexion
Largest single vertical pocket	>2 cm	<2 cm

Table 11.2 Biophysical profile score, interpretations and pregnancy management

Biophysical profile score	Interpretation	Recommended management
10	Normal, non-asphyxiated fetus	No fetal indication for intervention, repeat test weekly, except in diabetics and post-term pregnancy (twice weekly)
8/10 normal fluid	Normal, non-asphyxiated fetus	No fetal indication for intervention; repeat testing per protocol
8/10 decreased fluid	Chronic fetal asphyxia suspected	Deliver
6	Possible fetal asphyxia	If amniotic fluid volume abnormal, deliver
		If normal fluid at >36 weeks with favourable cervix, deliver
		If repeat test >6, observe and repeat per protocol
4	Probable fetal asphyxia	Repeat testing same day; if biophysical profile score <6, deliver
0–2	Almost certain fetal asphyxia	Deliver

Note: The recommended management is only suggestive. Management should be case-specific.

differentiating healthy fetuses from hypoxic fetuses, especially in FGR. They are also helpful in deciding the timing of delivery. Arterial Doppler includes uterine artery Doppler, umbilical artery Doppler and middle cerebral artery Doppler. Venous Doppler measures blood flow in the ductus venosus.

- Doppler ultrasonography of the umbilical artery (Fig. 11.6) assesses the blood flow to the fetus via the umbilical artery.
- With normal placental function, in order to maintain the blood flow to the fetus, there is low-resistance flow and even during diastole, there is good flow to the fetus.
- The systolic–diastolic ratio (S/D) is the most commonly used index and is considered abnormal when it is more than the ninety-fifth percentile for the gestational age or if the diastolic flow is either absent or reversed.

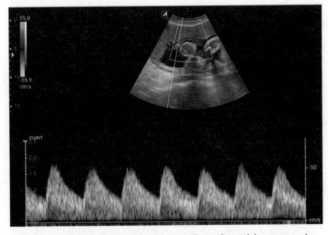

Fig. 11.6 Normal umbilical artery Doppler with sawtooth appearance indicating normal, low-resistance blood flow during systole and diastole (*Image courtesy:* Dr B H Parameshwar Keerthi, BM Scans, Kancheepuram)

- If the impedance to blood flow is increased, all the three indices are increased, followed by absent flow and then reversal of flow.

It has been reported that perinatal mortality for reversed end diastolic flow is approximately 33% and that for absent diastolic flow, it is about 10%. A detailed description of Doppler studies is provided in Chapter 10, *Imaging techniques*.

When the placental resistance increases, the diastolic flow is either absent or reversed (Fig. 11.7). Reversed diastolic flow warrants immediate termination of pregnancy irrespective of the period of gestation.

Middle Cerebral Artery (MCA) Blood Flow

In normal pregnancies, the diastolic flow in the cerebral arteries is lower than that in the umbilical arteries at

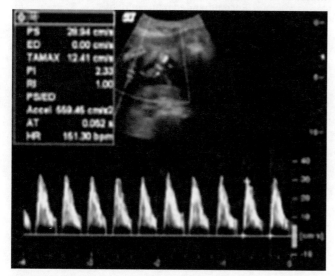

Fig. 11.7 Umbilical artery Doppler with absent diastolic flow

any gestational age. In the presence of fetal hypoxia, in order to maintain the blood flow to the vital organ—the brain—the blood is shunted to the cerebral arteries. This is called the **brain-sparing** effect. Increased diastolic flow in the middle cerebral arteries is an early sign of fetal hypoxia. In normal pregnancy, the pulsatility index of MCA and umbilical artery (MCA/UA) ratio (otherwise called cerebroplacental ratio [CPR]) is greater than 1. The index becomes less than 1 if the flow distribution is in favour of the brain in fetal hypoxia with pathological pregnancies.

Doppler changes develop in a sequential manner. Early changes occur in the peripheral vessels (umbilical and middle cerebral arteries) and late changes include umbilical artery reverse flow, abnormal changes in the ductus venosus and aortic and pulmonary outflow tracts.

Doppler studies have also been shown to be useful to identify at-risk patients for the future development of pre-eclampsia and fetal growth restriction by the identification of a 'notch' of the uterine artery waveform in the second trimester.

ANTENATAL TESTING RECOMMENDATIONS

Of all the tests available for antepartum surveillance, no single test has been found to be the best. The different tests are evaluated depending on the clinical situation. The testing usually begins around 32–34 weeks and is repeated at weekly intervals. However, pregnancies with severe complications might require earlier and more frequent tests.

KEY POINTS

✓ *The goal of antepartum surveillance tests is to identify fetuses at high risk of intrauterine hypoxia and acidosis and to prevent fetal death.*

✓ *These tests depend upon fetal parameters like breathing movements, fetal movement, amniotic fluid production and fetal heart rate.*

✓ *No single test has been found to be superior to the others.*

✓ *Antenatal testing usually begins around 32–34 weeks and is repeated at weekly intervals. However, pregnancies with severe complications might require earlier and more frequent tests.*

Essay question

1. What are the indications for antepartum fetal surveillance? Discuss the techniques used.

Short answer questions

1. Write a short note on fetal movement counting protocols.
2. What are the types of fetal breathing movements?

3. What do you understand by the non-stress test?
4. Describe the components of the biophysical profile.
5. What is the role of umbilical artery Doppler velocimetry?

MCQs

1. Which of the following is not a fetal well-being test?
   a) Non-stress test
   b) Fetal movement count

c)   Amniotic fluid volume
d)   Uterine artery Doppler

2.   How many movements should a pregnant woman perceive in 12 hours to be considered normal as per the Cardiff kick count?
a)   6   b)   8   c)   10   d)   12

3.   Which of these is not required to call a reactive NST?
a)   Variability of ≥5 bpm
b)   ≥2 accelerations
c)   Peak of ≥30 bpm
d)   Duration of acceleration ≥15 seconds

4.   Oligohydramnios is defined as AFI less than which of the following values?
a)   2   b)   5   c)   10   d)   15

5.   Which of the following is not a component of the Manning biophysical score?
a)   Non-stress test
b)   Amniotic fluid volume
c)   Fetal movement
d)   Uterine contractions

6.   Which of the following predicts the risk of future pre-eclampsia?
a)   Uterine artery Doppler
b)   Umbilical artery Doppler
c)   Non-stress test
d)   Biophysical profile

7.   When do you start testing for fetal surveillance antenatally?
a)   20 weeks
b)   32 weeks
c)   34 weeks
d)   37 weeks

Answers
1. (d), 2. (c), 3. (c), 4. (b), 5. (d), 6. (a), 7. (b)

Fill in the blanks

1.   A modified biophysical profile includes a _____ and _____.

2.   Amniotic fluid index of less than 5 is known as _____.

3.   AFI of more than 25 is known as _____.

Answers
1. non-stress test, amniotic fluid volume, 2. oligohydramnios, 3. polyhydramnios

Case scenario-based questions

1.   A primigravida is referred at 32 weeks of gestation with fetal growth restriction. She does not have any antenatal risk factors for FGR.
a)   When would you initiate antenatal fetal surveillance in this case and how would you monitor the well-being of the fetus?
b)   What is a reactive CTG?
c)   What is oligohydramnios?
d)   How is a woman with a normal biophysical profile monitored?

Answers
a) Fetal well-being is monitored by modified biophysical profile immediately.
b) A reactive CTG is one in which there are at least 2 fetal heart rate accelerations in response to a fetal movement or an acoustic stimulation over a period of 20 minutes.
c) AFI of less than 5 is known as oligohydramnios.
d) Biophysical profile is repeated once or twice a week and if necessary, Doppler studies are carried out.

Causation and Stages of Labour

Learning Objectives

» To describe the causes and initiation of labour
» To differentiate true labour pains from false labour pains
» To describe the stages of labour
» To describe the events occurring in the first stage of labour
» To describe uterine contractions and cervical dilatation in labour

DEFINITION OF LABOUR

Labour is the physiologic process by which the fetus, membranes, umbilical cord and placenta are expelled from the uterus. The WHO defines normal labour as follows—'Normal labour is spontaneous in onset, low-risk at the start of labour and remains so throughout labour and delivery. The infant is born spontaneously in the vertex position between 37 and 42 completed weeks of pregnancy. After birth, the mother and infant are in good condition.' Premature or preterm labour refers to labour that sets in before 37 weeks of gestation.

The spontaneous expulsion of the products of conception before the period of viability of the fetus is termed abortion or miscarriage. At present, the period of viability of the fetus is defined as 20 weeks in the USA, 24 weeks in the UK and 24–26 weeks in developing countries including India.

MECHANISM OF LABOUR

In order to understand the mechanism of labour, it is important to understand the architecture of the myometrium, the physiological changes in the uterus during pregnancy and labour, and the factors influencing the initiation of labour.

ARCHITECTURE OF THE MYOMETRIUM

The uterine wall consists of three layers, namely the thin serosa on the outside, the thick myometrium in the middle and the endometrium forming the inner layer.

The Serosa

It is a thin peritoneal layer firmly covering the uterus, extending anteriorly to the uterovesical junction where it becomes loose to form the uterovesical fold of the peritoneum. While performing a cesarean section, this fold is opened to mobilise the bladder down to reach the lower uterine segment. Posteriorly, it is firmly attached to the uterus up to the level of the cervix and then extends as the pouch of Douglas.

The Myometrium

The myometrium is thick and is composed of smooth muscle fibres. This is the most important layer in the mechanism of labour. It is made up of three layers.

* The outer longitudinal layer is thin and lies beneath the serosa and consists of delicate longitudinal fasciculi, which are continuous with the longitudinal layer of the tubes.
* The middle layer is made up of interlacing smooth muscle fibres, through which the blood vessels pass from the external vascular zone to the endometrium. This is the most important layer and plays a major role during labour in contraction and retraction. Following delivery, after the fetus and placenta are expelled, the uterus contracts and retracts and these kinked-up fibres constrict the blood vessels passing through this area. This results in the control of bleeding from the placental bed. Hence, the muscles of this layer are called '**living ligatures**'.
* The inner layer is made up of a thin, circular muscle layer.

The Endometrium

The inner layer is the endometrium or mucosa, which is continuous with the mucosa of the tube and the endocervix.

THE CHARACTERISTIC FEATURES OF UTERINE CONTRACTIONS

The anatomical and physiological features of the myometrial smooth muscles play a major role in the delivery of the fetus.

Contraction and Retraction

- During a uterine contraction, the smooth muscle fibres shorten to a greater extent than the striated muscles. While in the skeletal muscle, the force generated by contraction is always aligned with the axis of the muscle fibres, in the smooth muscle, the contractile force spreads to the adjacent areas also, thereby resulting in the contraction of the uterus.

- The musculature of the upper segment undergoes a type of contraction in which the muscle, after contraction, does not relax to get back to its original length. Instead, it becomes relatively fixed at a shorter length, with the tension remaining the same as before contraction. This is called **retraction**. This ability of the musculature to retract helps to maintain the uterine musculature in firm contact with the intrauterine contents and helps to prevent the fetus from slipping back. As a result of the shortening of the muscle fibres, the upper segment becomes progressively thicker with each contraction throughout the first and second stages of labour and is tremendously thick after the birth of the baby.

- At the same time, the lower segment relaxes and dilates. However, this is not a complete relaxation; rather, it is the opposite of retraction. The fibres of the lower segment become stretched with each contraction of the upper segment and do not subsequently return to their previous length. As a result, they remain relatively fixed at the greater length.

- The lengthening of the muscle fibres of the lower segment is accompanied by the thinning of the lower uterine segment, normally to only a few millimetres. As a result of the thinning of the lower uterine segment and the concomitant thickening of the upper segment, a ridge is formed on the inner uterine walls, which is known as the **physiological retraction ring**.

Polarity of Uterine Contractions

In order to expel the uterine contents, the upper segment should contract and retract, whereas the lower segment including the cervix should dilate to allow the passage of the fetus. This intrinsic property is termed '**polarity**'.

Gradient of Diminishing Physiological Activity

Tocodynamometer studies have shown a diminishing gradient of the strength of uterine contractions, starting from the fundus, through the body and to the lower uterine segment. For labour to progress, the contractions of the fundus must be strong and sustained (fundal dominance), with less strong, simultaneous contractions of the middle zone and relative inactivity of the lower parts. This is called the 'gradient of diminishing physiological activity'. These contractions must also be coordinated and simultaneous.

> **Characteristics of labour contractions**
> - In labour, there is fundal dominance with a diminishing gradient of activity from the fundus through the body to the lower uterine segment.
> - Polarity is maintained.
> - The contractions are accompanied by retractions.

UTERINE CONTRACTIONS DURING PREGNANCY AND LABOUR

- Starting from early pregnancy, uterine contractions known as Braxton Hicks contractions occur, which are painless, irregular and intermittent. These occur after long intervals, last for a shorter period of time than the contractions of true labour and are not associated with the dilatation of the cervix or descent of the presenting part. These contractions do not show any coordination or diminishing gradient. As pregnancy advances, there is a gradual increase in muscle tone and sensitivity. Nearer to term, these contractions become more frequent, regular and coordinated. They last longer and are converted into true labour pains at the onset of labour.

- The uterus has a baseline intrauterine pressure of 5–10 mmHg at term. Any pressure exceeding this will be felt as a contraction on abdominal palpation. Intrauterine pressure exceeding 15 mmHg produces pain.

- In early labour, contractions occur approximately every 3–5 minutes with a pressure of 20–30 mmHg above the resting tone. In active labour, the contractions usually occur every 2–4 minutes with pressures that are 30–50 mmHg above the resting tone. Between contractions, the pressure comes back to the normal base-level tone. With pushing, the pressure may rise to 100–150 mmHg.

- In addition to increased frequency and tone, the duration of contractions lengthens from 30–60 seconds in early labour and to 60–90 seconds at the end of the first stage and in the second stage of labour.

- Contractions are also coordinated by fundal dominance; the upper segment contracts, while the lower segment dilates to receive the presenting part. In normal progressive labour, the contractions of the fundus rise quickly to a maximum and are strong and sustained. The middle zone of the uterus contracts simultaneously, but less intensely and for a shorter time. The lower segment remains inactive, and its tone is low.

- In the second stage of labour, the expulsive pressure of an average uterine contraction amounts to about 7 Kg and the expulsive pressure exerted by the parturient by using the abdominal wall equals to another 7 Kg. Thus, the total expulsive force is 14 Kg. Occasionally, the expulsive force of uterine contractions stimulated by oxytocin reaches 14 Kg or more so that the fetus may, in exceptional cases, receive a total thrust of nearly 23 Kg. In forceps delivery, the average force exerted by traction is said to be about 16 Kg.

▌ RECORDING OF UTERINE ACTIVITY

In routine practice, uterine activity is assessed by the abdominal palpation of contractions. The frequency, baseline tone and the duration of contractions can be recorded using a cardiotocography (CTG) machine. These machines are very useful in induced and augmented labours to diagnose hyperstimulation. Recording of the intrauterine pressure can also be carried out using internal tocography, which involves placing a sensor-tipped catheter inside the uterus. However, this is not a routine method given its invasive nature.

▌ FACTORS INFLUENCING THE INITIATION OF LABOUR (Fig. 12.1)

In pregnancy, there is a balance between the forces that keep the uterus quiescent and those that produce coordinated uterine contractions. There is also a balance between the forces that keep the cervix closed to prevent the premature expulsion of the uterine contents and those that soften and dilate the cervix to allow the expulsion of the products. For delivery to occur, these balances should be in favour of active uterine emptying, and the uterus should be released from the inhibitory effects. For parturition to occur, the two important changes that should take place in the pregnant uterus are as follows:

- First, the pregnant uterus must be converted from a quiescent organ with uncoordinated, irregular and weak contractions to an actively contracting organ with coordinated contractions in labour.
- Secondly, there should be changes in the cervical connective tissue and smooth muscle resulting in the softening and dilatation of the cervix to allow the passage of the fetus from the uterus.

These changes are achieved by coordinated endocrine, biochemical and mechanical events in the fetoplacental and maternal units. The final pathway in the onset of labour is the release of prostaglandins, which occurs following a series of events taking place in the fetus, the placenta and in the mother.

▌ SEQUENCE OF EVENTS FOR THE INITIATION OF LABOUR (Fig. 12.1)

- Shift from progesterone to estrogen dominance
- Increased responsiveness to oxytocin by increasing myometrial oxytocin receptor
- Increased prostaglandin (PG) synthesis in the uterus

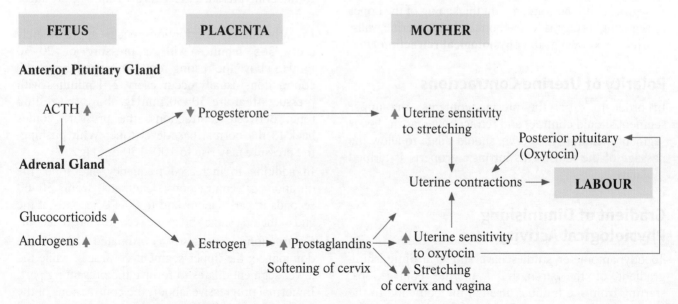

Fig. 12.1 Interaction between fetal, placental and maternal factors in the initiation of labour

- Increased myometrial gap junction formation
- Decreased nitric oxide (NO) activity
- Increased influx of calcium into myocytes inducing myometrial activity

The Fetal Contribution

Studies have shown that the fetus plays an important role in controlling the timing of labour. As the fetus matures, there is activation of the fetal hypothalamic–pituitary–adrenal (HPA) axis, which leads to a surge in adrenal cortisol production. The fetal cortisol acts by producing the following effects:

- It stimulates the activity of placental 17-α-hydroxylase/17,20 lyase enzyme, which catalyses the conversion of pregnenolone to estradiol. As a result, there is an increase in the levels of estrogen, which leads to the synthesis of uterine PG, culminating in labour.
- Fetal cortisol also promotes the expression of a number of placental genes for corticotropin releasing hormone (CRH), oxytocin and prostaglandins. The released CRH enhances prostaglandin production by the amnionic, chorionic and decidual cells. At term, the amnion and chorion, both of which are of fetal origin, occupy a large surface area in the uterine cavity and communicate with the maternal decidua and myometrium. Prostaglandin synthesis occurs in the amnion, chorion and decidua complex.
- Besides, fetal cortisol also prepares the fetal organs (fetal lung maturation) for extrauterine life.
- In women with anencephalic fetuses, the pregnancy is prolonged due to the hypoplastic adrenals.

HORMONAL CHANGES IN THE INITIATION OF LABOUR (TABLE 12.1)

- Progesterone causes the uterus to be quiescent by decreasing the myometrial contractility and inhibiting the formation of the myometrial gap junction. It acts by down-regulating prostaglandin production, oxytocin receptors and calcium channels. Progesterone also stimulates the uterine NO synthetase activity, which is a major factor in uterine quiescence. In the cervix, it maintains cervical integrity by inhibiting collagenase.
- In order to initiate labour, progesterone's effects on the uterus and cervix should be overcome. This is achieved by the alteration of the estrogen/progesterone ratio in favour of estrogen, which is brought about by fetal cortisol production.
- The resultant increase in the levels of estrogen promotes a series of myometrial changes. There is increased production of PGE_2 and $PGF_{2\alpha}$, increased expression of PG and oxytocin receptors and formation of calcium channels. There is also increased synthesis of connexin and gap junction formation in the myometrium.
- Estrogen, in addition to increasing the vascularity and growth of the uterus, induces uterine contractions and sensitises the uterine musculature to the action of oxytocin.

Release of Oxytocin

- The concentration of uterine oxytocin receptors increases towards the end of pregnancy, and estrogen increases. Progesterone suppresses oxytocin receptor expression in myometrial cells.
- Oxytocin release is seen towards the end of labour and is probably required for the final expulsive efforts. Oxytocin induces uterine contractions either by stimulating the release of PGE_2 and prostaglandin $F2_\alpha$ or by directly acting on the myometrial cells, activating the release of calcium from intracellular stores.
- Calcium is necessary for the activation of smooth muscle contraction.

Table 12.1   Role of hormones in labour

Estrogen	Progesterone
• Estrogen lowers the resting potential and increases the contractility of the muscle	• Progesterone raises the membrane potential and makes the muscle quiescent
• Estrogen, along with prostaglandins (PG), stimulates the formation of gap junctions	• Progesterone down-regulates prostaglandin production, oxytocin receptors and calcium channels
• Estrogens have been shown to labilise the intracellular lysosomes and increase the release of the phospholipase A2 enzyme, which is essential for the initiation of prostaglandin synthesis	• Progesterone lowers gap junction formation
• Estrogen increases the formation of oxytocin receptors in the myometrium	

Release of Prostaglandins

- Prostaglandins play an important role in the initiation of labour and delivery. PGE_2 and $PGF2_\alpha$ cause uterine contractions at any stage of pregnancy and also affect cervical softening and effacement. In these respects, PGE_2 is five to ten times more potent than $PGF2_\alpha$.

- Prostaglandins are produced in the placenta and fetal membranes, amnion and chorion from arachidonic acid and are stored as glycerophospholipids. The signal from the fetus stimulates a chain of metabolic reactions that release arachidonic acid from the glycerophospholipids by the activation of the enzyme, phospholipase.

- Prostaglandin levels are increased before and during labour in the uterus and membranes. $PGF2_\alpha$ is produced primarily by the maternal decidua and acts on the myometrium to up-regulate oxytocin receptors and gap junctions, thereby promoting uterine contractions. PGE_2 is primarily of fetoplacental origin and is likely more important in promoting cervical ripening (maturation) associated with collagen degradation and dilatation of the cervix and spontaneous rupture of the fetal membranes. Many factors affect the production of prostaglandins. PG levels are decreased by progesterone and increased by estrogens. Inflammatory factors such as interleukins also result in an increase in prostaglandin production.

> Prostaglandin plays a major role in the formation of gap junctions in the myometrial cells which are essential for coordinated uterine contractions in labour, activation of contractions and cervical ripening.

Formation of Gap Junctions

- Gap junctions are cell-to-cell contacts at the plasma membranes of adjacent cells that have pores that allow communication between the cytoplasm of both cells. They facilitate the passage of currents (electrical or ionic coupling) or metabolites (metabolic coupling) between cells. These gap junctions are absent throughout pregnancy until term. At term, the gap junctions increase, and continue to do so, peaking during labour. They begin to disappear within 24 hours of delivery. Gap junctions are present in preterm, induced and spontaneous labour.

- Prostaglandins are important in the formation of gap junctions (PGE_2, $PGF_{2\alpha}$, thromboxane and endoperoxides stimulate gap junctions, whereas prostacyclin inhibits them).

MECHANICAL FACTORS IN THE INITIATION OF LABOUR

Uterine Distension

It has been shown that as pregnancy nears term, uterine growth slows down, whereas the rate of fetal growth increases. This results in a rapid increase in intrauterine pressure. The resultant tension exerted on the uterine muscle fibres may by itself initiate labour. The myometrial excitability is also increased when the uterus is overdistended due to multiple pregnancy or polyhydramnios, which results in an increase in intrauterine pressure and preterm labour.

Mechanical Stretching

The stretching of the lower uterine segment by the fetal head and the pressure exerted by it on the paracervical nerve ganglia are also implicated as important factors in the onset of labour. This theory is supported by the efficacy of artificial rupture of membranes in the induction of labour at term.

NERVOUS CONTROL OF LABOUR

The uterus is supplied by both sympathetic and parasympathetic nerves. The sympathetic adrenergic nerves travel via the superior and inferior hypogastric plexus. The motor fibres of these nerves appear to be largely inhibitory, for their stimulation produces contractions of the circular muscle fibres and the lower segment.

The parasympathetic nerves travel from the second, third and fourth sacral nerve roots through the inferior hypogastric plexus to reach the uterus. The stimulation of these nerves is said to cause contractions of the uterus.

Though the uterus is richly supplied by the autonomic nervous system, it does not play a major role in the initiation and progression of myometrial contractions. However, nervous control plays a major role in the transmission of labour pains. Uterine contractions result in visceral pain, which is mediated by T10–L1. During descent, the fetal head exerts pressure on the mother's pelvic floor, vagina and perineum, causing somatic pain, which is transmitted by the pudendal nerve (innervated by S2–4).

Adrenaline

A sudden surge of adrenaline release may have an inhibitory effect on uterine contractions and may cause a temporary cessation of labour pain. Emotion or fright adversely affects a woman in labour; this may be due to the flooding of the system with adrenaline as a result of sympathetic stimulation by emotions.

CERVICAL CHANGES IN THE INITIATION OF LABOUR

During pregnancy, the cervix protects the fetus by remaining closed. This prevents ascending infection and also provides resistance to the pressure produced by Braxton Hicks contractions and the upright position. However, nearing labour, the cervix becomes soft, shortens in length (effacement) and dilates prior to the expulsion of the fetus. This process is known as cervical ripening.

The Structure of the Cervix

The cervix is made up of three components, namely smooth muscle, collagen and the connective tissue forming the ground substance.

1. Smooth muscle: The smooth muscle content of the cervix varies from 6–25% and does not play a role in the 'ripening of the cervix' during pregnancy.
2. Collagen
3. Connective tissue: It is the ground substance made up of glycosaminoglycans.

The Process of Cervical Ripening

With ripening, cervical softening and flexibility increase, and collagen and protein concentrations decrease. Glycosaminoglycans (dermatan sulphate and hyaluronic acid) are important in the process of cervical ripening, which is associated with collagen breakdown. The loss of collagen is due to the proteolytic digestion brought about by the action of collagenases. Near term, the relative amount of hyaluronic acid in the cervix increases with a concomitant decrease in dermatan sulphate. The water content of the cervix also increases. These changes are brought about by a decrease in progesterone levels and the action of prostaglandins and relaxin, leading to connective tissue alterations and the breakdown of collagen.

PREGNANCY MAINTENANCE/ TERMINATION FACTORS

Factors involved in the maintenance of pregnancy
- Myometrial growth and increased myometrial compliance to accommodate the growing fetus
- Increased placental progesterone
- Resistance offered by the cervix due to the collagen content

Factors that bring about termination of pregnancy
- Increasing uterine volume
- Decrease of placental progesterone along with estrogen dominance
- Increase in prostaglandins and oxytocin receptors
- Cervical ripening due to decreasing collagen content

STAGES OF LABOUR

The labour process may be divided into the prelabour and labour stages.

Prelabour

Prelabour is referred to as the period of increased uterine activity that takes place a few weeks before the onset of labour and is associated with some cervical softening and effacement, and slight to modest cervical dilatation. This preparatory stage of labour may begin about two or three weeks before the onset of labour in a primigravida and a few days before in a multigravida.

The events comprising the prelabour stage are as follows:
- Cervical ripening
- Descent of the fetal head into the pelvis

The descending fetal head exerts pressure on the bladder. This results in increased frequency of micturition. When the head descends, the pressure on the diaphragm is relieved and the woman feels light—this is called '**lightening**'. On examination, the falling forward of the uterus and **shelving** (ability to insinuate a hand behind the fundus) can be demonstrated. During this time, the engagement of the fetal head may take place in a primigravida.

Labour

Labour is characterised by uterine contractions that bring about demonstrable effacement and progressive dilatation of the cervix, culminating in labour.

The following events take place in this stage:
- Strong uterine contractions
- Progressive dilatation of the cervix

- Bloodstained show
- Rupture of the membranes
- Descent of the presenting part

True and False Labour Pains

In women presenting with labour pains, true labour pains should be differentiated from false labour pains.

False pains are more often caused by temporary indigestion or by a loaded rectum (Table 12.2); a relatively strong Braxton Hicks contraction may also be interpreted as pain. These pains are relieved by either a laxative or an enema. They are distinguished from true labour pains by their temporary character, irregularity, and the fact that they are generally felt over the abdomen instead of in the lumbosacral region or just above the pubis. They do not progress, are not associated with progressive uterine contractions or cervical dilatation. 'False' or spurious labour pains are seen more frequently in primigravidas than in multiparas.

Braxton Hicks contractions must be differentiated from true contractions. Typical features of Braxton Hicks contractions are as follows:

- Usually occur no more than a few times per day
- Irregular and do not increase in frequency with increasing intensity
- Resolve with ambulation or a change in activity

On the other hand, the contractions that lead to labour have the following characteristics:

- May start as infrequently as every 10–15 minutes, but usually accelerate over time, increasing to contractions that occur every 2–3 minutes
- Tend to last longer and are more intense than Braxton Hicks contractions
- Lead to cervical changes

Table 12.2 differentiates between true and false labour pain.

True Labour

With the onset of true labour pains, labour is divided into three stages, which are as follows:

1. The first stage or the stage of dilatation
2. The second stage or the stage of expulsion
3. The third stage or the stage of placental delivery and uterine contraction and retraction

Besides the three classic stages, a fourth stage of labour is also described—the two hours that follow placental expulsion, during which there is effective myometrial contraction and retraction along with vessel thrombosis to control bleeding from the placental site.

The first stage of labour

The first stage begins with regular uterine contractions and ends with complete cervical dilatation at 10 cm. The duration of the first stage is variable; on an average, it extends to about 12 hours in a primigravida, while in a multigravida, the average is about 6–8 hours. The first stage of labour is divided into a latent phase and an active phase.

- The latent phase of labour precedes the active phase by several hours and is associated with discomfort and mild and irregular uterine contractions that soften and shorten the cervix, resulting in cervical dilatation of up to 4 cm (5 cm according to recent guidelines).
- In the active phase, the contractions become progressively more rhythmic and stronger, starting at about 4 cm of cervical dilation (6 cm as per recent guidelines), This phase is characterised by rapid

Table 12.2 Differences between true and false labour pain

True labour pain	False labour pain (Braxton Hicks contractions)
The contractions are regular and persistent and gradually increase in frequency, duration and strength	The contractions are irregular and stop on lying down or walking; they do not increase in frequency or duration
	The contractions subside altogether on changing the position or on taking fluids.
The pain begins in the lower back and spreads to the abdomen; it may also radiate to the top of the legs	The pain is centred in the lower abdomen rather than the lower back
Show is present and is either pinkish or bloodstained	Show is usually not present and if at all present, it is brownish rather than pinkish
Membranes are likely to rupture	Membranes are intact
The membranes release a colourless fluid or 'waters' ('waters broken')	
Associated with cervical changes	Not associated with cervical changes

cervical dilatation and descent of the presenting fetal part.

The events comprising the first stage are as follows:

A. Uterine contractions

Uterine contractions or true labour pains occur at intervals of half an hour at the commencement of the first stage, but gradually become more frequent. By the end of the first stage, they may occur every three minutes. Each contraction lasts for about 45–60 seconds, and at the end of the first stage of labour, for as long as 60–90 seconds. Between contractions, the uterus relaxes. Each contraction gradually increases in intensity until it reaches an acme, and then diminishes in intensity.

Intrauterine pressure

The uterus has a baseline intrauterine pressure of 5–10 mmHg in early labour. Any pressure exceeding this is felt as a contraction on abdominal palpation. Pain is felt by the woman if the intrauterine pressure exceeds 15–20 mmHg. In early labour, contractions occur approximately every 5–10 minutes, with a pressure of 20–30 mmHg above resting tone. In active labour, contractions usually occur every 2–4 minutes with pressures 30–50 mmHg above resting tone. In between contractions, the pressure comes back to normal base-level tone.

Nature of labour pain

The labour pains are initially felt in the lower back, in the region of the sacrum, but may later radiate to the lower abdomen, and sometimes down the legs. In some cases, they may be associated with a feeling of nausea or actual vomiting, and urine may be passed frequently. Uterine contractions are involuntary and independent of extrauterine control.

B. Formation of the lower uterine segment

The lower uterine segment is developed from the isthmus and is defined as the portion of the non-pregnant uterus situated between the anatomical internal os and the histological internal os, the former being higher. This area is said to grow and stretch during pregnancy. The lower segment starts to form around 28 weeks of gestation. At term, it measures 7–10 cm and develops from the isthmus and the effaced and dilated cervix (Fig. 12.2).

The lower segment is formed by the retraction of the upper segment, which pulls up and thins out the intervening tissue between itself and the fixed cervix. The thinning of the lower segment that occurs in labour is due to the downward and outward thrust of the descending fetus. The upper margin of the lower segment is at about the level of the upper border of the symphysis pubis in late pregnancy and is indicated roughly by the line of close attachment of the uterovesical fold of the peritoneum on the uterus.

Lower segment in labour

During labour, under the influence of uterine contractions, the uterus gradually becomes differentiated into two distinct portions. The upper segment is thicker and more active and becomes progressively thicker as labour advances. The lower portion, that is, the lower segment with the cervix, is passive and becomes thinner and stretched out to receive the descending fetus as labour advances.

The junction between the upper and lower segments is characterised by a ring of circular muscle fibres, the so-called **physiologic retraction ring or Bandl's ring**. Above this level is the contracting thick upper segment, and below, the dilatating and stretching lower segment and cervix. This ring becomes prominent in obstructed labour.

C. Cervical changes

Cervical effacement

Cervical effacement is the progressive shortening of the cervical canal until it becomes a thin, circular opening at the external os. During the process of effacement, the cervix is incorporated into the lower segment.

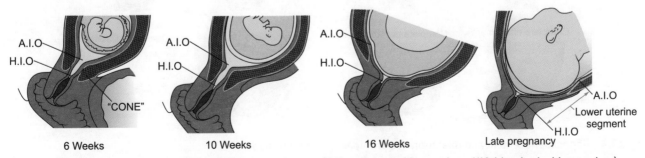

Fig. 12.2 Formation of the lower segment in late pregnancy (*AIO*, anatomical internal os; *HIO*, histological internal os)

Effacement takes place from above downwards. In a primigravida, the effacement starts even prior to labour, whereas in a multigravida both dilatation and effacement occur simultaneously.

Dilatation of the cervix

Dilatation of the cervix is the result of the contracting and retracting upper segment. It results in the lifting up and thinning out of the lower segment, and ultimately, the pulling of the cervix over the advancing presenting part without significantly altering the level of the external os in the pelvis. A well-fitting presenting part favours good uterine action and smooth dilatation of the cervix. The uterine contractions exerting pressure on the membranes and the hydrostatic action of the amniotic fluid also facilitate the dilatation of the cervical canal (Fig. 12.3).

The bag of forewaters is not essential to the process of the dilatation of the cervix. After the rupture of the membranes, the pressure exerted by the presenting part on the cervix induces reflex uterine contractions, which are more powerful than they are before the rupture of the membranes. This aids in more rapid dilatation. The dilatation of the external os, therefore, depends not only on the strong and coordinated action of the muscles, but on its own capacity to soften and stretch. This, in turn, depends on its intrinsic development and on its preparation during pregnancy. Estrogen and progesterone play a part in this preparation. Prostaglandins also play an important role.

The process of cervical dilatation

The process of cervical dilatation differs somewhat between a primipara and a multipara. At the commencement of labour in a primipara, the entire cervical canal is closed, with both the internal and external os being occluded. The dilatation occurs progressively from above downwards, the internal os dilating first, then the cervical canal, and last of all, the external os. In a multipara, on the other hand, at the commencement of labour, the external os is patulous, usually admitting one finger freely, sometimes more. The internal os is not quite completely occluded as in a primigravida. The process of dilatation, therefore, is a little more rapid and easier, so much so, that the dilatation of the internal os brings about a simultaneous dilatation of the entire cervical canal (Fig.12.4).

Pattern of cervical dilatation

Friedman explained that the cervical dilatation that takes place during labour, if plotted against time, takes the shape of a sigmoid curve (Fig. 12.5). The cervical dilatation curve can be divided into the following parts:

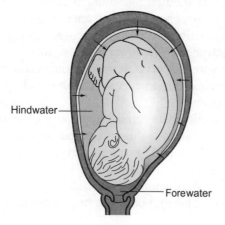

Fig. 12.3 Fore and hindwaters

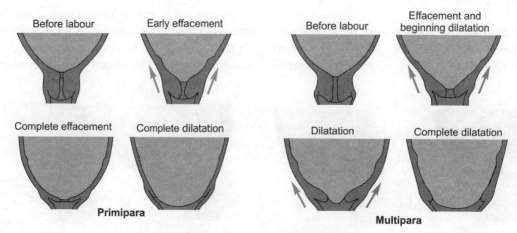

Fig. 12.4 Cervical effacement and dilatation in a primipara and a multipara

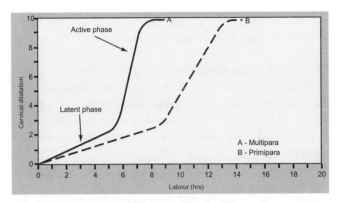

Fig. 12.5 First stage of labour: Friedman's curve

1. A relatively flat latent phase
2. A rapidly progressing active phase
   — The duration of the latent phase is variable; it precedes the active phase by several hours and is associated with cervical dilatation of up to 4 cm (5 cm according to recent guidelines). This stage is susceptible to factors like sedation and anesthesia.
   — The active phase is subdivided into the acceleration phase, during which the cervical dilatation begins to increase; the phase of maximum slope, in which there is rapid dilatation of the cervix; and the deceleration phase, during which there is slowing down of the cervical dilatation. The outcome of labour is determined by the characteristics of the acceleration phase. In the active phase of labour, the cervix is expected to dilate at a rate of 1 cm/hour.

D. Mucosanguineous bloodstained discharge or 'show'

With cervical effacement and dilatation, the mucus in the cervical canal separates and is passed. This mucus is bloodstained due to the disruption of the capillaries. This blood-tinged mucus is called 'show'. The presence of show is the evidence of cervical dilatation and effacement, and frequently, the descent of the presenting part.

E. Rupture of membranes

The spontaneous rupture of membranes usually occurs during the course of active labour. It manifests as a sudden gush of nearly colourless fluid. During labour, the stretching of the lower segment results in the detachment of the membranes from the decidua, which bulges into the cervical canal as the cervix dilates. Due to the pressure exerted by the uterine contractions, it becomes tense and dilates the cervical canal. With the increasing hydrostatic pressure, the membrane eventually ruptures. In vertex presentation, as the head fits well into the lower segment, the membrane is well-applied to the head. Whereas, in malpresentations, the membrane will be hanging loose.

F. Fetal descent

In nulliparas, the engagement of the fetal head usually takes place before the onset of labour. Non-fixation of the head in cephalic presentation suggests the possibility of abnormalities. Active descent occurs during the phase of maximum slope of cervical dilatation and continues in the second stage of labour until the head reaches the perineum.

The second stage of labour

The second stage is the stage of expulsion and extends from the complete dilatation of the cervix to the expulsion of the fetus or fetuses. This stage may last from one to two hours in a primigravida, and from half to one hour in a multipara. If regional anesthesia is used for pain relief, the duration of the second stage may be 2–3 hours in primigravidae and 1–2 hours in multis.

- The second stage of labour is divided into the pelvic phase and the perineal phase. In the pelvic phase, the fetal head reaches the pelvic floor, and the maximum fetal descent occurs. In the perineal phase, bearing down contractions occur, and the head reaches the perineum.

- The nature of the uterine contractions gradually changes, getting stronger in the second stage, occurring every 2–3 minutes and lasting from 60–90 seconds. They are more severe than in the first stage and are of a 'bearing down' character. The voluntary muscles, the accessory muscles of labour also begin to contract and exert their influence towards the end of the second stage. The diaphragm and the abdominal muscles begin to act. With pushing, the intrauterine pressure may rise to 100–150 mmHg.

- With each of these contractions, the fetus is pushed further down through the dilated cervical canal, and the vagina relaxes and dilates to receive it. When the fetal head reaches the perineum, it stretches, so that it begins to bulge with each uterine contraction.

- When the head reaches the perineum, the vulva begins to widen, exposing the fetal head. The term '**crowning of the head**' is used when the maximum transverse diameter of the fetal head stretches the vulval outlet and does not recede between contractions. At this stage, the woman feels an inclination to micturate and defecate. This is due to the pressure of the presenting part on the bladder and rectum.

- Finally, the head passes through the outlet, with a series of almost continuous uterine contractions, helped by involuntary straining efforts on the part of the woman due to the action of the accessory muscles of labour. As the expulsion of the head takes place, the woman exerts one last effort, delivering the rest of the fetus.

The third stage of labour

- The third stage is the stage of placental delivery, which is very important and should be carefully managed. This extends from the complete expulsion of the fetus to the complete expulsion of the placenta and membranes, and firm contraction and retraction of the uterus subsequently. The average duration of this stage, when spontaneously completed, may extend from a few minutes to fifteen minutes.
- The third stage of labour is considered prolonged if the placental delivery does not take place in 30 minutes. In such cases, active interventions should be undertaken.

Events occurring in the third stage of labour

- Characteristic uterine contractions
- Separation of the placenta
- Expulsion of the placenta
- Control of hemorrhage
- Permanent contraction and retraction of the uterus

Uterine contractions
After the completion of the second stage, the uterus is almost at the level of the umbilicus, and is firm, round and hard. Rhythmic contractions occur at this time, and the woman may sometimes feel pain.

Placental detachment
As the fetus is being delivered, the separation of the placenta may take place. The shrinkage of the placental site and the forcing downward of the entire placental mass by uterine contractions may cause this separation.

There are two methods by which placental separation and expulsion may occur.

1. *Duncan's method:* Due to the contractions of the uterus, the placenta may fold on itself, the separation beginning at the periphery. The placenta descends sidewards so that the long axis of the placenta corresponds to the long axis of the uterus, and the lower margin of the placenta presents at the cervix or vagina (Fig. 12.6).

2. *Schultze's method:* In this method, the placenta separates at its centre (Fig. 12.7). Due to the separation, retroplacental hematoma develops which, with each contraction of the uterus, forces more of the placenta to separate. The placenta thus separated presents itself at the vaginal outlet, with the centre of its fetal surface with the attached cord, like an inverted umbrella. It is of little significance as to which method of separation is responsible for the final delivery.

Expulsion of the placenta
This usually occurs within a few minutes after the birth of the fetus. During this period, the uterus should be moderately hard in terms of tonicity, so that when the placenta separates, the contractions and retractions of the uterus arrest hemorrhage by closure of the placental sinuses.

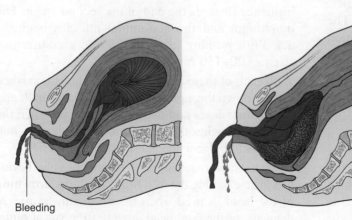
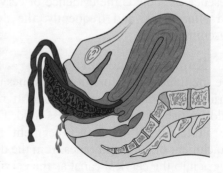

Bleeding

Fig. 12.6 Mechanism of expulsion of the placenta—Duncan's method

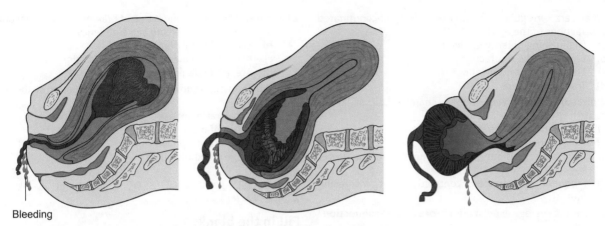

Fig, 12.7 Mechanism of expulsion of the placenta—Schultze's method

Control of hemorrhage

After the separation and expulsion of the placenta, the control of hemorrhage is due to three factors, which are as follows:

1. Contraction and retraction of the uterus, causing the constriction of the vessels passing through the uterine wall to the placental site
2. Occlusion of the torn vessels themselves
3. Formation of blood clots, which favour the closure of the lumen of the vessels

During the third stage and immediately after, there is always a moderate amount of bleeding, which normally does not exceed 250 mL. Following labour, the woman may occasionally have an episode of rigor, which is a purely vasomotor phenomenon and is not indicative of infection; this is generally of no particular significance. It is termed 'physiological chill' (apyrexial shivering).

KEY POINTS

✓ *Labour is the physiologic process by which the fetus, placenta, umbilical cord and membranes are expelled from the uterus.*

✓ *The initiation of labour is brought about by a complex dynamic interaction of the endocrine, biochemical and mechanical factors of the fetal, placental and maternal units.*

✓ *For labour to occur, the quiescent pregnant uterus must be converted to one capable of actively contracting. Cervical changes such as softening and dilatation should also take place.*

✓ *Labour is divided into three stages, the first stage—the stage of dilatation; the second stage—the stage of expulsion and the third stage—the stage of placental delivery.*

✓ *The first stage of labour extends from the onset of true labour pains to full cervical dilatation.*

✓ *The events taking place in the first stage of labour are effective uterine contractions, cervical dilatation, formation of the lower segment, show, rupture of membranes and descent of the fetal head.*

✓ *The second stage is the stage of expulsion and extends from full cervical dilatation to the delivery of the fetus.*

✓ *The third stage is a stage of placental expulsion extending from the delivery of the fetus to the delivery of the placenta.*

Essay questions

1. Discuss the causes and initiation of labour.
2. Describe the events that comprise the first stage of labour?

Short answer questions

1. Define 'normal labour'
2. What do you understand by cervical ripening?
3. What are gap junctions?
4. Describe the methods of placental expulsion.
5. Write a short note on hormonal control of uterine action.

6. Describe the pattern of cervical dilatation during the first stage of labour.
7. Differentiate between true and false labour pains.

MCQs

1. Which of these terms is NOT included in the WHO's definition of normal labour?
   a) Induction of labour
   b) Low risk
   c) Vertex presentation
   d) 37–42 weeks gestation

2. What are irregular, intermittent and uncoordinated contractions of the uterus called?
   a) Diminishing polarity gradient
   b) Braxton Hicks contractions
   c) Threatened preterm labour
   d) True labour pains

3. Which of the following is not a characteristic of labour pain?
   a) Contraction and retraction
   b) Fundal dominance
   c) Increasing gradient from the fundus to the lower segment
   d) Frequent coordinated contractions of increasing intensity

4. What is the average expulsive force of a uterine contraction?
   a) 7 Kg
   b) 14 Kg
   c) 16 Kg
   d) 23 Kg

5. Which of the following changes are not noticed in labour?
   a) Increased dermatan sulphate and decreased hyaluronic acid in the cervix
   b) Breakdown of cervical collagen by collagenase
   c) Release of arachidonic acid from the amnion elicited by the fetus
   d) Formation of gap junctions in the myometrium

6. Which of these is not noted in the first stage of labour?
   a) Uterine contractions
   b) Discharge of show
   c) Rupture of membranes
   d) Crowning of the head

7. Which is not true of cervical dilatation?
   a) Controlled by uterine contractions and hormones
   b) Progressive from below upwards with patulous external os
   c) Explained by the Friedman curve
   d) Acceleration phase determines the duration of labour

8. Which of these do not determine the progress of labour?
   a) Cervical dilatation
   b) Uterine contraction
   c) Rupture of membranes
   d) Fetal heart rate

9. Which of the following is not noted in the third stage of labour?
   a) Uterine contraction
   b) Separation of the placenta
   c) Routine manual removal of the placenta
   d) Physiological chill after delivery

10. Which of the following is NOT a parameter to assess the progress of labour?
    a) Cervical dilatation
    b) Descent of fetus
    c) Fetal heart rate
    d) Uterine contractions

11. Which of the following is true of Braxton Hicks contractions?
    a) Irregular in intensity and frequency
    b) Exhibit fundal dominance
    c) Are accompanied by cervical dilatation
    d) Are accompanied by retraction

12. Which of the following is NOT a component of the active phase?
    a) Acceleration phase
    b) Phase of maximum slope
    c) Deceleration phase
    d) Stage of expulsion

Answers
1. (a), 2. (b), 3. (c), 4. (a), 5. (a), 6. (d), 7. (b), 8. (d), 9. (c), 10. (c), 11. (a), 12. (d)

Fill in the blanks

1. The process of the cervix becoming soft, yielding and more easily dilatable before the onset of labour is called _____.

2. During labour, the thinning of the lower uterine segment and the thickening of the upper segment lead to the formation of a ridge known as the _____.

3. The irregular, intermittent and painless uterine contractions that occur during pregnancy are known as _____.

Answers
1. cervical ripening, 2. physiological retraction ring, 3. Braxton Hicks contractions

Case scenario-based discussion

1. A 24-year-old primigravida is seen in the casualty at 38 weeks of gestation with pains. On examination, she has contractions once in 10 minutes, each lasting for 15 seconds and the head is 4/5th palpable per abdomen. The fetal heart rate is good. On vaginal examination, the cervix is soft, at mid-position, about 2 cm long and admitting a finger. The head is above the brim. There is no discharge per vaginum.
   a) Is this woman experiencing true labour pain?
   b) When would you expect her to go into active labour?
   c) What is the rate of cervical dilatation you expect in this woman?
   d) How would you diagnose engagement of the fetal head?

Answers
Answers
a) As the contractions are weak and accompanied by some cervical changes, this woman may be in the latent phase of labour or false labour. This woman should be observed for 2–4 hours for progressive cervical changes which would indicate true labour.

b) The woman will enter into the active phase of labour at a cervical dilatation of 4 cm.

c) Since she is a primigravida, her cervix should dilate at least 1 cm per hour.

d) By abdominal palpation, the head should be 1/5th palpable with only the sinciput felt; the occiput should not be felt. On vaginal examination, the denominator, the occiput should be at or below the level of the ischial spines.

The Mechanism of Labour

Learning Objectives

» To know the cardinal movements of the fetus in labour
» To describe engagement and its different types
» To know the mechanism of labour in occipitoanterior presentation

INTRODUCTION

The mechanism of labour is defined as the process by which the fetus adjusts itself to the pelvic architecture and manoeuvres itself through the parturient canal with minimal difficulty to achieve a safe vaginal delivery. If this process of adjustment is arrested at any stage, then labour does not progress as expected.

THE CARDINAL MOVEMENTS OF THE FETUS

In the mechanism of labour, the fetus undergoes certain positional movements to pass through the maternal pelvis. These are called the cardinal movements, and comprise the following:

- Engagement
- Descent
- Flexion
- Internal rotation
- Extension
- Restitution
- External rotation
- Expulsion

All these movements occur simultaneously; however, for the sake of clarity, they are described separately here.

The following three factors influence labour:

1. The pelvis and soft parts—the passage
2. The fetus—the passenger
3. The uterine forces—the force

Variations from the normal in any of these factors may affect the mechanism of labour.

MECHANISM OF LABOUR IN VERTEX PRESENTATION

Definition of Vertex

Vertex is a diamond-shaped or rhomboid area of the fetal skull that is bound anteriorly by the anterior fontanelle, posteriorly by the posterior fontanelle and laterally by the parietal eminence on either side (Fig. 13.1).

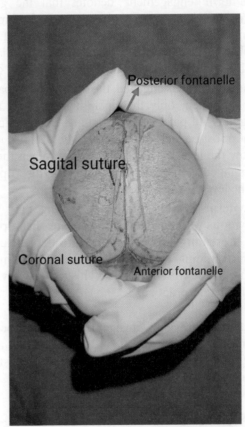

Fig. 13.1 The boundaries of the vertex (Dr K Jayashree Srinivasan, Saveetha Medical College, Chennai)

At the onset of labour, the vertex presentation is the most common presentation, occurring in about 95% of pregnancies. In a vertex presentation, the occiput enters the pelvis first and is called the denominator. Depending on the relationship of the occiput to the pelvis, various positions can occur. The most common position by which the fetus enters the pelvis is the left occipitotransverse (LOT) position, which occurs in 40% of pregnancies. The right occipitotransverse (ROT) occurs in 20%, the occipitoposterior (OP) in

20% of pregnancies and right occipitoanterior (ROA)/ left occipitoanterior (LOA) can occur in another 20%.

MECHANISM OF LABOUR IN THE OCCIPITOANTERIOR POSITION

At the pelvic inlet, the transverse and oblique diameters are the largest, and therefore, the head has to enter the pelvis with its engaging diameter, **the sub-occipitobregmatic diameter** (in the occipitoanterior position), which measures 9.4 cm, **in the transverse/ oblique diameter**.

Engagement

- The term 'engagement' denotes that the greatest transverse diameter of the fetal head (the biparietal diameter) has passed through the pelvic inlet. In all cephalic presentations, the greatest transverse diameter is always the **biparietal diameter**, which is 9.4 cm.

- When the head is engaged, the occiput is not palpable per abdomen; only the sinciput is palpable at this stage (1/5th palpable). On vaginal examination, the lowermost portion of the vertex, the occiput, is at or below the level of the ischial spines. When the head is engaged, it indicates that there is no disproportion at the level of the brim.

The term **fixation** of the presenting part is not synonymous with engagement. It means that a portion of the presenting part is entering into the pelvic brim. The surrounding structures and abdominal muscles help in fixing a presenting part. This term is very rarely used in current practice.

> In a primigravida, engagement usually occurs during the last few weeks of pregnancy. i.e., at or after 38 weeks, whereas in a multigravida, it usually occurs at the onset of labour.

Types of engagement

There are two types of engagements, namely **synclitic** and **asynclitic** engagements. In most normal labours, there is some amount of asynclitism. When the asynclitism is severe, labour may get arrested.

Synclitic engagement

Synclitic engagement is said to occur when the sagittal suture lies in the transverse diameter of the pelvic inlet and the head descends directly. When the descent occurs, the sagittal suture remains midway between the sacral promontory and the symphysis pubis (Fig. 13.2). This usually occurs when the head is small.

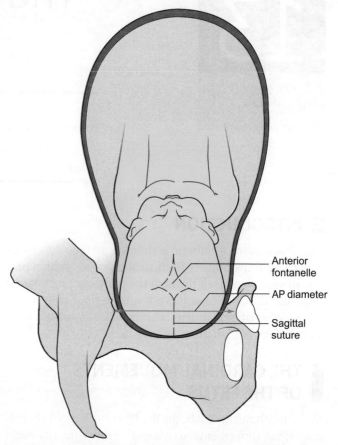

Anterior fontanelle

AP diameter

Sagittal suture

Fig. 13.2 Synclitic engagement at the inlet with the sagittal suture lying midway between the sacral promontory and the symphysis pubis

Asynclitic engagement

Usually, engagement occurs by the lateral tilting of the head—called asynclitism—wherein instead of the biparietal diameter, **the subparieto-supraparietal diameter enters the pelvis** (which is smaller than the biparietal diameter). In such cases, while the sagittal suture remains parallel to the transverse axis of the pelvic inlet, it may not lie exactly midway between the sacral promontory and the symphysis pubis. The sagittal suture is deflected either towards the symphysis pubis or the sacral promontory. Asynclitism plays a major part in engaging a large fetal head or a deflexed head or in a contracted pelvis. There are two types of asynclitism, namely posterior and anterior.

Posterior asynclitism

When the sagittal suture is deflected towards the pubic symphysis, the posterior parietal bone becomes the leading part. This is called the **posterior parietal presentation/posterior asynclitism or Litzman's obliquity** (Fig. 13.3). Posterior parietal presentation has a poor prognosis as the fetal head has to negotiate the entire depth of the symphysis pubis.

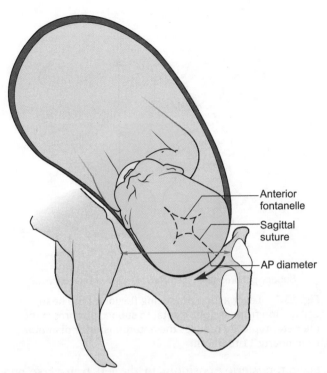

Fig. 13.3   Posterior asynclitism with the sagittal suture deflected towards the symphysis pubis and posterior parietal bone at a lower level

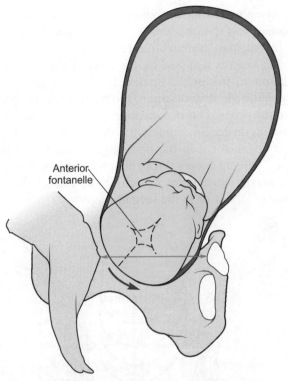

Fig. 13.4   Anterior asynclitism with the sagittal suture directed towards the sacral promontory

Anterior asynclitism

If the sagittal suture is directed towards the sacral promontory, the anterior parietal bone becomes the leading part, resulting in **anterior parietal presentation or anterior asynclitism**. This is called **Naegle's obliquity** (Fig. 13.4). Anterior asynclitism occurs when there is an anterior obliquity of the uterus as in the case of a pendulous abdomen.

Descent

Descent is the continuous downward movement of the fetus through the birth canal and it is brought about by four important factors, which are as follows:

- Direct downward pressure of the fundus of the uterus on the breech during uterine contractions (fetal axis pressure)
- Hydrostatic pressure of amniotic fluid
- Extension and straightening of the fetal body
- Abdominal muscle contractions during bearing down in the second stage of labour

By abdominal palpation (Fig. 13.5), the descent of the head is assessed and described as the number of fifths of the fetal head palpable per abdomen above the symphysis pubis. In the common occipitotransverse position, for descent to occur, the fetal neck bends sideways and the anterior parietal bone slips behind

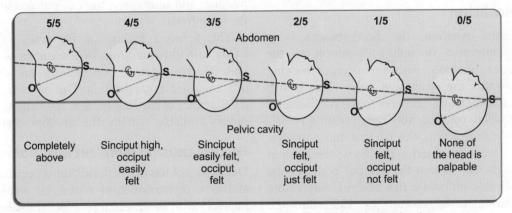

5/5	4/5	3/5	2/5	1/5	0/5
Completely above	Sinciput high, occiput easily felt	Sinciput easily felt, occiput felt	Sinciput felt, occiput just felt	Sinciput felt, occiput not felt	None of the head is palpable

Fig. 13.5   Assessment of the descent and engagement of the fetal head by abdominal palpation

the symphysis while the posterior parietal bone remains more or less stationary or below the promontory.

By vaginal examination (Fig. 13.6), the descent of the head is assessed by the level of the occiput in relation to the ischial spines. In the absence of any cephalopelvic disproportion, the head descends deeply into the pelvis. This occurs prior to or early in labour in a primigravida. In a multipara, descent usually begins with engagement in the first stage of labour. In both cases, descent occurs throughout the process of labour, but maximum descent is seen at the end of the first stage of labour or in the second stage.

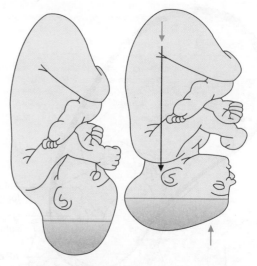

Suboccipitobregmatic diameter   Occipitofrontal diameter

Fig. 13.7   Lever action producing flexion of the head; conversion from occipitofrontal to suboccipitobregmatic diameter typically reduces the anteroposterior diameter from nearly 11 to 9.5 cm

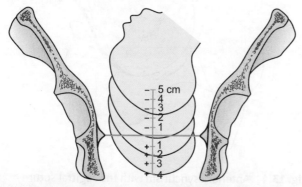

Fig. 13.6   Assessment of the descent of the fetal head by vaginal examination

Flexion

At the beginning of labour, the fetal head is not well-flexed and the engaging diameter is occipitofrontal, which is 11 cm. As the head descends, the fetal neck is flexed, and the chin touches the chest. Flexion is caused by the shape of the uterus, the resistance of the pelvic floor and the pressure exerted by the uterine wall and cervix. Flexion allows the smallest diameter of the fetal head to descend into the pelvis. While flexion is taking place, the engaging diameter—the shorter suboccipitobregmatic diameter (9.4 cm)—is substituted for the longer occipitofrontal diameter (Fig. 13.7).

Internal Rotation

During internal rotation, the head moves from the occipitotransverse or oblique position to the occipitoanterior position, with the occiput moving anteriorly towards the symphysis pubis. This brings the suboccipitobregmatic diameter to the AP diameter of the cavity. This rotation may range from 45–90°. In the transverse position, the occiput has to rotate through 90°, while in anterior positions, the occiput rotates through 45° so that the occiput is under the symphysis. Less commonly, the occiput may rotate posteriorly towards the sacrum by 135° into the

occipitoposterior position. In the left transverse and anterior positions, it occurs from left to right, and from right to left in the right transverse or anterior position. Internal rotation is not accomplished until the head has reached the spines.

The movement of internal rotation is caused by the levator ani muscles, which form a V-shaped gutter. The tonic resistance of this muscle rotates the vertex anteriorly. According to this view, the occiput is forced into a gutter, the sides of which are formed by the two halves of the levator ani muscle. The direction of the gutter is downward and forward, ending beneath the pubic arch. During a uterine contraction, the head is pushed down, stretching the levator ani muscle. As the occiput is at a lower level, the part of the levator ani that is in relation to the occiput is stretched more. Elastic recoil of the muscle follows at the end of the uterine contraction. The occiput, at each contraction and relaxation, is thus pushed inward towards the midline, and ultimately, the occiput lies directly under the symphysis.

The forward incline of the walls of the pelvic cavity, the impetus given by the spines of the ischium and effective uterine contractions are other factors influencing internal rotation. This movement brings the AP diameter of the fetal head to the longest of the pelvic outlets available, namely, the anteroposterior diameter.

Factors causing deficient internal rotation

Deficiency of the pelvic floor from a previous laceration and lack of uterine contractions or weak pains may interfere with the internal rotation of the head.

Extension and Birth of the Fetal Head

When internal rotation is complete, the occiput comes to lie underneath the inferior margin of the symphysis pubis, and the head is in an attitude of flexion. Subsequent uterine contractions favour the next movement, namely extension, which is essential for the birth of the head.

During the process of extension, the largest diameter of the fetal head is encircled by the vulvar ring. This is called '**crowning**' (Fig. 13.8).

At this stage, the perineum is stretched. If proper support is not available or if the head descends too rapidly in the process of extension, the perineum may tear. The degree of tearing depends upon the force with which the perineum is stretched and the particular diameter of the head that stretches the perineum.

The vulvar outlet is directed upward and forward, therefore extension of the head must occur before the head can pass through. The head is born by further extension with the occiput, vertex, bregma, forehead, nose, mouth and chin passing successively over the perineum. Immediately after birth, the head drops downwards so that the chin lies over the maternal anal region.

Extension is the result of two forces, which are as follows:

1. The effect of the uterine contractions from above
2. The elastic resistance of the pelvic floor from below

Restitution

At the time of internal rotation, the head gets twisted on the shoulder by 45°. It subsequently gets untwisted once the head is delivered. This is called restitution. After its delivery, the head returns to the position it occupied at engagement—the natural position relative to the shoulders (oblique position). This restitutional movement results in the occiput turning to the mother's left thigh in the LOA position. The chin rotates towards the right side in left occipitoanterior positions, and towards the left in right occipitoanterior positions.

The fetal body then rotates to bring one shoulder behind the symphysis pubis (the biacromial diameter into the anteroposterior diameter of the pelvic outlet).

External Rotation

After the neck has untwisted, the next movement is the internal rotation of the shoulders, which brings the bisacromial diameter into the anteroposterior diameter of the pelvic outlet. The anterior shoulder is now underneath the symphysis pubis.

As the shoulder undergoes internal rotation, in order to maintain its alignment with the shoulder, the head rotates another 45°. With the external rotation of the head to the transverse position, the occiput lies next to left maternal thigh (Fig. 13.9). Restitution and external rotation frequently occur in such quick succession that they may practically appear to be one continuous movement (Fig. 13.10). However, careful observation shows that restitution occurs first and after a short interval, external rotation takes place.

Expulsion

Once the shoulders have rotated into the anteroposterior diameter of the outlet, the descent continues with the uterine contractions until the anterior shoulder hitches under the symphysis pubis and the posterior shoulder sweeps over the perineum by a process of lateral flexion of the spine and is delivered first. This is followed by a slight slipping forward of the anterior shoulder from underneath the symphysis pubis. After the expulsion of the shoulders, the fetal body slips down through the pelvic cavity. The rest of the body is thus delivered.

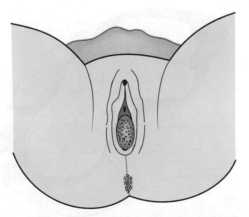
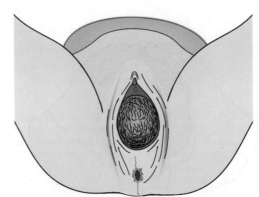
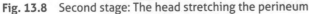

Fig. 13.8   Second stage: The head stretching the perineum

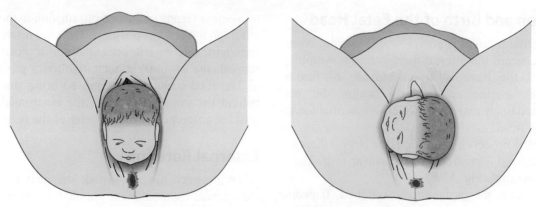

Fig. 13.9   Delivery of the head—extension completed and external rotation occuring

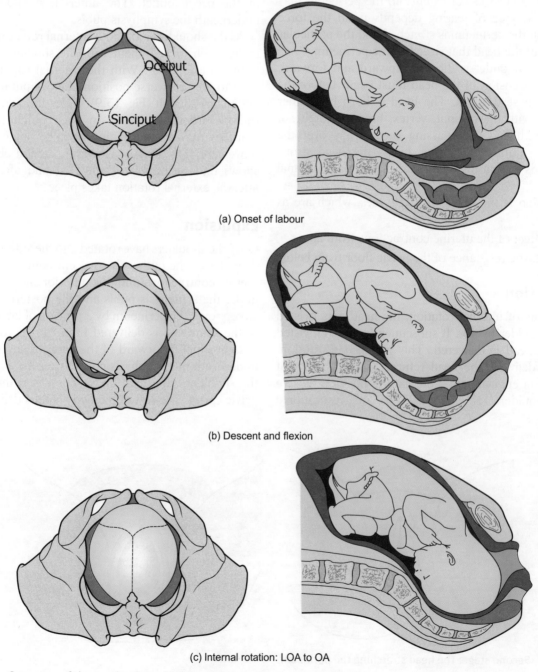

(a) Onset of labour

(b) Descent and flexion

(c) Internal rotation: LOA to OA

Fig. 13.10   Summary of the mechanism of labour

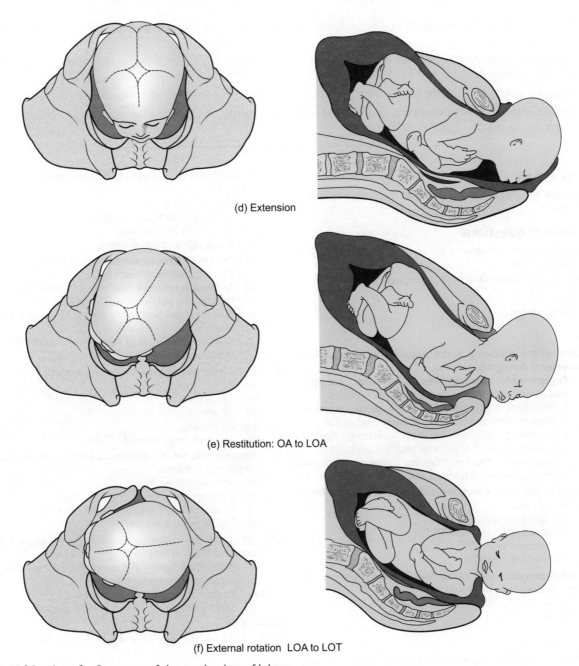

(d) Extension

(e) Restitution: OA to LOA

(f) External rotation LOA to LOT

Fig. 13.10 (*Continued*)   Summary of the mechanism of labour

■ SEPARATION OF THE PLACENTA

During the next stage, the placenta and membranes become separated from the uterine wall and are then extruded through the vaginal outlet by one of the two methods of expulsion described earlier.

With the separation of the placenta, and sometimes with its extrusion, some bleeding occurs and is associated with slight pain. Once the placenta has been expelled, the uterus contracts and retracts until it becomes as hard as a cricket ball, and bleeding stops completely.

KEY POINTS

✓   *The mechanism of labour is defined as the process by which the fetus adjusts to the pelvic architecture and manoeuvres itself through the parturient canal with minimal difficulty to achieve a safe vaginal delivery.*

✓   *The cardinal movements in the mechanism of labour are engagement, descent, flexion, internal rotation, extension, restitution, external rotation and expulsion.*

✓ The head is engaged if the greatest transverse diameter of the fetal head, i.e., the biparietal diameter, has passed through the brim of the pelvis.

✓ The most common position in which the fetus enters the pelvis is the left occipitotransverse (LOT) position, which occurs in 40% of pregnancies.

✓ When the head is engaged, the occiput is not palpable per abdomen; only the sinciput is palpable (1/5th palpable).

✓ The movement of internal rotation is caused by the levator ani muscles, which form a V-shaped gutter. The tonic resistance of this muscle rotates the vertex anteriorly.

Essay question

1. Describe the mechanism of labour in the occipitoanterior position.

Short answer questions

1. What do you understand by the term 'engagement' of the presenting part?
2. What do you understand by the term asynclitism?
3. Define restitution.
4. Describe vertex.

MCQs

1. Which of the following is the sequence of the cardinal movements during normal labour?
    a) Engagement, descent, flexion, internal rotation, extension, restitution, external rotation, expulsion
    b) Engagement, descent, flexion, internal rotation, restitution, extension, external rotation, expulsion
    c) Engagement, internal rotation, descent, flexion, restitution, extension, external rotation, expulsion
    d) Engagement, descent, flexion, internal rotation, restitution, external rotation, extension, expulsion
2. Which is the most common position by which the fetus enters the pelvis?
    a) Left occipitotransverse (LOT)
    b) Right occipitotransverse (ROT)
    c) Occipitoposterior (OP)
    d) Occipitoanterior (OA)
3. In what percentage of cases does the fetus present by vertex at the onset of labour?
    a) 95%
    b) 85%
    c) 75%
    d) 65%
4. Which of the following is not one of the factors causing deficient internal rotation?
    a) Deficient flexion of the head
    b) Deficient pelvic floor
    c) Lack of uterine contractions
    d) Premature rupture of membranes
5. What is the sequence of the delivery of the head in the occipitoanterior position?
    a) Chin, brow, vertex, occiput
    b) Occiput, vertex, brow, face, chin
    c) Face, brow, vertex
    d) Vertex, face, chin, occiput
6. To which of the following is engagement of the fetal head related?
    a) Biparietal diameter
    b) Suboccipitobregmatic diameter
    c) Occipitofrontal diameter
    d) Suboccipitofrontal diameter
7. Which of the following is not true of engagement?
    a) First cardinal movement of labour
    b) Greatest transverse diameter of the fetal head passes through the pelvic brim
    c) Portion of the presenting part enters into the superior strait
    d) Lowermost portion of the vertex is at the level of the ischial spine
8. In multiparous women, when is engagement expected to occur?
    a) 37 weeks
    b) 38 weeks
    c) 40 weeks
    d) At the commencement of labour
9. Which of the following is not a factor contributing to the descent of the fetus?
    a) Uterine contractions
    b) Bearing down efforts of the mother
    c) Extension and straightening of the fetus
    d) Position of the mother
10. Which of the following is not a factor responsible for deficient internal rotation?
    a) Inadequate flexion and occiput not the presenting part
    b) Inadequate maternal efforts
    c) Inadequate uterine contractions
    d) Inadequate pelvic floor due to lacerations

Answers
1. (a), 2. (a), 3. (a), 4. (d), 5. (b), 6. (a), 7. (c), 8. (d), 9. (d), 10. (b)

Fill in the blanks

1. At the time of engagement, if the sagittal suture lies close to the symphysis pubis, it is termed _____.
2. At the time of engagement, if the sagittal suture lies close to the sacral promontory, it is termed _____.
3. The descent of the fetal head is assessed by _____.

Answers
1. posterior asynclitism, 2. anterior asynclitism, 3. abdominal palpation

Conduct of Normal Labour

Learning Objectives

» To differentiate true labour pains from false labour pains
» To describe the monitoring of labour
» To describe a partograph and its components
» To describe the conduct of normal labour
» To discuss pain relief in labour
» To know the management of the third stage of labour
» To know the indications for an episiotomy
» To know how to perform an episiotomy and suture it

Though labour is a normal physiological process, assistance and careful monitoring during labour are important to achieve a successful pregnancy outcome. The first steps in the management of a pregnant woman in labour are to provide support, maintain privacy and confidentiality, alleviate her apprehensions and assure her that she and her child will receive the best possible care during labour. This approach will enable her to cope with the process of labour and delivery and have a positive childbirth experience.

ASSESSMENT OF A WOMAN ADMITTED IN LABOUR

In a pregnant woman admitted in labour, the first step is to confirm true labour pains. Thereafter, an initial assessment is carried out to assess the stage and phase of labour.

1. Diagnosis of Labour

In women admitted with labour pains, the diagnosis of true labour should be confirmed. This is very important from the standpoint of avoiding unnecessary interventions. True labour pains are characterised by their progressively increasing frequency and duration of uterine contractions; the pain is located in the back and lower abdomen and is associated with cervical changes, i.e., effacement and dilatation. 'Show' may or may not be present in early labour (differences between true and false labour pains are detailed in Chapter 12, *Causation and stages of labour*).

2. Initial Assessment

The initial assessment of labour should include a review of the woman's antenatal case record for a confirmation of the estimated date of delivery and to identify antenatal risk factors. After a detailed history and examination, an intrapartum risk assessment should be performed.

3. History

Focused history taking should elicit the following information:

- The frequency of contractions, the timing of their onset, their intensity, whether they are progressive in nature with regards to frequency, duration and intensity and location of the pain
- The status of the amniotic membranes (whether spontaneous rupture of the membranes has occurred, and if so, its duration and whether the amniotic fluid is clear or meconium-stained)
- Fetal movements
- Presence or absence of vaginal bleeding
- Any other specific complaints

4. Physical Examination

Physical examination should include the documentation of vitals, abdominal palpation and vaginal examination.

General examination

- Level of consciousness and orientation
- Presence of pallor and edema
- Blood pressure, pulse, temperature
- Examination of the cardiovascular, respiratory and central nervous systems and gait
- Examination of thyroid and breasts

Abdominal examination

- Height of the uterus (whether appropriate for gestation)
- Whether the uterus is overdistended or small for the gestational age

- Lie of the fetus, presentation and position of the fetus
- Abdominal examination with Leopold manoeuvres
- Frequency, duration and intensity of uterine contractions
- Whether the head is free, has entered the pelvis or is engaged
- Whether liquor is adequate clinically
- Auscultation of the fetal heart

Vaginal examination

- The woman should be asked to empty her bladder before the vaginal examination is performed.

> When the woman presents with bleeding, vaginal examination should not be performed unless placenta previa is excluded.

- After the vagina and the perineum are cleaned, the woman is positioned with her legs flexed.
- The presence of any discharge or bleeding or liquor in the vulva is noted.
- Vaginal examination is carried out with sterile gloves and using sufficient lubricating antiseptic gel. Digital examination allows the clinician to determine the cervical findings, status of the membranes, presentation, position and the station of the presenting part and architecture and adequacy of the pelvis for the fetus.

Cervical findings

The following cervical changes are noted:

- The degree of dilatation, which ranges from 0 cm (closed or fingertip) to 10 cm (complete or fully dilated)
- Effacement (assessment of the cervical length, which can be reported as a percentage of the normal [3–4 cm long] cervix or as the actual cervical length)
- Position of the cervix—whether it is anteriorly or posteriorly placed
- Consistency of the cervix—whether it is soft or firm

Status of the membranes and the nature of the amniotic fluid

- The presence or absence of the membranes and the colour of the amniotic fluid are noted.

Assessment of the presenting part

- On vaginal examination, the presentation, the position in relation to the pelvis and the station of the presenting part are noted.
- The station of the presenting part is ascertained by quantifying the distance of the occiput (−5 to

+5 cm), which is the presenting part, relative to the maternal ischial spines, where 0 station is in line with the plane of the maternal ischial spines.

Assessment of the pelvis

- The pelvis is examined for shape and adequacy.
- The mobility of the coccyx is also evaluated.
- Pelvic assessment is usually done after 38 weeks of gestation or in early labour.
- The anterior surface of the sacrum is palpated from below upwards and its vertical and lateral curvatures are noted. In a normal pelvis, only the last three sacral vertebrae can be felt without difficulty. In a contracted pelvis, the sacral promontory may be reached.
- The sacrosciatic notch is felt laterally and should normally admit two fingers.
- The side walls of the pelvis are usually parallel. If they are convergent, the space in the midcavity will be reduced.

Measurement of the diagonal conjugate and the obstetric conjugate

- In order to measure the diagonal conjugate (Fig. 14.1), the sacral promontory must be reached. This measurement is taken by inserting the middle and index finger of the right hand into the vagina until the middle finger touches the sacral promontory. With the finger closely applied to the most prominent part of the upper sacrum, the examining hand is elevated until it contacts the pubic arch and is marked by the index finger of the left hand. The distance between the two points—the sacral promontory and the undersurface of the pubic arch—is the diagonal conjugate. The obstetrical conjugate is arrived at by subtracting 1.5–2 cm from the diagonal conjugate.

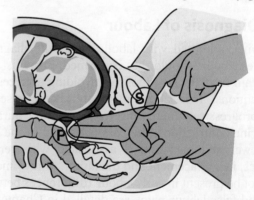

Fig. 14.1   Vaginal examination to determine the diagonal conjugate (P–sacral promontory; S–symphysis pubis)

- The mobility of the coccyx is then evaluated.
- The transverse diameter of the outlet is measured by placing the knuckles of the right hand between the

ischial tuberosities—four or more knuckles should be admitted.

- The assessment of cephalopelvic disproportion (CPD) is discussed in Chapter 45, *Cephalopelvic disproportion and obstructed labour.*

FETAL HEART RATE ASSESSMENT

On admission, all labouring mothers are monitored with electronic fetal monitoring (EFM) for a 20-minute period. Thereafter, all low-risk mothers can be monitored intermittently with a Pinard fetoscope or fetal Doppler. All high-risk mothers would need continuous EFM.

INVESTIGATIONS

All recent investigations are reviewed, and if postpartum hemorrhage (PPH) is anticipated, compatible blood is kept in reserve. Depending on the maternal complications, further investigations are carried out.

GENERAL PRINCIPLES OF LABOUR MANAGEMENT

- All labouring women should be provided with a supportive and encouraging atmosphere for birth. A birth companion should be encouraged; this could be the woman's partner, friend, relative or any trained person.
- The privacy and confidentiality of the woman are paramount.
- Cleanliness and sterile precautions should be maintained in the labour room. The cleanliness of the woman and her environment is also important. The woman should be encouraged to wash herself at the onset of labour. The personnel examining the woman should wash their hands with soap before and after each examination. The vulval and perineal areas should be cleaned before each examination. The cleanliness of labouring and birthing areas should be ensured, and all spills should be cleared immediately.

Ensuring Mobility

On admission to the labour room, a woman having normal labour should be encouraged to assume the position that she finds most comfortable such as walking, lying down, sitting or resting in a left–lateral decubitus position. Walking in early labour should be encouraged in uncomplicated cases. Women diagnosed with hypertension, antepartum hemorrhage, mobile head or polyhydramnios are advised to rest in bed. Lying supine on the back should be avoided as it can lead to supine hypotension syndrome due to the compression of the inferior vena cava. This manifests with fetal heart rate abnormalities and hypotension in the woman.

Enema

- Enema is not given routinely to women in labour unless the rectum is loaded.
- In women planned for elective cesarean sections, enema is not routinely given in the morning; rather, a laxative given the previous night can help the woman to empty her bowel with ease.

Attention to Bladder Emptying

A distended bladder will interfere with the descent of the presenting part and after delivery, can cause atonicity of the uterus. Therefore, a woman in labour should be encouraged to void regularly. Occasionally, catheterisation may be required, especially when the head descends into the pelvis.

Perineal Shaving

Routine shaving of the perineum is not advocated anymore. Occasionally, perineal hair may interfere with the delivery or an episiotomy; in such cases, the perineal hair may be clipped with scissors with the consent of the woman.

Nutrition

In early labour, unless contraindicated, oral fluids can be given. Nutritious drinks are important even in late labour. Solids are avoided as gastric emptying is delayed in labour, and this can precipitate aspiration if general anesthesia is required. If the woman is very tired and dehydrated/when there is poor progress in labour/there is a possibility that the woman may require anesthesia, intravenous fluids are given, preferably with dextrose with Ringer's lactate solution.

MANAGEMENT OF THE FIRST STAGE OF LABOUR

In any woman in labour, whether normal or complicated. the general principle is to monitor the following:

- Maternal condition
- Progress of labour
- Fetal condition
- Complications that may develop in labour

MONITORING OF MATERNAL CONDITION

- Temperature, pulse and blood pressure should be monitored.
- Signs of dehydration should be looked for. If the woman looks dehydrated, her urine should be tested for ketones. If urine is positive for acetone, it is corrected with IV dextrose.
- It is important to look for signs of distress such as increasing pulse rate, which may indicate dehydration or pain. This can be corrected with adequate hydration and adequate analgesia. Hemorrhage should also be suspected.
- If the woman's BP decreases, hemorrhage should be looked for and corrected promptly.

MONITORING THE PROGRESS OF LABOUR

After confirming the true labour pains, the stage and phase of labour are assessed. Labour can be divided into three functional divisions, which are as follows:

1. **Preparatory division:** This comprises the latent and acceleration phases, during which considerable changes take place in the connective tissue and collagen of the cervix, resulting in the effacement of the cervix. However, there is minimal cervical dilatation. This phase is affected by sedation and anesthesia.

2. **Dilatation division:** This comprises the phase of maximum slope, during which, cervical dilatation occurs at a maximum rate of 1.0 cm/hour in the primigravida and 1.5 cm/hour in the multigravida. This phase is not affected by sedation and anesthesia as labour is well-established by then.

3. **Pelvic division:** This comprises the deceleration phase of cervical dilatation and the maximum slope of descent of the fetus. In this division, full dilatation of the cervix occurs with the descent and delivery of the fetus. The cardinal movements of the fetus principally take place during this phase. The onset of this phase is not clearly identifiable.

Once the stage of labour is assessed, the progress of labour is evaluated based on the rate of cervical dilatation and descent of the presenting part using a partograph.

Partograph

The partograph is a graphical record of the progress of labour, wherein cervical dilatation and descent of the fetal head are plotted against time. Friedman was the first person to plot the progress of labour on a chart. The method was later developed by Studd. Philpott and Castle developed the idea of the alert line and the action line.

- The conventional partograph was a graphical representation of both latent and active phases of labour; the active phase was marked by a cervical dilatation of 3 cm.
- As a part of the Safe Motherhood initiative, the WHO developed a partograph to improve labour management. The main purpose of the partograph is to avoid prolonged labour and to initiate timely interventions. In the WHO partograph, the plotting starts in the active phase of labour at 4 cm cervical dilatation.
- Besides the cervical dilatation and descent of the fetal head, maternal and fetal conditions are also recorded on the partograph.
- Plotting in a partograph (Fig. 14.2) begins in the active phase when the cervix is 4 cm dilated.

Information recorded in the partograph

- **Patient information:** This includes the woman's name, age, gravidity, parity, date and time of admission and time of rupture of membranes.
- **Status of membranes:** At every vaginal examination, the status of the membranes should be noted. If the membrane is ruptured, the colour of the liquor should be noted. The observations are graded as follows:
  — I   : Membrane intact
  — C   : Membrane ruptured with clear liquor
  — M   : Membrane ruptured with meconium-stained liquor
  — B   : Membrane ruptured with bloodstained liquor
- **The degree of moulding:** The fetal cranial bones are connected by a membrane. This allows considerable shifting or sliding of each bone in order for the fetal head to be accommodated into the maternal pelvis. In normal labour, moulding results in a reduction of 0.5–1 cm of the biparietal and suboccipitobregmatic diameters without any brain damage. This reduction disappears a few hours after birth. Moulding is recorded as 1+, 2+ and 3+; 0 represents the absence of moulding.
  — 1 : Sutures apposed
  — 2 : Sutures overlapped but reducible
  — 3 : Sutures overlapped but irreducible
- **Fetal heart:** The fetal heart rate is recorded and documented every half hour.

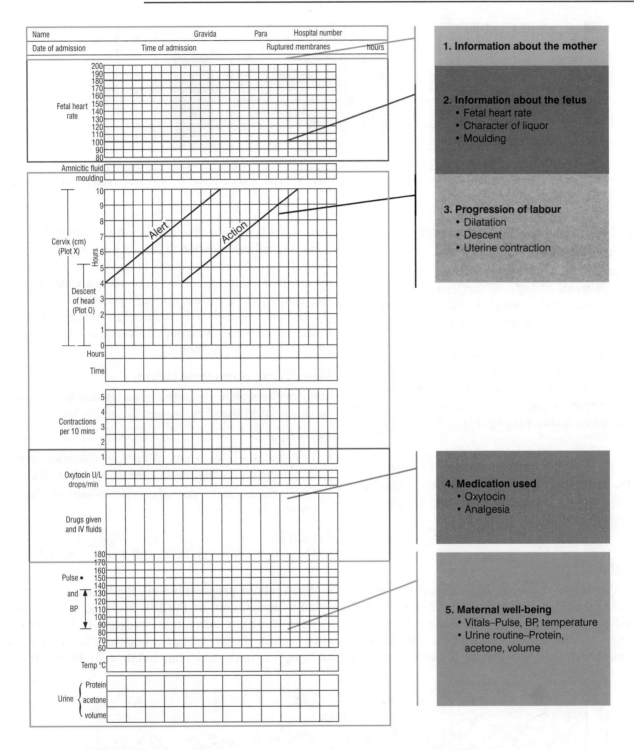

Fig. 14.2 Components of a partograph

- **Uterine contractions:** The uterine contractions are noted by palpating the uterus with the palm of the hand. The intensity of the contractions is gauged by the degree of firmness of the uterus. The frequency, duration and intensity of uterine contractions are noted at regular intervals. For a woman on electronic monitoring, the uterine contractions can be monitored on the trace. The contractions are marked every half hour (Fig. 14.3). The number of contractions in 10 minutes and their duration are noted.

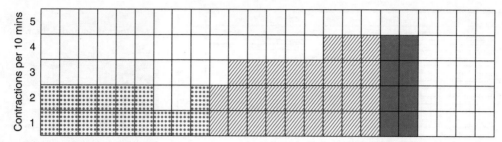

Fig. 14.3 Uterine contractions plotted on a partograph: Dotted boxes indicate contractions lasting less than 20 seconds; boxes with slanting lines indicate contractions lasting for 20–40 seconds and shaded boxes indicate contractions lasting for more than 40 seconds

Descent of fetal head by abdominal palpation (Fig. 14.4)

The descent of the fetal head is assessed by abdominal palpation in terms of fifths of the fetal head palpable above the symphysis pubis. If necessary, vaginal examination findings may be used to assess the descent of the presenting part of the fetus in relation to the ischial spines of the maternal pelvis. The number of fifths of the fetal head palpable above the symphysis pubis is noted and marked as a circle (O). When the head is completely above the symphysis pubis, it is graded 5; when no head is palpable, it is graded 0.

> When there is a significant degree of caput or moulding, assessment by abdominal palpation using fifths of the head palpable is more useful than assessment by vaginal examination.

Cervical dilatation

During the active phase of labour, routine vaginal examination should be performed every 2–4 hours and cervical dilatation at each exam is marked on the time scale with a cross (×). The time at which there is a dilatation of 4 cm is marked as the 0 hour and the actual time at the 0

hour is marked in the time column. After a dilatation of 8 cm, vaginal examination is carried out every 2 hours. Vaginal examination should also be carried out whenever the membrane ruptures or whenever there are fetal heart rate abnormalities to rule out cord prolapse. It should also be performed when the woman has an urge to push. In the active phase of labour, the cervix is expected to dilate at least 1 cm per hour.

Identifying abnormal labour

Abnormal labour in the active phase is demarcated by two lines called the alert line and the action line.

Alert line

- This line starts at 4 cm of cervical dilatation and shows the cervix dilating at 1 cm./hour up to 10 cm.
- This is the normal expected cervical dilatation in any labour.

Action line

- The action line is parallel to and 4 cm to the right of the alert line.
- When **labour progresses well,** the labour curve will fall to the left of or on the alert line (Fig. 14.5).
  When there is a delay in the progress of labour for some reason, the labour curve will cross the alert line to the right. Prolonged labour and delay in the progress

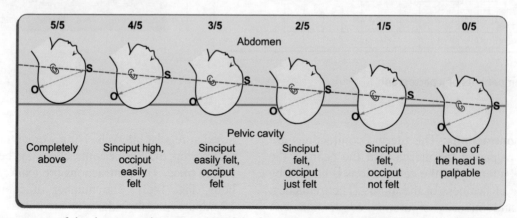

Fig. 14.4 Assessment of the descent and engagement of the fetal head by abdominal palpation

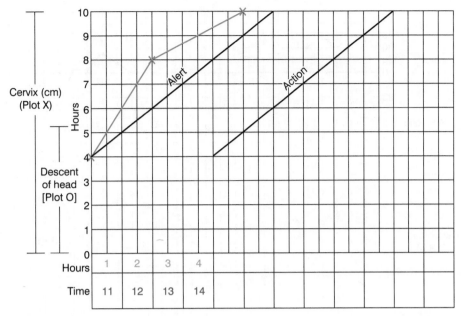

Fig. 14.5   Normal progress of labour with the labour curve on the left of the alert line

may be due to inadequate uterine contractions, malpositions, malpresentations or CPD (Fig. 14.6).

> In a primary healthcare setting, if the labour curve crosses the alert line, immediate referral/action to be initiated.

Monitoring of fetal heart rate

- In low-risk women, the fetal heart rate should be checked immediately after a contraction and every 15–30 minutes in the first stage of labour.
- For high-risk women, auscultation is performed every 15 minutes. In most obstetric units, the fetal heart is assessed continuously by electronic fetal heart monitoring.

Oxytocin infusion

- The dose of oxytocin, i.e., the amount of oxytocin and quantity of fluid in which it is added, is noted.
- At each examination, the flow rate of fluid (drops/minute) is also noted.

Drugs administered

- A record of any additional drugs that are used is also maintained.

Monitoring maternal condition

- Temperature : Checked every 2 hours
- Pulse : Checked every 30 minutes and marked as a dot (.)
- Blood pressure : Checked every 4 hours and marked with arrows; in hypertensive women, the BP is checked every hour
- Urine : Checked for acetone, protein and volume whenever urine is passed

Advantages of a partograph

- By using a partograph, the abnormal progress of labour can be detected early. By preventing prolonged labour, the risk of postpartum hemorrhage, sepsis, obstructed labour, uterine rupture and their sequelae can be significantly reduced.
- Late referrals of intrapartum cases from rural health centres can be avoided by using this tool.
- It is a low-cost tool and can be used in PHCs also.
- It can significantly reduce the cesarean section rate and maternal and perinatal morbidity and mortality.

■ PAIN CONTROL IN LABOUR

Labouring women often experience intense pain. Uterine contractions result in visceral pain, which is transmitted by T10–L1. When fetal descent is taking place, the fetal head exerts pressure on the mother's pelvic floor, vagina and perineum, causing somatic pain, which is transmitted by the pudendal nerve (innervated by S2–4). Therefore, pain control during labour should optimally relieve both sources of pain. The available methods for pain relief in labour include the following:

- **Systemic opioids**: Opioids such as meperidine (pethidine), tramadol and fentanyl are used in

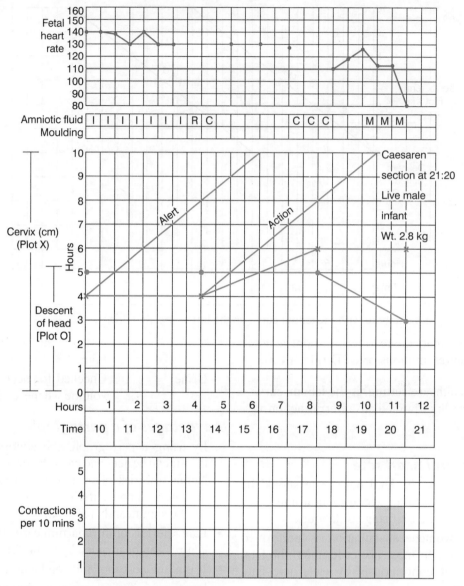

Fig. 14.6   Labour graph crossing the alert and action lines

labour for pain relief. They act as sedatives, and their analgesic effect is limited. Their major disadvantage is that they can delay gastric emptying and can cross the placenta to cause FHR abnormalities and respiratory depression in the neonate. Meperidine is used in a dose of 50 mg IM along with promethazine to reduce nausea and vomiting. The drug is administered in the active phase of labour when the cervix is >4 cm dilated. Babies born within 1–3 hours of administering the drug suffer from respiratory depression, which can be reversed with naloxone.

- **Inhalational agents:** Entonox is a mixture of 50% oxygen and 50% nitrous oxide. It exerts an analgesic effect when inhaled 3–4 times during a contraction. It has no effect on the uterine activity and fetal respiratory status.

- **Nerve blocking techniques:** Epidural analgesia is used for labour analgesia in facilities where round-the-clock anesthesia services are available. Epidural analgesia aims to provide effective lumbar and sacral sensory analgesia with minimal motor blockade. In epidural analgesia, the sensory fibres travelling through T11 and 12 and L1 from the body of the uterus and the pain sensation from the cervix, vagina and perineum—which is transmitted by S2–4—are blocked. The block is administered in the active phase of labour in the L1–2 epidural space with bupivacaine. Pain control maintenance can be achieved by administering intermittent boluses or by controlled infusion. The major advantages of this technique are its long duration of action and that it can be continued for instrumental deliveries/cesarean section if necessary. Disadvantages include transient hypotension, which can lead to FHR abnormalities and a prolonged second stage, which can lead to an increase in instrumental deliveries.

- Other modalities used for pain relief in labour are transcutaneous nerve stimulation (TENS) and relaxation and breathing techniques taught at antenatal classes.
- For vaginal delivery, local infiltration of the perineal area and pudendal block are administered. The pudendal nerve is blocked as it curves around the ischial spine. Along with pudendal block, perineal and vulval infiltration is also performed to block the ilioinguinal and genital branches of the genitofemoral nerve.

INDICATIONS FOR AMNIOTOMY IN THE FIRST STAGE OF LABOUR

- In the active phase for active management of labour
- When there is abnormal fetal heart rate, to note the colour of the liquor
- When there is unsatisfactory progress in the active phase of labour

Artificial rupture of membranes (ARM) should be deferred in early labour, in the occipitoposterior position, when the head is high and in case of fetal death. After performing an ARM, the FHR should be observed for abnormalities. Though transient FHR changes may be seen due to cord compression, it is important to rule out cord prolapse. If there is bleeding associated with FHR changes, placental abruption/vasa previa should be suspected. The advantage of ARM is that it promotes labour progression by inducing the release of prostaglandin. It also allows the stretching of the cervix by the fetal head. The colour of the liquor can also be noted. The risks associated with ARM are cord prolapse, infection and rapid release of liquor in polyhydramnios, which can lead to abruption.

MANAGEMENT OF THE SECOND STAGE OF LABOUR

The second stage of labour begins with complete dilatation of the cervix and ends with the complete expulsion of the fetus or fetuses.

DURATION

- The median duration of the second stage is 50 minutes in a nullipara and 20 minutes in a multipara without regional analgesia.

- In nulliparous women, the second stage should be considered prolonged if it exceeds 3 hours with regional analgesia or 2 hours without regional analgesia.
- In multiparous women, the second stage should be considered prolonged if it exceeds 2 hours with regional anesthesia or 1 hour without it.
- Satisfactory progress in the second stage of labour is indicated by the following:
  - Steady descent of the fetus through the birth canal
  - Onset of the expulsive (pushing) phase
  - No evidence of maternal or fetal distress
- In the second stage of labour, the fetal heart rate should be monitored or auscultated at least every 5 minutes or after each contraction. During a contraction, the fetal heart may slow down due to head compression. If after the contraction, the fetal heart rate becomes normal, labour is allowed to continue.
- Vaginal examination is carried out once every hour. Ironing and stretching of the perineum should be discouraged.
- Fundal pressure should not be applied.
- The second stage of labour has two phases— the phase of descent and the perineal phase.

PHASE OF DESCENT

In this phase, the baby's head is high in the pelvis, the occiput is transverse, the vagina is not stretched and there is no effort on the part of the mother to push.

- At this stage, the woman should not be urged to push.
- No attempt should be made to achieve vaginal delivery by traction with forceps.
- When the need arises for urgent delivery, this should be done by cesarean section.
- When there is no descent in one hour, the woman should be assessed carefully to exclude cephalopelvic disproportion (CPD).
- After ruling out CPD, if uterine contractions are not effective, oxytocin infusion can be given carefully.
- If there is still no descent, then delivery should be expedited by cesarean section.

PERINEAL PHASE

- This phase begins when the baby's head reaches the pelvic floor.

- It is accompanied by an urge to push.
- Maternal effort should not be encouraged until either the presenting part is visible or the anus is bulging. When the need arises to intervene, forceps can be used.
- The duration of active pushing must be restricted because prolonged pushing may lead to maternal and fetal distress. In the primigravida, this time should be restricted to one hour provided there is progress and the FHR monitoring and maternal conditions are satisfactory. In the multiparous woman, this time limit is usually 30 minutes.

■ DELIVERY OF THE FETUS

The woman can be positioned in any of the following ways for delivery:

- Supine with her knees bent (i.e., dorsal lithotomy position, which is the usual choice)
- Lateral (Sims) position
- Partial sitting or squatting position

At this stage, the woman should be encouraged to 'bear down' during the pains. She should be instructed to hold her breath and bear down as a contraction reaches its height and to relax after the completion of each contraction. When the pains become more frequent, they last much longer. The head presses against the perineum, and the anus begins to dilate. It is now that the obstetrician should provide the necessary assistance. Before doing so, she should put on a sterile mask, gown and gloves after proper scrubbing and washing of hands. The vulva and the perineum should be cleaned, and sterile draping should be done in such a way that only the area around the vulva is exposed.

Delivery of the Head (Fig. 14.7)

- The perineum bulges with each contraction and the vulvovaginal opening becomes dilated under the pressure of the fetal head. Ultimately, the vulvovaginal opening encircles the largest transverse diameter of the fetal head; this is known as crowning.
- When the vaginal introitus dilates to a diameter of 5 cm or more, a gloved hand is used to exert forward pressure on the fetal chin through the perineal skin just in front of the anus (Fig. 14.7a). The other hand exerts pressure against the occiput. This manoeuvre is described as the modified Ritgen manoeuvre (Fig. 14.7b). It allows the controlled delivery of the head and prevents perineal lacerations. Then, the chin is hooked out (Fig. 14.7c).

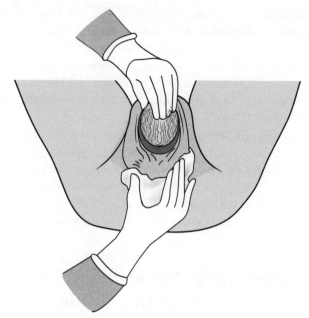

(a) Providing perineal support

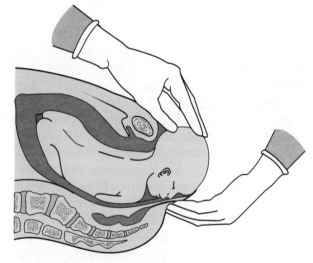

(b) Ritgen manoeuvre

(c) Hooking out of chin

Fig. 14.7 Dilatation of the introitus and birth of the head: (a) providing perineal support, (b) Ritgen manoeuvre and (c) hooking out of the chin

- The pressure applied by the hand placed over the vertex prevents the head from being pushed down during a contraction, while the hand over the perineum helps to ease the vertex out of the vulval outlet.
- At the time of extension and crowning of the fetal head, a pad is used to provide perineal support.
- The birth of the head should be controlled to keep it flexed.
- The baby's head should be allowed to turn spontaneously.
- After the delivery of the head, the obstetrician should ensure that the cord is not around the baby's neck. If the cord is around the neck, it may be slipped over the head, down the shoulder or cut between the clamps. If the cord is wrapped too tightly to be removed, the cord can be double-clamped and cut.
- The eyelids of the newborn should be cleaned with soft linen. Separate wipes should be used for each eye and the lids should be cleaned. A piece of gauze should then be used to wipe the lips and nose. Where secretions need to be aspirated, the use of a disposable **De Lee mucus sucker** or similar extractor is recommended.
- In some cases, an episiotomy is required.

Episiotomy

- Episiotomy is a surgical incision made at the perineum and vulva to increase the space available at the time of labour. It is equivalent to a **second-degree tear** and involves incising the vaginal mucosa and superficial and deep perineal muscles.
- It should not be performed routinely in all cases and should be considered only in cases of complicated vaginal delivery (breech, shoulder dystocia, forceps, vacuum), for the delivery of a big baby, when there is scarring from female genital cutting or poorly healed previous third- or fourth-degree tears. The advantages of an episiotomy are that it can prevent third- and fourth-degree lacerations, it increases the space at the time of delivery, and it is easier to suture than perineal tears.
- The types of episiotomy are lateral, mediolateral and central (Fig. 14.8a and b). Of these, mediolateral episiotomy is the most preferred. Though central episiotomy is associated with good healing, there is a risk of the incision extending while delivering the baby; in such cases, it may involve the anal sphincter, especially when the length of the perineum is short. Lateral episiotomy is not recommended.

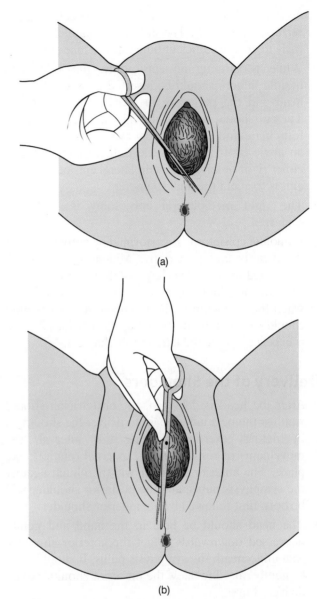

(a)

(b)

Fig. 14.8   Episiotomy: (a) mediolateral and (b) midline

- The timing of episiotomy is very important. It should be performed only when the head is crowning at the vulva without receding into the vagina when the contractions cease. At the time of episiotomy, the perineum should be thinned out and 3–4 cm of the head should be visible during a contraction. An episiotomy performed too early will cause excessive bleeding.

Procedure

- An episiotomy is carried out under aseptic precautions. Local infiltration with 1% lignocaine is given after administering a test dose. While giving the infiltration, the plunger is pulled back and aspirated to ensure that no vessel has been penetrated. If blood is drawn into the syringe with aspiration, the needle should be removed. IV injection of lignocaine can result in seizures and death. The infiltration should be given early to ensure sufficient time for it to take effect.

- While performing an episiotomy, the index and middle fingers should be inserted between the fetal head and the perineum to protect the fetal scalp. The cut should begin in the middle of the posterior fourchette and continue downwards and laterally at an angle of 45° towards the ischial tuberosity, and either right or left for a mediolateral episiotomy. The aim is to avoid the anal sphincter.

- The right mediolateral episiotomy is the most preferred.

- A midline episiotomy is performed by cutting directly downwards and posteriorly. Midline episiotomy is associated with good healing, but there is always a risk of third- and fourth-degree perineal tears, especially when the perineum is short. The episiotomy wound should be carefully sutured in layers after the placenta is expelled (discussed later in this chapter).

Delivery of the Shoulders

- After the head is delivered, the obstetrician should wait for the next labour pain to deliver the shoulders by natural exertion. During this interval, the movements of restitution and external rotation take place. The anterior shoulder will then hitch against the symphysis pubis, and the posterior shoulder will be born first followed by the anterior shoulder.

- The head should be held in the hand and gently depressed downwards to get the anterior shoulder well underneath the symphysis pubis. It should then be gently raised to allow the posterior shoulder to be delivered first.

- Traction should not be applied to the axilla, as doing so increases the chances of fracturing the humerus and injuring the nerve roots (Fig. 14.9a, b and c).

- The delivery of the shoulders should be delayed until the complete rotation of the bisacromial diameter has taken place.

- It is necessary to take care of the perineum during the delivery of the shoulders as perineal lacerations can occur due to rapid delivery or because of the larger bisacromial diameter of large babies.

Delivery of the Body

- After the delivery of the shoulders, the body is rapidly delivered and should be supported as it slides out. If there is a delay, the thorax may be held by the obstetrician and gentle traction applied.

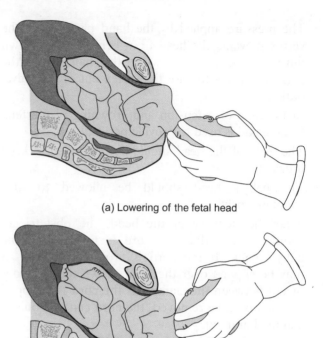

(a) Lowering of the fetal head

(b) Delivery of posterior shoulder

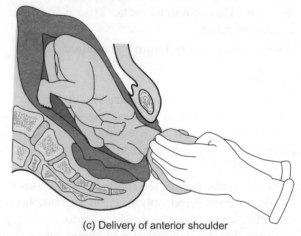

(c) Delivery of anterior shoulder

Fig. 14.9 Delivery of the shoulders: (a) lowering of the fetal head, (b) delivery of the posterior shoulder and (c) delivery of the anterior shoulder

- As soon as the baby has been delivered, it should be placed on its side between the mother's legs and covered with a dry towel.

- Routine suctioning of the baby's nose and mouth is not required. However, if there is delay in the initiation of respiration or in the presence of liquor, mucus or meconium in the pharynx, the air passages should be carefully cleared by aspiration with a plastic mucus catheter.

- The baby must be kept warm and in skin-to-skin contact on the mother's chest/abdomen.

The one delivery–one kit principle should be followed with autoclaved and pre-packed delivery sets and suture trays kept available for each case.

Ligation of the Cord

- If the cord is not clamped for three minutes after the delivery, the fetus receives 80–100 mL of maternal blood during this period. This amount of blood contains 50 mg iron, which reduces the incidence of iron deficiency anemia in the newborn. Therefore, the umbilical cord should be clamped and cut after 1–3 minutes.
- The cord should be ligated in two places—one ligature about 3–4 cm from the fetal umbilicus and the second as close to the vulval outlet as possible. The second ligature prevents the possibility of hemorrhage from the cord in twins. It also helps to determine the extravulval lengthening of the cord, which indicates placental separation in the third stage of labour. The cord is then divided close to the umbilical ligature. This is best done by taking the cord in the hollow of the palm and cutting it with scissors passed between the second and third fingers to avoid injury to the actively moving extremities of the child.
- After cutting the cord, the stump is examined for the presence of bleeding.
- The cord is left to dry on its own. There is no need to bandage and cover the cord as a routine.
- After the baby is delivered, the eyes and lids are wiped clean again and the baby wiped with a dry pre-warmed towel. This towel is then discarded, and the baby covered with another dry, pre-warmed towel. This technique is called the 'two-towel technique.'

Early cord clamping is advised in the following situations
- Birth asphyxia
- Cord wrapped tightly around the neck
- HIV-positive mothers
- Rh-isoimmunisation
- IUGR and preterm babies, to avoid cardiac overload
- Maternal complications such as PPH

MANAGEMENT OF THE THIRD STAGE OF LABOUR

The delivery of the placenta usually occurs within 5–10 minutes after the delivery of the fetus. Occasionally, it may take up to 30 minutes. If the third stage exceeds 30 minutes, active intervention is required. This is an important stage, during which the mother's condition, tonicity of the uterus and the amount of bleeding should be carefully observed. The third stage comprises two significant events—placental separation and placental expulsion.

■ PLACENTAL SEPARATION

As described in the previous chapter, signs of placental separation should be looked for. Without placental separation, the delivery of the placenta should not be attempted. When there is placental separation, the woman complains of pain associated with uterine contractions. The signs of placental separation are as follows:
- There will be a slight amount of fresh vaginal bleeding.
- The fundus of the uterus rises above the umbilicus and becomes globular and firmer. There will be a soft elevation above the symphysis with a depression immediately above, indicating that the placenta has separated from the fundus and is lying in the lower uterine segment (Fig. 14.10).

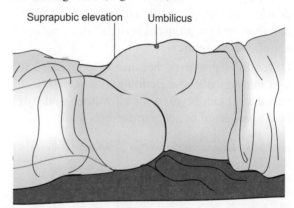

Suprapubic elevation   Umbilicus

Fig. 14.10   The third stage of labour (note the slight suprapubic elevation due to the expulsion of the placenta into the lower uterine segment)

- There is extravulval lengthening of the umbilical cord.
- If the fundus of the uterus is gently grasped and raised, the cord will not recede if the placenta has separated, whereas, if the placenta is still adherent to the uterus, the portion of the cord just outside the vulva will be drawn into the vagina.

■ DELIVERY OF THE PLACENTA

Normally, the placenta separates within 2–5 minutes of the birth of the baby. The features listed above as signs of placental separation are really signs of placental descent. In other words, the placenta separates some time before signs of descent are detected. The main objective of the management of the third stage of labour is to promote the separation of the placenta and membranes and their complete expulsion and to reduce bleeding by promoting permanent contraction and retraction of the uterus.

ACTIVE MANAGEMENT OF THE THIRD STAGE OF LABOUR (AMTSL)

The active management of the third stage of labour (Fig.14.11) reduces the amount of blood loss in the third stage by 33% and also prevents postpartum hemorrhage. Therefore, in all deliveries, the third stage should be managed by AMTSL.

Components of AMTSL

- Administration of oxytocic agents
- Delivery of placenta by controlled cord traction
- Uterine massage after the delivery of the placenta

Use of oxytocic agents

- In a singleton pregnancy, within one minute of the delivery of the placenta, 10 units of oxytocin are administered intramuscularly (this does not apply to a multiple pregnancy).
- Oxytocin is preferred because it is effective within 2–3 minutes of the injection and its side effects are minimal. It can be used for all women and can also be administered by the paramedical staff.

- If oxytocin is not available, ergometrine 0.2 mg is given IM or IV. Alternatively, syntometrine IM can be given. However, ergometrine is contraindicated in pre-eclampsia, eclampsia, hypertension and cardiac disease because it increases the risk of convulsions and cerebrovascular accidents. There is also a risk of retained placenta due to hourglass contractions of the uterus.
- At the PHC level, if oxytocin is unavailable, 600 μg of oral misoprostol is given within one minute of delivery of the baby. It can be given even by healthcare workers.
- In women in whom oxytocin was used for induction or augmentation of labour, the IV infusion of oxytocin should be continued for one hour post-delivery.
- Prostaglandins are reserved for the management of PPH.
- Oxytocin and ergometrine should be stored in the refrigerator to maintain efficacy.

Controlled cord traction (Brandt–Andrews manoeuvre)

- Before performing controlled cord traction, one should ensure that the placenta has separated.
- On confirming the placental separation, the clamped cord is held with one hand. The other hand is placed just above the symphysis pubis and used to apply counterpressure upwards and backwards (Fig. 14.12).
- This helps to prevent the inversion of the uterus.

Step 1: Administer uterotonic within 1 minute of delivery
Delivery of baby
Rule out presence of additional baby(s)
Uterotonic of choice; oxytocin 10 units IM as soon as the baby is delivered
Dry and warm the newborn
Put baby to breast
Wait till pulsation of cord stops
Clamp and cut the cord

Step 2: Controlled cord traction
Clamp cord close to perineum
Stabilise uterus using counter-pressure and gently pull downward on the cord
Encourage mother to push
Continue applying counter-pressure
Gently hold cord and await next contraction
Repeat controlled cord traction
As placenta delivers, hold in two hands and gently turn until membranes are twisted on themselves and they slowly deliver

Step 3: Massage the uterus
Immediately massage fundus of the uterus until it contracts
If membranes tear: gently examine cervix; remove any pieces of membrane visible
Ensure none of the placenta is missing
Take appropriate action if retained placenta fragments suspected
Palpate for contracted uterus every 15 minutes
Repeat uterine massage as needed during first 2 hours
Ensure uterus does not become soft after stopping massage
Teach mother to massage her own uterus as needed

Fig. 14.11 Algorithm for the AMTSL

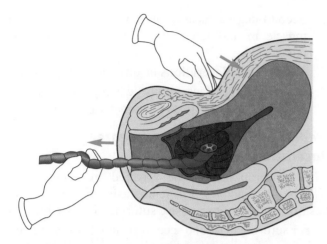

Fig. 14.12 Controlled cord traction (Brandt–Andrews manoeuvre)

EXAMINATION OF THE PLACENTA AND MEMBRANES

As soon as the placenta and membranes have been delivered, they are received in a basin, washed with water and examined (Fig. 14.13).

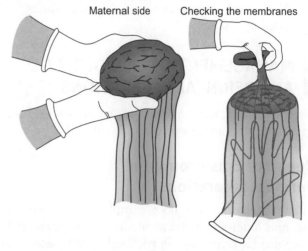

Maternal side   Checking the membranes

Fig. 14.13 Examination of the placenta: Maternal surface

- With the first strong uterine contraction, the mother should be instructed to push, and the placenta should be delivered by controlled cord traction. Cord traction should be applied only with the uterine contractions.
- Cord traction (pull) should never be applied without applying counter traction (push) above the pubic bone on a well-contracted uterus.
- As the placenta delivers, it is gently turned until the membranes are twisted. It is then slowly pulled to complete the delivery. The placenta and the membranes should be carefully checked for missing cotyledons and membrane bits.
- The woman should be carefully examined. Any tears to the cervix or vagina or episiotomy should be repaired.
- If the membranes start tearing, they should be grasped with a clamp and removed by applying gentle traction. If, at any time, there is brisk bleeding and the placenta cannot be delivered by these techniques, manual removal of the placenta is indicated.

Uterine massage
- After the delivery of the placenta, the uterus is massaged until the uterus is contracted. Thereafter, the uterus is palpated every 15 minutes for 2 hours to ensure that the uterus is contracted. Uterine massage can be performed by the woman herself.
- One should ensure that the uterus is not relaxed after the uterine massage is stopped.
- The mother should be encouraged to empty her bladder frequently in the immediate postpartum period, as a full bladder can displace the uterus backwards and result in uterine atonicity and PPH.

- The uterine surface of the placenta should first be examined to see that the cotyledons lie in close apposition. There should be no defect on the uterine surface at the grooves between the cotyledons or at the margin of the placenta.
- The membranes are then examined carefully to see that both the amnion and the chorion have been removed completely. Any small deficiency in the membranes should be carefully noted, as it may be due to the retention of a succenturiate lobe of the placenta.
- The umbilical cord should be examined for the presence of a single umbilical artery.

Retained Placenta or Membranes

If any portion of the placenta or the membranes is retained, there is a risk of hemorrhage and sepsis. If a large bit of placenta is retained, it should be removed immediately. However, small bits of the placenta and membranes may be managed conservatively under antibiotic cover as these may be passed in the lochia during the puerperium. These women should be observed for bleeding and sepsis and a USG may be carried out after 1–2 weeks to confirm the expulsion of the retained bits.

In a PHC setting, if there is any doubt about the completeness of the separated placenta, two IV lines should be instituted with large-bore (16 or 18 G) cannulae. Normal saline (NS) or Ringer's lactate (RL) should be started in one line and 10 units of oxytocin in RL should be started in the other line. Then, the Comprehensive Emergency Obstetric Care (CEmOC) centre should be informed, and the woman should be transferred in an ambulance. If facilities are available, grouping and cross-matching should be done at the PHC itself (management of retained placenta is discussed in Chapter 42).

MANAGEMENT OF EPISIOTOMY AND PERINEAL LACERATIONS

Lacerations of the vagina and perineum and the episiotomy should now be carefully sutured.

Repair of Episiotomy and Perineal Lacerations

After the placenta has been completely removed and the same ascertained, the perineum should be carefully examined for lacerations in good light, with the woman in the dorsal position. Following any instrumental delivery or any difficult procedure such as shoulder dystocia, the vagina, cervix and fornices should be examined for the presence of lacerations. Episiotomy is sutured at this point in time.

Lacerations of the vagina and perineum are classified as first-, second-, third- and fourth-degree lacerations.

1. **First-degree lacerations** involve the perineal skin and vaginal mucous membrane but not the underlying fascia and muscle.

2. **Second-degree lacerations** involve the fascia and muscle in addition to the skin and the mucous membrane.

3. **Third-degree lacerations** involve the anal sphincter.

4. **Fourth-degree lacerations** extend through the rectal mucosa to expose the lumen of the rectum.

Repair of first- and second-degree lacerations

These lacerations can be repaired in many ways. The basic principles are **hemostasis** and anatomical restoration without excessive suturing (Fig. 14.14a–c).

- For suturing first- and second-degree tears, adequate local infiltration should be given.
- First, all the freely bleeding points should be ligated using chromic 2-0 or 3-0 catgut or 1-0 or 2-0 polyglactin suture (vicryl).
- Chromic 2-0 or 3-0 suture is used as a continuous suture to close the vaginal mucosa and submucosa. The fascia and muscles are sutured by interrupted 2-0 and 3-0 chromic catgut. Closing all the layers together and applying tension on sutures should be avoided.
- The sutures must not be tied too tightly as this may result in pain. A few interrupted sutures of 3-0 chromic catgut are placed through the skin and subcutaneous fascia.
- In the PHC, only first- and second-degree tears can be sutured. Third- and fourth-degree tears should be referred to a CEmOC centre after ensuring hemostasis.

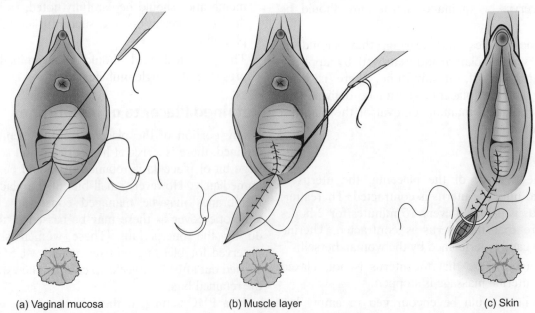

(a) Vaginal mucosa   (b) Muscle layer   (c) Skin

Fig. 14.14 Repair of a midline episiotomy: (a) Continuous locked 2-0 or 3-0 absorbable sutures are used to close the vaginal epithelium from the apex to the hymeneal ring; (b) interrupted sutures are used to close the superficial and deep perineal muscles and (c) a continuous suture is used to close the superficial fascia and a subcuticular stitch is applied to the skin

Repair of third- and fourth-degree lacerations

In third- or fourth-degree perineal lacerations, in which the anal sphincters and the anterior rectal wall are torn, repair should be carried out under anesthesia by experienced persons and under good light.

- First, the torn ends of the sphincter are localised. Then, the tear in the anterior rectal wall is closed with fine, interrupted catgut sutures tied within the lumen of the bowel.
- The ends of the rectal sphincter are reapproximated with interrupted catgut sutures.
- Then, the lacerations in the more superficial structures are sutured, and the skin closed over it.

■ POST-DELIVERY CARE

- The external genitalia should be carefully cleaned with antiseptic lotion. The cleaning should include the thighs, buttocks and the lower parts of the abdomen, since these are usually soiled with blood.
- A sterile or antiseptic pad of some absorbent material should be applied to the vulva.
- After suturing the episiotomy/perineal lacerations, the swabs and vaginal packs that were used should be checked and counted.

- The sphincter and rectal wall should be checked to see whether they are intact.
- In order to reduce pain, perineal care should be given with antiseptic wash and if necessary, with an ice pack. Analgesics may be required for pain. In the presence of acute pain and urinary retention, vulval and vaginal hematoma should be looked for.

THE FOURTH STAGE OF LABOUR

- The fourth stage of labour extends for one hour after the delivery of the placenta. During this period, the woman should be kept in the labour ward and observed for vitals and evidence of bleeding. Her bladder should be kept empty.
- Complications such as PPH, postpartum collapse and vulval hematoma may arise during this period and should be looked for.
- The woman may sleep at this stage, after light nourishment.
- Breastfeeding can be started as early as possible after a normal vaginal delivery but should always be within half an hour of delivery.
- Before leaving the woman, the obstetrician must make sure that the uterus is well-contracted, there is no undue bleeding and her vitals are stable.

KEY POINTS

- ✓ As soon as the woman reports to the labour room, a diagnosis of labour is made.
- ✓ True labour should be differentiated from false labour.
- ✓ During the first stage, the progress of labour is assessed, and fetal heart rate is monitored. A partograph should be used to monitor labour.
- ✓ A partograph is a graphic representation of the progress in labour in which cervical dilatation and the descent of the fetal head are plotted against time.
- ✓ In the active phase of labour, the cervix is expected to dilate 1 cm per hour.
- ✓ Controlled delivery of the head by using the modified Ritgen manoeuvre helps to prevent perineal lacerations.
- ✓ Active management of labour should be done in the third stage of labour.
- ✓ The basic principles of repair of perineal lacerations or episiotomy are hemostasis and anatomical restoration.
- ✓ Perineal lacerations are classified as first-, second-, third- and fourth-degree perineal tears.
- ✓ The placenta should be expressed only after one is certain that the placenta has completely separated from the upper uterine segment.
- ✓ The placenta should be carefully examined after delivery.
- ✓ The obstetrician should watch the woman for at least an hour after the completion of the third stage.

Essay questions

1. What information should be ascertained by vaginal examination at the onset of labour?
2. Describe the management of the first stage of labour.
3. Describe the management of the second stage of labour.
4. Describe the management of the third stage of labour.

5. A 30-year-old gravida 2, para 1 is admitted at 38 weeks of gestation with lower abdominal pain associated with mucoid discharge per vaginum. The pain occurs once in 10 minutes and is progressively increasing in severity.
   a) How would you differentiate true labour pains from false labour pains?
   b) What initial assessment should be carried out?
   c) What is a partograph and what are the components of a partograph?
   d) How will you assess the progress of labour? How do you diagnose abnormal labour?

6. A 28-year-old primigravida is admitted at 40 weeks of gestation with labour pains. She is getting contractions once in 3 minutes, each contraction lasting for 30–45 seconds. On examination, she is in the second stage of labour; the fetal head is engaged and the FHR is good.
   a) After delivery, what are the signs of placental separation?
   b) What is the active management of the third stage of labour?
   c) What is the fourth stage of labour?
   d) Describe the degrees of perineal tears.

Short answer questions
Write short notes on the following:
1. Repair of episiotomy
2. Partograph
3. The modified Ritgen manoeuvre
4. Midline versus mediolateral episiotomy
5. Active management of the third stage of labour
6. Retained placenta

MCQs
1. Which of the following is not a characteristic feature of true labour contractions?
   a) Increase in intensity of contractions
   b) Increase in duration of contractions
   c) Increase in interval between contractions
   d) Pain not relieved by sedation

2. Which of the following is not a characteristic feature of false labour pain?
   a) Irregular uterine contractions
   b) Pain in the lower abdomen
   c) Associated with cervical changes
   d) May be relieved by enema

3. An episiotomy is a planned perineal tear of the following degree:
   a) First
   b) Second
   c) Third
   d) Fourth

4. Which of the following is not part of the signs and symptoms of placental separation?
   a) Vaginal bleeding
   b) Extravulval lengthening of the cord
   c) Fundus of the uterus descends below the umbilicus
   d) The cord does not recede on raising the uterine fundus

5. Which of the following is not included in the active management of the third stage of labour (AMTSL)?
   a) Uterotonic agent
   b) Controlled cord traction
   c) Uterine massage
   d) Early cord clamping

6. How is the obstetric conjugate calculated?
   a) Direct measurement by vaginal examination
   b) X-ray pelvimetry
   c) 1.5–2 cm less than the measured diagonal conjugate
   d) 1.5–2 cm more than the measured diagonal conjugate

7. What is the rate of cervical dilatation in a primigravida?
   a) 0.5 cm/hr
   b) 1 cm/hr
   c) 1.5 cm/hr
   d) 2 cm/hr

8. In which phase of labour are cardinal movements of labour noted?
   a) Preparation phase
   b) Dilatation phase
   c) Pelvic phase
   d) Acceleration phase

9. What is the mean duration of second stage of labour in a primigravida?
   a) 20 mins
   b) 30 mins
   c) 50 mins
   d) 60 mins

10. Which of the following is not a sign of placental separation?
    a) Pain and slight fresh vaginal bleeding
    b) Extravulval lengthening of the cord
    c) Retraction of the cord
    d) Suprapubic bulge

11. AMTSL reduces blood loss by:
    a) 15%
    b) 20%
    c) 33%
    d) 50%

12. Which of the following refers to a perineal laceration involving the internal anal sphincter?
    a) First-degree tear
    b) Second-degree tear
    c) Third-degree tear
    d) Fourth-degree tear

Answers
1. (c), 2. (c), 3. (b), 4. (c), 5. (d), 6. (c), 7. (b), 8. (c), 9. (c), 10. (c), 11. (c), 12. (c)

Fill in the blanks
1. The encircling of the largest diameter of the fetal head by the vulvovaginal opening is known as _____.
2. _____ are the best parameters to indicate the progress of labour.

Answers
1. crowning, 2. Cervical dilatation and descent of the fetus

15

AN 49.5, OG 5.1, 13.1, 15.1 and 15.2, PE 18.4 and 18.5, PH 1.41, PY 9.8

Intrapartum Fetal Surveillance

Learning Objectives

» To describe the methods of fetal heart rate monitoring during labour
» To describe the normal and abnormal CTG findings in labour
» To be able to interpret abnormal CTG findings and understand their management
» To describe the management of fetal distress in labour

■ INTRODUCTION

Intrapartum fetal surveillance is the monitoring of the fetus in labour to ensure that the baby is delivered in good health. The aim of intrapartum surveillance is to detect fetal hypoxia early so that timely intervention can be undertaken to prevent fetal and neonatal complications.

Pathophysiology of Fetal Hypoxia

- In labour, during a uterine contraction, there is a transient reduction in blood flow through the placental bed. This results in decreased fetal oxygenation, which is well-tolerated by healthy fetuses. Oxygenation to the fetus is restored when the uterus relaxes between contractions.

- However, when the fetus is already compromised due to placental insufficiency or when there is a repetitive reduction in oxygenation to the fetus due to acute events, it is unable to tolerate the reduction in the oxygen supply and develops hypoxia. In response to hypoxia, the cardiac output is initially maintained and there is redistribution of blood to the brain at the expense of non-vital organs.

- These changes in blood flow manifest as fetal heart rate (FHR) changes long before there is sufficient hypoxia to result in brain injury. This forms the basis for intrapartum fetal monitoring. If the hypoxia is prolonged, it leads to metabolic acidosis which results in multi-organ dysfunction. The brain is damaged directly as a result of compromised blood flow or due to metabolic acidosis. These events can result in fetal distress and intrauterine/intrapartum or neonatal death. The babies that survive may exhibit severe neurological sequelae.

Fetuses at Risk of Developing Intrapartum Hypoxia

In the following instances, fetuses are particularly at risk of developing hypoxia:

- Growth-restricted and preterm fetuses and post-term pregnancies

- When there are pre-existing antenatal medical complications that predispose to placental insufficiency such as pre-eclampsia, type I diabetes mellitus, severe anemia/GDM, APLA, chronic renal insufficiency, etc.

- Even fetuses with a normal reserve may develop hypoxia in labour due to the hyperstimulation of the uterus, supine hypotension, epidural analgesia or acute events such as abruption or cord prolapse, cord compression, etc.

Besides these conditions, high-risk pregnancies such as those with a previous cesarean section should also be monitored in labour.

MONITORING IN LABOUR

Various techniques are available to detect evolving fetal hypoxia so that the fetus may be delivered before the development of permanent brain damage. The components of intrapartum surveillance include fetal surveillance and monitoring of uterine activity. In labour, the uterine activity is monitored simultaneously with FHR tracing as the fetal heart rate changes are interpreted in relation to the uterine activity.

■ FETAL SURVEILLANCE

The methods of assessing FHR include the following:

- FHR monitoring by intermittent auscultation (IA) with traditional methods and electronic fetal monitoring (EFM)
- Fetal acid–base measurement from fetal scalp pH
- Fetal pulse oximetry
- Fetal scalp lactate testing
- ST waveform analysis of the fetal heart

INTERMITTENT FETAL HEART RATE MONITORING

- This is the traditional method of monitoring FHR. The heart sounds are heard through a fetoscope (Pinard), stethoscope or a handheld fetal heart monitor. The number of heartbeats heard over a minute is used to calculate the heart rate (heart rate should be counted for a minimum of 60 seconds).
- The procedure is performed 30–45 seconds after a uterine contraction (so that the hypoxia due to the contraction is reversed).
- The procedure is repeated every 15 minutes during the first stage and every five minutes during the second stage of labour.
- As the woman pushes, the fetal heart is heard after every contraction.
- This technique is adequate for a low-risk pregnancy without complications. However, the fetus may be evaluated with CTG on admission which is called the **admission test**. If the fetal status is normal, intermittent monitoring may then be continued.
- The limitation of this method is that intermittent auscultation with a fetoscope may be difficult in very obese individuals.

ELECTRONIC FETAL MONITORING (EFM)

- The cardiac function of the fetus is controlled by the parasympathetic and sympathetic systems. Normal physiological events such as fetal movements, uterine contractions and stimulation as well as adverse events such as fetal hypoxia alter the sympathetic and parasympathetic activity. These alterations manifest as fetal heart rate changes.
- Electronic fetal monitoring (EFM) involves using external and internal FHR monitoring with cardiotocography (CTG). It can be used continuously and intermittently.
- This method allows for the assessment of sequential information regarding the fetal condition.
- In external monitoring, the fetal heart rate is detected by placing the ultrasound transducer on the maternal abdominal wall, at a site where the fetal heart is best heard. A coupling gel is applied between the transducer and the abdominal wall and the transducer is held in position by a belt.
- The fetal heart rate is obtained as a trace.
- CTG also records the uterine contractions in labour (Fig. 15.1).

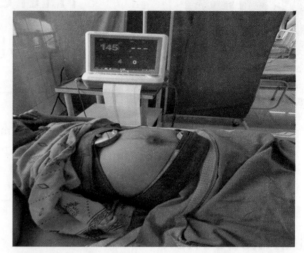

Fig. 15.1   External monitoring and recording of FHR and uterine contractions

- Internal FHR monitoring may be very useful in very obese individuals. It is performed by fixing a spiral electrode on the fetal scalp with a connection to the FHR monitor. The signals are processed and recorded as a graph. For internal monitoring, the fetal membranes must be ruptured and the cervix must be at least partially dilated before the electrode can be placed on the fetal scalp (Fig. 15.2). Internal FHR monitoring is not a routine procedure.

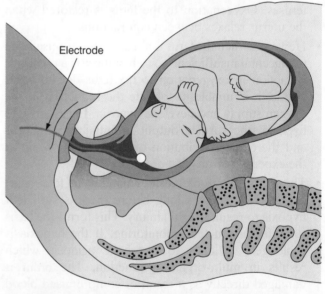

Fig. 15.2   Internal fetal heart monitoring with a scalp electrode

INDICATIONS FOR CONTINUOUS FHR MONITORING

Continuous fetal heart rate monitoring should be considered whenever risk factors exist. Risk factors may be present prior to labour or may develop during labour.

Antepartum risk factors

- Reduced fetal movement
- Abnormal umbilical artery Doppler velocimetry
- Suspected IUGR
- Antepartum hemorrhage
- Hypertension/pre-eclampsia (current pregnancy)
- Multiple pregnancy
- Overt diabetes mellitus/GDM
- Previous CS with VBAC
- Rh-isoimmunisation
- Oligohydramnios/polyhydramnios
- Maternal medical conditions (including severe anemia, cardiac disease, hyperthyroidism, vascular disease, renal disease)
- Preterm labour
- Post-term pregnancy

Risk factors in labour

- Prolonged rupture of membranes (>24 hours)
- Meconium-stained or bloodstained liquor
- Maternal pyrexia >38°C
- Chorioamnionitis
- Vaginal bleeding in labour
- Prolonged active first stage of labour
- Prolonged second stage of labour

Other indications

- Any use of oxytocin, whether for induction or augmentation of labour
- Before and for at least 20 minutes after the administration of prostaglandin
- Epidural analgesia (immediately after inserting an epidural block)

FETAL HEART RATE (FHR) CHANGES IN LABOUR

The FHR changes that occur in labour are classified into baseline changes and periodic changes. The baseline changes include the baseline heart rate and the variability. The periodic changes are the changes that occur in relation to stimulation and uterine contractions.

Baseline Changes

Normal baseline fetal heart rate

The normal baseline heart rate is 110–160 beats/minute (bpm) depending on the gestational age. It indicates the balance between the sympathetic and parasympathetic systems controlling the fetal heart. In mature fetuses, the heart rate is closer to the lower end of the spectrum—usually <130–140 bpm—which indicates the maturity of the parasympathetic system. In preterm fetuses, the control by the sympathetic system predominates, and the fetal heart rate is usually >140 bpm (Fig. 15.3). Changes in the baseline rate are an important indicator of developing hypoxia.

Abnormal baseline fetal heart rate patterns

The normal FHR is 110–160 bpm. Abnormal baseline fetal heart rate patterns are tachycardia and bradycardia.

Tachycardia (Fig. 15.4)

A baseline FHR of more than 160 bpm is termed tachycardia. It is classified as follows:

- Non-reassuring : 160 180 bpm
- Abnormal   : >180 bpm

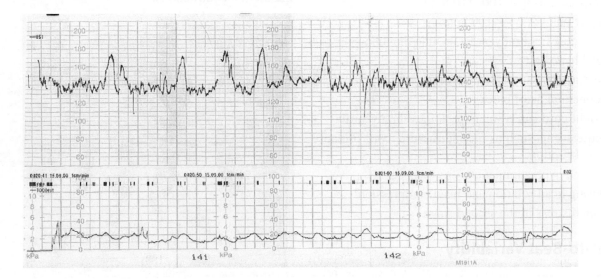

Fig. 15.3   Cardiotocograph: Baseline fetal heart rate of around 140 bpm

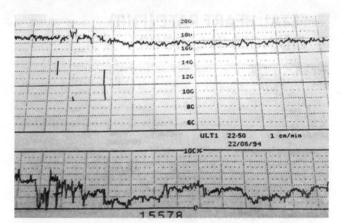

Fig. 15.4 CTG: Tachycardia with baseline heart rate above 170 bpm

The causes of tachycardia include the following:
• Prematurity
• Maternal tachycardia, fever
• Pain, anxiety, dehydration
• Maternal hyperthyroidism
• Fetal and intrauterine infections
• Acute and sub-acute fetal hypoxia and fetal distress due to the release of catecholamines
• Fetal cardiac arrhythmias
• Use of sympathomimetic drugs such as terbutaline, salbutamol, tocolytics such as ritodrine and hydralazine
• Fetal anemia due to abruption, vaso previa or fetomaternal hemorrhage

Bradycardia
A baseline FHR of less than 110 bpm is termed bradycardia. It is classified as follows:
• Non-reassuring : 100–110 bpm
• Abnormal : <100 bpm
   The causes of bradycardia include the following:
• Fetal hypoxia
• Epidural bolus with hypotension
• Congenital heart block
• A tight cord can result in prolonged bradycardia
• Acute events such as uterine rupture, cord prolapse and abruption
• Uterine hyperstimulation
• During head rotation and head compression
• Fetal distress in the second stage

Beat-to-Beat Variability
• Beat-to-beat variability is a function of the fetal autonomic nervous system. The fetal heart rate is not fixed; it keeps fluctuating above and below the

baseline for 5–25 beats. This is called variability. As it is not possible to measure the beat-to-beat variability, baseline variability is measured (the difference between the highest peak and lowest trough around the baseline). Diminished baseline variability is seen in fetal compromise and with the administration of drugs such as pethidine and magnesium sulphate to the mother. When the fetus is in the sleep phase, the variability may be reduced. In these instances, the fetus is stimulated, and the trace is repeated.
• Normal baseline variability is 6–25 bpm. If the variability is <5, it is considered reduced (Fig. 15.5). Variability of >25 beats (saltatory) is also abnormal. This may be seen in acute hypoxia, indicating excessive catecholamine secretion. Baseline variability rather than baseline rate is the best indicator of fetal well-being.

Causes of reduced baseline variability
Reduced variability up to 40 minutes can be seen when the fetus is in the rest phase (fetal sleep cycles). It is also seen in the following scenarios:
• Medications such as narcotics, anesthetic drugs, epidural and anti-hypertensives
• Fetal hypoxia
• Congenital malformations of the fetus
• Prematurity and fetal tachycardia

Periodic Changes
Periodic changes are accelerations and decelerations above and below the baseline that occur in relation to the uterine contractions.

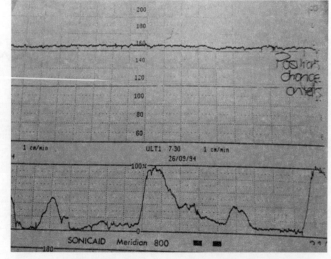

Fig. 15.5 CTG: Reduced variability (baseline heart rate is 160 bpm and the variability is <5)

Acceleration

It is a transient episode of an increase in fetal heart rate above the baseline. The FHR increases >15 bpm above the baseline for >15 seconds and then returns to the normal baseline rate. Fetal accelerations are seen with fetal movements, uterine contractions and stimulation. The presence of acceleration indicates reassurance. However, its absence does not indicate that the trace is abnormal.

Deceleration

It is a transient episode of slowing of the FHR below the baseline by >15 bpm for >15 seconds. It is divided into early, late and variable decelerations.

Early deceleration

- Early deceleration is synchronous with uterine contractions. Its onset, nadir and recovery are symmetrical with uterine contractions. The peak of the contraction is associated with the nadir of the FHR, but the FHR returns to the normal baseline value once the contraction passes. The FHR rarely falls below 20–30 bpm from its baseline value (Fig 15.6a and b).
- The **causes of early deceleration** are head compression in the late first stage and the descent of the head in the second stage of labour. With head compression, the intracranial pressure increases, which stimulates the vagus, leading to deceleration. ARM, vaginal examination and rarely, cord compression, cord presentation and cord prolapse can also cause early deceleration.

Late deceleration

- A late deceleration is late in timing with respect to the uterine contractions. It is usually pathological, indicating fetal distress.

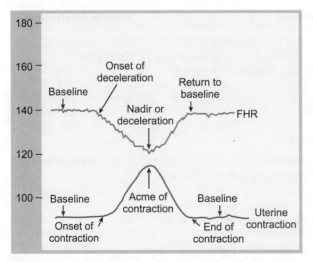

Fig. 15.6a   Diagrammatic representation of early deceleration

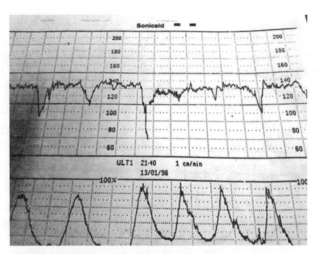

Fig. 15.6b   CTG sowing early deceleration

- The deceleration begins after the uterine contraction has reached its peak. FHR returns to baseline only after the uterine contraction has completely subsided. The FHR falls by 30–40 bpm from its baseline value (Fig 15.7a and b).

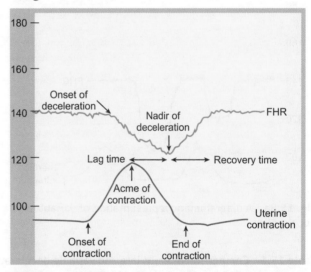

Fig. 15.7a   Diagrammatic representation of late deceleration

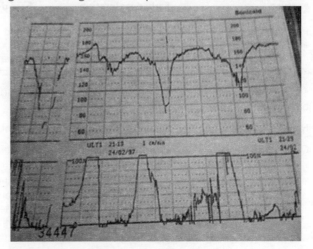

Fig. 15.7b   CTG showing late decelerations

Any process that causes maternal hypotension, uterine hyperactivity, acute events or placental dysfunction can produce late decelerations.

- **The causes of late deceleration** are as follows:
  — Epidural analgesia
  — Uterine hyperactivity due to oxytocin stimulation
  — Maternal diseases such as hypertension and diabetes
  — Severe fetal hypoxia
  — Acute events such as abruption, cord prolapse, and rupture of the uterus
  — Prolonged deceleration lasting for >3 minutes is due to an acute event

Variable decelerations

- In variable deceleration, the deceleration is variable in shape, size and occurrence in relation to uterine contractions (Fig. 15.8a and b).

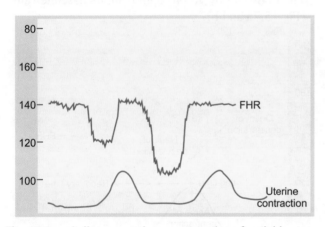

Fig. 15.8a A diagrammatic representation of variable deceleration

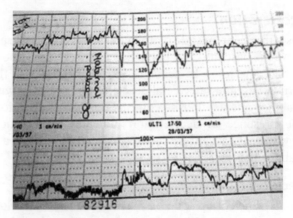

Fig. 15.8b CTG showing variable deceleration

- These decelerations occur due to umbilical cord compression. Variable deceleration is considered ominous if the FHR falls to >60 bpm and lasts >60 seconds or if it is associated with abnormal baseline and reduced variability.

The differences between the different types of decelerations are listed in Table 15.1.

▌ INTERPRETATIONS OF FETAL HEART RATE PATTERNS

CTG findings are interpreted as follows (Table 15.2):

Reassuring FHR

The FHR is considered reassuring if the baseline rate is 110–160 bpm and baseline variability is between 6 and 25, accelerations are present, decelerations are absent or there are early or variable decelerations for <90 minutes without any other concerning features. CTG is continued in these cases and routine care is given.

Table 15.1 Comparison of early, late and variable decelerations

Feature	Early deceleration	Late deceleration	Variable deceleration
Relationship between FHR and uterine contraction	Peak of the contraction and nadir of FHR coincide—'**mirror image**'	The drop in FHR begins almost after the peak of the contraction and recovery is long after the uterine contraction has subsided	No demonstrable correlation
FHR variability from baseline	20–30 bpm	30–40 bpm	
Nature of deceleration	Smooth and gradual	Smooth and gradual	Erratic
Common cause(s)	Head compression	• Epidural analgesia • Uterine hyperactivity due to oxytocin stimulation • Placental insufficiency due to maternal diseases like hypertension, diabetes and collagen vascular disease • Acute onset due to abruption	Cord compression

Table 15.2 Interpretation of CTG findings and management (RCOG guidelines)

Interpretation	Baseline (bpm)	Baseline variability (bpm)	Decelerations	Management
Reassuring	110–160	• 5–25	• None/early/variable without any concerning features <90 minutes	• Continue CTG/routine care
Non-reassuring	• 100–110 Or • 160–180	• <5 for 30–50 minutes • >25 for 30 minutes	• Variable decelerations without any concerning features >90 minutes	• Correct underlying cause such as hypotension and uterine hyperstimulation • Review entire clinical picture and CTG findings
Abnormal	<100–>180	• <5 for >50 minutes • >25 for >30 minutes • Sinusoidal	• Variable with concerning features for 30 minutes • Late decelerations for 30 minutes • Single prolonged deceleration for 3 minutes	• Exclude cord prolapse, placental abruption, uterine rupture • Correct underlying causes like hypotension and uterine hyperstimulation • If delivery is possible within a short period of time • Fetal blood sampling • Expedite delivery

Non-reassuring FHR

The FHR is considered non-reassuring if the baseline rate is 100–110 or 160–180 bpm and baseline variability is <5 bpm for 30–50 min and >25 for 30 minutes and if there are variable decelerations without any other concerning features but lasting >90 minutes. Underlying causes such as hypotension and uterine hyperstimulation should be looked for and corrected. The whole clinical picture and CTG findings should be reviewed.

Abnormal FHR

If the baseline rate is <100 or >180 bpm and the baseline variability is <5 or >25 and lasting for >30 minutes or if there is a sinusoidal pattern, variable decelerations with concerning features lasting >30 minutes or late/prolonged decelerations lasting >3 minutes, the FHR is considered abnormal. In such cases, cord prolapse, placental abruption and uterine rupture should be excluded. When present, the underlying causes like hypotension and uterine hyperstimulation should be corrected. If delivery is possible within a short period of time, fetal blood sampling can be done to determine the metabolic status of the fetus. If delivery is not imminent or the fetus is compromised with low pH, delivery should be expedited.

• A normal fetal heart pattern has a high negative predictive value, indicating that a normal pattern is reliably associated with good fetal outcome.

• An abnormal fetal heart pattern does not have a high positive predictive value—only 50% of abnormal traces are associated with significant acidosis.

• In order to avoid medicolegal issues, CTG traces should be preserved on record for a minimum of 25 years.

• All CTG traces should contain the woman's identity and the date and time of the test. All intrapartum events such as vaginal examination, rupture of the membrane, oxytocin infusion, epidural and mode of delivery should be recorded; the record should be duly signed.

▌ MANAGEMENT OF ABNORMAL FETAL HEART RATE PATTERNS

Abnormal fetal heart rate patterns are managed as follows:

1. The woman is moved to the left lateral position.

2. Maternal hypotension is corrected with IV fluids.

3. Uterine stimulants such as oxytocin infusion are discontinued.

4. Oxygen is administered to the woman.

5. Vaginal examination is performed to assess cord prolapse and to look for cervical dilatation and the descent of the fetal head.

6. Uterine contractions are assessed. If there is tachysystole associated with FHR changes, tocolytics should be administered. Amnioinfusion

may be carried out if there are recurrent variable decelerations.

7. Depending on the cervical dilatation/stage of labour, delivery should be promptly carried out by instrumental vaginal delivery or cesarean section.

8. In selected cases, abnormal CTG should be backed up by fetal scalp blood sampling.

9. The newborn may need to be resuscitated.

FETAL ACID–BASE MEASUREMENTS

The measurement of fetal acid–base levels is not a routine modality because not all medical centres are equipped with the required facilities. When there is an abnormal CTG finding, the purpose of assessing fetal pH is to ensure that the metabolic status of the fetus is normal so that vaginal delivery can be allowed, thereby reducing unnecessary cesarean sections. pH measurement is carried out only in women with 'abnormal' fetal heart rate tracings in whom the cervix is >4–5 cm dilated and Vx is at −1 or below so that rapid delivery is possible. Fetal blood sampling (FBS) should not be performed when the clinical picture demands early delivery due to ominous FHR.

Procedure

1. Fetal blood sampling should be performed with the woman in the left lateral position to prevent supine hypotension syndrome.

2. With an assistant holding up the woman's left leg, the perineum is cleaned. The position and dilatation of the cervix are then assessed by vaginal examination.

3. The fetal head is visualised through the amnioscope (Fig. 15.9). Before inserting the amnioscope, it should be cleaned and then coated with silicone grease.

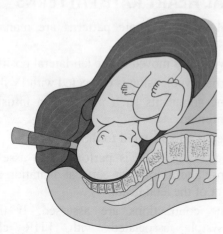

Fig. 15.9 Fetal scalp sampling using an amnioscope

4. Ethyl chloride is sprayed onto the fetal scalp, which causes hyperemia. A guarded blade is then pushed into the scalp to a depth of 2 mm, rotated through 90 degrees and then removed. On doing so, a bleb of blood appears, which is collected in a capillary tube.

5. Normal fetal pH is >7.25. A pH value of 7.2–7.24 indicates pre-acidosis. In such cases, the test should be repeated in 30 minutes; if the drop in pH is rapid, the baby should be delivered immediately.

6. A value of <7.2 indicates significant acidosis, which necessitates immediate delivery.

Contraindications for fetal blood sampling
- Maternal infection (HIV, hepatitis, HSV)
- Fetal bleeding disorders (e.g., hemophilia)
- Prematurity <34 weeks
- Face presentation

FETAL DISTRESS

Fetal distress in labour is diagnosed by abnormal CTG changes and by the passage of meconium in amniotic fluid, which indicates hypoxia and the relaxation of the anal sphincter. Thin, yellowish meconium is common in post-term pregnancies. Breech presentations also manifest with meconium-stained liquor. In the event of fetal distress, the baby should be delivered within 20–30 minutes.

OTHER METHODS OF ASSESSING FETAL HEALTH

Admission Test

When a woman is admitted in labour, continuous fetal monitoring is performed for 20 minutes.

- Normal tracing is indicated by the presence of a normal baseline, acceptable variability and two accelerations. This implies that the chance of the fetus developing hypoxia is small.

- A CTG in which there are no accelerations or in which there are abnormalities such as decreased variability, tachycardia, bradycardia or decelerations is considered a **suspicious tracing**.

- A CTG with two or more abnormalities is considered an **ominous or pathological tracing**.

- A combination of amniotic fluid volume assessment in early labour and an admission test may be used to identify fetuses at risk of hypoxia.

Fetal Stimulation Tests

Vibroacoustic stimulation test

In this test, the fetus is stimulated with a device such as an acoustic stimulator. The device is placed over the region of the fetal head on the maternal abdomen. The sound produced by the device causes a reflex in the fetus, resulting in fetal heart acceleration.

- **Normal result:** Prolonged acceleration for three minutes, two accelerations or one acceleration lasting for more than one minute
- **Abnormal result:** No response or acceleration, followed by a deceleration

Scalp Stimulation Test

The presence of fetal heart rate acceleration in response to fetal scalp stimulation is taken as normal.

Pulse Oximetry

When the cervix is dilated and when the membrane has ruptured, a sensor is placed against the fetal cheek, and the fetal arterial oxygenation is measured (SpO_2). Fetal oximetry values greater than or equal to 30% are indicative of fetal well-being and are rarely associated with fetal metabolic acidosis.

▌ SURVEILLANCE OF UTERINE ACTIVITY

The measurement of uterine activity is not routinely carried out.

Intrauterine Pressures in Labour

- The baseline pressure increases from 8 mmHg to 10 mmHg.
- The intrauterine pressure increases progressively during the first stage of labour from 25 mmHg to 50 mmHg.

- During the second stage of labour, the intrauterine pressure increases to 100 mmHg.
- Uterine contractions become painful when the intrauterine pressure exceeds 15 mmHg

Techniques of Measuring Intrauterine Pressure

Internal monitoring

An intrauterine catheter is placed in the amniotic fluid above the presenting part to measure intrauterine pressure. It measures the exact intensity of uterine contractions. This is not a routine method of monitoring intrauterine pressure.

External monitoring

A transducer is placed on the abdominal wall to measure the strength of uterine contractions. It measures the onset, peak and end of contractions.

Manual evaluation

In practice, uterine contractions are evaluated manually. With the palm of the hand resting lightly on the uterus, the time of the onset of contractions is determined. The intensity of a contraction is proportionate to the degree of firmness of the uterus. At the peak of effective contractions, the finger cannot readily indent the uterus. The time of disappearance of contractions is then noted. In this way, the frequency, duration and intensity of uterine contractions are determined.

▌ MANAGEMENT IN THE PRIMARY HEALTH CENTRE

If persistent FHR abnormality is detected, the woman is turned to the left lateral position and the oxytocin drip (if on flow) is stopped. The woman is given nasal oxygen and transferred to a Comprehensive Emergency Obstetric Care (CEmOC) centre with a Ringer's lactate (RL) infusion.

KEY POINTS

✓ Intrapartum fetal surveillance is the monitoring of the fetus in labour to ensure that the baby is delivered in good health.

✓ Transient reduction in blood flow through the placental bed results in decreased fetal oxygenation, which is well-tolerated by healthy fetuses. In cases of fetal compromise or in the presence of acute events, the fetus is unable to tolerate the reduction in the oxygen supply. In such cases, the fetus develops hypoxia, which manifests as FHR changes.

✓ The FHR changes that occur in labour are classified into baseline changes and periodic changes. The baseline changes comprise baseline heart rate and variability. Abnormal baseline changes are fetal tachycardia, fetal bradycardia and reduced baseline variability.

✓ Decelerations occurring in labour are classified into early, variable and late.

✓ Early decelerations develop as a result of head compression in the second stage of labour.

✓ Late deceleration indicates severe hypoxia and necessitates immediate delivery.

✓ Fetal distress in labour is diagnosed by abnormal CTG changes and the passage of meconium in amniotic fluid.

✓ In the event of fetal distress, the baby should be delivered within 20–30 minutes.

Essay questions

1. Describe the methods of fetal heart rate monitoring during labour.
2. Describe the normal and abnormal CTG findings seen in labour.
3. How would you interpret abnormal CTG findings in labour? Discuss the management of abnormal CTG.
4. A 30-year-old gravida 2, para 1 was admitted at 39 weeks of gestation with labour pains. The labour was augmented with oxytocin infusion as there was slow progress of labour in the active phase. The CTG shows a baseline rate of 100 bpm with variable decelerations up to 80 bpm. The cervix is 5 cm dilated and the fetal head is at the –2 station.
   a) What is the CTG finding in this case?
   b) What are the causes of this abnormal CTG finding?
   c) What is the immediate action you will take?
   d) How would you deliver the woman?

Short answer questions

Write short notes on the following:

1. Indications for continuous fetal heart rate monitoring
2. Indications of fetal blood sampling and the technique
3. Contraindications for fetal blood sampling
4. Monitoring of uterine activity

MCQs

1. Which of the following is not included in fetal surveillance?
   a) Fetal heart rate
   b) Fetal acid–base status
   c) Uterine activity
   d) Cervical dilatation
2. Which of the following is not a cause of fetal tachycardia?
   a) Maternal fever
   b) Fetal compromise
   c) Fetal head compression
   d) Maternal intake of terbutaline
3. Which of these conditions causes variable deceleration?
   a) Head compression with uterine contraction
   b) Epidural analgesia causing maternal hypotension
   c) Umbilical cord compression
   d) Placental abruption
4. Fetal blood sampling is contraindicated in all except:
   a) Maternal HIV infection
   b) Variable decelerations >45 minutes
   c) Face presentation
   d) Impending delivery
5. Painful uterine contractions are noted when minimum intrauterine pressure is more than:
   a) 10 mmHg
   b) 15 mmHg
   c) 25 mmHg
   d) 50 mmHg
6. Which of the following is not associated with diminished beat-to-beat variability?
   a) Fetal breathing
   b) Epidural analgesia
   c) Mother on magnesium sulphate
   d) Fetal compromise
7. Which of the following causes early decelerations?
   a) Fetal head compression
   b) Umbilical cord compression
   c) Fetal hypoxia
   d) Congenital heart block
8. What is the normal fetal heart rate response to fetal stimulation?
   a) Acceleration
   b) Acceleration followed by deceleration
   c) Deceleration followed by acceleration
   d) Deceleration
9. Immediate delivery is indicated if the scalp pH is:
   a) <7.2
   b) >7.25
   c) <7.25
   d) >7.2
10. During labour, which one of the following fetal heart rate patterns is ominous?
    a) Variable deceleration
    b) Early deceleration
    c) Tachycardia
    d) Persistent late deceleration

Answers

1. (d), 2. (c), 3. (c), 4. (b), 5. (b), 6. (a), 7. (a), 8. (a), 9. (a), 10. (d)

Fill in the blanks

1. The normal baseline fetal heart rate at term is _____.
2. The normal beat-to-beat variability is _____.
3. Normal fetal pH is _____.
4. Uterine contractions become painful when the intrauterine pressure exceeds _____ mmHg.
5. The fetal heart rate is monitored every _____ minutes during the first stage and every _____ minutes during the second stage of labour.

Answers

1. 110–160, 2. 6–25, 3. 7.25, 4. 15, 5. 15, 5

Case scenario-based discussion

1. A 27-year-old primigravida is admitted at 38 weeks of gestation with labour pains, which she has been experiencing for the past 6 hours. On examination, she is in the active phase of labour with 4 cm cervical dilatation.
   a) How would you monitor the fetal condition?
   b) How often should you auscultate the fetal heart in the first and second stages of labour?
   c) What are the indications for continuous CTG monitoring?
   d) What are the causes of fetal tachycardia?

Answers

a) In low-risk cases, following an admission test, fetal heart rate can be monitored intermittently with a fetoscope or a fetal Doppler. In high-risk cases, continuous CTG monitoring is required.

b) If intermittent auscultation is used, the fetal heart is auscultated every 15 minutes during the first stage and every five minutes during the second stage of labour. As the woman is pushing, the fetal heart is heard after every contraction.

c) Continuous fetal heart rate monitoring should be considered whenever risk factors exist such as reduced fetal movement, abnormal umbilical artery Doppler velocimetry, suspected IUGR, antepartum hemorrhage, associated medical conditions, previous CS with VBAC, oligohydramnios, prolonged rupture of membranes (>24 hours), meconium-stained or bloodstained liquor and the use of oxytocin for the augmentation of labour.

d) The causes of tachycardia include prematurity, maternal tachycardia, fever, pain, anxiety, dehydration, maternal hyperthyroidism, fetal and intrauterine infections and fetal hypoxia. The use of sympathomimetic drugs such as terbutaline, salbutamol and tocolytics such as ritodrine and hydralazine also cause fetal tachycardia.

16

OG 13.1

Induction of Labour

Learning Objectives

» To know the principles of induction of labour
» To know the indications and contraindications for the induction of labour
» To know the methods and complications of the induction of labour

■ INTRODUCTION

- **Induction of labour** is defined as the process of initiating labour by artificial means prior to its spontaneous onset at a viable gestational age with the aim of achieving vaginal delivery in a pregnant woman.
- **Augmentation of labour** is the stimulation of already established spontaneous contractions that are considered inadequate for successful delivery.

- **Induction of labour:** Stimulating the uterus to begin labour
- **Augmentation of labour:** Stimulating the uterus during labour to increase the frequency, duration and strength of contractions

■ INDICATIONS FOR INDUCTION OF LABOUR (IOL)

Induction of labour is indicated when the risk to the mother and/or fetus from the continuation of pregnancy outweighs the risk of terminating the pregnancy. The goals of induction of labour are to eliminate the potential risk to the mother and/or the fetus and to achieve vaginal delivery. Induction should be performed only for a specific medical and/or obstetric indication and the induction process should reproduce spontaneous labour as closely as possible without subjecting the mother or fetus to risks.

Indications for IOL
- Prolonged pregnancy
- Prelabour rupture of membranes
- Fetal growth restriction
- Rhesus-isoimmunisation
- Medical diseases such as pre-eclampsia, eclampsia, diabetes, chronic hypertension, chronic kidney disease, autoimmune diseases, etc.
- Oligo/Polyhydramnios

- Bad obstetric history/previous unexplained intrauterine death
- Intrauterine fetal demise (IUFD) in current pregnancy
- Congenital malformations of the fetus
- Non-medical indications—on maternal request (elective induction)

Induction of Labour in Post-Term Pregnancy

The International Classification of Diseases defines term pregnancy as delivery between 37 weeks and 0 days and 41 weeks and 6 days. Post-term pregnancy is one where the pregnancy extends beyond 42 weeks of gestation. If pregnancy is allowed to go beyond term, the following complications may occur:
- Liquor volume reduces
- Placental insufficiency
- Incidence of meconium staining of liquor is higher
- Fetal heart rate variations during labour may increase
- Macrosomia
- Fetal and neonatal death
- Dysfunctional labour
- Shoulder dystocia

Because of these risks, the WHO recommends induction of labour at 41 weeks of gestation.

Before induction, the accurate estimation of gestational age is crucial in order to diagnose and manage late-term and post-term pregnancies.

- EDD is calculated based on the reliable LMP, regularity of cycles and the first- and early second-trimester USG findings.
- If the EDD calculated by the LMP and USG fall within 10 days of each other, the LMP is used to calculate the EDD.

- For women with uncertain dates or an unknown LMP, the first-trimester scan at 11–13 weeks is recommended for dating.

Prerequisites to wait until 40 weeks + 7 days

- There should not be any high-risk factors such as pre-eclampsia, GDM, IUGR, oligohydramnios, Rh-incompatibility, short stature of the mother or PROM.
- There should not be any CPD.
- The fetus should be in good health.

Premature Rupture of Membranes

When a woman presents with premature rupture of membranes, the two options are expectant management or immediate induction of labour. Immediate induction is required when it is associated with maternal or fetal complications or to reduce maternal and perinatal morbidity associated with infection.

Rh-Incompatibility

In an Rh-negative woman who is carrying an Rh-positive fetus, the indirect Coombs test is carried out periodically to identify antibodies produced against fetal cells. This is called isoimmunisation. In isoimmunised pregnancies, these antibodies cause hemolysis of fetal red blood cells, leading to fetal anemia. In order to shorten the exposure of the fetus to maternal antibodies, induction of labour may be required. In any Rh-negative woman, pregnancy is not allowed to go beyond 40 weeks of gestation so as to reduce the chances of fetomaternal hemorrhage.

Pregnancy-Induced Hypertension

One of the most common indications for induction of labour is pre-eclampsia. The indications include mild/severe pre-eclampsia at >37 weeks of gestation, associated IUGR, severe pre-eclampsia at any gestational age not responding to treatment, and eclampsia. In these cases, induction of labour is required in order to prevent maternal and fetal morbidity and mortality.

Diabetes

- Uncomplicated GDM patients are induced at 40 weeks, and they are not allowed to go beyond 40 weeks because of the risk of intrauterine fetal death (IUFD).
- GDM patients on insulin therapy with well-controlled blood sugar are induced at 39 weeks of pregnancy.

- In uncontrolled gestational diabetes mellitus/ macrosomic fetus or in the presence of diabetic vasculopathy, induction may be indicated by 38 weeks to prevent sudden intrauterine death of the fetus. Earlier induction may also be required depending on the fetomaternal condition.

Deteriorating Maternal Illness

In certain maternal conditions such as hypertension, renal disease, liver disease and autoimmune disorders, induction may be required in the interest of the mother.

Fetal Malformations

When lethal and non-correctable fetal malformations such as severe hydrocephalus, anencephaly or meningo myelocele are identified, the woman may be given the option to terminate the pregnancy by inducing labour.

Intrauterine Death of the Fetus (IUFD)

The expulsion of the dead fetus can occur spontaneously. However, if it is retained for more than two weeks, there is a risk of sepsis and coagulation failure. In order to avoid these complications, induction of labour is performed in cases of IUFD.

Elective Induction (Social Induction)

Elective induction refers to the induction of labour at full term in a woman in whom there are no maternal or fetal indications or clear health benefits to induce labour; rather, IOL is carried out for the convenience of the obstetrician or the pregnant woman. Elective induction is not recommended as induced labour is associated with increased cesarean rates.

■ CONTRAINDICATIONS FOR IOL

The contraindications to induction of labour include those that would preclude spontaneous labour and vaginal delivery.

Absolute Contraindications for IOL

- Contracted pelvis
- Placenta previa
- Uterine scar–classical CS or inverted T-shaped incision
- Myomectomy scar
- Hysterotomy/unification surgery in a bicornuate uterus

- Floating presenting part, abnormal fetal lie
- Compromised fetus that cannot withstand the stress of labour
- Cord presentation
- Vasa previa
- Active genital herpes
- Invasive cervical carcinoma
- Fever due to general medical causes
- Previous pelvic surgeries—VVF, RVF, third- and fourth-degree perineal tear repair

Relative Contraindication

- Previous lower segment cesarean section scar

PREINDUCTION ASSESSMENT

- It is important to perform a thorough evaluation of the maternal and fetal condition before undertaking labour induction in order to make sure there are no contraindications to labour or vaginal delivery. A maternal and fetal risk vs. benefit analysis should also be performed. Counselling and informed written consent are important.
- The favourability of the cervix should be assessed for the likelihood of successful induction.

Assessing the Favourability of the Cervix for Induction

The success of induction of labour is related to the condition of the cervix at the beginning of induction and the gestational age (the higher the better). To assess the condition of the cervix, a cervical examination is performed, and a score is assigned based on Bishop's criteria. When the Bishop score was introduced in 1964, cervical effacement was noted as the percentage of effacement—a score 0 denoted 0–30% effacement; 1 denoted 40–50% effacement; 2 denoted 60–70% effacement and 3 denoted 80% effacement. In 1974, the modified Bishop score (Table 16.1) was introduced; in this system, the cervical effacement was reported in terms of cervical length, which is more objective.

- If the cervix is favourable (has a score of 6 or more), labour is usually successfully induced by artificial rupture of the membranes (ARM) or ARM with oxytocin infusion.
- If the cervix is unfavourable (has a score of 5 or less), the cervix is ripened using prostaglandins. Alternatively, a Foley catheter is used for induction.

Table 16.1 Modified Bishop score

Findings	0	1	2	3
Cervical dilatation (cm)	0	1–2	3–4	5+
Cervical effacement (cm)	4	3–4	1–2	<1
Consistency	Firm	Medium	Soft	
Position	Posterior	Central	Anterior	
Decent by station of the head (cm from the ischial spines)	–3	–2	–1, 0	+1, +2

Total score: 13
Favourable score: 6–13
Unfavourable score: 1–5
Modifiers:
Add 1 point for pre-eclampsia
Add 1 point for each previous vaginal delivery
Subtract 1 point for postdated pregnancy, nulliparity and PPROM

METHODS OF LABOUR INDUCTION

Broadly, the following methods are used for the induction of labour.

1. Prostaglandins: Dinoprostone vaginal gel (PGE$_2$)/ misoprostol (PGE$_1$) tablets can be used by the oral, buccal and vaginal routes
2. Mechanical methods: Insertion of a Foley catheter and membrane sweeping or a hygroscopic or osmotic dilator (laminaria tent, Dilapan)
3. Artificial rupture of membranes (ARM)
4. Oxytocin infusion

THE UNFAVOURABLE CERVIX (SCORE <6)

The unfavourable cervix is associated with a high chance of unsuccessful induction. Therefore, many techniques have been described to ripen the cervix before stimulating uterine contractions.

Pharmacological Techniques— Prostaglandins

Prostaglandin E$_2$ (Dinoprostone)

- *Dinoprostone gel:* 0.5 mg (3 g gel) is commonly used for cervical ripening prior to induction. It is instilled into the endocervix and not beyond the internal cervical os. The dose can be repeated every 6 hours. If there is inadequate cervical change and minimal uterine activity, the dose can be repeated up to three times in 24 hours. The fetal heart should be monitored by continuous CTG for 15–30 minutes following each insertion and thereafter, periodically. The interval between the final dose and the initiation of oxytocin should be >6 hours to prevent uterine hyperstimulation (Fig. 16.1). The induction is considered a failure if there is no response to this regimen. The side effects of prostaglandins include GI upset such as diarrhea, vomiting, hyperpyrexia and hypertonus of the uterus. PGE_2 should be used cautiously in patients with glaucoma, severe hepatic or renal dysfunction or asthma. The gel should be stored in a refrigerator at 2–8°C.

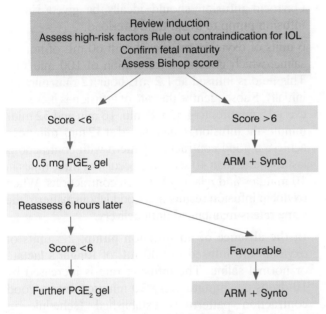

Review induction
Assess high-risk factors Rule out contraindication for IOL
Confirm fetal maturity
Assess Bishop score

Score <6 → 0.5 mg PGE_2 gel → Reassess 6 hours later → Score <6 → Further PGE_2 gel

Score >6 → ARM + Synto

Favourable → ARM + Synto

Fig. 16.1 Induction of labour with PGE_2 gel

Misoprostol (synthetic analogue of PGE_1)

It is given in a dose of 25 µg vaginally or orally every 6 hours. The dosage should not exceed four doses in 24 hours. The major advantage of misoprostol is that it is stable at room temperature. However, this drug is not yet FDA approved, and therefore, should be used with caution. It can be used for the induction of IUFD/ severe pre-eclampsia occurring in the second trimester. Though many organisations recommend the use of misoprostol for inducing labour in a term pregnancy with a viable fetus, caution should be exercised. Side effects include diarrhea, nausea, vomiting, febrile illness, tachysystole and meconium-stained liquor. Uterine rupture can occur if used for women who have a scarred uterus.

Mifepristone

Mifepristone is an antiprogesterone. It acts on the cervix and softens it, thereby making it sensitive to prostaglandins. It converts the quiet pregnant uterus into an organ of spontaneous activity. Mifepristone is not used alone for the induction of labour. A single oral tablet of 200 mg is used 24 hours before administering PGE_2 gel or PGE_1.

Mechanical Techniques

Mechanical methods release prostaglandins, thereby, stimulating uterine contractions. These techniques include the following:

- Membrane sweeping
- Hygroscopic cervical dilators, e.g., laminaria tent
- Balloon catheter (transcervical Foley catheter)

Membrane sweeping

The procedure involves separating the fetal membranes from the lower uterine segment digitally through a partially dilated cervix, which releases prostaglandins from the membranes. The procedure can cause discomfort, a small amount of bleeding and occasionally, the rupture of membranes. The option of membrane sweeping can be offered at 40 weeks for nulliparous women and at 41 weeks for multiparous women.

Hygroscopic cervical dilator

Both synthetic and natural dilators are available. Natural dilators are made from seaweed; the synthetic one is the Dilapan. These are rigid rods that are inserted into the cervix, whereupon, they absorb the local moisture and swell up to exert mechanical pressure on the cervix. This helps in the release of prostaglandins.

Foley catheter

The Foley catheter is an effective alternative to prostaglandins for cervical ripening and labour induction, especially in cases of previous cesarean section. 14–18 F catheters are used. The catheter is placed in such a way that the bulb rests against the internal cervical os. Then, the bulb is inflated with 30–60 mL of sterile water. This method is contraindicated in women with absent membranes, cervicitis or vaginitis. The catheter is left in place until the contractions begin or for 12–24 hours.

Advantages of mechanical methods

- The risks of uterine hyperstimulation and fetal heart abnormalities are lesser than with other methods.
- These methods are suitable for inducing women who have had a previous cesarean section, those who have oligohydramnios, in cases of FGR and in multiparous women.

◼ THE FAVOURABLE CERVIX (SCORE >6)

When the cervix is favourable, all the methods of induction are equally effective. Oxytocin infusion and artificial rupture of membranes (ARM) are used when the cervix is favourable.

Amniotomy

- Amniotomy or artificial rupture of membranes (ARM) stimulates uterine activity by causing uterine decompression and local prostaglandin release. Usually, after amniotomy, there is a variable interval (the latent period) before labour starts. Amniotomy may be followed by oxytocin infusion if the labour does not start within 1–2 hours in a multiparous woman or when the cervix is very favourable. If labour is induced because of severe maternal disease (e.g., eclampsia) oxytocin infusion should be started at the same time as (ARM).

- The procedure should be carried out under sterile precautions. Prior to the procedure, the FHR should be noted. Following the ARM, the amount and colour of the liquor should be noted. The obstetrician should also look for excessive bleeding and ensure that there is no cord prolapse. The fetal heart and fetal lie should also be checked.

- In cases of polyhydramnios, fluid should be let out very slowly to prevent placental abruption. If delivery is not anticipated within 12 hours, prophylactic antibiotics are given—ampicillin 2 g IV every 6 hours until delivery.

Contraindications for ARM

AROM is contraindicated if the head is high, in the presence of malpresentation or unstable lie, when the cervix is unfavourable and in the presence of cord presentation. If a woman is HIV-positive, the membranes should be left intact for as long as possible to reduce the perinatal transmission of HIV.

Risks of amniotomy

The main risks of amniotomy are cord prolapse and infection.

Oxytocin Infusion

- It is a synthetic analogue of endogenous oxytocin and is very potent. Oxytocin stimulates receptors in the uterus directly, thus, stimulating uterine contractions.

- The response to oxytocin increases after 20 weeks of gestation until the middle of the third trimester and then remains stable until term, after which it increases dramatically.

- The goal of oxytocin infusion is to induce uterine activity that can produce cervical dilatation and fetal descent without causing uterine hyperstimulation or fetal distress.

- Oxytocin infusion is not started within six hours of using prostaglandins. In order to avoid the risk of amniotic fluid embolism, oxytocin infusion should be avoided before rupturing the membranes.

Procedure

- Each ampoule contains 5 units (1 mL) of oxytocin.
- Oxytocin infusion should ideally be given via an infusion pump to avoid fluid overload.

- 6 units of oxytocin are mixed with 60 mL of normal saline, which gives a concentration of 100 miu/mL. This fluid is infused at 1.2 mL/hour (2 miu/minute) initially. Subsequently, the rate of infusion is increased every 15 minutes to 4 miu, 8 miu, 16 miu and 32 miu/minute; the infusion is maintained at 32 miu/minute to achieve a good contraction pattern with contractions lasting more than 40 seconds, occurring three times in 10 minutes and relaxing between contractions. When oxytocin infusion results in a good labour pattern, the same rate is maintained until delivery.

- **In the absence of an infusion pump,** 2.5 units of oxytocin are infused in 500 mL of Ringer's lactate or normal saline. The infusion rate is increased by 10 drops per minute every 30 minutes until a good contraction pattern is established (schedule in Table 16.2).

Table 16.2 Oxytocin infusion rates for the induction of labour

Time (hours)	Drops/ minute	2.5 units/500 mL* (5 miu/minute)	Volume infused
0.00	10	2.5	0
0.30	20	5	15
1.00	30	7.5	30
1.30	40	10	45
2.00	50	12.5	60
2.30	60	14.5	75

*(1 mL = 20 drops)

- If there aren't three contractions in 10 minutes, each lasting more than 40 seconds with the infusion rate at 60 drops per minute, oxytocin concentration may be increased to 5 units in 500 mL of fluid in a primi. Alternatively, delivery by cesarean section should be undertaken. (The total dose of oxytocin should not exceed 5 units.)

Monitoring a woman on oxytocin infusion

- Women receiving oxytocin should never be left alone.
- The woman is nursed on her left side.
- Her pulse, blood pressure and uterine contractions and the fetal heart rate are carefully monitored. A medical officer stays with the woman, watching the contractions, adjusting the rate of the drip and recording the fetal heart rate every half hour; preferably, continuous electronic monitoring is used.
- The oxytocin drip is discontinued if there are more than 5 uterine contractions in 10 minutes or when there are fetal heart irregularities. Uterine hypersensitivity usually gets corrected once the infusion is stopped.

Risks associated with oxytocin infusion

- Uterine hyperstimulation and uterine rupture can occur, especially in multiparous women.
- Water intoxication can occur if a large dose of oxytocin is infused in a large volume of fluid. This could result in convulsions, coma and death.
- Fetal distress/fetal death can occur from hyperstimulation.

■ RISKS OF IOL

- Failure of induction—20%
- Prolonged labour
- Hyperstimulation (tachysystole or hypertonus)—tachysystole is defined as the presence of 5 contractions in 10 minutes and hypertonus refers to contractions lasting >60 seconds

- Abruption/Rupture/Laceration of the cervix due to tumultuous uterine contractions
- With hyperstimulation, amniotic fluid embolism can occur
- Cord prolapse
- Intrauterine infection
- Iatrogenic prematurity
- Fetal distress
- If oxytocin infusion was used in labour, it should be continued after delivery to prevent PPH

Management of Hyperstimulation

Hyperstimulation is defined as a contraction lasting more than 60 seconds or more than 5 contractions in 10 minutes. If hyperstimulation occurs, the infusion is stopped and the woman is turned to the lateral position. Oxygen is then administered at 4 litres/minute and tocolytics are used to relax the uterus (terbutaline inhalation [2 puffs]/terbutaline 250 µg IV slowly over 5 minutes/salbutamol 10 mg in 1 litre IV fluid [NS or RL] run at 10 drops/minute).

> **Recent developments**
> Long-acting dinoprostone preparations are available. Dinoprostone vaginal insert contains 10 mg of dinoprostone, which is designed to release at approximately 0.3 mg/hour over a 12-hour period. Dinoprostone vaginal insert should be removed upon the onset of active labour or 12 hours after insertion.

KEY POINTS

✓ *Induction of labour is defined as the initiation of labour by artificial means prior to its spontaneous onset at a viable gestational age, with the aim of achieving vaginal delivery.*

✓ *Induction of labour is indicated when the risk to the mother and or fetus from the continuation of pregnancy outweighs the risk of terminating the pregnancy.*

✓ *The cervix can be ripened by prostaglandins and by mechanical methods.*

✓ *Oxytocin infusion, amniotomy and prostaglandins are the methods used for the induction of labour.*

Essay questions

1. Define 'induction of labour'. What are the indications for the induction of labour?
2. A 32-year-old primigravida presents with BP 170/110 and c/o headache at 36 weeks pregnancy. She has 3+ albuminuria. On examination, her cervix is in the mid-position, is of medium consistency, 3 cm long and 1 cm dilated with head at −3 station.
   a) What is the Bishop score? What is this woman's score?
   b) What are the indications for inducing labour?
   c) What are the various available modes of induction?

Short answer questions

1. What are the techniques used for the ripening of the cervix?
2. Describe the methods of inducing labour when the cervix is favourable.
3. Write short notes on the following:
   a) Bishop score
   b) Preinduction assessment

MCQs

1. Which of the following is NOT a contraindication for the induction of labour?
   a) Previous lower segment cesarean section
   b) Transverse fetal lie
   c) Umbilical cord prolapse
   d) Non-reassuring fetal heart rate pattern

2. Which of the following agents is NOT used for cervical ripening?
   a) Hygroscopic cervical dilators
   b) Prostaglandin F_2
   c) Prostaglandin E_2
   d) Balloon catheter

3. Which of the following is NOT associated with the risks of oxytocin infusion?
   a) Uterine rupture
   b) Water intoxication
   c) Uterine hyperstimulation
   d) Exacerbation of bronchial asthma

4. Which of the following is not included in the modified Bishop score for assessing cervical ripeness?
   a) Cervical length
   b) Cervical dilatation
   c) Station of the fetal head
   d) Position of the fetal head

5. Which of these cannot be used for induction of labour?
   a) Prostaglandin E_2
   b) Balloon catheter
   c) Membrane sweeping
   d) Prostaglandin F_2

6. Which of these is not an indication for the induction of labour?
   a) Severe pre-eclampsia
   b) Ruptured membranes without pains
   c) Intrauterine fetal death
   d) 36 weeks uncomplicated pregnancy

7. The induction of labour should be avoided in all except:
   a) Active genital herpes
   b) Transverse lie
   c) Uncontrolled GDM at term
   d) Contracted pelvis

8. In which of the following is the induction of labour contraindicated?
   a) Ruptured membranes
   b) 41 weeks of gestation
   c) Previous classical cesarean section
   d) HELLP syndrome

9. What is the main risk of performing amniotomy?
   a) Uterine rupture
   b) Fetal tachycardia
   c) Cord prolapse
   d) Failure of progress of labour

10. Prostaglandin E_2 gel is applied for induction at what intervals and to a maximum of how many doses?
    a) 2 doses 6 hours apart
    b) 2 doses 12 hours apart
    c) 3 doses 6 hours apart
    d) 3 doses 12 hours apart

11. Which of the following methods of induction cannot be used in a woman with previous lower segment cesarean section?
    a) Prostaglandin E_1 tablet
    b) Prostaglandin E_2 gel
    c) Oxytocin infusion
    d) Membrane sweeping

Answers

1. (a), 2. (b), 3. (d), 4. (d), 5. (d), 6. (d), 7. (c), 8. (c), 9. (c),
10. (c), 11. (a)

Fill in the blanks

1. Membrane sweeping releases _____.
2. The WHO recommends induction of labour at _____ of gestation.
3. The induction of labour is the _____.
4. Augmentation of labour is the _____.

Answers

1. prostaglandins, 2. 41 weeks, 3. stimulation of the uterus to begin labour, 4. stimulation of the uterus during labour

Case scenario-based discussion

1. A 28-year-old gravida 2, para 1 is induced at 41 weeks of gestation for postdated pregnancy. On examination, the cervix is in mid-position, soft, 1 cm long, 2 cm dilated and the head is at 0 station.
   a) What is her Bishop score?
   b) What is the best method of inducing her and what is the advantage of this method?
   c) What are the contraindications for ARM?
   d) If the woman develops hyperstimulation with oxytocin infusion, how would you manage it?

Answers

a) The Bishop score is 8.
b) As the cervix is favourable, ARM with oxytocin infusion is the best method of inducing labour in this woman.
c) ARM is contraindicated when the head is high, in the presence of malpresentation or unstable lie, and in the presence of cord presentation.
d) The infusion should be stopped, the woman should be turned to lateral position, oxygen should be administered at 4 litres/minute, the uterus should be relaxed using tocolytics and labour should be expedited.

Normal Puerperium

Learning Objectives
» To describe the physiological changes taking place during the puerperium
» To know the care of the mother in the postnatal period and to identify postpartum complications
» To understand the physiology of lactation
» To know how to counsel mothers on breastfeeding
» To identify complications related to breastfeeding

■ INTRODUCTION

Puerperium is the period during which the anatomical and physiological changes of pregnancy revert to the non-pregnant state. The puerperal period extends from the end of the third stage of labour, i.e., from expulsion of the placenta to six weeks postpartum.

■ ANATOMICAL CHANGES IN THE UTERUS IN THE PUERPERIUM

Uterine Size (Involution)

The most striking features of the puerperium are the changes that take place in the uterus. Involution is the process of gradual reduction in the size of the uterus to reach the non-pregnant state. Involution is an autolytic process in which the protein of the uterine musculature is broken down into simpler components which are then absorbed and excreted in the urine.

- Immediately after delivery, the uterus is hard and very much reduced in size. The fundus lies just below the umbilicus—about 10–12 cm above the symphysis pubis.
- During puerperium, the uterus gradually diminishes in size, and by the tenth or twelfth day, it can no longer be felt by abdominal palpation. This process is known as involution of the uterus. Normally, the uterus reduces in size by 1 cm/day.
- The uterus never actually returns to its original state, and in a parous woman, it always remains a little bigger and more freely movable than that in a nulliparous woman.
- Though the total number of muscle cells that formed the pregnant uterus does not decrease appreciably, the size of the individual muscle fibres decreases markedly. It is to be noted that the involution of the

surrounding connective structures also occurs as rapidly as that of the uterus.
- The rate of involution of the uterus varies with different individuals, but it should generally be progressive from the first day onwards. Immediately postpartum, the uterus weighs approximately 1,000 g; 4–6 weeks after delivery, it weighs the same as the pre-pregnant uterus—around 100 g.

Subinvolution of the Uterus

In certain situations, the expected reduction in the size of the uterus does not occur, and there may be a delay in the process of involution. This is called subinvolution. This is diagnosed by the delay in the reduction of the uterine size as well as by the presence of prolonged lochial discharge and bleeding in the puerperal period.

The causes of subinvolution of the uterus are as follows:

- Retained bits of placental tissue or membranes
- Endometritis and puerperal sepsis
- Distorted uterine anatomy, resulting in the collection of lochial discharge in the cavity and preventing involution
- Presence of fibroids

Uterine Vessel Changes

Soon after delivery, the uterine blood vessels—which are markedly hypertrophied during pregnancy—are obliterated by thrombosis and later, are degenerated. Hyaline changes completely obliterate the larger vessels. New and smaller vessels develop in the surrounding area. Eventually, the blood clot in the lumen of the vessels gets absorbed. The vessel walls are then represented by a solid or thinly canalised mass of hyaline tissue. The placental site vessels also undergo thrombosis and hyalinisation.

Endometrial Changes

The superficial layer of the endometrium degenerates and sheds as lochia, whereas the deeper basal layer remains, and from it, the endometrium develops in the future.

Lochia—Discharge from the Uterus

Lochia is a discharge from the uterus that is seen in the puerperal period. After delivery, the endometrial surface of the uterus is thick and rough, especially over the placental site. Degenerating decidua, blood clots and bits of fetal membrane may be present in the uterus. Gradually, these undergo degeneration and are usually cast off in the lochial discharge.

- After the greater part of the surface has been thus shed, regeneration takes place from the remains of the mucous membrane and from the epithelium of the deeper portions of the uterine glands. The process closely resembles that of the healing of a granulating surface on a mucous membrane. The regeneration generally begins in the first week after labour and is complete in a month, except over the placental site.
- The lochia is generally red for the first three days due to the presence of blood (lochia rubra). It becomes pink (lochia serosa) gradually, and after about the tenth day, it becomes pale due to the presence of leukocytes and reduced fluid content (lochia alba). The discharge of lochia lasts for ten to twelve days and may recur after 2–3 weeks when the woman begins to move about freely.
- Lochia may persist for up to 6 weeks after delivery.
- The healthy lochia has a sweetish–mawkish odour, but it becomes offensive if there is an infection.
- Healthy lochia stains the diaper dark in the centre and pale in the periphery. In infected lochia, due to the degeneration of the red cells by the infective process, the periphery stains dark and the centre is pale. This is one of the earliest signs of puerperal infection.

■ CHANGES IN THE CERVIX, VAGINA AND EXTERNAL GENITALIA

Cervix

Along with the uterus, the cervix also undergoes involution and becomes smaller. The cervix, which is thin and 10 cm dilated at the time of delivery, gradually becomes thicker and smaller. However, the size and appearance never return to the non-gravid state. The external os of the cervix is always patulous in a multipara, while it is closed in a nullipara. In a multigravida, the cervix appears wide, the external os appears as a transverse slit and there are bilateral depressions on either side due to lacerations. In a nullipara, the cervical os is round. Multiparous women who have only had elective cesareans in the past also have a small cervix with a narrow external os.

Vagina

- The vagina takes some time to recover from the distension caused by the descent of the fetal head. The vaginal opening becomes markedly relaxed and may show signs of laceration.
- The hymen completely disappears; its place is taken by a number of small tags of tissue which undergo cicatrisation. These tags are known as **carunculae myrtiformes**. This is a characteristic sign of parity. The vascularity of the vagina decreases gradually, and vaginal rugosity appears.

Perineum

- The pelvic floor and the perineum are stretched during the process of delivery, resulting in relaxation.
- The levator ani muscle tone is also reduced due to pudendal neuropathy caused by the compression of the pudendal nerves between two bony structures, namely the ischial spine and the fetal head. Though some amount of 'gaping of the vulva' usually remains in a parous woman, the pelvic floor and perineal muscle tone can be improved by postnatal pelvic floor exercises.

Abdominal Wall and Peritoneum

Synchronous with the changes taking place in the uterus and vagina, the pelvic peritoneum and the structures of the broad ligament also reduce in size to accommodate the diminishing size of the pelvic organs.

The striae gravidarum do not disappear because the elastic fibres of the skin have ruptured. As a result of continued distension during pregnancy, the abdominal wall remains flat and flabby for some time. A certain amount of this laxity and flabbiness will remain permanently unless abdominal exercises are performed regularly.

Occasionally, there may be divarication of the recti muscles, so that one can easily insinuate the fingers in the median line between the two recti muscles. Here again, proper exercise is required to regain the tone of these muscles.

PHYSIOLOGICAL CHANGES IN THE PUERPERAL PERIOD

Fluid Balance Changes

- Following delivery, the average woman loses about 3–4 Kg as a result of the excretion of fluids and electrolytes through increased diuresis.
- These changes mostly occur in the first two weeks, after which the values return to pre-pregnant levels.

Hormonal Changes

- The levels of hCG, estrogen and progesterone fall abruptly to normal non-pregnant levels within a week of delivery.
- In lactating women, the prolactin level increases, whereas gonadotrophin and estrogen levels are low. During lactation, there is suppression of gonadotrophins as the suckling stimulus renders the HPO axis more sensitive to negative feedback. In breastfeeding mothers, there is initially a phase of complete ovarian suppression during which conception cannot take place. When ovarian activity returns during lactation, the cycles are frequently anovulatory or associated with defective luteal function. Once sucking is greatly reduced or stopped altogether, normal ovulation and fertility are restored. 1–10% of nursing mothers may conceive during lactational amenorrhea.
- In the absence of breastfeeding, there is early restoration of ovarian activity and ovulation. In non-lactating women, the hormone levels normalise in 2–3 weeks.

Cardiovascular Changes

- In the puerperium, the cardiac output, which increases during pregnancy, remains high for another 24 hours. Then, there is a steady decline, and cardiac output reverts to non-pregnant levels in two weeks.
- Heart rate and blood pressure reach the non-pregnant values 1–2 days after delivery. The cardiac size also reduces.

Urinary Tract Changes

- The urinary tract also undergoes changes in the puerperal period. Soon after delivery, there is edema and congestion of the bladder mucosa and at times, the trigone may be markedly edematous.
- The puerperal bladder has increased capacity and is relatively insensitive. The bladder can, therefore, get over-distended. Incomplete emptying is common in the puerperium, resulting in urinary retention. The insensitivity of the bladder is due to the trauma sustained by the nerve plexus during delivery, which heals quickly. Urinary retention is more common after episiotomy (due to the pain associated with suturing and urethral spasm), instrumental delivery and epidural analgesia. As a result of overdistension and the presence of residual urine, infection of the urinary tract is common in the puerperium.
- If a woman is not able to void within four hours of delivery, vulval, vaginal or genital tract hematoma should be ruled out. If no demonstrable cause can be made out, and if conservative measures fail, an indwelling catheter is left in place for 24 hours and the urine output is noted. Before removing the catheter, it should be ensured that there is only minimal residual urine. In all women who have to be catheterised, antimicrobial therapy is indicated.
- The dilatation and tortuosity of the ureters that occurs during pregnancy disappears completely in the puerperium within 4–6 weeks. There is pronounced diuresis on the second or third day of the puerperium. The increased glomerular filtration that occurs during pregnancy reduces to normal in 6–8 weeks.

Hematological Changes

- The blood volume increase that occurs during pregnancy returns to normal in 4–6 weeks. The blood volume is reduced by about 20% by the fifth day.
- After a normal vaginal delivery, the hematocrit rises by about 5% above the pre-delivery value.
- There is marked leukocytosis and thrombocytosis during and after labour. The leukocyte count sometimes reaches 30,000/mm^3 and reduces 7–10 days after delivery.
- The platelet count and the adhesiveness of the platelets are increased.
- The raised ESR returns to normal in 4 weeks.
- Fibrinogen and other coagulation factors remain elevated during the puerperium, which may predispose to thrombotic manifestations.

Changes in the Gastrointestinal System

In the puerperal period, there is reduced motility of the bowel, which results in constipation. Reflex pain from episiotomy and perineal lacerations also contribute to constipation. This can be corrected by maintaining a high residual diet, increasing the fluid intake and by early ambulation.

Resumption of Ovulation and Menstruation

- In non-lactating women, menstruation resumes in >40% of cases by the 6th week; >80% menstruate by the third month.
- In women who breastfeed, there is great variation in the resumption of menstruation and ovulation. It may occur as early as 8–10 weeks or as late as 18 months after delivery. Therefore, even in exclusively breastfeeding women, contraception is advised after three months. However, ovulation is less frequent in breastfeeding mothers. This is due to the lowered responsiveness of the ovaries to FSH, which is inhibited by prolactin. Breastfeeding increases the duration of postpartum amenorrhea.

Weight Loss in the Puerperium

Following delivery, a woman loses 6–7 Kg of weight due to the delivery of the fetus, placenta, amniotic fluid and the loss of water due to diuresis in the puerperal period.

NORMAL EVENTS IN THE PUERPERIUM

- **Puerperal chill or postpartum chill:** Nearly 25% of mothers may experience shivering as soon as they have delivered. The etiology of this phenomenon is not known. This shivering may last up to one hour. The chill is self-limiting, and temperature usually returns to normal afterwards.
- **After-pain:** Due to the uterine contractions associated with suckling or in an effort to expel the collected blood from the uterus, the uterus contracts intermittently in a manner similar to labour, resulting in pain. The after-pain usually disappears within one week.
- **Transient urinary and fecal incontinence:** Transient urinary or fecal incontinence may be noted in some women in the puerperal period. This is mainly due to the transient pudendal neuropathy caused by the compression of the pudendal nerve by the fetal head. These symptoms can also occur due to levator ani muscle damage resulting from a prolonged second stage, the delivery of a big baby, etc.

CARE OF THE MOTHER DURING PUERPERIUM

The care of a pregnant woman does not end with the delivery of the child and the conclusion of the third stage of labour. The woman and her child should receive adequate care after delivery. It is important to monitor their well-being and to watch for evolving complications. Following a normal delivery, the woman is kept in the hospital facility for a minimum of 48 hours and if necessary, for a longer period of time. At each examination, the general condition of the woman and her temperature and pulse are checked. Lochia, the involution of the uterus, the perineum (in those with sutures) and the state of the bladder and bowel should be assessed. The condition of the newborn should also be monitored. In women who have had a cesarean section, one should specifically look for wound site pain, infection, post-spinal headache and bowel-related problems such as paralytic ileus.

Early Ambulation

Following normal delivery, the woman is encouraged to mobilise as soon as she feels comfortable. Early ambulation reduces the frequency of puerperal venous thrombosis and pulmonary embolism. Bladder complications leading to urinary retention, catheterisation and constipation are also less frequent. Not only does the woman feel stronger, but early ambulation also induces a feeling of well-being.

Monitoring of After-Pains

The uterus often contracts vigorously to go back to its pre-pregnant size, resulting in after-pains that may be severe enough to require analgesics. After-pains are more likely to occur in a multipara, in women who have had precipitate labour, in a primipara whose uterus has been overdistended, and in cases where clots are retained inside the uterus. After-pains are particularly noticeable when the infant suckles as this results in the release of oxytocin. These pains generally become mild by the third postpartum day. The woman should be reassured and given analgesics to alleviate the pain.

Monitoring of Temperature

The normal puerperium should be apyrexial. Temperature should be recorded at four-hour intervals and any rise above 100°C should be specially noted. It is not infrequent for a slight rise of temperature to be present within the first 24 hours after delivery; occasionally, the woman may even get a chill with rigor, and her temperature may shoot up to 101–102°C. Generally, within 24 hours, the temperature comes back to normal and stays normal. Any rise in temperature thereafter must be viewed with suspicion, and all causes of infection should be ruled out.

Rest

The delivered mother should be encouraged to get adequate rest and sleep as and when she finds time.

Advice on Diet

If the woman has had a normal vaginal delivery, she can be given something to eat and drink two hours after delivery, according to her desire. The diet of a lactating woman should be fairly liberal and of a varied nature; it should contain plenty of proteins, meat, fish, fresh fruit and green vegetables. The diet should have an additional 400–700 Kcal to cover the energy requirements of lactation. If the woman does not breastfeed, her protein and calorie requirement are the same as that of a non-pregnant individual. Iron supplementation should be continued for at least three months after delivery. There is a tendency, particularly in rural areas, to restrict the water intake of the puerperal mother. Therefore, the woman and her family should be counselled about the need for adequate hydration. Inadequate hydration in the puerperal period is one of the precipitating factors for thromboembolic diseases.

Regulating Bladder and Bowel Movements

Early ambulation and early feeding can reduce the incidence of constipation. If required, mild, non-cathartic laxatives may be given to promote bowel movement, though they are better avoided. The genitalia should be cleaned and kept dry after every evacuation of the bowels.

Care of the Perineum

In cases where the perineum has been sutured, it should be kept clean and dry. The perineum should be attended to in the morning and evening and after each urination or defecation. The woman should be instructed to cleanse the vulva from the anterior to the posterior. Glycerine magsulph fomentation has proven valuable in reducing edema and discomfort. Warm sitz baths also help in alleviating pain and discomfort. Where a complete perineal tear has been repaired, a **non-residual diet** should be given for 4–5 days. Laxatives should then be given to permit a soft motion. If the perineum has not healed satisfactorily, the woman is advised to seek further treatment at the end of the third month after delivery for further repair of the complete perineal tear.

Care of the Breasts

The care of the breasts must begin during the antenatal period. Early identification of retracted nipples during the antenatal period makes it easier to manage than when it is recognised during lactation. If sufficient care is taken to keep the breasts clean and to draw out the nipples, no problem should arise during the puerperium. The nipples may develop fissures requiring treatment with emollients after each feed. Since dried milk is likely to accumulate and irritate the nipples, cleansing the areolae with water is recommended after each nursing. Occasionally, with irritated nipples, it is necessary to resort to the use of a nipple shield for 24 hours or longer.

Breastfeeding

The mother should be advised to feed the baby on demand. Rooming-in should be encouraged, wherein the baby stays with the mother and is nursed in the same cot. Breastfeeding and lactation are detailed later in this chapter.

Advice on Postnatal Exercise

Women should be given advice on exercise in the postnatal period. Women who have had a normal vaginal delivery can undertake low-impact activities such as walking, abdominal tightening and pelvic floor exercises in 1–2 weeks after delivery. The main purpose of postnatal exercise is to restore the tone of the abdominal and pelvic floor muscles. Pelvic floor exercises, i.e., contracting and relaxing the pelvic floor, improves the vaginal tone and helps in the prevention of stress urinary incontinence and prolapse at a later date.

Sexual Activity

Most couples resume sexual activity within 3–4 weeks. However, sexual activity may be affected by a loss of libido or dyspareunia due to an episiotomy wound.

Immunisation

All Rh-negative women who have an Rh-positive baby should be given 300 µg of anti-D immunoglobulin within 72 hours of delivery, provided isoimmunisation has not taken place (negative direct Coombs test). Any woman who has not been immunised against rubella should be given the rubella vaccine in the postpartum period with concurrent use of contraception. If required, catch-up vaccination against cervical carcinoma can be given in the postpartum period to women up to 26 years of age.

Puerperal Complications

The complications one can encounter in the puerperal period are postpartum psychological changes, puerperal fever due to various causes, breastfeeding difficulties, secondary postpartum hemorrhage, thromboembolic manifestations and problems related to the skeletal and nervous systems. Puerperal fever is discussed in detail in (Chapter 49, *Puerperal infection and other postpartum complications*).

Recognising Postpartum Depression

During the puerperal period, besides physiological changes, postpartum mothers experience psychological changes and are vulnerable to psychological disturbances. Mild, transient depression, known as **postpartum blues**, is common in the first few days after delivery. Postpartum blues is a very common but self-limiting condition that begins shortly after childbirth and lasts up to two weeks. The symptoms include tearfulness or crying 'for no apparent reason', mood swings, irritability, anxiety, loss of appetite and sleep and fatigue. The symptoms are generally mild and do not affect everyday activities. Treatment is supportive with adequate sleep and emotional support. If symptoms are severe enough to affect daily functioning or if they last longer than two weeks, the woman should be evaluated for postpartum depression.

Pelvic Arthropathy

During pregnancy, there is softening and relaxation of the joints of the pelvis. This may sometimes be excessive and may give rise to pain over the symphysis pubis and one or both sacroiliac joints. The condition is aggravated by walking and relieved by rest. Wearing a supporting corset for two to three months helps in curing this condition. Though the symptoms disappear rapidly after delivery in most women, some may suffer from persistent backache.

Maternal Palsies

The lumbosacral cord may be bruised at the brim of the pelvis by the fetal head during labour. This is more so in cases of prolonged labour (due to disproportion) or instrumental delivery. It may also occur in spontaneous labour. As a result, in the postnatal period, unilateral paralysis of the lower extremity can occur. The fourth and fifth lumbar nerve roots and first and second sacral trunks are commonly affected. These muscles are the extensors of the foot and toes and the evertors of the foot. There is numbness over the skin of the lower part of the leg, the ankle and the foot.

The symptoms, usually noted soon after delivery, are numbness and weakness of one or both lower extremities. In a day or two, foot-drop develops and there is an inability to evert the foot. Ankle jerks may be absent. Both sides may be involved. Treatment consists of keeping the foot dorsiflexed with the help of a splint to prevent overstretching of the muscles. Gentle massage and passive and active movements are helpful.

Timing Discharge From Hospital

- Following an uncomplicated delivery, the woman can be discharged within 48 hours.
- She should be advised regarding normal physiological puerperal changes including lochia and milk 'let-down' and the significance of symptoms like fever, excessive vaginal bleeding, and leg pain and swelling.
- Following a cesarean section, the woman is discharged after 4–5 days and should be reviewed in the clinic in two weeks' time.
- All women, after confinement, must be given definite appointments to attend the postnatal clinic.
- The woman should be advised to report immediately if she develops symptoms such as fever, excessive vaginal bleeding, leg pain or swelling.

■ POSTNATAL CARE

- Though the sixth-week postnatal visit is the traditional approach, it is recommended to have two visits—the first at 2–3 weeks and the second at 12 weeks to check for early problems and discuss contraception.
- Postnatal care includes the evaluation of general health—including BP and sugar wherever indicated—and recovery from the effects of childbirth, discussion on contraception and the vaccination of the mother.
- Postnatal clinics should ideally be set up along with child welfare clinics, where the mother can be evaluated at the same time as her baby.
- At this time, the mother's general physical condition, Hb and blood pressure should be checked, her urine should be examined for protein, the condition of her abdominal wall should be noted, her breasts should be inspected, and a thorough pelvic examination should be carried out.
- Ideally, Hb should be more than 10 g%. If the mother was anemic during delivery or puerperium, her Hb should show an increasing tendency. Otherwise, the reason for continuing anemia should be investigated.
- In those diagnosed with GDM during pregnancy, oral GTT should be carried out.
- In those diagnosed with pre-eclampsia, BP should be checked to see whether the level has returned to normal.

- There should be discussion on contraception and suitable advise is given at the first postnatal visit. In order to avoid unplanned pregnancy, effective contraception should be offered to all women from day 21 postpartum.

- In non-lactating women, ovulation and menstruation resume in 6–8 weeks. In those who are breastfeeding, menstruation may occur any time from 2 months to 18 months. Therefore, an effective contraceptive method should be followed even if the woman is exclusively breastfeeding. In those who have completed the family, postpartum sterilisation can be offered within 72 hours of delivery. IUCD and progestogen-only pills and injectables are suited for breastfeeding women as they do not interfere with the quantity and quality of milk production, unlike combined pills with estrogen and progesterone, which can affect the quality and the quantity of milk production and are best avoided for 6 months. In non-lactating women, combined oral contraceptive pills can be prescribed after 3 months.

■ BREASTFEEDING AND LACTATION

Physiology of Lactation

The basic component of the breast lobule is the alveolus, which is surrounded by the contractile myoepithelial cells. The alveolus is the milk-secreting gland. It is lined with a single layer of milk-secreting epithelial cells. The alveoli open into ductules which unite to form intralobular ducts—the lactiferous ducts. These lactiferous ducts open on the alveoli through small openings. The growth of the breasts and milk production are dependent on numerous hormonal factors which appear in two sequences—at puberty and then, during pregnancy. The most important stimulus for the development of the breast at puberty is estrogen. Several hormones influence the further development of the breast.

- Estrogen stimulates the growth of the ductal system.
- Progesterone influences the development of the alveolar component (should be primed with estrogen).
- Neither estrogen nor progesterone alone can induce optimum breast growth and development. Both require other hormones such as insulin, cortisol, thyroxine, prolactin and growth hormones.

Lactogenesis (Milk Production)

- During pregnancy, in addition to estrogen and progesterone, prolactin levels increase to very high levels—>200 ng/mL—reaching a peak at parturition. There is also an increase in the availability of free cortisol and insulin and increased production of human placental lactogen (HPL) from the placenta. All these factors influence breast development and milk production.

- Though all the hormones necessary for breast growth and milk production are available in pregnancy, milk secretion does not occur during pregnancy because high levels of estrogen inhibit the action of prolactin on the target tissue (estrogen has dual action; it increases the prolactin secretion and at the same time, prevents the full effect of prolactin on the breast tissue).

- With the delivery of the placenta, the levels of estrogen fall tremendously, resulting in the removal of the inhibitory effect of estrogen on prolactin. This, in turn, results in the initiation of milk secretion.

- Suckling sends afferent impulses to the hypothalamus, resulting in further release of prolactin, which also helps in the initiation of lactation (Fig. 17.1). Women with extensive pituitary necrosis, as in Sheehan's syndrome, do not lactate.

- Once milk production is initiated, its maintenance at high levels is dependent on the combined action of the anterior and posterior pituitaries stimulated by suckling. The anterior pituitary secretes prolactin and the posterior pituitary secretes oxytocin. Oxytocin, by acting on the contractile myoepithelial cells, empties the alveolar lumen and helps in alveolar refilling.

Ejection or 'Letting Down' of Milk

During suckling, the tactile sensors concentrated in the areola activate the afferent sensory neural arc, which stimulates the paraventricular and supraoptic nuclei of the hypothalamus, stimulating the release of oxytocin. This oxytocin release causes the myoepithelial cells surrounding the glandular tissue to contract and increase the milk flow to the baby (Fig. 17.2). This is called the milk ejection reflex ('let-down' reflex). Besides suckling, other stimuli such as the cry of the child, handling the baby and thinking of feeding can also stimulate the release of milk. This neural arc is extremely sensitive to emotional disturbances, fright or stress, which can adversely affect lactation.

Types of Breast Milk

There are three types of breast milk, which are as follows:

- **Colostrum or early milk,** which is produced in the late stages of pregnancy and until 4 days after delivery; it is rich in antibodies

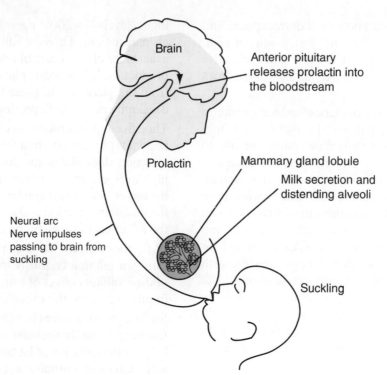

Fig. 17.1 The prolactin reflex

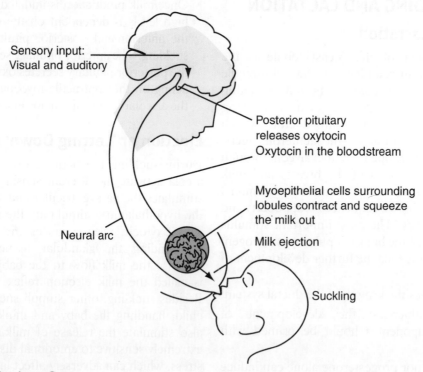

Fig. 17.2 The milk ejection reflex

- **Transitional milk**, which is produced from day 4–10 postpartum; its protein content is lower than that of colostrum
- **Mature milk**, which is produced from approximately 10 days after delivery and until the termination of breastfeeding

Colostrum or early milk

- For the first 48 hours after delivery, a thin liquid is secreted from the breasts, which is known as **colostrum**. The breasts become larger and fuller, the veins become more prominent, and the woman has the feeling that the secretion of milk is beginning.

If the child is put to the breasts regularly, milk begins to be secreted gradually and in increasing quantities.

- Colostrum is of a deep yellow colour and alkaline in nature. If a drop of it is examined under the microscope, it will be found to contain fat globules, a watery fluid and some corpuscles known as **colostrum corpuscles**. These corpuscles are round, ovoid or stellate cells. Colostrum contains very little casein, sugar and fat, but a great proportion of lactalbumin and lactoglobulin and more minerals.
- Antibodies are demonstrable in the colostrum. Both colostrum and mature milk are rich in immunoglobulin A (IgA), which offers protection to the newborn against enteric pathogens.

There is a tendency amongst some people to avoid feeding the baby with colostrum. This is an unhealthy practice. The expectant mother and her family should be counselled during the antenatal period about the benefits of colostrum for the baby.

Mature milk

The milk that is secreted after 48 hours differs from the colostrum. Mature milk is an opaque, slightly yellowish liquid, with a sweetish taste and characteristic odour. It is slightly alkaline and has a specific gravity of 1.025–1.035. The fluid portion of the milk is transudate and consists of protein material, milk, sugar, salts and water.

The protein in milk is one-third casein and two-thirds lactalbumin. The protein content of breast milk is low. In addition to fat and lactose (or milk sugar), milk contains a considerable amount of minerals, half of which comprises calcium phosphate and potassium carbonate, while the remainder is made up of sodium chloride and minute quantities of several other salts, including iron.

Composition of Human Milk

- Carbohydrates constitute nearly 7–8% of human milk. Lactose is present in a high concentration, which enhances the growth of *Lactobacillus* in the GI tract.
- Since the baby cannot metabolise a high concentration of protein, the protein content of human milk is low—1–2%. The proteins that are present in human milk are lactalbumin and lactoglobulin.
- The fat content of breast milk is 3–5%. It is rich in polyunsaturated fatty acids needed for myelination.
- Adequate vitamins and minerals are present in human milk.

- Water and electrolytes constitute 88% of breast milk.
- Breast milk has immunogenic properties. It contains IgA, lymphocytes and interferons.

Human milk has a slight laxative action on the newborn baby, which helps to clear the meconium from the intestines. All vitamins except vitamin K are found in human milk. The administration of vitamin K to the newborn after delivery is recommended to prevent hemorrhagic disease of the newborn.

Factors Affecting Milk Secretion

It is estimated that the rate of secretion of mature milk flow is about 850 mL per day, representing a net energy loss of about 600 calories for the mother. Secretion is influenced by various factors such as diet, hormones and emotional status. Most drugs given to the mother are secreted in milk. Among them are antibiotics, sulphonamides, most alkaloids, salicylates and bromides, cathartics, purgatives, iron, opium, arsenic, lead and mercury. Several factors influence the volume of milk production. They include age, parity and the state of health of the mother as well as the age and weight of the infant. Emotional disturbances and stress can have a negative effect on milk secretion.

Advantages of Breastfeeding

Breastfeeding has numerous benefits for both mothers and children. It not only provides nutrition essential for the growth and development of the newborn but also has significant emotional and psychological benefits.

Benefits of breastfeeding for the infant

- Human milk is the ideal and complete food for the neonate. In addition to the right balance of nutrients, it stimulates biological signals that promote cellular growth and differentiation.
- There is no need for preparation. It is hygienic, readily available, free of cost, easily digested and convenient.
- It helps in the development of the immune system and reduces the risk of infection, allergies and diarrheal and respiratory diseases.
- It stimulates cognitive development.
- Breastfeeding helps in reducing the chances of childhood obesity and adult-onset diseases such as diabetes.

Benefits of breastfeeding for the mother

- Breastfeeding strengthens the emotional bond between the mother and the neonate.

- It reduces blood loss after delivery and helps in involution.
- Long-term breastfeeding may help in weight reduction.
- It is associated with a reduced risk of breast, ovarian and endometrial cancers.
- It helps in child spacing and may act as a natural method of contraception.

Contraindications to Breastfeeding

- When the mother is critically ill
- Puerperal psychosis
- Active tuberculosis with multi-drug resistance; herpes lesions on mother's breasts
- Infant born with an inborn error of metabolism
- When the baby has a cleft lip/cleft palate
- When the mother is on anti-cancer therapy or radioactive isotopes

Lactation Suppression

Lactation suppression is required when there are contraindications to breastfeeding and in cases of perinatal death. Non-pharmacological methods such as cold fomentations and the use of tight breast binders help in the prevention of the accumulation of milk. The pharmacological agents used are dopamine agonists such as bromocriptine and cabergoline, which act by inhibiting prolactin secretion from the pituitary. Bromocriptine (parlodel) is given in a dose of 2.5 mg twice daily for 3–5 days. Ice packs and analgesics may be required for 12–24 hours.

Breastfeeding Recommendations

Breast milk should be the baby's first feed. There should be no pre-lacteal feeding with honey, water or any other liquids as these may affect the baby's desire to suckle. Breast milk completely satisfies the baby's nutritional and fluid needs for the first six months. Exclusive breastfeeding is recommended until 6 months of age. After this, complementary foods are introduced with continued breastfeeding until 2 years of age or longer.

> **Optimal breastfeeding practices**
> - Exclusive breastfeeding is the practice of feeding the baby only breast milk for the first 6 months of life (no other food or water is given).
> - Breastfeeding should be initiated within one hour of birth and be continued for up to 2 years of age or beyond.

Feeding Techniques

- The mother should be seated with her back well supported. The baby should be facing the mother, with its head, neck and back in the same plane and supported by the mother's arm.
- Proper latching-on is important, wherein the entire nipple and most of the areola are covered by the baby's mouth.
- The baby should be fed from one breast completely before moving to the other so that baby gets both foremilk and hindmilk. Hindmilk is rich in fat, and therefore, calories.
- After feeding, the baby should be burped by holding it upright until the swallowed air comes out.

Average Milk Requirement

In the early days, the baby requires 100 mL/Kg of body weight/24 hours. By the tenth day, the requirement increases to 150 mL/Kg of body weight/24 hours.

Common Problems with Breastfeeding

- **Insufficient milk production:** Mothers may complain of an insufficient supply of milk. In these instances, if the infant is gaining adequate and expected weight (on an average 15–30 g per day), passing 3–4 stools, voiding 6–8 times, reassurance is all that is required. The mother may be encouraged to increase the frequency of feeding to 8–12 times a day. However, nearly 5% of mothers may not produce adequate amounts of milk. This may be due to poor latching techniques, the use of pacifiers, stress and pain, maternal medications, previous breast surgery, breast hypoplasia and Sheehan's syndrome. Management in such cases consists of reassurance, good diet and sufficient fluids, adequate rest and emotional support.
- **Breast engorgement:** This usually occurs on the third day after delivery, when the secretion of milk begins. It may be due to a sudden increase in milk production or due to the baby not feeding properly due to sickness or retracted nipples. On examination, the breasts are overdistended with visible and dilated veins. The breasts are painful and tender, and fever may develop. In the presence of breast engorgement, secretions must be let out gently either manually or by using a breast pump. Warm water fomentation may be required for pain relief. Analgesics are also given for pain relief.
- **Mastitis:** Organisms such as *Staphylococcus aureus* and *viridans* from the infant's nose and mouth can infect the breast tissue, resulting in mastitis. The

mother presents with pain due to breast engorgement and there is evidence of inflammation and associated symptoms such as fever with rigors. The breast is hard, red and tender. Infection is usually unilateral. Breastfeeding is stopped on the affected side and treated with analgesics and antibiotics, and the engorgement is relieved by expressing the milk. If necessary, a sample of milk may be sent for culture and sensitivity. Flucloxacillin 500 mg/6 hours is usually effective. Once the acute phase is over, breastfeeding can be resumed. If not adequately treated, it may progress to a breast abscess, wherein fluctuant swelling can be felt and can be confirmed by USG.

- **Breast abscess:** Here, a segment of the breast becomes painful and tender and fluctuation can be detected. The skin over the affected area is edematous. There is fever, and the axillary lymph nodes are enlarged. In women presenting with mastitis, USG may be performed to rule out a breast abscess. Treatment involves incision and drainage of the abscess under general anesthesia.
- **Cracked nipple:** This can occur due to improper attachment of the newborn's mouth during suckling or biting at the nipple or leaking breasts. Lack of cleanness and dryness of the nipples, leaving the baby too long at the breast and monilial infection are the other causes of cracked nipples. Cracked nipples are very painful and are treated with proper cleaning, antibiotics and emollient application. The baby should not be put on the affected breast until the nipple has healed. During this time, the breast should be emptied manually. If severe, a breast pump can be used until the pain subsides. Left unattended, a cracked nipple may progress to mastitis and breast abscess formation.
- **Inverted or retracted nipples:** Flat and retracted nipples should be looked for in the antenatal period

and corrected. If diagnosed in the postnatal period, a flat nipple can be pulled out so that the baby is able to suckle. However, there may be severely retracted nipples, which may not get corrected by suckling. In these cases, either a breast pump or the syringe method can be used to relieve the retracted nipple. For the latter, the nozzle of a 20 cc syringe is cut off, and the smooth end of the syringe is applied over the areola. The plunger is inserted into the cut end and gentle suction is applied to pull out the nipple (Fig. 17.3).

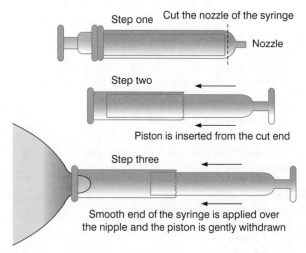

Fig. 17.3 Syringe method for the correction of a retracted nipple

Storage of Breast Milk

Breast milk can be expressed manually or by using a breast pump and stored at room temperature for 6–8 hours. It can be stored in the refrigerator for 24 hours and in the freezer for up to three months. Milk that has been stored in the refrigerator/freezer should not be boiled. Instead, the container/bottle should be placed in warm water at 40°C and gently shaken.

KEY POINTS

- ✓ *The normal duration of the puerperium is six weeks following delivery.*
- ✓ *Puerperium is the period after delivery during which the changes that occur during pregnancy regress. The involution of the uterus occurs and lactation is established.*
- ✓ *Prolactin is responsible for milk formation. Oxytocin released from the posterior pituitary in response to suckling is responsible for milk ejection.*
- ✓ *Breastfeeding has many advantages and should be encouraged unless it is contraindicated.*
- ✓ *Women should be instructed and counselled regarding the normal physiological changes of the puerperium including the normal pattern of the lochia, after-pains, milk 'let-down' and weight loss.*
- ✓ *Women presenting with fever, excessive vaginal bleeding, leg pain or chest discomfort and persistent depression should receive prompt medical attention.*

Essay questions

1. Describe the physiology of lactation, the composition of human milk and the advantages of breastfeeding.
2. Define 'puerperium' and describe the anatomical and physiological changes occurring in this period.
3. A 25-year-old para 1 who had a vaginal delivery by outlet forceps and episiotomy 2 days ago is seen in the postnatal ward.
   a) How do you evaluate a postnatal woman?
   b) What is the involution of the uterus?
   c) Describe lochia.
   d) What is the postnatal advice you would give this woman?
   e) Describe the complications that may arise in the first two days of delivery.

Short answer questions

1. Write short notes on the following:
   a) Uterine involution
   b) Lochia
   c) Exclusive breastfeeding
   d) Contraindications to breastfeeding
   e) Management of mastitis
2. Describe the humoral mechanisms involved in lactation.
3. What are the advantages of breastfeeding?
4. Define puerperium.

MCQs

1. What is the duration of the puerperium?
   a) 2 weeks
   b) 4 weeks
   c) 6 weeks
   d) 8 weeks
2. Following delivery, the uterus becomes a pelvic organ at:
   a) 24 hours post-delivery
   b) 48 hours post-delivery
   c) 1 week post-delivery
   d) 2 weeks post-delivery
3. Which of the following does not cause the subinvolution of the uterus?
   a) Retained placental fragments
   b) Pelvic infection
   c) Anemia
   d) Complete perineal tear
4. Which of these is not true of lochia?
   a) Initially, it is lochia rubra
   b) After 10–12 days, it is lochia alba
   c) Healthy lochia stain is dark at the centre and pale at the periphery
   d) Infective lochia stain is dark at the centre and pale at the periphery
5. The hymen is replaced by tags of tissue after delivery called carunculae myrtiformis.
   a) True
   b) False
6. Cardiac output is high for how long after delivery?
   a) 2 hours
   b) 12 hours
   c) 24 hours
   d) 48 hours
7. Which is not true of lactation?
   a) Lactation failure is noted with Sheehan syndrome.
   b) Pulsatile oxytocin secretion causes contraction of myoepithelial cells.
   c) Suckling leads to the letting down reflex.
   d) It is unaffected by stress.
8. After-pains are increased in all except:
   a) Precipitate labour
   b) Multiple pregnancy
   c) Preterm delivery
   d) Retained clots in the cavity
9. How much additional energy does lactation require?
   a) 100 Kcal
   b) 200 Kcal
   c) 300 Kcal
   d) 400 Kcal
10. Which of the following vitamins is not found in human milk?
    a) A
    b) D
    c) E
    d) K

Answers
1. (c), 2. (d), 3. (d), 4. (d), 5. (a), 6. (d), 7. (d), 8. (c), 9. (d), 10. (d)

Fill in the blanks

1. The thin fluid secreted from the breast within the first 24–48 hours of delivery is known as _____.
2. The uterine contractions in the puerperium are known as _____.
3. During the puerperium, the uterus gradually diminishes in size. This process is known as _____.
4. Vaginal discharge during the puerperium is known as _____.
5. After delivery the hymen is replaced by a number of small tags of tissue, which are known as _____.
6. Mild transient depression after delivery is known as _____.

Answers
1. colostrum, 2. after-pains, 3. involution, 4. lochia, 5. carunculae myrtiformes, 6. postpartum blues

Case scenario-based discussion

1. A 22-year-old para 1 had a spontaneous vaginal delivery two hours ago. She has already started breastfeeding and she has some queries about breastfeeding.
   a) What is exclusive breastfeeding?
   b) What are the benefits of breastfeeding?
   c) Describe the technique of breastfeeding.
   d) Describe the diagnosis and management of mastitis and breast abscess.

Answers
a) Exclusive breastfeeding is the practice of giving only breast milk to the infant for the first six months of life (no other food or water is given).
b) Breast milk is the ideal and complete food for the neonate. There is no need for preparation; it is hygienic, readily available, involves no cost and is easily digested. It reduces the risk of infection, allergies and diarrheal and respiratory diseases. In the mother, it reduces blood loss after delivery, helps in involution and strengthens the emotional bond between the mother and the neonate. It also reduces the risk of breast, ovarian and endometrial cancers and is a natural method of contraception.
c) The mother should be seated with her back well supported. The baby should be facing the mother, with its head, neck and back in the same plane and supported by the mother's arm. Proper latching on is important, wherein the entire nipple and most of the areola are covered by the baby's mouth.
d) Mastitis is treated with analgesics and antibiotics and the engorgement is relieved by expressing the milk. Flucloxacillin 500 mg/6 hours is usually effective. Breastfeeding is stopped on the affected side. Once the acute phase is over, breastfeeding can be resumed. Breast abscess is treated by incision and drainage.

18 Hyperemesis Gravidarum

OG 9.5

Learning Objectives

» To be able to differentiate hyperemesis from morning sickness
» To know the etiopathology of hyperemesis
» To enumerate the complications of hyperemesis
» To know the investigations to be ordered in hyperemesis
» To know the principles of management of hyperemesis

INTRODUCTION

Hyperemesis gravidarum is defined as **vomiting in pregnancy** that is severe enough to produce dehydration, weight loss and ketosis from starvation and warrants hospitalisation.

FEATURES OF PHYSIOLOGICAL VOMITING IN PREGNANCY

Pregnancy is essentially a physiological process and vomiting in the early weeks of pregnancy is very common. In some individuals, however, the physiological symptoms may be exaggerated, necessitating special attention. The vomiting of pregnancy usually starts early in pregnancy—at around 4–6 weeks of gestation. In some, it may be one of the earliest symptoms of pregnancy. In most cases, the vomiting wanes by week 12, whereas in others, it may persist in the second trimester as well. Pregnancy-related vomiting episodes are often mild, their frequency being once or twice in the morning and the quantity small. Such vomiting does not affect the woman's health. The woman is able to retain enough food, and there is no appreciable weight loss.

ETIOLOGY OF HYPEREMESIS

Excessive vomiting in pregnancy is more common in a primigravida than in a multigravid woman. It may sometimes recur in successive pregnancies. The possible causes of hyperemesis include the following:

- Hyperemesis or excessive vomiting appears to be related to high or rapidly rising levels of **human chorionic gonadotropin (hCG)**. Excessive vomiting often occurs in patients with a vesicular mole or in multiple pregnancies, where the levels of hCG are very high.
- It has been noted that almost all cases of hyperemesis have a **psychological basis**. This theory has been substantiated to a great extent by the rapid improvement noted in women who were removed from their surroundings and isolated in an institution. Hence, psychological assessment of the woman is very useful.
- Women who experience motion sickness are prone to hyperemesis.
- Women who have a history of excessive vomiting in previous pregnancies are predisposed to hyperemesis.
- It may be genetically determined, as is indicated by similar history among family members (mother and sisters).
- Hyperemesis is more common in women who have vestibular disturbances.
- In women who have **previous history of gastrointestinal dysfunction,** the impaired motility of the bowel and relaxation of the esophageal sphincter get aggravated in pregnancy due to high progesterone levels.
- In women with previous history of hepatic dysfunction, there is impaired fatty acid oxidation leading to excessive vomiting.
- *Helicobacter pylori* infection has also been implicated as one of the causes of excessive vomiting.

SIGNS AND SYMPTOMS

- The primary symptoms of hyperemesis are **nausea and vomiting**. Over a period of time, the vomiting gets worse—it persists throughout the day and the woman is unable to retain both solids and liquids.
- The woman may present with **excessive salivation (ptyalism)** and her sense of taste may be distorted.
- **Due to dehydration, hypotension and hypoglycemia,** the woman feels tired, weak and dizzy.
- There may be sleep disturbances, depression, anxiety and irritability.
- There is a gradual loss of weight.

- Due to continuous vomiting and retching, the woman may present with hematemesis due to tears in the esophagus. In such cases, the woman can also develop pneumothorax.
- If the woman presents with depression, peripheral neuritis, confusion, ataxia, nystagmus and psychotic features, Wernicke's encephalopathy due to thiamine deficiency should be suspected.
- If the woman develops starvation ketoacidosis, she may present with ketotic breath.

METABOLIC CHANGES ASSOCIATED WITH HYPEREMESIS GRAVIDARUM

- Starvation and depletion of glycogen stores lead to increased production of ketone bodies
- Hypoglycemia, hypoproteinemia, hypovitaminosis
- Hypokalemia, hyponatremia
- Hemoconcentration due to dehydration
- Hepatic dysfunction and elevated liver enzymes

INVESTIGATIONS

1. Urinalysis for ketones and specific gravity: These are the most important investigations since the presence of ketone bodies and high specific gravity indicate the severity of the condition. The specific gravity of urine increases in cases of hyperemesis due to dehydration and volume depletion. If the urine is positive for ketone bodies, the test should be repeated every 12–24 hours until the ketones disappear.
2. Blood sugar levels
3. Serum electrolytes
4. Liver enzymes and bilirubin
5. Urine culture to rule out urinary tract infection
6. Hematocrit
7. Other investigations:
   - Serum amylase/lipase to rule out pancreatitis
   - Viral markers for infective hepatitis may be tested in women with intractable vomiting
   - Thyroid stimulating hormone (TSH), free thyroxine to rule out hyperthyroidism and serum calcium level
   - Ultrasonography to rule out molar and multiple pregnancy and surgical causes such as gallbladder disease

MANAGEMENT

In managing women who have hyperemesis, it may not be possible to achieve complete relief of nausea and vomiting. However, the unpleasantness and discomfort can usually be minimised. At times, it is difficult to evaluate whether the woman is exaggerating her symptoms or if she is genuinely vomiting excessively. Outpatient management can be attempted first; if there is no relief, hospitalisation may be required to prevent serious complications.

Outpatient Treatment

Reassurance

It is important to reassure the woman that vomiting in early pregnancy is normal and very common. The woman should be assured that this symptom usually reduces gradually and disappears by about 12–14 weeks of pregnancy.

Simple dietetic regulations

- The woman should be advised to consume small quantities of food at frequent intervals.
- Foods whose odour precipitates or aggravates symptoms should be avoided. The woman can eat whatever appeals to her.
- Fatty and spicy food should be avoided.
- The woman should be asked to avoid an empty and a full stomach. Pregnant women are prone to gastric acidity, which is aggravated by an empty stomach; regurgitation can occur on a full stomach.
- The woman's diet should be high in protein and low in fat.
- Between meals, the woman can be advised to consume bland snacks.
- Iron supplements should be avoided.
- The woman should avoid lying down after meals; instead, she should be advised to rest in the reclining position.
- Traditional remedies such as the chewing of ginger have also been shown to be effective in some situations.

Medications

Drugs with antiemetic properties such as antihistamines and vitamins and metoclopramide are commonly used.

Antiemetic drugs
- Meclizine, 25 mg, at bedtime and during the day if needed
- Doxylamine, 10 mg, up to a maximum of four times a day
- Prochlorperazine, 5 mg, may be given twice daily
- Metoclopramide, 20 mg, three to four times a day
- Vitamins—vitamin B_6 has been tried with varied success (10–30 mg/day)

Hospitalisation

Uncontrolled vomiting could result in **starvation**, at which stage, the body's carbohydrate stores are used up for its immediate needs. When the carbohydrate stores are depleted, the body's fat stores are utilised (which gives rise to **ketosis**), and symptoms of toxic manifestation follow. In order to avoid ketosis, a woman with intractable vomiting may need to be hospitalised.

The primary aim of management is to **correct the electrolyte imbalance** and supply the body with easily assimilable carbohydrates in the form of glucose in sufficient quantities to replace the depleted **glycogen stores** and correct the **acidosis**.

- The woman should be asked to rest, and all feeding by mouth must be stopped for at least 24–48 hours to relieve the gastrointestinal system.
- The woman's vitals and urine output should be monitored continuously.
- Urine ketones and blood sugar levels should be checked every 12 hours and electrolytes, every 24 hours.
- An intravenous infusion should be started and approximately three litres of fluid should be administered over 24 hours. The solutions used for this purpose are 5% dextrose, normal saline and Ringer's lactate. Intravenous solutions are used to correct dehydration, electrolyte deficits and acid–base imbalances. This requires appropriate amounts of sodium, potassium, chloride, lactate or bicarbonate, glucose and water, all of which should be administered parenterally until vomiting has been controlled. Unless ketosis is corrected, the vomiting will continue in a vicious cycle. Therefore, when ketones are present in the woman's urine, 10% dextrose infusion should be administered to correct ketosis. If only dextrose solutions are used in cases of prolonged vomiting, it may precipitate Wernicke's encephalopathy due to thiamine deficiency. Therefore, thiamine is administered in a dose of 100 mg daily intravenously. Once ketosis sets in, the medical team should also be involved in the management.
- Multivitamins (IV preparation) can be added to the infusion.
- Antiemetics—promethazine and metoclopramide—are administered by the parenteral route.
- If vomiting persists despite these measures, methylprednisolone can be used.
- Periodic checking of electrolytes is also important as hypokalemia is common in these women and needs to be corrected.

- With this simple line of treatment, marked improvement is seen in most cases in 24–48 hours.
- This clinical improvement is associated with increased urinary output, fast-disappearing ketonuria and a steady normal pulse rate.
- Oral intake can be started if vomiting has been controlled for 24 hours.
- To begin with, the woman can be given small quantities of fluids at frequent intervals. Within a few days, she may be brought back to a solid diet regimen.
- Very rarely, the deteriorating condition of the woman may require the termination of pregnancy.

Fig. 18.1 presents an algorithmic approach to the management of vomiting in pregnancy.

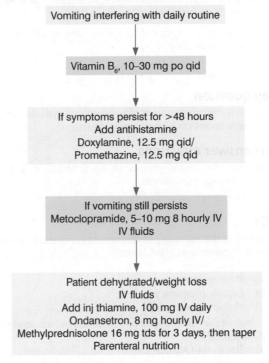

Fig. 18.1 Flowchart showing the management of vomiting in pregnancy

■ DIFFERENTIAL DIAGNOSIS

In some pregnant women, the vomiting may be due to some underlying disease and not due to the pregnancy itself. In such cases, the woman may not respond to the aforementioned regimen. The following conditions should be considered in such cases:

- Gastroenteritis
- Cholecystitis
- Pyelonephritis
- Hepatitis
- Any other medical and surgical condition

■ COMPLICATIONS

The complications of hyperemesis include the following:

- Liver dysfunction
- Renal failure
- Electrolyte imbalance
- Ketosis
- Stress ulcers
- Hematemesis due to Mallory–Weiss tears (tears in the esophagus)
- Pneumothorax
- Wernicke's encephalopathy due to thiamine deficiency

KEY POINTS

✓ *Hyperemesis is the exaggeration of a physiological symptom of pregnancy. It occurs commonly in primigravidae and with pregnancy complications such as molar pregnancy and multiple pregnancy.*

✓ *Urine should be checked for ketones periodically and electrolyte imbalance should be looked for.*

✓ *The presence of ketones necessitates hospitalisation and active management.*

✓ *Management involves fluid replacement, correcting electrolyte imbalance, maintaining blood sugar levels and controlling vomiting with antiemetics.*

✓ *If the woman does not respond to treatment, her vomiting may not be pregnancy-related. In such cases, one should look for other underlying causes.*

Essay question

1. Discuss the management of hyperemesis gravidarum. What complications could the woman develop?

Short answer questions

1. Discuss the investigations to be ordered in a case of hyperemesis gravidarum.
2. List the complications of hyperemesis.

MCQs

1. Which of the following conditions does not usually manifest with hyperemesis gravidarum?
   a) Primigravida
   b) Molar pregnancy
   c) Ectopic pregnancy
   d) Multiple pregnancy
2. Which of the following complications is not associated with hyperemesis?
   a) Electrolyte imbalance
   b) Renal failure
   c) Wernicke's encephalopathy
   d) Anemia
3. Which of the following causes Wernicke's encephalopathy?
   a) Electrolyte imbalance
   b) Ketosis
   c) Thiamine deficiency
   d) Dehydration
4. A 25-year-old primigravida presents at 8 weeks of gestation with hyperemesis. Which of these is not included in the triad of hyperemesis?
   a) Dehydration
   b) Weight loss
   c) Ketosis
   d) Increased appetite

5. Which is the most important investigation to be done in hyperemesis?
   a) Renal function test
   b) Serum calcium
   c) Random blood sugar
   d) Urinalysis for ketones
6. A pregnant woman presents at 8 weeks of gestation with vomiting and asking for dietary advice. Which of the following is not advisable in women who have hyperemesis?
   a) Frequent intake of small quantities of food
   b) Dry foods
   c) Foods without a strong odour
   d) Fat-rich food
7. A 30-year-old primigravida with a history of infertility treatment presents at 10 weeks of pregnancy with c/o vomiting—10 episodes/day for the previous 2 days. She is not tolerating solids or liquids; and is fatigued. On examination, she is dehydrated, and USG shows viable DCDA twins at a gestational age of 10 weeks. What should be the course of management?
   a) Outpatient doxylamine 10 mg bd
   b) Outpatient diet advice, antacids, doxylamine 10 mg bd
   c) Admission, food restriction, IV fluids, antiemetics
   d) Terminate pregnancy

Answers
1. (c), 2. (d), 3. (c), 4. (d), 5. (d), 6. (d), 7. (c)

Fill in the blanks

1. The physiological vomiting of pregnancy usually passes by _____ weeks.
2. The most important investigation that helps in the management of hyperemesis gravidarum is _____.

Answers
1. 12,   2. urine analysis for ketones

Case scenario-based discussion

1. A 22-year-old primigravida presents at 9 weeks of gestation with intractable vomiting for three days. On examination, her eyes are sunken, her pulse is 96/mt, her BP is 90/70 mm of Hg and she is dehydrated.
    a) What are the investigations to be ordered?
    b) How would you treat this woman?
    c) What are the commonly used antiemetics?
    d) Name three complications this woman can develop.

Answers

a) The immediate investigations required are assays for urine ketones, electrolytes and blood sugar levels. Subsequently, renal and liver function tests can be carried out. This woman would also require investigations to rule out urinary infection and hepatitis.

b) The woman should be hospitalised and given parenteral fluids to correct dehydration, hypoglycemia and ketosis. Antiemetics should be given to stop the vomiting.

c) Commonly used antiemetics are meclizine, 25 mg; doxylamine, 10 mg, up to a maximum of four times a day; prochlorperazine, 5 mg; metoclopramide, 20 mg, three to four times a day and vitamin B6.

d) Common complications are electrolyte imbalance, ketosis and stress ulcers.

19

Miscarriage (Abortion)

OG 1.3, OG 6.1, OG 9.1, OG 37.7, AN 78.5

Learning Objectives

» To know the definition and types of miscarriages
» To discuss the causes of first- and second-trimester miscarriages
» To describe the clinical features of different types of miscarriages and their management
» To discuss the etiology and management of recurrent miscarriage
» To discuss the diagnosis and management of cervical insufficiency
» To know how to counsel patients who have had a miscarriage

■ INTRODUCTION

Spontaneous miscarriage is defined as the spontaneous termination of pregnancy before 20 weeks of gestation. The WHO defines miscarriage as 'a spontaneous expulsion of the conceptus weighing 500 grams or less'.

■ CLASSIFICATION

Miscarriages are classified as follows:
- **Spontaneous (sporadic/recurrent)**
  ❖ Threatened miscarriage
  ❖ Inevitable miscarriage
  ❖ Complete miscarriage
  ❖ Incomplete miscarriage
  ❖ Missed miscarriage
  ❖ Septic abortion
- **Induced**
  ❖ Legal (MTP)
  ❖ Illegal (criminal abortion)

■ INCIDENCE

The incidence of spontaneous miscarriage ranges from 10–15% of all recognised pregnancies. Approximately 15–20% of couples trying to conceive have at least one miscarriage, 5% have two consecutive miscarriages and 1% of couples have three or more consecutive losses. Nearly 80% of all spontaneous miscarriages occur in the first trimester. The risk of spontaneous miscarriage rates is higher in the following situations:

- Maternal age >35 years
- History of miscarriages in the previous pregnancies

- Multiple pregnancy
- Pregnancy following assisted reproductive techniques

■ ETIOLOGY OF SPONTANEOUS MISCARRIAGES

The etiology of spontaneous miscarriage may be due to fetal factors or maternal factors.

Fetal Factors

Intrinsic defects of varying degrees in the fertilised ovum may result in clinical abortions. Chromosomal aberrations have been demonstrated in 40–50% of cases of spontaneous miscarriages. These chromosomal defects are more commonly seen with blighted ova (anembryonic pregnancy) and advanced maternal age. There may be numerical defects in the chromosomes such as trisomy 16, 21 and 22, monosomy 45 XO, triploidy, etc., or there may be structural defects in the chromosomes with translocations and inversion. Chromosomal aberrations occur due to errors during gametogenesis or non-disjunction in paternal or maternal meiosis.

Maternal Factors

Maternal infections

Acute infections such as pneumonia, malaria, acute appendicitis and pyelonephritis can cause miscarriages as a result of **hyperpyrexia and toxins** in the mother, leading to fetal anoxia and fetal death. **Viral infections** such as rubella, herpes simplex and cytomegalovirus infection and toxoplasmosis can also result in abortions.

Syphilis is another important infection that can result in miscarriages. Chorioamnionitis caused by listeriosis, and mycoplasma infections are other causes.

Maternal systemic diseases

Spontaneous abortion and major congenital malformations are more common in women with **insulin-dependent diabetes**. The risk is related to the degree of metabolic control in the first trimester of pregnancy. Chronic hypertension and renal disease can also result in miscarriages due to vascular pathology.

Uterine causes

- **Congenital malformations of the uterus** play an important role in causing abortions, especially second-trimester and recurrent miscarriages. While a mild degree of malformations may not interfere with pregnancy, severe degrees may result in abortion.
- **Cervical insufficiency (formerly called cervical incompetence)**, either congenital or acquired as a result of obstetric or surgical trauma, is an important factor in repeated abortions. The commonest cause of second-trimester abortions is cervical insufficiency. Other uterine causes are submucous myomas and Asherman's syndrome. Most often uterine causes result in second-trimester miscarriages.

Endocrine causes

Endocrine causes such as hypothyroidism, hyperthyroidism, progesterone deficiency and luteal phase defects associated with abnormal ovulation with polycystic ovaries, and hyperprolactinemia can lead to spontaneous miscarriages. Corpus luteum is essential for the survival of pregnancy up to 8 weeks of gestation. If the corpus luteum is removed inadvertently before 8–10 weeks during surgical procedures, miscarriage will ensue.

Immunological factors

Autoimmune diseases such as antiphospholipid antibody syndrome (APLA), systemic lupus erythematosus (SLE) and inherited thrombophilia are also causes of spontaneous miscarriage.

Maternal habits

Smoking, the use of habit-forming drugs and the excessive consumption of alcohol also lead to abortions.

Exposure to toxic agents

Exposure to anesthetic gases and radiation may result in miscarriages.

Iatrogenic causes

Procedures such as amniocentesis and chorion villus sampling can result in abortions.

Causes of spontaneous miscarriage
- *Fetal factors*
  - ❖ Chromosomal aberrations
- *Maternal factors*
  - ❖ Infections: Hyperpyrexia, viral infections
  - ❖ Systemic disease: Diabetes, renal disease, hypothyroidism, autoimmune disorders such as antiphospholipid antibody syndrome
  - ❖ Uterine causes: Congenital malformations of the uterus, cervical insufficiency, submucous fibroid, Asherman's syndrome (presence of uterine synechiae)
  - ❖ Maternal habits: Smoking, excessive alcohol consumption
  - ❖ Pregnancy-related: Insufficient progesterone secretion by corpus luteum or placenta

---

■ CLINICAL FEATURES

The woman generally has a history of amenorrhea, followed by more or less severe pain in the lower abdomen and back accompanied by vaginal bleeding. The extent of hemorrhage varies and may sometimes be so profuse as to cause severe collapse. Usually, the hemorrhage continues for some days, the quantity varying from day to day.

The signs and symptoms of miscarriage
- Amenorrhea
- Abdominal pain due to uterine contractions
- Bleeding per vagina due to the separation of the ovum
- Dilatation of the cervix due to uterine contractions
- Partial or total expulsion of the products of conception

■ TYPES OF SPONTANEOUS MISCARRIAGE

The different types of abortion (Fig. 19.1) are classified (Table 19.1) depending on the signs and symptoms.

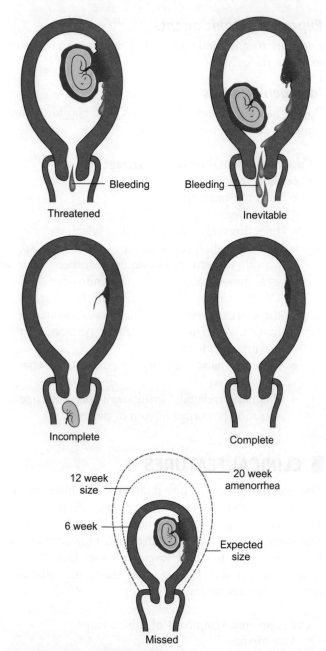

Fig. 19.1 Types of abortion

Table 19.1 Classification of abortions (Copyright © 2010–2014 Merck Sharp & Dohme Corp., a subsidiary of Merck & Co., Inc., Whitehouse Station, N.J., U.S.A)

Type	Definition
Early	Abortion before 12 weeks of gestation
Late	Abortion between 12 and 20 weeks of gestation
Spontaneous	Non-induced abortion
Induced	Termination of pregnancy for medical or elective reasons
Therapeutic	Termination of pregnancy because of threat to woman's life or health or because the fetus is dead or has malformations incompatible with life
Threatened	Vaginal bleeding before 20 weeks' gestation without cervical dilatation and indicating that spontaneous abortion may occur
Inevitable	Vaginal bleeding or rupture of the membranes accompanied by dilatation of the cervix
Incomplete	Expulsion of some of the products of conception
Complete	Expulsion of all products of conception
Recurrent/ habitual	Three consecutive spontaneous abortions
Missed	Undetected death of an embryo or a fetus that is not expelled and that causes no bleeding (also called blighted ovum, anembryonic pregnancy or intrauterine demise)
Septic	Serious infection of the uterine contents during or shortly before or after an abortion

Threatened Miscarriage

Definition

Threatened miscarriage is one where there is vaginal bleeding before 20 weeks of gestation with a viable fetus, uterine size corresponding to the period of gestation and no cervical dilatation.

Clinical features

Symptoms

- Amenorrhea
- Slight colicky pain in the lower abdomen or/and backache
- Slight vaginal bleeding
- Sometimes, frequency of micturition

Signs

- No pallor, unless woman was anemic before this problem
- General condition—there is no hypotension; mild or no tachycardia
- On clinical examination, uterus size corresponds to the period of amenorrhea and the cervical os is closed with slight bleeding through the os
- On a gentle bimanual pelvic examination (Fig. 19.2), the cervix will be soft, and the size of the uterus will correspond to the period of amenorrhea

Confirmation of diagnosis

This is always done by an ultrasound examination, which will reveal a viable pregnancy, indicating that the amount of bleeding has not affected the fetus. There may be small areas of sub-chorionic hematoma.

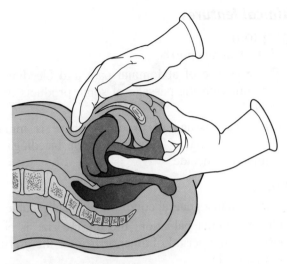

Fig. 19.2 Bimanual examination

Management

- Once the ultrasound confirms the fetal viability, it is important to **reassure** the woman about fetal well-being and explain to her that the chances of the pregnancy continuing are between 70 and 80 per cent.
- **Bed rest** is advised, though it does not alter the course of the condition.
- A **repeat ultrasound** is performed after a week to confirm the continuation of pregnancy. In about 75% of cases, the pregnancy continues normally.
- If fetal cardiac activity is not seen on repeat ultrasound and the woman is not bleeding, a diagnosis of **missed abortion** is made, and she is treated accordingly.
- If bleeding continues, the woman may abort partially or completely and is managed according to the clinical features.
- In a pregnancy continuing after a threatened abortion, there seems to be a slightly higher incidence of premature labour, intrauterine growth restriction and antepartum hemorrhage. It is, therefore, advisable to place these women in the **high-risk category** and monitor them for all these complications during the antenatal period.
- All Rh-negative pregnant women should be given anti-D immunoglobulin in a dose of 50 µg for pregnancies <12 weeks and 300 µg for pregnancies >13 weeks.

Inevitable and Incomplete Miscarriage

Definition

This term denotes that the ovum has separated from the uterine wall and is, therefore, bound to be expelled.

An abortion is called an **inevitable abortion** when the products of conception have not been expelled. When the products of conception are partially expelled and partially retained, it is called an **incomplete abortion**.

Clinical features

Symptoms

- History of amenorrhea
- Lower abdominal pain that is moderate to severe
- Bleeding from the vagina, which is usually heavy (more than a normal period)
- History of expulsion of products of conception

Signs

- Tachycardia and hypotension may be present depending on the amount of bleeding.
- On abdominal palpation, the uterine size may correspond to (inevitable abortion) or may be lesser than (incomplete abortion) the period of amenorrhea.
- On vaginal examination, the cervical os is dilated and products of conception may be felt in the uterine cavity or cervical canal in cases of inevitable abortion.
- In incomplete abortion, the products of conception may be protruding through the cervical canal in the process of expulsion.

Ultrasound

Ultrasound determines whether the products of conception (POC) have been expelled fully or if they are retained within the uterine cavity or the cervical canal in the process of being expelled. No fetal cardiac activity is seen in inevitable and incomplete miscarriages.

Management

Most often, the woman expels the products of conception (POC) by herself. However, intervention may be required when the bleeding is severe or persistent or when there is bleeding even after the expulsion of the POC. Very often, a 'check curettage' is done to remove any retained bits of POC and to ensure complete emptying of the uterine cavity.

General management

- An IV line is started with NS or RL.
- If the bleeding is severe, blood should be arranged.
- A single dose of parenteral antibiotic may be given as a prophylactic measure against infection (usually, 1 g of inj. ampicillin is given IV after the test dose).
- If the woman is not already immunised, inj. tetanus toxoid is given.

- In those presenting with inevitable abortion, if the pregnancy is <12 weeks, suction evacuation is performed under anesthesia. If the uterine size is >12 weeks, oxytocin infusion is given.
- When a woman presents with incomplete abortion and is hemodynamically stable, tablet misoprostol can be given in a dose of 400–600 µg orally or vaginally to hasten the process of expulsion. These women should be given adequate pain relief and measures to prevent vomiting. If the woman is hemodynamically unstable, immediate suction evacuation is carried out.

Surgical evacuation of the uterus

1. *Evacuation of the uterus when the cervix is sufficiently dilated*
   - If the POC are protruding from the external os, they can be removed by gently introducing sponge-holding forceps and twisting the POC with them.
   - **Manual vacuum aspiration (MVA)** can be used for emptying the uterine cavity. The exact technique is described in Chapter 63, *Medical termination of pregnancy;* the same method can be followed here. MVA is a safe procedure, and the chances of perforation are minimal. It also ensures complete evacuation.
   - If MVA is not available, suction evacuation should be performed.
2. *When the cervix is not sufficiently dilated*
   - *If the cervix is not sufficiently dilated*, *either* the MVA technique or suction evacuation is carried out.

Post-evacuation care
- Oral antibiotics should be continued along with analgesics such as paracetamol 500 mg.
- The woman can be given oral fluids after two hours, following which soft solids can be given after 6 hours.
- She should be counselled regarding family planning methods and advised to plan pregnancy after three months.
- Anti-D should be given whenever indicated.

Complete Abortion

Definition
In a complete abortion, the entire products of conception are expelled.

Clinical features
Symptoms
- History of amenorrhea
- The presence of abdominal pain and bleeding per vaginum with the passage of some products or big clots
- After the passage of products, there is minimal bleeding or pain, following which bleeding may completely subside

Signs
- The woman's general condition is usually stable.
- On abdominal palpation, the uterine size is either less than the period of amenorrhea, or the uterus is not palpable.
- On vaginal examination, the cervical os is closed, the uterus is smaller than the period of gestation, and there is no significant bleeding.
- An ultrasound examination will confirm the diagnosis in doubtful cases.

Missed Abortion

Definition
In this condition, symptoms of abortion appear and subsequently subside without any products of conception being expelled. The ovum dies but is retained in the uterus.

Clinical features
Symptoms
- In a woman who had amenorrhea and pregnancy symptoms earlier, the symptoms gradually disappear.
- History of threatened abortion may or may not be present.
- Brownish discharge may be present.

Signs
- The uterus does not enlarge in size; instead, it becomes smaller.
- On vaginal examination, bleeding is minimal or absent and the uterine size is smaller than the period of gestation.

Management
- If a missed abortion terminates spontaneously—and most do—the process of expulsion is the same as in any abortion.
- If a missed abortion occurs early in pregnancy, the entire contents of the uterus transform into a dark red or brownish shaggy mass known as a **carneous mole**.

- If a missed abortion occurs late in pregnancy, it becomes a shrivelled sac containing a macerated fetus, depending on the time of fetal death.
- The pregnancy test is usually negative at this stage.
- An ultrasound examination will confirm the non-viability of the fetus.

The minimal criteria for diagnosing miscarriage are as follows:

- **Crown–rump length** of at least 7 mm and no heartbeat
- Mean **gestational sac** diameter of at least 25 mm and no embryo (anembryonic pregnancy)
- Absence of embryo with heartbeat at least two weeks after an ultrasound scan that showed a gestational sac **without a yolk sac**
- Absence of embryo with a heartbeat at least 11 days after an ultrasound scan that showed a gestational sac **with a yolk sac**
- Embryo without cardiac activity

Management

If the dead fetus is retained for more than 5–6 weeks, the woman is at risk of developing coagulation disorders; there is also a risk of sepsis. Therefore, all women presenting with missed abortion should be evaluated for coagulation defects. Blood and blood products are made available before the termination of pregnancy and precautions are taken to prevent infection.

If the size of the uterus is less than 12 weeks of gestation, evacuation can be done using **medical methods of abortion (MMA)**. Misoprostol tablets, 600–800 µg, inserted vaginally every three hours are very effective in bringing about the expulsion of the POC. Alternatively, surgical evacuation using MVA can be performed. A prophylactic antibiotic should be given. If the uterine size is >12 weeks, medical termination of pregnancy is performed. Anti-D should be given whenever indicated.

FOLLOW-UP AFTER MISCARRIAGE

The woman should be reviewed after one month to discuss contraception and the prognosis of future pregnancies. She should also be offered emotional support and extensive counselling.

COMPLICATIONS FOLLOWING MISCARRIAGE MANAGEMENT

Complications include incomplete abortion and infection due to retained products, uterine perforation during surgical evacuation and delayed complications such as Asherman's syndrome due to vigorous curettage.

CERVICAL INCOMPETENCE (CERVICAL INSUFFICIENCY)

Definition

Cervical incompetence is defined as the inability of the uterine cervix to retain a pregnancy in the absence of uterine contractions in the second trimester of pregnancy. It is a condition characterised by painless cervical dilatation in the second trimester or later with the membranes bulging through the cervical canal followed by the expulsion of a fetus that is apparently normal and may show signs of life.

> With cervical incompetence, this sequence of events tends to repeat itself in subsequent pregnancies. Hence, it is important to diagnose the condition and to treat it early in subsequent pregnancies.

Etiology

Cervical insufficiency is due to the lack of sphincteric action of the internal cervical os.

The causes of cervical insufficiency are as follows:

- Congenital: This is rare.
- Acquired: This may develop due to surgical operations on the cervix.
  - Forcible dilatation of the cervix in dilatation and curettage
  - Cone biopsy of the cervix
  - Large loop excision of the transformation zone (LLETZ) of the cervix in cervical intraepithelial neoplasia (CIN) lesions
  - Amputation of the cervix during Manchester operation for genital prolapse

Clinical Features

Cervical insufficiency does not produce any symptoms in the non-pregnant state. However, those who have had a previous fetal loss due to insufficiency give a typical history of the following:

- Painless expulsion of the fetus
- Fetus expelled along with intact membranes
- No uterine contraction and pain
- There may be premature rupture of membranes
- Occasionally, abdominal cramping, with or without vaginal discharge
- Most often, the fetus is born alive

Diagnosis

During pregnancy: Diagnosis is made by transvaginal ultrasound. A cervical length of less than 25 mm is suggestive of insufficiency. There would also be dilatation of the cervix from the internal os downwards resulting in **'funnelling', and protrusion** of the membranes through the cervical os may be seen.

In those with a previous history of cervical insufficiency, weekly ultrasounds are done between weeks 16 and 24. Cervical length <2.5 cm or the presence of funnelling is considered abnormal. However, the diagnosis remains difficult in most women and is often based on history alone.

In the non-pregnant state: The following investigations are essential in the non-pregnant state in women who have had second-trimester miscarriages/recurrent miscarriage:

- A detailed history should be taken regarding the pregnancy that resulted in abortion. Investigations should include screening for diabetes and serological tests for syphilis and other infections.
- Karyotyping of the parents may be indicated in repeated early abortions.
- Autoimmune disorders such as APLA and inherited thrombophilia should be ruled out in women presenting with recurrent miscarriage.
- A hysterogram is indicated whenever uterine malformation or cervical insufficiency is suspected (Fig. 19.3a and b).

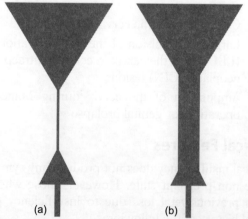

(a) (b)

Fig. 19.3 Diagrammatic representation of the shadow obtained on hysterography in the premenstrual phase using a cannula (a) with a normally competent cervix and (b) with an incompetent cervix showing the classic funnelling

The diagnostic methods described to diagnose cervical insufficiency in the non-pregnant state are as follows:

- Hysterography in the premenstrual phase to demonstrate funnelling and widening of the internal os

- Easy passage of a No. 8 or No.10 Hegar's dilator in the premenstrual phase
- Easy pulling of a Foley catheter with an inflated balloon through the cervical os

Management

The treatment of cervical insufficiency is surgical and consists of reinforcing the weak cervix with a suture. The suture is placed after week 14 of gestation, by which time, early abortions due to other causes are ruled out, but not later than week 24. Ultrasound is done to confirm fetal viability and to exclude congenital malformations prior to the procedure. Any obvious cervical infection should be treated.

Cerclage procedures

These include the McDonald's suture and Shirodkar suture.

- **A McDonald's suture** is simple (Fig. 19.4a–d). A No. 2 monofilament, non-absorbable purse-string suture is placed by taking 4–6 bites into the body of the cervix above the external os and tightening the knot posterior to the cervix. When the purse-string suture is in place, it encircles the cervix and tightens the internal os.
- The **Shirodkar stitch** involves dissecting the bladder and is more complicated. Hence, it is not frequently used.

Complications of cerclage procedure

The incidence of complications increases with advancing gestation. The common complications associated with cerclage procedures include **rupture of membranes, chorioamnionitis** and **intrauterine infections**. When these complications occur, or if the suture fails, or if there are signs of imminent abortion or delivery, the suture should be removed. Otherwise, the suture is removed after 36 weeks of gestation.

Success rates

In 80–90% of cases, success has been reported with the application of suture.

■ RECURRENT MISCARRIAGE

Definition

Recurrent miscarriage is described as three or more consecutive pregnancy losses at 20 weeks or less or at fetal weights less than 500 g.

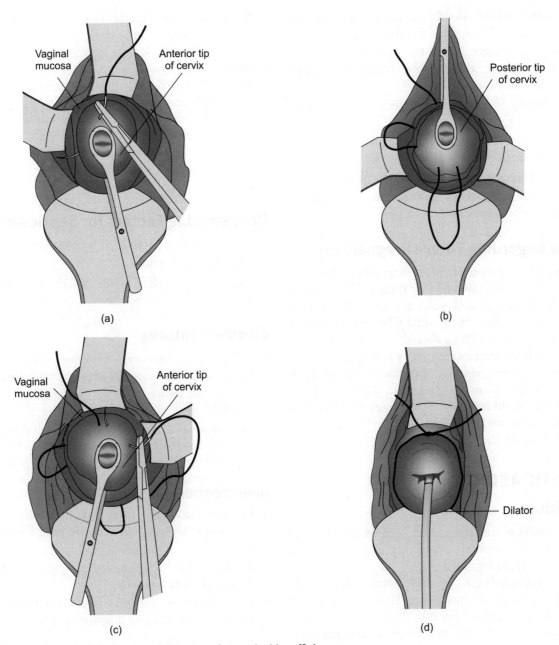

Fig. 19.4 (a–d)   *Application of McDonald's suture for cervical insufficiency*

Etiology

There are several etiological factors associated with recurrent pregnancy loss. These include the following:

- Parental chromosomal and genetic abnormalities due to abnormal oogenesis and errors in fertilisation
- Defects in coagulation factors such as thrombophilias and antiphospholipid antibodies
- Endocrine factors such as PCOS, luteal phase defects, hypothyroidism and diabetes mellitus
- Anatomical defects such as uterine anomalies, cervical insufficiency, fibroids and intrauterine adhesions

Nearly 70% of miscarriages that occur in the first 12 weeks are due to chromosomal anomalies and losses due to APLA. Cervical insufficiency tends to occur in the second trimester of pregnancy. In the majority of cases, no etiology may be found for recurrent miscarriage.

Counselling and Investigations After Recurrent Miscarriages

Though the definition of recurrent abortions is three or more consecutive losses, it is better to counsel the woman and order investigations after two abortions since the pregnancy loss is high after two losses.

- A **detailed history** should be taken regarding the pregnancies which resulted in miscarriage.
- Investigations depend on the gestation at which pregnancy losses occurred and whether the fetuses were viable or not.
- **Karyotyping** of partners is indicated in repeated early abortions.
- Investigations for **cervical insufficiency and uterine malformations** are indicated if history is suggestive.
- **Autoimmune disorders** may need to be ruled out.
- Screening for **diabetes** and serological tests for **syphilis** may be indicated.

Advice Regarding Future Pregnancies

Following investigations, treatable conditions should be corrected before planning further pregnancies. Obesity should be managed, and women with PCOS should be advised to reduce their weight before attempting another pregnancy. Women should be advised to report to a specialist as soon as pregnancy is diagnosed since they may require treatment for conditions such as antiphospholipid antibody syndrome, diabetes and so on. Women should receive antenatal care in a high-risk pregnancy clinic and deliver in a centre fully equipped to care for the mother and newborn.

■ SEPTIC ABORTION

Definition

Septic abortion usually results from a criminal intervention to terminate pregnancy and, to a much lesser extent, from legal abortions.

The infection begins as endometritis due to the retained products of conception. If not treated, the infection may spread further into the myometrium and parametrium. Parametritis may progress to **peritonitis**.

Septic abortion is one of the most common causes of morbidity and mortality, especially in the developing countries. According to the **World Health Organization**, approximately 68,000 women die each year due to complications from unsafe abortions, with sepsis as the main cause of death.

The etiology of septic abortion is usually **polymicrobial**, the common pathogens being gram-positive and gram-negative aerobes and facultative or obligate anaerobes. Sepsis is often caused by a variety of organisms—*Escherichia coli, Enterococcus, Pseudomonas, Streptococcus* and *Proteus* are the ones commonly involved. Rarely, the infection may be caused by *Clostridium welchii* or *C. tetani*. Pregnancy

induces alterations in the maternal immune system, which could be an important contributory factor in endotoxic shock following gram-negative infection in septic cases.

Severe hemorrhage, sepsis, bacterial shock and acute renal failure are the dangerous complications that could result. Alterations in coagulation factors during pregnancy predispose to increased risk of intravascular coagulation, consumptive coagulopathy and renal shutdown. *C. welchii* infection can cause hemolysis and jaundice.

Predisposing Factors for Septic Abortion

- Illegal abortion performed by unqualified persons
- Incomplete abortion
- Uterine perforation with injury to surrounding viscera such as the bowel

Clinical Features

- Following a history of recent pregnancy and termination, the woman presents with fever, chills, abdominal pain, vaginal discharge and vaginal bleeding.
- **Septicemia** is suggested by high fever and prostration, tachycardia, tachypnea, respiratory difficulty and hypotension; there may be evidence of peritonitis.

Investigations

- Routine blood and urine investigations, CBC and liver and renal function tests are performed.
- Blood, urine, high vaginal swab and cervical cultures are taken, and high-dose broad-spectrum antibiotics are begun intravenously.
- USG abdomen and pelvis are carried out to detect retained products and diagnose pelvic abscess.

Management

According to the degree of severity, septic abortion is graded as follows:

- **Grade 1:** The infection is limited to the uterine cavity. The woman's general condition is stable. There is pyrexia of varying degrees and offensive vaginal discharge. Vaginal examination may show a partially open or closed cervix with a bulky, tender uterus. The fornices are free.
- **Grade 2:** The infection has spread beyond the uterus to the parametrium. The woman is more acutely ill. The lower abdomen is slightly rigid, and tenderness is present over the hypogastrium and on either side.

Vaginal examination reveals a tender adnexal region and diffuse fullness with a tender, bulky uterus.

- **Grade 3:** The infection has spread beyond the pelvis. In this group, the woman is very ill with signs of peritonitis—fever, dry tongue, rapid pulse and distended and tender abdomen.

General principles of treatment

- Patients of all three grades should be hospitalised, and prompt and aggressive therapy must be instituted. The aims of treatment are to control infection with empirical broad-spectrum antibiotic therapy, correct electrolyte imbalance and blood volume, remove the infected products and prevent further bleeding. Depending on the sensitivity of the organism, the antibiotic can be changed later on.
- Two large-bore IV lines should be started with NS/ RL.
- Oxygen should be instituted.
- The drug therapy should cover gram-positive and -negative aerobic organisms and anaerobic organisms. The initial regime consists of a combination of ampicillin (1 g IV every 6 hours) combined with an aminoglycoside (e.g., gentamicin, 2 mg/Kg loading dose, followed by 1.5 mg/Kg every 8 hours) and metronidazole, 500 mg, IV every 8 hours. This is subsequently changed according to the culture reports. Ceftriaxone, 1 g, IV every 12 hours can also be given to cover gram-negative organisms.
- Blood and blood components should be kept ready.
- An ultrasound examination would reveal the presence or absence of retained POC.
- In case perforation of the bowel is suspected, X-ray abdomen erect view is taken to demonstrate air under the diaphragm.
- Removing the focus of sepsis is the primary aim of treatment.
- If retained POCs are demonstrated in the uterine cavity, then the evacuation of the uterine cavity may be done by either MVA or suction evacuation, preferably under USG guidance.
- If perforation of the bowel or rupture/perforation of the uterus is suspected, then laparotomy under antibiotic cover is mandatory.
- Hysterectomy may be required in some septic abortion patients.

Management of grade I cases

Empirical antibiotic therapy followed by surgical evacuation within 24 hours is recommended.

Management of grade 2 cases

More aggressive management is required. IV fluids and broad-spectrum antibiotics are administered. In addition, patients may require prophylactic anti-gas gangrene serum and blood transfusion. The patient should be carefully monitored for impending shock and other complications. Besides monitoring vital parameters, the progression of the disease and deterioration of the condition should be looked for. Evacuation can be carried out under good antibiotic cover in 12–24 hours.

Pelvic abscess

If the infection is localised in the POD, a pelvic abscess can develop. Pelvic abscess causes a spiky rise in temperature with rectal tenesmus. A boggy mass is felt through the posterior fornix or by rectal examination. The diagnosis can be confirmed by USG. Pelvic abscess is treated by draining the pus through a posterior colpotomy (by making an incision in the posterior fornix).

Management of grade 3 cases

These patients are at great risk and should be given immediate and aggressive treatment to prevent vasomotor shock and renal failure. Monitoring of the blood pressure, pulse rate, central venous pressure and urine output is essential.

Most of these patients need to be given intravenous infusions to combat shock and electrolyte imbalance; some may require blood transfusion. Broad-spectrum antibiotics, covering both aerobes and anaerobes, should be given intravenously. High doses should be continued, unless the woman's clinical response or culture and sensitivity tests provide an indication for changing the antibiotic regimen after 48–72 hours. Early evacuation should be carried out under antibiotic cover. Rarely, if the infected products of conception cannot be easily removed per vaginum, hysterectomy may be required. Currently, the indications for hysterectomy are non-responsiveness to medical management, traumatic uterine perforation that cannot be repaired and *C. welchii* infection.

Indications for exploratory laparotomy

- Uterine perforation with bowel injury is suspected
- Not responding to evacuation and medical therapy
- General peritonitis with pelvic abscess

Prevention of Septic Abortion

Primary prevention of septic abortion includes access to effective and acceptable contraception and access to safe, legal abortion in case of contraceptive failure.

If a suspected case of septic abortion is received in the PHC, the following measures should be undertaken:

- Start two IV lines
- Monitor the vitals
- Start oxygen
- Give the initial dose of antibiotic and transfer the woman to the next level of care where further management is available

Differential Diagnosis of Septic Abortion

The **differential diagnosis** includes:

1. Acute appendicitis
2. Ectopic pregnancy
3. Twisted ovarian tumours
4. Acute pelvic inflammatory disease
5. Shock due to other non-obstetric conditions

Long-term sequelae of septic abortion are chronic pelvic pain, chronic PID and infertility due to tubal block.

KEY POINTS

✓ Spontaneous abortion or miscarriage is the termination of pregnancy before 20 weeks of gestation.

✓ Etiology of abortion is varied, but early abortions are usually due to chromosomal abnormalities of the fetus.

✓ Clinically, abortion may present as threatened, incomplete, complete or missed abortion.

✓ When a spontaneous abortion is complicated by infection, it is known as a septic abortion.

✓ The minimal criteria for diagnosing miscarriage are: 1. Crown–rump length of at least 7 mm and no heartbeat, 2. mean gestational sac diameter of at least 25 mm and no embryo (anembryonic pregnancy) and 3. embryo without cardiac activity.

✓ Recurrent abortions need to be investigated to determine the possible etiology. This helps in the management of a subsequent pregnancy.

✓ Cervical insufficiency is the main cause of second-trimester miscarriage.

Essay question

1. Enumerate the causes of first and second-trimester miscarriages. How do you diagnose and manage a case of cervical insufficiency?

Short answer questions

1. Enumerate the causes of miscarriage.
2. Outline the diagnosis and management of a missed miscarriage.
3. Discuss the management of an incomplete miscarriage.
4. Discuss the management of a septic miscarriage.

MCQs

1. What is the incidence of spontaneous miscarriage?
   a) 5–10%
   b) 10–15%
   c) 15–20%
   d) 20–30%

2. Which of the following is the commonest cause of first-trimester miscarriages?
   a) Chromosomal cause
   b) Infection
   c) Cervical os insufficiency
   d) Uterine anomalies

3. Which of the following is not a criterion for the diagnosis of a missed abortion?
   a) ≥7 mm CRL with no heartbeat
   b) ≥25 mm gestational sac with no embryo
   c) Absence of embryo two weeks after the scan with gestational sac but no yolk sac
   d) Absence of heartbeat one week after scan with gestational sac and yolk sac

4. Which of the following is not a cause of recurrent miscarriage?
   a) APLA
   b) TORCH
   c) Diabetes
   d) Cervical insufficiency

5. Which of the following are the clinical features of cervical insufficiency?
   a) Cervical length <2.5 cm
   b) Funnelling of cervical canal
   c) Easy passage of No. 8 Hegar dilator
   d) All of the above

6. At what gestational age is cervical cerclage for cervical insufficiency usually placed?
   a) 6–8 weeks
   b) 10–12 weeks
   c) 12–14 weeks
   d) 24–28 weeks

7. If not expelled, the contents of a missed abortion become a dark red mass. What is this mass known as?
   a) Gestational trophoblastic disease
   b) Carneous mole
   c) Red degeneration
   d) Lithopedion

8. When the products of conception have separated from the uterine wall but are not expelled, this is called:
   a) Threatened abortion
   b) Inevitable abortion
   c) Missed abortion
   d) Incomplete abortion

9. A 31-year-old G2A1 at 15 weeks of gestation reports with a history of previous PPROM at 24 weeks and painless expulsion of products. On examination, her uterus is palpable one inch above the symphysis pubis. On USG, there is a viable fetus corresponding to 15 weeks, no anomalies detected as of now and a cervical length of 20 mm. What is your plan of action?
   a) Reassurance
   b) Bed rest
   c) Progesterone supplementation
   d) McDonald's suture

Answers
1. (b), 2. (a), 3. (d), 4. (b), 5. (d), 6. (c), 7. (b), 8. (b), 9. (d)

Fill in the blanks

1. A woman with six weeks amenorrhea, mild bleeding, uterus size corresponding to six weeks and a closed cervical os is diagnosed with _____.
2. A cervical length of less than _____ is suggestive of cervical insufficiency.

Answers
1. threatened abortion, 2. 2.5 cm

Case scenario-based discussion

1. A 21-year-old G2P1L1 at 8 weeks of pregnancy presents with pain abdomen and bleeding pv. On examination, her uterus is found to be corresponding to the period of pregnancy and her cervical os is closed with mild bleeding through the os.
   a) What investigation would you advise for this patient?
   b) If cardiac activity is absent, what would your diagnosis be?
   c) If cardiac activity is present, what would your diagnosis be?
   d) Mention two methods of managing missed miscarriage.

Answers
a) Ultrasound of the pelvis should be carried out.
b) Missed miscarriage would be the diagnosis.
c) Threatened miscarriage would be the diagnosis.
d) Medical methods with misoprostol and suction evacuation are used in the management of missed miscarriage.

2. A 32-year-old G3A2 has a history of spontaneous expulsion of fetuses between 16 and 20 weeks. She visits the antenatal OPD at 12 weeks.
   a) What is your probable diagnosis?
   b) How will you confirm your diagnosis?
   c) Mention two conditions that can predispose to this problem.
   d) What surgery would you plan for this patient?

Answers
a) This is a most likely a case of cervical insufficiency.
b) The diagnosis can be confirmed by USG—cervical length of <2.5 cm.
c) Forcible cervical dilatation and cone biopsy of the cervix.
d) McDonald's suture should be performed.

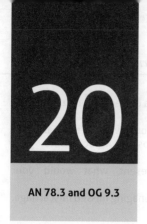

Ectopic Pregnancy

Learning Objectives

» To describe the various causes of acute abdomen in early pregnancy
» To discuss the etiology, clinical features and differential diagnosis of ectopic pregnancy
» To discuss the medical and surgical management of ectopic pregnancy
» To know the different types of ectopic pregnancy

■ INTRODUCTION

Ectopic pregnancy is the leading cause of maternal death in early pregnancy. In recent years, the incidence of ectopic pregnancy has increased from 1% to nearly 2.5%. This rise is attributed to an increase in the prevalence of sexually transmitted infections and pelvic inflammatory disease (PID), the increased use of assisted reproductive techniques and better means of diagnosing ectopic pregnancy using transvaginal ultrasound and serum β-hCG estimation.

Definition

Ectopic pregnancy refers to the implantation of the zygote (fertilised ovum) outside the uterine cavity or at an abnormal location within the uterus.

■ SITES OF ECTOPIC PREGNANCY (TABLE 20.1; Fig. 20.1)

* 95–96% of all ectopic pregnancies occur in the fallopian tubes. The ampulla is the commonest site—nearly 70% of ectopic pregnancies occur in the ampullary region. 12% occur in the isthmus,

11% are seen in the fimbrial end and the interstitial portion is involved in 2–3% of cases. Rarer are the ovarian ectopic (3% of cases), cervical ectopic (<1%), cesarean section scar pregnancy (<1%) and abdominal pregnancy (1%).

* Abdominal pregnancy could be primary or secondary.
* Very rarely, ectopic pregnancy has been reported following subtotal or total hysterectomy. It occurs either in the prolapsed fallopian tube, at the vault, following abdominal hysterectomy or in the cervical stump following subtotal hysterectomy.

Table 20.1 Sites of ectopic pregnancy

Site of ectopic pregnancy	%
Fallopian tube	95–96%
Ampullary region	70%
Isthmus	12%
Fimbrial end	11%
Interstitial portion (cornual)	2–3%
Ovarian ectopic	3%
Cervical ectopic	<1%
Ectopic in cesarean section scar	<1%
Abdominal pregnancy	1%

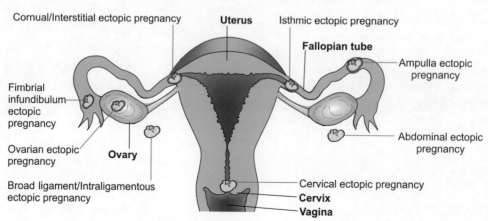

Fig. 20.1 Sites of ectopic pregnancy

INCIDENCE

The incidence of ectopic pregnancy (Table 20.2) varies depending on the type of ectopic pregnancy. The incidence of ectopic pregnancy in the fallopian tube is 2–2.5%. The incidence of ovarian pregnancy is reported to vary from 1 in 7,000 to 1 in 40,000 deliveries; abdominal pregnancy ranges from 1 in 10,000 to 1 in 30,000 deliveries and cervical pregnancy ranges from 1 in 9,000 to 1 in 95,000 deliveries.

A heterotopic pregnancy is a condition in which there is normal intrauterine pregnancy along with an extrauterine pregnancy. This condition was rare in the past with an incidence of 1 in 30,000 spontaneous pregnancies. However, with the advent of assisted reproductive techniques (ART), its incidence has increased to 1 in 4,000 pregnancies.

Table 20.2 Incidence of ectopic pregnancy

Site of ectopic pregnancy	Incidence
Tubal ectopic pregnancy	2–2.5%
Ovarian pregnancy	1 in 7,000 to 1 in 40,000 deliveries
Abdominal pregnancy	1 in 10,000 to 1 in 30,000 deliveries
Cervical pregnancy	1 in 9,000 to 1 in 95,000 deliveries
Heterotopic pregnancy	1 in 4,000 in ART pregnancies and 1 in 30,000 in spontaneous pregnancies

ETIOLOGY

Any factor that affects the transport of the fertilised ovum through the fallopian tube leads to ectopic pregnancy. In nearly 50% of cases, no risk factors are identified.

- **Congenital/developmental anomalies of the fallopian tubes**, e.g., congenital diverticula or the tube being tortuous and long, results in ectopic pregnancy.
- **Premature development of the trophoblast** could result in the premature embedding of the fertilised ovum in the tube, and thereby, ectopic pregnancy.
- **Tubal infections and pelvic inflammatory disease (PID)** are the most important etiological factors for ectopic gestation. PID increases the risk of ectopic pregnancy 7–10-fold. The inflammatory process in the fallopian tube may be caused by gonococcal and chlamydial infection post-abortion and puerperal infection or secondary to peritonitis caused by appendicitis. Pelvic tuberculosis is also an important cause of ectopic pregnancy. The resulting endosalpingitis leads to the agglutination of the mucosa, loss of ciliary function or formation of diverticula which interfere with the transport of the fertilised ovum. There are also peritubal adhesions affecting the peristalsis of the tube which is important for the transport of the ovum.
- **Peritubal adhesions** due to a previous surgery such as that performed for appendicitis, pelvic infections and endometriosis could lead to an ectopic pregnancy.
- **Prior tubal surgery** such as tuboplasty for infertility, tubectomy procedures and reversal of sterilisation are associated with an increased risk of ectopic pregnancy. The risk of developing an ectopic pregnancy following reversal of sterilisation is 3–4%.
- When there is a **history of ectopic pregnancy**, the chance of recurrence in subsequent pregnancies is 10–20 % as tubal disease is always bilateral.
- **Contraceptive use**
  - **IUCD** users are 50% less likely to have ectopic pregnancy than women using no contraception. Ectopic pregnancy in IUCD users is rare and ranges from 0.25–1.5 per 1,000 women-years. However, when pregnancy occurs, the chance of ectopic pregnancy is 30% higher than in the general population.
  - Progestogen-only contraceptives have been shown to cause an increase in the incidence of ectopic pregnancy by slowing the ovum transport.
- With the widespread use of **assisted reproductive techniques** (ART), the incidences of ectopic and heterotopic pregnancies have increased. The occurrence of ectopic pregnancy following ART depends on the number of embryos transferred, and the indication for ART. The incidence is higher when the indication for ART is a tubal factor. To reduce the risk of ectopic pregnancy, salpingectomy or proximal tubal occlusion is carried out before in vitro fertilisation.
- Conditions distorting the anatomy of the fallopian tubes such as tumours that distort the tubes, e.g., fundal myoma, adnexal cysts and ventro suspension with shortening of the round ligaments can also lead to ectopic pregnancy.

MODE OF IMPLANTATION OF THE OVUM IN TUBAL PREGNANCY

- Fertilisation normally takes place in the lumen of the fallopian tube. Aided by the ciliated epithelium of the tube, the fertilised ovum makes its way into the uterine cavity, where it gets implanted on the already prepared endometrium.
- When the fertilised ovum is arrested in any portion of the tube, it burrows into the wall of the tube

because of the eroding and penetrating properties of the chorionic epithelium.

- There is no decidual formation or reaction in the stroma of the tubal mucosa. There is, however, increased congestion and softening of the tissues.
- The ovum, after burrowing rapidly into the softened and highly vascularised tissue, is encapsulated within the muscular tissue of the tubal wall.
- As the ovum grows in size, the muscular wall of the fallopian tube is unable to accommodate the growing ovum.
- There is mechanical distension of the fallopian tube along with the thinning of the wall due to trophoblastic invasion. These result in the early rupture of the tube.

CHANGES IN THE UTERUS

As the aforementioned changes occur in the fallopian tube, the uterus too undergoes a number of changes. It enlarges, but not to the same extent as in an intrauterine pregnancy. The endometrium undergoes decidual changes; it becomes thick and spongy like the decidua vera in a uterine pregnancy. However, it does not contain any chorionic tissue. This decidual tissue is either expelled as a cast (**decidual cast**) or as piecemeal at the time of termination of ectopic pregnancy.

OUTCOMES OF TUBAL PREGNANCY (Fig. 20.2)

Tubal Abortion

In tubal abortion, the products of conception separate from the endosalphinx and then extrude through the fimbrial end. When there is complete extrusion of the products, it is called a complete abortion; the products of conception then get absorbed. Tubal abortion commonly occurs when an ectopic pregnancy occurs in the ampullary or fimbrial region.

Incomplete abortion may occur when the products reach the fimbria and partially extrude through it. When the fimbrial end is occluded, the tube may gradually become distended to form a hematosalphinx. Occasionally, there is repeated slow trickling from the implantation site, through the tubal wall and into the peritoneal cavity. The collected blood surrounds the tube and the ovary to form a peritubal hematocele, and later, a pelvic hematocele.

Tubal Rupture

There is marked increase in vascularity—arteries and veins are dilated. There is hypertrophy of the musculature

except at the placental site. As the tube is only capable of limited distension, there is inadequate placentation, and eventually, rupture occurs. Tubal rupture occurs between 6 and 8 weeks if the isthmus is the site of ectopic pregnancy, and between 8 and 10 weeks if it is in the ampullary region. When there is a cornual pregnancy, because of the greater distensibility of the myometrium, pregnancy can continue up to 14–16 weeks before rupture occurs. In cases where a rupture occurs and only the villi protrude, the woman continues to bleed and presents with signs and symptoms of intraperitoneal bleeding and shock. Occasionally, there is complete extrusion of the products; in such cases, the rent in the tube retracts and the bleeding stops.

Fate of the Fetus

If there is complete extrusion of an undamaged pregnancy, the fetus can implant anywhere in the pelvic or abdominal cavity. It gets adequate blood supply from the surrounding organs to form a secondary abdominal pregnancy. The fetus may continue to grow, or there may be placental insufficiency, malformations or intrauterine death.

If the extruded fetus does not get adequate blood supply, it either gets absorbed or undergoes mummification and forms a calcified lithopedion. If fetal development is advanced, its bones remain while other tissues get degenerated. These fetal bones may extrude through the bladder or rectum POD even after a year.

Occasionally, if the implantation is towards the mesosalphinx, rupture occurs between the layers of the broad ligament. One layer of broad ligament may give way, subsequently resulting in a tertiary pregnancy. The possible terminations vary with the **site** of the gestation (Table 20.3).

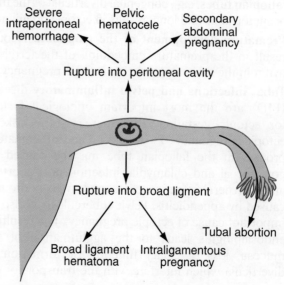

Fig. 20.2 The outcomes of tubal pregnancy

Table 20.3 Various modes of termination depending on site of ectopic gestation

Type of tubal gestation	Mode of termination
Interstitial pregnancy	• Rupture occurs at around 12–14 weeks of gestation with severe intraperitoneal hemorrhage • Pregnancy at the cornual end of the tube may grow into the uterus and develop as tubouterine pregnancy • Very rarely gets aborted into the uterine cavity
Isthmic pregnancy	• Rupture occurs much earlier—by 6–10 weeks of pregnancy and severe intraperitoneal hemorrhage can occur • If the fetus is viable after rupture, secondary abdominal pregnancy can occur • The **tubal rupture** may occur between the layers of the broad ligament to cause broad ligament hematoma
Ampullary pregnancy	• Tubal abortion • Tubal rupture
Fimbrial ectopic	• Complete/incomplete abortion

CLINICAL FEATURES OF TUBAL PREGNANCY

The clinical manifestations of tubal pregnancy are diverse and can be atypical. A high index of suspicion should be there to diagnose ectopic pregnancy.

Symptoms

The **classic triad of symptoms of ectopic pregnancy** are the following:

1. Amenorrhea
2. Abdominal pain
3. Irregular vaginal bleeding

However, only about 45–50% of women present with these classical symptoms. Most cases present with atypical presentation.

Amenorrhea/menstrual disturbances

A history of amenorrhea is seen only in 80% of cases of ectopic pregnancy. Most women interpret the irregular bleeding which occurs in ectopic pregnancy as normal menstruation. The absence of a missed period does not rule out an ectopic pregnancy. Because of the atypical bleeding, the woman may think that she is having normal menstruation. It is important to enquire about the LMP, onset, character, duration and amount of

bleeding. Profuse bleeding occurs only in 5% of cases. A decidual cast is passed in 5–10% of cases.

About a fourth of women do not report amenorrhea and mistake the uterine bleeding that occurs with tubal pregnancy for true menstruation.

Pain and irregular bleeding

Pain is reported by 90% of women, and irregular bleeding is seen in 70% of cases due to the intermittent shedding of the decidua. Pain can be acute and may be associated with fainting spells. With a history of amenorrhea or delayed periods, if the woman experiences severe lower abdominal pain, an ectopic pregnancy must be suspected. With abdominal pain, the woman may experience vasomotor disturbances ranging from vertigo to syncope.

Other symptoms include the following:

• Fainting spells are typical but rare; dizziness, weakness, nausea and vomiting are more common
• Symptoms of shock in acute rupture
• Shoulder pain
• Urge to defecate—10–15% of cases

UNRUPTURED ECTOPIC

Among women with an unruptured ectopic (Fig. 20.3), a history of amenorrhea is present only in 75–80% of cases. Others have atypical presentations with on-and-off irregular spotting. When the ectopic is unruptured, the woman may present with a vague, colicky pain on the affected side due to the stretching of the broad ligament and the tube. Besides the symptoms of pregnancy, the woman may develop malaise, discomfort and uneasiness.

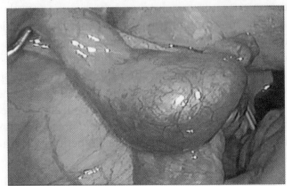

Fig. 20.3 Laparoscopic picture of an unruptured ectopic pregnancy

Clinical Features

Before the rupture of an ectopic pregnancy, **blood pressure** and **pulse** may be normal or there may be slight tachycardia.

Abdominal examination may not reveal any significant findings. On deep palpation, there may be tenderness on the affected side. On examination, the uterus may be slightly enlarged, not corresponding to the period of amenorrhea. A tender unilateral pulsatile mass may be palpable on one side or in the POD. The movement of the cervix may be painful due to the stretching of the broad ligament. This is called a positive cervical excitation.

TUBAL ABORTION

Tubal abortions can manifest with acute or chronic presentations.

Acute Presentation

Tubal abortion is associated with intermittent pain in the lower abdomen due to the irritation of the peritoneum by the trickling blood. Tubal abortion is more of a chronic picture when the intraperitoneal bleeding is small and recurrent. More often, after a period of amenorrhea, the woman presents with pain in one or both iliac fossa—a sharp, stabbing pain due to chorio-decidual hemorrhage and peritoneal irritation. There may be associated syncope, pallor and increased pulse rate. Abdominal examination reveals distension, guarding and tenderness.

On pelvic examination, the uterus is bulky to feel, the movement of the cervix is painful and an ill-defined mass can be felt in the POD or the adnexal region.

Chronic Presentation

Following a tubal abortion, a pelvic hematocele can develop and present as chronic rupture. The tubal abortion goes unrecognised, and the woman complains of chronic intermittent pelvic pain, generalised malaise, urinary frequency, rectal symptoms, diffuse lower abdominal pain and low hemoglobin with leukocytosis. On vaginal examination, there is a tender, boggy swelling in the POD extending to the lateral fornices. Sometimes, this hematocele gets absorbed; alternatively, it results in permanent residual disease, presenting with chronic pelvic pain, menorrhagia, infection, PID and abscess formation.

RUPTURE OF ECTOPIC PREGNANCY

Symptoms of Rupture

Depending on the site of ectopic pregnancy, tubal rupture occurs at different periods of gestation. Ectopic at the isthmic site ruptures at 8–10 weeks of gestation;

ectopic at the ampullary region ruptures at 6–12 weeks and an interstitial ectopic usually ruptures at 14–16 weeks of gestation. The rupture may be spontaneous or it could be precipitated by straining at stools, coitus, coughing, sneezing, vaginal examination, etc.

In women with rupture, the intermittent pain will become continuous, and due to the rupture and peritoneal irritation, the pain is stabbing or tearing in nature. Pain is the most common symptom—it may be unilateral or bilateral, may be present in the lower abdomen or may involve the upper abdomen too. The woman may present with shoulder pain due to the irritation of the diaphragm by the intraperitoneal bleeding. There may be associated vaginal bleeding. The intensity of pain may not be related to the amount of intraperitoneal bleeding as a person in shock will not be able to appreciate the pain. The woman could also present with dizziness, fainting spells and signs of shock such as sweating, dulling of the sensorium, pallor, restlessness and air hunger.

Signs of Rupture

On examination, the woman is pale and tachycardic. Her temperature may be low and she may have severe hypotension.

On abdominal palpation, there is guarding and rigidity due to peritoneal irritation. The abdomen is distended and tender on palpation. On percussion, the abdomen is dull, and a shifting dullness may be present. Rebound and cough tenderness may also be elicited.

Cullen's sign is rarely seen in thin women and in those with umbilical hernia. In such cases, there is a bluish discolouration on the periumbilical skin due to the connection between the broad ligament and umbilical veins.

On pelvic examination, there may be adnexal masses and fullness in the POD. Cervical excitation may be elicited due to the stretching of the broad ligament. Occasionally, it may not be elicited when the woman is in shock. In some cases, due to defects in the diaphragm, hemoperitoneum may leak into the pleural cavity and cause hemothorax.

Danforth's sign—shoulder pain elicited due to subdiaphragmatic irritation—can be seen in 10% of patients.

DIAGNOSIS OF ECTOPIC PREGNANCY

Early diagnosis of ectopic is important in order to avoid maternal morbidity and mortality. One should have a high index of suspicion to diagnose an ectopic pregnancy. In any woman of the reproductive age with or without amenorrhea presenting with abdominal pain, ectopic pregnancy must first be ruled out. In any woman presenting with acute abdomen with hemodynamic instability, ectopic pregnancy should be ruled out.

Culdocentesis

Culdocentesis was a common practice before the advent of USG. The procedure involved inserting a wide-bore needle through the posterior fornix into the POD (Fig. 20.4). Aspirating non-clotting blood was diagnostic of an intraperitoneal bleed due to a ruptured ectopic pregnancy. A dry tap did not rule out an ectopic. With the availability of USG, this procedure has now become outdated.

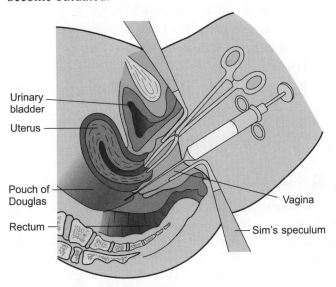

Fig. 20.4 Procedure of culdocentesis

The foremost investigations for the diagnosis of ectopic are the detection of serum β-hCG level and a transvaginal ultrasound.

Serum hCG

Serum hCG determination should be the first step in evaluating women suspected of having an ectopic pregnancy.
- If the hCG is negative, the test rules out the possibility of intra and extrauterine pregnancy.
- If positive, the test could indicate one of the following—a viable intrauterine pregnancy, threatened abortion, missed abortion or an ectopic pregnancy.

The next step is to perform a transvaginal scan (TVS). The use of TVS permits the gestational sac to be consistently identified as early as at 33–34 days of conception.

Transvaginal USG

- The presence of a gestational sac with a yolk sac or an embryo within the uterine cavity confirms a diagnosis of an intrauterine pregnancy.
- However, it is important to remember that heterotopic pregnancy may occur in rare cases. There should be a high index of suspicion in women conceiving through in vitro fertilisation or when, in the presence of an intrauterine pregnancy, there is echogenic fluid in the posterior cul-de-sac.
- TVS is 96% sensitive and 97% specific for the diagnosis of ectopic pregnancy.

USG features of ectopic pregnancy

- On USG, ectopic pregnancy appears as an intact, well-defined tubal ring (the '**bagel sign**') in which the yolk sac and/or embryonic pole, with or without cardiac action, is/are seen within a completely sonolucent sac.
- An empty uterine cavity (Fig. 20.5) and the presence of an adnexal mass and/or fluid in the POD confirms ectopic pregnancy.

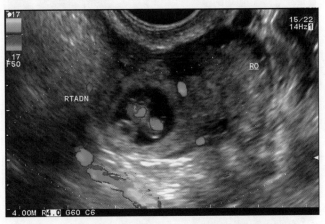

Fig. 20.5 USG showing an empty uterine cavity with the right adnexa showing a large, irregular heterogenous lesion with internal anechoic cystic areas extending to the pouch of Douglas (*Image courtesy*: Mediscan systems, Chennai)

Doppler

- With colour Doppler (Fig. 20.6), it is possible to visualise high velocity and low impedance signals with a 'ring of fire' appearance around the gestational sac.
- In patients in whom expectant management is planned, the decision is based on the findings on Doppler. Conservative management is undertaken only on hypoperfused and avascular ectopics.

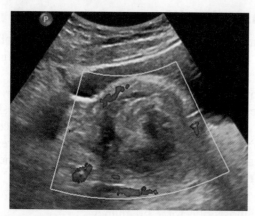

Fig. 20.6 'Ring of fire' appearance on colour Doppler (*Image courtesy:* Dr B H Parameshwar Keerthi, Consultant Radiologist, BM Scans, Kancheepuram)

Transabdominal Scan

In a ruptured ectopic pregnancy, hemoperitoneum may extend to the perihepatic and perisplenic areas (Fig. 20.7).

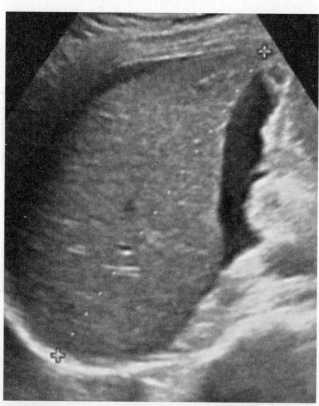

Fig. 20.7 Gross hemoperitoneum extending to the perihepatic area *(Image courtesy:* Dr B H Parameshwar Keerthi, Consultant Radiologist, BM Scans, Kancheepuram)

Laparoscopy

- As most ectopics are diagnosed with the combined use of serum β-hCG and TVS, laparoscopy is not used for the sole purpose of diagnosis. Its main use is in the management of ectopic pregnancies.

Additional Investigations

- Additional investigations are required to prepare the patient for surgery or methotrexate therapy.
- Grouping, cross-matching and reserving adequate quantities of blood is important.

■ DIFFERENTIAL DIAGNOSIS

Around 25% of ectopic pregnancies are falsely diagnosed as such. The differential diagnosis include the following:

- Pelvic inflammatory disease
- Abortion—threatened or incomplete
- Ovarian cyst—persistent corpus luteum with delayed period (Halban syndrome)
- Rupture of follicular/corpus luteum cyst
- Acute appendicitis
- Rupture of an endometriotic cyst
- Dysmenorrhea
- Bleeding episode of abnormal uterine bleeding (AUB)
- Renal colic
- Other GI conditions

■ MANAGEMENT

The management of ectopic pregnancy should be tailored to the clinical condition and future fertility requirements of the woman. Tubal pregnancy can be managed by laparotomy, operative laparoscopy, and medical methods. The management of ectopic pregnancy should begin with appropriate resuscitative measures and in all patients, blood should be grouped and cross-matched. The management of ruptured ectopic pregnancy is only surgical, whereas the management of unruptured ectopic pregnancy affords the medical option in selected cases.

Medical Management

Medical therapy with methotrexate (MTX) can be offered to suitable women. Methotrexate is an antimetabolite, which acts as a folic acid antagonist. It can be given intramuscularly or can be injected into the ectopic site under ultrasound or laparoscopic guidance. Only 25% of cases are suitable for this therapy.

Selection criteria

Medical management can be undertaken only when the following criteria are fulfilled:

- It should be an unruptured ectopic pregnancy

- The size of the mass should be <3–4 cm
- The β-hCG level should be <5,000 miu/mL (preferably <3,000 miu/mL)
- There should not be any cardiac activity
- There should not be any hemoperitoneum
- The woman should be hemodynamically stable
- The woman should be adequately counselled and should understand the need for follow-up

Medical therapy cannot be applied to women who are not compliant.

Methotrexate contraindications

Methotrexate is contraindicated in intrauterine and heterotopic pregnancy (discussed later). Also, when there is a known renal, hepatic or active pulmonary disease or hematological disorders, or when any of the baseline hematologic, renal or hepatic laboratory values are abnormal, methotrexate cannot be used.

Methotrexate can cause the suppression of the bone marrow. Therefore, it cannot be used in immunodeficiency states. It is contraindicated during breastfeeding.

Contraindications to the use of methotrexate
- β-hCG level of >5,000 miu/mL
- Fetal cardiac activity
- Free fluid in the cul-de-sac
- Documented hypersensitivity to methotrexate
- Breastfeeding
- Immunodeficiency
- Liver disease
- Blood dyscrasias including thrombocytopenia
- Anemia
- Active pulmonary disease
- Acid peptic disease

Side effects of methotrexate

Methotrexate can cause the suppression of the bone marrow and inflammation of mucosal surfaces. In the presence of renal insufficiency, even a single dose of MTX can lead to death or severe complications such as bone marrow suppression, ARDS, and bowel ischemia. Patients may develop hypersensitivity and consequently, conjunctivitis, stomatitis and gastrointestinal upset.

Management regimens

For the medical management of ectopic pregnancy, single-dose and multiple-dose regimens are available. The multiple-dose regimen is ideally suited for interstitial and cervical pregnancies.

Single-dose regimen

The most widely used medical treatment is intramuscular methotrexate given as a single dose that is calculated (Fig. 20.8) based on the woman's body surface area (50 mg/m^2). **For most women, this will be between 75 and 90 mg.** The single-dose regimen has been found to be as efficacious as the multiple-drug regimen and is being widely followed.

The following measures are taken before initiating therapy:

- Initial β-hCG levels are taken.
- Levels of SGOT, SGPT, urea, creatinine and full blood count are measured.
- Blood grouping and Rh typing are performed. If the woman is Rh-negative, she is given anti-D immunoglobulin.
- Day 1: Inj. methotrexate, 50 mg/m^2 of body surface is given deep IM. The woman is advised not to take folic acid either singly or in combination with other vitamins until the ectopic pregnancy is resolved completely.
- Day 4: β-hCG levels are measured; this forms the baseline level.
- Day 7: β-hCG level is measured again.
- If the decrease in β-hCG level is ≥15% of the day 4 level, it indicates response to treatment. In such a case, β-hCG is repeated weekly until it becomes undetectable (<10 miu/mL).

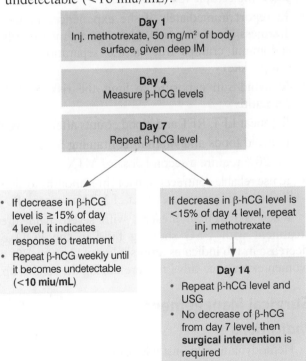

Fig. 20.8 Flowchart of medical management of ectopic pregnancy with methotrexate

- If the decrease in β-hCG level is <15% of the day 4 level, then inj. methotrexate is repeated and the woman is monitored as if from day 1. It is advisable to do a TVS to rule out significant hemoperitoneum before administering the second dose.
- Day 14: β-hCG level and ultrasound are repeated. If there is no decrease in β-hCG from day 7, then surgical intervention is required.

Multiple-dose regimen

The treatment involves giving MTX 1 mg/Kg IM on day 1, 3, 5 and 7 and leucovorin in a dose of 0.1 mg/Kg IM on days 2, 4, 6 and 8. β-hCG level should be checked every 48 hours until it decreases by 15%. Thereafter, it should be checked weekly. If the expected response is not seen with the first course, either surgical intervention is required or a second course can be attempted after normal lab test results are obtained.

Precautions

During methotrexate therapy, it is important to look for the rupture of the ectopic and any side effects of methotrexate. Outpatient treatment can be undertaken only if the woman is compliant and has easy access to emergency services. The following instructions should be given to the woman:

- To not have sexual intercourse as doing so could cause the ectopic to rupture
- To report immediately if she experiences fainting, dizziness or severe pain (the woman may develop abdominal cramps due to the separation of the ectopic site)
- To avoid sun exposure to limit the risk of MTX dermatitis
- To repeat LFT, RFT and blood counts after one week
- To avoid foods and vitamins containing folic acid
- 15–20% require a second dose of MTX
- To use reliable contraception for three months to allow the possible teratogenic effect of MTX to wean off

When the woman presents with severe pain after treatment with USG showing fluid in the POD or decrease in Hb indicates a possibility of rupture; 7% of women experience tubal rupture during the follow-up.

Surgical Management

Indications

- Hemodynamically unstable patient
- Hemodynamically stable patient with tubal rupture or abortion as evidenced by hemoperitoneum on USG

- Unruptured ectopic pregnancy where methotrexate is contraindicated
- Heterotopic pregnancy with coexisting viable intrauterine pregnancy
- When medical management of unruptured ectopic has failed
- In the management of ovarian pregnancy, secondary abdominal pregnancy and interstitial pregnancy

Surgical approach

The surgical approach to the management of ectopic pregnancy is either by conventional laparotomy or by laparoscopic approach.

- Laparotomy is indicated in a hemodynamically unstable patient diagnosed with or suspected of having ectopic with USG showing evidence of hemoperitoneum.
- Laparoscopic approach is indicated in patients with an unruptured pregnancy. Tubal abortions and rupture can be managed by experienced laparoscopic surgeons. Laparoscopy is preferable because the hospital stay is decreased and patient comfort is increased. It is contraindicated in an unstable patient in whom extensive intra-abdominal adhesions are present and when there are medical problems such as cardiac and respiratory disease.

Surgical method

The surgical methods available for the management of ectopic pregnancy are as follows:

1. Removal of the tube (salpingectomy)
2. Conservative surgery and preserving the fallopian tube (salpingotomy)

The decision about the method depends on the woman's desire for future fertility, the condition of the contralateral tube and the condition of the tube at the time of surgery.

Salpingectomy

Indications for salpingectomy

- Women who do not wish to have any more children
- When there is tubal rupture with a moderately or severely damaged tube
- Inability to control bleeding at conservative surgery
- When the size of the ectopic site is more than 3 cm
- When there is recurrent ectopic pregnancy on the same side

Procedure

At laparotomy, as soon as the abdomen is opened, a hand is slipped into the pelvis, the uterus is located and brought out. Then, the ectopic side is identified. The tube is lifted with the fingers, and clamps are applied on either side of the ectopic—on the mesosalpinx and at the uterine end. Then, the abdomen is cleared of blood before proceeding with the required surgery. In the past, partial salpingectomy was carried out by excising only the ectopic site. Total salpingectomy is preferable as it prevents the occurrence of ectopic in the remaining stump and also prevents the development of ovarian cancer in future. The removed portion of the tube should be sent for HPE to confirm an ectopic and to identify any underlying cause for ectopic such as tuberculosis.

Autotransfusion

Blood from the peritoneal cavity is collected in a sterile solution containing 2% sodium citrate, filtered and transfused. This can be done if the blood has not accumulated for >24–36 hours. Autotransfusion may be very useful in situations where appropriate blood is not available.

Advantages of salpingectomy

- It avoids the need for further treatment for persistent trophoblast at the ectopic site.
- If IVF is chosen for future conceptions, salpingectomy will be helpful in preventing future ectopic pregnancies.

Indications for conservative surgery

- The woman desires to conserve her fertility
- She is hemodynamically stable
- The gestational sac is unruptured and <5 cm in size
- The contralateral tube is absent or damaged—if salpingectomy is performed in these women, IVF would be the only choice available to them in the future

Procedure

- The options available are salpingotomy and end-to-end anastomosis.
- This can be undertaken by the laparoscopic approach.

Salpingotomy

An incision is made on the anti-mesenteric surface of the tube, over the ectopic site. The ectopic contents are shelled out gently and hemostasis is obtained with electrocoagulation or fine sutures. The incision can either be sutured or left unsutured to heal by secondary intention. All efforts should be made to prevent adhesions. If the bleeding is heavy, the procedure may have to be converted to salpingectomy.

Following salpingotomy, there is a possibility of a persistent trophoblast, which is detected by the failure of serum hCG to decrease as expected. These cases may present with delayed hemorrhage. Therefore, following surgery, serial weekly measurement of hCG is important. Methotrexate may be administered—at a dose of 50 mg/m²—if the levels fail to decrease as expected.

Resection and end-to-end anastomosis

Tubal segmental resection and end-to-end anastomosis can be performed, if the pregnancy is in the isthmic region or if the bleeding is heavy with the ruptured tube and where tube has to be preserved.

> **Anti-D immunoglobulin**
> Anti-D immunoglobulin at a dose of 250 IU (50 micrograms) should be given to all non-sensitised women who are rhesus-negative and have an ectopic pregnancy.

PREGNANCY IN A RUDIMENTARY UTERINE HORN

During development, the uterus develops as two horns and fuses. In some conditions, there may be only one well-developed horn, with the other horn being rudimentary. This rudimentary horn may or may not communicate with the well-developed uterine horn. Occasionally, the fertilised ovum migrates into this sac, develops there and causes the same difficulties as tubal gestation.

The development of the ovum in the rudimentary horn is associated with the formation of a **false decidua** in the uterine cavity proper. In such cases, the uterus increases in size. As the muscular tissue of the horn is poorly developed and cannot keep pace with the progressively enlarging ovum, a rupture occurs.

This may occur at any time within the first 16 weeks of pregnancy. At times, however, the pregnancy may progress further.

Diagnosis

It is difficult to diagnose this condition with any degree of certainty. When a pulsating mass corresponding in size to the duration of pregnancy is detected alongside the slightly enlarged uterus, the possibility of a pregnancy in a rudimentary horn is suspected. Before the operation, it is almost impossible to differentiate this condition from the more common tubal gestation.

> The round ligament is lateral to the gestational sac when the pregnancy is in a rudimentary horn, whereas in a tubal gestation, it is on the medial side.

Treatment

The only option is to remove the pregnant horn of the uterus, conserving the main body of the uterus, if possible.

ABDOMINAL PREGNANCY

Primary implantation of the fertilised ovum on the peritoneum is extremely rare. Almost all cases are, therefore, secondary to early rupture of a tubal pregnancy into the peritoneal cavity. After penetrating the tubal wall, the ovum maintains its tubal attachment, but gradually encroaches upon and gets implanted in the neighbouring serosa. Meanwhile, the fetus continues to grow in the peritoneal cavity. In some cases, after tubal rupture, the conceptus reimplants itself elsewhere in the peritoneal cavity. Rarely, abdominal pregnancy may result from the silent dehiscence of a classical cesarean scar.

> **Primary abdominal pregnancy** is diagnosed by **Studdiford's criteria**, which are as follows:
> * Presence of normal tubes and ovaries with no evidence of recent or past pregnancy
> * No evidence of uteroplacental fistula
> * The presence of a pregnancy related exclusively to the peritoneal surface and early enough to eliminate the possibility of secondary implantation after primary tubal nidation

Clinical Features

Signs and symptoms

Since early rupture of a tubal pregnancy is the usual cause, a history suggestive of tubal pregnancy can be obtained in retrospect. Nausea, vomiting, flatulence, constipation, diarrhea and abdominal pain may be present in varying degrees. Late in pregnancy, fetal movements can be felt with great ease, and these movements cause pain in the patient. Braxton Hicks contractions are absent.

On pelvic examination, the cervix is usually displaced; depending partly on the position of the fetus, the presenting part is unusually high. Fetal heart sounds, if present, appear to be quite superficial.

USG diagnosis

No clear uterine shadow is seen around the gestational sac. The uterus may be seen as a separate mass in relation to the gestational sac. There is an absence of myometrial tissue between the bladder and the pregnancy.

X-ray examination

X-ray evaluation often reveals the fetus in a transverse or oblique lie and in an unusual attitude and location. A lateral view shows fetal parts overlying the maternal vertebra.

Treatment

Surgery is the only treatment for an abdominal pregnancy.

Principles of surgical management

The following principles of surgical management must be followed:
* Before submitting the patient to surgery, it is essential to have adequate **blood cross-matched** and made available.
* The massive **hemorrhage** that often occurs with surgery for abdominal pregnancy is related to the lack of constriction of hypertrophied, opened blood vessels after placental separation.
* At laparotomy, care should be taken in the **management of the placenta**. Since its removal is always associated with severe hemorrhage, it should not be attempted unless it is possible to ligate all the blood vessels supplying the placenta. In those rare instances where the placenta can be easily removed without provoking hemorrhage, it may be removed.
* **The best policy is to avoid unnecessary exploration, remove the fetus, tie the cord close to the placenta and close the abdomen.** In the majority of cases, the placenta may get absorbed. However, these patients need good antibiotic cover and methotrexate. Uterine artery embolisation has also been attempted.

Maternal morbidity and mortality are increased in abdominal pregnancy.

Fetal salvage in an abdominal pregnancy is exceedingly precarious, and the great majority of fetuses die even prior to removal or in the neonatal period. The incidence of congenital malformations is also higher in these pregnancies.

OVARIAN PREGNANCY

Primary ovarian pregnancy (Fig. 20.9) is one of the rarest types of extrauterine pregnancy. It constitutes 3% of all ectopics, with an incidence of 1 in 25,000–40,000 of all pregnancies. Here, the fertilisation occurs in the Graafian follicle and the fertilised ovum gets implanted directly into the ovarian tissue. Except in few cases, the final diagnosis is made at laparotomy and final confirmation is by histopathology.

Spiegelberg criteria for the diagnosis of ovarian pregnancy

- The fallopian tube on the affected side must be intact.
- The gestational sac must occupy the position of the ovary, and there should be no separate ovary on the affected side.
- The gestational sac must be connected to the uterus by the ovarian ligament.
- A histological examination must reveal the presence of definite ovarian tissue in the wall of the gestational sac.

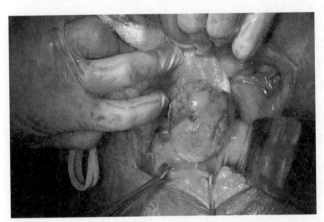

Fig. 20.9 Ovarian pregnancy with normal fallopian tube

CERVICAL PREGNANCY

Important Facts Regarding Cervical Pregnancy

Cervical pregnancy was a rare event in the past; however, since the advent of assisted reproductive techniques, its incidence is increasing. The following are features of a cervical pregnancy:

- The endocervix is eroded by the trophoblast.
- The duration of pregnancy depends on the site of implantation.
- The higher the implantation, the greater is the capacity to grow.
- Painless vaginal bleeding occurs, and at times, there is massive hemorrhage.
- Diagnosis is made on ultrasound examination—the uterus is empty and a gestational sac is seen in the cervical canal.
- Treatment is usually surgical. However, medical treatment with methotrexate or the injection of potassium chloride in the gestational sac has been attempted.

Diagnosis is by Rubin's criteria

- The uterus is smaller than the distended cervix.
- The internal os is not dilated.
- The external os opens earlier than it does in spontaneous abortion.
- Curettage of the endometrial cavity is non-productive of placental tissue.

CESAREAN SCAR ECTOPIC PREGNANCY

Cesarean scar ectopic is one of the rarest of all ectopic pregnancies. Here, the blastocyst gets implanted in a microscopic or macroscopic tract on the uterine scar or in a niche or dehiscence left behind by a previous cesarean delivery. The incidence of cesarean scar ectopics is increasing due to a rise in number of cesarean deliveries.

USG Features

- Empty uterine cavity and closed, empty endocervical canal
- Chorionic/gestational sac and/or placenta located low in the anterior wall of the uterus, below the bladder, in close proximity and at the level of the internal os, at the site of the previous hysterotomy scar/niche, with or without fetal or embryonic pole and/or yolk sac and with or without heartbeats (depending on gestational age)
- Absent or thin myometrial layer between the chorionic/gestational sac and unusually close proximity to the bladder wall

The treatment options include medical, surgical and less invasive methods. The cesarean scar pregnancy can be managed medically using systemic or intragestational injection of methotrexate. Minimally invasive methods such as uterine artery embolisation have also been attempted. Surgical options include hysterectomy, excision and suction aspiration.

COMBINED EXTRAUTERINE AND INTRAUTERINE PREGNANCIES

A **tubal gestation** is sometimes associated **with an intrauterine pregnancy (heterotopic ectopic pregnancy).** This diagnosis should be considered after assisted reproductive techniques and can be confirmed by sonography when in doubt. After excision of the extrauterine pregnancy, in most instances, the intrauterine pregnancy continues to grow without many complications, provided a timely diagnosis is made.

KEY POINTS

✓ *Ectopic pregnancy is defined as the development of a fertilised ovum outside the uterine cavity or in an abnormal location within the uterine cavity.*

✓ *Around 95% of ectopic pregnancies occur in the fallopian tube.*

✓ *Risk factors such as pelvic inflammatory disease that cause tubal damage or dysfunction predispose to ectopic tubal pregnancy.*

✓ *A ruptured ectopic pregnancy presents as acute abdomen with classical features of amenorrhea, abdominal pain and shock. With the help of ultrasound and β-hCG estimations, it is possible to make a diagnosis.*

✓ *Early unruptured tubal pregnancies can be treated medically by careful selection of cases.*

✓ *Diagnosis of cervical ectopic pregnancy is made on ultrasound examination, when the uterus visualised as being empty and a gestational sac is seen in the cervical canal.*

✓ *Cesarean scar ectopic pregnancy is rare. Here, the blastocyst gets implanted in a tract on the uterine scar or dehiscence left behind by a previous cesarean delivery. USG features are an empty uterine cavity and closed, empty endocervical canal with a gestational sac located low in the anterior wall of the uterus.*

✓ *Simultaneous occurrence of intrauterine and extrauterine pregnancy is known as heterotopic pregnancy.*

Essay question

1. Describe the symptoms and signs of a ruptured tubal gestation and its management.

Short answer questions

1. What are the various sites of ectopic pregnancy?
2. What are the risk factors for ectopic pregnancy?
3. What criteria should be fulfilled for medical management of an ectopic pregnancy?

MCQs

1. Which is the commonest site of ectopic pregnancy?
   a) Fallopian tube
   b) Ovary
   c) Cervix
   d) Rudimentary horn
2. Which of the following is not a risk factor for ectopic pregnancy?
   a) Prior PID
   b) Previous sterilisation
   c) OCP
   d) IUCD
3. A tubal pregnancy that is expelled through the fimbria is called:
   a) Tubal abortion
   b) Tubal mole
   c) Decidual cast
   d) Rupture
4. Which of the following is not included in the classical triad of ectopic?
   a) Amenorrhea
   b) Mass abdomen
   c) Abdominal pain
   d) Vaginal bleeding
5. What is the name of the test that is done by aspirating collected blood from the pouch of Douglas?
   a) Chorionic villous sampling
   b) Amniocentesis
   c) Culdocentesis
   d) Biopsy

6. Which of these is not an indication for methotrexate?
   a) Patient hemodynamically unstable
   b) β-hCG <5,000 miu/mL
   c) Gestational sac <4 cm
   d) Absent FH
7. What percentage of decrease in β-hCG requires repeat dose of methotrexate?
   a) 10%
   b) 20%
   c) 30%
   d) 40%
8. Primary abdominal pregnancy is identified by which of the following criteria?
   a) Amsel criteria
   b) Studdiford criteria
   c) Spiegelberg criteria
   d) Rubin criteria

Answers
1. (a), 2. (c), 3. (a), 4. (b), 5. (c), 6. (a), 7. (a), 8. (b)

Fill in the blanks

1. Adequate response to methotrexate treatment in ectopic pregnancy is indicated by a decrease in β-hCG level between day 4 and day 7 of _____.
2. A normal intrauterine pregnancy along with an extrauterine pregnancy is known as a _____.

Answers
1. >15%, 2. heterotopic pregnancy

Case scenario-based discussion

1. A 32-year-old female with two previous LSCS and sterilisation done three years ago presents with abdominal pain. Her last menstrual period was two months ago. She has pallor, tachycardia and hypotension. She has no other comorbidities.
   a) What investigations would you perform?
   b) If the pregnancy test was positive with an adnexal mass and free fluid in the abdomen by USG, what would the diagnosis be?
   c) What would be your line of management?

Answers

a) A pregnancy test and USG abdomen and pelvis should be performed.

b) If the urine pregnancy test is positive and there is free fluid in the abdomen with an adnexal mass, it confirms the diagnosis of ectopic pregnancy.

c) The woman should be resuscitated and an emergency laparotomy, and a salpingectomy should be performed.

2. A 24-year-old gravida 2, para nil, previous 1 spontaneous miscarriage presents with five weeks of amenorrhea with throbbing pain in her right lower abdomen. On examination she is not pale, there is no tachycardia and abdominal palpation reveals deep tenderness.

   a) What investigations would you perform?
   b) Serum β-hCG is positive, and the scan shows an empty uterus with a complex mass in the adnexal region. There is no free fluid in the abdomen. What is your diagnosis?

c) How would you manage this patient?

d) What are the criteria for medical management?

Answers

a) Serum β-hCG and TVS of the pelvis should be performed.

b) The diagnosis is an unruptured ectopic pregnancy.

c) Conservative management by medical/surgical methods is recommended.

d) The criteria for medical management are as follows:
   i. Patient hemodynamically stable
   ii. β-hCG <5,000 miu/mL
   iii. Gestational sac <4 cm
   iv. Absent FH

21

Hydatidiform Mole (Vesicular Mole)

OG 4.3, OG 9.4, PA 30.5

Learning Objectives

» To discuss the spectrum of gestational trophoblastic disease and the types of hydatidiform moles

» To discuss the risk factors, genetics and pathological features of hydatidiform moles

» To discuss the clinical presentation, investigations, USG features and differential diagnosis of trophoblastic disease

» To discuss the management and follow-up of trophoblastic disease

» To discuss diagnosis and management of gestational trophoblastic neoplasia

INTRODUCTION

Vesicular moles or hydatidiform moles are grouped under gestational trophoblastic diseases (GTD) which are pathological conditions affecting the placenta caused by the abnormal differentiation and proliferation of the trophoblastic tissue. GTD includes a spectrum of disorders, ranging from benign non-neoplastic lesions to malignant conditions of the trophoblast. The benign conditions within the GTD spectrum are complete hydatidiform mole (CHM) and partial hydatidiform mole (PHM). Recently, placental site nodule (PSN) has been included in the GTD spectrum. The malignant conditions arising from the trophoblast are invasive mole, choriocarcinoma (CC) and placental site trophoblastic tumour (PSTT) (Table 21.1).

Table 21.1 Spectrum of gestational trophoblastic disease (GTD)

Benign conditions	Malignant conditions
Complete hydatidiform mole (CHM)	Invasive mole
Partial hydatidiform mole (PHM)	Choriocarcinoma (CC)
Placental site nodule (PSN)	Placental site trophoblastic tumour (PSTT)

DEFINITION OF HYDATIDIFORM MOLE

The hydatidiform mole is a benign condition with malignant potential. It can locally proliferate, invade into the myometrium and metastasise to distant organs. It occurs due to the **cystic degeneration of the chorionic villi**, which results in the death of the fetus and the conversion of chorionic villi into a large number of vesicles, varying in size from that of a pea to a large-sized grape. They resemble hydatid cysts, and hence the name, hydatidiform mole.

INCIDENCE

The incidence of hydatidiform moles varies across the world—in most parts of the world it is 1 per 1,000 pregnancies. Prevalence varies with race and ethnic groups; there is a high prevalence in Asian countries and studies have shown that women in most Asian countries have a two-fold increased risk than most white populations. Unpublished data from the Institute of Obstetrics and Gynaecology, Chennai, have shown the incidence of GTD to be 1 per 314 live births.

RISK FACTORS

Maternal Age

The occurrence of a molar pregnancy strongly correlates with maternal age and is more common in the extremes of age. Teenagers have a two-fold increased risk of having a molar pregnancy. The risk of complete moles also increases with advancing maternal age >35 years.

Paternal Age

Increasing paternal age may also be a risk factor for developing GTD, perhaps due to the defective gametogenesis at the extremes of reproductive life which predisposes to the androgenic conceptus, giving rise to complete moles.

Previous History of Hydatidiform Mole

It is well-recognised that a history of prior hydatidiform mole is associated with a near ten-fold increase in the risk of a subsequent mole. The risk of recurrence is

0.5–2% after one hydatidiform mole and 15–20% after two prior molar pregnancies.

TYPES OF HYDATIDIFORM MOLE

There are two types of hydatidiform moles, namely the complete and the incomplete (partial) moles. Although the histology and the morphology of these two types of tumours differ, their clinical features and management are similar.

- In a **complete hydatidiform mole**, there is diffuse trophoblastic proliferation. Fetal blood vessels are not seen in the villi and there is no evidence of the existence of a fetus.
- In a **partial mole**, there is focal trophoblastic proliferation with cystic degeneration mixed with areas of normal chorionic villi. A normal or abnormal fetus may be present.

PATHOGENESIS

Pathology and Genetics (Fig. 21.1)

In GTD, there is defective fertilisation, which results in an abnormal karyotype and consequently, abnormal proliferation of placental villi. Molar pregnancies are subdivided into complete (CM) and partial moles (PM) based on genetic and histopathological features (Table 21.2).

- **Complete moles:** Complete moles are diploid and androgenic in origin, with no evidence of fetal tissue. Genetically, a complete mole is totally paternal in origin and has no maternal DNA. Complete moles are usually homozygous XX and less commonly, heterozygous XY (5–10% of cases).
  - In a homozygous complete mole, an empty ovum is fertilised by a haploid sperm, which then duplicates its own chromosomes after meiosis, resulting in the 46 XX chromosomal pattern.
  - Occasionally, a heterozygous complete mole occurs when two spermatozoa, each with 23 X and 23 Y components, fertilise an empty ovum.
- **Partial mole:** The fertilised egg contains the normal set of maternal DNA but double the number of paternal DNA. As a result, the embryo only develops partially and does not become a viable fetus. Partial moles are usually (90%) triploid in origin, with two sets of paternal haploid genes and one set of maternal haploid genes, producing the 69 XXY pattern. In a partial mole, there is usually evidence of a fetus or fetal red blood cells.

Moles are considered a premalignant condition. Around 2% of partial and 15% of complete moles develop into persistent trophoblastic disease or choriocarcinoma and hence it is important to differentiate between the two.

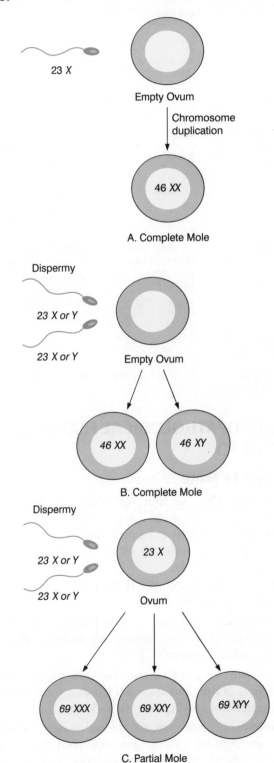

Fig. 21.1 Genetic basis of trophoblastic disease

Table 21.2 Differences between complete and partial moles

Features	Complete mole	Partial mole
Karyotyping	46 XX and occasionally, 46 XY pattern is seen All chromosomes are paternally derived	Triploid with 69 chromosomes Two paternal sets and one maternal complement is seen
Origin	Only paternal origin	Paternal plus maternal origin
Embryo/fetus/amnion/fetal red blood cells	Absent	Fetal or embryonic tissues are usually identified Fetal blood vessels and RBCs are present
Histopathological examination	Diffuse hydropic swelling of the chorionic villi with diffuse trophoblastic proliferation	Focal lesions with varying sized chorionic villi with focal hydropic changes as well as trophoblastic hyperplasia
Malignant propensity	15%	2%
Metastasis	Metastasis common	Non-metastatic

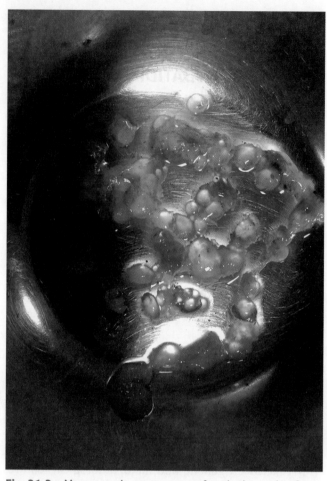

Fig. 21.2 Macroscopic appearance of vesicular mole after evacuation

HISTOPATHOLOGICAL FEATURES OF GTD

Complete Mole

Macroscopically, vesicles of different sizes are formed, giving the mole a typical 'bunch of grapes' appearance. The cyst is formed due to the failure of villus circulation, resulting in villus edema and fluid collection (Fig. 21.2).

Microscopically, a complete mole is characterised by the following features:

- Generalised diffuse hyperplasia of both cytotrophoblast and syncytiotrophoblast and an intact villous pattern (Fig. 21.3)
- Generalised edema of the chorionic villi (hydropic swelling of the villus stroma) including the formation of vesicles of varying sizes (0.1–3 cm)
- Absence of fetal stromal blood vessels, absence of an embryo (which gets absorbed before the development of the cardiovascular system), and absence of nucleated fetal erythrocytes in the villous capillaries

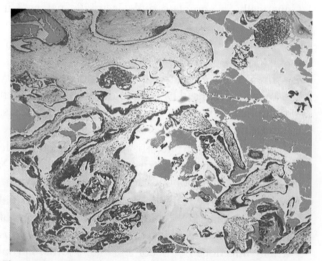

Fig. 21.3 Microscopic view of complete hydatidiform mole—the chorionic villi are enlarged and edematous with circumferential trophoblastic proliferation (H&E-stained; 10X magnification) (*Image courtesy*: Dr M P Kanchana, Professor of Pathology, Institute of Obstetrics and Gynecology and Madras Medical College)

Partial Mole

A partial mole is characterised by the following features:

- Focal hydropic villi changes and focal and minimal trophoblastic hyperplasia; because of the focal trophoblastic proliferation and hydropic change in partial hydatidiform moles, malignant sequelae are fewer than those associated with complete moles
- Frequently, there is macroscopic or microscopic evidence of a fetus; fetal vessels are often identified and usually contain nucleated fetal erythrocytes
- The embryo survives much longer than it does in complete moles; embryonic deaths typically occur at or before approximately eight weeks of gestational age

Theca Lutein Cysts

The ovaries contain multiple **theca lutein cysts,** which result from overstimulation of lutein elements by large amounts of chorionic gonadotropin.

CLINICAL MANIFESTATIONS OF HYDATIDIFORM MOLES

- **Bleeding following a period of amenorrhea** is the most common clinical presentation and is seen in nearly 90% of cases. The woman presents with irregular vaginal bleeding following a period of amenorrhea. The amount of bleeding varies and may be interspersed with dark brown vaginal discharge called 'prune juice' discharge. There may be only spotting at times, lasting for weeks. In between, there may be serosanguineous discharge. Occasionally, the bleeding may be very heavy and life-threatening. Along with blood, the woman may pass vesicles. In nearly 10% of cases, the diagnosis is made by USG in early pregnancy even before the bleeding starts.
- All pregnancy symptoms are exaggerated in GTD, and the woman may look ill.
- **Hyperemesis gravidarum** occurs in approximately 25% of women due to the raised levels of β-hCG. It can lead to severe dehydration and electrolyte imbalance.
- **Pre-eclampsia** may manifest early when pregnancy progresses to the second trimester, as seen in 12–54% of cases. The development of **hypertension and albuminuria** prior to 20 weeks of gestation should alert the clinician as to the possibility of vesicular mole. Even eclampsia has been observed in molar pregnancy.

- **Severe anemia** may be present and may be disproportionately high for the amount of bleeding.
- Signs and symptoms of **hyperthyroidism** are seen in 10% of cases due to elevated chorionic thyrotrophin. In severe cases, the woman may present with thyroid storm, which manifests as the rapid enlargement of the thyroid, fine tremor, weight loss and supraventricular tachycardia.
- **Disseminated intravascular coagulation (DIVC)**—in long-standing cases of hydatidiform mole or during the evacuation of the uterus, there may be embolisation of the trophoblastic tissue into the general circulation, releasing thromboplastin, which triggers disseminated intravascular coagulation.
- **Manifestations due to metastatic disease** rarely include acute respiratory failure or neurological symptoms such as seizures. There may be hemoptysis from lung metastasis and neurologic manifestations from brain metastasis.

Examination

- On general examination, the woman usually looks ill and pale; goitre may be present. With hyperemesis, the woman may present with evidence of dehydration and other signs of metabolic derangement. There may be signs of thyrotoxicosis. There may be tachycardia with or without hypotension. Monitoring of vitals is important, as the patient may go into sudden acute respiratory failure or hemodynamic instability. The respiratory system should be thoroughly examined for evidence of metastasis.
- On abdominal examination, there may be abdominal distension in the presence of large theca lutein cysts. The uterus is large for the period of amenorrhea and boggy in consistency. The fetal parts are not palpable, nor can a fetal heart (FH) be heard. In a partial mole, the uterine size may not be large and one may be able to appreciate the FH rarely.
- Local and speculum examinations may reveal vaginal and suburethral nodules.
- On vaginal examination, the uterus is larger than the period of amenorrhea. There is no internal ballottement, and theca lutein cysts may be palpable.

DIFFERENTIAL DIAGNOSIS OF GESTATIONAL TROPHOBLASTIC DISEASE

- Since vesicular mole is one of the complications of early pregnancy, the other pregnancy-related conditions such as miscarriages and ectopic pregnancy should be ruled out.

- A patient with a partial hydatidiform mole usually presents with clinical and ultrasound features of a missed or threatened spontaneous abortion.

- Degenerating fibroids may be reported as hydatidiform mole by USG.

DIAGNOSIS

USG Examination

- In women who have already started expelling the vesicles, the diagnosis is easy.
  - The diagnosis of hydatidiform mole is made by USG when the patient presents with early pregnancy bleeding.
  - As most patients have an early USG nowadays, the diagnosis of hydatidiform mole is made even before the onset of symptoms such as bleeding, anemia and hyperemesis.

- The classic finding in a complete mole is the 'snowstorm' appearance; theca lutein ovarian cysts may or may not be present (Fig. 21.4). Though USG examination is helpful in making a pre-evacuation diagnosis, histological examination of the products of conception is required to make a definitive diagnosis.

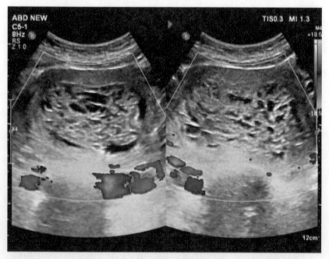

Fig. 21.4 USG picture showing complete hydatidiform mole—uterine cavity filled with multiple cystic spaces of varying sizes with intervening echogenic areas, giving it a characteristic 'snowstorm appearance'; there is internal and peripheral vascularity (*Image courtesy:* Dr B H Parameshwar Keerthi, Consultant Radiologist, BM Scans, Kancheepuram)

- Besides confirming the diagnosis of a hydatidiform mole, it is important to exclude the presence of a

fetus, which may indicate a partial mole, and to look for the presence and size of theca lutein cysts of the ovaries.

MANAGEMENT

- Despite the differences between partial and complete hydatidiform moles, the initial management and subsequent surveillance of patients with partial or complete molar gestations are similar.

- After the diagnosis has been confirmed, the evaluation of a patient with a molar gestation is directed towards screening for metastatic disease and stabilisation of the patient for evacuation.

Preoperative Evaluation

- Preoperative evaluation consists of a complete physical examination, baseline serum hCG level, chest roentgenogram to pick up pulmonary lesions, hematologic profile, renal and liver function tests, blood sugar, screening for pre-eclampsia, coagulation profile, electrolytes and thyroid function tests. CT and MRI are not required to confirm the diagnosis.

Preoperative investigations
- Baseline serum hCG level
- Complete hemogram
- Renal function test
- Liver function test
- Coagulation profile
- Electrolytes
- Thyroid function test
- Chest roentgenogram

The management of a hydatidiform mole involves two phases, which are as follows:

1. Immediate evacuation of the mole
2. Meticulous follow-up to identify and treat gestational trophoblastic neoplasia

Evacuation of the Uterus

- Before surgical evacuation, it is important to stabilise the patient, treat hypertension, correct anemia by blood transfusion and components and correct coagulation profile where and when necessary.

- Since complete molar pregnancies are not associated with fetal parts, suction evacuation is the method of choice for uterine evacuation even if the uterus is large. After the cervix is dilated, suction evacuation is performed with a No. 10 or No. 12 cannula.

- The use of oxytocic infusion prior to the completion of the evacuation is not recommended because uterine contractions before evacuation may promote the entry of trophoblastic tissue into the circulation. However, in order to control life-threatening bleeding or to control bleeding after evacuation, oxytocic infusions may be administered.
- The material obtained is sent for histopathological examination.

Anti-D Immunoprophylaxis

All rhesus D-negative women should be given prophylactic anti-D rhesus immunoglobulin to counter the expression of the rhesus D factor on trophoblasts.

Follow-Up After Evacuation of Molar Pregnancy

Follow-up is very important as there is a 20% incidence of persistent trophoblastic disease after evacuation and 10% chance of a persistent lesion developing into choriocarcinoma.

FIGO recommendations for the follow-up of molar pregnancy

- Surveillance (Fig. 21.5) using serial, highly sensitive and accurate quantitative serum hCG levels is the only reliable means for the early detection of malignant sequelae after the evacuation of a hydatidiform mole.
- At every visit, symptoms such as irregular bleeding, persistent cough, dyspnea and hemoptysis should be enquired about.
- Pelvic examinations should be repeated every two weeks to identify the subinvolution of the uterus and persistent theca lutein cysts.
- Chest roentgenograms should be carried out in the presence of respiratory symptoms to detect pulmonary metastasis.

Monitoring of serum β-hCG levels

- After 48 hours of evacuation, serum β-hCG levels are obtained.
- Thereafter, the test is repeated every week until the levels are normal. After three consecutive normal values are obtained, serum β-hCG levels are measured monthly for six months.
- Normal levels are usually reached within 8–12 weeks after evacuation. As long as the levels are decreasing, there is no need for any intervention.

- If the levels plateau or rise, the patient is considered to have gestational trophoblastic neoplasia and is managed as described later on in this chapter.
- If there is persistent bleeding or if the β-hCG levels are increasing and the USG showing a lesion, then there is a need for curettage and histopathological confirmation of the diagnosis.
- The routine 'basal curettage' is not advocated anymore.

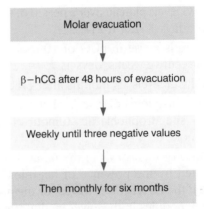

Fig. 21.5 Surveillance following the evacuation of a molar pregnancy

The purpose of meticulous follow-up is to identify persistent trophoblastic disease early and to provide appropriate management for GTN.

CONTRACEPTION FOLLOWING MOLAR PREGNANCY

- In order to avoid confusion caused by an elevated hCG level associated with an intercurrent pregnancy, the woman should be prescribed contraception following the evacuation of a vesicular mole.
- Oral contraceptives with low estrogen content are the most effective means of reversible contraception. They are started immediately post-evacuation and should be used at least for a year for complete moles to enable adequate follow-up.
- Intrauterine devices (IUDs) should not be used for contraception as they may result in the perforation of the uterus. Moreover, occasionally, there may be irregular bleeding, which can cause confusion.
- The barrier method of contraception may be used until β-hCG levels are normal. However, as the failure rate with barrier method is high, there are chances of pregnancy.

GESTATIONAL TROPHOBLASTIC NEOPLASIA (GTN)

GTN can develop following the evacuation of a molar pregnancy or it can develop after a non-molar pregnancy, abortion, ectopic pregnancy or live birth. Approximately half to two-thirds of cases of GTN follow molar pregnancies.

Criteria for Diagnosis of Postmolar GTN

- When hCG levels plateau over a period of three weeks or longer; days 1, 7, 14, 21
- When there is a rise in hCG of 10% or greater for three consecutive weeks; days 1, 7, 14, 21
- Elevated hCG levels six months after evacuation
- If there is a histologic diagnosis of choriocarcinoma, placental site trophoblastic tumour (PSTT) or invasive mole
- Appearance of metastasis in the brain, liver or lung as indicated by the presence of neurological signs, jaundice if the GI tract is involved, or the presence of blue-black nodules in the lower genital tract

GTN after Non-molar Pregnancy

Only around 50% of GTN follows molar pregnancy; the rest can occur after a spontaneous abortion, ectopic pregnancy, or a term pregnancy. Irregular vaginal bleeding is the most common presenting symptom of GTN diagnosed after miscarriage, therapeutic termination of pregnancy or postpartum. Amenorrhea may also be observed. Most often, women present with non-gynecologic signs and symptoms, including gastrointestinal or urologic hemorrhage, hemoptysis or cerebral hemorrhage. In order to diagnose non-molar GTN, one should have a high index of suspicion. hCG levels should be checked.

The spectrum of gestational trophoblastic neoplasia includes the following:
- Invasive hydatidiform mole
- Choriocarcinoma
- Placental site trophoblastic tumours
  All of the above are malignant conditions.

Invasive Hydatidiform Mole

An invasive mole is characterised by pathologic features of a complete hydatidiform mole and in addition, invasion from the normal placental site directly into the myometrium. There is often invasion into the venous system. Metastasis to the lower genital tract and to the lungs can occur. Invasion through the entire thickness

of the myometrium can lead to the rupture of the uterus, leading to massive intraperitoneal hemorrhage. Microscopically, the villi pattern is maintained.

Choriocarcinoma

Macroscopically, the tumour is bulky with hemorrhagic and necrotic areas. Apart from the uterus, it can be found in the tubes, ovaries, lung, liver, spleen, kidneys, bowel or brain. Microscopically, choriocarcinoma is characterised by the presence of cytotrophoblast and syncytiotrophoblast elements showing varying amounts of pleomorphism and anaplasia with areas of hemorrhage and necrosis. Typically, the chorionic villi are absent even at the primary uterine sites of disease (Fig. 21.6).

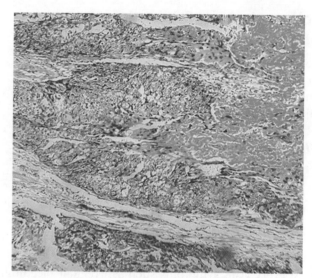

Fig. 21.6 HPE of choriocarcinoma with closely placed neoplastic syncytiotrophoblasts and cytotrophoblasts without the formation of villi (H&E 10X) (*Image courtesy:* Dr M P Kanchana, Professor of Pathology, Institute of Obstetrics and Gynecology and Madras Medical College)

Placental Site Trophoblastic Tumours

Placental site trophoblastic tumours should be considered to be locally invasive with a low malignant potential because a minority of patients will develop extrauterine metastasis.

Investigations

Once the diagnosis of GTN is established, a complete metastatic work-up is done to assign a prognostic score to the patient, which helps in choosing the treatment modality. This consists of the following:

- Detailed history and physical examination
- Pelvic examination (labial, vaginal, suburethral nodules)

- Complete blood count/liver and renal function test/coagulation studies
- Immediate pre-treatment serum β-hCG values
- Sonography—pelvis and abdomen (size of the uterus, size of the tumour, abdominal organ metastasis)
- Chest X-ray for typical 'cannonball' appearance and number of lung metastasis
- CT chest may be required to pick up small lesions
- CT/MRI—abdomen and brain metastasis
- CSF analysis (in suspected brain metastasis, the ratio of serum β–hCG values to the concentration of β–hCG in cerebrospinal fluid [normal ≥ 60:1])

Management of GTN

The prognosis of a patient with GTN can be calculated by using the FIGO/WHO prognostic score (Table 21.3) in combination with an anatomical staging system (Table 21.4).

Table 21.3 Modified WHO Prognostic Scoring System (2002)

Scores	0	1	2	4
Age	<40	>40	-	-
Antecedent pregnancy	Mole	Abortion	Term	-
Interval months from index pregnancy	<4	4–6	7–12	>12
Pre-treatment serum hCG IU/L	<10^3	10^3–10^4	10^4–10^5	≥10^5
Largest tumour size (including uterus)	-	3 cm	3–4 cm	>5 cm
Site of metastases	Lung	Spleen, kidney	Gastrointestinal	Liver, brain
Number of metastases	-	1–4	5–8	>8
Previous failed chemotherapy	-	-	Single drug	Two or more drugs

Table 21.4 FIGO anatomic staging

Stage	Description
Stage I	Disease confined to the uterus
Stage II	GTN extends outside the uterus but is limited to the genital structures (adnexa, vagina and broad ligament)
Stage III	GTN extends to the lungs, with or without known genital tract involvement
Stage IV	All other metastatic sites

The scoring system predicts the possibility of developing a single-drug chemotherapy resistance and identifies those who will require intensive therapy. A score less than 6 indicates a low risk and a score ≥7 suggests a high risk for primary resistance to monochemotherapy.

Women with GTN may be treated either with single-agent or multi-agent chemotherapy for GTN based on the FIGO 2002 scoring system.

Treatment of low-risk disease

- Patients having less than 6 points based on the FIGO scoring system fall in the low-risk group. In this group, a nearly 100% cure rate is achieved by single-agent systemic chemotherapy.
- Various single-agent chemotherapy regimens are available to treat low-risk GTN. Of all approved agents, methotrexate (MTX) is the most commonly used drug with a good therapeutic index. Single-agent intramuscular methotrexate is alternated with folinic acid for a week, followed by six rest days (Table 21.5). The 'folinic acid rescue' is crucial to prevent negative side effects of MTX such as mouth ulcers, sore eyes and pleuritis, which occur due to the inhibition of folate metabolism by MTX.
- Another agent used in single-agent chemotherapy for low-risk disease is actinomycin D, an antitumour antibiotic. Actinomycin D is approved for patients resistant to MTX treatment or in cases where toxicity precludes the use of MTX. If actinomycin D is used, it is given in a dose of 0.5 mg intravenously for five days every two weeks.

Table 21.5 MTX regimen in the treatment of low-risk GTN

Agent	Regimen	Frequency
Methotrexate (MTX)	50 mg IM (day 1, 3, 5, 7)/ (1 mg/Kg)	biweekly repeated
Folinic acid	15 mg p.o. (30 hours after each MTX injection)	biweekly repeated

- After the hCG level has returned to normal, consolidation with 2–3 more cycles of chemotherapy decreases the chance of recurrence.

Management of high-risk gestational trophoblastic neoplasia (Table 21.6)

- Patients with a FIGO score greater than 6 points have a high risk of developing resistance to single-agent systemic chemotherapy. Therefore, a polychemotherapy regimen with etoposide,

MTX and actinomycin D alternated with cyclophosphamide plus vincristine (EMA-CO) is used as the first line of therapy for patients with high-risk disease.

- These patients require specialised care by medical oncologists.
- The treatment is repeated every two weeks.

Table 21.6   Treatment regimen for high-risk GTN patients

Day	Drug	Dose
1	Etoposide	100 mg/m² (infused over 30 minutes)
	Actinomycin D	0.5 mg IV bolus
	Methotrexate	100 mg/m² IV bolus
		200 mg/m² (infused over 12 hours)
2	Etoposide	100 mg/m² (infused over 30 minutes)
	Actinomycin D	0.5 mg IV bolus
	Folinic acid	15 mg IM every 12 hours for four doses beginning 24 hours after starting methotrexate
8	Cyclophosphamide	600 mg/m² IV infusion
	Vincristine	1 mg/m² bolus

Fig. 21.7 presents an algorithm of the optimum treatment of GTN (RCOG Guideline No: 38, 2010).

Follow-Up of Patients With GTN

Patients should be kept in long-term follow-up. Careful surveillance with serum β-hCG is crucial. Most relapses occur within a year of the completion of the first chemotherapy. USG and other imaging modalities would be required periodically.

- **Low-risk patients:** Serum β–hCG weekly until three negative values are obtained, and one cycle of chemotherapy is given after the last normal value; thereafter, β–hCG testing is repeated monthly for a year
- **High-risk patients:** Serum β–hCG weekly until three negative values are obtained, and two to three cycles of chemotherapy are given after the last normal value; thereafter, β–hCG levels are checked monthly for two to five years followed by yearly β–hCG lifelong

A subsequent pregnancy can be planned one year after completing the chemotherapy. Women who received chemotherapeutic treatment are fertile in up to 80% of cases without an increased rate of infants with congenital anomalies. In the meantime, effective contraception should be used. Low-dose oral contraceptives can be safely used.

> Choriocarcinoma can be treated and cured by chemotherapy. This is one of the malignancies where treatment and follow-up reduces mortality. Pregnancies have been reported after the treatment of choriocarcinoma.

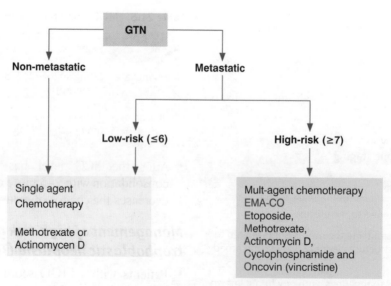

Fig. 21.7   Flowchart showing the optimum treatment of GTN (Adapted from RCOG Guideline NO. 38, 2010)

KEY POINTS

✓ *Hydatidiform mole is a benign neoplasm of the chorion with malignant potential.*

✓ *The most common presentation of a molar pregnancy is vaginal discharge, bleeding or passage of vesicles after a period of amenorrhea.*

✓ *Diagnosis is based on ultrasound findings and β-hCG levels.*

✓ *Follow-up is mandatory to diagnose GTN early.*

✓ *GTN is staged according to the FIGO classification; the WHO's scoring system helps in choosing the appropriate chemotherapy.*

Essay questions

1. Discuss the diagnosis and management of molar pregnancy. What is the importance of post-evacuation follow-up? How is it done?

2. A 27-year-old G2P1 presents with a history of two months of amenorrhea and bleeding per vaginum. She has vague discomfort in the lower abdomen and is hemodynamically stable.
   a) What differential diagnosis would you consider in this woman and what investigations would you order?
   b) What are the clinical features of molar pregnancy?
   c) How do you manage a case of hydatidiform mole?
   d) What is the surveillance required in this woman following the evacuation and why?

Short answer questions

1. List the clinical features of molar pregnancy.
2. Describe the management of molar pregnancy.
3. Detail the follow-up of a patient after the evacuation of a molar pregnancy.
4. Discuss the modified WHO prognostic scoring system.
5. What is the chemotherapy regimen for low-risk non-metastatic GTN?

MCQs

1. What is the recurrence rate of hydatidiform moles?
   a) 1–2%
   b) 2–3%
   c) 3–5%
   d) 5–10%

2. Which of these conditions is not associated with hydatidiform moles?
   a) Hyperemesis gravidarum
   b) Gestational diabetes
   c) Hyperthyroidism
   d) Pre-eclampsia

3. 'Snowstorm' appearance on ultrasound is suggestive of which of the following?
   a) Ectopic pregnancy
   b) Threatened abortion
   c) Hydatidiform mole
   d) Placenta previa

4. Which of the following is characteristic of lung metastasis in gestational trophoblastic neoplasia?
   a) 'Snowstorm' appearance
   b) 'Ring of fire' appearance
   c) 'Cannonball' appearance
   d) Decidual ring

5. Which of these doesn't include malignant gestational trophoblastic neoplasia?
   a) Hydatidiform mole
   b) Invasive mole
   c) Choriocarcinoma
   d) Placental site trophoblastic tumour

6. Which of these are not included in the modified WHO prognostic scoring system for GTN?
   a) Age
   b) hCG
   c) Tumour size
   d) CA 125

7. Which of the following is the recommended management for a patient scoring 10 on the WHO scoring system?
   a) Expectant management
   b) Methotrexate
   c) MAC regimen
   d) EMA-CO regimen

8. When GTN extends to the lungs, what is the stage of the disease?
   a) Stage 1
   b) Stage 2
   c) Stage 3
   d) Stage 4

Answers
1. (a), 2. (b), 3. (c), 4. (c), 5. (a), 6. (d), 7. (d), 8. (b)

Fill in the blanks

1. Hydatidiform mole is a _____ neoplasm of the chorion.

2. Genetically, a complete mole is totally _____ in origin.

Answers
1. benign, 2. paternal

Case scenario-based discussion

1. A 25-year-old primigravida with a diagnosis of molar pregnancy is referred for termination. On admission, the patient is hemodynamically stable with a β-hCG of 10,000 IU/L.
   a) What mode of treatment would you choose for this patient?
   b) How would you follow-up the patient?
   c) What are the criteria to diagnose GTN?
   d) How do you treat GTN?

Answers
a) Termination by suction evacuation is the treatment of choice.
b) Follow-up is by serial β-hCG measurements every week until three consecutive negative results are obtained, then monthly for six months.
c) The criteria are β-hCG levels plateauing or increasing or not coming back to normal in six months or evidence of metastasis.
d) The treatment of GTN is based on the FIGO 2002 scoring system. If the score is <6, single-agent chemotherapy with either methotrexate or actinomycin is given; if the score is >7, the EMA-CO regimen with multiple drugs is given.

22 Antepartum Hemorrhage— Abruptio Placentae

OG 10.1

Learning Objectives

» To know the causes of antepartum hemorrhage
» To describe the etiology, pathology and causes of abruptio placenta
» To discuss the clinical features, diagnosis and differential diagnosis of abruption
» To know the maternal and perinatal complications associated with abruptio placenta
» To discuss the management of abruptio placenta

■ INTRODUCTION

Antepartum hemorrhage is defined as bleeding from the genital tract occurring after 24 weeks of gestation (after the period of viability and prior to the birth of the baby).

■ CAUSES OF BLEEDING IN THE ANTEPARTUM PERIOD

A pregnant woman may bleed due to causes associated with pregnancy (antepartum hemorrhage) or occasionally, due to coincidental factors unrelated to pregnancy.

Causes of Antepartum Hemorrhage (Table 22.1)

- Premature separation of the normally situated placenta or abruptio placentae
- Placenta previa—bleeding from the placenta implanted in the lower segment
- Circumvallate placenta
- Rupture of the marginal sinus of the placenta
- Vasa previa—hemorrhage from the fetal blood vessels due to velamentous insertion of the umbilical cord
- Unclassified or indeterminate—if no cause for bleeding can be identified and all the above causes are excluded

Coincidental or Local Factors

These include local factors such as a benign cervical polyp, cervical erosion, or rarely, carcinoma cervix.

Table 22.1 Causes of bleeding in the antepartum period

Pregnancy-related factors (antepartum hemorrhage)	Coincidental or local factors
• Placenta previa • Abruptio placentae • Unclassified or indeterminate causes • Circumvallate placenta • Rupture of the marginal sinus of the placenta • Vasa previa	• Cervical polyp • Bleeding cervical erosion • Carcinoma cervix (rare)

A pregnancy in which bleeding occurs remains at an increased risk of poor outcomes even if the bleeding stops and no cause is identified. Therefore, pregnancy should be terminated in any woman at term with unexplained bleeding.

■ ABRUPTIO PLACENTAE

Definition

The term **accidental hemorrhage** or abruptio placenta refers to a condition in which hemorrhage occurs as a result of premature separation of a normally situated placenta after 24 weeks of gestation but before the delivery of the fetus. Incidence varies from place to place and occurs in approximately one per cent of pregnancies. The Institute of Obstetrics and Gynaecology, Chennai, has reported an incidence of 0.71% for the period from 2001–2010.

Etiology

A number of risk factors and pathogenic mechanisms have been implicated as possible causes of abruptio placenta. The causes of abruption may be attributed to defective placentation or sudden uterine decompression.

Age and parity

The condition is more common with increasing age and parity. This has been attributed to defective placentation.

Race

Abruptio placenta is reported more commonly among African-American and Caucasian women.

Maternal smoking and substance abuse

Cigarette smoking is an important etiological factor for abruptio placenta. A two-fold increased risk for abruption has been reported in smokers. Smoking has a vasoconstrictive effect on the uteroplacental circulation, leading to necrosis of the decidua basalis and associated large placental infarcts. A sudden release of spasms with surging of blood results in arteriolar rupture. Substance abuse, especially with cocaine, has been shown to be associated with an increased risk of abruption.

Maternal hypertension

Maternal hypertension due to pre-eclampsia, gestational hypertension or chronic hypertension is associated with a three- to five-fold increase in the risk of abruption.

Sudden uterine decompression

- In pregnancies complicated by hydramnios, the rupture of the membranes could result in the sudden decompression of the uterus, resulting in the shearing of the placenta from the uterine attachment.
- At the time of spontaneous or artificial rupture of membranes, there could be sudden uterine decompression leading to abruption.
- A three-fold increase in the incidence of abruption has also been reported in women with preterm premature rupture of membranes, which is managed conservatively.
- In women with multiple pregnancy, after the delivery of the first baby, abruption can occur due to uterine decompression.

Defective placentation

Defective placentation can occur due to endothelial dysfunction caused by various conditions such as:

- Folate deficiency resulting in hyperhomocysteinemia
- Unexplained elevation of alpha-fetoprotein (above two multiples of median) in the second trimester indicating a compromised placenta

- Inherited or acquired thrombophilia
- First-trimester bleeding

Uterine fibroids complicating pregnancy

If the fibroids are located behind the placental implantation site, they can predispose to abruption.

External trauma

Motor accidents with or without the use of a seat belt, a fall from a height and blunt trauma can result in abruption.

Iatrogenic causes

Procedures such as external cephalic version and cordocentesis can induce the separation of the placenta from its attachment.

Recurrent abruption

Recurrent abruption is seen in 4.4% of women; there is a 20–25% risk of recurrence in a woman who has had two previous abruptions. Antenatal fetal surveillance tests are not predictive of recurrent abruption in those who have a past history of abruption.

Others

A short umbilical cord is occasionally responsible for abruption.

Pathology and Mechanism

Placental separation or abruption begins with uterine vasospasm, which is followed by relaxation and subsequent venous engorgement and arteriolar rupture into the decidua. The blood escaping under the decidua basalis can follow one of four courses:

- The blood can dissect under the membranes where a large volume of blood may be concealed
- It can break through the membranes into the amniotic cavity
- It can dissect under the placenta, separating it from the maternal surface
- It can infiltrate into the myometrium, causing the uterus to contract and take on a purple colour (Couvelaire uterus); the uterine contractions may be localised or diffuse and tetanic

Effect of Abruption

- Because of abruption, fetal hypoxia, acidosis and death can occur due to compromised uteroplacental circulation, non-relaxation of the uterus or the increase in intra-amniotic pressure secondary to tetanic contraction.

- The woman develops hemorrhagic shock.
- Since the decidua is rich in thromboplastin, it releases thromboplastin into the maternal circulation, triggering **disseminated intravascular coagulation** (DIVC).

Types of Abruptio Placentae

Concealed variety

In this type, blood is retained within the uterine cavity and is not visible externally (Fig. 22.1a). The concealed type is likely to occur when blood collects behind the placenta as a retroplacental clot but the placental margins remain adherent. The placenta is almost completely separated, but the membranes retain their attachment to the uterine wall; alternatively, blood enters the amniotic cavity but is unable to get past the fetal head, which is closely applied to the lower uterine segment.

Revealed variety

This type of bleeding is seen in nearly 80% of cases. In this condition, the blood collected due to placental separation escapes by dissecting under the membranes and is seen externally (Fig. 22.1b). Bloodstained liquor is a frequent finding in abruptio placenta when the membrane ruptures.

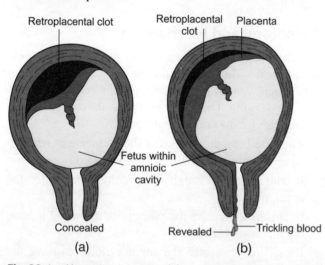

Fig. 22.1 Abruptio placentae: (a) concealed and (b) revealed

Mixed type

This is the most common type. Bloodstained liquor reveals abruption but there is still concealed bleeding within the uterine cavity.

Clinical Features

Clinical features vary according to the degree of separation and the type and amount of bleeding.

Symptoms

- Symptoms may appear either before or after the onset of labour.
- Abdominal pain and bleeding per vaginum are the most common symptoms with which the woman presents.
- The majority of women are asymptomatic until they experience sudden-onset abdominal pain, vaginal bleeding or both. A woman with severe abruption presents with vaginal bleeding, a tonically contracted uterus, uterine tenderness and fetal distress or absent fetal heart tones. Even if bleeding is minimal, the woman may present with shock, rapid and weak pulse, hypotension and cold, moist skin. In some cases, bleeding may not be revealed. Hence, the mere absence of bleeding does not rule out abruption.
- **Vaginal bleeding** is the most common symptom. However, there is little correlation between the amount of visible bleeding and the degree of placental separation. The amount of visible bleeding may be minimal even when the fetus is dead or when the woman is in shock.
- **Abdominal pain** is the second most common symptom. It may occur due to the disruption of the myometrial fibres and intravasation of blood from the site of abruption.
- There may be a history of fainting attacks and blackouts.

Signs

- Vaginal bleeding is noted in the revealed and mixed varieties, but the amount of bleeding noted may not correlate with the severity of the condition. The blood is dark red and may even come in 'spurts' corresponding to uterine contractions.
- Bleeding results in tachycardia, hypotension and alterations in the level of consciousness.

Physical examination

- Uterine height is usually greater than the period of amenorrhea, especially in the concealed variety.
- There is uterine tenderness and difficulty in palpating fetal parts in the concealed variety.
- Uterine contractions may be present.
- Uterine hypertonus and non-relaxing uterus may be present.
- The fetal heart may be normal, abnormal or absent.
- There could be features of pregnancy-induced hypertension (PIH)/pre-eclampsia/eclampsia.
- In severe abruption, the woman may present with shock and DIVC.

- Intense systemic vasospasm may mask the hypovolemia in the woman, and her BP may be falsely elevated.

Grades of Abruption

Depending on the severity of clinical findings, abruption is graded as shown in Table 22.2.

Table 22.2 Grades of abruption

Grade	Features
Diagnosed after delivery/grade 0	In this, the diagnosis is not suspected clinically before delivery; the diagnosis is made after seeing a retroplacental clot.
Mild types/grade I	• Pain precedes external vaginal bleeding. • There are no signs of shock. • Mild uterine tenderness may be present. • On palpation, the uterus is of normal tone, and the fetal heart is usually unaffected. These women may go into labour spontaneously and deliver live babies. If they do not go into labour, the bleeding may stop or recur later. Examination of the placenta after delivery shows dark adherent clots, which on removal may reveal depressed areas over the placenta.
Moderate/grade II	• There is mild vaginal bleeding. • The uterus is tender. • There is no maternal shock. • Fetal distress is invariably present.
Severe/grade III	• Vaginal bleeding is moderate to severe. • The uterus is tender. • Maternal shock is present. • There is fetal distress or fetal death. • There are associated complications like renal failure and consumptive coagulopathy.

Investigations

- Complete blood count (CBC) as a baseline indicator for hemoglobin, hematocrit and platelet count
- Urine analysis, particularly if there is associated PIH
- Serum fibrinogen <100 mg is suggestive of severe abruption
- Coagulation profile—prothrombin time (PT), activated partial thromboplastin time (aPTT) and fibrinogen and fibrinogen degradation products to know the coagulation status
- Blood grouping and Rh typing, if the status was not known earlier
- Renal function tests are useful, especially in severe abruption

- USG is mainly useful to rule out placenta previa. The presence of a retroplacental clot confirms diagnosis but the absence of a clot does not rule out abruption. The retroplacental clot appears isoechoic or hyperechoic.

Diagnosis

The diagnosis of placental abruption is mainly clinical.

- Diagnosis is not difficult in the presence of the classical symptoms and signs of abruptio placentae, i.e., pain, bleeding and a tetanically contracted, tender uterus.
- If bleeding is the only symptom, it is important to rule out placenta previa.
- In abruption, retroplacental hematoma is visualised as an anechoic collection between the placenta and the uterine wall. Ultrasound has a sensitivity of 70% in diagnosing abruptio placentae. The following differential diagnosis has to be considered to differentiate it from other conditions.

Differential diagnosis

Placenta previa

In placenta previa, the bleeding is painless and stops spontaneously. However, it can recur at a later date. The uterus is soft and non-tender and the fetal parts are easily palpable. The degree of shock is proportional to the amount of bleeding seen outside. Fetal heart sounds are often present unless the hemorrhage is profuse. The presenting part is high, and malpresentation may be present. Ultrasound examination will confirm or exclude the diagnosis of placenta previa. Coagulopathy is rare with placenta previa.

Acute hydramnios

This is not a very common condition. In acute hydramnios, the sudden distension of the abdomen may give rise to pain and an increased pulse rate. There is no associated bleeding. The fetal parts may not be easily palpable and the fetal heart sounds may not be heard clearly. Again, an ultrasound examination will help in diagnosis.

Ruptured uterus

In women with a previous cesarean section scar and in those who have a risk of uterine rupture (transverse lie in labour, major cephalopelvic disproportion), the presentation may be abdominal pain and bleeding. In cases of complete rupture, fetal parts may be more easily palpable in contrast to abruptio placentae.

Other acute abdominal conditions

Sometimes, other acute abdominal emergencies may be confused with abruptio placentae. These include torsion of an ovarian cyst, degeneration of a uterine fibroid and acute appendicitis. A careful history and examination will confirm or exclude these conditions.

Management

Principles of management

Placental abruption needs active management with prompt diagnosis and early delivery. The longer the abruption delivery interval, the worse will be the maternal and fetal prognosis. Adequate blood transfusion should be given.

Main goals of treatment

- Restoration of effective circulation to prevent hemorrhagic shock and renal failure
- Early delivery
- Continued surveillance of the coagulation status to prevent DIVC

Mild cases

In most of the mild cases, premature separation results in spontaneous delivery with little risk to the mother and a slightly higher risk to the fetus. It must be borne in mind that once premature separation starts, even a mild case may turn into a serious one at any stage. Hence, all cases require careful observation and active management.

Severe cases

- In severe cases, measures should be taken to combat shock, and the blood loss should be adequately replaced.
- Uterine distension should be relieved by promoting uterine contractions and hastening delivery.
- Early detection and prompt management of complications such as renal failure and consumptive coagulopathy are important. The prognosis would be worse if there is a delay in the management of complications.

General management

- Two large-bore intravenous lines are set up. Initial resuscitation should be with crystalloids, preferably, NS or RL.
- A venous sample should be collected to check the hemoglobin status and coagulation profile. Serum fibrinogen should be estimated along with PT and aPTT.
- Adequate amounts of blood and blood products should be ordered and transfused as soon as possible.

If the facilities required for checking the coagulation profile are not available, a quick bedside clotting test can be performed. 10 mL of blood is drawn into a clean, dry test tube and the following observations are made:

- Failure of the blood to clot within 8–10 minutes indicates hypofibrinogenemia.
- By the end of one hour, the clot should retract from the sides of the tube. If not, thrombocytopenia should be suspected.
- If the clot dissolves within one hour and breaks down, it is likely that the patient has excessive fibrinolysis. This test should be repeated hourly or once in two hours.

- Ultrasound examination should determine the status of the fetus. It may also show the presence of the retroplacental clot.
- Urine output should be monitored carefully with an indwelling catheter. The excretion of at least 30 mL/hour indicates adequate renal perfusion; lower rates indicate the possibility of inadequate renal perfusion.
- In hemodynamically unstable women, blood and component transfusion should be started without delay. Since a large volume of fluid and blood may have to be given, central venous pressure monitoring should ideally be done.
- Two important points to be remembered during the resuscitation of the patient:
  - The blood loss may be much greater than evident on vaginal examination.
  - Coagulopathy may be present even when clinical evidence is lacking.

Obstetric management

Fig. 22.2 presents a flowchart representing the obstetric management of abruptio placenta.

- If the fetus is alive, cesarean delivery should be undertaken unless vaginal delivery is imminent.
- If vaginal delivery is imminent, delivery is conducted with continuous CTG monitoring. Assistance may be required in the second stage of labour with outlet forceps/vacuum extraction. The third stage of labour is managed by AMTSL. The placenta should be examined for retroplacental clots.
- If the fetus is dead, vaginal delivery is preferable, especially in the presence of coagulation defects, unless there is persistent hemorrhage or a deterioration in the general condition. Labour is augmented with ARM and oxytocin infusion to facilitate vaginal delivery.

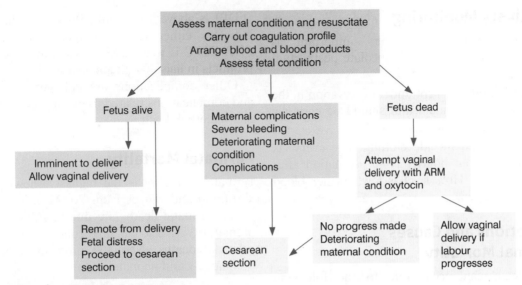

Fig. 22.2 Obstetric management of abruptio placenta

- Immediate amniotomy is important to hasten delivery, to decrease the intervillous space pressure, to reduce the bleeding from the placental site and to prevent the entry of thromboplastin into the maternal circulation.

- During the course of vaginal delivery, if the expected progress is not made or if there is a deterioration of the maternal condition, cesarean section may have to be performed immediately to reduce maternal morbidity.

- If a cesarean section is necessary for a live or dead fetus, in the presence of obvious bleeding, the amount of bleeding can be greatly reduced with sufficient cryoprecipitate given prior to the cesarean section to increase the fibrinogen concentration to 150 mg/dL. This can be achieved by infusing 10 units of cryoprecipitate, which increases the plasma concentration of fibrinogen by 100 mg/dL and also increases the factor VIII level. Prior to the cesarean section, it is mandatory that the patient be stabilised with fluids and blood/blood products. In those with associated pre-eclampsia, blood pressure should be controlled prior to cesarean section.

Indications for cesarean section

Cesarean section is indicated in the following situations:

- With a live and mature fetus, if the vaginal delivery is not imminent

- If the labour is not progressing satisfactorily after ARM and oxytocin infusion, even in the case of a dead fetus

- When the maternal condition is deteriorating with continued bleeding, reducing urine output and impending hemodynamic instability

- In the presence of Couvelaire uterus

Couvelaire uterus

Couvelaire uterus, which is also known as uteroplacental apoplexy, was first described by Couvelaire. It is a severe form of placental separation associated with widespread extravasation of blood into the uterine musculature and below the serous coat of the uterus (Fig. 22.3). Sometimes, blood is seen in the broad ligament and beneath the tubal serosa and in the peritoneal cavity. The degree of separation is severe, resulting in uterine tetany, shock and the death of the fetus.

Clinically, Couvelaire uterus is suspected when there is no uterine response to artificial rupture of the membranes and oxytocin infusion and the woman does not show improvement (as judged by blood pressure and pulse) despite blood transfusion. There are complications such as clotting defects and renal failure.

Couvelaire uterus is an indication for cesarean section but is not an indication for a hysterectomy as the uterus can contract sufficiently so that severe PPH may not occur.

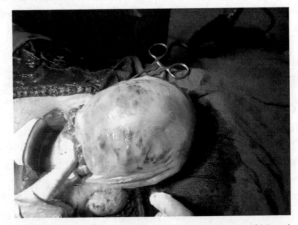

Fig. 22.3 Couvelaire uterus with extravasation of blood into the musculature beneath the serosa

Post-Delivery Monitoring

Post-delivery management is very important as complications can arise in the immediate postpartum period.

- The woman should be kept under observation in the labour ward for 48 hours and should be carefully watched for the development of PPH.
- Monitoring should include clotting time every six hours, urine output hourly, Hb% estimation after 24 hours—if the Hb% level is low, further blood transfusion is given.

Complications and Causes of Maternal Mortality

Maternal death can occur due to the following complications.

Hypovolemic shock

The blood loss in cases of abruptio placentae is nearly always underestimated. This is because of the concealed bleeding behind the placenta and into the myometrium. Moreover, in the presence of pre-eclampsia and eclampsia, hypovolemia may be masked, and the BP falsely elevated.

Postpartum hemorrhage

PPH can occur due to atonicity of the uterus caused by the intravasation of blood into the myometrium or high circulating levels of fibrin degradation products which have an inhibiting effect on the myometrium. Postpartum hemorrhage coupled with consumptive coagulopathy may be fatal.

Renal failure

Renal cortical necrosis of the kidney is a serious complication of abruptio placenta. The most likely cause of this is inadequate perfusion during the phase of acute blood loss. 'Shock proteinuria' is seen in women with abruption, wherein the proteinuria is not associated with hypertension and subsides soon after delivery. Renal failure is largely preventable by appropriate fluid management or blood replacement.

Consumptive coagulopathy

Placental abruption is one of the most common causes of significant consumptive coagulopathy. Thromboplastin enters the maternal circulation from the placental bed and triggers DIVC. There is a drop in fibrinogen levels, platelet count and the levels of factors VII and VIII. In cases of DIVC, there is prolonged bleeding from the venipuncture sites and the serum fibrinogen level is <100 mg/dL or the level of fibrin degradation products (FDP) is above 10 µg/mL. Prolonged thrombin time indicates either low fibrinogen level or increased FDP. DIVC is treated with adequate blood and blood products in liaison with a hematologist.

Other complications are emergency hysterectomy and complications related to massive blood transfusion and maternal death.

Perinatal Mortality

Perinatal mortality is the highest following placental abruption and ranges from 20–25%. More than half of the perinatal deaths are due to stillbirth. Associate prematurity is also an important cause of increased perinatal deaths. Neonatal problems are related to prematurity and neonatal anemia.

Management in the PHC

- In a PHC, if abruption is diagnosed, the pregnant woman should be started on two IV lines using large-bore cannulae.
- Blood for grouping and typing is taken and if the facilities are available, appropriate compatible blood transfusion can be started.
- An indwelling urinary catheter is introduced and connected to a urobag.
- If delivery is not imminent, the woman should be transferred to a higher centre in an ambulance.
- If she comes to the PHC in the late stages of labour, delivery should be conducted with all the above supportive measures.
- Active management of the third stage of labour should be followed and the placenta removed.
- Retroplacental clots, if present, should be weighed and removed.
- The woman should be watched carefully for PPH and transferred to a higher centre in an ambulance.
- The higher centre to which the woman is being transferred should be informed well in advance that she is being sent to that facility.

Prevention

- Patients at risk of abruption should be identified. Because of the risk of recurrence in subsequent pregnancies, women who have had abruptio placenta in previous pregnancies should be evaluated for hyperhomocysteinemia and APLA.
- Advice on the cessation of smoking should be given to those who smoke.
- Folate administration during early placentation and in the preconception period should be advocated.

■ VASA PREVIA

Vasa previa is one of the causes of antepartum hemorrhage. In this condition, the bleeding is of fetal origin. In vasa previa, the fetal vessels (umbilical vessels) run along the membrane below the presenting part before reaching the placenta. The vessels may be inserted at the margin of the placenta—this is called velamentous insertion. Bleeding occurs when the membrane ruptures, leading to severe fetal hypoxia. It is difficult to diagnose antenatally; if it is diagnosed by Doppler study, elective cesarean section should be undertaken.

KEY POINTS

✓ Antepartum hemorrhage is defined as bleeding from the genital tract occurring after 24 weeks of gestation (after the period of viability) and prior to the birth of the baby.

✓ Bleeding during pregnancy may be due to pregnancy-related factors such as placenta previa, abruptio placentae, unclassified or indeterminate causes, circumvallate placenta or rupture of the marginal sinus of placenta. Coincidental or local factors include cervical polyp, bleeding cervical erosion and carcinoma cervix.

✓ The term accidental hemorrhage or abruptio placentae refers to a condition where hemorrhage occurs as a result of the premature separation of a normally situated placenta after 24 weeks of gestation but before the delivery of the fetus.

✓ The bleeding may be revealed, concealed or of the mixed variety.

✓ The maternal complications are hemorrhagic shock, renal failure and coagulation failure.

✓ Fetal distress and fetal death are common.

✓ The main presenting symptom is painful vaginal bleeding.

✓ Risk factors such as hypertension, multiparity, hydramnios and maternal smoking are associated with abruption.

Essay questions

1. Define abruption. Describe the pathology, types, grades and clinical features of abruption.
2. Discuss the investigation, differential diagnosis and management of abruption.

Short answer questions

1. Define antepartum hemorrhage and enumerate its causes.
2. What is the differential diagnosis of abruptio placentae?
3. Define Couvelaire uterus.
4. What are the complications of abruption and how are they managed?
5. What are the causes of maternal mortality in abruptio placentae?
6. How would you differentiate between abruptio placentae and placenta previa?
7. What are the different grades of placental abruption?
8. What investigations are carried out in cases of abruptio placenta?

MCQs

1. Antepartum hemorrhage is defined as bleeding from or into the genital tract occurring after:
   a) 22+0 weeks of pregnancy
   b) 24+0 weeks of pregnancy
   c) 26+0 weeks of pregnancy
   d) 28+0 weeks of pregnancy
2. Which of the following does NOT result in antepartum hemorrhage?
   a) Circumvallate placenta
   b) Placenta previa
   c) Vasa previa
   d) Retained placenta

3. What is the incidence of abruption in pregnancy?
   a) <1%
   b) 2%
   c) 5%
   d) 10%
4. Which of the following is NOT a risk factor associated with abruption?
   a) Smoking
   b) Hypertension
   c) PPROM
   d) Hypothyroidism
5. What is the percentage of risk of recurrent abruption?
   a) 2%
   b) 4.4%
   c) 10%
   d) 20%
6. Which of these is not a pathophysiology of abruption?
   a) Uterine vasospasm
   b) Venous engorgement and arteriolar rupture
   c) Rupture of decidual spiral arteries and extension into uterine musculature
   d) Never causes bloodstained liquor
7. Abruption with fetal death is classified as:
   a) Minimal
   b) Mild
   c) Moderate
   d) Severe
8. What urinary output indicates adequate renal perfusion?
   a) 10 mL/hr
   b) 30 mL/hr
   c) 50 mL/hr
   d) 70 mL/hr

9. Which of these complications is not associated with abruption?
   a) Couvelaire uterus
   b) Hypovolemic shock
   c) Acute kidney injury
   d) Ketoacidosis

10. Perinatal mortality with abruption is:
    a) 5–10%
    b) 10–15%
    c) 20–25%
    d) 30–35%

11. Which of the following is not an indication for emergency cesarean in abruption?
    a) Nil urine output
    b) No progress of labour in a stable mother with a live fetus at 38 weeks
    c) Grade 1 abruption in a live fetus at 36 weeks, imminent to deliver
    d) Fall in maternal vital parameters

Answers
1. (b), 2. (d), 3. (a), 4. (d), 5. (b), 6. (d), 7. (d), 8. (b), 9. (d), 10. (c), 11. (c)

Fill in the blanks

1. Hemorrhage occurring from a fetal blood vessel due to a velamentous insertion of the umbilical cord is called _____.

2. When hemorrhage occurs as a result of premature separation of a normally situated placenta it is called _____.

Answers
1. vasa previa, 2. abruption

Case scenario-based discussion

1. A 30-year-old G4P3 presents at 36 weeks of gestation with complaints of abdominal pain and bleeding per vaginum. She has soaked two pads in one hour. She also complains of fainting attacks for the last two hours with reduced fetal movements. In her past obstetric history, she had similar bleeding, for which she was given blood transfusion. On examination, there is mild pallor, her pulse rate is 90/minute and BP is 110/70 mmHg. On abdominal examination, the uterus is contracting and tender. The fetal head is 3/5th palpable and the FHR is 120 bpm. The woman's previous records do not show evidence of placenta previa.
   a) What is the probable diagnosis and what action should be taken?
   b) What investigations would this woman require?
   c) On vaginal examination, if the cervix is 1 cm long and 2 cm dilated with intact membranes and the fetal head is in the −2 station, what is the course of action?
   d) What are the complications you expect in this case?

Answers
a) The probable diagnosis is abruptio placenta as the woman has presented with painful bleeding per vaginum associated with reduced fetal movements, the head is fixed in the pelvis and the review of her records does not show placenta previa. Therefore, vaginal examination should be carried out. IV fluids should be started immediately, blood samples should be collected for investigations and the bladder should be catheterised.
b) Please refer to the section on *Investigations*.
c) As the fetus is still alive and since vaginal delivery may take longer, cesarean delivery is the preferred method of delivery in this case.
d) Please refer to the section on *Complications*.

Placenta Previa

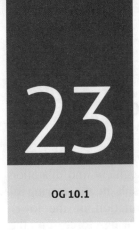

Learning Objectives

» To know the types and etiologies of placenta previa
» To know the clinical presentation and USG features of placenta previa
» To know the differential diagnosis of placenta previa
» To know the management of placenta previa

INTRODUCTION

Placenta previa is defined as the presence of the placenta over or adjacent to the internal os of the cervix. In placenta previa, the fertilised ovum is implanted very close to the internal os of the cervix so that the placenta develops in the lower segment, covering it either completely or partially. Placenta previa complicates around 0.5% of deliveries. The incidence of placenta previa reported by the Institute of Obstetrics and Gynecology, Chennai, between 2001 and 2010 was 0.63%.

TYPES OF PLACENTA PREVIA

Placenta previa is classified into four types (Fig. 23.1a–d).

- **Type I:** It is otherwise called low-lying placenta or lateral placenta. In this type, the placenta's edge does not actually reach the internal os but is in close proximity to it.

- **Type II:** It is otherwise called marginal placenta. Here, the edge of the placenta is at the margin of the internal os but does not cover it.

- **Type III:** It is otherwise called partial placenta previa. Here, the internal os is covered by the placenta, but only partially, when the cervix is dilated.

- **Type IV:** It is otherwise called total placenta previa/complete or central placenta previa. Here, the internal os is covered completely by the placenta even when the cervix is fully dilated.

Placenta previa can be anterior or posterior. All posterior placenta previa and types III and IV anterior placenta previa are considered major degrees. Types I and II anterior are considered minor degrees of placenta previa. Type II posterior is considered dangerous because the placenta can get compressed between the fetal head and the sacral promontory, predisposing to fetal distress; further, the spontaneous arrest of bleeding is reduced with this type as there is no effective compression by the fetal head.

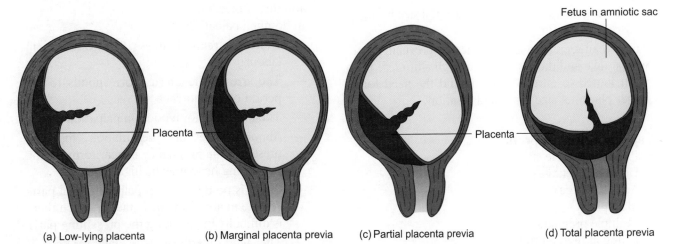

(a) Low-lying placenta   (b) Marginal placenta previa   (c) Partial placenta previa   (d) Total placenta previa

Fig. 23.1(a–d) Types of placenta previa

USG CLASSIFICATION OF PLACENTA PREVIA

With the advent of transvaginal USG, the distance between the edge of the placenta and the internal os can be easily measured. Based on the USG findings, placenta previa is classified as follows:

- Placenta previa—the placenta lies directly over the internal os.
- Low-lying placenta—the placental edge lies within 2 cm from the internal os but does not cover it (in a normally located placenta, the placental edge is located >2 cm from the cervical os).

ETIOLOGY

In the presence of a large placenta or when the vascularity of the placenta is compromised, the placenta tends to occupy a larger area. Any previous injury to the myometrium or endometrium can predispose to the development of placenta previa. The risk of placenta previa increases with the following factors:

- There is a two- to three-fold increased risk of placenta previa in women with a previous cesarean section (scarred uterus). This risk increases further as the number of previous cesarean deliveries increases. The risk of placenta previa is also increased in women who have had a myomectomy or repeated uterine curettage.
- Previous placenta previa increases the risk by 6- to 8-fold.
- Advancing maternal age >35 years and multiparity can predispose to placenta previa because of poor vascularisation and the larger surface required for implantation.
- Multifetal gestation, where the placental size is large, is also a risk factor.
- There is an increased risk of placenta previa in those who smoke and those who live at high altitudes. This is attributed to chronic hypoxia and the need for a larger placental size for vascularisation.

Causes of placenta previa
- Previous uterine surgery
- Uterine curettage
- Advanced age
- Multiparity
- Multiple pregnancy
- Living at high altitudes
- Smoking and drug abuse

CAUSES OF BLEEDING IN PLACENTA PREVIA

When the placenta is located over the internal os, the formation of the lower uterine segment and dilatation of the internal os invariably result in the tearing of placental attachments. The formation of the lower uterine segment exerts a shearing force on the inelastic placental attachment, resulting in the partial separation of the placenta. The bleeding is augmented by the inability of the myometrial fibres of the lower uterine segment to contract and thereby constrict the torn vessels. This bleeding is called **inevitable or unavoidable bleeding**.

CLINICAL FEATURES

Placenta previa presents with spontaneous, painless bleeding. Usually, bleeding occurs in the second or third trimester. The woman presents with recurrent episodes of bleeding which may stop spontaneously.

Symptoms
- Painless bleeding
- Spontaneous bleeding not related to any activity
- Bleeding may stop spontaneously but tends to recur
- The first bleeding episode may occur at any time; usually occurs at the end of the second trimester, in the third trimester or during labour

Signs
- Tachycardia or hypotension, depending on the amount of blood loss
- The woman is anemic in proportion to the amount of bleeding
- Abdominal palpation
  - Uterus is relaxed unless the woman is in labour
  - The size of the uterus corresponds to the period of amenorrhea
  - The uterus is not tender on palpation
  - Abnormal lie or presentation may be present if the pregnancy is near term, or the presenting head may be high (floating)
  - There is no difficulty in palpating fetal parts (unlike in abruptio placentae, in which there is difficulty in palpating the presenting part)
  - The fetal heartbeat is usually present if bleeding is not excessive

— In cases of posterior placenta previa, Stallworthy's sign can be elicited by pressing the head down, which results in the slowing of the fetal heart and subsequent recovery on releasing the fetal head

— Presence or absence of vaginal bleeding must be noted

In any woman presenting with antepartum hemorrhage, vaginal examination should not be performed unless placenta previa has been ruled out.

DIFFERENTIAL DIAGNOSIS

Placenta previa should be differentiated from abruptio placentae based on the features listed in Table 23.1 (discussed in Chapter 22, *Antepartum hemorrhage—abruptio placentae*).

Table 23.1 Differences between abruptio placentae and placenta previa

Characteristic	Abruptio placentae	Placenta previa
Bleeding	May be revealed or concealed	Sudden onset; always revealed
	Dark red	Red
Pain	Always present	Generally painless
Clinical condition (pallor, vitals)	Usually disproportionate to the amount of blood loss	Proportionate to the amount of blood loss
Uterus	Tense and tender	Soft and non-tender
Height of the uterine fundus	More than the period of amenorrhea	Corresponds to the period of amenorrhea
Fetal parts	Difficult to palpate/non-palpable	Easily palpable
Presenting part	In the pelvis and very often fixed	High, mobile presenting part
Malpresentations	Uncommon	Common
Fetal heart	Difficult to auscultate/very often slow	Generally normal and easily heard
Associated problems	Very often associated with pre-eclampsia	No specific associated problems
Coagulation problems	DIVC is common in severe cases	No specific coagulation problems

ULTRASOUND EXAMINATION FOR CONFIRMING DIAGNOSIS

USG examination is the simplest, most precise and safest method of placental localisation (Fig. 23.2). However, false-positive results can occur as a result of bladder distension. Therefore, placenta previa diagnosed by USG should be repeated after emptying the bladder.

Poor imaging can also occur in a posterior placenta previa due to the absence of an anatomical landmark posteriorly. Besides, the acoustic shadow from the fetal presenting part may obscure the placental view. If a transabdominal scan shows a placenta previa, it should be confirmed by TVS, which is also useful in measuring the distance between the placental edge and the internal os. Transvaginal sonography has been shown to be safe in placenta previa. Transperineal sonography is also reasonably accurate in diagnosing placenta previa. The use of transvaginal USG is superior to transabdominal sonography in the diagnosis of placenta previa for the following reasons:

- The transabdominal approach requires bladder filling, which results in the approximation of the anterior and posterior walls of the lower uterine segment. As a result, a normally situated placenta may appear to be a previa.
- As vaginal probes are closer to the lower segment and have a higher frequency, they produce higher resolution images.
- The internal cervical os and the lower placental edge frequently cannot be imaged adequately by the transabdominal approach. The position of the internal os is usually assumed rather than actually seen.

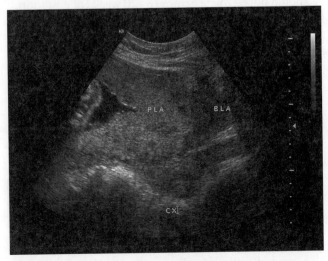

Fig. 23.2 USG picture showing placenta in the lower uterine segment

- The fetal head may obscure views of the lower placental edge in the transabdominal approach. In addition, posterior placenta previa may not be adequately imaged.

  In all women diagnosed with placenta previa, colour Doppler USG should be carried out to rule out placenta accreta. It is also useful to rule out vasa previa when the umbilical cord is noted in the lower segment.

> During ultrasound examination for placenta previa, the sonologist should specifically look for any evidence of placenta accreta or percreta.

MAGNETIC RESONANCE IMAGING (MRI)

MRI is not routinely used for the diagnosis of placenta previa. However, it is useful in obese women, in cases of posterior placenta previa or when adherent placenta is suspected.

MIGRATION OF THE PLACENTA

In some cases, placenta previa is reported during the anomaly scan, but USG at a later date may not show its presence. This phenomenon is called 'placental migration'. This is commonly seen when a low-lying placenta or marginal placenta is reported. This is due to the differential growth of the upper and lower segments as pregnancy advances. Migration is less likely in cases of previous cesarean section and when the placenta covers the os.

> The diagnosis of placenta previa or low-lying placenta should not be made before 18–20 weeks of gestation, and the provisional diagnosis made at anomaly scan must be confirmed after 32 weeks of gestation or earlier if the clinical situation warrants it.

> All placenta previa reported at the anomaly scan between 18–20 weeks of gestation should be confirmed at 32 weeks of gestation.

COMPLICATIONS OF PLACENTA PREVIA

- Though small warning hemorrhages may occur repeatedly, the bleeding may occasionally be very heavy, leading to shock.

- The risk of developing adherent placenta (placenta accreta, increta and percreta) is increased and is reported to occur in 1–4% of cases and could be as high as 10–20% in those with previous cesarean section.
- PPH may occur due to uncontrollable bleeding from the placental site.
- Chronic repeated hemorrhage may lead to IUGR.
- Acute fetal distress or even fetal death can occur in the presence of heavy bleeding.
- Preterm labour can occur.
- In women with placenta previa or a low-lying placenta, the presence of a marginal/velamentous cord insertion close to the cervical os or a succenturiate placental lobe increases the risk of vasa previa, which is dangerous to the fetus.
- Maternal mortality may be due to hemorrhage, especially in the presence of adherent placenta.

MANAGEMENT OF PLACENTA PREVIA

The routine use of USG in pregnancy has made it possible to diagnose or suspect a low-lying placenta/placenta previa in asymptomatic pregnant women. Though it is not possible to predict the migration of placenta, measuring the distance between the placental edge and the internal os by ultrasound helps in predicting the outcome.

- On USG, if the placenta overlies the internal os by >20 mm before 20 weeks of gestation, it is unlikely to migrate and needs to be followed up and managed as a major-degree placenta previa until proven otherwise on subsequent ultrasound examination at 32 weeks of gestation.
- Before 20 weeks of gestation, if the placenta is overlying the internal os by 0–20 mm, USG repeated at a later date may show migration.

GENERAL MANAGEMENT

In all cases presenting with antepartum hemorrhage, the initial management is as follows:
- The woman is admitted.
- Two IV lines are started with large-bore cannulae (size 14 or 16) and NS/RL is infused rapidly until blood transfusion is available.
- Blood samples are collected to test for Hb and hematocrit, blood grouping and typing and cross-matching. A coagulation profile is also performed if abruption is suspected.
- Oxygen is made available.

- The woman's vitals are monitored.
- The woman is given a clean diaper, and the presence or absence of vaginal bleeding is noted.
- If there is bleeding, the colour of the blood (bleeding in placenta previa is usually red) is noted and visual estimation of blood loss is made.
- The woman may require catheterisation and continuous bladder drainage.
- History and clinical examination are carried out to make the diagnosis of placenta previa. The woman's previous scan records should also be reviewed. A detailed and clear history should be obtained with regard to when the bleeding started, how many pads were soaked, any triggering factors, similar past history, associated pain abdomen and presence or absence of fetal movements.
- The abdomen is palpated to determine whether the uterus is relaxed or tender, to look for contractions and to know the presentation (Table 23.1). In placenta previa, the uterus is relaxed, and there may be malpresentation or a floating head.
- Fetal heart monitoring is performed to see whether the fetal condition is good and whether there is fetal distress or death. In placenta previa, the fetal heart is generally good unless there is heavy bleeding.
- Vaginal examination should never be performed in suspected cases of placenta previa.
- A speculum examination may be required after 48 hours, after bleeding stops, to rule out cervical pathology.
- Urgent USG is carried out to confirm placenta previa and fetal well-being.

SPECIFIC MANAGEMENT

Depending on the gestational age, the condition of the fetus and the amount of bleeding, placenta previa is managed either conservatively or by active management.

Expectant Line of Management—McAfee–Johnson Regimen

Conservative management of placenta previa by the McAfee–Johnson regimen prevents the risks of prematurity without compromising the maternal or fetal status. Conservative management is carried out in a hemodynamically stable woman in whom the gestational age is <36 weeks. This is based on the fact that, in most cases of placenta previa, the first episode

of bleeding is not heavy and stops spontaneously but may recur at a later date.

Prerequisites for conservative management

- The woman should be hemodynamically stable.
- Bleeding should not be ongoing and should stop early.
- The fetus should be in good condition and the gestational age should be <36 weeks.
- The woman should not be in labour.
- Facilities for emergency cesarean section and blood transfusion should be readily available.

The protocol for the expectant management of placenta previa is as follows (Fig. 23.3):

- The woman is put on complete bed rest with bedside toilet facilities; the woman is allowed to go to the toilet only after the bleeding has stopped.
- If the woman is anemic, the necessary blood transfusion is given with the aim to achieve a PCV of 30%.
- Cross-matched blood should always be kept ready.
- Antenatal steroids are given to promote lung maturity of the fetus.
- If the woman is Rh-negative, she is given anti-D immunoglobulin.
- Routine antenatal care of the pregnancy is continued until the pregnancy advances to 37 weeks, at which time, the pregnancy is terminated, usually by cesarean section.

Conservative management is discontinued, and pregnancy is terminated in the following scenarios:
- There is recurrent bleeding, leading to hemodynamic instability in the woman
- There is fetal distress or fetal death
- Suspicion of intrauterine growth restriction (IUGR)
- Rupture of membranes
- The pregnancy has reached term
- The woman goes into labour

Domiciliary Treatment

- All major degrees of placenta previa diagnosed at 32 weeks of gestation should be hospitalised.
- In minor-degree placenta previa, after the bleeding stops, there may be a place for domiciliary treatment provided the woman lives close to the hospital and can reach the hospital within 10 minutes of further episodes of bleeding.

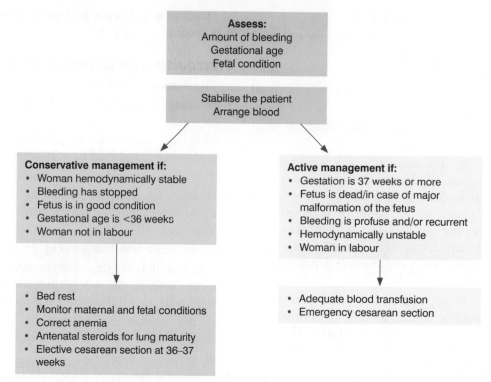

Fig. 23.3 Management of a woman diagnosed with placenta previa

Active Line of Management

The indications for the active line of management are as follows:

- The gestation is 37 weeks or more
- The fetus is dead or there is a major malformation of the fetus
- The bleeding is profuse and/or recurrent, thus compromising the hemodynamic status
- The woman goes into shock—irrespective of the gestational age, the pregnancy has to be terminated; after stabilising the mother and with adequate blood, an emergency cesarean section is performed; this should be done by a senior obstetrician
- The woman is in labour

Mode of delivery

- Most cases of placenta previa are delivered by performing a cesarean section.
- However, there is a place for vaginal delivery in a hemodynamically stable woman with an anterior low-lying or marginal placenta previa. When such a woman is at term with the fetal head fixed and spontaneous onset of labour, vaginal delivery may be considered in a well-equipped facility. The delivery should be planned in a setting that is suited for both vaginal and ceserean delivery. In the theatre, a gentle vaginal examination is first carried out. Initially,

the fornices are felt; if there is bogginess through the fornices, suggesting a major degree, a cesarean section is performed. If the fetal head is felt through all the fornices, the fingers are inserted into the cervix and the membranes are ruptured. The labour is allowed to progress provided there is no bleeding.

Cesarean section in placenta previa

Cesarean section should be performed in a setting where a senior obstetrician and all ancillary facilities, such as blood transfusion and neonatal care, are available. Adequate blood should be made available. A cesarean section should always be performed by an experienced obstetrician as an elective procedure. As the procedure is associated with a risk of massive obstetric hemorrhage and hysterectomy, informed consent should be obtained from the woman beforehand.

The lower segment section is the choice in all varieties of placenta previa.

- Placenta previa is not a contraindication for the lower segment operation. When the placenta is anterior, large vessels may be seen over the lower segment. These vessels can be tied off before performing the lower segment operation.
- Sometimes, the incision may have to be made through the placenta, resulting in severe hemorrhage of both

maternal and fetal origins. Under these circumstances, after the delivery of the fetus, the umbilical cord should be clamped immediately to decrease fetal bleeding, resulting in fetal anemia. There are also high chances of the uterine incision extending laterally into the vessels and causing severe hemorrhage.

- The other way is to deliver around the placental edge, avoiding an incision over the placenta (Ward technique). After the uterine incision, a cleavage plane is created digitally between the uterus and the placenta until the membranes are reached and ruptured. The fetus is then delivered through the site of rupture of the membranes.
- A low vertical or classical cesarean would be required if large vessels are encountered in the lower segment or adherent placenta is suspected.
- Profuse hemorrhage may occur from the placenta site. This is more common with posterior placenta previa. The hemorrhage may be due to the poor contractile nature of the lower uterine segment. Additional purse-string suture/Cho's sutures may be required at the implantation site to achieve hemostasis.
- In some cases of uncontrollable hemorrhage, bilateral internal iliac ligation, or even hysterectomy may be necessary. If a hysterectomy is undertaken, it should be a total hysterectomy to control bleeding from the lower segment.
- Placenta previa may also be associated with placenta accreta, increta or percreta. These cases are delivered by cesarean section at 34–35 weeks of gestation.
- Cases complicated by adherent placenta may require uterine artery embolisation. However, this procedure necessitates an experienced interventional radiologist and the necessary infrastructure.

MANAGEMENT OF ASYMPTOMATIC PLACENTA PREVIA

Occasionally, placenta previa may be diagnosed at the anomaly scan, but the woman may not experience any bleeding episodes. Approximately 10% of women may have asymptomatic presentation and reach term without any bleeding. In these patients, the following protocol should be followed:

- Placenta previa should be confirmed at 32 weeks of gestation.
- Morbidly adherent placenta should be ruled out by Doppler USG.
- The woman should be counselled regarding the risks associated with placenta previa and advised to report to the hospital immediately whenever there is bleeding.

- The woman should be advised against sexual intercourse, which can precipitate bleeding.
- She should be asked to avoid heavy lifting, straining at stools and moderate to heavy exercise and travel.
- Speculum and vaginal examinations should not be performed.
- The woman should be given antenatal steroids at 30–32 weeks of gestation.
- All major degrees of placenta previa should be hospitalised at 32 weeks of gestation.
- Women with a minor degree of placenta previa can be managed as OP cases. However, they should be asked if they live close to the hospital and if they will be able to reach the hospital at the earliest in the event of an episode of bleeding.
- Elective cesarean is carried out at 36–37 weeks of gestation.

Management at the primary health centre

All cases of antepartum hemorrhage seen at a primary health centre should be transferred as early and as speedily as possible to the nearest referral hospital. The following protocol is recommended:

- Two IV lines should be started with NS and/or RL.
- Blood grouping, typing and if possible, cross-matching should be performed.
- Oxygen SOS should be initiated.
- The woman should be transferred along with a hospital staff member to the nearest functional higher centre.
- The higher centre should be informed about the transfer beforehand.
- In case a woman diagnosed with placenta previa delivers in the PHC, the delivery is conducted with two IV lines. After the delivery of the baby, active management of the third stage of labour should be performed. 20 units of oxytocin should be added to one of the IV fluids and infused at the rate of 20–30 drops per minute. A woman who has delivered vaginally is unlikely to have had a major degree of placenta previa. However, the woman should be monitored carefully for bleeding and transferred to a higher centre after one hour even if there is no excessive bleeding.

MATERNAL AND FETAL MORTALITY

With the early detection of placenta previa due to the liberal use of ultrasound, the better availability of blood and components and better anesthesia and surgical techniques and skill, maternal and fetal mortality associated with placenta previa have reduced in recent times. The mortality rate can be reduced further with early diagnosis by ultrasound examination and by advising women to visit a hospital for antenatal supervision and delivery. Maternal mortality is usually due to massive obstetric hemorrhage, especially if there is associated adherent placenta. Preterm delivery is a major cause of perinatal death, even though expectant management of placenta previa is practiced.

KEY POINTS

✓ Placenta previa is categorised into four types depending on the relation of the placenta to the internal os.

✓ The diagnosis of placenta previa is made by ultrasound examination. TVS is superior to TAS in the diagnosis of placenta previa.

✓ In all cases diagnosed with placenta previa, adherent placenta should be ruled out by Doppler study.

✓ A low-lying placenta diagnosed in the early weeks of pregnancy needs to be confirmed in the third trimester, since some of these may migrate in the latter half of pregnancy.

✓ Depending on the maternal and fetal condition, either conservative or active line of management can be undertaken.

✓ Cesarean delivery is indicated in all patients with third- or fourth-degree placenta previa, and in some cases of first- and second degrees.

✓ Cesarean section must be performed by an experienced surgeon in a well-equipped hospital.

Essay questions

1. Describe the management of a woman at 37 weeks of gestation with placenta previa.
2. Describe the symptoms and signs of placenta previa. How is the diagnosis confirmed?
3. Describe the types of placenta previa and the clinical features and investigation of placenta previa.

Short answer questions

1. What are the risk factors for placenta previa?
2. What are the differences between abruption and placenta previa?
3. Describe the expectant management of placenta previa.
4. What are the degrees or varieties of placenta previa?
5. Compare transabdominal and transvaginal sonography in placenta previa.

MCQs

1. The expectant line of management is not recommended in placenta previa in which of the following conditions?
   a) Gestation is less than 36 weeks
   b) Vaginal bleeding is not excessive
   c) The fetus is alive
   d) The woman is in labour

2. A 32-year-old woman was diagnosed with placenta previa at 37 weeks of gestation. What is the best management for her?
   a) Induction of labour
   b) Cesarean section
   c) Tocolysis
   d) Conservative management

3. A 28-year-old woman was diagnosed with complete placenta previa at 30 weeks of gestation. Which of the following is a risk factor for her condition?
   a) Polyhydramnios
   b) Hypertension
   c) Multiple gestation
   d) Prior salpingitis

4. Which of these is not a feature of placenta previa?
   a) Relaxed uterus
   b) Painless bleeding
   c) Recurrent bleeding
   d) Tense and tender uterus

5. Which of the following is not true of USG in diagnosing placenta previa?
   a) Done on an empty bladder
   b) Transabdominal approach has better sensitivity
   c) Transvaginal approach has better sensitivity
   d) Placenta accreta can be picked up on ultrasound and confirmed by MRI

6. Which of the following is not a component of the McAfee–Johnson regimen?
   a) Premature pregnancy with one episode of bleeding
   b) Hemodynamically stable patient
   c) Anemia correction to achieve 30% PCV
   d) Conservative management till 40 weeks

7. Active management of placenta previa is indicated if:
   a) Gestational age is <37 weeks
   b) The woman is hemodynamically stable
   c) The bleeding episode is resolved
   d) The fetus is dead

8. Perinatal mortality is highest in:
   a) Low-lying placenta
   b) Marginal placenta previa
   c) Anterior placenta previa
   d) Vasa previa

9. A condition where the placenta reaches the edge of the internal os is called:
   a) Low-lying placenta
   b) Marginal placenta previa
   c) Partial placenta previa
   d) Total placenta previa

10. Which of these is not true of cesarean section in placenta previa?
    a) Needs to be performed in silent placenta previa at 34 weeks
    b) Ward technique for delivery of the fetus

c) Additional sutures in placental implantation site

d) Should be done by a senior obstetrician

Answers

1. (d), 2. (b), 3. (c), 4. (d), 5. (b), 6. (d), 7. (d), 8. (d), 9. (b), 10. (a)

Fill in the blanks

1. Expectant line of management in placenta previa is called _____.

2. In all women diagnosed with placenta previa, _____ should be ruled out.

Answers

1. McAfee–Johnson regimen, 2. adherent placenta

Case scenario-based discussion

1. A 28-year-old G3P1, abortion 1, attends the casualty with eight months of amenorrhea and complains of painless bleeding per vaginum since one hour. She says that the episode occurred while she was asleep and that the bleeding subsequently stopped. There are no labour pains or leaking per vaginum. There is no history of trauma or recent sexual intercourse. The woman is able to perceive the fetal movements well. She had one full-term normal delivery 3 years ago, followed by a spontaneous miscarriage at 8 weeks which was surgically evacuated. As per her dates, she is 32 weeks pregnant. On examination, there is mild pallor, the BP is 110/70 mmHg and pulse is 80 bpm. Her uterus is 32 weeks in size, well-relaxed and non-tender, the fetal head is in the lower pole and the fetal heart rate is 150 bpm.

a) What is the most likely diagnosis in this case?

b) How would you manage this case?

c) What are the indications for the active line of management?

Answers

a) The most likely diagnosis is placenta previa, which should be confirmed by USG examination. Doppler study should also be carried out to rule out adherent placenta.

b) Since the woman is hemodynamically stable, the fetal heart rate is normal and the bleeding has stopped, conservative management should be undertaken at 32 weeks of gestation to avoid the risk of prematurity. The woman should be hospitalised, her vitals monitored, anemia corrected, and antenatal steroids given to enhance fetal lung maturity. If no further bleeding occurs, elective cesarean should be carried out at 36–37 weeks of gestation.

c) The following are the indications for active management:

- Due to bleeding, if maternal and/or fetal condition is compromised
- If the woman is in labour
- If the gestational age is >36 weeks
- If the fetus is dead or if there are fetal malformations

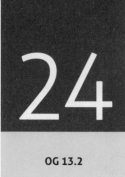

24

OG 13.2

Preterm Labour

Learning Objectives

» To define preterm labour and preterm premature rupture of membranes
» To discuss the complications of preterm labour
» To discuss the causes and pathophysiology of preterm labour
» To describe the diagnosis and prevention of preterm labour
» To discuss the management of preterm labour
» To discuss the diagnosis and management of PPROM

■ INTRODUCTION

Preterm labour is defined as the presence of painful uterine contractions associated with progressive effacement and dilatation of the cervix occurring any time after the period of viability (24 weeks of gestation) and before the completion of 37 weeks of gestation. The lower limit to define preterm labour depends on the period of viability. In the developed nations, the lower limit ranges from 20–24 weeks, whereas in India, the lower limit to define preterm labour is 24–26 weeks of gestation. According to the WHO, any child born at 20–37 weeks of gestation (141–259 days) should be called preterm.

■ INCIDENCE

In 2005, the WHO estimated that 9.6% of births were preterm. The incidence of preterm deliveries is increasing due to artificial reproductive technology (ART) and due to the increase in the incidence of multiple pregnancies. The incidence of preterm labour depends on the population studied. In developing countries like India, it is as high as 20–30%. Deliberate medical interventions account for nearly 30% of preterm deliveries. Approximately 30–40% of cases of preterm labour are preceded by premature rupture of membranes (PROM).

COMPLICATIONS OF PRETERM DELIVERY

Preterm births are associated with increased perinatal morbidity and mortality. 85% of neonatal deaths occurring in the structurally normal infant are due to

preterm delivery. The risks associated with preterm births are as follows:

- Respiratory distress syndrome (RDS)
- Sepsis
- Patent ductus arteriosus
- Necrotising enterocolitis
- Intraventricular hemorrhage
- Hypothermia, hypoglycemia, hypocalcemia, hyperbilirubinemia
- Delayed sequelae of preterm deliveries—rise in the incidence of cerebral palsy, retinopathy of prematurity, low IQ, higher incidence of neurological abnormalities, learning disabilities, chronic pulmonary disease, visual defects such as blindness, refractory errors, astigmatism, myopia, hearing loss and behavioural problems

ETIOLOGICAL FACTORS FOR PRETERM LABOUR

A number of factors may contribute to the occurrence of preterm labour. However, in 20–30% of cases, no cause may be found despite thorough investigations. Factors that could contribute to preterm labour are discussed in this section.

■ MATERNAL CHARACTERISTICS

Age

Preterm labour is more common in pregnancies at the extremes of maternal age. Both teenage pregnancies and pregnancies after the age of 35 are associated with an increased risk of preterm labour.

Socio-economic Status

Poor socio-economic status, which is associated with maternal malnutrition, is an important risk factor for preterm deliveries. Pre-pregnancy weight of <45 Kg and poor weight gain during pregnancy have a strong correlation to preterm labour. The risk of preterm delivery is higher among unmarried pregnant women.

Physical Activity

Increased physical work, hard labour, ambulatory occupations, long hours of commutation and prolonged working hours may result in inadequate rest during pregnancy, which can contribute to preterm labour.

Maternal Habits

Cigarette smoking as well as the use of drugs such as cocaine and alcohol consumption have been reported to play an important role in the etiology of preterm labour. Smoking increases carboxyhemoglobin levels, which results in maternal and fetal hypoxia.

Psychological Stress

Psychological stress has also been implicated as an important cause of preterm labour.

Past Obstetric History

- A history of spontaneous preterm birth is an important indicator of the increased risk of preterm labour in the current pregnancy. In such cases, the risk of recurrence is 25–50%. The mechanism of recurrence is not known; there may be an inherent error in the timing of delivery of either fetal or maternal etiology. The tendency for repeat preterm delivery may also be due to underlying infection, uterine abnormalities, cervical incompetence or leiomyoma of the uterus.
- A history of multiple induced abortions also indicates a risk of preterm labour.
- Previous second-trimester losses are associated with a risk of preterm labour as well.
- An interpregnancy interval of <18 months has been shown to be associated with an increased risk of preterm labour.

Present Pregnancy Complications

- **Maternal weight:** Both inadequate and excessive weight gain are associated with preterm labour.
- **Medical conditions:** A number of medical conditions complicating pregnancy lead to a rise in the incidence of spontaneous or induced preterm labour. In nearly 30% of cases, pregnancy is terminated either in the interest of the mother or that of the fetus. These include hypertensive disorders of pregnancy with pre-eclampsia and eclampsia, chronic renal disease, diabetes—both GDM and pre-gestational diabetes, Rh-isoimmunisation, the presence of severe FGR and congenital anomalies of the fetus. Spontaneous preterm labour can occur due to the above causes or as a result of other medical conditions such as urinary tract infections, bronchial asthma, heart disease, severe anemia and immunological disorders such as systemic lupus erythematosus (SLE), sickle cell disease and antiphospholipid syndrome.
- **Pregnancy complications:** Certain pregnancy complications are known to be associated with preterm labour. These are as follows:
  — Threatened miscarriage in the first trimester of pregnancy is associated with an increased of risk preterm delivery.
  — Due to the over-distension of the uterus, women with multiple pregnancies go into preterm labour. The average gestational age for twins is 35 weeks and that of quadruplets is 33 weeks. Selective reduction of triplets may result in a small increase in gestational age by 2 weeks.
  — Depending on the degree of hydramnios, the risk of preterm labour increases as the liquor volume increases.
  — In placenta previa or abruptio placentae, preterm labour starts spontaneously or is induced for medical reasons.
  — Premature calcification or fibrinoid degeneration of the placenta may be associated with preterm labour.
  — Pregnancies following assisted reproductive techniques are prone to preterm labour.
- **Maternal infections:**
  — Either systemic or intrauterine infection can lead to preterm labour. Systemic infections release endotoxins, which can stimulate uterine activity. In the presence of intrauterine infections, the cell wall of the infecting organism stimulates the fetal membranes to secrete inflammatory cytokines, tumour necrosis factor-alpha and interleukins, which in turn stimulate prostaglandin synthesis, triggering uterine activity.
  — Febrile illnesses such as malaria, pyelonephritis, pneumonia and other conditions that cause high fever and result in the release of endotoxins stimulate myometrial activity, resulting in preterm labour.

— Sexually transmitted infections caused by *Treponema pallidum*, *Neisseria gonorrhoeae* and *Trichomonas vaginalis* and chlamydia are important causes of preterm labour. Bacterial vaginosis, *Mycoplasma*, toxoplasmosis and periodontal diseases are other causes of preterm labour. In certain unexplained cases of preterm labour, chorioamnionitis caused by a variety of microorganisms emerged as a possible explanation.

- **Surgical causes, including appendicectomy**
- **Uterine factors:**
  — Mullerian anomalies, submucous fibroids and intrauterine synechiae interfere with the enlargement of the uterus. They can also cause abnormal placentation.

Anatomical Defects of the Uterus and Cervix

The presence of abnormal anatomic conditions due to internal os insufficiency or septate or bicornuate uterus can predispose to preterm labour.

Mullerian duct anomalies

Congenital anomalies of the uterus such as bicornuate uterus, septate uterus and unicornuate uterus can predispose to preterm delivery. A bicornuate uterus is associated with high rates of preterm labour (80%). A history of diethylstilboestrol (DES) exposure may be associated with abnormal uterine shapes, predisposing to preterm labour.

Cervical incompetence (insufficiency)

Incompetence of the cervix, whether inherent or acquired, increases the risk of preterm labour. The cause of an incompetent cervix may be developmental abnormalities such as Mullerian duct abnormalities, diethylstilboestrol (DES) exposure, cervical laceration following previous deliveries, trauma to the cervix or inherited collagen diseases.

■ IATROGENIC PREMATURITY

Iatrogenic prematurity can occur due to the induction of labour or elective cesarean section performed based on an incorrect date.

■ FETAL FACTORS

Fetal factors such as fetal growth restriction and anomalous babies are associated with preterm delivery.

PATHOGENESIS OF PRETERM LABOUR

Though the exact mechanism is not understood, the fetus appears to play a synergistic role in the initiation of preterm birth due to bacterial infection. The decidua and fetal membranes are the sites of the synthesis of prostaglandins. Raised prostaglandin activity may be stimulated by intrauterine infection, hemorrhage, overdistension of the uterus by polyhydramnios or multiple gestation and the rupture of membranes.

PREDICTION OF PRETERM LABOUR

Prediction of preterm labour involves identifying at-risk patients and carrying out necessary investigations as and when necessary. In order to prevent preterm birth, it is important to identify the possible underlying cause of preterm birth. In nearly 1/3rd of cases, iatrogenic preterm birth may be required because of medical and obstetrical complications. In 2/3rd of cases, preterm delivery is spontaneous.

- A detailed history of socio-economic status, nutrition, work, personal habits and past and current genital infections should be elicited.
- Previous obstetric history is important. History related to previous preterm birth and the possible cause, induced miscarriages and second-trimester losses should be elicited.
- A rapid and painless delivery resulting in second-trimester pregnancy losses or the delivery of a live fetus with or without an intact sac would indicate the possibility of internal os insufficiency.
- Poor nutrition, anemia, urinary tract/reproductive tract infections and smoking should be eliminated.
- Specific problems such as hypertension, diabetes, anemia and other medical disorders should be identified and effectively treated prior to embarking on pregnancy.
- Diagnosis of internal os insufficiency—in the non-pregnant state, a few tests can be carried out to diagnose cervical incompetence:
  — In the presence of internal os insufficiency, a No. 8 Hegar dilator can be passed into the cervical canal and internal os easily without pain or resistance.
  — Traction test with Foley catheter—an inflated Foley catheter with 1 mL of water can be easily removed in the presence of cervical incompetence.

— In the premenstrual period, a hysterogram may show a pencil line due to the effect of progesterone, whereas in the presence of incompetence, the internal os widens and becomes funnel-shaped.

- A hysterogram or hysteroscopy may be required to diagnose uterine anomalies.
- Investigations such as APLA may be required in certain situations with recurrent fetal losses.

PREVENTION OF PRETERM LABOUR

- General advice on rest and diet is important.
- Manual labour should be avoided. Women should be advised regarding pelvic rest and avoiding standing for long hours.
- Commuting long distances should be avoided.
- Women should be advised about the warning signs of preterm labour such as abdominal cramps, backache, pelvic pressure, mucoid discharge per vaginum with instructions to report immediately to the hospital in case of any of these.
- Frequent attendance to the AN clinic is recommended to identify complications such as anemia or UTI at the early stages.
- Sexual activity—during pregnancy, restriction of sexual activity and avoiding nipple stimulation should be advised. The use of condoms may reduce the bacterial load and exposure to seminal prostaglandins.
- Screening for infections—aggressive treatment of cervicovaginal infections is important. In women who had unexplained preterm labour in the previous pregnancy, screening for bacterial vaginosis should be carried out in early pregnancy and if positive, should be treated with clindamycin and metronidazole. Urine should be screened for asymptomatic bacteriuria periodically. One should also look for GBS and *Ureaplasma* infections. Vaginal gels can also be used in the management of infections.
- The assessment of gestational age should be done correctly in cases of induction of labour and elective cesarean section.
- Serial assessment of the cervix by USG—attempts have been made to predict preterm labour by measuring the cervical length using transvaginal sonography. The mean cervical length at 24 weeks is about 35 mm. Women with progressively shorter cervices (less than 25 mm), cervical funnelling (occupying 50% of the cervix) and a U-shaped cervix have a higher risk of preterm birth.

- Management of internal os insufficiency—if a specific problem such as cervical incompetence is suspected based on a history of previous mid-trimester miscarriages, history of cervical injury, uterine anomalies or USG findings showing short cervical length <25 mm, encirclage should be carried out after 14 weeks of gestation (after excluding the majority of anomalies). Different techniques are available for the treatment of cervical incompetence. The Shirodkar's stitch involves tightening the cervix at the level of the internal os. In the McDonald's technique, circumferential bites are taken into the body of the cervix, avoiding entry into the endocervical canal. Occasionally, emergency cerclage may be required when the cervix is getting dilated. The sutures are removed at 34 weeks of gestation to avoid rupture of the uterus. If the cervix is badly torn, its repair can be undertaken in the non-pregnant state by the Lash procedure, in which the cervix is tightened after mobilising the bladder adequately.
- Biochemical markers—a number of biochemical markers are available for the prediction of preterm labour. An increased level of fetal fibronectin in cervicovaginal secretions is the most sensitive and is used to predict preterm birth. Fetal fibronectin comes from the choriodecidual membrane and is not normally seen in the cervicovaginal discharge between 24 and 34 weeks. The levels increase in the presence of infection or uterine contraction. The fibronectin levels are measured every 2 weeks from 24 weeks onwards. Its presence indicates the possibility of preterm labour in 14 days. Salivary estriol and relaxin are other biochemical markers used for the prediction of preterm labour.
- Inflammation–related markers with elevated C-reactive protein >60 mg/litre also may predict preterm labour.
- Continuous monitoring of the uterine activity (home uterine activity monitoring) has also been attempted to predict and detect preterm labour early.
- Progesterone in the prevention of preterm labour:
  - In asymptomatic women with previous preterm births, weekly IM injections of 250 mg of 17 alpha-hydroxy progesterone caproate from 16–20 weeks of gestation to 37 weeks have been shown to be beneficial. 100 mg of vaginal micronised progesterone daily has also been used.
  - It has been recommended that high-risk women should be screened. If the cervical length is <25 mm between 16 and 24 weeks of gestation, progesterone supplementation may be given.

— In an asymptomatic woman, if the USG shows a short cervix <20 mm, micronised progesterone is given in a dose of 200 mg vaginally to prevent preterm labour.

DIAGNOSIS OF PRETERM LABOUR

Patients may present with early warning signs of preterm labour or they may present with established preterm labour.

SYMPTOMS OF THREATENED PRETERM LABOUR

The diagnosis of preterm labour is often difficult, and Braxton Hicks contractions may be interpreted as labour pains. The early warning symptoms of preterm labour are as follows:

- Uterine irritability presenting as menstrual-like cramps (constant or intermittent)
- Low, dull backache radiating to the suprapubic region
- Feeling of heavy pressure in the pelvis, rectum and perineum
- Abdominal cramping
- Increased mucoid vaginal discharge
- Fluid leaking into the vagina
- Irregular and intermittent uterine contractions
- No cervical changes

DIAGNOSIS OF ESTABLISHED PRETERM LABOUR

Early differentiation between true and false labour is difficult prior to demonstrable cervical effacement and dilatation. The following criteria may be used to document preterm labour:

- Contractions occurring at a frequency of 4 in 20 minutes or 8 in 60 minutes with changes in the cervix
- Cervical dilatation >1 cm
- Cervical effacement of 80% or greater

MANAGEMENT OF PRETERM LABOUR

An algorithm of the approach to the management of preterm labour is presented in Fig. 24.1.

The management of preterm labour is categorised as follows:

- Management of women with warning signs of preterm labour (threatened preterm labour)

- Suppressing established preterm labour
- Conduct of preterm labour and delivery of the preterm infant

MANAGEMENT OF WOMEN WITH WARNING SIGNS OF PRETERM LABOUR

- An initial evaluation of the woman should be conducted.
- The woman should be evaluated for progressive cervical changes as she may progress to established labour.
- Urine should be sent for investigations.
- A high vaginal swab (HVS) should be taken for microscopy, culture and Gram's stain.
- A vaginal swab should be sent for fibronectin testing.
- USG assessment for cervical length should be performed.
- If the woman is febrile, the source of infection should be identified.
- Bed rest should be initiated.
- Hydration therapy with 1 litre of 5% dextrose should be run for 6 hours to suppress oxytocin release. Fluid therapy increases AFI by 0.5–1 cm.
- Antibiotics are given only if there is evidence of infection or premature rupture of membranes.
- As these women may progress to established labour, antenatal corticosteroids are given.
- Prophylactic tocolytic drugs are not used in threatened preterm labour.
- Progesterone therapy is useful in high-risk women in the presence of a positive fibronectin assay or a short cervix.
- The woman should be observed to determine whether she is progressing to established labour.
- If there are no further uterine contractions or cervical changes following observation, the woman is discharged for normal antenatal care.

MANAGEMENT OF WOMEN WITH ESTABLISHED PRETERM LABOUR

When a woman presents with established preterm labour, one has to decide whether the woman has to be delivered immediately or if labour can be suppressed to prolong the pregnancy to facilitate the administration of corticosteroids. The management depends on the gestational age and the available facilities for neonatal care. The aim of management is to identify women who may benefit from steroid therapy.

Conditions Warranting Immediate Delivery

- Advanced labour with the cervix dilated >3 cm
- Fetal death or congenital anomalies incompatible with life
- In the presence of clear clinical chorioamnionitis
- Maternal diseases requiring immediate delivery such as hyperthyroidism, pre-eclampsia, chronic renal disease, SLE, sickle cell disease, diabetes, Rh-incompatibility and antepartum hemorrhage
- Fetal conditions necessitating immediate delivery such as fetal growth restriction and multiple pregnancy with complications

Suppressing Labour

In the absence of the above conditions, labour can be suppressed with tocolytic drugs to prolong pregnancy. All tocolytic drugs are given for a period of 48–72 hours to give time for the corticosteroids to act. Tocolytic drugs are given for gestational ages between 28 and 34 weeks of gestation.

Before suppressing labour, the following prerequisites should be met:

- Live fetus with no signs of fetal distress
- Cervix should be <3 cm dilated
- No medical or obstetrical contraindications such as pre-eclampsia or antepartum hemorrhage
- No intrauterine infection

Tocolytic therapy to arrest labour

Drugs used in the prevention of preterm labour are as follows:

- Beta-adrenergic agents
- Ritordine, salbutamol, terbutaline
- Calcium channel blockers
- Nifedipine
- Prostaglandin inhibitors
- Indomethacin
- Magnesium sulphate
- Nitroglycerin transdermal patch
- Oxytocin receptor antagonist–atosiban

The choice of therapy depends on the maternal condition, e.g., beta-mimetics are contraindicated in cardiac diseases; in diabetic patients, the control of blood sugar may be difficult. If there is polyhydramnios, indomethacin may be used as it reduces fetal urine output.

Calcium channel blocking agents

- Nifedipine is the first-line tocolytic therapy in the prevention of preterm labour.
- Calcium channel blockers act by relaxing the uterine smooth muscles. The co-administration of nifedipine and magnesium sulphate is not recommended as both are calcium channel blocking agents.
- A 20 mg loading dose of nifedipine is given orally followed by 10–20 mg 4–6 hourly.
- The side effects are minimal with a rise in heart rate and minimal decrease in BP which does not produce symptoms. There may be flushing, headache and sweating.

Prostaglandin inhibitors

- Anti-prostaglandin agents act by inhibiting the synthesis of prostaglandins or by blocking the action of prostaglandins on target organs. Indomethacin inhibits cyclo-oxygenase, thereby causing a decrease in prostaglandin levels and producing tocolysis.
- It is given in a dose of 50 mg orally as a loading dose, and then, 25 mg every 6 hours for 48 hours.
- The drug is not commonly used as there is an increased risk of premature closure of the neonatal ductus arteriosus and neonatal pulmonary hypertension. It may be useful in cases of polyhydramnios.
- Side effects include IVH, PDA and renal artery spasm. It can also cause PPH because of the antiplatelet activity of NSAIDs and the anti-prostaglandin effect on the myometrium.

Beta-adrenergic drugs

- These drugs are not commonly used nowadays because of their side effects.
- Drugs used in this category are ritodrine, salbutamol and terbutaline. They act by inhibiting uterine contractions by stimulating myometrial beta-2 receptors.
- Before initiating beta-adrenergic agonists, it is important to evaluate the cardiovascular system, ECG, hematocrit and electrolytes. These drugs should be used with caution in multiple pregnancy. They are absolutely contraindicated in cardiovascular diseases.
- Maternal side effects include palpitation, tremor, restlessness, glucose intolerance, hypokalemia, myocardial ischemia and pulmonary edema.
- Ritodrine is given in a dose of 50 mg in 500 mL of 5% dextrose through an infusion pump.
- While on these drugs, the following monitoring should be undertaken:
  — Pulse and BP should be recorded every 15 minutes

— Strict intake–output chart should be maintained
— Lung fields should be auscultated every 4 hours
— Blood glucose levels should be measured initially, then every 4 hours
— Urea and electrolytes should be measured every 2 hours

Magnesium sulphate

• Magnesium sulphate in high concentrations can alter myometrial contractility. It may be a useful choice in women in whom other agents are contraindicated, e.g., those with insulin-dependent diabetes. The drug is given in a loading dose of 4–6 g IV in 5% dextrose to run at 1–2 g per hour for not more than 48 hours.

• Careful monitoring of urine output, reflexes and respiratory depression is important.

Nitroglycerine transdermal patch

• It is a powerful smooth muscle relaxant. Though it has very few side effects such as hypotension, it is not widely used.

• A 50 mg patch is used and can be repeated in 2 hours if necessary.

• Monitoring of BP is important. No more than 2 patches are used in 24 hours.

• Side effects include headache and tachycardia.

Oxytocin receptor antagonist

• Atosiban selectively inhibits oxytocin receptors.

• The drug is given as an IV infusion of 300 micrograms/minute via an infusion pump.
The disadvantages of this drug are that it is expensive and can cause PPH.

All tocolytic drugs are administered for a period of 48–72 hours to give time for the corticosteroids to act.

Strategies to Improve Neonatal Outcomes

Besides tocolytic therapy, the following measures should be taken to improve the neonatal outcome.

• If facilities for neonatal care are inadequate, in utero transfer to a higher centre should be advised.

• Administration of corticosteroids—if the duration of pregnancy is less than 36 weeks, corticosteroid administration is indicated to prevent respiratory distress in the newborn. Corticosteroids enhance the production and release of pulmonary surfactants. The other beneficial effects of steroid use are reduced risk of necrotising enterocolitis, IVH, patent ductus arteriosus and periventricular leukomalacia. 24 mg

of betamethasone or dexamethasone is given in divided doses for 24 hours. Corticosteroids are contraindicated in the presence of GI bleeds, chorioamnionitis, tuberculosis, herpes and other viral infections. Caution should be exercised in diabetic and hypertensive pregnancies.

— Neuroprotection by magnesium sulphate—in order to reduce the risk of cerebral palsy, magnesium sulphate is given to the woman before 32 weeks of gestation for neuroprotection. A 4 g loading dose of a 10–20% solution is administered IV over 30 minutes. This is followed by a maintenance IV infusion of 1 g/hour over 24 hours. This is given between the gestational ages of 24–32 weeks. The infusion should not be continued for >24 hours. The monitoring is the same as that for pre-eclampsia, with careful monitoring of urine output, respiratory rate and reflexes.

— Antibiotics are prescribed in the presence of UTI or group B streptococcal infection, which is treated when the labour is established. However, antibiotics are not effective in preventing labour in women with preterm labour with intact membranes.

• Two doses of 12 mg betamethasone are given IM 24 hours apart.
OR
• Four doses of 6 mg dexamethasone are given 12 hours apart.

If there are no further changes and contractions stop, normal care is continued for the woman, and the baby is delivered at 37 weeks. Women are advised to return to the clinic in the case of contractions or rupture of membranes.

■ CONDUCT OF PRETERM DELIVERY

• Preterm infants require neonatal intensive care. If such facilities are not available and if the woman is not in active labour, she may be given corticosteroids and referred to a centre where neonatal facilities are available.

• Intrapartum management—preterm fetuses tolerate hypoxia poorly. Neonatal morbidity and mortality can be reduced by proper intrapartum fetal monitoring and care.

— Precipitate and prolonged labour should be avoided.

— Maternal hypotension should be avoided.

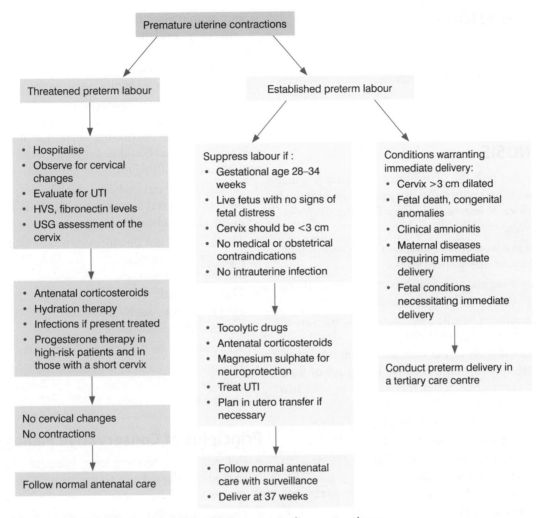

Fig. 24.1 Management of a woman presenting with preterm uterine contractions

— Hyperstimulation with oxytocin drugs should be avoided.

— Narcotics, sedation and analgesics should be avoided as they can depress the baby.

— The membranes should be kept intact as long as possible to prevent infection.

— CTG may show abnormal findings.

— A neonatologist should be available at the time of delivery.

— Episiotomy may be required when the fetal head reaches the perineum.

— The use of outlet forceps may be beneficial when epidural analgesia is used and if there are poor voluntary expulsive efforts in the second stage of labour.

— Vacuum should be avoided.

• Care of the newborn—this is described in Section VII.

PRETERM PREMATURE RUPTURE OF MEMBRANES (PPROM)

DEFINITION

Preterm premature rupture of membranes (PPROM) is defined as the rupture of membranes before 37 weeks of gestation and before the onset of labour. It accounts for 50% of all preterm births.

ETIOLOGY

• Increased intrauterine pressure as in multiple pregnancy, hydramnios, malpresentation
• Infections
• Procedures such as amniocentesis, fetoscopy
• Inherent weakness in the membranes as a result of collagen deficiency

■ COMPLICATIONS

The complications associated with PPROM are chorioamnionitis, abruption, increased induction and cesarean section rates and puerperal sepsis. The fetal complications include pulmonary hypoplasia, fetal and neonatal infection and cord compression in labour.

■ DIAGNOSIS

Sometimes, the passage of urine or excessive vaginal discharge may be confused with leakage of amniotic fluid. Therefore, it is essential to confirm the diagnosis by the following methods:

- Based on the woman's description of a gush of fluid followed by an intermittent trickle
- By placing a vaginal pad over the vulva and examining it (visually and by odour) after 1–2 hours
- By performing a sterile speculum examination to visualise the leakage of amniotic fluid—fluid may be seen coming from the cervix or forming a pool in the posterior fornix; there may be a gush of fluid from the cervical os when the woman is asked to cough
- By examining a smear of the fluid under the microscope to look for the presence of fine, floating vernix
- A few tests may be performed on the fluid to confirm the presence of amniotic fluid:
  — A simple dipstick assessment of pH >7.1 confirms alkalinity.
  — Nitrazine test to check the alkalinity of the amniotic fluid: Nitrazine yellow paper turns dark blue in the high pH range. If the fluid is alkaline (pH of 7.3–7.4), it is suggestive of amniotic fluid. Blood and some vaginal infections may give false-positive results.
  — Ferning test: A few drops of the fluid are spread on a slide and allowed to dry; the slide is then viewed under a microscope. Amniotic fluid crystallises, forming a fern-leaf pattern. False negatives are common.
  — Ultrasound examination may show decreased liquor or absence of liquor.
  — Fetal fibronectin: If negative, it is highly unlikely that the membranes have ruptured.

■ MANAGEMENT

The management of PPROM (Fig. 24.2) can be either conservative or active. Most women will go into labour within 4–7 days of PPROM. In the absence of infection, evidence of fetal distress and maternal contraindications, conservative management can be undertaken to delay delivery so that corticosteroids can be given to enhance fetal lung maturity. The aim of conservative management is to continue the pregnancy to near-34 weeks to improve the perinatal outcome without increasing maternal morbidity. The following criteria should be fulfilled for the conservative management of PPROM:

- A vaginal examination should not have been performed as it is associated with a four-fold increase in the risk of chorioamnionitis.
- There should not be any evidence of infection in the form of tachycardia, fever, foul-smelling discharge, uterine tenderness, etc.
- There should be no associated complications of pregnancy such as severe pre-eclampsia or antepartum hemorrhage.
- There should be no fetal malformations.
- The maternal risks and neonatal benefits should be explained to the woman and her informed consent obtained.

Principles of Conservative Management

- Referral to a tertiary care hospital: The woman should be referred to a centre with neonatal intensive care facilities.
- Use of antibiotics: Antibiotics are beneficial for decreasing maternal and fetal infective morbidity. Intravenous antibiotics are given for three days, followed by oral administration for four days (a total of seven days). The preferred drugs are amoxicillin and erythromycin.
- Corticosteroids: They are administered in the dosage described earlier for preterm labour. The only absolute contraindication of steroid use is suspected chorioamnionitis.
- Tocolysis: In the case of established labour, tocolytic agents may be used when indicated.
- Monitoring for the onset of sepsis: While the woman is on conservative management, efforts should be made to diagnose the onset of sepsis early. Her temperature should be recorded at least four times a day and her leukocyte count should be estimated twice weekly to look for leukocytosis. A cervical swab (once weekly) should be taken to detect pathogenic organisms. The presence of any unhealthy vaginal discharge indicates sepsis.

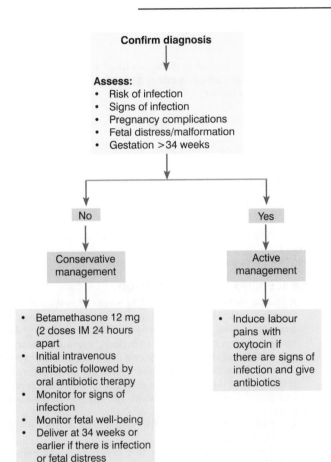

Assess:
- Risk of infection
- Signs of infection
- Pregnancy complications
- Fetal distress/malformation
- Gestation >34 weeks

No → Conservative management

- Betamethasone 12 mg (2 doses IM 24 hours apart
- Initial intravenous antibiotic followed by oral antibiotic therapy
- Monitor for signs of infection
- Monitor fetal well-being
- Deliver at 34 weeks or earlier if there is infection or fetal distress

Yes → Active management

- Induce labour pains with oxytocin if there are signs of infection and give antibiotics

Fig. 24.2 Management of preterm premature rupture of membranes

- Assessment of fetal well-being: The non-stress test should be performed daily. USG assessment is important to identify the presentation and to assess the growth, amniotic fluid volume and fetal breathing movement and to rule out anomalies.
- Indications for delivery: At any time, if there is a suspicion of sepsis or if the period of gestation reaches 34 weeks, conservative management must be abandoned, and the woman should be delivered with oxytocin infusion.

Active Management

Active management is undertaken when the woman establishes labour or when there is evidence of sepsis, fetal distress or CTG abnormalities.

- When a woman is unsuitable for conservative management, labour pains should be induced with oxytocin after administering corticosteroids for fetal lung maturation.
- Cesarean section is reserved for obstetric indication only.

KEY POINTS

✓ *Preterm labour is defined as the presence of painful uterine contractions associated with progressive effacement and dilatation of the cervix occurring after the period of viability (24 weeks of gestation) and before the completion of 37 weeks of gestation.*

✓ *Preterm births are associated with increased perinatal morbidity and mortality.*

✓ *Maternal systemic diseases, infections, uterine malformations and pregnancy complications such as multiple pregnancy, hydramnios and antepartum hemorrhage contribute to preterm labour.*

✓ *In nearly 1/3rd of cases, preterm birth is indicated because of medical and obstetrical complications that necessitate delivery. In 2/3rd of cases, preterm delivery is spontaneous.*

✓ *The criteria for preterm labour are contractions occurring at a frequency of 4 in 20 minutes or 8 in 60 minutes with changes in the cervix, cervical dilatation greater than 1 cm and cervical effacement of 80% or more.*

✓ *In women presenting with established labour, one has to make a decision whether labour should be allowed to progress or if it should be suppressed to prolong pregnancy.*

✓ *Nifedipine is the first-line tocolytic drug used to suppress preterm labour.*

✓ *Labour should be conducted in a setting where neonatal facilities are available.*

✓ *Preterm premature rupture of membranes (PPROM) is defined as the rupture of membranes before 37 weeks of gestation and before the onset of labour. It accounts for 50% of all preterm births.*

Essay questions

1. Discuss in detail the etiology, diagnosis and management of preterm labour with intact membranes.
2. Discuss the causes, diagnosis and management of preterm premature rupture of membranes.

Short answer questions

1. What is the role of the administration of corticosteroids in the management of preterm labour?
2. What is the role of tocolytic agents in the management of preterm labour?

3. What are the indications and contraindications of tocolytic use?
4. Define preterm labour and enumerate its causes and risk factors.
5. Describe the diagnosis of preterm premature rupture of membranes.
6. Discuss the predictors, diagnosis and prevention of preterm labour.
7. Define PPROM and discuss its diagnosis and management.

MCQs

1. Preterm labour is defined as regular uterine contractions with dilatation of the cervix after:
   a) 12 weeks
   b) 20 weeks
   c) 24 weeks
   d) 28 weeks
2. Raised prostaglandin activity leading to preterm labour is noted in all except:
   a) Intrauterine infection
   b) Oligohydramnios
   c) Multiple pregnancy
   d) Antepartum hemorrhage
3. The risk of preterm labour at 24 weeks is more with a cervical length of:
   a) <25 mm
   b) <30 mm
   c) <35 mm
   d) <40 mm
4. Which of the following is not a diagnostic criterion of preterm labour?
   a) Four uterine contractions in 20 minutes
   b) Cervical dilation >1 cm
   c) Engaged head
   d) Cervical effacement >80%
5. Which of the following is the most sensitive marker to predict preterm birth?
   a) Fibronectin
   b) Serum ferritin
   c) hCG
   d) Salivary estriol
6. Which of these is not a tocolytic agent?
   a) Atosiban
   b) Labetalol
   c) Magnesium sulphate
   d) Nifedipine
7. In which of the following conditions is tocolysis not recommended?
   a) Gestational age <37 weeks
   b) Cervical dilatation <3 cm
   c) Evidence of chorioamnionitis
   d) No sign of fetal distress
8. Which of the following is not recommended for the delivery of a preterm infant?
   a) Episiotomy
   b) Vacuum delivery
   c) Forceps delivery
   d) Epidural analgesia
9. Which of the following pH is suggestive of amniotic fluid?
   a) 5.5
   b) 6.5
   c) 7.0
   d) 7.5
10. Which of the following tocolytics has the least side effects?
    a) Beta-sympathomimetic drugs
    b) Indomethacin
    c) Nifedipine
    d) Magnesium sulphate

Answers
1. (c), 2. (b), 3. (a), 4. (c), 5. (a), 6. (b), 7. (c), 8. (b), 9. (d), 10. (c)

Fill in the blanks

1. In the management of preterm labour, the main aim of the administration of corticosteroids is _____.
2. The drug used for neuroprotection is _____ .

Answers
1. improving lung maturity,   2. magnesium sulphate

Case scenario-based discussion

1. A 28-year-old G2P1 presents at 32 weeks of gestation with intermittent lower abdominal pain and pelvic pressure with a mucoid vaginal discharge. In her past obstetric history, she had a full-term normal vaginal delivery without antenatal and intrapartum complications and delivered at term. In the present pregnancy, she has been suffering from recurrent urinary tract infections. On vaginal examination, the cervix was 1 cm long and 2 cm dilated, and the membranes are intact.
   a) What is the probable diagnosis? What could be the etiological factor involved?
   b) How would you manage this pregnancy? Enumerate the tocolytic drugs you would use.
   c) What are the other medications used to improve the neonatal prognosis?
   d) If the labour does not get arrested, how would you conduct the delivery?
   e) What are the complications of preterm delivery?

Answers
a) The woman is exhibiting signs of preterm labour—the cervix is nearly 80% effaced and 2 cm dilated. Therefore, she is in established labour. The probable cause could be recurrent urinary tract infection.
b) One has to make a decision whether labour should be allowed to progress or if it should be suppressed to prolong pregnancy. Conditions warranting immediate delivery are: a cervix >3 cm dilated, fetal death, congenital anomalies, amnionitis and maternal and fetal indications necessitating deliveries. In all other cases, labour can be suppressed. The medications used in the suppression of labour are beta-adrenergic agents such as ritodrine, salbutamol, terbutaline, calcium channel blockers, nifedipine, prostaglandin inhibitors such as indomethacin, magnesium sulphate and nitroglycerine transdermal patch and oxytocin receptor antagonists such as atosiban.
c) Antenatal corticosteroids should be administered to enhance lung maturity and magnesium sulphate should be prescribed for neuroprotection.
d) Labour should be conducted in a setting where neonatal facilities are available. Care should be taken to avoid precipitate, prolonged labour, hypotension and hyperstimulation of the uterus. Narcotics, sedation and analgesics should be avoided as they can depress the baby. A neonatologist should be available at the time of delivery.
e) The risks associated with preterm births are RDS, sepsis, hypothermia, hypoglycemia, hypocalcemia, hyperbilirubinemia, PDA, IVH, necrotising enterocolitis and delayed sequelae such as neurological deficits and hearing and visual disturbances.

25 Fetal Growth Restriction

OG 4.1, OG 8.3,
OG 8.4, OG 16.3

Learning Objectives

» To know the phases of normal fetal growth
» To know the definitions of small-for-gestational age (SGA), average-for-gestational age (AGA) and large-for-gestational age (LGA) babies
» To know how to differentiate between fetal growth restriction and the constitutionally small baby
» To know the types and causes of fetal growth restriction
» To know the assessment of fetal growth and well-being during pregnancy
» To know the management of FGR

■ INTRODUCTION

Fetal growth restriction (FGR), which was previously known as intrauterine growth restriction (IUGR), is a condition wherein the fetus fails to reach its genetic growth potential and consequently, is at an increased risk of perinatal morbidity and mortality. This may result in a fetus that is small for gestational age (SGA). It is estimated that 3–10% of infants are growth-restricted.

■ DEFINITIONS

- Fetuses whose weight is between the 10th and 90th percentile for their gestational age are called average-for-gestational age (AGA) fetuses.
- Fetuses whose weight is above the 90th percentile for their gestational age are called large-for-gestational age (LGA) fetuses.
- Fetuses whose weight is below the 10th percentage for the gestational age are called small-for-gestational age (SGA). SGA includes fetuses that are genetically small (normal small fetus) and growth-restricted fetuses (FGR).
- The most common definition of SGA is EFW or AC below the 10th percentile for the gestational age (of the given reference ranges).

Constitutionally Small Fetus

This is a normal fetus that is genetically small but has achieved its growth potential. This is constitutional as fetal growth may be influenced by maternal build and ethnicity.

Fetal Growth Restriction

This refers to a fetus that has failed to achieve its genetic growth potential due to some underlying pathological process. Fetal growth restriction is defined as a condition wherein the fetal weight is below the tenth percentile or two standard deviations for gestational age. The appropriate reference is to use the 'normal' ranges for the local population since there may be ethnic variations. Fetuses whose birth weight is below the 10th percentile are at an increased risk of stillbirth and perinatal mortality; among these, fetuses whose birth weight is below the 3rd percentile are at the highest risk. Therefore, some organisations use the fetal size at the lower extreme of the growth charts, for example, AC or EFW below the 3rd percentile, as an isolated criterion to define FGR.

■ THE GROWTH PATTERN OF A NORMAL FETUS

Fetal growth occurs in three phases, which are as follows:

- **Phase I:** The cellular hyperplasia phase is characterised by an increase in cell number and new cell formation and lasts for the first 16 weeks of gestation.
- **Phase II:** It is the phase of concomitant hyperplasia and hypertrophy and occurs between weeks 16 and 32 of gestation. In this phase, there is continuous multiplication of new cells as well as an increase in the size of the existing cells.
- **Phase III:** The cellular hypertrophy phase, which occurs between weeks 32 and term, is characterised by a rapid increase in cell size. During this phase, most of the fetal glycogen and fat deposition takes place. The corresponding growth rates during these three phases are 5 g/day at 15 weeks, 15–20 g/day at 24 weeks, and 30–35 g/day at 34 weeks.

THE EFFECTS OF FETAL GROWTH RESTRICTION

Fetal growth restriction is one of the major causes of perinatal deaths. FGR babies have significant morbidity due to hypoglycemia, hypothermia, thrombocytopenia, polycythemia, hyperbilirubinemia, hypocalcemia and perinatal asphyxia. Neurodevelopmental delay can occur as a delayed complication.

TYPES OF FETAL GROWTH RESTRICTION

FGR is classified depending on the pathological process and the time of onset.

Type I or Symmetrical or Intrinsic IUGR

- It accounts for 20–30% of FGR and occurs as a result of factors affecting the growth of the fetus early in pregnancy, during which time, hyperplasia predominates.
- Here, the sizes of the fetal organs are decreased proportionally due to impairment of early fetal cellular hyperplasia and growth.
- These neonates have anthropometric measurements below the tenth percentile for the gestational age.
- The majority of these babies have some intrinsic pathology such as intrauterine infections (TORCH), chromosomal disorders and congenital malformations. Twenty-five per cent of those with severe, early-onset FGR have aneuploidy.
- This is called symmetrical growth restriction since all organs including the brain are equally affected. The head and abdominal size are proportionately decreased. There is a decrease in the overall size of the fetus.
- This type of growth restriction is usually evident in the second or early third trimester.

Type II or Asymmetrical or Extrinsic FGR

- It accounts for 70–80% of FGR and occurs as a result of uteroplacental insufficiency. In this type, there is brain-sparing growth restriction.
- It is characterised by a relatively greater decrease in abdominal size than in head circumference. Asymmetric growth occurs due to the redistribution of blood flow in favour of the vital organs (e.g., brain, heart and placenta) at the expense of non-vital fetal organs (e.g., abdominal viscera, lungs, skin and kidneys).

- The causes of type II FGR are chronic hypertension, vasculopathy and renal diseases. This type leads to chronic hypoxia and fetal death.
- Asymmetrical FGR is recognised only in the third trimester.

The differences between symmetrical and asymmetrical FGR are listed in Table 25.1.

Table 25.1 Differences between symmetrical and asymmetrical FGR

Characteristic	Symmetrical FGR	Asymmetrical FGR
Incidence	20–30%	70–80%
Growth inhibition	Occurs early in pregnancy—in the hyperplastic stage	Usually occurs late in the pregnancy—28 weeks and after, in the hypertrophic stage
Number of cells	Reduced	Near-normal number of cells but smaller in size
Growth parameters	HC/AC ratio and weight/length ratio are below tenth percentile	Brain-sparing effect and hence HC/AC ratio altered
Ponderal index	Normal	Low
Associated with	• Early intrauterine infections like cytomegalovirus, rubella and toxoplasmosis • Chromosomal abnormalities • Anemia • Maternal substance abuse	• Chronic high blood pressure (pre-eclampsia/PIH) • Severe malnutrition • Genetic mutation, • Ehlers–Danlos syndrome
Baby size	Uniformly small	Head is normal; the rest of the body is thin and small

Intermediate FGR

In this type of FGR, both the types of growth restriction are seen. Intermediate FGR occurs in approximately 5–10% of all cases of IUGR.

FGR is also classified as **early-onset** or **late-onset**, depending on the time of onset, whether before 32 weeks or after 32 weeks of gestation respectively.

ETIOLOGY

FGR can be caused by genetic and environmental factors or due to a decrease in the supply of oxygen and nutrients from the mother. This interferes with cell proliferation, organ differentiation and maturation. There are several maternal, fetal and placental complications known to be associated with fetal growth restriction. However, in about 20–30% of cases, no risk factor may be identified. Table 25.2 lists the various causes of FGR.

Maternal Factors

Maternal nutrition

Malnutrition is an important cause of FGR. A woman should consume an additional 300 Kcal/day during pregnancy to gain the adequate amount of weight. Protein intake should also be adequate. Being underweight before pregnancy and poor weight gain during pregnancy are associated with FGR.

Substance abuse and cigarette smoking

Maternal cigarette smoking, alcohol consumption and illicit drug use can cause FGR. Smoking causes increased carboxyhemoglobin, which reduces the release of oxygen to the fetus. Cocaine causes vasoconstriction, which has deleterious effect on the fetus.

Uteroplacental insufficiency

A low impedance of blood flow is necessary for the developing fetus to receive an adequate supply of nutrients and gas exchange. Uteroplacental insufficiency could be caused by a number of medical conditions affecting the mother and leading to FGR.

Chronic hypertension, pre-eclampsia, pregestational diabetes, collagen vascular disorders, renal conditions and immunological causes such as antiphospholipid antibody (APLA) syndrome are associated with uteroplacental insufficiency. In pre-eclampsia, there is a failure of trophoblastic invasion of the spiral arteries, which leads to a failure of dilation of these vessels. This results in increased resistance to blood flow and diminished uteroplacental perfusion. In APLA syndrome, there is thrombosis of the intervillous space, which results in a decrease in the uteroplacental perfusion.

Chronic maternal hypoxia

There could be chronic maternal hypoxia due to pulmonary diseases such as bronchial asthma, cyanotic heart disease, hemoglobinopathies and severe anemia which are often associated with FGR. People living in high altitudes also suffer from chronic hypoxia.

Maternal medications

Drugs such as anticonvulsants, anticoagulants, folic acid antagonists and antineoplastic agents can adversely affect the fetal growth.

Uterine factors

Sub-optimal placentation can occur in cases of fibroids complicating pregnancy and congenital malformations of the uterus such as bicornuate and unicornuate uterus.

Others

- Socio-demographic variables: Various demographic variables are associated with an increased risk of delivering growth-restricted fetuses; these include race and pregnancy at the extremes of reproductive ages.
- Obstetric history: A previous delivery of a growth-restricted neonate increases the risk of FGR in the current pregnancy. The risk of recurrence of FGR is nearly 30% here.
- Raised alpha-fetoprotein levels: Raised alpha-fetoprotein levels at 16 weeks of gestation in the absence of the congenital anomalies increases the risk of FGR.

Fetal Factors

Chromosomal abnormalities

Nearly 25% of fetuses with severe early-onset FGR are chromosomally abnormal. Autosomal trisomies account for >80% of chromosomal abnormalities of FGR; trisomy 21 is the commonest.

Congenital malformations

Around 20–25% of fetuses with major congenital malformations are associated with growth restriction.

Multiple pregnancy

Pregnancies with two or more fetuses are more likely to be complicated by the diminished growth of one or more fetuses than singleton pregnancies. More than 15% of FGR is reported in multiple pregnancy. In multiple pregnancy, there is a decrease in the placental mass in relation to the fetal mass.

Pregnancy following assisted reproductive techniques

Even singleton pregnancies conceived via assisted reproductive technologies have a higher prevalence of low birth weight due to prematurity and FGR.

Fetal infections

Viral, bacterial, protozoan and spirochetal infections have been known to affect intrauterine fetal growth in approximately 5–10 % of cases. Among viral infections, cytomegalovirus and rubella are the important ones. The important protozoal infections include toxoplasmosis and malaria. Listeriosis, tuberculosis, chickenpox and syphilis have also been reported to cause fetal growth restriction. Maternal infections that develop early in pregnancy have the maximum adverse effects on the fetus.

Placental Factors

Circumvallate placenta, placenta previa, placental infarction and chorioangioma of the placenta are likely to be associated with FGR due to the decreased surface area available for the exchange of nutrients. Abnormal cord insertion such as marginal insertion of the cord/velamentous insertion may be associated with FGR.

Table 25.2 The etiological factors responsible for FGR

Maternal causes	Fetal causes	Placental causes
Maternal nutrition	Chromosomal abnormalities	Placenta previa
Smoking and substance abuse	Congenital malformations	Circumvallate placenta
Uteroplacental insufficiency	Fetal infections	Placental infarction
Maternal chronic hypoxia	Multiple pregnancy	Chorioangioma of the placenta
Maternal medications	Pregnancy following assisted reproductive techniques	Abnormal cord insertions
Uterine causes		
Others		

▌ DIAGNOSIS OF FETAL GROWTH RESTRICTION

In the First Trimester

Women at risk of FGR should be identified in the first booking visit. Risk factors include the following:

- Extremes of maternal age
- Low BMI at booking
- Previous FGR infant, stillbirth, pre-eclampsia
- Maternal habits—smoking and substance abuse
- Maternal medical conditions—essential hypertension, pregestational diabetes, renal disorders, anemia, cardiac disease, thrombophilia
- Early trimester bleeding
- Investigations showing raised alpha-fetoprotein before 16 weeks of pregnancy with a normal fetus

Estimation of gestational age

- The accurate estimation of the gestational age is critical for the diagnosis of FGR.
- If the gestational age is unknown, measurements of fetal long bones, orbital diameters, and the transverse cerebellar diameter can assist the clinician in evaluating gestational age and growth.

Accuracy of the methods used to assess the gestational age

- IVF: <1 day
- Crown–rump length by USG between 6–14 weeks: ±5–7 days
- BPD before 20 weeks: ±5–7 days
- BPD between 20 and 26 weeks: ±1.6 weeks
- BPD after 26 weeks: 3–4 weeks

Identification of Fetal Growth Restriction

Fetal growth assessment is important for the diagnosis of FGR. Clinical methods and biometric assessment by USG are used to diagnose FGR.

Clinical parameters to suspect growth restriction of the fetus

- Static weight or weight loss during pregnancy
- Reduced liquor volume by clinical examination
- Height of the uterus by abdominal palpation
- Symphysiofundal height measurement

Uterine fundal height

- The serial measurement of fundal height performed carefully throughout pregnancy is a simple, safe, inexpensive and reasonably accurate screening method to detect small-for-gestational age (SGA) fetuses.
- On abdominal palpation, if the height of the uterus is less by 4 weeks than the expected gestational age, growth restriction should be suspected.

Measurement of symphysiofundal height

Symphisiofundal height measurement can be taken serially to screen for FGR. The technique for the measurement of symphysiofundal height is as follows:

- The woman is asked to empty her bladder.
- Dextrorotation, if present should be corrected.
- The fundus of the uterus is identified by the ulnar border of the left hand.
- A non-elastic tape calibrated in centimetres is placed over the abdominal curvature from the fundus to the upper edge of the symphysis (Fig. 25.1).
- The uterine height in centimetres coincides with the weeks of gestation between 18 and 34 weeks. If there is a discrepancy of 2–3 cm, inadequate fetal growth may be suspected. The serial fundal height is plotted on a graph and is known as a **gravidogram** (Fig. 25.2).

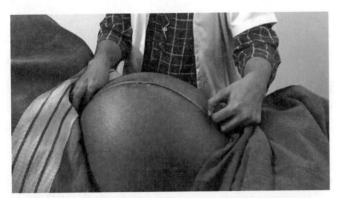

Fig. 25.1   Measurement of the symphysiofundal height

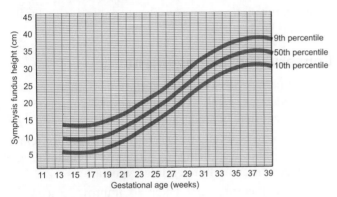

Fig. 25.2   A gravidogram

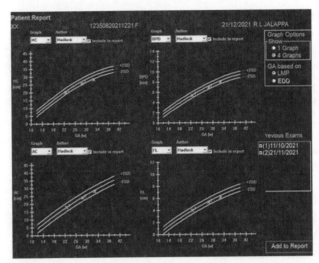

Fig. 25.3   Fetal growth chart with head circumference, BPD, abdominal circumference and femur length serially measured and plotted on a graph (*Image courtesy:* Dr B H Parameshwar Keerthi, Consultant Radiologist, BM Scans, Kancheepuram)

Fetal biometric measurements by USG

When FGR is suspected on clinical grounds based on risk factors and physical examination, biometric measurements by USG are carried out to diagnose SGA and FGR fetuses.

Diagnosis and evaluation for FGR in low-risk patients

Routine growth scan and EFW at 32–34 weeks of gestation in all low-risk pregnancies help in the early diagnosis of FGR.

Diagnosis of FGR in high-risk patients

For all pregnancies with high-risk factors, serial biometric assessment of the fetus is done from 26–28 weeks onwards. In general, measurements are taken every 3–4 weeks and plotted on a chart. Customised charts suitable for the particular population should be used (Fig. 25.3).

- In cases where FGR is diagnosed or suspected, serial scans are necessary every 2 weeks.
- The biometric parameters used for the diagnosis of FGR are as follows:
  — Head circumference (HC)
  — Biparietal diameter (BPD)
  — Abdominal circumference (AC)
  — Femur length (FL)
  — Estimated fetal weight (EFW)
  — HC/AC, FL/AC ratio
  — Assessment of the interval growth
- In a fetus with normal growth, the measurements will fall between the 10th and the 90th percentile and the interval growth will be maintained.
- In an SGA fetus, the measurements fall below the 10th percentile. However, the interval growth is maintained in a fetus that is constitutionally small, whereas in a growth-restricted fetus, the interval growth may be reduced.

Abdominal circumference (AC)

AC is the most sensitive indicator of fetal growth and fetal restriction. AC is the most affected parameter in FGR because of the reduction in the adipose tissue and depletion of glycogen in the fetal liver. AC below the 10th percentile is suspicious and below the 3rd percentile is diagnostic of FGR.

Femur length (FL)

In situations where early gestational age assessment was not possible, femur length measurement can be used for gestational age assessment and to diagnose FGR.

Estimated fetal weight (EFW)

Computer-based estimation of the fetal weight is achieved using the biometric parameters AC, BPD, HC and FL. EFW below the 10th percentile is suggestive of SGA/FGR.

HC/AC ratio

The HC/AC ratio is useful for the diagnosis of FGR and to differentiate asymmetrical growth restriction from symmetrical growth restriction. The HC/AC ratio decreases linearly throughout normal pregnancy. In a normal fetus, the HC/AC ratio is >1 before 32 weeks of gestation, nearly 1 between 32–34 weeks of gestation and, due to the rapid growth of the liver, <1 after 34 weeks of gestation. In growth-restricted fetuses, the size of the liver tends to be disproportionately small as compared to the circumference of the head or the length of the femur, which are initially spared from the effects of nutritional deficiency. In these cases, the HC/AC is more than normal. A ratio of greater than two standard deviations (SD) above the mean for gestational age suggests asymmetric FGR. In symmetric FGR, the ratio remains the same as both HC and AC are affected equally.

FC/AC ratio

The femur length is also spared in asymmetric FGR. Therefore, increasing FL/AC ratio suggests asymmetrical growth restriction.

Amniotic fluid volume measurements

Oligohydramnios refers to amniotic fluid volume that is less than expected for the gestational age. Oligohydramnios occurs in FGR due to reduced renal blood flow and diminished fetal urine production. Pregnancies with the most severe oligohydramnios have the highest perinatal mortality rate.

Doppler velocimetry studies

Abnormal umbilical artery Doppler velocimetry, as characterised by increased systolic–diastolic ratio and absent or reverse end-diastolic flow, is correlated with poor perinatal outcome. Amniotic fluid volume measurement and Doppler studies are more valuable for the assessment of well-being of the fetus. Constitutionally small babies can also be diagnosed at this stage based on the presence of normal interval growth, normal amniotic fluid volume and normal Doppler indices.

■ MANAGEMENT OF FGR

Management should be tailored to the individual. Delay in delivery increases the risk of intrauterine death, whereas early intervention might lead to death from prematurity. It is important to decide the timing of delivery before fetal deterioration. The management of FGR (Fig. 25.4) depends on the following factors:

- Gestational age at diagnosis
- Estimated fetal weight
- The underlying etiology and the associated morbidity
- The severity of FGR

Indications for Immediate Delivery

- If the woman has severe pre-eclampsia, hypertension, uncontrolled bleeding or other morbidities necessitating delivery, irrespective of the period of gestation, the baby should be delivered immediately.
- If the fetus is severely compromised, as shown by Doppler velocimetry studies, it should be delivered without delay.
- All mature fetuses >37 weeks diagnosed with FGR should be delivered.

Conservative Management

- In fetuses <37 weeks of gestation, if there is no maternal or fetal contraindication, conservative treatment may be undertaken.
- These fetuses should be carefully monitored for fetal growth and well-being to diagnose deteriorating fetal condition and impending hypoxia.
- General measures are taken to improve placental blood flow.
- The decisions on the timing and mode of delivery should be made carefully.

General Measures

Rest

Bed rest in the left lateral position is believed to increase the uteroplacental flow. This is particularly important in developing countries like India where women may not be able to get adequate rest during pregnancy. Theoretically, bed rest results in the diversion of blood flow from the periphery to the central circulation, which in turn, increases the uteroplacental circulation.

Maternal oxygen therapy

Maternal administration of 55% oxygen at the rate of 8 L/min continuously has been shown to improve fetal oxygenation and decrease perinatal mortality. It may be useful in medical conditions such as bronchial asthma and cyanotic heart disease to improve oxygenation.

Pharmacotherapy

Low-dose aspirin (1–2 mg/Kg/day), betamimetics, heparin and calcium channel blockers have all been attempted, but with no significant clinical improvement. The use of low-dose aspirin may improve placental circulation in cases of APLA syndrome.

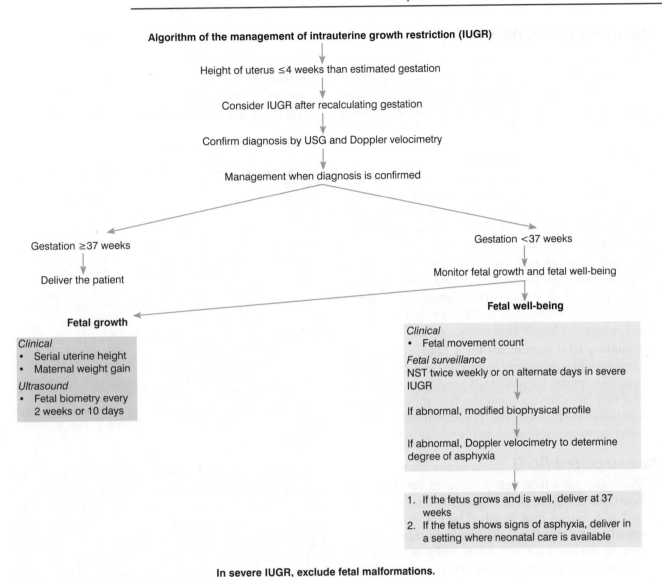

Fig. 25.4   Algorithm of the management of intrauterine growth restriction (IUGR)

Maternal nutrition supplementation

Poor nutrition resulting in poor weight gain during pregnancy leads to intrauterine growth restriction. Nutritional supplementation in the form of orally administered calories and protein supplements may have a modest effect on increasing birth weight. Hyperalimentation with 10% glucose and 12% amino acids may increase the fetal weight. Zinc supplementation and fish oil supplementation have also been tried.

Treatment of Associated Maternal Conditions

Maternal factors such as anemia and hypertension that contribute to FGR should be treated.

Monitoring Fetal Growth

Once the diagnosis of FGR is made, fetal growth needs to be monitored by clinical and ultrasound parameters serially.

- Fetal growth is assessed based on weekly maternal weight gain and fundal height measurement plotted on a gravidogram (Fig. 25.2).
- Ultrasound assessment, the more objective method of assessing fetal growth, should be continued. The biparietal diameter, head circumference, femur length and abdominal circumference should be measured serially every 10–14 days and plotted on a chart to see if there is any improvement in fetal growth (Fig. 25.3). It is also important to exclude any fetal malformations that may be associated with FGR.

Monitoring Fetal Well-Being

IUGR fetuses are more prone to fetal hypoxia and fetal death. Therefore, the careful serial monitoring of fetal well-being by antepartum fetal surveillance is important. Timely intervention should be undertaken when hypoxia is suspected.

Daily fetal movement count

The ability of the pregnant woman to feel the fetal movement is a reassuring indicator of fetal well-being. Therefore, the woman may be advised to keep track of the fetal movements. There are several methods by which fetal movements can be counted.

- **Cardiff count to ten:** The woman records the time taken each day to feel 10 movements. Usually, this takes 2–3 hours. The failure to perceive 10 movements during a 12-hour period needs assessment by biophysical methods.
- **Counting fetal movements for 1 hour everyday:** As the pregnant woman may find it cumbersome to count fetal movements for prolonged periods or repeatedly, she may be asked to count the fetal movements for one hour every day. The perception of 3–4 fetal movements in a 1-hour period is reassuring.

Non-stress test (NST)

- The term non-stress test is used to describe fetal heart rate acceleration in response to fetal movement and is a sign of fetal health. The non-stress test is based on the hypothesis that the heart rate of a fetus that is not acidotic will temporarily accelerate in response to a fetal movement. This is recorded with the help of a cardiotocograph.
- A normal or reactive non-stress test is defined as one in which there are two or more accelerations of the heart rate (15 beats or more), each lasting 15 seconds or more, with fetal movements within 20 minutes of testing. To account for fetal sleep cycles, the recording may have to be continued for 40 minutes before diagnosing non-reactive CTG.
- Although a normal number and amplitude of accelerations seem to reflect fetal well-being, 'insufficient accelerations' do not necessarily predict fetal compromise. Whenever the non-stress test is non-reactive, further evaluation by other methods needs to be done.

Biophysical profile (Manning's score)

The combined use of fetal biophysical variables is a more accurate means of assessing fetal health than a single parameter used alone. The variables used are presented in Table 25.3.

- Fetal heart rate accelerations (non-stress test)
- Fetal breathing fetal movements
- Fetal tone
- Amniotic fluid volume
  A score of 2 or 0 is assigned to each variable.

Table 25.3 Biophysical profile

Variables	Score 2	Score 0
Non-stress test	Reactive	Non-reactive
Fetal breathing	One or more episodes of rhythmic breathing lasting 30 seconds or more within 30 minutes	Less than 30 seconds of breathing in 30 minutes
Fetal movement	Three or more body or limb movements in 30 minutes	Two or less movements within 30 minutes
Fetal tone	One or more episodes of movements or extension of a fetal extremity with return to flexion, or closing or opening of hand	No extension/flexion
Amniotic fluid volume	Single vertical pocket >2 cm	Largest single pocket of 2 cm or less

A biophysical score of zero is invariably associated with significant fetal acidemia, whereas normal scores of 8 or 10 are associated with normal pH. Of all the variables in the biophysical profile, amniotic fluid volume is the most important. Occasionally, a modified biophysical profile is used, wherein only the non-stress test and the measurement of amniotic fluid volume alone may be done.

Amniotic fluid volume (AFV) measurement

AFV is an important parameter to assess fetal well-being as it is a reflection of fetal urine production. Oligohydramnios occurs due to decreased renal perfusion with a resultant chronic reduction in urine production. In FGR, blood is deviated from the kidney to other organs, resulting in reduced urine production. Decreasing AFV indicates a deteriorating intrauterine environment.

Diagnosis of oligohydramnios

- A vertical pocket of <1 cm
- AFI—the sum of four quadrant vertical pockets of <5 cm

Doppler velocimetry of umbilical arteries

With the deterioration of the fetal condition, the first abnormality to manifest is an abnormal Doppler study of the umbilical and cerebral arteries. This is followed by variations in fetal heart rate and body movements; the breathing movements are the last to become abnormal.

Doppler assesses the hemodynamic status of the fetus and is useful for assessing the well-being of the baby. The blood flow studies of the umbilical arteries not only differentiate healthy fetuses from those with impending hypoxia, but they can also help in the identification of SGA fetuses that are constitutionally small.

Umbilical artery blood flow studies

- In a healthy pregnancy, the umbilical artery blood flow is characterised by minimal vascular resistance. There is a high diastolic flow, and by the end of pregnancy, the end-diastolic flow is increased.
- When there is uteroplacental insufficiency, there is increased impedance, resulting in decreased blood flow with elevated systolic/diastolic (S/D) ratio. SGA fetuses with normal S/D ratio may be constitutionally small and do not suffer from the morbidity of FGR.
- With increasing impedance in the umbilical artery blood flow, absent end diastolic volume (AEDV) and reverse diastolic flow (RDF) develop.
- The following indices are calculated from the Doppler studies:
  - S/D ratio
  - Pulsatility index: S-D/mean velocity
  - Resistance index: S-D/S
- If the impedance to blood flow is increased, all three indices are increased, followed by absent flow and then, reversal of flow.

Cerebral circulation

In healthy pregnancies, the resistance to flow is greater in the cerebral vessels than it is in the umbilical vessels. In growth-restricted fetuses with hypoxia, the diastolic blood flow increases and therefore, the resistance indices decrease.

Obstetric Intervention

If the fetal growth is satisfactory and the fetal surveillance tests indicate that the fetus is not in distress, the pregnancy is allowed to continue until 37 weeks. However, if the fetus is not in good condition, early delivery is indicated. Management should be in a place where there are adequate facilities for cesarean and neonatal care and experienced personnel are available.

Management of Late-Onset Growth Restriction

- In any pregnancy that has advanced to 37 weeks or more at the time of the diagnosis of FGR, delivery of the fetus is required.

- FGR fetuses diagnosed before 37 weeks are monitored for interval growth and fetal well-being. BPP is performed 1–2 times a week and umbilical artery Doppler is performed 1–3 times a week. To enhance lung maturity, corticosteroids are administered to fetuses <36 weeks of gestation. Many guidelines and studies recommend magnesium sulphate prophylaxis for neuroprotection in growth-restricted fetuses.
- If the growth restriction is mild and uncomplicated and the antepartum fetal testing results are reassuring, the fetus can be delivered at 37 weeks. At any gestational age, if one of the following is present at a follow-up, the baby should be delivered immediately:
  - Arrest of growth over a 2–4-week interval
  - Spontaneous repeated persistent unprovoked fetal heart rate decelerations
  - Altered BPP (score ≤ 4)
  - Maternal indication (e.g., severe pre-eclampsia, HELLP syndrome) or obstetric emergency requiring delivery

Mode of delivery

The mode of delivery depends on the severity of growth restriction and the assessment of fetal well-being.

- If it is diagnosed as mild IUGR, where the fetus is not under stress as determined by tests of fetal well-being, labour can be induced, and vaginal delivery attempted.
- However, if the fetus is severely growth restricted, then cesarean section with good neonatal back-up would improve the chances of fetal survival.

Induction of labour

In the absence of contraindications, the induction of labour can be undertaken. It is preferable to induce labour with a Foley catheter, as pharmacological agents may cause hyperstimulation of the uterus.

Labour management

- Continuous CTG monitoring is important in the management of FGR. Because of oligohydramnios, there is a risk of cord compression. FHR abnormalities may be noted due to cord compression and meconium-stained liquor.
- Oxygen therapy and maternal hydration during labour may be helpful.

Indications for cesarean section in FGR

- Severe fetal compromise diagnosed at any period of gestation

- Fetal compromise/distress diagnosed in labour
- Other obstetric indications such as malpresentations

Management of Early-Onset Growth Restriction

Early-onset growth restriction includes the following:

- Asymmetrical FGR diagnosed before 32 weeks of gestation
- Symmetric growth restriction at any gestational age

In the absence of maternal systemic diseases or risk factors, one should consider congenital infection and chromosomal and congenital abnormalities as the possible causes. The investigations required in such cases are fetal blood sampling to rule out chromosomal abnormalities and infection and careful screening for structural defects. The presence of intracranial and liver calcification indicates fetal infection. The rest of the management is similar to that of late-onset FGR.

▌ PREVENTION

- Women should be educated regarding the adverse effects of alcohol consumption and smoking.
- Teenage pregnancies should be prevented.
- Pre-pregnancy counselling should be instituted to identify risk factors based on previous obstetric history and family and medical history.
- Those diagnosed with APLA syndrome should be started on low-dose aspirin prior to pregnancy.
- Women who are at risk of developing FGR should be identified during the first antenatal visit.
- At-risk women should be carefully monitored during the antenatal period.

ANTIPHOSPHOLIPID SYNDROME

Antiphospholipid syndrome (APS) is an immunological condition characterised by the occurrence of venous or arterial thrombosis or specific pregnancy complications in the presence of laboratory evidence of antiphospholipid antibodies (APLA). Pregnancy-related complications associated with APLA syndrome are recurrent miscarriages, unexplained second- and third- trimester losses, unexplained fetal growth restriction, intrauterine death, severe early-onset eclampsia, abruption and postpartum thrombosis.

▌ CLINICAL CRITERIA TO DIAGNOSE APS

- One or more unexplained fetal deaths of a morphologically normal fetus at gestation >10 weeks
- Preterm delivery of a morphologically normal infant before 34 weeks of gestation due to severe pre-eclampsia, eclampsia or features consistent with placental insufficiency
- Three or more unexplained, consecutive and spontaneous pregnancy losses <10 weeks of gestation after the exclusion of maternal anatomic and hormonal abnormalities and paternal and maternal chromosomal abnormalities
- Unexplained arterial or venous thrombosis in pregnancy or puerperium

▌ DIAGNOSTIC EVALUATION FOR APS

- IgG and IgM anticardiolipin antibodies (aCL)
- IgG and IgM anti-β_2-glycoprotein (GP) antibodies
- Lupus anticoagulant testing

These tests should be done twice, 6–8 weeks apart, because a low-to-mid positive level could be due to viral illness and may revert to normal.

▌ MANAGEMENT

- Low-dose aspirin (50–100 mg per day) is started when conception is attempted and a prophylactic dose of low-molecular-weight heparin (LMWH) or unfractionated heparin is given on confirmation of intrauterine pregnancy.
- As in all pregnancies at increased risk of complications, close antenatal fetal surveillance is performed to allow timely intervention in the event of maternal or pregnancy-related complications.
- The delivery is scheduled at 39 weeks of gestation or earlier depending on fetal surveillance tests. Heparin should be discontinued before labour and delivery to minimise delivery-related bleeding. Low-dose aspirin can be stopped any time after 36 weeks of gestation and, ideally, should be stopped 7–10 days before delivery.
- Preventive measures should be taken in the postpartum period also to prevent deep vein thrombosis (DVT) and cortical vein thrombosis.
- Women with APLA should avoid estrogen-containing hormonal contraceptives.

KEY POINTS

✓ *Fetal growth restriction (FGR) is a condition wherein the fetus fails to reach its genetic growth potential and, consequently, is at an increased risk of perinatal morbidity and mortality.*

✓ *Fetuses whose weight is below the 10th percentile for the gestational age are considered small for gestational age (SGA).*

✓ *SGA also refers to fetuses that are genetically small (constitutionally small fetus) and growth-restricted fetuses (FGR).*

✓ *FGR babies have significant morbidity due to hypoglycemia, polycythemia, hyperbilirubinemia and asphyxia, which begin before birth.*

✓ *IUGR is classified as type I and type II depending on the pathological process and the time of onset.*

✓ *The accurate estimation of the gestational age is critical for the diagnosis of FGR.*

✓ *Fetal growth assessment is done by clinical methods and by biometric assessment using USG.*

✓ *The USG parameters used for the diagnosis of FGR are head circumference (HC), biparietal diameter (BPD), abdominal circumference (AC), femur length (FL), estimated fetal weight and HC/AC and FL/AC ratios.*

✓ *AC is a good indicator of fetal weight and fetal growth.*

✓ *The combined use of fetal biophysical variables is a more accurate means of assessing fetal health than any one used alone.*

✓ *Pregnancy with suspected IUGR needs to be carefully monitored for fetal growth and fetal well-being. Tests of fetal well-being include fetal movement count, non-stress test, fetal biophysical profile and Doppler studies.*

Essay questions

1. Define intrauterine growth restriction (IUGR). What are the factors that contribute to IUGR?

2. How would you manage a case of IUGR at 34 weeks of gestation?

3. A 26-year-old para 1 is seen at the clinic. She had a cesarean delivery 6 months ago and the baby died 3 days later. During the antenatal period, the woman was diagnosed with pre-eclampsia and severe fetal growth restriction at 34 weeks of gestation. She is worried about her future pregnancies.
   a) Define FGR and describe the types of FGR.
   b) Enumerate the causes of FGR.
   c) What preventive measure can be taken before and during future pregnancies?
   d) How would you monitor this woman in pregnancy?

Short answer questions

Write short notes on the following:

1. Biophysical profile
2. Fetal biometry
3. Classification of IUGR
4. Umbilical artery Doppler

MCQs

1. Which of the following is not a cause of FGR?
   a) Pre-eclampsia
   b) Heart disease
   c) GDM
   d) Fetal infection

2. Which of the following is not a neonatal complication of FGR?
   a) Hyperglycemia
   b) Hypothermia
   c) Hyperbilirubinemia
   d) Hypocalcemia

3. Which of the following is NOT a cause of type II or asymmetric or extrinsic FGR?
   a) Hypertension
   b) Cyanotic heart disease
   c) Renal diseases
   d) Chromosomal abnormalities

4. FGR is defined as fetal weight below the:
   a) 5th percentile
   b) 15th percentile
   c) 10th percentile
   d) 20th percentile

5. FGR is classified as late onset after:
   a) 12 weeks
   b) 22 weeks
   c) 32 weeks
   d) 10 weeks

6. FGR is suspected on palpation if the height of uterus is:
   a) Less than 2 weeks to estimated GA
   b) Less than 4 weeks to estimated GA
   c) More than 2 weeks to estimated GA
   d) More than 4 weeks to estimated GA

7. Which of the following is the best morphometric test to diagnose FGR?
   a) BPD measurement
   b) FL measurement
   c) Sonographic estimation of fetal weight
   d) Head circumference

8. If no fetal compromise is noted in FGR, delivery is conducted at:
   a) 32 weeks
   b) 34 weeks
   c) 37 weeks
   d) 40 weeks

9. Which of the following is an indication for immediate termination of pregnancy with FGR?
   a) Reverse end diastolic flow
   b) Mild IUGR
   c) Reactive biophysical profile
   d) None of the above

10. What is the approximate incidence of FGR?
    a) 5–10%
    b) 15–20%
    c) 10–15%
    d) 20–25%

11. Which of the following is used for the lab diagnosis of APLA syndrome?
    a) IgG and IgM anticardiolipin antibodies
    b) IgG and IgM anti-β_2-glycoprotein (GP) I antibodies
    c) Lupus anticoagulant testing
    d) All of the above

Answers

1. (c), 2. (a), 3. (d), 4. (c), 5. (c), 6. (b), 7. (c), 8. (c), 9. (a), 10. (a), 11. (d)

Fill in the blanks

1. Fetal growth restriction is defined as a condition wherein the fetal weight is below the _____ for the gestational age.

2. Fetal growth restriction should be suspected if, on abdominal palpation, the height of the uterus is _____ than the estimated gestation.

Answers

1. 10th percentile, 2. 4 weeks less

Case scenario-based discussion

1. A 22-year-old primigravida presents to the clinic at 11 weeks of gestation. Her prepregnancy weight was 42 Kg and she is a known case of bronchial asthma. She is found to be at a high risk of developing FGR.
    a) How would you monitor this woman?
    b) How would you monitor this woman clinically?
    c) How would you monitor this woman using USG?
    d) How would you monitor this woman once growth restriction is diagnosed?

Answers

a) Dating of pregnancy is crucial in the diagnosis of FGR. Therefore, CRL measurement should be taken between 6 and 14 weeks of gestation. Careful anatomic screening should be carried out at 18–20 weeks of gestation. Since this woman is at high risk of developing fetal growth restriction because of inadequate prepregnancy weight and chronic hypoxic state due to bronchial asthma, her nutritional status should be improved, and hypoxic episodes should be avoided.

b) Her weight gain should be monitored, and the growth of the fetus should be assessed by serial measurement of the symphysiofundal height.

c) Serial fetal biometry should be carried out from 24 weeks onwards at 4-week intervals. Fortnightly scans may be required if the growth velocity is not maintained and if the AC falls to the 3rd percentile.

d) As the fetus has developed growth restriction, growth scans and well-being assessment should be carried out. Doppler study of the umbilical artery should be carried out to assess placental function, AFI for renal function, DFMC and BPP for neural function and CTG for the metabolic state of the fetus.

Prolonged Pregnancy (Post-Term Pregnancy)

Learning Objectives

» To know how to accurately assess gestational age
» To know the causes of post-term pregnancy
» To know the risks associated with prolonged pregnancy
» To know the management of late-term and post-term pregnancies

INTRODUCTION

According to the International Federation of Gynecology and Obstetrics (FIGO), post-term (prolonged) pregnancy is defined as a pregnancy that has extended to or beyond 42 weeks (294 days) from the first day of the last normal menstrual period.

Using Naegele's rule, the expected date of delivery (EDD) is calculated, which is 280 days or 40 weeks from the first day of the last menstrual period. The International Classification of Diseases has classified the duration of pregnancy as follows:

- Term pregnancy is one that extends between 37 weeks 0 days and 41 weeks 6 days. It is sub-classified as follows:
  — Early term: 37 weeks to 38 weeks and 6 days
  — Full term:　39 weeks to 40 weeks and 6 days
  — Late term:　41 weeks to 41 weeks and 6 days
- Post-term pregnancy is one that extends to 42 weeks and beyond.

INCIDENCE

It is estimated that when no induction methods are adopted, 50% of women will deliver spontaneously in the early term at 37–39 weeks, 20% will deliver at full term at 39–41 weeks, 10% will deliver late-term at 41–42 weeks and 7% will continue to post-term >42 weeks.

CAUSES OF PROLONGED PREGNANCY

The most common causes of prolonged pregnancy are as follows:

- Incorrect calculation of EDD—the most common cause of prolonged pregnancy is an error in gestational age dating
- Nulliparity

- Previous post-term pregnancy
- Male fetus
- Obesity
- Anencephaly without hydramnios
- Genetic factors—if a woman's mother had a history of a prolonged pregnancy while delivering the woman, then the woman's risk of post-term pregnancy is two- to three-fold higher than a woman without such a familial history
- Ethnicity—Italians are more predisposed to post-term pregnancies
- Rarer causes include placental sulfatase deficiency and fetal adrenal hypoplasia; fetal cortisol plays an important role in the initiation of labour; in anencephaly and fetal adrenal hypoplasia, fetal cortisol is absent, which predisposes the woman to post-term pregnancy

COMPLICATIONS ASSOCIATED WITH POST-TERM PREGNANCY

After 36 weeks of gestation, there is a gradual decline in placental function and the placenta starts showing infarcts and calcification. When pregnancy is prolonged, placental function may either remain unaffected or, due to placental ageing with calcification and infarcts, placental insufficiency may set in, leading to a compromised fetus—this is called the post-maturity syndrome.

Effects of Placental Insufficiency and Placental Ageing

- Liquor volume gets reduced due to fetal hypoxia and diminished renal blood flow. The resultant oligohydramnios leads to cord compression and fetal heart rate abnormalities. Fetal heart rate variations may increase during labour.

- There is increased meconium staining of liquor due to fetal hypoxia (meconium staining can also occur due to cord compression or increasing vagal tone associated with fetal maturity relaxing the anal sphincter).
- Because of placental insufficiency, the infant is born with typical features of 'postmaturity syndrome', which is described in the latter half of this chapter.

If the Placental Function is Unaffected

- The fetus continues to grow in utero and progresses to macrosomia
- Moulding in labour is reduced, leading to CPD
- As a result of the large size of the baby, the woman goes into dysfunctional labour, with increased chances of operative deliveries and shoulder dystocia

Maternal and Fetal Complications

In late-term and post-term pregnancies, both the fetus and the mother are at risk in the antepartum and intrapartum periods. The neonatal complications are also increased.

- There is increased perinatal morbidity and mortality.
- Post-term infants are more likely to be admitted to intensive care units.
- Due to fetal hypoxia and cord compression associated with oligohydramnios, there is fetal distress. As a result, intrapartum deaths could occur.
- Meconium aspiration syndrome is more common in post-term pregnancies, presenting with respiratory distress due to mechanical obstruction or chemical pneumonitis.
- Macrosomia leads to labour dystocia, operative deliveries, shoulder dystocia and birth trauma.
- The incidences of neonatal seizures and death are doubled at 42 weeks.
- The baby may develop cerebral palsy.
- There is increased maternal morbidity due to instrumental deliveries, cesarean section, perineal trauma and PPH.

Late-term and post-term pregnancies are associated with increased perinatal morbidity and mortality.

DIAGNOSIS OF POST-TERM PREGNANCY

The accurate estimation of gestational age is crucial for the diagnosis and management of late-term and post-term pregnancies.

Estimating Gestational Age

EDD is calculated based on a reliable LMP, the regularity of cycles and first- and early second-trimester USG findings.

- If LMP is taken for calculating EDD, the woman should have had at least three regular menstrual cycles prior to conception.
- If the EDD calculated by the LMP and USG fall within 10 days, LMP is taken for calculating the EDD.
- For women with uncertain dates/irregular periods or unknown LMP, a first-trimester scan at 11–13 weeks is recommended for dating.
- The crown–rump length measured in the first trimester is an accurate measure of EDD with an error of 5–7 days.
- Occasionally, a pregnant woman may report late in the second trimester for antenatal care. If LMP is not known or is unreliable, then a second-trimester ultrasound can still be used for EDD calculation, though it is not as reliable as a first-trimester ultrasound.

All pregnant women should be offered a first-trimester ultrasound examination between 11 and 13 weeks, as this provides a more accurate assessment of gestational age.

MANAGEMENT OF PROLONGED PREGNANCY

Although the risk to the fetus generally increases after 42 weeks of gestation, fetal compromise may occur between 40 and 42 weeks of gestation as well. Therefore, it is important to initiate fetal surveillance from 40 weeks onwards so as to reduce perinatal morbidity and mortality.

The aim of fetal surveillance is to identify fetuses at risk, where the early induction of labour may be beneficial for the fetus.

Induction of Labour

Because of the risks associated with post-term pregnancy, the WHO recommends induction of labour at 41 weeks of gestation. However, there are certain prerequisites that need to be met before taking the decision to wait until 41 weeks of gestation.

Prerequisites to wait until 40+7 days

- There should not be any high-risk factors such as pre-eclampsia, GDM, IUGR, oligohydramnios,

Rh-negative mother, short stature, history of first-trimester bleeding, pregnancy following infertility treatment or PROM.

- There should not be any CPD.
- The fetus should be in good health, and fetal surveillance should be carried out until delivery.
- The woman should be counselled about the benefits of waiting. It should be explained to her that by waiting, she may establish spontaneous labour, which increases the chances of vaginal delivery.
- The process of induction and the probable time that it may take to initiate labour should also be explained to the couple.

Antepartum Fetal Surveillance

- The mother can be asked to monitor the fetus by counting fetal movements daily. Daily fetal movement counting (DFMC) or a kick count is valuable in evaluating the fetal condition. This has been described in detail in Chapter 11, *Antepartum fetal surveillance*.
- The fetus is monitored by bi-weekly non-stress test (NST), biophysical profile and modified biophysical profile (non-stress test and amniotic fluid index).
- Doppler ultrasonography does not seem to provide any advantage in evaluating prolonged pregnancies and hence is not recommended as a routine testing modality.
- While awaiting the induction of labour at 41 weeks of gestation, membrane sweeping can be done at 40 weeks of gestation if the cervical os is opened. This elicits the release of endogenous prostaglandins, which may aid the spontaneous onset of labour.

  During fetal surveillance, if fetal compromise is indicated by decreased fetal movements, compromised non-stress test or biophysical profile, the pregnancy should be terminated immediately either by induction or by cesarean section, depending on the findings. The methods of induction are described in Chapter 16, *Induction of labour.*

> Induction of labour at 41 weeks has been found to decrease perinatal mortality and morbidity without increasing the maternal risks of cesarean section.

Intrapartum Problems and their Management

- The chances of fetal distress are higher in prolonged pregnancies due to fetal hypoxia and reduced liquor, which predisposes to cord compression.

- Meconium may become a frequent problem since all fetuses of this gestational age have a readily activated vagal system. Since the liquor volume may be low, the meconium will become thick and tenacious.
- Large babies are more likely to have prolonged labour.
- Fetal head moulding is reduced in late-term and post-term pregnancies, which may lead to dystocia.

Management in Labour

- Labour in prolonged pregnancy needs to be closely monitored.
- Continuous electronic fetal heart monitoring is ideal for monitoring the fetus in labour to diagnose fetal distress early.
- Fetal heart sounds must be heard during and immediately after a uterine contraction if facilities for electronic monitoring are not available.
- Once the woman is in labour, early amniotomy should be carried out to detect meconium in the liquor.
- Immediate delivery of the fetus is indicated in the presence of fetal heart rate abnormalities.
- The progress of labour should be watched carefully (using a partograph).
- Labour dystocia should be detected early, and traumatic vaginal delivery should be avoided.
- Shoulder dystocia should be anticipated, and a senior obstetrician should be present at the time of delivery to manage shoulder dystocia.
- At the time of delivery, care should be taken to prevent meconium aspiration syndrome.
- Current evidence does not support routine amnioinfusion or deep oropharyngeal suctioning to prevent meconium aspiration syndrome (MAS).

Postnatal Management

The newborn should be monitored for hypoxia, hypoglycemia and birth injuries. If meconium aspiration has occurred, intubation and tracheal suctioning should be carried out. Gastric lavage may be required to remove the swallowed meconium to prevent vomiting and aspiration later on.

▪ POSTMATURITY SYNDROME

The term postmature is used to describe an infant with recognizable clinical features indicating a prolonged pregnancy, wherein the fetus suffers from malnutrition. Only a few infants from prolonged pregnancies are postmature, and therefore, the use of the term postmature in all post-term pregnancies may falsely imply a pathologically prolonged pregnancy. A postmature infant has quite a characteristic 'old man' appearance. Such an infant has the following features:

- Wrinkled, patchy, peeling skin, particularly on the palms and soles
- Absence of vernix
- Meconium staining of skin, nails and amnion

- Well-developed palmar creases
- Long nails
- The eyes are open and alert
- A long and thin body
- Has an 'old-man' and worried look
- Skin changes may occur due to the loss of the protective effect of the vernix caseosa

KEY POINTS

✓ Post-term (prolonged) pregnancy is defined as a pregnancy that has extended to or beyond 42 weeks (294 days) from the first day of the last normal menstrual period.

✓ The most common cause of prolonged pregnancy is an error in gestational age dating.

✓ Accurate estimation of gestational age is crucial for the diagnosis and management of late-term and post-term pregnancies.

✓ Accurate dating and the use of early-trimester ultrasonography may decrease the incidence of prolonged pregnancy and help in avoiding unnecessary induction.

✓ Late-term and post-term pregnancies are associated with increased perinatal morbidity and mortality.

✓ The WHO recommends induction of labour at 41 weeks of gestation.

✓ Post-term pregnancies require antepartum surveillance from 40 weeks of gestation so that interventions can be performed at the appropriate time.

✓ Sweeping or stripping the membranes may reduce the prolongation of pregnancy after term.

✓ Induction of labour at the optimum time and careful monitoring of labour help to reduce the perinatal morbidity/mortality associated with prolonged pregnancy.

Essay questions

1. How is prolonged pregnancy diagnosed?
2. Discuss the management of a woman presenting at 41 weeks of gestation.

Short answer questions

Write short notes on the following:

1. Estimation of gestational age
2. Causes of prolonged pregnancy
3. Postmaturity syndrome
4. Management of prolonged pregnancy

MCQs

1. Which of the following is the definition of prolonged pregnancy endorsed by FIGO and ACOG?
   a) Completion of 40 weeks
   b) Completion of 37 weeks
   c) Completion of 42 weeks
   d) Completion of 41 weeks
2. Which of the following is a common cause of prolonged pregnancy?
   a) Obesity
   b) Wrong dates
   c) Previous post-dated pregnancy
   d) Any of the above
3. Which of the following is a characteristic of postmaturity syndrome in newborns?
   a) 'Old man' appearance
   b) Long nails
   c) Open eyes
   d) All of the above

4. Which of the following is the most reliable for antepartum surveillance in postdated pregnancy?
   a) NST test
   b) Kick count
   c) Biophysical profile
   d) Modified biophysical profile
5. Stripping (membrane sweeping) is done at:
   a) 38 weeks
   b) 38–40 weeks
   c) <38 weeks
   d) 37 weeks
6. Which of the following are methods of induction of labour?
   a) PGE$_2$ gel
   b) Foley catheter
   c) Membrane sweeping
   d) All of the above
7. What of the following are complications of prolonged pregnancy?
   a) Cord compression
   b) Fetal distress
   c) Meconium-stained liquor
   d) All of the above
8. At what gestation age should fetal surveillance begin?
   a) 42 weeks
   b) 41 weeks
   c) 40 weeks
   d) 37 weeks
9. Which of the following is NOT a usual modality for monitoring prolonged pregnancy?
   a) Fetal movement count
   b) Biophysical profile
   c) Doppler sonography
   d) Non-stress test

10. In prolonged pregnancy, perinatal morbidity/mortality is more due to the increased incidence of all the following EXCEPT:
    a) Cesarean delivery
    b) Forceps delivery
    c) Malpositions of the vertex
    d) Meconium aspiration syndrome
11. Prolonged pregnancy is associated with:
    a) Inaccurate dating of pregnancy
    b) Fetal anencephaly
    c) Nulliparity
    d) All of the above

Answers

1. (c), 2. (d), 3. (d), 4. (d), 5. (b), 6. (d), 7. (d), 8. (c), 9. (c), 10. (c), 11. (d)

Fill in the blanks

1. The duration of pregnancy according to Nagele's rule is about _____ from the first day of the last menstrual period.
2. The definition of prolonged pregnancy is _____ or more from the first day of the last menstrual period.

Answers

1. 280 days or 40 weeks,   2. 42 completed weeks (294 days)

Case scenario-based discussion

1. A 26-year-old primigravida reports at 40 weeks of gestation on her EDD for safe confinement. She does not have any complaints.
   a) How would you manage this case?
   b) The woman's dates were confirmed, and she has completed 40 weeks of gestation. When would you deliver her and what advice would you give her?
   c) The woman goes into spontaneous labour at 40 weeks +6 days. What complications should be anticipated in labour?

Answers

a) Accurate assessment of the gestational age should be done based on the woman's LMP and her first- and second-trimester USG results. The presence of high-risk factors should be looked for, which would indicate immediate delivery. These factors include pre-eclampsia, GDM, Rh-incompatibility, CPD and fetal compromise.

b) The woman should be delivered at 41 weeks of gestation. In the meantime, if the cervical os opens, membrane sweeping should be performed, and fetal surveillance with DFMC, bi-weekly CTG and biophysical profile should be carried out. The benefit of waiting until 41 weeks is that the woman may go into spontaneous labour, which increases the chances of a vaginal delivery; this should be explained to the woman.

c) The risk of fetal distress is high due to fetal hypoxia and cord compression caused by oligohydramnios. There may also be dysfunctional labour due to the large size of the baby, and reduced moulding of the fetal head. There may be meconium-stained liquor, which predisposes to meconium aspiration syndrome. Shoulder dystocia should also be anticipated.

27

Multiple Pregnancy

Learning Objectives

» To know the types of multiple gestation
» To discuss the etiology and clinical features of multiple pregnancy
» To describe the diagnosis of multiple pregnancy
» To discuss the maternal and fetal complications of multiple pregnancy
» To discuss the antenatal care and monitoring of multiple pregnancy
» To know the intrapartum management of multiple pregnancy

■ INTRODUCTION

In humans, conception usually results in only one fetus. Sometimes, however, conception may result in two or more fetuses growing simultaneously, resulting in twins, triplets, quadruplets, quintuplets, sextuplets and more. With the increased use of assisted reproductive techniques, the incidence of multiple pregnancy is on the rise. Multiple pregnancy is associated with high rates of fetal losses due to prematurity, growth restriction, fetal congenital malformations and twin-to-twin transfusion syndrome. The risk of all pregnancy complications is also higher when there is more than one fetus.

Definition

Multiple pregnancy is the simultaneous development of more than one fetus in the uterus.

■ TYPES OF TWINS

When multiple pregnancy occurs, it may result from one of two types of twinning—dizygotic twinning or monozygotic twinning (zygosity refers to the type of conception). The differences between these two types are presented in Table 27.1.

Dizygotic twinning is the commonest type of twinning (two-third of all cases) and results from the fertilisation of two ova by two sperms. In dizygotic twinning, the developing fetuses have their own membranes, chorion, amnion and placenta (**diamniotic dichorionic [DCDA] placentation**). When the placentation sites are close, the placentae may get fused. The fetuses may be like or unlike in sex and have different genetic constitutions.

Monozygotic twins (one-third of all cases) result from the fertilisation of a single ovum, which splits after conception. Monozygotic twins are otherwise known as uniovular twins. In monozygotic twins, depending

Table 27.1 Differences between monozygotic and dizygotic twins

Monozygotic twins	Dizygotic twins
Uniovular	Binovular
Known as identical twins	Known as fraternal twins
Both fetuses are always of the same sex	Twins may be of the same or different sexes
Twins resemble each other	Twins may or may not bear a resemblance
Placental characteristics depend on when the twinning occurs	Two separate placentae though they may appear as one due to fusion
Type depends on the period of twinning	Always diamniotic dichorionic

on the time at which division occurs, different varieties (Fig. 27.1; Table 27.2) are seen (chorionicity refers to the type of placentation).

• If the division occurs within the first 72 hours of fertilisation (before the 8-cell stage), the cells retain their full potential to develop two separate blastocysts, each with its own membrane. This results in a **dichorionic and diamniotic monozygotic twin pregnancy.** There may be two placentae or a single, fused placenta. The fetuses are identical, are of the same sex, and possess the same genetic markers. This accounts for nearly 1/3rd of monozygotic twinning.

• If the division occurs between the fourth and seventh day, a **monochorionic diamniotic** (MCDA) pregnancy results. This accounts for nearly 2/3rds of monozygotic twinning.

• If the division occurs between the eighth and thirteenth day after fertilisation, the result is a **monochorionic monoamniotic** (MCMA) pregnancy. This accounts for 1% of all monozygotic twinning.

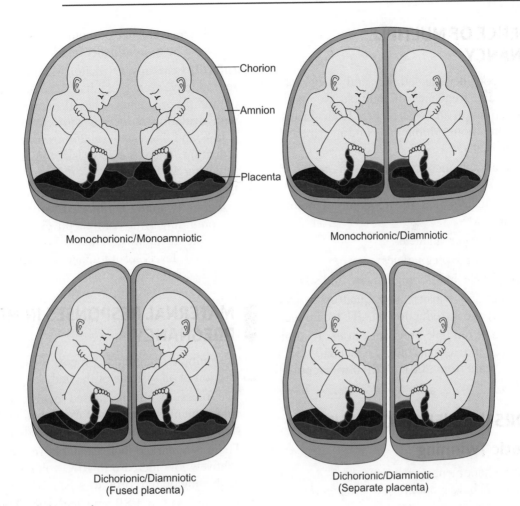

Fig. 27.1 Types of placentation

Table 27.2 Types of division of monozygotic twins

Period of division	Outcome of division
Within 72 hours of fertilisation	Dichorionic diamniotic (nearly 30%)
4–7th day after fertilisation	Monochorionic diamniotic (nearly 70%)
8–13th day after fertilisation	Monochorionic monoamniotic (rare, accounts for 1% of monozygotic twins)
Division after the 14th day	Conjoined twins

- If the division occurs even later (> the fourteenth day), conjoint twins or Siamese twins are formed (Fig. 27.2).
- Beyond the fifteenth day after fertilisation, twinning does not occur.

Superfetation is the fertilisation of two ova at an interval longer than a menstrual cycle. It has not been proven to occur in humans. **Superfecundation** is the fertilisation of two ova within the same cycle but not at the same coitus.

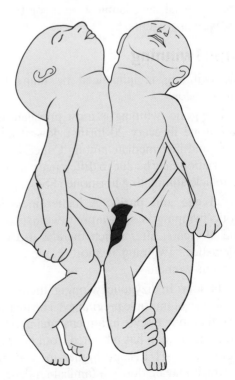

Fig. 27.2 Conjoined twins

INCIDENCE OF MULTIPLE PREGNANCY

- There are considerable ethnic and geographic variations in the frequency of multiple pregnancy. It is most common in Nigeria (45/1,000 births), least common among Mongolians and intermediate among Caucasians.
- There is remarkably a constant rate of monozygotic twinning across the world—1 in 250 births.
- According to Hellin's rules, the frequency of multiple births is as follows:
  — Twins: 1 in 80 pregnancies
  — Triplets: 1 in 80^2 pregnancies
  — Quadruplets: 1 in 80^3 pregnancies, and so on
- The incidence of triplets and quadruplets has increased since the introduction of ART techniques.
- The incidence of multiple pregnancy at the Institute of Obstetrics and Gynaecology, Chennai, for a period of 10 years from 2001 to 2010 was reported to be 1.62%.

FACTORS INFLUENCING TWINNING

Monozygotic Twinning

It is a chance phenomenon occurring in 3–4/1,000 births. Women who have monozygotic twin pregnancies do not have any particular features; the twinning is not related to maternal age, family history or the use of ovulation-inducing agents.

Dizygotic Twinning

Dizygotic twinning is influenced by many factors, which are as follows:

- **Race:** Dizygotic twinning is most prevalent among Africans (one in every 20 births), lowest amongst Mongols and intermediate among Caucasians. This racial variation may be due to differences in the levels of the follicle stimulating hormone (FSH).
- **Maternal age and parity**: A higher incidence of dizygotic twinning is seen among women between 35 and 39 years, after which there is a decline in the incidence. Twinning is more common among multiparous women.
- **Family history:** In dizygotic twinning, there may be a family history of multiple pregnancy. The maturation of more than one oocyte in a menstrual cycle might be a trait the woman has inherited from her mother. The levels of FSH/LH are higher in women with twins, which may be due to a familial tendency.

- **Build:** The incidence of multiple pregnancy has been shown to be more in taller and heavier women.
- **Infertility therapy**: Ovulation induction and assisted reproductive technology has increased the incidence of multiple pregnancy. The risk of multiple pregnancy with ovulation induction with clomiphene therapy is 8% and increases to 25% with gonadotrophin induction. There is a 20% risk of multiple pregnancy following ART techniques.
- **Use of oral contraceptives**: A higher incidence of dizygotic twinning is reported within one month of discontinuing oral contraceptives, but not during subsequent months. This is mainly due to the increased levels of pituitary gonadotropins soon after discontinuing OC pills.

MATERNAL RESPONSES IN MULTIPLE PREGNANCY

In a multiple pregnancy, there is an exaggerated adaptation of all systems of the body.

- The pressure effects caused by excessive uterine enlargement results in the exacerbation of varicose veins, hemorrhoids and dependent edema.
- There is a marked increase in plasma volume with a relatively low increase in RBC volume. This causes the hemoglobin to drop to <10 g% by 30 weeks.
- The increase in ESR and leukocyte count is also greater in multiple pregnancy as compared to the singleton pregnancy.
- The cardiac output is increased, and the second-trimester fall in BP is greater in multiple pregnancy.
- There is an increase in body water which facilitates weight gain.
- There is a greater increase in GFR.
- There is an increase in tidal volume.
- Due to increased placental mass, placental hormones are 50% above the singleton values. Due to this, the interpretation of hormone results in twin pregnancies can be difficult.
- There is decreased gastric motility, hypochlorhydria and esophageal reflex. Constipation is also more marked.

DIAGNOSIS OF MULTIPLE PREGNANCY

Early diagnosis of multiple pregnancy is important for assessing the gestational age of the fetuses and the chorionicity of the placenta.

Clinical Diagnosis

- Family history of twin pregnancy, advanced maternal age, high parity, previous history of twins, a history of clomiphene or gonadotropin intake or assisted reproductive techniques should raise a suspicion of multiple pregnancy.

- On examination, inspection may show fundal height of the uterus to be larger than the period of gestation. Palpation of too many fetal parts with at least two fetal heads or three identifiable fetal poles will help to make a diagnosis of multiple pregnancy. There may be associated polyhydramnios. Incorrect dates associated uterine fibroids and ovarian cysts are the differential diagnoses when the uterine size is larger than the period of gestation.

- The time-tested auscultatory criteria for the diagnosis of multiple pregnancy are as follows:
  1. Two independent observers should auscultate simultaneously.
  2. Two fetal heart sounds should be heard separately in two different areas, which are at least 10 cm from one another.
  3. There should be an echo-free area between the two fetal heart sounds.
  4. There should be a difference of at least 10 beats per minute between the two fetal heart rates.

- It is unwise to rely on the auscultatory findings alone to make a diagnosis.

- Before the advent of USG, multiple pregnancy was diagnosed by clinical examination or X-rays. Based on the clinical examination findings alone, up to 20% of cases of multiple pregnancy may remain undiagnosed until delivery.

USG Diagnosis of Multiple Pregnancy

- At the time of USG examination, the number of fetuses and their chorionicity must be determined. In early pregnancy, the role of ultrasound is crucial.

- Ultrasound scanning provides a definite method of diagnosing multiple pregnancies as early as 6 weeks. However, difficulties may be encountered in higher-order multiple pregnancies and in late gestation.

- Two gestational sacs can be identified very early in gestation, as early as 6 weeks, by transvaginal sonography (Fig. 27.3, 27.4 and 27.5).

- The optimum time to determine chorionicity is 6–9 weeks. As pregnancy advances, diagnosis is more difficult due to the fusion of the placenta, thinning of the dividing membranes and intrauterine crowding.

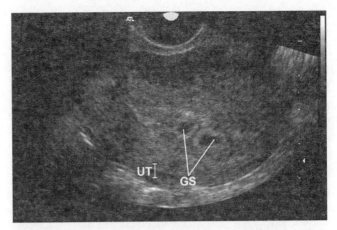

Fig. 27.3 Early twin pregnancy—two intrauterine gestational sacs (*UT*, uterus; *GS*, gestational sacs)

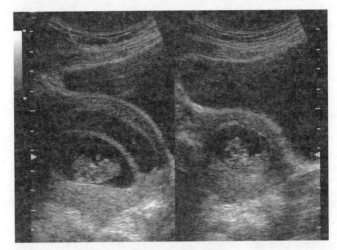

Fig. 27.4 Two intrauterine gestational sacs

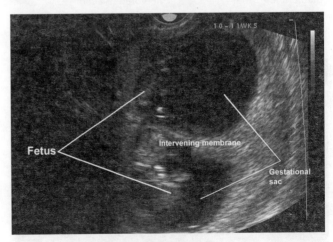

Fig. 27.5 Twin pregnancy at 11 weeks

- Monochorionicity is associated with a higher incidence of fetal growth restriction, congenital anomalies and intrauterine demise. Determination of chorionicity by USG helps clinicians to provide counselling, identify the high-risk group and plan management. Chorionicity should be determined in the first trimester of pregnancy.

USG assessment of chorionicity

USG assessment of chorionicity (Table 27.3) involves the assessment of the thickness of the membranes and the assessment of the junction of the membranes with the placental site.

Assessment of the thickness of the membranes

- Dichorionicity is associated with a thick membrane of >2 mm.
- In monochorionic twins, the width of the inter-twin membrane is <2 mm.

Assessment of the junction of the membrane with the placental site

- The lambda sign or twin peak sign (V-shaped projection of tissue between the dividing membranes at insertion) is seen in the dichorionic placenta (Fig. 27.6).
- A 'T' insertion is seen in the monochorionic type of twins.

Table 27.3 USG diagnosis of dichorionic and monochorionic twinning

Dichorionicity	Monochorionicity
Width of inter-twin membrane >2 mm	Width of inter-twin membrane <2 mm
Twin peak sign or lambda sign	T sign

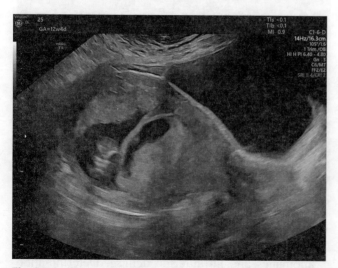

Fig. 27.6 Two gestational sacs with lambda sign in a dichorionic placenta (*Image courtesy:* Dr B H Parameshwar Keerthi, BM Scans, Kancheepuram)

Characteristic features of different types of placentation

Dichorionic twins

- Dichorionic diamniotic twinning occurs in all dizygotic twinning and in some monozygotic twinning where the division occurs within 72 hours of fertilisation.
- There are separate gestational sacs with the chorion extending between them (<10 weeks).
- The twin peak sign or lambda sign is present (>10 weeks)—thick intertwin membrane with more than two layers.
- Separate placental masses can be visualised.
- Twins may be of different genders in dizygotic twinning. However, if the twins are of the same sex, genetic testing is required after birth to determine the zygosity.

Monochorionic diamniotic twins

- There is a single gestational sac.
- Two yolk sacs are present.
- T sign—a thin inter-twin membrane—is present.
- A single placental mass is present.

Monochorionic monoamniotic twins

- There is a single gestational sac.
- There is no inter-twin membrane.
- There is usually only one yolk sac.

Whenever there is a single chorion, there is almost always vascular anastomosis connecting the circulation of the two fetuses—artery to artery, vein to vein and artery to vein—which can be demonstrated by Doppler studies.

Examination of the Placenta

In women who present in late pregnancy, placental examination after birth, and if required, histopathology helps to identify the chorionicity. After delivery, in all cases of multiple pregnancy, the placenta should be examined for chorionicity.

- **Number of placentae:** Two separate placentae denote dichorionicity.
- **Number of layers visualised:** In dichorionic twins, there are either three or four layers, whereas, in monochorionic twins, there are only two layers.
- **Sex of the fetus:** Twins of different sexes denote dichorionicity.

MATERNAL AND FETAL COMPLICATIONS OF TWIN PREGNANCY

Antenatal Complications

- The incidence of **hyperemesis** is increased in the first trimester, which may be due to the higher levels of pregnancy hormones.
- Because of the unduly enlarged uterus, there is a greater tendency for some of the subjective symptoms of pregnancy to be exaggerated in cases of twin pregnancy. The **pressure symptoms** of multiple pregnancy include edema of the lower extremities, varicosity of the veins, constipation and breathlessness.
- The woman may experience a greater amount of fatigue, backache, indigestion, sleepiness and difficulty in walking on account of the distension. All these symptoms will be exaggerated in cases where hydramnios coexists with twin pregnancy.
- Pregnancy-specific complications are more frequently seen and tend to be more severe in multiple pregnancy.

Anemia

Anemia is more frequent in multiple pregnancies than in singleton pregnancies. Due to a greater increase in plasma volume as compared to the red cell mass, there is pronounced 'physiological anemia'. There is also an increase in fetal demand for iron and folic acid, and as a result, the woman may present with both iron deficiency and megaloblastic anemia. The problem is further exaggerated when the woman begins her pregnancy with poor iron reserves. In all women diagnosed with multiple pregnancy, prophylactic iron and folic acid requirements are more because the iron stores are inadequate and as there is megaloblastic erythropoiesis.

Pregnancy-induced Hypertension

The incidence of pre-eclampsia is increased four-fold in multiple pregnancy. It also tends to develop early and can be more severe.

Antepartum Hemorrhage

Both placenta previa and placental abruption are more common in twin pregnancy. A large placental mass can predispose to placenta previa. Increased incidence of pre-eclampsia contributes to abruptio placentae.

Gestational Diabetes Mellitus

There is a two- to three-fold increase in the incidence of gestational diabetes mellitus due to the increased hormones secreted by the large placental mass.

Hydramnios

Polyhydramnios is more common in multiple pregnancy than in singleton pregnancies. The incidence of chronic polyhydramnios is the same in both monozygotic and dizygotic twins. However, monoamniotic twins have a higher risk of acute polyhydramnios, suggesting twin-to-twin transfusion syndrome. The possibility of fetal anomalies should also be considered.

Labour and Third Stage Complications

Malpresentations

Malpresentations are more frequent in multiple pregnancies. In 70% of cases, the first fetus is vertex. In most instances, the fetuses present as both vertex or as vertex and breech. The combinations of the presentations, in their order of frequency, are cephalic–cephalic (40%), cephalic–breech, cephalic–transverse, breech–breech and both transverse.

Prolonged labour

Due to uterine distension, there may be inadequate uterine contractions, leading to labour dystocia.

Interlocking of twins

When the after-coming head of the first twin gets interlocked with the head of the second twin, it is referred to as the interlocking of twins. It is a rare occurrence.

Cord prolapse

Due to various types of malpresentations, cord prolapse is more common in multiple pregnancies than it is in singleton pregnancies.

Operative deliveries

There is a higher rate of operative vaginal delivery and manipulations like versions. There is also increased likelihood of cesarean section.

Postpartum Complications

There is an increased risk of atonic postpartum hemorrhage because of the increased area of the placental site, uterine overdistension and uterine atony. During the puerperium, there could be subinvolution of the uterus, infection and lactation failure.

Fetal Complications

- **Spontaneous abortion** is more common in twins.
- The term **'vanishing twin syndrome'** describes a situation wherein the identification of two viable fetuses in the first trimester is followed by the intrauterine demise of one of the twins at a later point. As a result, the number of twins detected in the first trimester may be higher than the number at birth. At the time of initial diagnosis in early pregnancy, there could be two normal pregnancies or one normal pregnancy accompanied by a blighted ovum or missed abortion. There may not be any symptoms associated with vanishing twins; in 25% of cases, there may be first-trimester bleeding. The fetus may be completely absorbed, or if the loss occurred in the second trimester, the fetus may get compressed into the uterine wall, resulting in fetus papyraceous. Whenever a diagnosis of a twin pregnancy is made early in pregnancy, the mother should be appraised of the possibility of the loss of one conceptus later on.
- **Congenital anomalies** such as anencephaly, PDA, exomphalos, hydrocephalus and atresia of the GI tract are more common in multiple pregnancies, more so in monozygotic twins. Anomalies unique to monochorionic twins include acardiac twins and conjoined twins. The most common type of conjoined twins is the thoracopagus twin. Acardiac twins may be associated with the twin reversed arterial perfusion (TRAP) sequence, wherein there is a normally formed donor twin, who has heart failure, and a recipient twin with a missing heart. When there is persistent polyhydramnios, there is 50% incidence of malformation in one of the twins.
- **Premature labour and preterm prelabour rupture of membranes** is one of the most important complications of multiple pregnancy and is seen in nearly 30% of pregnancies. The major cause is overdistension of the uterus. The mean duration of pregnancy decreases as the number of fetuses increases. In monozygotic twinning, there is a higher incidence of preterm delivery.
- **Fetal growth restriction**—multiple gestations are more likely to result in low-birth-weight babies. The low-birth-weight may be due to restricted fetal growth as well as preterm delivery.
- The greater the number of fetuses, the greater is the degree of growth restriction. Nearly 20–25% of twins are small for gestational age. This is seen in

both monozygotic and dizygotic twins but is more common among monochorionic twins.

- **Discordant twins** are twins that differ considerably in size. This may occur due to a relatively large amount of blood supply passing to one fetus at the expense of the other. The difference in the growth of the fetuses is due to cord abnormalities, vascular anastomosis and unequal placental mass. A diagnosis of growth discordancy is made if the difference in the AC measurement is >20 mm or the fetal weight difference between the twins is >15% in the absence of any major congenital anomalies in either of the twins and in the absence of twin-to-twin transfusion syndrome. This disproportion in the placental circulation may sometimes be so extreme that one fetus practically monopolises the entire supply of blood, and consequently, the second twin dies. In such cases of intrauterine death, one fetus gradually becomes dried up and mummified. The pressure exerted by the living and growing fetus so compresses and flattens the mummified one that it forms a **fetus papyraceus.**
- Fetal distress and **birth asphyxia** are more common in multiple pregnancy. Delayed complications such as cerebral palsy can also occur.
- Perinatal morbidity and mortality are six times more common in multiple pregnancies than they are in singletons, especially in cases of monochorionic twins.

A summary of maternal and fetal complications of multiple pregnancy is presented in Table 27.4.

Table 27.4   Antenatal and postpartum complications of multiple pregnancy

Antenatal complications	Postpartum complications
- Hyperemesis - Pressure symptoms - Anemia - Hypertension - GDM - Antepartum hemorrhage - Hydramnios	- PPH - Subinvolution - Failure of lactation
Labour and third stage complications	**Fetal complications**
- Malpresentations - Prolonged labour - Interlocking of twins - Cord prolapse - Increased operative deliveries	- Increased spontaneous abortions - Vanishing twins - Congenital malformations - Preterm labour, PPROM - Fetal growth restriction - Discordant growth - Single fetal demise - Birth asphyxia - Increased perinatal mortality

Complications of Monochorionic Twin Pregnancy

- Certain complications are unique to monochorionic twins such as twin-to-twin transfusion, acardiac twin, single fetal demise and conjoint twins.
- Monochorionic and monoamniotic placentation is the least common type of twinning, accounting for only 1% of all cases. It is associated with high perinatal mortality of 30–70% due to cord entanglements, which is seen in 60% of monoamniotic twins.
- Monochorionic placentation is associated with the increased incidence of congenital malformations, fetal death and complications due to the presence of vascular anastomosis connecting the circulation of the two twins.

Twin-to-twin transfusion

Twin-to-twin transfusion manifests in the second trimester of pregnancy as growth discordancy. Here, there is arteriovenous vascular communication between the two fetuses. As a consequence of arteriovenous anastomoses, blood is pumped from the artery of one fetus to the vein of the other. One fetus gets most of the nutrition and blood supply from the 'donor fetus', which suffers from chronic malnutrition in utero. Hypervolemia and hyperviscosity of the blood in one and hypovolemia and growth restriction in the other are the net result. The donor twin is anemic and growth restricted, the sac shows oligohydramnios, and the twin is stuck. This condition is unique to monochorionic pregnancies. At birth, the birth weight difference between the twins is >20% and the hemoglobin difference is >5 g/dL.

Single fetal demise

Single fetal demise is more common in monochorionic twins than it is in dichorionic twins. The death of one twin (2–7%) is associated with a poor outcome of the co-twin (25%), especially in monochorionic placenta. The surviving twin runs the risk of cerebral palsy, microcephaly, renal cortical necrosis and DIC. This is due to the thromboplastin liberated from the dead twin, which crosses via placental anastomosis to the living twin. This occurs predominantly in the late second trimester and in the third trimester. After the death of one fetus, repeated USG assessment should be performed and the surviving fetus may be delivered at 34 weeks.

Twin reversed arterial perfusion (TRAP)

Acardiac twins manifest a spectrum of abnormalities; they may appear as amorphous masses or with a poorly developed head and thorax with well-formed limbs.

This acardiac twin receives its blood supply from a normal co-twin via large arterioarterial anastomosis. Poorly oxygenated blood from the normal twin passes in a pulsatile and retrograde fashion through the umbilical artery to the acardiac twin. This is called reversed perfusion.

Conjoint twin

This is a very rare occurrence, which is seen in 1 in 50,000 to 1 in 100,000 deliveries. It occurs due to monoamniotic placentation. In conjoined twins, four types of fusion may occur:

- Thoracopagus (commonest)
- Pycopagus (posterior fusion)
- Craniopagus (cephalic)
- Ischiopagus (caudal)

Ventral fusion is more common than dorsal fusion. Perinatal survival depends upon the type of fusion. Major cardiovascular anastomosis leads to mortality.

■ MANAGEMENT OF MULTIPLE PREGNANCY

The goals of the management of multiple pregnancy are the following:

- Accurate diagnosis of chorionicity
- Detection and management of abnormal consequences of monochorionic placentation
- Detection and correction of anemia, maternal hypertension and GDM
- Prediction and prevention of preterm labour
- Detection of fetal growth restriction

Management During Pregnancy

- Because of the increased risk and complications associated with multiple pregnancy, a woman with multiple pregnancy should be—seen more frequently—once in 15 days between 20 and 30 weeks and thereafter weekly to diagnose and treat anemia, pre-eclampsia and fetal growth restriction.
- These women should have increased rest at home and earlier cessation of employment. Routine hospitalisation is not required before 34 weeks unless complications arise. There should be limited physical activity.
- Women should be educated about the risks of preterm labour. Adequate rest may diminish the chance of premature labour and improve fetal birth weight. In cases of three or more fetuses, hospitalisation is advised from 26 weeks onwards.

- Coital activity may be restricted.
- Calorie and protein requirements are further increased in women with a twin pregnancy. The calorie requirement is 300 Kcal/day more than that recommended for a singleton pregnancy. The prophylactic iron and folic acid supplementation should be more than that prescribed for singleton pregnancies.
- The woman should be carefully monitored for evolving anemia and pre-eclampsia.
- First-trimester ultrasound helps in the identification of chorionicity and to assess the gestational age.
- Ultrasound should be done at 16–18 weeks to rule out congenital malformations.
- Ultrasound should be performed once in 4 weeks for dichorionic and diamniotic twins, and once in 2 weeks for monochorionic twins starting from 16 weeks to diagnose complications earlier.
- Antepartum fetal surveillance should be started from 28 weeks.
- In women diagnosed with monozygotic twinning, Doppler studies should be carried out from 28 weeks onwards to diagnose twin-to-twin transfusion and TRAP syndrome.
- Serial growth scans should be carried out to diagnose growth restriction and discordancy. When there is discordant growth, Doppler studies should be carried out to differentiate idiopathic growth restriction from twin-to-twin transfusion.
- Cervical length assessment also helps in predicting preterm labour.
- In order to improve neonatal prognosis, corticosteroids should be given at the appropriate time to accelerate fetal lung maturity.

Intrapartum Management

As multiple pregnancy is associated with numerous intrapartum complications, the following arrangements should be made for optimal maternal and neonatal outcomes:

- An intravenous line should be established.
- Blood and blood products should be kept ready.
- Delivery should be performed in a well-equipped hospital.
- Epidural analgesia, if available, reduces the risk of the woman pushing prior to full cervical dilatation and ensures adequate analgesia during labour and birth. If there is a need for operative vaginal delivery, for internal podalic version for the second of the twins or for cesarean section, epidural can be easily converted to anesthesia.

- A skilled obstetrician, two neonatal personnel skilled in neonatal resuscitation and an anesthesiologist trained in obstetric anesthesia should be available.
- A cesarean section may be preferred if the first twin is non-cephalic and in cases of higher-order multiple pregnancies (triplets or quadruplets).
- In view of the high risk of intrapartum asphyxia, the fetal heart of both fetuses should be monitored continuously. The first fetus can be monitored with an internal scalp electrode, if it is available, and the second baby can be monitored by external monitoring. Care should be taken to ensure that the traces are not obtained from the same fetus.
- Malpresentations are common, especially of the second twin. However, mechanical difficulty is rare as the fetuses are small.
- The second of the twins is more at risk of intrapartum hypoxia than the first.
- In 70% of twin pregnancies, the first fetus presents by vertex. In 40% of cases, both babies present as cephalic.

Conduct of Vaginal Delivery (Fig. 27.7)

If the presentation of the first twin is cephalic, it should be delivered as in singleton pregnancies. Occasionally, where the first stage is prolonged, artificially rupturing the membranes may help in augmenting the labour. If required, oxytocin may be used for augmentation. Care should be taken to avoid cord prolapse.

- After the delivery of the first child, the cord is ligated at two places and cut in between. Oxytocic medications should not be given after the delivery of the first twin.

It is advisable to apply one clamp on the maternal side for the first twin and two clamps for the second twin so as to easily recognise which cord belongs to which twin and to identify chorionicity.

- After the delivery of the first twin, the abdomen is palpated to ascertain the lie, presentation, size and fetal heart of the second baby. Vaginal examination is subsequently carried out to confirm the abdominal findings and to exclude cord prolapse.
- It is advisable to complete the delivery of the second twin within half an hour of the delivery of the first, as delays can result in intrauterine hypoxia, birth asphyxia and sepsis.
- If the second fetus is presenting as a vertex or breech, the membranes are ruptured soon after the fetal head or breech is fixed in the pelvis. At this stage, it is important to rule out prolapse of the cord. If uterine

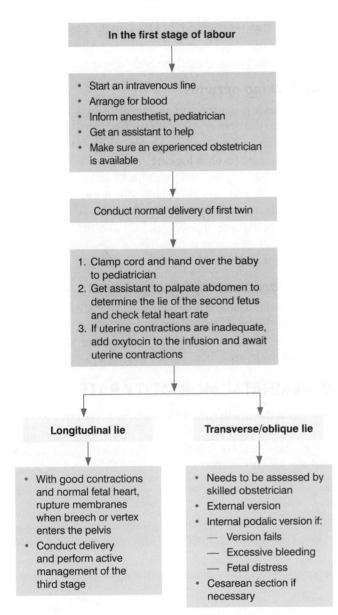

In the first stage of labour

- Start an intravenous line
- Arrange for blood
- Inform anesthetist, pediatrician
- Get an assistant to help
- Make sure an experienced obstetrician is available

Conduct normal delivery of first twin

1. Clamp cord and hand over the baby to pediatrician
2. Get assistant to palpate abdomen to determine the lie of the second fetus and check fetal heart rate
3. If uterine contractions are inadequate, add oxytocin to the infusion and await uterine contractions

Longitudinal lie

- With good contractions and normal fetal heart, rupture membranes when breech or vertex enters the pelvis
- Conduct delivery and perform active management of the third stage

Transverse/oblique lie

- Needs to be assessed by skilled obstetrician
- External version
- Internal podalic version if:
  — Version fails
  — Excessive bleeding
  — Fetal distress
- Cesarean section if necessary

Fig. 27.7 Algorithm for conducting twin delivery (first twin in vertex)

inertia sets in, an intravenous infusion is started with 2.5 units of oxytocin in 500 mL of Ringer's lactate to augment labour. There is no need to hasten the delivery unless there is non-reassuring fetal heart rate or bleeding due to premature separation of the placenta. In the presence of fetal distress, cord prolapse or abruption, labour should be expedited. If the presenting part of the second twin is high, cesarean section should be done. If the presenting part is engaged and well in the pelvis, vacuum is applied for vertex presentation and for breech presentation, breech extraction is done.

- In cases where the second of the twin is presenting in a transverse lie, an external cephalic version is carried out, and the presenting part is guided into the pelvis. The membranes can then be artificially ruptured, leaving labour to natural efforts. If ECV is not successful, the patient is anesthetised, internal podalic version is performed and breech extraction is carried out.

In modern obstetrics, the only indication for internal podalic version is second of the twins presenting in a transverse lie.

- Cesarean section for the second twin may be necessary if the second twin is much larger than the first and is in a non-cephalic presentation or if the cervix promptly thickens and closes after the delivery of the first twin.

Management of the Third Stage of Labour

The management of the third stage of labour is very important. Postpartum hemorrhage should be anticipated, and all precautions should be taken to prevent it. Active management of the third stage of labour with an oxytocic agent should be carried out after the birth of the second twin or the last one in a higher-order multiple pregnancy. Continuous oxytocin infusion should be given for one to two hours after the delivery of the second baby. The woman should be carefully observed for PPH in the postpartum period.

Indications for Cesarean Section

- Malpresentation of the first fetus such as breech or transverse
- Both fetuses with non-cephalic presentation
- Twins with complications such as IUGR, conjoint twins, monoamniotic twins and monochorionic twins with TTS
- Higher-order multiple births such as triplets and quadruplets
- Conjoined twins
- Fetal distress in either of the twins in the first stage of labour
- If there is cord prolapse and delivery is not imminent
- Abnormal uterine contractions
- Associated obstetric causes such as placenta previa, severe pre-eclampsia, previous cesarean section

Special Situations in Multiple Pregnancy
Management of single fetal demise

- When one of the twins dies in utero, the management depends on the type of twinning (whether monochorionic or dichorionic) and the period of gestation.

- All single fetal demise should be managed in a tertiary care centre with access to blood and blood products, neonatal care and round-the-clock specialist care of an obstetrician, anesthesiologist and neonatologist.
- The woman and her family should be supported emotionally and psychologically, and the situation should be clearly explained to them.
- The coagulation profile should be checked periodically every 15 days, particularly when the single fetal demise had occurred early in pregnancy.
- In dichorionic twins, fetal surveillance should be continued for the surviving twin.
- In monochorionic twins, fetal status should be assessed by biophysical profile. Doppler velocimetry of the umbilical and middle cerebral arteries should be carried out for anemia which may indirectly predict brain damage. Wherever possible, ultrasound of the fetal brain and MRI are carried out to check for brain damage.
- If all maternal and fetal parameters continue to be normal, delivery is conducted at 37 weeks by cesarean section.

- The mother is observed for DIVC in the postoperative period also.
- Conjoined twins are delivered by cesarean section.

Interlocking of twins

- Interlocking is rare and occurs in 1 in 1,000 twins (1 in 90,000 deliveries), with the first fetus presenting as breech and second as vertex. With interlocking, there is chin-to-chin locking.
- If interlocking is encountered, after instituting anesthesia and uterine relaxation, an attempt must be made to dislodge the head of the second baby out of pelvis and then, to deliver the first twin as a breech. If this is not possible, a classical cesarean section is performed.

Higher-order multiple pregnancies

Higher-order multiple pregnancies (triplets, quadruplets and above) are usually delivered by cesarean section by 32–34 weeks in a tertiary care centre with good neonatal back-up.

■ PERINATAL MORTALITY RATE

The perinatal death rate with multiple pregnancy is 5–6 times higher than with singleton pregnancies. Among these, the rates are higher among monozygotic twins and the second of the twins.

KEY POINTS

✓ *Multiple pregnancy means the simultaneous development of more than one fetus in the uterus.*

✓ *Its incidence is highest in Nigeria (45/1,000), intermediate among Caucasians (12/1,000) and lowest among the Japanese (<5/1,000).*

✓ *The incidence of dizygotic twins increases with increasing maternal age and parity, family history and the use of ovulation-inducing agents.*

✓ *Monozygotic twinning occurs at random.*

✓ *Fetal complications in twin pregnancies include increased incidence of miscarriage, congenital malformations, abnormal presentation, cord prolapse, twin-to-twin transfusion syndrome and low birth weight.*

✓ *Preterm labour occurs in 30% of cases and fetal growth restriction in 20%.*

✓ *Maternal complications include higher incidence of anemia, pre-eclampsia, GDM and postpartum hemorrhage. Pre-eclampsia is 3–5 times more common.*

✓ *It is essential that the chorionicity of a twin pregnancy is determined as early as possible in the pregnancy as it influences the management of discordant growth or anomalies.*

✓ *Monozygotic twins are associated with an increased risk of congenital malformations and fetal death.*

✓ *Monoamniotic and monochorionic presentation is the least common type, but the perinatal mortality associated with it is as high as 30–70%.*

✓ *The intrapartum complications to be anticipated in twin pregnancy include abnormal presentations, uterine dysfunction, cord prolapse, premature separation of the placenta, interlocking of twins and postpartum hemorrhage.*

✓ *In 70% of cases, the first fetus is in vertex and in 40% of cases, both are vertex.*

✓ *The second twin is at risk of hypoxia.*

✓ *Elective cesarean section is carried out if there is malpresentation of the first fetus (transverse/breech) and in cases of monozygotic twins, higher order multiple births such as triplets and conjoined twins.*

✓ *A multiple pregnancy is a high-risk pregnancy and should be managed in a specialised unit.*

✓   *Perinatal mortality is 6 times higher than that of singletons.*
✓   *20% of pregnancies following IVF are multiple.*

Essay questions

1. Describe the intrapartum management of a woman with multiple pregnancy.
2. Discuss the maternal and fetal complications associated with multiple pregnancy.

Short answer questions

1. What are the differences between monozygotic and dizygotic twins?
2. What are the complications of multiple pregnancy?
3. Describe the twin-to-twin transfusion syndrome.
4. What are discordant twins?
5. Describe the determination of chorionicity of the placenta in twin pregnancy.

MCQs

1. If the division of fertilised ova occurs within 72 hours, it is called:
    a) Dichorionic diamniotic twins
    b) Conjoined twins
    c) Diamniotic monochorionic twins
    d) Monochorionic monoamniotic twins
2. In which of the following types of twins does division occur after 14 days?
    a) Monochorionic monoamniotic twins
    b) Diamniotic monochorionic twins
    c) Dichorionic diamniotic twins
    d) Conjoined twins
3. Which of the following is the most common type of presentation in twin pregnancy?
    a) Cephalic–breech
    b) Cephalic–transverse
    c) Breech–breech
    d) Cephalic–cephalic
4. Which of the following is a maternal complication of twin pregnancy?
    a) Anemia
    b) PIH
    c) Hydramnios
    d) All of the above
5. In which of the following is the twin peak or lambda sign seen?
    a) Dichorionic placenta
    b) Monochorionic placenta
    c) Triplet pregnancy
    d) Singleton pregnancy
6. Which of the following is the only indication for internal podalic version?
    a) Cephalic presentation of the second fetus
    b) Breech presentation of the second fetus
    c) First fetus presenting in a transverse lie
    d) Second fetus presenting in a transverse lie
7. Which of the following is not seen in dichorionic twin pregnancy?
    a) Lambda sign on ultrasonography
    b) Twin-to-twin transfusion syndrome
    c) Babies of different sexes
    d) Inter-twin membrane thickness of more than 2 mm

8. A diamniotic dichorionic twin will result if a fertilised egg divides:
    a) Within 3 days
    b) Between the 4th and 8th day
    c) After the 8th day
    d) After the 15th day
9. Which of the following USG signs is seen in monochorionic diamniotic twins?
    a) T sign
    b) Lambda sign
    c) Twin peak sign
    d) Membrane thickness >2 mm
10. Which of the following statements about twinning is true?
    a) The incidence of monozygotic twinning varies with race.
    b) Conjoined twinning occurs if division occurs after 14 days.
    c) The incidence of the monozygotic and dizygotic twins is the same.
    d) Perinatal mortality rate is more with dizygotic twins as compared to monozygotic twins.

Answers
1. (a), 2. (d), 3. (d), 4. (d), 5. (a), 6. (d), 7. (b), 8. (a), 9. (a), 10. (b)

Fill in the blank

1. In modern obstetrics, the only indication for internal podalic version is _____.

Answers
1. transverse lie of the second twin

Case scenario-based discussion

1. A 27-year-old G3P2 presents to the antenatal clinic at 6 weeks of gestation. Her first-trimester scan shows two gestational sacs.
    a) What is the diagnosis? What further history you would like to elicit?
    b) What further information you would like to obtain from the first-trimester USG?
    c) What are the USG features of monozygotic twins?
    d) What are the unique complications associated with monozygotic twins?
    e) What are the other maternal and fetal complications associated with multiple pregnancy?

Answers
a) The diagnosis is multiple pregnancy. It is important to elicit family history of twins or the use of ovulation-inducing agents, which may suggest dizygotic twinning.
b) There is a possibility of a vanishing twin, and complications are more common in monozygotic twins. Thus, it is important to know the gestational age and chorionicity of the pregnancy. This information would help in counselling the mother regarding the risks associated with multiple pregnancy.
c) In monozygotic twinning, there is a single gestational sac. Two yolk sacs are seen in MCDA twins. MCDA twinning is characterised by the T sign—a thin inter-twin membrane; there is no such membrane in MCMA twinning. There is a single placental mass.
d) The unique complications associated with monozygotic twins are twin-to-twin transfusion, acardiac twin, single fetal demise, conjoint twins and cord entanglement. Cord entanglement is the most common complication seen in 60% of monoamniotic twins.

e) The maternal complications include anemia, pre-eclampsia, antepartum hemorrhage, exaggerated pressure symptoms and polyhydramnios. Malpresentations and PPH are also more common. There is an increased risk of preterm labour, discordant fetal growth, increased congenital malformations and perinatal mortality rate.

2. A 24-year-old G2P1 is admitted at 36 weeks of gestation with labour pains of 6 hours duration. She is a known case of twin gestation. She is in active labour with 6 cm dilatation and the first fetus is in cephalic presentation.
   a) How would you conduct her labour?
   b) How would you conduct the delivery of the second twin?
   c) What are the indications for cesarean section in multiple pregnancy?
   d) What are the postpartum complications associated with multiple pregnancy?

Answers

a) As the first fetus is presenting in the vertex position, vaginal delivery can be allowed. Blood and blood components should be kept ready. An IV line should be established, and labour progress should be monitored with a partograph. Fetal heart rate should also be monitored. As soon as the first baby is delivered, the cord should be clamped in two places.

b) The management of the second twin depends on the presentation. If the second baby is presenting in the vertex, the membrane is ruptured, and vaginal delivery is conducted. If the second of the twin is presenting as a breech, assisted breech delivery is conducted. If the second of the twins is transverse, external cephalic version is attempted. If ECV fails, internal podalic version is carried out under anesthesia and the baby is delivered by breech extraction.

c) Malpresentation of the first twin with a breech or transverse lie, monozygotic twins, higher-order multiple pregnancy and other associated obstetrical conditions such as pre-eclampsia, antepartum hemorrhage are indications for cesarean section in multiple pregnancy. In labour, fetal distress and cord prolapse are indications for cesarean section.

d) The postpartum complications in multiple pregnancy are atonic PPH, traumatic PPH due to operative interventions and manual removal of the placenta.

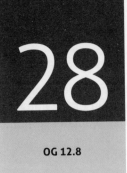

28

OG 12.8

Rh-Isoimmunisation

Learning Objectives

» To know the factors influencing Rh-isoimmunisation and the mechanism of isoimmunisation
» To understand the pathogenesis of hemolytic disease of the fetus and the newborn
» To know the methods of identifying Rh antibodies
» To describe the methods of diagnosing fetal anemia
» To discuss the prevention of Rh-isoimmunisation
» To know the management of Rh-immunised pregnancy

■ INTRODUCTION

• The RBCs carry a number of surface antigens. These antigens are—C, c, D, d, E and e—and are collectively called the Rh factor. These antigens are inherited from both parents. It is the presence of the D antigen (either one or two) that determines the Rh positivity of the individual. The presence of two 'D' antigens makes an individual homozygous for the trait, whereas the presence of only one D antigen makes the individual heterozygous. If the individual has not inherited even a single D, she is Rh-negative.

• Rh incompatibility is an immunological disorder, wherein the mother produces antibodies against this blood group factor present in the red cells of the fetus, which she does not possess. When an Rh-negative woman is exposed to Rh-positive blood cells from the fetus, the mother's immune system can be stimulated to produce antibodies against the fetal cells. These Rh antibodies can freely cross the placenta to destroy the fetal RBCs. The production of these Rh antibodies is called Rh-isoimmunisation.

■ INCIDENCE

The incidence of Rh negativity varies with race. In Caucasians, the Rh-negative genotype is seen in 15% of the population; in India, 5–10% are Rh-negative. Very low incidence is seen among the Japanese. Whenever an Rh-negative woman becomes pregnant with an Rh-positive fetus, there is always a risk of isoimmunisation. However, not all women develop anti-D antibodies.

■ FACTORS INFLUENCING RH-ISOIMMUNISATION

Small amounts of fetomaternal hemorrhage (FMH) are common in pregnancy right from the first trimester onwards and the following factors determine whether an Rh-negative pregnant woman is likely to develop anti-D antibodies when she carries an Rh-positive fetus.

Duration of pregnancy

The Rh antigen expression is well developed at as early as 32 days of gestation. Fetomaternal hemorrhage (FMH) is a normal occurrence during pregnancy, which facilitates the entry of fetal blood cells into the maternal circulation. Both the frequency and the magnitude of bleeding increase as pregnancy advances, and maximum fetomaternal hemorrhage is seen at the time of delivery. In the first trimester of pregnancy, nearly 5% and in the second trimester, 5–15% may have fetomaternal hemorrhage. However, the amount of bleeding is always less than 0.1 mL. In the third trimester, nearly 20–40% develop FMH. This increases to 100% at the time of delivery. As fetal Rh-antigen can be detected in the embryo when it is only 32 days old, sensitisation can occur as early as 7 weeks of gestation.

Events that Precipitate FMH During Pregnancy

• Following spontaneous and therapeutic miscarriages, if anti-D immunoglobulin is not given to the woman, the risk of Rh-isoimmunisation is 3–4% following a spontaneous miscarriage and 5.5% following therapeutic terminations. The risk increases to 12%

in the second trimester and 46% with the delivery of the fetus in the third trimester.

- Ectopic pregnancy and molar pregnancy also precipitate FMH.
- Pre-eclampsia/eclampsia also increases the risk of FMH.
- Antepartum hemorrhage due to abruptio placenta and placenta previa increase the risk of FMH. A large amount of fetomaternal hemorrhage can occur following abruptio placenta.
- In multiple pregnancy, the amount of FMH is more.
- Invasive procedures such as chorion villus sampling, amniocentesis and cordocentesis are associated with increased risk of FMH.
- External cephalic version can result in fetomaternal hemorrhage.
- Fetal demise and maternal trauma are other precipitating factors.

In labour

With the delivery of the placenta, during separation and expulsion, large amounts of fetal cells are liberated into the maternal venous sinuses. This can be further aggravated in the following situations:

- Cesarean section
- Manual removal of the placenta
- Massage of the uterus
- Early ligation of the cord
- Use of ergometrine, which may squeeze the fetal cells into the maternal circulation

Quantum of Transplacental Hemorrhage

The occurrence of Rh-isoimmunisation also depends on the quantity of fetomaternal hemorrhage. The critical sensitising volume that can trigger isoimmunisation is 0.25 mL. The volume of fetal blood cells entering the maternal circulation is not uniform in all pregnancies. It may vary from 0.1 mL to more than 5 mL. In the first and second trimesters, the amount of bleeding is always less than 0.1 mL. On average, the bleed may not be more than 15 mL in a term pregnancy. The risk of immunisation is 3% with 0.1 mL of fetal red cells, 25% with 0.25–1 mL and increases to 65% with more than 5 mL.

ABO Incompatibility

ABO incompatibility between the mother and the fetus protects against Rh-isoimmunisation. In the presence of ABO incompatibility, there is rapid clearance of fetal cells from the maternal circulation so that they are no longer immunogenic.

Other Factors

The other factors that can influence the occurrence of Rh-isoimmunisation are the repetition of the antigenic stimulus and the capacity of the woman's immune response to produce antibodies.

MECHANISM OF RH-ISOIMMUNISATION

Primary Immune Response

When the ABO-compatible Rh-positive RBCs from the fetus enter the maternal circulation of an Rh-negative woman, they circulate for 120 days, then undergo degeneration and are then removed by the maternal reticuloendothelial system, where antigens are released. The released antigens stimulate the maternal immune response, thereby releasing antibodies.

> Because of the time taken for fetal antigens to reach the reticuloendothelial system, the first pregnancy does not get sensitised unless there is substantial fetomaternal hemorrhage or if RBCs are removed faster than usual.

The development of Rh antibodies requires 8–9 weeks and may extend up to 6 months. The initial antibody response is weak with IgM antibody, which does not cross the placenta because of its larger molecular weight. Later, IgG is produced, which traverses the placenta easily.

Secondary Immune Response

After the primary immune response, which has a long incubation period and weak antibody levels, when the woman is exposed to a second dose of antigen in the next pregnancy, the secondary immune response is produced, which is stronger, with a sharp rise in IgG levels.

EFFECT OF ISOIMMUNISATION ON THE FETUS

- The first infant is invariably unaffected, provided the mother was not exposed to Rh-positive cells previously (e.g., from transfusion with Rh-positive blood/blood products, miscarriages or other triggers).
- Less than 1% of Rh-negative women can still get immunised during the first Rh-positive pregnancy without any other triggering factors due to antenatal isoimmunisation.

- The risk of Rh-isoimmunisation is greatest with the second pregnancy.
- With a Rh-negative mother and a Rh-positive fetus, in 0.75% of women, antibodies are seen at the time of delivery due to antenatal isoimmunisation. In 8–10% of cases, the woman is positive for antibodies at 6 months if immunoprophylaxis was not given. If there is a second Rh-positive pregnancy, another 8% are sensitised.

PATHOGENESIS OF HEMOLYTIC DISEASE OF THE FETUS AND THE NEWBORN (HDFN)

Effect on the Fetus

- This disease was previously called erythroblastosis fetalis.
- When these maternal antibodies (anti-D IgG) cross the placenta, this causes hemolysis of fetal Rh-positive red cells, leading to fetal anemia. When fetal anemia becomes severe, it leads to **hydrops fetalis** and stillbirth.
- Hydrops fetalis is invariably fatal, presenting with edema, anasarca, anemia and ascites.
- Due to severe hemolysis, there is extramedullary erythropoiesis, resulting in hepatosplenomegaly and portal obstruction. Consequently, hydrothorax and cardiac failure occur.
- Fetuses presenting with mild to moderate anemia without hydrops can develop severe jaundice and kernicterus after birth.
- The placenta is pale and edematous with swollen villi.

Effect on the Newborn

- Due to the severe hemolysis, the bilirubin level increases. This does not affect the fetus in utero as it is removed by the maternal circulation. However, after birth and especially in a premature baby, the high levels of bilirubin are not effectively removed from the circulation.
- This excess unconjugated bilirubin diffuses into tissues with high lipid content such as the neurons. After crossing the blood–brain barrier and binding with the neurons, bilirubin interferes with the mitochondrial function, leading to neuronal cell death.
- The basal ganglia is most commonly affected. This is called **kernicterus**.

- The chances of kernicterus developing depends on the bilirubin content at birth (the normal level is 30 micromol/lit; icterus is seen at 50–100 micromol/lit and the danger level is 275 micromol/lit). The newborn presents with cerebral irritation, convulsions, twitching and spasticity. Other minor defects are difficulties with fine motor skills due to bilirubin toxicity.

METHODS TO IDENTIFY FETOMATERNAL HEMORRHAGE DURING PREGNANCY

There are a number of techniques to detect fetal cells in maternal circulation.

Kleihauer Acid Elution Technique

The presence of fetal cells in the maternal circulation may be detected by applying the acid elution principle, which was first described by Kleihauer. The test is based on the fact that fetal erythrocytes contain hemoglobin F, which is more resistant to acid elution than adult hemoglobin A. When a blood smear is exposed to a pH of 3.3 (by adding acid citrate phosphate buffer) adult hemoglobin elutes from the red cells, leaving behind non-staining 'ghost' cells. Fetal hemoglobin, on the other hand, does not elute from red cells at this pH (Fig. 28.1). Hence, red cells containing fetal hemoglobin stain bright red with eosin. The Kleihauer-Betke test is chiefly used to evaluate for large-volume fetomaternal hemorrhage as seen in abruptio placenta to decide the dose of anti-D immunoglobulin to be given. It is not recommended for routine administration of anti-D in the postpartum period.

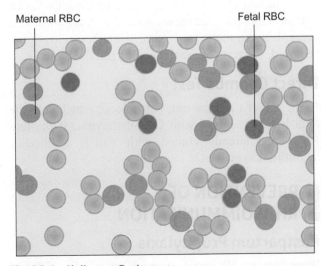

Fig. 28.1 Keihauer–Betke test

> **Calculating the amount of fetomaternal hemorrhage**
> - 5 fetal cells in 50 low-power fields represent 0.25 mL of fetomaternal hemorrhage.
> - 80 fetal cells represent 4 mL of fetomaternal hemorrhage.
> - 100 µg of anti-D would be required to neutralise this 4 mL of FMH.

Rosetting Test

This test is based on the principle that Rh-positive cells coated with antibodies form rosettes when Rh-positive indicator cells are added.

Flow Cytometry

Flow cytometry is an alternative method to detect fetal cells in the maternal circulation.

METHODS TO ASSESS THE PRESENCE OF RH ANTIBODIES (ISOIMMUNISATION)

- The direct and indirect Coombs tests are used to identify unbound circulating antibodies in the maternal circulation. The indirect test is carried out in maternal serum and the direct test on cord blood.
- Both indirect and direct tests use Coombs serum, which contains antiglobulin antibodies which are capable of enhancing the agglutination of red cells coated with incomplete antibodies (IgG) or complement.

Indirect Coombs Test

Known Rh-positive red cells are incubated with the serum which is to be tested for Rh antibody. The agglutination of incubated red cells by Coombs serum indicates that the red cells are coated with the antibodies present in the maternal serum. If antibody titration is required, the test can be done after serial dilution.

Direct Coombs Test

In the direct Coombs test, cord blood, which contains fetal RBCs, is mixed with Coombs serum. If the fetal RBCs are already coated with anti-D antibodies, agglutination occurs.

PREVENTION OF RH-ISOIMMUNISATION

Postpartum Prophylaxis

Whenever an Rh-negative pregnant woman delivers, a cord blood sample is taken to determine the baby's blood group. If the baby is Rh-negative, anti-D is not administered to the mother. However, if the baby is Rh-positive, it is necessary to administer anti-D immunoglobulin to prevent isoimmunisation (Coombs test should be negative before administering anti-D immunoglobulin). Since the amount of fetal blood entering the maternal circulation is usually not more than 15 mL, a dose of 300 µg of anti-D immunoglobulin is considered adequate to neutralise the cells. It has been shown that the administration of anti-D immunoglobulin within 48–72 hours of delivery decreases the incidence of isoimmunisation.

Antepartum Prophylaxis

- **In uncomplicated pregnancy:** It has been shown that in nearly 1–2% of Rh-negative mothers with an Rh-positive fetus, sensitisation can occur due to silent fetomaternal hemorrhage, especially during the third trimester. Therefore, in order to prevent this isoimmunisation, the administration of anti-D immunoglobulin to a Rh-negative mother with uncomplicated pregnancy has been recommended. A dose of 300 µg is given IM at week 28, and a repeat dose is given within 72 hours after the delivery of an Rh-positive infant. As the anti-D immunoglobulin provides protection only for 12 weeks, a second dose is administered if the woman does not deliver at 40 weeks. However, if the woman delivers within three weeks of receiving the anti-D, then it is not repeated in the postpartum period.
- **First-trimester pregnancy wastage:** Following an induced/spontaneous miscarriage, ectopic pregnancy or trophoblastic disease, the Rh-negative mother should receive anti-D immunoglobulin. A dose of 50 µg is adequate to prevent sensitisation in pregnancies that terminated prior to 13 weeks of gestation. A higher dose may be required following surgical evacuations.
- **Following second-trimester miscarriage:** A dose of 300 µg of Rh anti-D immunoglobulin is administered following second-trimester miscarriages.
- **Following amniocentesis:** Following amniocentesis to study genetic abnormalities, 300 µg of anti-D immunoglobulin is given IM. A dose of 300 µg is repeated 12 weeks later if the woman has not yet delivered. A third dose is given as postpartum prophylaxis.
- **Antepartum hemorrhage:** If significant fetomaternal hemorrhage is suspected following abruptio placenta, abdominal trauma, placenta previa or fetal demise, the dose of Rh Ig should be determined after estimating the amount of fetomaternal hemorrhage

by flow cytometry or the Kleihauer test. 300 μg of anti-D immunoglobulin is administered for every 30 mL of fetal whole blood or 15 mL of fetal RBCs. The administration of anti-D immunoglobulin may increase the antibody levels in the maternal circulation, but the titre should be <1:4 due to passively acquired antibodies. If the titre is >1:4, the woman is probably actively immunised.

■ MANAGEMENT

The management of an Rh-negative pregnancy depends on whether the woman is immunised (has antibodies) or non-immunised. Therefore, management will be discussed under two headings:

- Pregnant Rh-negative non-immunised woman
- Pregnant Rh-negative immunised woman

Management of Rh-negative Non-immunised Woman (Fig. 28.2)

This includes primigravidae who are Rh-negative and Rh-negative multigravidae who do not have detectable antibodies in the initial antenatal evaluation.

- Blood grouping and Rh-typing are routine investigations done for all pregnant women.

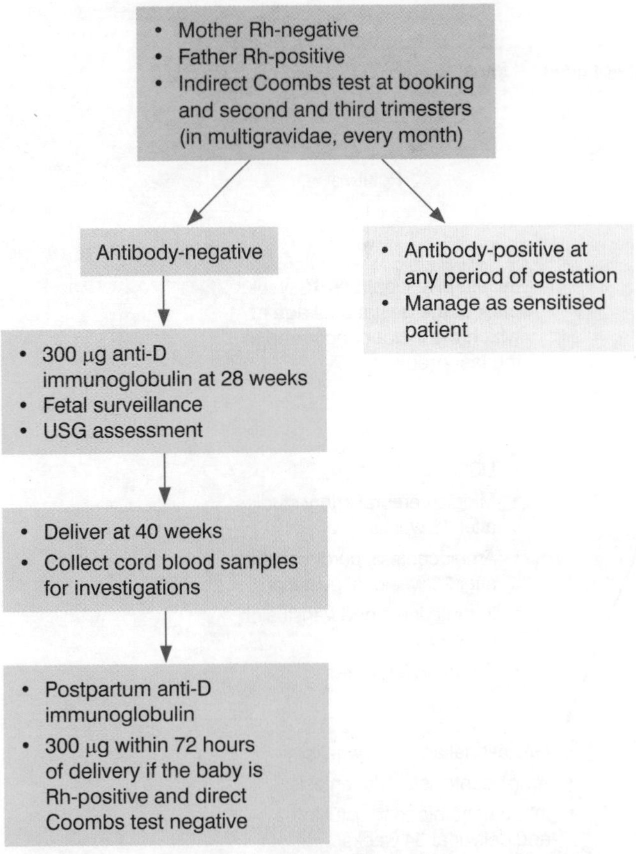

- Mother Rh-negative
- Father Rh-positive
- Indirect Coombs test at booking and second and third trimesters (in multigravidae, every month)

Antibody-negative

- Antibody-positive at any period of gestation
- Manage as sensitised patient

- 300 μg anti-D immunoglobulin at 28 weeks
- Fetal surveillance
- USG assessment

- Deliver at 40 weeks
- Collect cord blood samples for investigations

- Postpartum anti-D immunoglobulin
- 300 μg within 72 hours of delivery if the baby is Rh-positive and direct Coombs test negative

Fig. 28.2 Management of Rh-negative woman diagnosed at booking

- If the pregnant woman is Rh-negative, then the father's blood group is checked. If the father is also Rh-negative, no further investigation is required, and the pregnancy is managed as a normal one, which does not need any additional care.
- If the pregnant woman is Rh-negative and the father is Rh-positive, then at the first visit, an indirect Coombs test is performed to detect anti-D antibodies in maternal serum.
- If antibodies are not detected, the test is repeated in the second and third trimesters of pregnancy. In multigravidae, the indirect Coombs test is repeated every month.
- The indirect Coombs test is also repeated following any event that precipitates fetomaternal hemorrhage.
- Antenatal prophylaxis with 300 μg of anti-D immunoglobulin is given at 28 weeks of gestation in those who have not produced antibodies.
- It is not necessary to perform further indirect Coombs testing after administering anti-D immunoglobulin (antibody titre may become positive to 1:2).
- Serial USG assessment is carried out to diagnose fetal anemia.
- Fetal surveillance is carried out periodically.

Delivery

- An Rh-negative pregnant woman should not be allowed to go beyond 40 weeks of gestation as this increases the chances of fetomaternal hemorrhage.
- At the time of vaginal delivery, precautions should be taken to prevent fetomaternal hemorrhage. Though labour can be induced, hyperstimulation should be avoided. After delivery, the cord should immediately be clamped. Milking of the cord and manual removal of the placenta should be avoided. Blood should not be allowed to spill into the episiotomy wound. Ergometrine should be avoided in the third-stage management.
- During the cesarean section, care should be taken to avoid spillage of blood into the peritoneal cavity; this can be done by proper packing of the peritoneal cavity.

Cord blood samples are collected for the following investigations:

- Blood group and Rh typing of the newborn
- Hemoglobin and hematocrit levels
- Serum bilirubin level
- Direct Coombs test
- Peripheral smear for immature red cells and spherocytes, which are commonly seen in affected babies

- After delivery, if the baby is Rh-positive and the direct Coombs test is negative, then 300 µg of anti-D immunoglobulin is administered within 72 hours of delivery (this will neutralise 30 mL of fetal blood/15 mL of fetal cells). In women who have abruption/traumatic deliveries with the possibility of large fetomaternal hemorrhage, the Kleihauer test is carried out to decide on the dose of anti-D immunoglobulin.
- If the indirect Coombs' test is positive during pregnancy, then it is diagnosed as an Rh- immunised pregnancy and the pregnant woman should be referred to a tertiary care centre for further management.
- When the indirect Coombs titre is >1:4, the pregnancy is Rh-sensitised. If the titre is >1:16 (critical antibody titre), the pregnancy is at risk of hemolytic disease.

Management of Rh-negative Isoimmunised Woman (Fig. 28.3)

The severity of fetal disease in a sensitised woman depends on the past obstetric history of erythroblastosis with neonatal jaundice/stillbirth and the critical level of the antibody titre in the current pregnancy.

- Recognition of fetal anemia is the first step in the management of isoimmunised pregnancy.
- The timing of the first intervention as well as the diagnostic intervention varies with each patient.
- In those with past history of erythroblastosis, investigations are initiated 10 weeks prior to the last pregnancy complication. Non-invasive testing such as middle cerebral artery studies indicate the presence of fetal anemia early. To assess the severity of anemia, amniocentesis/fetal blood sampling (FBS) is carried out from 26 weeks onwards.
- When there is no past history of erythroblastosis and isoimmunisation is diagnosed at the first antenatal visit, antibody levels are checked every month. As long as the antibody levels are below the critical level, the pregnancy can be allowed to continue until term. In these women, antenatal care includes serial USG assessment for evidence of impending fetal hydrops, middle cerebral artery studies to diagnose worsening anemia, routine fetal surveillance and antenatal corticosteroids. NST may show a sinusoidal pattern due to fetal anemia.
- The woman may also develop complications such as pre-eclampsia, hydramnios and PPH due to the large size of the placenta.

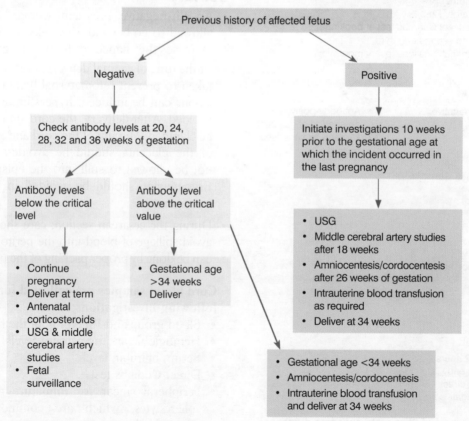

Fig. 28.3 Management of Rh-negative immunised woman

- If the antibody level is above the critical level, the management depends on the period of gestation. If the gestational age is >34 weeks of gestation, the baby can be delivered.
- If the gestational age is <34 weeks of gestation, invasive investigations are required (FBS and amniocentesis). Depending on the severity of anemia, intrauterine transfusion is given.

In an Rh-immunised pregnancy, the maternal blood contains anti-D antibodies. These enter fetal circulation and destroy Rh-positive fetal red blood cells, resulting in fetal anemia. It is necessary to diagnose the degree to which the fetus has been affected and treat the fetus in utero or deliver it depending on the period of gestation. Various diagnostic modalities are used to diagnose the severity of isoimmunisation and fetal anemia. These are described below.

Non-invasive methods

Rh antibody titre
The maternal antibody titre is the first step in the evaluation of the RhD-sensitised patient. The human antiglobulin titre (indirect Coombs) is used to determine the degree of isoimmunisation. A critical titre is defined as the titre associated with a significant risk of fetal hydrops (in most centres, it is taken as 1:16 or 1:32).

- If the Coombs test is positive in a dilution of 1:16 or more, further evaluation of the fetus is required.
- If the titre is less than the critical titre, the test is repeated every four weeks. In the third trimester, the titres are repeated every two weeks to determine whether there is a rising trend.

Actual antibody levels
Besides the titres, the actual antibody levels can be measured.
- If the level is <4 IU/mL, fetal hemolysis is mild and pregnancy can be allowed to continue to term.
- If the level is 4–8 IU/mL, this indicates moderate hemolysis and warrants delivery by 38 weeks of gestation.
- Levels >8 IU/mL indicate severe hemolysis and indicate immediate intervention with either intrauterine transfusion or preterm delivery depending on the gestational age.

Ultrasound evaluation of the fetus
- This is performed early in pregnancy to establish the correct gestational age, as it becomes important in determining laboratory values such as amniotic fluid bilirubin levels (ΔOD450) for a particular gestation

as well as to study the middle cerebral artery (MCA) Doppler values.
- USG also helps in the diagnosis of evolving fetal anemia.

Early signs of fetal anemia
1. Hepatosplenomegaly
2. Polyhydramnios
3. Increase in umbilical and intrahepatic portal vein diameter—in order to maintain oxygenation of the fetus, there is increased blood flow through the umbilical vein as a compensatory mechanism
4. Large placenta

Late findings of fetal anemia
1. Pleural and pericardial effusions
2. Enlargement of the heart
3. Scalp edema
4. Increased skin thickness

Hydrops fetalis (Fig. 28.4) can be detected easily by ultrasonography. Fetal ascites may be the earliest marker of the development of fetal hydrops. However, this is a late sign of fetal anemia when hemoglobin values have already declined to more than 7 g/dL below the norm for gestational age.

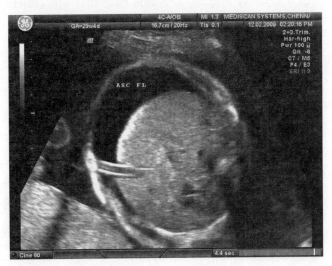

Fig. 28.4   Hydrops fetalis

Doppler velocimetry of umbilical and portal veins
Normal portal venous flow is smooth, whereas in the presence of anemia, the venous waveform bears a 'saw-toothed' appearance.

Middle cerebral arterial Doppler

The assessment of MCA peak systolic velocity has been shown to be accurate in the determination of fetal anemia. A value above 1.5 multiples of the median (MOM) for gestational age is diagnostic of anemia, with a low false-positive rate. Measurements can be initiated as early as week 18 of gestation and should be repeated at 1–2-week intervals for upto 35 weeks of gestation.

Invasive methods to assess the severity of fetal anemia

Since the antibody titre may not accurately reflect the severity of anemia, in addition to antibody levels, the degree of hemolysis is assessed by measuring the AF bilirubin level and the hematocrit and hemoglobin concentrations of fetal blood following fetal blood sampling by cordocentesis.

Amniocentesis and the examination of amniotic fluid

- An indirect method of diagnosing the severity of fetal anemia is by the spectrophotometry analysis of amniotic fluid for bilirubin levels. The amount of amniotic fluid bilirubin correlates roughly with the degree of hemolysis, and thus indirectly indicates the severity of fetal anemia.

- Analysis of amniotic fluid may be required if the antibody titre is >1:16 or when there is a history of a severely affected previous baby that was either stillborn or required blood transfusion.

- This investigation used to be the principal tool in the determination of fetal anemia in the past. Currently, it has been replaced by MCA Doppler.

- The amount of bilirubin present in the amniotic fluid can be quantified by spectrometric scanning with a large wavelength ranging from 300–700 mμ. In the presence of bilirubinoid substances, absorption takes place at the optical density of 450 mμ. In the absence of bilirubinoid-like pigments, the spectrometric analysis shows a smooth, unbroken line, whereas when such pigments are present, there is a typical humping of the line, beginning at 375 mμ, peaking at 450 mμ and returning to normal slope at 525 mμ. The difference between the expected slope and the peak of deformation at 450 mμ is proportional to the amount of pigment present and the degree of abnormality can be graded. The result is plotted on a **Liley's graph** (Fig. 28.5 and 28.6).

- The original Liley curve was divided into three zones and provided values to be used from week 27 of gestation to term. Later, Queenan proposed a modified curve consisting of four zones, with data for earlier gestations. A rising or plateauing trend of OD values that reaches the 80th percentile of zone two on the Liley curve or enters the intrauterine transfusion zone of the Queenan curve necessitates investigation by fetal blood sampling.

  — Zone I: The baby is either unaffected or mildly affected and can be allowed to go to term.

  — Zone II: The baby can be allowed to develop in utero until 34 weeks of gestation.

  — Zone III: The fetus is severely affected, and intrauterine death is imminent. Immediate delivery should be performed if the gestational age is >34 weeks. If the gestational age is <34 weeks, intrauterine transfusion should be planned.

- Values in zone 1 or 2 should be followed by a repeat sampling in 1 or 2 weeks, and the trend of the two values used to estimate the severity of the hemolytic process.

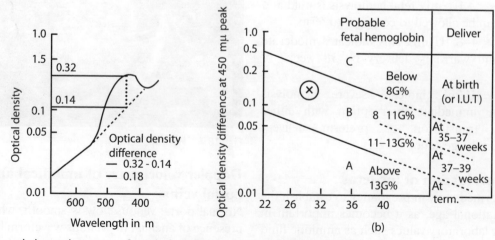

Fig. 28.5 Spectral absorption curve of amniotic fluid in hemolytic disease

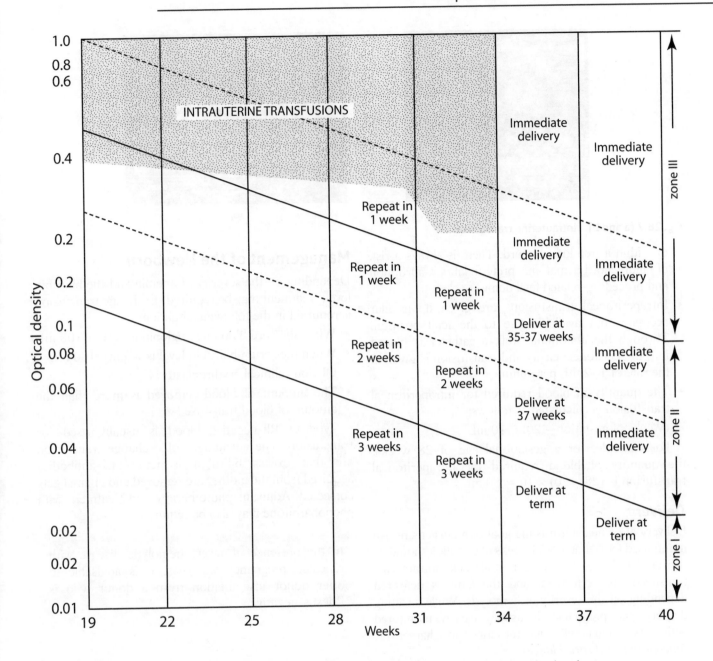

Fig. 28.6 Modified Liley chart used to determine the appropriate management of an isoimmunised patient

Fetal blood sampling

The most accurate method of assessing fetal anemia is by fetal blood sampling after cordocentesis. Normally, this is carried out along with intrauterine transfusion.

Intrauterine transfusion

It is generally performed between 18 and 34 weeks. The most common indication is to treat fetal anemia caused by hemolytic disease of the fetus. If the fetal hemoglobin concentration reduces before 34 weeks (below 10 gm/dL) fetal transfusion is indicated. This is done under ultrasound guidance (Fig. 28.7a and b).

- The mother is given a local anesthetic. The movement of fetus is reduced by agents like vecuronium.
- Currently, intravascular transfusion is favoured over intraperitoneal transfusion.
- The red cells for intrauterine transfusion are typically blood type O, RhD-negative, cytomegalovirus-negative, cross-matched against maternal blood and collected in the previous 72 hours.
- Cells are packed to a hematocrit of 75–85% to prevent volume overload in the fetus. The aim is to increase the hematocrit to 40%. The transfusion is given through the umbilical vessel at its insertion into the placenta

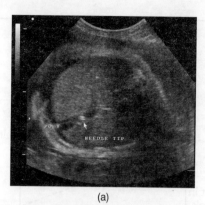
(a)

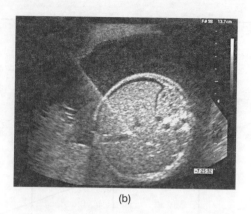
(b)

Fig. 28.7 (a and b) Intrauterine transfusion

or within a free loop of cord. There is always a risk of failure, cord hematoma, preterm labour, abruption and procedure-related fetal demise.

- Intraperitoneal transfusions are given if vascular access is not available due to the fetal position. Through the abdominal wall, a catheter is placed into the peritoneal cavity and transfusion is given at the rate of 1–2 mL per minute.-

- The quantity of blood required for intraperitoneal transfusion is calculated as follows:

(Weeks of gestation – 20) × 10 mL

For example, for a gestational age of 28 weeks, the quantity of blood required for intraperitoneal transfusion is (28 – 20) × 10 = 80 mL

Delivery

Delivery at or near term is the goal of management. An immunised fetus that is >34 weeks of gestation should be delivered. If the gestational age is <34 weeks, intrauterine transfusion is performed, and the fetus is delivered depending on the severity of hemolysis. While awaiting delivery, the pregnancy is usually closely monitored with tests of fetal well-being (described in Chapter 11, *Antepartum fetal surveillance*).

Management of the Newborn

Depending on the severity of anemia and the bilirubin level, treatment may be required. Exchange transfusion is required in the following situations:

- When the cord blood hemoglobin is <10 g/100 mL
- When the serum bilirubin level is >5 mg/100 mL
- Obvious clinical erythroblastosis
- The amount of blood removed is more than the amount of blood transfused

Type O Rh-negative blood is usually used for transfusion. The advantages of exchange transfusion are that excess bilirubin is removed, antibodies acquired from the mother are removed and anemia gets corrected. Adjuvant phototherapy and treatment with phenobarbitone may also be required.

In the presence of severe hemolytic disease with repeated pregnancy wastages, it is advisable to offer donor insemination from a donor who is Rhesus-negative.

KEY POINTS

✓ *It is the presence of the D antigen that determines the Rh-positivity of the individual.*

✓ *An Rh-negative woman can develop antibodies when she carries an RhD-positive fetus.*

✓ *The formation of antibodies in the woman can be prevented by the administration of anti-D immunoglobulin at 28 weeks of gestation.*

✓ *All Rh-negative women delivering an Rh-positive infant with a negative direct Coombs test should be given prophylactic anti-D immunoglobulin within 72 hours of delivery.*

✓ *Rh-isoimmunisation is indicated by the presence of Rh antibodies in maternal serum.*

✓ *Circulating antibodies are detected by indirect and direct Coombs tests.*

✓ *The circulating antibodies cross the placenta to cause fetal anemia. If severe, this results in fetal hydrops.*

✓ *In the newborn, the high levels of bilirubin due to hemolysis leads to kernicterus.*

✓ *If antibodies are detected in the maternal circulation, delivery should be undertaken in a tertiary care centre where facilities for intrauterine transfusion and specialised neonatal care are available.*

Essay question

1. What is Rh-isoimmunisation? How would you manage an Rh-immunised pregnancy?

Short answer questions

Write short notes on the following:

1. Factors influencing Rh-isoimmunisation
2. Prevention of Rh-isoimmunisation
3. Indirect Coombs test
4. Kleihauer test
5. Middle cerebral arterial Doppler in the evaluation of fetal anemia
6. Hydrops fetalis
7. Neonatal management in the case of an Rh-negative mother

MCQs

1. The maximum risk of Rh-isoimmunisation occurs after:
   a) First-trimester abortion
   b) Ectopic pregnancy
   c) Second-trimester abortion
   d) Term delivery

2. At what gestational age is antenatal anti-D prophylaxis given?
   a) 20 weeks
   b) 24 weeks
   c) 28 weeks
   d) 32 weeks

3. What is the dosage of antenatal anti-D prophylaxis?
   a) 50 µg
   b) 100 µg
   c) 200 µg
   d) 300 µg

4. What is the dosage of postpartum prophylaxis?
   a) 50 µg
   b) 100 µg
   c) 200 µg
   d) 300 µg

5. Rh-isoimmunisation occurs in pregnancy when:
   a) Both the pregnant woman and her partner are Rh-negative
   b) The pregnant woman is Rh-negative and the fetus is Rh-positive
   c) The pregnant woman is Rh-positive and the fetus is Rh-negative
   d) Both the pregnant woman and the fetus are Rh-positive

6. Which of the following is not a cause of fetomaternal hemorrhage?
   a) Abruptio placentae
   b) Intrauterine death of the fetus
   c) Procedures such as external cephalic version
   d) Bleeding disorders in the pregnant woman

7. Which of the following tests is used to identify fetal cells in maternal circulation?
   a) Indirect Coombs test
   b) Direct Coombs test
   c) Kleihauer–Betke test
   d) Amniocentesis and cytology of liquor

8. Which of the following is a sign of hydrops fetalis?
   a) Fetal ascites
   b) Scalp edema
   c) Fetal anemia
   d) All of the above

9. Fetomaternal hemorrhage is precipitated by:
   a) Abruption
   b) Fetal demise
   c) Ectopic
   d) All of the above

10. Which of the following statements regarding Rh-isoimmunisation is false?
    a) Leads to hemolysis of fetal RBCs
    b) Occurs in Rh-negative woman pregnant with an Rh-positive fetus
    c) IgG antibodies are produced against fetal RBCs
    d) More severe in the first pregnancy

11. What is the dose of anti-D immunoglobulin in a woman with ectopic pregnancy at 6 weeks on medical management?
    a) 50 µg
    b) 100 µg
    c) 200 µg
    d) 300 µg

12. Which of the following does not cause Rh-isoimmunisation in an Rh-negative woman?
    a) APH
    b) ECV
    c) Postdated pregnancy
    d) Advanced maternal age

Answers
1. (d), 2. (c), 3. (d), 4. (d), 5. (b), 6. (d), 7. (c), 8. (d), 9. (d), 10. (d), 11. (a), 12. (d)

Fill in the blanks

1. It is recommended that anti-D should be administered within _____ of delivery.
2. The volume of fetomaternal hemorrhage can be evaluated by _____.

Answers
1. 72 hours,   2. Kleihauer test

Case scenario-based discussion

1. A 26-year-old primigravida presents at 10 weeks of gestation for antenatal booking. On investigations, she is found to be Rh-negative.
   a) What is the first investigation you will perform in this case?
   b) The woman's husband is found to be Rh-positive. What further measures should be taken?
   c) What measures should be taken to prevent Rh-isoimmunisation?
   d) What precautions will you take to prevent Rh-isoimmunisation in labour?

Answers

a) The woman's husband's blood grouping and Rh typing should be done.

b) An indirect Coombs test should be performed to detect sensitisation. In the absence of previous triggering episodes such as blood transfusion, antibody production in the first trimester is rare. The indirect Coombs test should be repeated in the second and third trimesters also.

c) Following any triggering events for fetomaternal hemorrhage such as miscarriages, ectopic pregnancy, invasive procedures such as amniocentesis, external cephalic version and antepartum hemorrhage, the woman should be given anti-D immunoglobulin. She should also be given anti-D immunoglobulin at 28 weeks of gestation and the dose should be repeated after delivery if the newborn is positive and the direct Coombs test is negative.

d) The following precautions should be taken:
- The pregnancy should not be allowed to go beyond 40 weeks.
- Ergometrine should not be used for third-stage management.
- The cord should be clamped immediately after delivery.

- Manual removal of the placenta should be avoided.
- Cord blood samples should be collected for investigations.

2. A 30-year-old G2P0 presents at the clinic at 9 weeks of gestation. She is Rh-negative and her husband is Rh-positive. In her past obstetric history, she had a spontaneous miscarriage at 10 weeks of gestation for which surgical evacuation was performed. She does not remember whether anti-D immunoglobulin was given at the time. On investigation, the indirect Coombs test is positive.
   a) How would you manage this case?
   b) What are the risks associated with Rh-isoimmunisation?
   c) What are the features of hydrops fetalis?
   d) How do you diagnose fetal anemia and its severity?
   e) What is kernicterus and how is it treated?

Answers

a) This woman has already developed antibodies against Rh-positive cells and Rh-isoimmunisation has already taken place. Therefore, the fetal RBCs can be destroyed by the maternal antibodies.

b) Due to the destruction and hemolysis of the RBCs, the fetus can develop fetal anemia and hyperbilirubinemia. This is known as the hemolytic disease of the fetus and the newborn (HDFN). Because of the ongoing severe anemia, fetal hydrops or intrauterine death can occur. After birth, the newborn will present with anemia, icterus and kernicterus.

c) Hydrops fetalis is invariably fatal. It presents with edema, anasarca, anemia and ascites. Due to severe hemolysis, there is extramedullary erythropoiesis, resulting in hepatosplenomegaly and portal obstruction. There is also hydrothorax and cardiac failure. The placenta is pale and edematous with swollen villi.

d) In this woman, the antibody titres should be ascertained every 4 weeks. The critical value of the antibody titre is 1:16, above which the fetus will be in danger. In order to know the severity of fetal anemia, middle cerebral artery peak systolic velocity is measured periodically. This is a non-invasive method.

If the levels are abnormal, invasive methods such as assessment of the bilirubin level in the amniotic fluid and/or FBS after cordocentesis should be undertaken. A hematocrit value of <30% indicates severe anemia. If the gestational age is >34 weeks, the baby is delivered, and exchange transfusion given. If the gestational age is <34 weeks, intrauterine transfusion is given.

e) The newborn is severely anemic and jaundiced. Jaundice manifests within 24 hours of delivery. Due to excessive hemolysis, the bilirubin level is high, and it crosses the blood–brain barrier and binds to the neurons. Clinically, the child presents with cerebral irritation, convulsions, twitching and spasticity. The danger level for developing kernicterus is 275 micromol/lit. The child is treated with exchange transfusion to correct anemia, to remove the circulating antibodies and to reduce the bilirubin levels. Phototherapy is also given.

29 Anemia Complicating Pregnancy

OG 12.2

Learning Objectives

» To define and classify anemia

» To know the causes of anemia

» To discuss the diagnosis and investigations performed in suspected cases of anemia

» To describe the effect of anemia on the mother and the fetus

» To know the management of anemia in pregnancy and labour

■ INTRODUCTION

The World Health Organization (WHO)/World Health Statistics' data show that 40.1% of pregnant women worldwide were anemic in 2016. The condition is prominent in Southeast Asian countries. The incidence of anemia ranges from 40–90% in India. A marginal decrease in its prevalence has been noted in pregnant women in India—from 58% in the NFHS-3 (National Family Health Survey, 2005–06) to 50% in the NFHS-4 survey (2015–16).

Anemia has a major impact on maternal and child health and is associated with a number of maternal and fetal complications. It decreases the woman's reserve to tolerate bleeding during or after childbirth and also makes her prone to infections. Anemia is also associated with an increased risk of fetal growth restriction, premature delivery, low birth weight (LBW) and maternal and perinatal mortality.

Anemia is one of the major causes of maternal deaths worldwide. According to the World Health Organization (WHO), anemia contributes to 40% of maternal deaths in third world countries, a sizeable percentage of which are from India. In India, anemia contributes to 10–15% of direct maternal deaths.

■ DEFINITION

Anemia is defined as a decrease in the oxygen-carrying capacity of the blood due to low hemoglobin (Hb) concentration or a decrease in the number of RBCs.

- According to the WHO, an Hb level <11 g/dL is considered as anemia during pregnancy. In the postpartum period, a hemoglobin level <10 g/dL is considered as anemia.
- The Centers for Disease Control and Prevention define anemia as Hb less than 11 g/dL in the first

and third trimesters and less than 10.5 g/dL in the second trimester (to make an allowance for physiological anemia).

■ DEGREE OF ANEMIA

Anemia is graded based on hemoglobin levels, as shown in Table 29.1.

Table 29.1 Degrees of anemia

Degree of anemia	WHO	ICMR
Mild	10–10.9 g/dL	10–10.9 g/dL
Moderate	7–9.9 g/dL	7–10 g/dL
Severe	<7 g/dL	<7 g/dL
Very severe		<4 g/dL
Postpartum	<0 g/dL	

■ PHYSIOLOGICAL ANEMIA OF PREGNANCY

During pregnancy, the plasma volume increases by 40–45%. This increase starts in the 6th week of pregnancy and peaks at 32 weeks. The increase of plasma volume is greater than that of the red cell mass, which increases to 15–20%. This disproportionate increase of the plasma volume and red cell mass results in physiological anemia of pregnancy. The lower limits of hematological criteria to diagnose physiological anemia are as follows:

- Hb level is 10 g/dL
- RBC count is 3.2 million/mm^3
- PCV is 30%
- Peripheral smear shows normal morphology of RBC

The reduced viscosity of blood in physiological anemia allows adequate placental perfusion.

ETIOLOGY

The causes of anemia can be broadly classified as follows:

Nutritional anemia
- Iron deficiency
- Folate and vitamin B12 deficiency

Anemia due to chronic blood loss
- Hookworm infestation
- Heavy periods antedating pregnancy
- Hemorrhoids

Hereditary anemia and anemia due to increased cell destruction
- Thalassemia
- Sickle cell anemia
- Hereditary spherocytosis and elliptocytosis
- Malaria

Anemia due to bone marrow insufficiency
- Decreased production of blood cells as in aplastic anemia
- Bone marrow suppression due to radiation, drugs, etc.
- Hematological malignancies causing bone marrow suppression

Nutritional Causes of Anemia

In India, nutritional causes contribute to nearly 50–55% of cases of anemia during pregnancy. An active bone marrow requires not only iron but also traces of copper and zinc, folic acid, vitamin B, vitamin C and protein for hemoglobin formation. In pregnancy, though iron deficiency is the commonest cause of nutritional anemia, folic acid or vitamin B12 deficiency are also frequently reported. More often, one encounters a combined deficiency of iron and folic acid known as dimorphic anemia.

Iron deficiency anemia (IDA)

It is the commonest cause of nutritional anemia in pregnancy. The iron deficiency may pre-exist and worsen during pregnancy, or it may develop during pregnancy.

Causes of iron deficiency anemia in pregnancy

- **Poor intake of dietary iron due to non-availability:** The average Indian diet contains 20–22 mg of iron, of which only 10% is absorbed. This is adequate for a non-pregnant adult woman. In a pregnant woman, at least 4–6 mg of iron should be absorbed daily, which necessitates a daily dietary intake of 40–60 mg. During pregnancy, the demand for iron increases, which may not be met due to non-availability/poor nutrition or due to reduced intake of food owing to nausea and vomiting of pregnancy. The iron content in the diet of women in lower socio-economic groups may also be very low.

- **Poor absorption and bioavailability:** There are two types of iron—heme iron and non-heme iron. The bioavailability of heme iron found in animal protein is greater than that of non-heme iron found in a vegetarian diet. Nearly 30–40% of heme iron is absorbed whereas, only 10% of non-heme iron is absorbed.

  — Factors influencing absorption: Absorption of iron is regulated by the state of the body stores. Iron absorption is rapid in the presence of diminished reserves. Poor absorption can also occur due to worm infestation and malabsorption due to intestinal factors.

  — Iron enhancers and iron inhibitors: There are a number of dietary substances that act as 'iron enhancers' and 'iron inhibitors'. Iron enhancers are foods rich in vitamin C, such as citrus fruits, meat and fish; these enhance the absorption of iron. Iron inhibitors are substances that inhibit iron absorption, e.g., tannins (found in tea and coffee), phytates (found in wheat and maize products), phosphates in egg, dairy products and antacids and calcium tablets, when used concurrently.

- **Increased demand during pregnancy:** The physiological demand for iron during pregnancy is three times higher than in non-pregnant women and it increases as pregnancy progresses. The increased demand for iron requirements in a singleton pregnancy has been calculated to be 900–1,000 mg, taking into account the requirements for the fetus, placenta, expansion of maternal erythrocyte mass and final losses due to delivery (Table 29.2). The daily requirement of iron during pregnancy is 4–6 mg in the second trimester and 6–8 mg per day in the third trimester. The demand further increases in the presence of multiple pregnancy.

- **Loss of iron:** Excessive iron loss—as in hookworm infestation (ancylostomiasis), dysentery, chronic malaria, bleeding piles, previous menorrhagia, chronic intake of drugs such as NSAIDs, excessive sweating (as in tropical countries)—contributes to iron deficiency anemia. Infestation with *Ancylostoma* can result in a blood loss of 0.2 mL per worm per day.

Table 29.2   Iron requirement during pregnancy

Requirement	Amount of iron
To meet the increase in RBC mass	500 mg
Transplacental transport to the fetus	300 mg
For the enlarging uterus, breast and placenta	150 mg
To meet the blood loss at delivery	150–200 mg
Iron saved due to amenorrhea in pregnancy	200 mg

- **Inadequate transport:** Protein deficiency can lead to poor transport of iron from blood to the bone marrow.
- **Poor reserve:** This may be seen in women entering their first pregnancy with inadequate iron reserves due to pre-existing adolescent anemia or in multiparous women who have repeated pregnancies without spacing (less than two years between pregnancies), in women who have prolonged lactation and those with a previous PPH. These are important factors predisposing to iron deficiency anemia.
- **Chronic illness:** Chronic illnesses such as recurrent urinary tract infections, renal failure with erythropoietin deficiency and achlorhydria are contributing factors for iron deficiency anemia.

Stages of iron deficiency anemia

Iron deficiency anemia evolves through three distinct stages (Fig. 29.1). Depletion of storage iron occurs in the first phase (stage I), wherein the total iron of the body decreases but red cell indices and hemoglobin (Hb) synthesis remain unchanged. Both these indices change when the supply of iron to the bone marrow is reduced (stage II or iron-deficient erythropoiesis). Eventually, IDA develops due to an insufficient supply of iron to sustain a normal Hb; this is stage III.

Iron metabolism

Absorption of iron

Iron is absorbed in the duodenum and upper jejunum. Dietary iron is mainly in the ferric form and has to be reduced to ferrous iron before absorption. Food has two types of iron:

- **Heme iron** is present in a non-vegetarian diet. It is a divalent iron with a ferrous molecule, and therefore, is easily absorbed. The composition of food has little effect on its absorption.
- **Non-heme iron** (makes up 90% of dietary iron) found in a vegetarian diet is mostly in the ferric form, which has to be reduced to the ferrous form by gastric acidity or by reducing substances such as ascorbic acid before absorption. The absorption of non-heme iron is affected by inhibitors.

Transport

After absorption, the iron is oxidised back to the ferric form in the mucosal cells and then transported to the blood. In blood, it binds to transferrin, an iron-binding protein and transported to various parts of the body.

Storage

After combining with apoferritin, iron is stored in the liver, spleen and bone marrow as ferritin or an aggregate of ferritin called hemosiderin.

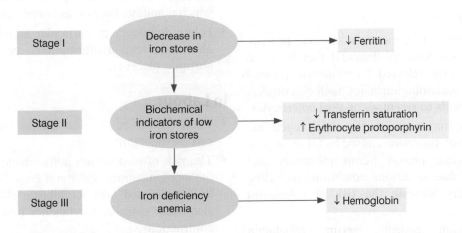

Fig. 29.1   Stages of iron deficiency anemia

- The average diet contains 20–22 mg of iron/day, of which only 10% is absorbed.
- The daily iron loss through urine, feces, sweat and mucosal surface is 1 mg/day.
- The daily iron requirement for non-pregnant women is 1.5–1.8 mg /day.
- During pregnancy, it increases by three times.

Vitamin B12 and Folate Deficiency

Besides iron, folic acid and B12 are other essential nutrients required for hemopoiesis, the deficiency of which leads to megaloblastic anemia. Folate and cobalamin are also necessary for DNA synthesis, and they influence the cell division and growth of cells in the mother and the fetus.

Folic acid deficiency

Green, leafy vegetables are rich in folic acid, which gets absorbed in the jejunum. Folate deficiency can occur due to poor nutrition, overcooking of food, alcoholism, intestinal malabsorption, and increased demands for folic acid, as seen in multiple pregnancy, hemolytic disorders, folate metabolism disorder, pregestational diabetes and in epileptic women on valproate or carbamazepine. For women who are at an increased risk of neural tube defects (NTD) because of personal or family history of NTD, the folic acid requirement is more. Pure folic acid deficiency is uncommon but is usually associated with iron deficiency anemia causing dimorphic anemia. The WHO recommends folate supplementation for all pregnant women—400 µg per day from early pregnancy to three months postpartum. A higher supplementation dose—5 mg per day—is recommended for women who have increased demands and those who are in deficient states.

B12 deficiency

- Cobalamin, which is present in animal protein, is absorbed in the terminal ileum. It then binds to the intrinsic factor released from gastric parietal cells. The cobalamin–intrinsic factor complex subsequently binds to receptors on ileal enterocytes.
- B12 deficiency may occur with a strict vegetarian diet or due to malabsorption caused by GI disorders. Atrophic gastritis, proton pump inhibitors and malabsorption due to various conditions including bariatric surgery increase the risk of cobalamin deficiency.
- In non-pregnant patients, serum cobalamin <200 pg/mL is diagnostic of cobalamin deficiency, whereas levels above 300 are considered normal.

CLINICAL FEATURES

- In mild anemia, there may be a few non-specific symptoms such as fatigue, weakness, light-headedness, headache and mild dyspnea during exertion. Alternatively, anemia may be diagnosed during routine antenatal investigations.
- Late features include dizziness, breathlessness, palpitation, anorexia, swelling of the legs and trouble with concentrating.
- Signs of anemia include pallor of skin, lips, nails, conjunctiva and mucous membrane, glossitis, stomatitis, tachycardia, high-volume pulse and ankle edema. There is systolic murmur on cardiac evaluation. Specific signs of iron deficiency anemia are koilonychia and brittle nails and hair. In severe anemia, there are features of cardiac failure.
- Besides anemia, folic acid and B12 deficiencies also present with vomiting, anorexia, glossitis, weight loss and neurological symptoms.

EFFECTS OF ANEMIA ON PREGNANCY

Antenatal Period

- During the antenatal period, anemia is associated with increased susceptibility to infections and asymptomatic bacteriuria and increased risk of preterm labour. Severe anemia is associated with an increased risk of cardiac failure at 32–34 weeks of gestation.
- Anemic women have a three times greater risk of delivering a low-birth-weight baby due to prematurity or fetal growth restriction than women who are not anemic. The risk of perinatal deaths also increases with anemia. The iron stores in the neonate are reduced, which manifests later on as anemia in the neonate.
- Folate deficiency in particular increases the risk of abortions, fetal malformations, pre-eclampsia and abruptio placenta.

In Labour

- There could be uterine inertia due to impaired myometrial contractions.
- The risk of postpartum hemorrhage is increased as the woman cannot withstand even the normal blood loss associated with childbirth. Atonic PPH can also occur since iron deficiency impairs myometrial contractions.
- The woman may present with postpartum collapse and shock.

- In severe anemia, cardiac failure may be precipitated by uterine contractions and is an important cause of maternal mortality.

Postpartum Complications

- During the puerperium, anemic mothers are prone to puerperal sepsis.
- There is an increased risk of deep venous thrombosis and cortical vein thrombosis.
- Anemia may lead to subinvolution of the uterus due to infection.
- There may be failure of lactation.
- In operative deliveries, there may be delayed wound healing.
- Cardiac failure can occur in the puerperium also. Anemic women are prone to myocardial depression and congestive cardiac failure (CCF).

Maternal mortality in anemia is due to cardiac failure, hemorrhagic shock and severe puerperal sepsis.

■ INVESTIGATIONS

In a pregnant woman presenting with anemia, investigations are required for the following purposes:

- To confirm the diagnosis of anemia
- To determine the severity of anemia
- To diagnose the type of anemia
- To determine the cause of anemia
- To evaluate response to treatment

1. Diagnosis, Confirmation and Assessment of Severity Of Anemia

The woman's hemoglobin level is estimated to confirm the diagnosis and to assess the severity of anemia. The test is carried out by a semi-autoanalyser or by the calorimetric method.

2. To Determine the Type of Anemia

Several blood parameters are available to assess the iron status of the individual.

- **Peripheral blood smear:** By examining a peripheral blood smear, the morphology of the blood cells is studied, which is very useful to determine the type of anemia and its cause. In a healthy individual without anemia, the smear is normochromic and normocytic.

Iron deficiency anemia

In iron deficiency anemia, the characteristic findings include smaller than normal RBCs (microcytosis), anisocytosis (variation in cell size), poikilocytosis (variation in cell shape) and pale-staining (hypochromic) vacuolated red cells in abundance. This is called **hypochromic, microcytic anemia**. Microcytosis in the peripheral smear may be seen even before abnormalities in complete blood count (CBC) develop. The presence of microcytic, hypochromic red cells and long, thin hypochromic cells called 'photo pencil cells' is indicative of iron deficiency anemia. Other conditions in which microcytic RBCs are seen are anemias of chronic disorders, β-thalassemia, sideroblastic anemia, lead poisoning and alcoholism.

Folic acid and B12 deficiency

In folic acid and vitamin B12 deficiency, the erythrocytes are large with more hemoglobin. Therefore, the peripheral smear shows a macrocytic picture with hyperchromic anemia and nucleated RBCs.

The diagnosis of folic acid deficiency is also made by the presence of >4% neutrophils showing >5 lobes.

Aplastic anemia

In bone marrow aplasia and depression, the peripheral smear shows pancytopenia with a reduced number of all blood cells.

Cause of Anemia

A peripheral smear may show evidence of the malarial parasite, fragmented RBCs in hemolytic anemia and immature cells in leukemia.

Red cell indices

Besides hemoglobin, RBC count and hematocrit are checked, and from these three parameters, other indices such as mean corpuscular volume (MCV), mean corpuscular hemoglobin (MCH) and mean corpuscular hemoglobin concentration (MCHC) are calculated.

MCV is the measure of the average RBC volume and MCHC is the measure of the concentration of Hb in a given volume of packed RBCs. In iron deficiency anemia, the MCV is below 80 fl/cell and the MCHC is less than 30%. It is important to note that up to 40% of patients with true IDA have normocytic erythrocytes (i.e., a normal MCV does not rule out iron deficiency anemia). In megaloblastic anemia, the MCV is increased >100 fl/cell.

Red cell distribution width (RDW) has a better sensitivity than MCV for the diagnosis of iron deficiency anemia. The RDW is a measure of the change in RBC width. In the initial stages of iron deficiency anemia, there is a decrease in MCV, accompanied by increasing RDW values due to a preponderance of microcytes. Following treatment, marked reticulocytosis occurs in the first four weeks, which manifests as a sudden increase in RDW, sometimes to over 30%. Thus, decreasing MCV accompanied by a rising RDW should alert the clinician to the presence of possible iron deficiency anemia.

Serum ferritin

Ferritin is a sensitive indicator of iron deficiency anemia in pregnant women. Normal serum ferritin levels are 15–200 µg/L. A decrease in serum concentration below 15 µg/L indicates iron depletion in all stages of pregnancy. Treatment needs to be initiated when the concentration falls below 30 µg/L, as this indicates early iron depletion. In any woman diagnosed with iron deficiency anemia and not responding to iron therapy, it is mandatory to estimate serum ferritin before further iron therapy.

Serum iron, and total iron-binding capacity (TIBC)

In iron deficiency anemia, there is a characteristic decrease in the transferrin saturation (serum iron level is decreased, whereas the TIBC is increased; therefore, the transferrin saturation drops to <16%. (The normal percentage of saturation is 20–45%.)

Serum and RBC folic acid level and B12 levels

In women in whom folic acid/B12 deficiency is suspected, serum folic acid and B12 levels can be estimated. Serum folic acid concentrations <2 ng/mL are diagnostic of folic acid deficiency.

Besides serum B12 estimation, a fractional test meal is required to diagnose achlorhydria in B12 deficiency.

Other investigations to determine the cause of anemia

- Peripheral smear to detect the malarial parasite
- Stool examination may reveal *Ancylostoma duodenale* ova, which have a typical transparent outer membrane with four blastomeres, are non-bile-stained and float in normal saline; occult blood should be looked for
- Urine analysis and culture and sensitivity to diagnose asymptomatic bacteriuria and symptomatic urinary tract infection
- Serum proteins to diagnose hypoproteinemia
- Occasionally, the following special investigations may be required:
  — Serum bilirubin for hemolytic anemia

  — Fractional test meal for B12 deficiency
  — Bone marrow examination for aplastic and hypoplastic anemia

■ TREATMENT

In the management of anemia in pregnancy, apart from treating the cause of anemia, iron therapy should be given to correct the anemia and to replenish the iron stores.

Even milder forms of anemia should be treated, as the situation is likely to worsen into severe anemia, thereby increasing the maternal and perinatal risks. Management depends on the following factors:

- The period of gestation and the time remaining until delivery
- The severity of anemia
- Maternal co-morbid conditions
  The treatment options include the following:
- Oral iron
- Parenteral iron
- Stimulation of hemopoiesis with growth factors such as recombinant human erythropoietin
- Blood transfusion

Dietary Modification

This involves improving the intake of iron by increasing the quantity of iron-rich food and adopting practices that increase the absorption of iron. Non-heme iron, a poorly absorbed form of iron, derived from cereals, pulses, vegetables and fruits, contributes to about 90–95% of the total daily iron in Indian diets. Absorption is inhibited by phytic acid, which is found in whole grains, lentils, maize and nuts. In addition, tannins found in coffee and tea also inhibit iron absorption. Promoting the consumption of iron absorption enhancers like ascorbic acid is an effective way of increasing bioavailability of iron and results in an improvement in the Hb level.

Iron-rich foods include the following:

- Meat and poultry—beef, mutton, spleen and liver
- Green, leafy vegetables, greens such as drumstick leaves, fenugreek, spinach
- Raisins, jaggery
- Cereal grains and products—whole wheat, *ragi*, *jowar*
- Pulses and legumes—Bengal gram, green gram, horse gram, lentils, dry peas, soya beans, groundnuts and almonds
- Fruits—gooseberry (*amla*), dates and pomegranate
- Nuts and oil seeds

If the pregnant woman is severely anemic (Hb <7.0 g/dL irrespective of gestational age), she will require blood transfusion. However, if the anemia is not severe, iron therapy may be initiated.

Oral Iron Therapy

Indications, prescription of iron and assessment of response

- In pregnant women with established mild to moderate anemia and a period of gestation <30–32 weeks, oral iron can be given.
- 100 mg elemental iron is given twice daily with 500 µg of folic acid.
- A repeat hemoglobin test is recommended after four weeks of oral iron. After achieving the normalisation of hemoglobin, a prophylactic daily iron supplementation (60–100 mg of iron and 500 µg of folic acid) is recommended for at least six months during pregnancy and should be continued for another six months postpartum.
- Available preparations of oral iron are ferrous sulphate, carbonate, fumarate and gluconate. Ferrous ascorbate and bisglycinate have been found to be more effective and better tolerated than ferrous sulphate.
- Iron should be taken on an empty stomach, one hour before meals. Tea, coffee and other dairy products should be avoided within two hours of iron intake.
- Citrus fruits and vitamin C tablets enhance iron absorption. The concurrent consumption of iron preparations with calcium citrate and carbonate preparations and antacids should be avoided.
- Side effects include diarrhea, constipation, abdominal pain, flatulence, nausea, black or tarry stools and heartburn.
- Response to treatment is observed by an increase in reticulocytes within a week of starting iron therapy. The hemoglobin level also increases.

The Hb level begins to rise by 2–3 weeks. The expected rise in hemoglobin is 1 g/dL/week from the second week onwards.

- If there is no response despite treatment, one should look for non-compliance, poor absorption, continued loss of iron and an incorrect diagnosis, which mandates further investigations to exclude other causes of anemia.

Parenteral Therapy

Indications for parenteral therapy

- Insufficient or no response to oral iron
- Inability to tolerate oral iron
- Poor compliance because of side effects
- Moderate anemia between 30 and 36 weeks of gestation
- Need for rapid restoration of iron stores
- Poor absorption due to dysentery or malabsorption syndrome

Prerequisites for the use of parenteral iron

- Iron deficiency confirmed by serum ferritin levels of <15 µg/L
- No hemoglobinopathy
- No liver disease
- No known iron overload
- Oral iron should be stopped at least 24 hours prior to therapy to avoid toxic reaction

Contraindications

- A history of anaphylactic reactions to parenteral iron therapy—a sensitivity test is recommended prior to infusion

Adverse effects

- Mild symptoms include joint pains and discolouration at the injection site, headache and malaise.
- Severe reactions such as allergy, itching, fever, lymphadenopathy, arthralgia and anaphylaxis can occur.

Preparations

Both intravenous and intramuscular preparations are available.

Calculation of parenteral iron requirement

Required iron dose (mg) = (2.4 × [target Hb – actual Hb] × pre-pregnancy weight [Kg]) + 1,000 mg for replenishment of stores

Intravenous iron

- Iron sucrose is the most commonly used preparation for IV infusion; it is safe, has fewer adverse events and is well-tolerated. It is rapidly taken up by the bone marrow for erythropoiesis and the reticuloendothelial system for storage.
- Iron sucrose is available in 5 mL ampules containing 20 mg/mL each. The IV infusion is prepared by dissolving 100–200 mg of iron sucrose in 100 mL of normal saline and is administered over a period of 15–20 minutes.

It is important for the duration of IV infusion of intravenous iron to not exceed 30 minutes since prolonged administration of iron sucrose results in the release of free radicals, which can give rise to reactions.

- A maximum dose of 200 mg can be given, which can be repeated 2–3 times a week.
- Iron sucrose cannot be diluted in dextrose.
- Ferric carboxymaltose (FCM) is a dextran-free IV iron preparation that allows rapid administration of high doses of iron (up to 1,000 mg iron in 15 minutes). FCM administration in the postpartum period has been found to be safe and effective in improving the mean Hb level. It can be used during pregnancy also. Compared to other parenteral iron preparations, FCM has several advantages—it has fewer side effects; a single, high-dose administration is possible; and it can reduce the frequency of hospital visits. FCM is diluted in 250 mL of normal saline for administration; the dose should not exceed 15 mg/Kg body weight. Side effects include headache and swelling at the injection site.

Intramuscular preparations

- Intramuscular preparations are not commonly used nowadays due to the availability of effective intravenous preparations with minimal adverse effects.
- Previously, iron dextran and iron–sorbitol–citric acid complexes were used as parenteral therapy. However, the high incidence of anaphylactic reactions, occasionally leading to maternal death, has resulted in the discontinuation of these parenteral preparations.
- Intramuscular injections are given by the Z technique to avoid staining the skin. After injecting a 25 mg test dose intramuscularly, 100 mg of iron–sorbitol–citric acid complex can be given IM on alternate days. Side effects include pain at the injection site, discolouration of the skin and joint pains. Iron dextran preparations may be associated with thrombophlebitis, arthralgia, urticaria, fever and lymphadenopathy. Severe anaphylactic reaction may also occur.

Blood Transfusion

There are few indications for blood transfusion. Blood transfusion in anemic patients is associated with an increased risk of congestive cardiac failure and preterm labour. Therefore, while giving transfusion, packed red cells are transfused to avoid fluid overload.

Indications

- Severe anemia with Hb <7 g/dL at any gestational age
- Moderate anemia beyond 36 weeks of gestation
- Anemia due to thalassemia and sickle cell disease
- All pregnant women with moderate anemia facing labour and cesarean section
- Anemia with signs of shock/acute hemorrhage and signs of hemodynamic instability

Exchange transfusion

It is indicated in severe anemia with congestive cardiac failure. Packed cells are transfused through one antecubital vein, while withdrawing whole blood on the opposite side at the same time. The amount of blood withdrawn is 200 mL more than the amount of blood transfused to keep a negative balance.

Recombinant Human Erythropoietin (rHu EPO)

Recombinant human erythropoietin (rHu EPO) has been successfully given to patients with end-stage renal disease. Recently, this preparation has been tried in pregnant woman with resistant anemia, especially when it is due to renal disease. This is not recommended for routine use in pregnancy as it may be associated with complications such as hypertension and thrombotic manifestations.

The management of anemia has been summarised algorithmically in Fig. 29.2.

- In all cases of anemia, deworming should be done after 14 weeks of gestation.
- After treating anemia with iron, response to treatment should be checked in 3–4 weeks' time.
- After correcting anemia, the prophylactic dose should be continued.
- If there is no response, the woman should be evaluated for other causes of anemia.

Deworming

As per the national guidelines for deworming in pregnancy prescribed by the MoHFW, Government of India, a single dose of 400 mg of albendazole tablet should be given to the woman after the first trimester, preferably in the second trimester.

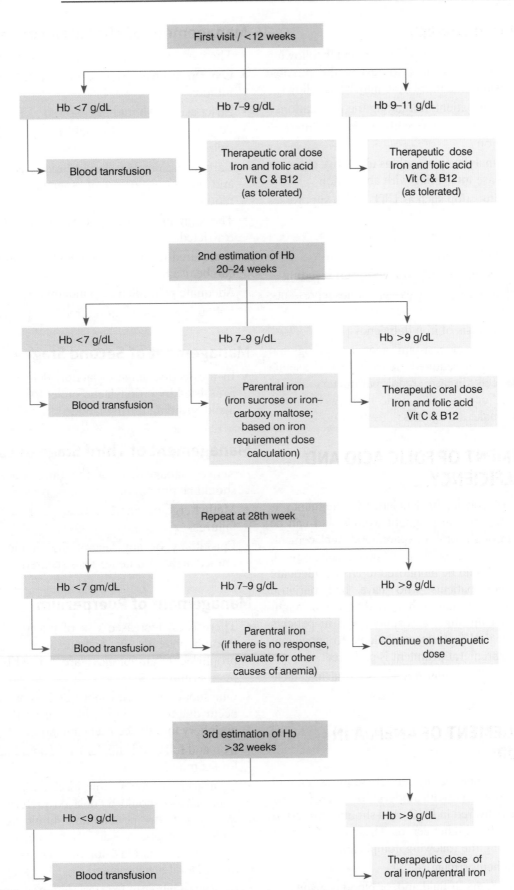

Fig. 29.2 Flowchart for the management of anemia based on gestational age and severity of anemia

Failure of Iron Therapy

In women not showing the expected rise in Hb following iron therapy, it is important to review the possible causes for resistant anemia. These may be as follows:

- Non-compliant patient, not taking the medications
- Taking medications along with foods that interfere with absorption
- Gastrointestinal diseases such as ulcerative colitis or Crohn's disease interfering with absorption
- Presence of infection such as UTI, which suppresses erythropoiesis
- Malabsorption of iron in coeliac disease
- Underlying kidney disease
- Ongoing bleeding due to parasites or GI bleeding
- Drugs inhibiting erythropoiesis—immunosuppressants, cytotoxic drugs
- Incorrect diagnosis of iron deficiency
- In the presence of resistant anemia, hemoglobin electrophoresis is required to exclude thalassemia and sickle cell disease; renal parameters should be assessed; occasionally, bone marrow biopsy is required to make a diagnosis

TREATMENT OF FOLIC ACID AND B12 DEFICIENCY

- Treatment of cobalamin deficiency in pregnancy is similar to that of non-pregnant women and can be achieved through oral or parenteral replacement. When oral vitamin cobalamin, 1,000 µg daily, is used, serum levels should be monitored to ensure adequate repletion. For patients who have had bariatric surgery, those who have other conditions that might interfere with intestinal absorption, and in patients with neurological features attributable to cobalamin deficiency, parenteral treatment is preferred.
- Folic acid is administered as oral/injectable preparations.

MANAGEMENT OF ANEMIA IN LABOUR

Management of anemia in labour requires careful monitoring. Any woman with moderate or severe anemia should not be delivered in PHCs and should be referred well in advance to a higher centre. These women are at risk of developing the following complications:

- Postpartum hemorrhage
- Pulmonary edema, if fluid and/or blood is given
- Cardiac failure

Management of First Stage of Labour

- The woman is nursed in the propped-up position.
- Oxygen is given by face mask at the rate of 4 L/minute.
- Strict asepsis should be followed.
- IV access and blood should be kept ready (packed cells).
- Careful monitoring should be carried out for CCF and in severe cases of anemia, digitalisation is required.
- The woman can be on clear liquids; IV fluids are restricted.
- If required to infuse medications, an infusion pump can be used.
- Adequate pain relief is mandatory.
- Labour progress is monitored by a partograph.

Management of Second Stage of Labour

- In the second stage of labour, delivery of the head is assisted by prophylactic outlet forceps/vacuum to avoid straining during labour.

Management of Third Stage of Labour

- Active management of the third stage of labour should be practised.
- Methyl ergometrine is avoided as it can precipitate failure.
- Episiotomy or any lacerations should be sutured immediately, and hemostasis secured.

Management of Puerperium

- There is an increased risk of puerperal sepsis and thrombophlebitis in anemic women. Therefore, prophylactic antibiotics are prescribed in the puerperium.
- One should be careful about CCF as overloading can occur due to shunting of blood from the uterus and periphery into the central circulation.
- Iron and folic acid supplements should be continued for six months.
- Contraception for anemic mothers is a challenging issue. IUCD should be delayed preferably until the woman gets her periods and should be introduced under antibiotic cover. The barrier method of contraception is ideal for the first 3–4 weeks until the Hb level has improved.
- In women who opt for sterilisation, it can be carried out after treating anemia and improving the Hb level.

PREVENTION

Preventive measures should focus on the following areas:

1. Dietary modification
2. Effective temporary methods of contraception to avoid pregnancy within 2–3 years
3. Improvement in health services
4. Control of hookworm, malaria and parasitic infestations
5. Sanitation
6. Measures to prevent adolescent anemia
7. Early diagnosis of anemia in pregnancy—hemoglobin level should be checked at booking visit, thereafter in every, trimester
8. Oral iron supplementation during pregnancy
   - Regular iron supplementation is necessary for pregnant women to prevent iron deficiency anemia. The 2013 Ministry of Health and Family Welfare (MoHFW) guidelines recommend 100 mg of iron and 500 µg of folic acid daily for at least 100 days, starting after the first trimester, at 14–16 weeks of gestation, followed by the same for six months in the postpartum period.
   - Woman should be advised to take the tablets on an empty stomach or at least one hour after a meal for better absorption. They should avoid consuming tea, coffee, milk or calcium tablets along with iron tablets.

National Anemia Prevention Programmes

1. **National Anemia Prophylaxis Programme:** Under this programme, all pregnant and lactating mothers should receive 100 mg of elemental iron and 0.5 mg of folic acid for at least 100 days.
2. **The 12-by-12 Initiative:** This initiative targeted all adolescents across the country. The aim was to achieve an Hb of 12 g/dL in every girl by the age of 12 years by 2012. Measures to achieve this target included better nutrition, iron and folic acid supplementation and deworming.
3. **Weekly Iron and Folic Acid Supplementation (WIFS) Programme:** In this programme, adolescent girls (and boys) across the country are given one iron tablet every Thursday.
4. **National Health Policy, 2017:** This policy addressed malnutrition and micronutrient deficiencies interventions.

5. **National Iron Plus Initiative**: It was launched in 2013 and was a comprehensive strategy to combat the public health challenge of iron deficiency anemia (IDA) prevalent across the life cycle.

HEMOGLOBINOPATHIES

Hemoglobinopathies are genetic disorders affecting hemoglobin synthesis, wherein the globin chains of the Hb molecule are affected. These disorders fall into two major categories: quantitative defect (thalassemia syndromes, in which production is affected) and qualitative defect (sickle cell syndrome, in which the structure of the globin chain is abnormal). These conditions result in anemia due to reduced erythrocyte life span, increased erythrocyte destruction, altered morphology of the erythrocyte and increased affinity of hemoglobin for oxygen, leading to poor oxygen delivery to the tissues.

Thalassemia

It is an inherited autosomal recessive hematologic disorder in which there are quantitative abnormalities in the synthesis of globin chain. Thalassemia is common in the northwestern part of India.

α-Thalassemia

Here, the four genes involved in the synthesis of α-globin chains are affected. The resulting deficit is compensated by an increase in either γ-globin or β-globin chains. When all the four genes are affected, the fetuses die in utero due to non-immune hydrops. α-Thalassemia major is otherwise called Bart disease.

β-Thalassemia

Here, the β-globin chain production is decreased, which is compensated by α chain production. The individual may be heterozygous or homozygous for this trait.

The heterozygous state is known as β-thalassemia minor and the homozygous state is known as β-thalassemia major (Cooley's anemia).

β-thalassemia minor (trait)

- Patients with the thalassemia trait have a normal life expectancy.
- If a woman who has a thalassemia trait has a partner who also has the trait, there is a 25% chance that the fetus will have thalassemia major. Such a couple should be offered prenatal diagnosis with amniocentesis and biochemical analysis.
- Individuals who have the minor trait commonly present with mild anemia or may remain asymptomatic.

- If anemia is present, the peripheral smear picture shows microcytic, hypochromic anemia.
- There may be a family history of anemia and repeated blood transfusions.
- In a woman with mild to moderate anemia, who is not responding to iron therapy, thalassemia should be suspected, and electrophoresis should be carried out to rule it out.
- There may be associated diabetes and hypothyroidism in these patients.
- They should never be treated with parenteral iron. Blood transfusions are required for the treatment of anemia.
- There may be mild splenomegaly.
- There may be relative folate deficiency.
- Thalassemia traits are associated with a reduced mean corpuscular volume (MCV), reduced mean corpuscular hemoglobin (MCH), and a normal to near-normal mean corpuscular hemoglobin concentration (MCHC). Of all these markers, the most accurate marker is MCH.
- Additionally, β-thalassemia is associated with elevated HbA$_2$ levels (>3.5 g/dL).
- High levels of serum iron and ferritin levels may be found.

Treatment
- Folic acid supplements should be prescribed during the preconception period and during pregnancy.
- With documented iron deficiency, oral iron can be given.
- Parenteral iron therapy is contraindicated.
- In the presence of anemia with hemoglobin <8 g/dL, and failure to respond to oral iron therapy, blood transfusion should be given.

β-Thalassemia major
- It is a homozygous state in which β-globin synthesis is affected, and there is an excess of free α chains. As a result, there is ineffective hemopoiesis, and subsequently, hemolysis. The resultant anemia stimulates increased erythropoietin, increased iron absorption and expansion of bone marrow, leading to various bony deformities such as frontal bossing, prominent zygomatic bone and expansion of metatarsals and metacarpals.
- Repeated blood transfusions are required in childhood, which further increases the risk of iron overload. Due to iron deposition (hemosiderosis), there is liver, cardiac and endocrine dysfunction.

- There could be thrombotic complications and gallstone formation.
- Individuals with β-thalassemia major generally die from cardiac complications due to iron overload by the time they reach 30 years of age.
- Pregnancy in a woman who has β-thalassemia major is rare due to its association with hypogonadotropic hypogonadism. However, with the advancement of treatment leading to the increased lifespan for these individuals, pregnancy is now possible, but needs careful antenatal monitoring. This includes screening for viral markers associated with repeated blood transfusions. These women have compromised cardiac function apart from diabetes and thyroid abnormalities. Clinically, they present with severe anemia and heart failure; there may be CPD.
- Preconception genetic counselling is strongly advised for all patients with thalassemia.
- Mortality may be high in these women. If there is severe organ damage, termination of pregnancy may be considered in early pregnancy.
- Desferrioxamine, the chelating agent used in iron overload, should be discontinued during pregnancy to prevent harmful fetal effects and iron deficiency in the fetus.
- Thalassemia major patients may require repeated blood transfusions during pregnancy. Labour management is similar to that for iron deficiency anemia.
- Desferrioxamine should be restarted within the first week postpartum. Breastfeeding is not contraindicated.
- Investigations:
  — The RBCs of thalassemia patients hemolyse in hypotonic saline
  — Hb electrophoresis findings (Table 29.3)
  — Patients suffering from β-thalassemia major disorder generally have a high percentage of HbF, whereas an increased fraction of HbA$_2$ levels is present in individuals having β-thalassemia minor

Table 29.3 Electrophoresis findings in β-thalassemia patients

	HbA	HbA$_2$ ($\alpha_2\delta_2$)	HbF ($\alpha_2\gamma_2$)
Normal adult	95%	2–3%	<2%
β-Thalassemia minor	80–95%	4–10%	1–5%
β-Thalassemia major	0%	4–10%	90–98%

Management

- Women who have thalassemia major are at an increased risk of various maternal complications such as cardiac failure, alloimmunisation, viral infection, thrombosis, osteoporosis, endocrine disorders like diabetes mellitus, hypothyroidism and hypoparathyroidism due to the increasing iron burden. They may develop early-onset pre-eclampsia. The risk of fetal hydrops is high.
- Iron supplementation is absolutely contraindicated.
- Blood transfusion is the mainstay of treatment.
- CBC is performed every two weeks to maintain Hb at 9.5–10 g/dL.
- High folic acid supplementation is prescribed.
- Iron overload should be checked for by evaluating serum ferritin levels.
- Stem cell or bone marrow transplants and gene therapy are upcoming treatment modalities.

Sickle Cell Anemia

- Sickle cell disease is a group of inherited single-gene autosomal recessive disorders. In this condition, there is a qualitative defect wherein glutamic acid is replaced by valine at position 6 of the β-globin chain. In the oxygenated state, the cell functions normally. Whereas in the reduced state, the RBCs form clumps, become rigid and sickle-shaped and break easily, causing hemolytic anemia and vaso-occlusion of blood vessels presenting with painful vaso-occlusive crisis.
- Pregnant women with sickle cell anemia are at a high risk of maternal anemia (folate deficiency is common), recurrent infections (respiratory, pyelonephritis and puerperal sepsis), sickle cell crisis, acute chest syndrome, sickle cell disease (proliferative retinopathy, renal and hepatic impairment and leg ulcers), thrombophlebitis and proteinuric hypertension. Fetal effects include recurrent abortions, intrauterine growth restriction and prematurity and intrauterine fetal death. There could be sickling crisis in the third trimester and in the postpartum period. These women may also develop CCF and pulmonary embolism.
- In the homozygous state, sickling occurs commonly. In the heterozygous state, whenever there is infection, hypoxia, acidosis or dehydration, there is a chance of sickling crisis.
- Patients present with mild to moderate anemia. On peripheral smear, normocytic, normochromic anemia, sickle cells and increased reticulocyte count are seen. Sickling can be demonstrated by placing a coverslip over a drop of blood to exclude oxygenation.
- Hemoglobin electrophoresis will confirm the diagnosis.
- Genetic counselling and prenatal diagnosis are very important.

Management

Management involves preventing dehydration, hypoxia and infection, timely blood transfusion to maintain hemoglobin at 60–70%, folic acid supplementation, prophylactic antibiotics, screening for UTI and treating the same. Labour should be managed carefully, and care should be taken to avoid dehydration and hypotension, and oxygen saturation should be adequately maintained. Oral contraceptive pills are contraindicated.

KEY POINTS

- ✓ *40% of pregnant women worldwide are anemic.*
- ✓ *Anemia is one of the major causes of maternal deaths.*
- ✓ *According to the WHO, an Hb level less than 11 g/dL is considered as anemia during pregnancy. In the postpartum period, a hemoglobin level of <10 g/dL is considered as anemia.*
- ✓ *During pregnancy, the plasma volume increases by 40–45% and the red cell mass increases by 15–20%. This disproportionate increase of the plasma volume and red cell mass results in physiological anemia of pregnancy.*
- ✓ *Nutritional deficiency is the commonest cause of anemia in pregnancy.*
- ✓ *The increased demand for iron for a singleton pregnancy is 900–1,000 mg.*
- ✓ *The daily requirement of iron during pregnancy is 4–6 mg in the second trimester, which increases to 6–8 mg per day in the third trimester.*
- ✓ *Peripheral blood smear testing is important to determine the type of anemia and its cause.*
- ✓ *Iron deficiency anemia presents with microcytic hypochromic anemia.*
- ✓ *Serum ferritin is a sensitive indicator of iron deficiency anemia.*

✓ The management of anemia depends on the period of gestation, the time remaining until delivery and the severity of anemia.

✓ If the pregnant woman is severely anemic (Hb <7.0 g/dL irrespective of gestational age), blood transfusion is given.

✓ There is an increased demand for folic acid in multiple pregnancy, hemolytic disorders, pregestational diabetes and in epileptic women on valproate or carbamazepine.

✓ B12 deficiency anemia is seen in women who maintain a strictly vegetarian diet, in those who have had bariatric surgery and in those who have malabsorption syndrome.

✓ Thalassemia is an inherited autosomal recessive hematologic disorder in which there are quantitative abnormalities in the synthesis of globin chains.

✓ Pregnant women with sickle cell anemia are at high risk of maternal anemia, recurrent infections and sickle cell crisis.

Essay questions

1. What are the causes of iron deficiency anemia? Discuss the diagnosis and management of iron deficiency anemia in pregnancy.

2. A 30-year-old G3P2 was admitted at 39 weeks of gestation with labour pains. Her hemoglobin was 8 g/dL. How would you manage her labour? What complications should one anticipate in such a case?

Short answer questions

1. List the effects of iron deficiency anemia on the mother and the fetus.

2. Define anemia and enumerate the causes of anemia.

3. What are the causes of resistant anemia?

4. Discuss the prevention of anemia in pregnancy.

5. What is β-thalassemia?

6. What is sickle cell disease? Enumerate the risks associated with this condition.

MCQs

1. As per the WHO, what percentage of maternal deaths are due to anemia?
   a) 10%
   b) 30%
   c) 40%
   d) 50%

2. According to ICMR, severe anemia in pregnancy is defined as hemoglobin below what value?
   a) 11 g/dL
   b) 10 g/dL
   c) 7 g/dL
   d) 4 g/dL

3. By what percentage does the plasma volume increase by week 32 of pregnancy?
   a) 10–15%
   b) 20–25%
   c) 30–35%
   d) 40–45%

4. What is the most common cause of anemia in India?
   a) Nutritional
   b) Hemoglobinopathy
   c) Heavy periods
   d) Aplastic anemia

5. What is the average requirement of iron in the third trimester?
   a) 2—4 mg/day
   b) 4—6 mg/day
   c) 6—8 mg/day
   d) 8—10 mg/day

6. Which of the following regimen is provided by the National Anemia Prophylaxis Programme?
   a) 60 mg elemental iron and 0.5 mg folic acid for 60 days
   b) 60 mg elemental iron and 0.5 mg folic acid for 100 days
   c) 100 mg elemental iron and 0.5 mg folic acid for 60 days
   d) 100 mg elemental iron and 0.5 mg folic acid for 100 days

7. Which of the following is not caused by folate deficiency?
   a) Neural tube defects
   b) Down syndrome
   c) Abruption
   d) Abortion

8. Which of the following is not one of the complications of anemia?
   a) Puerperal sepsis
   b) Subinvolution of the uterus
   c) Decreased risk of venous thrombosis
   d) Lactation failure

9. Which of the following is not a cause of microcytic hypochromic anemia?
   a) Iron deficiency
   b) Vit B12 deficiency
   c) Lead poisoning
   d) Thalassemia

10. Under the National Anemia Prophylaxis Programme, how much elemental iron should all pregnant and lactating mothers receive?
   a) 50 mg of elemental iron
   b) 80 mg of elemental iron
   c) 100 mg of elemental iron
   d) 150 mg of elemental iron

11. Which of the following is not one of the causes of anemia?
   a) Hookworm infestation
   b) Malaria infection
   c) Thalassemia
   d) High altitude

Answers
1. (c), 2. (c), 3. (d), 4. (a), 5. (c), 6. (d), 7. (b), 8. (c), 9. (b), 10. (c), 11. (d)

Fill in the blanks

1. The earliest response to the treatment of iron deficiency anemia is an increase in the number of _____.

2. The daily iron requirement in the third trimester of pregnancy is _____.

Answers
1. reticulocytes, 2. 6–8 mg

Case scenario-based discussion

1. A 30-year-old G3P2 presents at 28 weeks of gestation with complaints of lethargy, giddiness, tiredness

and breathlessness on exertion, which she has been experiencing for the past four weeks. She also reports bilateral swelling of the feet for the past two weeks. She had two full-term normal pregnancies, delivered at an interval of 18 months. Her last childbirth was two years ago. She was given blood transfusion in the last pregnancy 10 days prior to delivery. On examination, she was pale; there was bilateral pitting pedal edema, her pulse was 90/minute, BP was 100/70 mm of Hg, RS was clear and there was an ejection systolic murmur. On palpation, her uterus corresponds to 26 weeks of gestation, and a good fetal heartbeat is detected.

a) What is the probable diagnosis in this case?
b) What are the causes of anemia complicating pregnancy?
c) What immediate investigations would you order?
d) The woman's hemoglobin was 8 g/dL, the peripheral smear shows hypochromic microcytic anemia, the MCV and MCH were low and the urine and stool examinations are normal. What type of anemia does she have? What confirmatory test would you carry out?
e) How would you treat this woman?

Answers

a) The probable diagnosis is anemia complicating pregnancy.
b) The causes of anemia include nutritional anemia caused by iron, folic acid and B12 deficiency, anemia due to chronic blood loss caused by hookworm infestation and hemorrhoids, hereditary anemia and anemia due to bone marrow insufficiency.
c) The immediate investigations include complete hemogram, peripheral smear, red cell indices, stool examination and urine analysis.
d) The investigations are suggestive of iron deficiency anemia. If necessary, it can be confirmed by serum ferritin estimation.
e) As the woman is suffering from moderate anemia, she can be treated with therapeutic doses of oral iron. If she is intolerant to oral iron, parenteral iron with iron sucrose infusion should be given. The iron requirement should be calculated prior to the parenteral therapy. The response to treatment should be checked in 2–3 weeks' time by checking the reticulocyte count and hemoglobin level.

2. A 29-year-old primigravida presents at 32 weeks of gestation with complaints of breathlessness, lethargy and palpitation. On examination, she is pale and has swollen ankles; her pulse rate is 92 bpm.
   a) What is the possible cause for her symptoms?
   b) What investigations would you order?
   c) The woman's hemoglobin is 6 g/dL. What treatment does she require? How would you administer this treatment?
   d) What are the maternal and fetal complications you expect in this woman?

Answers

a) In the differential diagnosis, one should consider anemia and heart disease complicating pregnancy. However, the diagnosis is more in favour of anemia as there is associated pallor.
b) The investigations include blood investigations hemoglobin, hematocrit estimation, and peripheral smear and stool and urine examination. Cardiac status should also be assessed.
c) As the woman is suffering from severe anemia, she needs a blood transfusion, for which packed cell should be used. As the rise in hemoglobin level is 1 g% per unit of blood transfused, she would need at least 3–4 units of blood. Before starting blood transfusion, cardiac status should be evaluated, and measures should be taken to prevent failure.
d) The maternal complications include susceptibility to infections, preterm labour and CCF. In labour, there is an increased risk of failure and uterine inertia and in the postpartum period, the woman is prone to PPH and postpartum collapse. In the puerperium, she could develop puerperal sepsis and venous thrombosis. The fetal and neonatal complications include prematurity, growth restriction, low birth weight, congenital malformations and increased chances of perinatal death. The infant has low iron reserves. There may be failure of lactation in the mother.

30 Hypertensive Disorders of Pregnancy

OG 12.1

Learning Objectives

» To define and classify hypertensive disorders of pregnancy
» To describe the pathophysiology of pre-eclampsia/eclampsia
» To enumerate the complications of pre-eclampsia/eclampsia
» To discuss the investigations required
» To discuss the principles of management of pre-eclampsia and eclampsia
» To discuss the morbidity related to pre-eclampsia and eclampsia

■ INTRODUCTION

Hypertensive disorders of pregnancy constitute one of the leading causes of maternal and perinatal mortality worldwide. Globally, 42,000 deaths occur every year due to hypertensive disorders of pregnancy, which account for 14% of all maternal deaths. Besides maternal mortality, pre-eclampsia and eclampsia also cause significant maternal and perinatal morbidity worldwide.

■ CLASSIFICATION

The National High Blood Pressure Education Programme, 2000 (NHBPEP, 2000), classifies hypertensive diseases complicating pregnancy into five types, which are as follows:

1. Gestational hypertension, also known as pregnancy-induced hypertension (PIH)
2. Pre-eclampsia
3. Eclampsia
4. Chronic hypertension
5. Chronic hypertension with superimposed pre-eclampsia

In 2018, the International Society for the Study of Hypertension in Pregnancy (ISSHP) introduced a new classification and criteria for the diagnosis of hypertensive disorders of pregnancy (Table 30.1).

Gestational Hypertension (PIH)

Gestational hypertension is defined as hypertension that develops for the first time in pregnancy after 20 weeks of gestation, in the absence of proteinuria and without biochemical or hematological abnormalities. It is usually not accompanied by fetal growth restriction. Outcomes in pregnancies complicated by gestational

Table 30.1 Classification and definitions of hypertensive disorders of pregnancy (ISSHP, 2018)

Hypertension arising at or after 20 weeks of pregnancy	
Gestational hypertension	BP ≥140/90 mmHg diagnosed after 20 weeks of gestation without proteinuria, hematological or biochemical abnormalities
Pre-eclampsia	BP ≥140/90 mmHg diagnosed after 20 weeks of gestation with proteinuria and/or evidence of maternal organ or placental dysfunction
Other conditions	Transient gestational hypertension
Hypertension known before pregnancy or diagnosed in the first 20 weeks	
Chronic hypertension	BP ≥140/90 mmHg diagnosed before pregnancy or in the first 20 weeks
	May be essential hypertension or secondary to other causes such as renal conditions, vascular pathology, etc.
Chronic hypertension with superimposed pre-eclampsia	Worsening of blood pressure/new-onset proteinuria/evidence of dysfunction of any one of the maternal organs consistent with pre-eclampsia in a woman with chronic hypertension
Other conditions	White-coat hypertension, masked hypertension

Characteristics of gestational hypertension
- Hypertension develops after 20 weeks of gestation
- Not accompanied by proteinuria
- There are no biochemical or hematological abnormalities
- Blood pressure returns to normal within 12 weeks postpartum
- Final diagnosis is made only after 12 weeks postpartum
- Gestational hypertension may evolve into pre-eclampsia

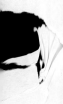

hypertension are normally good. However, about 50% of women with gestational hypertension may progress to pre-eclampsia and have a poor outcome. The blood pressure returns to normal within 12 weeks postpartum and hence, the **final diagnosis can only be made postpartum.**

Transient Gestational Hypertension

The ISSHP introduced the term 'transient gestational hypertension' to describe a de novo hypertension that develops in the second or third trimester and resolves without treatment during the pregnancy. Women diagnosed with transient gestational hypertension have a 20% chance of developing pre-eclampsia and another 20% chance of developing gestational hypertension. Therefore, these women should be monitored throughout their pregnancy. Ideally, home BP measurement should also be incorporated into their monitoring schedule.

Pre-eclampsia

As per the earlier diagnostic criteria, pre-eclampsia is the development of hypertension and significant proteinuria after 20 weeks of gestation. Although hypertension and proteinuria are considered to be the classical criteria to diagnose pre-eclampsia, in the current guidelines (ISSHP), proteinuria is not mandatory for a diagnosis of pre-eclampsia. In women presenting with hypertension in pregnancy, even in the

---

Current criteria to diagnose pre-eclampsia (ISSHP, 2018; ACOG, 2019)

New-onset hypertension after 20 weeks of gestation accompanied by ≥1 of the following new-onset conditions:

- Proteinuria
- Serum creatinine >1.1 mg/dL indicating renal insufficiency
- Elevated transaminases—alanine aminotransferase or aspartate aminotransferase indicating hepatic dysfunction (twice the upper limit of normal concentration)
- Platelet count <1,00,000/μL indicating hematological complication
- Neurological complications, including altered mental status, blindness, stroke, clonus, severe headaches and persistent visual scotomata
- Pulmonary edema
- Uteroplacental dysfunction presenting as fetal growth restriction, abnormal umbilical artery Doppler waveform analysis or stillbirth

---

absence of proteinuria, a diagnosis of pre-eclampsia is made if they present with evidence of maternal acute kidney injury (AKI), liver dysfunction, neurological features, hemolysis or thrombocytopenia, or fetal growth restriction. Besides the antenatal manifestation, pre-eclampsia may develop for the first time intrapartum or early postpartum in some cases.

Chronic Hypertension

A diagnosis of chronic hypertension complicating pregnancy is made when hypertension is diagnosed before pregnancy or is diagnosed before 20 weeks of gestation.

Chronic Hypertension with Superimposed Pre-eclampsia

About 25% of women with chronic hypertension will develop superimposed pre-eclampsia. These rates may be higher in women with underlying renal disease. A diagnosis of pre-eclampsia superimposed on chronic hypertension is made if there is worsening of blood pressure/in the presence of new-onset proteinuria/or if there is evidence of dysfunction of any one of the maternal organs, consistent with pre-eclampsia.

Eclampsia

Eclampsia is characterised by the occurrence of new-onset tonic–clonic seizures and/or coma during pregnancy, labour or the puerperium. In 80–90% of cases, eclampsia is preceded by pre-eclampsia. However, in a smaller proportion of cases, the presentation of eclampsia is atypical, without the classical signs of pre-eclampsia, hypertension and proteinuria.

The dictum is to consider any episodes of fits in a pregnant woman after 20 weeks of gestation as eclampsia unless proven otherwise.

■ PRE-ECLAMPSIA

Pre-eclampsia is a multi-organ disorder characterised by the development of hypertension and significant proteinuria and/or evidence of one of the maternal organ dysfunction after 20 weeks of gestation.

Incidence

There is a wide variation in the incidence of pre-eclampsia/eclampsia worldwide. The National Eclampsia Registry (NER) of India (FOGSI-ICOG) reported that the incidence of pre-eclampsia is 10.3%

(NER, 2013) and that of eclampsia is 1.9%. The incidences of pre-eclampsia and eclampsia reported by the Institute of Obstetrics and Gynaecology, Chennai, for the period from 2010 to 2017 were 11.3% and 0.86% respectively.

Criteria for Diagnosing Hypertension in Pregnancy

- Hypertension is diagnosed in pregnancy if the systolic blood pressure is ≥140 mmHg or if diastolic blood pressure is ≥90 mmHg or more on two occasions at least four hours apart after 20 weeks of gestation in a woman with previously normal blood pressure.
- Severe hypertension is diagnosed if the systolic blood pressure is ≥160 mmHg or diastolic blood pressure is ≥110 mmHg and can be confirmed within 15 minutes to facilitate timely antihypertensive therapy.

Criteria for Diagnosing Proteinuria

The gold standard for diagnosing abnormal proteinuria in pregnancy is a 24-hour urinary protein excretion of ≥300 mg per day. However, monitoring this is time-consuming, and therefore, proteinuria is assessed by screening urine with an automated dipstick. If positive (≥1+, 30 mg/dL), then a spot urine protein/creatinine (PCr) ratio should be performed. A PCr ratio of ≥30 mg/mmol is abnormal. Proteinuria is also considered significant if it is 2+ on the dipstick (>100 mg/dL); 3+ indicates that urinary protein is 300 mg/dL and 4+ indicates 1,000 mg/dL of urinary protein. Proteinuria is severe if the excretion is greater than 5 g in a 24-hour urine collection or more than 3+ on the dipstick in two random urine samples collected at least four hours apart.

Significance of Edema

The presence of edema is not an essential criterion to diagnose pre-eclampsia as it may occur in a normal pregnancy as well as other pathological conditions such as anemia, cardiac failure and renal disease. However, in patients with pre-eclampsia, when there is persistent pedal edema which does not resolve on taking rest, edema in dependent areas such as the vulva, pre-sacral edema or generalised edema, it indicates the severity of the condition. Edema of the face, vulva and pre-sacral edema are more ominous than pedal edema alone.

Assessment of Severity of Pre-eclampsia

Traditionally, pre-eclampsia is classified into mild and severe pre-eclampsia based on the degree of hypertension and proteinuria. However, in recent years, it has been recognised that even mild disease can take a severe turn. Therefore, mild disease is considered 'pre-eclampsia without severe features' and should be carefully monitored like severe disease. Both the ISSHP and the American College of Obstetricians and Gynaecologists recommend that the terms 'severe' and 'mild' pre-eclampsia should no longer be used, as all cases are potentially threatening clinically.

Pre-eclampsia without severe features (previously known as mild pre-eclampsia)

- Systolic BP is greater than 140 mmHg
- Diastolic BP is greater than 90 mmHg on two successive measurements 4–6 hours apart
- Proteinuria is >3 g in a 24-hour sample or 2+ in a random sample

Pre-eclampsia with severe features (previously known as severe pre-eclampsia)

- Systolic BP ≥160 mmHg
- Diastolic BP ≥110 mmHg
- Proteinuria greater than 5 g in a 24-hour collection or more than 3+ in two random urine samples

In the absence of proteinuria, any of the following clinical findings and investigations suggest organ involvement.

- Serum creatinine >1.1 mg/dL
- Platelet count <1,00,000/μL
- Liver enzymes >twice the normal
- Pulmonary edema
- New-onset visual and neurological disturbances
- Oliguria with less than 500 mL urine output in 24 hours

Imminent Signs and Symptoms

The following signs and symptoms, when present in a patient with pre-eclampsia, are considered danger signs and indicate the possibility of impending eclampsia. In these cases, the treatment should be as for eclampsia.

- Persistent maternal headache
- Visual disturbance
- Vomiting
- Epigastric pain
- Thrombocytopenia
- Impaired liver function test
- Presence of pulmonary edema or cyanosis
- Reduced urine output
- Evidence of hemolysis

Risk Factors for Pre-eclampsia

Though a number of risk factors (Table 30.2) can predispose a woman to pre-eclampsia and eclampsia, most cases of pre-eclampsia occur in healthy nulliparous women with no obvious risk factors.

Table 30.2 Risk factors that can predispose a woman to pre-eclampsia and eclampsia

Genetic predisposition—family history of pre-eclampsia in first-degree relatives

Medical conditions
- Chronic hypertension
- Type I and type II diabetes
- Chronic renal disease
- Pre-pregnancy obesity (BMI >30 Kg/m²)
- Autoimmune diseases—APLA syndromes and inherited thrombophilia, systemic lupus erythematosus
- Insulin resistance as in PCOS
- Hyperhomocysteinemia
- Nutritional deficiency—folic acid and calcium deficiency have also been implicated

Obstetrical conditions
- Pregnancy in the teenage or advanced maternal age (>35 years)
- First pregnancy
- Long interval between pregnancies >10 years
- Previous history of pre-eclampsia/eclampsia
- Previous placental abruption
- Having a new sexual partner
- Pregnancy following assisted reproductive techniques
- Multiple pregnancy
- Hydatidiform mole
- Large placenta due to hydrops fetalis

Pathogenesis of Pre-eclampsia

Although the exact pathophysiologic mechanism is not clearly understood, pre-eclampsia is primarily a disorder of placental dysfunction leading to endothelial dysfunction with associated vasospasm.

Normal placentation

The two objectives of implantation and placentation are to establish structural support for the embryo in the uterus and to bring maternal and fetal circulations close enough to allow an adequate transfer of gases, nutrients and waste products. This is achieved by unique vascular remodelling, resulting in a 10- to 12-fold increase in uterine blood flow.

In normal pregnancies, the cytotrophoblast cells of the developing placenta migrate through the decidua and part of the myometrium to invade both the endothelium and the highly muscular tunica media of the maternal spiral arteries. As a result, these vessels undergo transformation from small muscular arterioles to large-capacity vessels of low resistance, thus, greatly facilitating blood flow to the placenta compared to other areas of the uterus. This remodelling of the spiral arteries occurs in two phases. The 'first wave' of endovascular trophoblast migration occurs in the first trimester and involves the decidual segment of the spiral artery. The 'second wave' of trophoblast invasion occurs in the second trimester and involves the myometrial segments of the spiral arteries and is complete by weeks 18–20 of gestation.

Abnormal placentation in pre-eclampsia

In pre-eclampsia, the cytotrophoblastic cells invade only the decidual portion of the spiral arteries but fail to penetrate the myometrial segment. As a result, the spiral arteries (Fig. 30.1) fail to develop into large, tortuous vascular channels. Instead, they remain narrow, resulting in placental hypoperfusion. The hypoperfused, ischemic placenta releases a variety of factors into the maternal bloodstream, inducing a systemic inflammatory response that results in maternal endothelial dysfunction. Pre-eclampsia is considered a two-stage disorder. In stage I, there is poor placentation and inadequate uterine artery remodelling, resulting

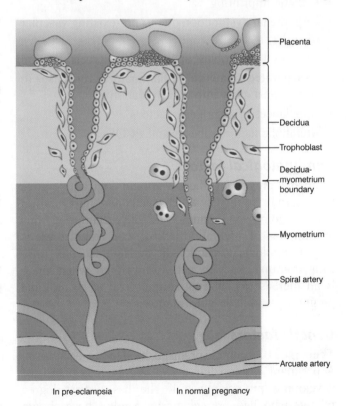

Fig. 30.1 Spiral arterioles in pre-eclamptic and normal pregnancy

in placental hypoxia. No symptoms are produced at this stage. The hypoxic placenta releases stress factors which, on entering the maternal circulation, induce endothelial dysfunction with the resultant signs and symptoms of pre-eclampsia in stage II.

Besides pre-eclampsia, abnormal placentation is seen in a spectrum of conditions such as IUGR, preterm labour, late spontaneous abortions and abruptio placentae. These conditions are collectively called the 'great obstetrical syndrome'.

What triggers abnormal placentation is not known. It has been postulated that genetic predisposition, pre-existing vascular pathology and immunological factors may be involved. Following abnormal placentation, other mechanisms are set in motion. The resultant increase in antiangiogenic factors, oxidative stress due to free radical release and lipid peroxidation and release of cytokines and interleukins lead to widespread endothelial cell damage. The final pathogenesis in the occurrence of pre-eclampsia is endothelial cell dysfunction and generalised vasospasm.

The following mechanisms have been proposed in the pathogenesis (Fig. 30.2) of pre-eclampsia:

- Chronic uteroplacental ischemia
- Immune maladaptation
- Genetic imprinting
- Endothelial dysfunction due to pre-existing vascular disorders
- Increased trophoblast apoptosis or necrosis
- Exaggerated maternal inflammatory response to trophoblast entry into the circulation
- Imbalances of angiogenic factors
- Metabolic factors, obesity and PCOS

Immunological factors

In normal pregnancy, there is immunological tolerance to paternal antigens, which facilitates implantation and ongoing pregnancy. In pre-eclampsia, this immunological adaptation is lost. As a result, there is an immunological reaction in the fetoplacental unit. This immune reaction gets exaggerated when there is an increase in paternal antigen load as in multiple pregnancy and hydatidiform mole.

Genetic factors

There may be a genetic predisposition to pre-eclampsia. A pregnant woman has a five-fold increased risk of developing pre-eclampsia if she has a first-degree relative who had pre-eclampsia. Studies have shown that a number of genes are implicated in the etiology of pre-eclampsia, including the genes responsible for the increase in antiangiogenic factors.

Increased production of antiangiogenic factors

A number of proangiogenic (vascular endothelial growth factor [VEGF], placental growth factor [PlGF]) and antiangiogenic factors (soluble FMS–like tyrosine kinase [sFLT-1] and soluble endoglins [sEng]) are released by the developing placenta. The balance between these factors is important for normal placental development. Increased production of antiangiogenic factors disturbs this balance and results in systemic endothelial dysfunction, characteristic of pre-eclampsia.

Imbalance in the prostaglandin milieu

Prostacyclin, which is produced by the endothelium, is a powerful vasodilator and prevents platelet aggregation. Thromboxane A2 is produced by platelets and is a potent vasoconstrictor; it causes platelet aggregation. In normal pregnancy, there is a delicate balance between the two prostaglandins, favouring prostacyclin production. In pre-eclampsia, due to endothelial cell dysfunction and injury, there is a decrease in prostacyclin and a shift towards an increase in thromboxane with resultant vasospasm, platelet activation and activation of the coagulation system.

Activation of the coagulation system

With endothelial cell damage, the tissue factors on the endothelium are activated. This triggers the coagulation system. As the clotting factors and platelets are used up, widespread microhemorrhages, fibrin deposition and disseminated intravascular coagulation ensue.

Changes in nitric oxide and endothelin levels

The endothelia of the arteries produce both nitric oxide (vasodilator) and endothelin (vasoconstrictor). Damaged endothelial cells result in the production of less nitric oxide and more endothelin, resulting in vasospasm.

Oxidative stress and free radical release

Hypoperfusion of the placenta also results in oxidative stress, leading to free radical release and lipid peroxidation. The free radicals damage the endothelial cells, activate the coagulation system, decrease the nitric oxide level and increase the capillary permeability.

Release of pro-inflammatory factors

As a result of hypoperfusion, there is also a release of cytokines, tumour necrosis factor and interleukins, all of which can injure the endothelial cells further.

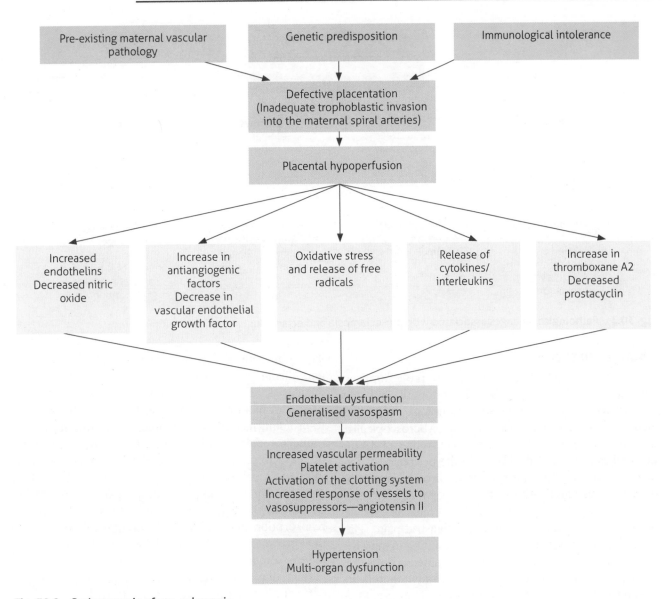

Fig. 30.2 Pathogenesis of pre-eclampsia

Metabolic factors

Obesity and PCOS result in hyperlipidemia due to insulin resistance. This can either occur directly or through oxidative stress, resulting in endothelial dysfunction.

Pathological Changes in Pre-eclampsia and Eclampsia (Fig. 30.3)

Pre-eclampsia/eclampsia has an impact on most organs.

Changes in the vascular system

The most significant change seen in the vascular system is intense vasospasm. This is due to the imbalance in the prostaglandin levels with an increase in thromboxane A2. Also, there is a decrease in nitric acid levels and an increase in the level of endothelin, which is a potent vasoconstrictor. This results in the narrowing of the intravascular space. Fluid therapy, if required, should be very carefully administered because the narrowing of the intravascular space and the tendency for the capillary leak could precipitate pulmonary edema in pre-eclampsia.

Hematological changes

The hematological changes seen in association with pre-eclampsia and eclampsia include hemoconcentration, thrombocytopenia and hemolysis. Thrombocytopenia is a common finding due to platelet activation and consumption and is a marker of disease severity. Due to the capillary leak and vasospasm, hemoconcentration occurs, which may mask underlying anemia. In the presence of hemolysis, the serum concentration of LDH is elevated to >600 IU/L.

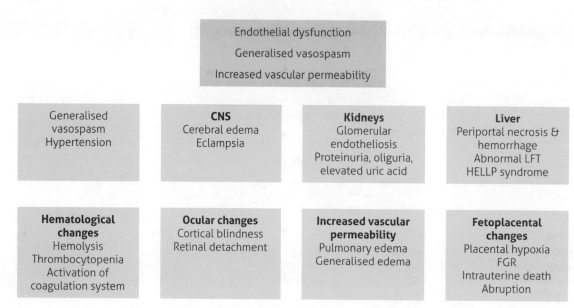

Fig. 30.3 Pathological changes associated with pre-eclampsia and eclampsia

Changes in the liver

Liver changes are characteristic of pre-eclampsia. The surface of the liver becomes smooth and the appearance mottled due to numerous scattered areas of subcapsular hemorrhage. Microscopically, the characteristic finding is the occurrence of fibrin thrombi in the portal capillaries in the periphery of the lobules. Surrounding the peripheral thrombi are areas of hemorrhage and necrosis; this is known as periportal hemorrhagic necrosis. The stretching of the liver capsule presents as nausea, vomiting and epigastric pain. The subcapsular hematoma can rupture, resulting in massive intraperitoneal hemorrhage and unexplained collapse.

Hepatic function may be significantly altered in women with pre-eclampsia with severe features. Due to the necrosis and infarctions of liver tissue, alanine aminotransferase (ALT) and aspartate aminotransferase (AST) may be elevated. Aspartate aminotransferase is the dominant transaminase released into the peripheral circulation in liver dysfunction due to pre-eclampsia and is related to periportal necrosis. Because of hepatic dysfunction and hemolysis, LDH levels are elevated. Other changes that can happen due to hepatic dysfunction are abnormalities of prothrombin time, partial prothrombin time and fibrinogen, which usually develop in advanced pre-eclampsia. The evaluation of these coagulation parameters is important when the platelet count is below 150,000/mm³, when there is significant liver dysfunction, or when placental abruption is suspected.

Renal changes

The characteristic histopathological finding described in pre-eclampsia is 'glomerular capillary endotheliosis'.

The glomeruli are enlarged, with swollen, vacuolated endothelial cells, which block the lumen of the capillaries. There is also fibrinoid deposition in the basement membrane. These pathological changes lead to proteinuria, decreased glomerular filtration rate and reduced renal blood flow. All these changes lead to an increase in creatinine and uric acid levels and proteinuria due to increased glomerular permeability. These changes that occur in pre-eclampsia are reversible. The cause of hyperuricemia in pre-eclampsia is increased reabsorption and decreased excretion of uric acid in the proximal renal tubules. In eclampsia, acute renal failure from tubular necrosis may develop. Rarely, renal cortical necrosis develops when a major portion of the cortex of both kidneys undergoes necrosis.

Changes in the central nervous system

The cerebral pathology noted in pre-eclampsia/eclampsia comprises diffuse cerebral edema and microhemorrhages. These neurological manifestations of eclampsia are due to cerebral vasospasm and failure of autoregulation of cerebral circulation, resulting in hyperperfusion and edema. Whenever there is an increase in blood pressure, the neurogenic response—which is controlled by the sympathetic system—is to prevent the rapid dilatation of vessels. In pre-eclampsia, there is a failure of this autoregulation, resulting in cerebral edema. This, along with increased blood–brain barrier permeability, hypercoagulability and inflammation, leads to complications such as arterial infarcts, intracerebral hemorrhage and cerebral venous sinus thrombosis (CVT). In recent years, a condition called posterior reversible encephalopathy syndrome (PRES) has been associated with eclampsia and its neurological manifestations. It is a neuroimaging diagnosis in which the posterior circulation is predominantly affected due to vasogenic edema.

Placental changes

Vasospasm leads to a decrease in uteroplacental blood flow, resulting in anoxia. As a result of anoxia, thromboplastic substances liberated by the placenta enter the bloodstream and initiate intravascular coagulation. The histological findings in a normal placenta are exaggerated in pre-eclampsia. These include increased syncytial knots, an increased number of true infarcts, increased loss of syncytium, proliferation of cytotrophoblasts, villous necrosis and acute fibrinoid degeneration of maternal decidual arteries.

Ocular changes

The fundal changes include arteriolar narrowing and the presence of exudates and hemorrhages. Due to petechial hemorrhages and focal edema in the parieto-occipital area, patients may present with cortical blindness. There may also be blindness due to retinal detachment when there is markedly elevated blood pressure.

Investigations

Apart from the routine investigations performed in a normal pregnancy, the following investigations are carried out to determine the severity of the problem and to choose the appropriate line of management.

Urine examination

All pregnant women should routinely undergo urinalysis for urine albumin. When there is persistent trace albuminuria or no albuminuria with other signs and symptoms of pre-eclampsia, then a 24-hour urine estimation for protein should be performed. A value of 300 mg or more of urinary protein indicates the presence of high albumin excretion. Urine should also be examined for pus cells and casts, which are indicative of renal disease.

Complete blood count

A complete blood count should include Hb, PCV, WBC-TC, DC, platelet count and RBC count. Platelet count is indicative of the presence or absence of thrombocytopenia. Overt thrombocytopenia, defined as a platelet count less than 1,00,000/mm³, indicates severe disease. Due to vasospasm, Hb and PCV may be falsely elevated. Low hemoglobin and PCV indicate possible hemolysis.

Peripheral smear

On peripheral smear, the presence of fragmented cells and schistocytes indicates hemolysis.

Renal function test

The estimation of blood urea, uric acid and creatinine is done when pre-eclampsia or eclampsia is diagnosed; it is repeated as and when necessary.

Liver function tests

For all pregnant women diagnosed with pre-eclampsia, a liver function test should be performed to check for indirect bilirubin levels and AST and ALT (SGOT and SGPT) levels, which are increased in severe eclampsia, especially in the HELLP syndrome.

Coagulation profile

When the platelet count is <1,50,000 or when HELLP syndrome or DIC is suspected, serum fibrinogen, prothrombin time (PT) and partial thromboplastin time (aPTT) are checked. A simple bedside test can be performed to check the bleeding time (BT), clotting time (CT) and clot retraction time (CRT).

Fundoscopy

In all cases of pre-eclampsia and eclampsia, the fundus should be examined for arteriolar spasm, exudates and hemorrhages. The presence of papilledema indicates raised intracranial tension, the need for anti-edema measures and urgent neuroimaging studies. In the presence of blindness, fundoscopy is important to diagnose retinal detachment.

Maternal and Fetal Complications of Pre-eclampsia

Maternal complications

- CNS complications:
  - Intracerebral hemorrhage (ICH), cerebrovenous thrombosis (CVT), arterial and venous infarcts
- Ocular complications:
  - Cortical blindness
  - Retinal detachment
- Renal system:
  - Acute tubular necrosis
  - Acute cortical necrosis
- Hepatic system:
  - HELLP syndrome
  - Hepatic hematoma
  - Rupture of the liver
- Respiratory system:
  - Pulmonary edema
  - ARDS
- Cardiovascular system:
  - Ischemia
  - Congestive cardiac failure

- Hematological:
  - DIC
  - Thrombocytopenia
- Placenta:
  - Abruption

Fetal complications

Fetal complications in pre-eclampsia are directly related to gestational age and the severity of maternal disease and are as follows:

- FGR
- Intrauterine death
- Prematurity
- Intrauterine asphyxia

Intrauterine death and perinatal death are related to premature delivery, placental abruption and intrauterine asphyxia.

Management of Pre-eclampsia

General principles of management

All women diagnosed with pre-eclampsia should be hospitalised.

Antihypertensives in the management of pre-eclampsia

- Regardless of the type of hypertensive disorder of pregnancy, BP consistently at or >140/90 mmHg in the clinic or hospital (or ≥135/85 mmHg at home) should be treated. In order to prevent the development of severe hypertension and its related complications, the diastolic BP should be kept below 85 mmHg and the systolic BP should be kept at 110–140 mmHg. The antihypertensive agents that can be used are oral methyldopa, labetalol and nifedipine. Medications can be reduced or stopped if the diastolic BP falls below 80 mmHg.
- When a pregnant woman presents with severe hypertension (>160/110 mmHg), she should be treated urgently with oral nifedipine or intravenous labetalol or hydralazine. Oral labetalol may also be used if parenteral preparations are not available. The rapid reduction of BP should be avoided.

Maternal monitoring in pre-eclampsia

- Depending on the severity of pre-eclampsia and the need for parenteral therapy, BP monitoring is required either continuously or every 2–4 hours.
- Tests to detect proteinuria should be performed every day.
- Daily clinical assessment for warning signs and symptoms (headache, vomiting, epigastric pain, giddiness, breathlessness, blurring of vision, reduced urine output, knee jerk, ankle jerk, plantar reflexes and clonus) should be performed.
- Blood tests for hemoglobin, platelet count, and tests of liver and renal function, including uric acid should be carried out at least twice weekly. Elevated uric acid levels are associated with worse maternal and fetal outcomes.
- Fundus examination should be performed to look for hypertensive retinopathy changes.

Fetal monitoring in pre-eclampsia

- An initial assessment by biophysical profile should be carried out to confirm fetal well-being.
- Serial fetal surveillance with biophysical profile and Doppler studies are carried out in cases without severe features and in severe pre-eclampsia, where expectant management is undertaken.

Delivery

The definitive management of pre-eclampsia is delivery. Delivery is indicated in the following situations:

- When the fetus has reached 37 weeks of gestation or
- If the woman develops any of the following:
  - Repeated episodes of severe hypertension despite treating with three classes of antihypertensive agents
  - Progressive thrombocytopenia
  - Progressively abnormal renal or liver enzyme tests and hematological parameters
  - Pulmonary edema or impending features
  - Abnormal neurological features such as severe intractable headache, repeated visual scotomata or convulsions
  - Evidence of fetal compromise by biophysical profile and Doppler studies

Convulsion prophylaxis

Women with pre-eclampsia who have proteinuria and severe hypertension or hypertension with neurological signs or symptoms should receive magnesium sulphate (MgSO$_4$) for convulsion prophylaxis.

> In the management of pre-eclampsia, there should be NO attempt to differentiate between mild and severe pre-eclampsia clinically as all cases may become emergencies, often rapidly.

Management of pre-eclampsia without severe features (Fig. 30.4)

- Women with pre-eclampsia without severe features can progress to severe pre-eclampsia rapidly.

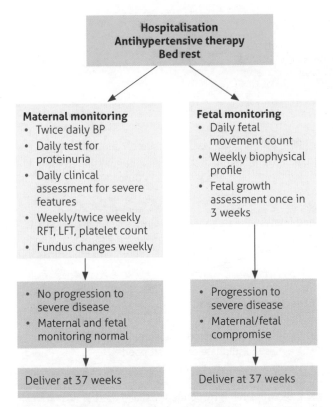

Fig. 30.4 Flowchart of the management of pre-eclampsia without severe features

Therefore, these women should be hospitalised to reduce physical activity and to enable close monitoring. Antihypertensives are given to maintain the BP at 110–140/85 mmHg. Besides daily clinical assessment, proteinuria is checked every day and hematological parameters and renal and liver function tests are carried out twice weekly.

- The fetal growth is monitored once in 2–3 weeks. Fetal surveillance is done by daily fetal movement count and weekly biophysical profile.

Women with pre-eclampsia without severe features should be delivered at 37 weeks of gestation to avoid progression to severe pre-eclampsia and eclampsia.

Management of pre-eclampsia with severe features (Fig. 30.5)

The definitive treatment of pre-eclampsia is delivery of the fetus and the placenta. Though immediate delivery in cases of severe pre-eclampsia prevents maternal complications, it may put the fetus at risk of prematurity and related complications. Therefore, the decision to deliver depends on the gestational age at presentation and the severity of pre-eclampsia.

- The immediate measures in the management of severe pre-eclampsia are to control hypertension, to give seizure prophylaxis, to administer corticosteroids for fetal lung maturity and to evaluate the maternal and fetal condition.
- Antihypertensives are administered, preferably by the parenteral route. If the facilities for this are unavailable, the oral route can be used. The commonly used drugs are nifedipine, labetalol and hydralazine.
- Women with pre-eclampsia who have proteinuria and severe hypertension or hypertension with neurological signs or symptoms should receive MgSO$_4$ for convulsion prophylaxis.
- If the gestational age is 26–34 weeks, corticosteroids should be administered to accelerate fetal lung maturity.
- Investigations are carried out to assess maternal and fetal conditions.

Indications for immediate delivery

After stabilising the woman, immediate delivery is undertaken in the following situations:

- Gestational age <26 weeks: The chances of fetal survival are poor and the maternal and perinatal complications are greater. Therefore, the pregnant woman and her partner should be counselled, and termination should be undertaken.
- Gestational age >34 weeks: The prognosis for the fetus is good and delaying delivery will put the mother and the fetus at risk of major complications. Therefore, pregnancy should be terminated.
- When the gestational age is between 26 and 34 weeks of gestation: The management and timing of delivery will depend on the maternal and fetal condition, response to antihypertensive medications and the presence or absence of renal, liver and hematological abnormalities. Based on these findings, either immediate delivery or expectant management may be undertaken.

Immediate delivery is indicated when the woman's condition is deteriorating, which is indicated by the following:

- Failure to control hypertension with effective antihypertensive therapy
- Symptoms imminent of eclampsia
- Presence of/impending pulmonary edema
- Intractable cerebral symptoms despite magnesium therapy
- HELLP syndrome/DIC
- Raised renal parameters
- Compromised fetus, as shown by abnormal biophysical profile and umbilical artery Doppler
- IUGR
- Woman already in labour
- In the presence of abruption and intrauterine death

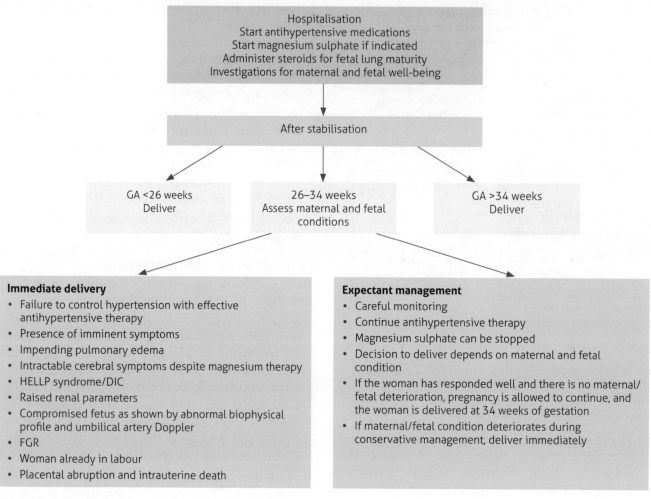

Fig. 30.5 Flowchart of the management of pre-eclampsia with severe features

Expectant management

Prolonging pregnancy by expectant management improves the chances of survival of the fetus. However, it puts the pregnant woman at considerable risk of major complications including severe hypertension, eclampsia, HELLP syndrome and placental abruption. Risks for the fetus include fetal growth restriction and fetal death. Therefore, expectant management warrants very careful monitoring and evaluation by hematological and biochemical parameters. Antihypertensives are continued and magnesium sulphate stopped.

- BP is checked every 2–4 hours.
- Tests to detect proteinuria are performed daily.
- Warning signs and symptoms are looked for.
- Urine output is monitored.
- RFT, LFT and platelet count are checked on alternate days/twice weekly.
- Fetal well-being is assessed.

If the woman responds well to medications and there is no maternal or fetal deterioration, the pregnancy is allowed to continue and the woman is delivered at 34 weeks of gestation. If the BP is not under control, and the woman is developing cerebral symptoms/pulmonary edema or if there are signs of fetal compromise, delivery should be undertaken immediately, irrespective of the gestational age.

Mode of delivery

The mode of delivery depends on the favourability of the cervix and any other contraindication for vaginal delivery.

- In multiparous women and in women with a favourable cervix, if the fetal condition is good, labour can be induced for a vaginal delivery.
- When the cervix is unfavourable, or if there is associated growth restriction or other evidence of fetal compromise, a cesarean section is undertaken. If hematological parameters are normal and there are

no other maternal complications, regional anesthesia can be used.

- There is a risk of convulsions and pulmonary edema in labour. If magnesium therapy was not started earlier, it should be initiated at this point. Some women may require parenteral antihypertensives. The total fluid intake should be limited to 60–80 mL/hour.
- The second stage of labour should be shortened by applying outlet forceps/vacuum.
- These women are prone to postpartum hemorrhage because of the medications used (both nifedipine and magnesium sulphate can relax the uterus) and the underlying abnormal clotting profile.
- Active management of the third stage should be practised to avoid PPH. Oxytocin is the preferred oxytocic agent. Ergometrine is contraindicated in hypertensive disorders as it causes vasoconstriction and elevation of blood pressure.

Postpartum management

- Monitoring of BP following delivery should be continued every 4–6 hours for 3–4 days. The BP will gradually normalise. Until then, antihypertensive medications should be continued.
- The general well-being and neurological status of the woman should be continuously monitored as she may have seizures in the postpartum period.
- Repeated tests for Hb, platelets, creatinine and liver transaminases should be performed the day after delivery and then every second day until the levels are stable (in cases where these levels were abnormal before delivery).
- Women with pre-eclampsia still requiring antihypertensives at discharge from the hospital should be reviewed within 1 week. All women should be reviewed 3 months postpartum, by which time BP, urinalysis, and all laboratory tests should have normalised.

Long-term risks associated with pre-eclampsia

- All women with chronic hypertension, gestational hypertension and pre-eclampsia require lifelong follow-up because of their increased cardiovascular risk.
- Women with pre-eclampsia have approximately a 15% risk of developing pre-eclampsia again and a further 15% risk of developing gestational hypertension in a future pregnancy. Such women should receive low-dose aspirin in future pregnancies.

- Women with gestational hypertension have approximately a 4% risk of developing pre-eclampsia and a further 25% risk for gestational hypertension in a future pregnancy.
- Women with gestational hypertension or pre-eclampsia have increased risks of small-for-gestational age babies in another pregnancy even if pre-eclampsia does not recur.

MANAGEMENT OF GESTATIONAL HYPERTENSION

- Antihypertensives are used to keep the BP at 110–140/85 mmHg.
- These women should be carefully monitored for the development of severe gestational hypertension. Periodic investigations are carried out to diagnose pre-eclampsia.
- Women with gestational hypertension can be managed as outpatients provided their BP is under control. If possible, home monitoring of BP should be advocated.
- Women with severe hypertension—systolic >160 and diastolic >110 mmHg—should be hospitalised and managed as for severe pre-eclampsia.
- Monitoring of fetal growth and well-being should also be carried out.
- Delivery can be delayed until 39+6 weeks if the BP is well under control, fetal monitoring is reassuring, and pre-eclampsia has not developed. Those with severe gestational hypertension should be delivered once fetal maturity is reached.
- The woman should be reviewed at 12 weeks postpartum.

MANAGEMENT OF CHRONIC HYPERTENSION

- Chronic hypertension may be essential or secondary to renal disease such as glomerulonephritis or polycystic kidney or a vascular disease such as coarctation of the aorta, renal artery stenosis or connective tissue disorders.
- If, prior to pregnancy, the woman is on angiotensin-converting enzyme (ACE) inhibitors, the antihypertensive should be replaced with a safer drug such as labetalol. ACE inhibitors will lead to congenital malformations. Investigations should be carried out to assess for the dysfunction of various organs before embarking on pregnancy.

These women should be started on low-dose aspirin to prevent pre-eclampsia.

• All women diagnosed with chronic hypertension in pregnancy should have the following investigations performed to provide baseline reference levels: full blood count, renal function test, liver function test, urinalysis and microscopy. Renal ultrasound is carried out if serum creatinine or any of the urine tests is abnormal. Antihypertensives are given to maintain BP in the range of 110–140/80–85 mmHg. Commonly used antihypertensives are labetalol, methyldopa and nifedipine. Hydralazine is used in emergencies. Women should be carefully monitored for developing pre-eclampsia based on blood pressure and urine analysis for proteinuria at each visit. In order to diagnose organ involvement, blood investigations such as Hb, platelet count, liver transaminases, uric acid, and creatinine should be carried out at least once in each trimester. Fetal well-being should be assessed from 26 weeks of gestation, and thereafter at 2–4 week intervals. If there is no superimposed pre-eclampsia, the woman is delivered at 38–39 weeks of gestation. If the woman develops superimposed pre-eclampsia, the timing of delivery should be as for pre-eclampsia.

◼ HELLP SYNDROME

HELLP syndrome is one of the more severe forms of pre-eclampsia and is associated with increased maternal morbidity and mortality. This condition is associated with hemolysis, elevated liver enzymes and low platelet count.

Pathogenesis

Due to endothelial dysfunction, there is platelet activation and consumption leading to ischemia and hepatocellular death. This may be segmental or may affect the entire liver. More commonly, the terminal arterioles are involved, leading to periportal or focal parenchymal disease. When large vessels are involved, hepatic infarct or subcapsular hematoma result.

Clinical Presentation

HELLP syndrome is mostly seen in the third trimester, but can also manifest in the postpartum period. It can also appear de novo without prior hypertension/proteinuria. In HELLP syndrome, the chief presenting symptoms are right upper quadrant pain and generalised malaise in up to 90% of cases and nausea and vomiting in 50% of cases.

Investigations

Hemolysis is evidenced by schistocytes on peripheral smear, elevated LDH >600 IU/L and elevated bilirubin >1.2 mg/dL. Due to hepatocyte destruction, AST (aspartate aminotransferase) is elevated >70 IU/L and LDH >600 IU/L. The platelet count is <1,00,000/mm^3.

The following are the criteria to diagnose HELLP syndrome:

• Lactate dehydrogenase (LDH) elevated to 600 IU/L or more (indicator of hemolysis)
• Liver enzymes aspartate aminotransferase (AST) and alanine aminotransferase (ALT) elevated more than twice the upper limit of normal
• Platelets count less than 1,00,000/mm^3

Management

Delivery is the definitive therapy. The woman should be stabilised and coagulation abnormalities corrected before delivery. Steroids and intravenous magnesium sulphate may be required to prevent intraventricular bleeding and respiratory distress syndrome in the fetus. The routine use of steroids in the management of HELLP syndrome is not recommended. However, the use of steroids has been shown to increase the platelet count.

Blood and blood component therapy

When the platelet count is <20,000 or if there is bleeding from a wound or puncture site or intraperitoneal ecchymoses, 6–10 units of platelet transfusion should be given. If a cesarean section is to be performed and if the woman's platelet count is <40,000, platelet transfusion is given. With severe coagulopathy, red cells and FFP are required. Postpartum plasmapheresis with FFP may be required if there is evidence of progressive hemolysis, thrombocytopenia and deterioration of renal function.

◼ ANTIHYPERTENSIVE THERAPY IN THE MANAGEMENT OF HYPERTENSIVE DISORDERS OF PREGNANCY

The objectives of treating severe hypertension are to prevent cerebral hemorrhage, congestive heart failure, myocardial ischemia, renal injury or failure and ischemic or hemorrhagic stroke.

Intravenous hydralazine and labetalol and oral nifedipine are the three agents most commonly used for this purpose. Although parenteral antihypertensive therapy may be needed initially for the acute control of blood pressure, oral medications can be used later. Oral labetalol and calcium channel blockers are commonly used for this purpose. Methyldopa can also be used in the management of chronic hypertension.

Oral Medication

- When the BP is not severely high, labetalol (tab) 200 mg is given orally every 12 hours; the dose can be increased to 800 mg orally every 8–12 hours, up to a maximum of 1,600 mg/day. If the maximum dose is inadequate to control the blood pressure or the woman develops undesirable side effects, then short-acting oral nifedipine can be added gradually.
- In the management of chronic hypertension, if the woman is already on α-methyldopa, it can be continued at a dose of 500 mg 4 times daily.
- Nifedipine is also used in the management of gestational hypertension, chronic hypertension and pre-eclampsia.

Urgent Control of Blood Pressure

For urgent control of blood pressure, the following antihypertensive medications can be used:
- Injection labetalol is given at a dose of 10–20 mg IV, every 20 minutes to a maximum cumulative dosage of 300 mg/day. It should be avoided in women who have asthma, pre-existing myocardial disease, decompensated cardiac function, heart block or bradycardia.

- Nifedipine (immediate release) 10–20 mg is given orally, repeated in 20 minutes if needed and then maintained at 10–20 mg every 2–6 hours upto a maximum daily dose of 120 mg. There may be reflex tachycardia, palpitation, flushing and headache.
- Hydralazine 5 mg IV or IM, then 5–10 mg IV every 20–40 minutes can be given upto a maximum cumulative dosage of 20 mg. Higher or more frequent dosages are associated with maternal hypotension, headaches and abnormal CTG.

The acceptable first-line antihypertensives include labetalol, methyldopa and nifedipine. Prazosin and hydralazine are usually used as second- or third-line agents. Table 30.3 summarises the antihypertensive drugs, their action, dosage and contraindications.

■ ECLAMPSIA

Eclampsia is an obstetric emergency and a potentially life-threatening condition. According to the WHO's estimation, eclampsia is responsible for 12% of all maternal deaths globally.

Definition

Eclampsia is defined as the development of convulsions and/or unexplained coma during pregnancy or during the postpartum period in women with signs and symptoms of pre-eclampsia after 20 weeks gestation and within 48 hours of delivery, where the cause is neither epilepsy nor any other convulsive disorder. Any pregnant woman presenting with seizures should

Table 30.3 Antihypertensive drugs

Drug	Action	Dosage	Side effects	Contraindications
Oral labetalol	Selective α-1 blocker and non-selective β blocker	200 mg orally every 12 hours; can be increased to 800 mg twice daily upto a maximum of 1,600 mg/day	Bronchoconstriction	Heart block, asthma
Injectable labetalol	Selective α-1 blocker and non-selective β blocker	20 mg IV bolus, repeated every 20 minutes to a maximum of 300 mg/day	Should be carefully used when combined with calcium channel blockers Postural hypotension	Asthma, pre-existing myocardial disease, decompensated cardiac function, and heart block and bradycardia
Nifedipine	Calcium channel blocker	10–20 mg orally, repeated every 20 minutes, then maintained with 10–20 mg every 2–6 hours	Unpredictable decrease in BP Reflex tachycardia, headache	Care is required when used concomitantly with magnesium sulphate
Hydralazine	Peripheral vasodilator	5 mg IV or IM, then 5–10 mg IV every 20–40 minutes to a maximum cumulative dosage of 20 mg	Reflex tachycardia, hypotension, tremors, abnormal CTG	Tachycardia
Methyldopa	Central action	500 mg 4 times daily	Depression, postural hypotension	

be considered as having eclampsia unless proven otherwise. In 80–90% of cases, eclampsia is preceded by pre-eclampsia. However, in a smaller proportion of cases, the presentation of eclampsia is atypical, wherein the classical signs of pre-eclampsia, hypertension and proteinuria, are absent and the timing of eclampsia may be before 20 weeks of gestation or 48 hours after delivery.

Pathogenesis

In the pathogenesis of pre-eclampsia/eclampsia, the final pathway is generalised vasospasm, which leads to multi-organ failure. In the brain, due to the spasm of the cerebral vessels and increased vascular resistance, there is tissue hypoxia. As the vascular permeability increases, there is leakage of fluid and shifting of fluid from the intravascular compartment to the interstitial spaces, leading to cerebral edema. With increasing hypoxia and cerebral edema, there is fibrinoid necrosis of the arterial wall, leading to perivascular microinfarcts and hemorrhages. These changes lead to abnormal signals from the brain, and consequently, convulsions.

The symptoms and signs of impending eclampsia include the following:

- Severe frontal headache
- Confusion and persistent visual disturbance
- Visual blurring
- Nausea/vomiting
- Epigastric pain/tenderness
- Hyperreflexia/sustained clonus

Timing of Eclampsia

Antepartum eclampsia

Seizures occur in the third trimester of pregnancy in more than 50% of cases. On rare occasions—as in the case of a hydatidiform mole—fits may occur in the early months. Sometimes, when seizures occur in the antenatal period, the woman may soon establish labour; in such cases, it may be difficult to differentiate antepartum eclampsia from intrapartum eclampsia.

Intrapartum eclampsia

In 30% of cases, seizures occur for the first time during labour.

Postpartum eclampsia

In 20% of cases, seizures occur for the first time in the puerperium, usually within 48 hours of delivery. Late postpartum eclampsia is where convulsions occur after 48 hours but less than 4 weeks after delivery.

Course of Convulsion

Eclamptic fits are epileptiform, lasting for 3–4 minutes and consisting of four stages, namely:

- Premonitory stage
- Tonic stage
- Clonic stage
- Stage of coma

The premonitory stage

The woman becomes unconscious; there is twitching of the muscles of the face and limbs. The eyeballs turn to one side and become fixed. This stage lasts for about 30 seconds.

The tonic stage

In this stage, the entire body goes into spasms called trunk opisthotonus. There is stiffening of the body and generalised muscle contraction. The limbs are flexed and hands clenched. Respiration ceases, and the tongue protrudes between the teeth. There is cyanosis and fixation of the eyeballs. This stage lasts for about 30 seconds.

The clonic stage

The phase of clonic convulsion lasts for 1–2 minutes. There is alternate contraction and relaxation of the voluntary muscles of the body in rapid succession, starting in the face and spreading throughout the body. There is bloodstained, frothy discharge at the mouth and laboured breathing. The woman may bite her tongue if it isn't protected. The cyanosis gradually disappears. The woman may fall from the bed.

The stage of coma

Following a seizure, the woman may go into a coma. The coma stage may last for a brief period or may persist until another convulsion occurs.

Occasionally, the patient recovers consciousness but appears to be in a confused state following the seizure with no memory of the happenings. The convulsions are usually multiple, recurring at varying intervals. When it occurs continuously, it is called status eclampticus. Rarely, coma occurs without prior convulsion.

The post-convulsive stage

The woman usually remembers nothing of the episode. Some patients also become restless and agitated, requiring sedation. Aspiration is possible during or after the convulsion. Apnea develops during and immediately after the convulsion, lasting about

120 seconds. A period of hyperventilation follows to compensate for the respiratory acidosis during the apnoeic period. Following the convulsion, temperature rises along with pulse and respiration rates. Blood pressure is also increased. The urinary output is markedly diminished, proteinuria is pronounced and blood uric acid is raised.

Management

In any pregnant woman with convulsions, the first diagnosis should be eclampsia unless proven otherwise. Based on a quick history/referral letter and after checking the blood pressure and urine for albumin, the diagnosis should be made within a minute.

Eclampsia is an obstetric emergency, for which a stepwise approach is important. All obstetric units should have up-to-date protocols and should conduct periodic drills to prepare the nursing staff, obstetric, anesthesia team and pediatric staff members working in these units to manage eclampsia. Inappropriate management during and after an eclamptic convulsion can be detrimental to the mother and fetus. A senior obstetrician and anesthesiologist should be involved in the management.

It is important to maintain an eclampsia tray in the labour room with the following:
- At least 14 amps of $MgSO_4$
- At least 2 amps of calcium gluconate (10 mL amps)
- 20 cc syringe
- Oxygen with face mask
- Airway
- Suction cannula
- Adult Ambu bag
- Knee hammer
- Injection labetalol
- Tablet nifedipine

The principles of management are as follows:
- General management
- Control of seizures
- Control of hypertension
- Anticipate complications
- Terminate pregnancy

General management

The initial response is not to panic and to call for help. Most eclamptic convulsions are self-limiting. Therefore, during a seizure, one must resist the impulse to administer anticonvulsive drugs.

- The woman should be turned on her side (recovery position), her airway should be secured and any vomitus should be cleared.
- It is vital to support maternal respiratory and cardiovascular functions to prevent hypoxia, acidosis and cardiorespiratory arrest and to prevent maternal injury and aspiration.
- The airway should be secured, and oxygen should be delivered via face mask at the rate of 8–10 L/minute. A multipurpose monitor should be connected to monitor the vitals and oxygen saturation.
- During the apnoeic period, the woman may develop hypoxia. Pulse oximetry should be used to monitor oxygen saturation with the goal of keeping it above 94%.
- During the convulsive phase, the woman may throw herself out of the bed and sustain injuries. To avoid this, the side rails of the bed should be secured by elevating them; further, they should be padded to prevent trauma during convulsions and afterward, when some women become agitated.
- The woman should be positioned in the lateral position to minimise aspiration of oral secretions. If any secretions or vomitus are present, they should be removed by suction.
- During the clonic phase, the woman may bite her tongue; therefore, an airway or padded mouth gag should quickly be inserted.
- Other measures are placing two IV cannulae and inserting a Foley's catheter to maintain an intake–output chart.
- Blood samples should be sent for investigations—CBC, RFT, LFT and coagulation profile.
- In eclampsia, meticulous monitoring is required. The heart rate should be monitored continuously with an ECG monitor as these women are prone to ventricular arrhythmias. Blood pressure and oxygen saturation should be monitored continuously and documented every 15 minutes. Invasive hemodynamic monitoring may be required in intractable cardiac failure, severe renal disease, refractory hypertension, pulmonary edema and oliguria.
- The woman may require muscle paralysis and assisted ventilation if she presents with status eclampticus or coma, when the arterial blood gas levels are compromised, in the presence of laryngeal edema/pulmonary edema or when there is respiratory arrest.

Anticonvulsant therapy

- In the past, Krishna Menon's regimen of using a combination of pethidine, phenergan and chlorpromazine was used to control convulsions in eclampsia. It is not used anymore.

- Currently, parenteral magnesium sulphate is the drug of choice for the control of convulsions in eclampsia. Magnesium sulphate is a potent vasodilator, particularly in the cerebral vasculature. In women with pre-eclampsia, magnesium sulphate has been shown to improve cerebral arterial circulation, and there is evidence to suggest possible neuroprotective effects. It also protects the endothelial cells from damage by free radicals, prevents calcium entry into the ischemic cells and acts as a competitive antagonist to the glutamate N-methyl–D-aspartate receptor (which is epileptogenic).

Preparation of 20% magnesium sulphate solution
- Each ampoule of magnesium sulphate contains 2 mL of the drug, with each mL having 500 mg of magnesium sulphate. Hence, one ampoule contains 1 g of magnesium sulphate.
- It is available as a 50% solution, which is used undiluted for IM injection. 1 mL of 2% lignocaine should be added to the IM doses to reduce pain at the injection site.
- For intravenous use, the 50% solution should be converted to a 20% solution. To make the 20% solution of $MgSO_4$, 12 mL of NS is added to 8 mL (4 amps) of 50% $MgSO_4$.

Regimens for magnesium sulphate administration

Pritchard's regimen
Magnesium sulphate is given as a loading dose intravenously followed by a maintenance dose intramuscularly. The treatment is continued for 24 hours after the last seizure or delivery, whichever occurs last.

Loading dose
- The total loading dose is 14 g of 50% $MgSO_4$.
- 4 g is given by the intravenous route as 20 mL of 20% solution given over a period of 20 minutes.
- This is followed by 5 g (5 amps) of the same solution in each buttock, deep IM (total of 10 g IM), with 1 mL of lignocaine in the same syringe. A large-bore needle may be required.

Maintenance dose
- 5 g (5 amps) of a 50% solution + 1 mL of 2% lignocaine IM is administered every 4 hours into alternate buttocks.

Alternatively, continuous infusion protocols are also available to avoid IM injections. In India, some centres use low-dose magnesium sulphate therapy using various regimens; these are found to be effective and safe. Myasthenia gravis is an absolute contraindication for magnesium therapy.

Monitoring of the woman while on magnesium sulphate

Careful monitoring is important while the woman is on magnesium therapy. The following parameters are monitored hourly before repeat administration:
- Deep reflexes hourly
- Respiratory rate >16/minute
- Urine output >30 mL/hour

The signs of hypermagnesemia are as follows:
- Respiratory rate <16/minute
- Knee-jerk reflexes absent

Urine output monitoring is important as impaired renal function can increase magnesium toxicity.

When there are clinical signs of hypermagnesemia, further doses of magnesium sulphate should be withheld, and an injection of 10% calcium gluconate should be given intravenously. Once the clinical signs of hypermagnesemia resolve, 2 g of $MgSO_4$ should be given IV over 5–10 minutes and followed-up with the maintenance dose. In case of respiratory depression, intubation and mechanical ventilation should be started without any delay.

Serum monitoring of magnesium levels is not routinely recommended as it is expensive and has not been shown to be superior to clinical monitoring. However, in certain situations, measuring serum levels may be required—in the presence of renal disease, when urine output is <100 mL/4 hours and there are signs of magnesium toxicity and in the presence of recurrent convulsions. The therapeutic range of serum magnesium is 4–7 mEq/L. Depending on the severity of hypermagnesemia, complications will manifest.

Other side effects of magnesium sulphate
Warmth, flushing, nausea, vomiting, diplopia, slurred speech, hypotension and arrhythmias can occur; it can also potentiate muscle relaxant activity. Magnesium sulphate may relax the uterus, and there may be fetal heart rate abnormalities. In women with elevated creatinine levels, the loading dose should be reduced to 4 g.

Control of Hypertension

- To avoid injury to the brain, heart and kidneys, it is essential to reduce the BP to a safe range gradually without compromising cerebral perfusion pressure and uteroplacental blood flow. The goal of antihypertensive therapy is to keep systolic BP between 140 and 155 mmHg and diastolic between 90 and 100 mmHg. While choosing an antihypertensive agent, the woman's vital parameters should be taken into account. Eclampsia patients have raised intracranial pressure, and therefore, it is important to lower the blood pressure gradually, otherwise the intracranial pressure will rise further.

- Hydralazine and nifedipine are associated with tachycardia and should be avoided in patients with a heart rate above 110 bpm; labetalol can be used instead. In patients with bradycardia (heart rate <60 bpm), asthma or congestive heart failure, labetalol should be avoided.
- Nifedipine is associated with improved renal blood flow and a resultant increase in urine output, making it preferable for patients with decreased urine output.

Differential Diagnosis

Occasionally, there may be other conditions presenting with seizures in pregnancy. Whenever there is atypical presentation of eclampsia or if the woman is in a deep coma presenting with recurrent seizures in spite of magnesium sulphate therapy or in the presence of neurological deficits, the following differential diagnosis should be considered:

- Cerebrovascular accidents
- Epilepsy
- Meningitis, encephalitis
- Intracerebral hemorrhage due to a ruptured aneurysm
- Cerebral venous thrombosis
- Arterial or venous infarcts
- Angiomas
- Hypertensive encephalopathy
- Previously undiagnosed brain tumours
- Metastatic gestational trophoblastic disease
- Metabolic diseases
- Postdural puncture syndrome

Delivery

The definitive treatment of eclampsia is delivery of the fetus and placenta irrespective of the gestational age. Delivery should take place as soon as the woman's condition is stable. Vaginal delivery is preferred for women with eclampsia. If the cervix is favourable,

labour should be induced with prostaglandins, ARM, oxytocin or a Foley's catheter. Eclampsia itself is not an indication for cesarean section. However, cesarean section is recommended in the following situations:

- When there is an obstetric indication for cesarean section
- When the cervix is unfavourable and the fetus is alive
- For all deeply unconscious patients, unless delivery is imminent
- For uncooperative, restless patients
- For a woman who is having convulsions continuously
- When vaginal delivery unlikely within 6–8 hours of the onset of seizures

Management of labour

The following measures must be taken during labour:
- Antihypertensives and anticonvulsants should be continued.
- Fluid should be restricted to 80 mL/hour unless there is ongoing blood loss. Infusion/syringe pumps should be used to regulate the fluid intake.
- In labour, the frequency and the tone of the uterine contractions are raised, and fetal heart rate changes are very common following a convulsion for 3–15 minutes.
- One should not rush into cesarean section for CTG changes as they are likely to return to normal after stabilisation. If the fetal heart rate changes persist, abruptio placenta should be suspected.
- The second stage of labour may be shortened with forceps to avoid the rise in maternal BP with each uterine contraction.
- Continuous epidural analgesia is beneficial for vaginal and operative delivery in pre-eclampsia and eclampsia provided there are no contraindications such as thrombocytopenia (platelets <75,000/mm³) or altered coagulation profile.

Third stage management

- The third stage should be actively managed with oxytocin 10 units IM/600 micrograms of misoprostol rectally.
- Ergometrine and syntometrine are contraindicated as these are potent vasoconstrictors.
- The development of PPH should be looked for in all cases of pre-eclampsia and eclampsia as magnesium sulphate and nifedipine are calcium channel blockers and both can relax the uterus. Further, these

women could have complications such as HELLP/coagulopathy.

- The patient can go into postpartum collapse due to electrolyte imbalance, PPH or a sudden fall of BP.

Postpartum management

- Continuous close monitoring is required as most deaths occur in the immediate postpartum period. The woman should be kept in the high-dependency unit for 48 hours following delivery.
- Fluid replacement should be restricted to 80 mL/hour.
- The anticonvulsant should be continued for 48 hours after delivery.
- The antihypertensive should also be continued and gradually weaned.

Indications for neuroimaging studies

In order to rule out ICH, CVT or infarcts, neuroimaging with CT scan/MRI may be required when there is atypical presentation or if the woman develops focal neurological deficits or blindness, if the woman goes into prolonged coma or if the convulsions are not responding to magnesium therapy.

Postnatal follow-up

At 6 weeks, postnatal follow-up is mandatory to look for hypertension and/or proteinuria.

In women with early-onset/severe eclampsia/eclampsia, it is important to investigate for APLA, hyperhomocysteinemia and renal disease so that preventive measures can be undertaken in the subsequent pregnancies. Advice should be given on early booking in subsequent pregnancies to evaluate the need to administer low-dose aspirin for prevention.

Contraception

Puerperal sterilisation should be avoided because of the risk of thromboembolism associated with pre-eclampsia/eclampsia. IUCD, progesterone-only pills and injectable progestogens are safe to use in women with hypertensive disorders of pregnancy.

Complications of Eclampsia

Besides the complications discussed under pre-eclampsia, women with eclampsia can develop life-threatening complications such as pulmonary edema, laryngeal edema, aspiration, aspiration pneumonitis, renal failure, cerebrovascular accidents, cardiopulmonary arrest and rupture of the liver. Maternal death can occur due to these complications.

Women may also sustain injuries during seizures, ranging from bruises to fractures. The tongue may sustain injuries from being bitten, or it may fall backward, occluding the glottis and leading to fatal asphyxia. Hyperpyrexia may develop, especially when there is a pontine hemorrhage.

Prevention

The ISSHP recommends that women with established clinical risk factors for pre-eclampsia should be prescribed preventive measures with aspirin and calcium supplementation. Low-molecular-weight heparin is not indicated to prevent pre-eclampsia, even when there is a history of prior early-onset pre-eclampsia.

Risk Factors for Pre-eclampsia (Table 30.4)

Table 30.4 Risk factors that predispose to pre-eclampsia

Major risk factors	Minor risk factors
• Prior pre-eclampsia • Chronic hypertension • Pregestational diabetes mellitus • Chronic renal disease • Maternal body mass index >30 Kg/m² • Antiphospholipid syndrome • Pregnancy following assisted reproduction techniques • Presence of ≥2 minor risk factors	• Advanced maternal age • Family history of pre-eclampsia • Short duration of sexual relationship • Connective tissue disorders
• Treated ideally before 16 weeks but definitely before 20 weeks • Low-dose aspirin is given in a dose of 75–150 mg/day • Calcium supplementation of 1,200 mg daily if dietary calcium intake is low	• Preferably starting before 16 weeks' gestation until 37 weeks, using 100–150 mg daily • Calcium supplements 1,200 mg daily if dietary calcium intake is low

Predictors of Pre-eclampsia

Many clinical, ultrasonographic and laboratory parameters have been explored during early pregnancy as tools for predicting who will later develop pre-eclampsia. These include uterine artery Doppler studies, measurement of angiogenic factors (such as soluble endoglin, PlGF, sFlt-1 and sFLt-1/PlGF ratio) and pregnancy-associated plasma protein A (PAPP-A). Uterine artery Doppler is carried out between 11 and 14 weeks of gestation to predict pre-eclampsia.

Referral to Higher Centres

When a woman with eclampsia is being referred to a tertiary care centre, the medical officer should ensure the following:

- Antihypertensive medication is started, preferably with 20 mg of oral nifedipine.
- A loading dose of magnesium sulphate is started; at least 4 g should be given intravenously before shifting the woman.

- The woman should be kept in the recovery position.
- The tongue should be protected with a padded mouth gag.
- An intravenous line should be in place with an RL/dextrose saline at 80 mL/hour.
- The woman should be accompanied by a doctor.

KEY POINTS

✓ Hypertensive disorders in pregnancy include gestational hypertension or PIH, pre-eclampsia, eclampsia and chronic hypertension with or without superimposed pre-eclampsia.

✓ Hypertension in pregnancy is defined as systolic BP of >140 mmHg and a diastolic BP of 90 mmHg checked twice 4–6 hours apart.

✓ Gestational hypertension develops after 20 weeks of gestation and there is no proteinuria.

✓ Pre-eclampsia is the development of new-onset hypertension after 20 weeks of gestation with or without proteinuria. In the absence of proteinuria, there is evidence of organ dysfunction.

✓ Eclampsia is a serious condition necessitating prompt management of convulsions and expediting delivery of the fetus. Magnesium sulphate has proved to be effective in controlling convulsions in eclampsia and is the preferred line of therapy. Eclampsia can be prevented if pre-eclampsia is diagnosed early and managed effectively.

✓ Antihypertensives used in the hypertensive disorders of pregnancy are labetalol, nifedipine, methyldopa and hydralazine.

✓ In high-risk women, low-dose aspirin is recommended at a dosage of 75–150 mg to prevent pre-eclampsia.

Essay questions

1. Discuss the risk factors and pathogenesis of pre-eclampsia.
2. Describe the pathological changes in various organs in eclampsia.
3. How would you manage a pregnant woman with pre-eclampsia presenting with severe features?
4. Describe the clinical features of eclampsia and the principles of management.

Short answer questions

1. Classify the hypertensive disorders of pregnancy.
2. List the antihypertensive drugs used in pregnancy.
3. What is the HELLP syndrome?
4. What are the complications of eclampsia?
5. List the differential diagnosis of eclampsia.

MCQs

1. Which of the following drugs is contraindicated in pre-eclampsia?
   a) Labetalol
   b) Nifedipine
   c) Methyldopa
   d) ACE inhibitor
2. To diagnose gestational hypertension, blood pressure should come back to normal within:
   a) 4 weeks postpartum
   b) 6 weeks postpartum
   c) 8 weeks postpartum
   d) 12 weeks postpartum
3. What should be the concentration of magnesium sulphate for intravenous use?
   a) 10%
   b) 20%
   c) 30%
   d) 50%
4. Which of these does not explain the pathophysiology of pre-eclampsia?
   a) Vasospasm
   b) Absence of spiral artery remodelling
   c) Decreased soluble fms-like tyrokinase 1 (sFlt1)
   d) Decreased PlGF
5. Which is a feature of gestational hypertension?
   a) Onset at >20 weeks of gestation
   b) Proteinuria
   c) Persistent elevated blood pressure after 6 months postpartum
   d) Blurring of vision
6. Which of the following is not one of the danger signs of pre-eclampsia?
   a) Persistent headache
   b) Vision disturbance
   c) Pain abdomen
   d) Pulmonary edema
7. Which of the following types of organ involvement is not commonly noted in pre-eclampsia?
   a) Subcapsular liver hemorrhage
   b) Glomerular endotheliosis
   c) Papilledema
   d) Autosplenectomy

Answers
1. (d), 2. (d), 3. (b), 4. (c), 5. (a), 6. (c), 7. (d)

Fill in the blanks

1. The characteristic lesion in the kidney in pre-eclampsia is _____.

2. The goal of antihypertensive therapy is to keep the diastolic BP between _____.

3. The antidote for magnesium sulphate toxicity is _____.

4. The route for the administration of nifedipine is _____.

Answers

1. glomerular endotheliosis, 2. 90 and 100 mmHg, 3. calcium gluconate, 4. per oral

Case scenarios-based discussions

1. A 35-year-old primigravida at 35 weeks of gestation reports to the casualty with c/o severe headache. On examination, her BP is 170/110 mmHg. She is not in labour, and the fetal heart rate is good. The dipstick analysis of her urine shows 3+ protein.
   a) What is the diagnosis?
   b) What investigations will you order?
   c) What are the medications you will prescribe?
   d) When would you deliver her?
   e) What is the anticonvulsant to be administered, its dosage and the monitoring required?

Answers

a) The diagnosis is pre-eclampsia with severe features.
b) Maternal assessment is based on LFT, RFT, hematological parameters, peripheral smear, coagulation profile, fundus examination and fetal assessment by biophysical profile and umbilical artery Doppler study.

c) Antihypertensives, preferably IV or oral labetalol/nifedipine, and an anticonvulsant should be given with magnesium sulphate.
d) Once the mother is stabilised, she should be delivered.
e) Magnesium sulphate should be administered as per the Pritchard regimen. Urine output, respiratory rate and the patellar reflex should be monitored.

2. A 21-year-old primigravida is brought to the casualty with a history of 32 weeks of gestation and having had 4 seizures at home. She is conscious, has pedal and facial edema and her BP is 150/100 mmHg. Her urine protein is 2+. Clonus is positive. She is not in labour and the FH is good.
   a) What is the diagnosis?
   b) What is the immediate measure you should take?
   c) What is the obstetric management?
   d) What preventive measure would you advise for subsequent pregnancies?

Answers

a) The diagnosis is antepartum eclampsia.
b) The woman should be nursed in the left lateral position in a railing cot, any secretions in her respiratory tract should be cleared, oxygen should be administered at 8–10 litres/minute, magnesium sulphate should be administered as per the Pritchard regimen, an antihypertensive should be administered and investigations should be ordered.
c) Once the woman is stabilised, she should be delivered. At 32 weeks of gestation, as the cervix is likely to be unfavourable, the woman should be delivered by cesarean section.
d) The woman is a high-risk candidate for recurrence in future pregnancies. Therefore, she should be advised to take tablet aspirin 75–150 mg/day before 16 weeks of gestation. She should also consume at least 1,000 mg of calcium every day.

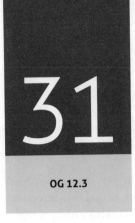

31 Diabetes Complicating Pregnancy

OG 12.3

Learning Objectives

» To discuss carbohydrate metabolism in pregnancy
» To describe the pathophysiology of GDM and pre-existing diabetes
» To know the screening methods to diagnose GDM
» To know the adverse effects of GDM and pre-existing diabetes on the mother and the fetus and the complications in the newborn
» To discuss the management of GDM during pregnancy and labour

INTRODUCTION

The prevalence of pre-existing diabetes and gestational diabetes among women of childbearing age is increasing throughout the world, particularly in south-east Asia. This rise in GDM and type II diabetes parallels the increasing incidence of obesity among women. Hyperglycemia in pregnancy is a medical condition resulting from either pre-existing diabetes or insulin resistance developing during pregnancy. Fetal and neonatal morbidity and mortality associated with diabetes in pregnancy can be prevented by meticulous prenatal and intrapartum care.

CLASSIFICATION OF DIABETES IN PREGNANCY

The International Association of Diabetes and Pregnancy Study Group (IADPSG) and the International Federation of Gynecology and Obstetrics (FIGO) divided hyperglycemia in pregnancy (HIP) into two distinct conditions—diabetes in pregnancy (DIP) and gestational diabetes mellitus (GDM).

DIABETES IN PREGNANCY (DIP)

DIP, which was previously known as overt or pregestational diabetes, refers to diabetes that was diagnosed before the onset of pregnancy. There are two types of pregestational diabetes:

- Type I: There is absolute insulin deficiency.
- Type II: There is defective insulin secretion or insulin resistance.

GESTATIONAL DIABETES MELLITUS (GDM)

GDM is defined as carbohydrate intolerance resulting in hyperglycemia of variable severity with onset or first recognition during pregnancy. (This does not exclude the possibility of unrecognised glucose intolerance, which may have been present before the onset of pregnancy.)

Incidence

Gestational diabetes mellitus (GDM) has emerged as a global public health problem. Globally, the prevalence of GDM ranges from 1–28% depending on the screening method used and the population studied. The incidence of gestational diabetes is high among Asian populations. Among Indian women, it is 10–11-fold higher than the Caucasian population. In India, the prevalence ranges from 3.8% in Kashmir to 17.9% in Tamil Nadu. A community-based study found the prevalence of GDM to be 17.8% in the urban, 13.8% in the semi-urban and 9.9% in the rural areas in Tamil Nadu.

Carbohydrate Metabolism in Normal Pregnancy

(Discussed in detail in Chapter 5, *Maternal changes during pregnancy*.)

- In a healthy pregnancy, the woman's body undergoes a series of physiological changes to support the growing fetal demands. A significant metabolic adaptation takes place in insulin sensitivity. During early gestation, insulin sensitivity increases, promoting the uptake of glucose into adipose stores to prepare for the energy demands of later pregnancy. However, as gestation advances, there is a surge of hormones including estrogen, progesterone, leptin, cortisol, placental lactogen and placental growth hormone, which promotes a state of insulin resistance. Human placental lactogen affects the carbohydrate, protein and fat metabolism, increasing the free fatty acids by lipolysis. As a result, blood glucose is slightly elevated, and this glucose is readily transported across the placenta to fuel the growth of the fetus.

This mild state of insulin resistance also promotes endogenous glucose production and the breakdown of fat stores, resulting in a further increase in blood glucose and free fatty acid (FFA) concentrations. During pregnancy, there is fasting hypoglycemia and postprandial hyperglycemia. In the fasting state, as there is hypoglycemia, triglycerides are broken down into fatty acids and ketones. So, in pregnancy, there is a shift in the source of fuel from glucose to lipids. If starvation is prolonged, it leads to ketosis.

- In short, pregnancy induces a diabetogenic state in the individual. This diabetogenic response is attributed to an increase in insulin-antagonising hormones like human placental lactogen, progesterone and cortisol and also the production of enzymes (placental insulinase) by the placenta, which results in an increase in the degradation of insulin.

Pathophysiology of GDM

GDM is a result of β-cell dysfunction and the chronic insulin resistance that develops during pregnancy. In most cases, these impairments exist prior to pregnancy and can be progressive, leading to an increased risk of the development of type 2 diabetes mellitus after pregnancy. Lowering of glucose uptake by the cells induced by insulin resistance of pregnancy further contributes to hyperglycemia, overburdening the β-cells, which have to produce additional insulin in response. Once β-cell dysfunction begins, there is a vicious cycle of hyperglycemia, insulin resistance and further β-cell dysfunction. GDM usually manifests in the latter half of pregnancy.

Risk Factors for GDM

There are a number of risk factors that predispose a woman to develop GDM; these are as follows:

- Overweight/obesity
- Excessive gestational weight gain
- Ethnicity
- Genetic polymorphisms
- Advanced maternal age
- Intrauterine environment (low or high birth weight)
- Family and personal history of GDM
- Diseases related to insulin resistance such as polycystic ovarian syndrome (PCOS)

Diagnosis of GDM

The World Health Organization (WHO) and Diabetes in Pregnancy Study Group, India (DIPSI), do not recommend a screening test for the diagnosis of GDM;

instead, they suggest a direct diagnostic test—the oral glucose challenge test (OGCT), which was used as a screening test in the past but is now considered both a screening and a diagnostic test.

Who should be screened?

In countries with a low prevalence of GDM, selective screening is carried out for women who are at a high risk of developing GDM. This includes Asian women, obese women, women of advanced maternal age and those who have a family history of diabetes or a past history of GDM, those who have a past history of delivering macrosomic babies, those who have had unexplained neonatal or intrauterine deaths or the birth of a malformed child in the past. However, in the Indian context, universal screening is essential in all pregnant women as Indian women have an 11-fold increased risk of developing glucose intolerance during pregnancy as compared to Western women.

When should screening be performed?

The ideal time to perform the diagnostic test for GDM is at 12–16 weeks of gestation or at the first visit to the antenatal (AN) clinic. If a woman's test results are normal at the first visit, the test is repeated between 24 and 28 weeks of gestation and later at 32–34 weeks. The schedule for the diagnostic tests is presented in Table 31.1.

Table 31.1 GDM—diagnostic test schedule

Diagnostic test	Week of gestation
I diagnostic test	Ideally, at 12–16 weeks or at the time of the first visit for an antenatal check-up
II diagnostic test	At 24–28 weeks
III diagnostic test	At 32–34 weeks

Screening methods

Different screening methods are used in different parts of the world. Either a single-step method or a two-step method is used to diagnose GDM.

Single-step methods

The International Association of Diabetes and Pregnancy Study Group (IADPSG), the WHO and the Government of India recommend a single-step method for the diagnosis of GDM as this is convenient for the woman, is economical and does not require the woman to be in the fasting state.

Diabetes in Pregnancy Study Group India (DIPSI) method

- The antenatal woman is given 75 g of glucose in 300 mL of water irrespective of the time of her last meal and whether she is in the fasting or the non-fasting state (the glucose water can be consumed slowly over about 5 minutes to avoid nausea and vomiting). Oral glucose does not cause nausea and vomiting if administered in the non-fasting state. Lemon juice can be added to make the oral glucose palatable. Two hours after the woman has consumed the glucose solution, venous blood is drawn and tested for plasma glucose. The plasma glucose can be tested by an autoanalyser/semi-autoanalyser. If these machines are not available, capillary blood may be tested by glucometers that are calibrated to plasma glucose.

• The test result is considered normal if the plasma glucose at 2-hour post-glucose load is <140 mg/dL. If the 2-hour post-glucose load is >140 mg/dL, the woman is considered positive for GDM. Women who

test normal at the first visit should undergo repeat testing at 24–28 weeks and if found normal, should be tested once again between 32 and 34 weeks (Fig. 31.1).

IADPSG criteria

• The woman comes after overnight fasting and her fasting plasma glucose level is checked.

• Then, the woman is given 75 g of glucose mixed in 150 mL of water or lime juice. The plasma glucose is checked at 1 and 2 hours.

• GDM is diagnosed if any one value is equal to or more than the cut-off values listed below:
  — Fasting plasma glucose: 92 mg/dL
  — 1-hour plasma glucose: 180 mg/dL
  — 2-hour plasma glucose: 153 mg/dL

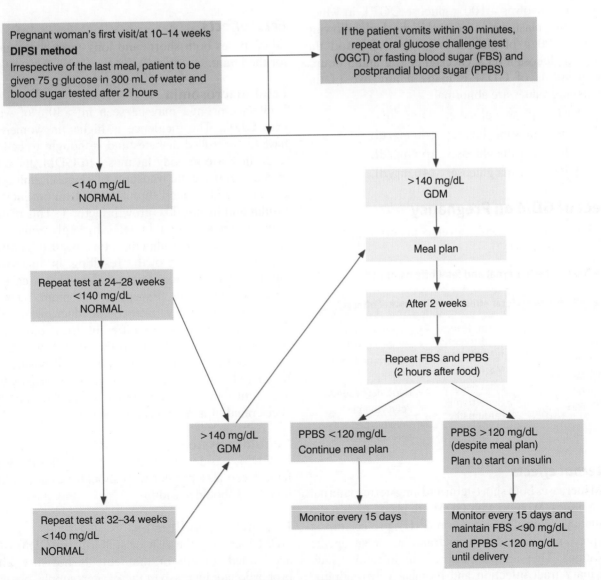

Fig. 31.1 Screening and management of gestational diabetes mellitus

The WHO method

The WHO also endorses universal screening for GDM at 24–28 weeks of gestation using the 75 g 2-hour glucose tolerance test (GTT). For this test, the woman comes in a fasting state and is given a 75 g glucose load. A 2-hour plasma glucose value of ≥140 mg/dL is diagnostic of GDM.

Two-step method

In the two-step method, first, a screening test is carried out and if it is positive, the second step, which is a diagnostic test, is performed.

- The first step is a 50 g glucose challenge test irrespective of the woman's last meal. It is performed at 24–28 weeks of gestation in women who do not have pre-existing diabetes. If the 1-hour plasma glucose is ≥140 mg/dL, then the second step is carried out.

- Step two involves a 100 g glucose OGTT, in which the fasting plasma glucose level is checked, following which, 100 g of glucose is given orally, and the plasma glucose level is checked at 1, 2 and 3 hours. A diagnosis of GDM is made if any two of the following values are abnormal:
  - Fasting plasma glucose: 95 mg/dL
  - 1-hour plasma glucose: 180 mg/dL
  - 2-hour plasma glucose: 155 mg/dL
  - 3-hour plasma glucose: 140 mg/dL

Effect of GDM on Pregnancy

GDM is associated with adverse maternal and fetal outcomes (Table 31.2).

Table 31.2 The maternal and fetal effects of GDM

Maternal effects	Fetal effects	Neonatal effects
• Preterm labour • Pre-eclampsia • Infections • Hydramnios • Operative delivery	• Second- and third-trimester fetal loss • Macrosomia • Fetal death • Hypertrophic cardiopathy	• Hypoglycemia • Hypocalcemia • Hyperbilirubinemia • RDS • Hypomagnesemia • Polycythemia • Unexplained neonatal death

Maternal effects

GDM increases both short-term and long-term maternal health issues. Women with GDM are prone to develop pregnancy-induced hypertension (PIH), pre-eclampsia and preterm labour due to hydramnios or iatrogenic indications. They are prone to various infections such as urinary tract infection and monilial vulvovaginitis.

In cases of uncontrolled GDM, hydramnios is often seen; this may be due to the large placenta or fetal polyuria secondary to fetal hyperglycemia. Operative deliveries are more common due to macrosomia of the baby, which can lead to poor progress in labour and obstructed labour. Therefore, there is an increased risk of cesarean and instrumental deliveries. There is also an increased risk of trauma to the genital tract if the labour is complicated by shoulder dystocia.

Long-term sequelae

Women with a prior history of GDM are at risk of recurrent GDM in subsequent pregnancies. Approximately 50% of women with a past history of GDM develop type II DM later in life. As the vasculature in GDM is permanently altered, these women are also prone to developing cardiovascular disease (CVD) later in life.

Fetal effects

GDM poses both short- and long-term consequences for the infant.

Fetal macrosomia

Fetal macrosomia may be seen in >30% of women with GDM. The incidence is higher in women who have uncontrolled diabetes and is thought to be linked to an increase in body fat mass. In GDM, there is an increase in placental transport of glucose, amino acids and fatty acids, which stimulate the fetal production of insulin and insulin-like growth factor 1. This maternal hyperglycemia results in fetal hyperglycemia, which causes fetal hyperinsulinemia; this, in turn, stimulates excessive somatic growth, resulting in macrosomia and birth weight exceeding 4,500 g. This is called the Pederson hypothesis. Except for the brain, most fetal organs are affected by macrosomia. Macrosomic infants of diabetic mothers are different from other large-for-gestational age infants in that they have excessive fat deposition on the shoulders, predisposing them to shoulder dystocia. Genetic and maternal obesity also contribute to macrosomia. Once fetal growth is accelerated, it is difficult to reverse it.

Shoulder dystocia

In GDM, besides macrosomic babies, normal-weight fetuses can also present with shoulder dystocia due to increased shoulder width.

Unexplained stillbirths

GDM increases the risk of stillbirth. In GDM, if the accelerated growth of the fetus is not met with a proportionate increase in the oxygen supply, especially in the presence of associated complications such as pre-eclampsia, it can result in fetal death. Both hyper- and hypoglycemia and associated ketoacidosis are dangerous for the fetus. Fetal hyperinsulinemia induced by maternal hyperglycemia can also cause hypokalemia leading to fetal arrhythmia and death. Fasting hyperglycemia, defined as more than 105 mg/dL, is associated with an increased risk of fetal death during the last 4–8 weeks of gestation.

Fetal losses and fetal malformations

First- and second-trimester fetal losses and fetal malformations are complications of uncontrolled, overt diabetes. However, if hyperglycemia is diagnosed for the first time in early pregnancy, it could have been a case of undiagnosed overt diabetes; in these women, there may be an increased risk of fetal loss and malformations.

Neonatal complications

- Infants born to women who have GDM are at an increased risk of hypoglycemia as maternal hyperglycemia stimulates fetal hyperinsulinemia. Such infants present with twitching, convulsions, hypotonia and tachypnea.
- Infants are prone to polycythemia due to the hypoxic status, which can lead to hyperviscosity of blood and renal vein thrombosis.
- Hyperbilirubinemia may develop due to the decreased life span of RBCs.
- Hypocalcemia may develop.
- Respiratory distress syndrome (RDS) may develop due to insulin antagonising the cortisol synthesis by fibroblasts.
- The infant of a woman with poorly controlled diabetes is increased in length; there is adiposity and organomegaly of the heart and liver due to increased glycogen storage.
- In the long term, babies born of GDM pregnancies are at increased risk of obesity, type II DM and cardiovascular disease.
- Babies born to mothers with GDM have almost double the risk of developing childhood obesity as compared with those born to non-diabetic women.
- Female infants are more likely to experience GDM in their own pregnancies in the future.

Effect of Pregnancy on GDM

Because of the diabetogenic response in pregnancy, the insulin requirement increases gradually from early pregnancy and continues until term. Because of constantly changing insulin requirements during

pregnancy, ketosis is more likely to develop in diabetic women. There is a lowered threshold for glucose excretion in pregnancy which is more marked in diabetic patients. This lowered renal threshold makes repeated blood sugar estimation imperative in the control of diabetes in pregnancy.

Management of GDM

A team approach is important in the management of women with GDM. The team would usually comprise an obstetrician, a diabetologist, a dietitian and a pediatrician. The principles of management include control of diabetes, obstetric management and decision on timing of delivery and specialised care for the newborn.

Medical management

Glycemic control

- In the management of GDM, the aim is to maintain the two-hour postprandial plasma glucose (PPPG) level in the range of 110–120 mg/dL and fasting plasma glucose <95 mg/dL. Good glycemic control is important to prevent perinatal complications.
- Medical management involves dietary management and insulin therapy.

Dietary management—meal plan (medical nutrition therapy [MNT])

- All women diagnosed with GDM should be advised to follow a meal plan and exercise for two weeks. A moderate exercise of at least 30 minutes daily should be prescribed. The food plan should provide adequate calorie intake to promote fetal/neonatal and maternal health, achieve glycemic goals and promote weight gain.
- Caloric intake should be adjusted to prevent weight loss or excessive weight gain. Calorie intake should start at 30 Kcal/Kg of the ideal body weight and carbohydrates should form 40–50% of the diet. In women who are overweight, the calorie intake may be restricted to 24 Kcal/Kg per day. They should take complex carbohydrates with high fibre content and avoid simple carbohydrates. Depending on the BMI, weight gain should be adjusted.
- The diet should include 80–100 g of protein/ day unless there is diabetic nephropathy (in overt diabetes), in which case, the protein intake should be limited to 60 g (1.1–1.5 g/Kg of body weight). 10–35% of the total energy per day should be provided by proteins.
- Fat intake should constitute 30% of the diet and should be made up of monounsaturated fats (>10%

of total daily energy) and polyunsaturated fats (up to 10%) and should be low in saturated fats (<10%). Trans or hydrogenated fat should be avoided.

- 30–35 g of natural fibres should be included.
- It is essential to divide the food intake into 3 meals and 3 snacks to avoid nocturnal and preprandial hypoglycemia. This also helps in preventing peaks in plasma glucose levels after the consumption of the total quantity of food.
- In a woman who has GDM, unlike non-diabetic women, there is a deficiency in insulin secretion following breakfast. Therefore, the quantity of breakfast taken should be adjusted and divided into portions.

The advice of splitting breakfast into two portions has a scientific basis as the peaking of plasma glucose is higher with breakfast (due to the dawn phenomenon) than it is with lunch and dinner.

- Sugar, sweets, fruit juices and tubers like potatoes, tapioca, beetroot and sweet potato should be avoided. Diabetic women should eat to satisfy their appetite and should avoid both fasting and feasting. They should be encouraged to eat more green, leafy vegetables.
- After 15 days of initiating the meal plan, FBS and two-hour postprandial glucose levels should be estimated, preferably after breakfast. If FBS is <95 mg/dL and PP glucose is <120 mg/dL, the woman is said to be under control by meal planning and the meal plan can be continued. While on a meal plan, two-hour PPPGs should be performed once every four weeks until delivery, provided the values are normal at each testing.

Pharmacotherapy

- Medications are required if the metabolic goals are not met with dietary management or if there are signs of excessive fetal growth clinically or by USG.
- Both metformin and insulin therapy are accepted in the medical management of pregnant women with GDM not controlled with medical nutrition therapy. Insulin is the first drug of choice if there is fasting hyperglycemia or complications such as evolving macrosomia and polyhydramnios. Metformin can also be considered after 20 weeks of gestation for the medical management of GDM.

Insulin

It is ideal to use human insulin for the management of GDM as it is the least immunogenic and reduces the risk of fetal beta-cell damage. Though insulin does not cross the placenta, insulin antibodies produced in response to animal-sourced insulin can cross the placenta and stress the fetal beta-cell, increase insulin production and induce macrosomia. Rapid-acting insulin analogues (novorapid/humalog) have been found to be safe and effective in achieving the targeted postprandial glucose value during pregnancy. Lispro is the first analogue to receive category B approval by US FDA for use in pregnancy. Intermediate-acting insulin (premixed insulin 30/70, which contains one-third of regular insulin and two-thirds of intermediate-acting insulin) can be used if pre-food values are high. Two-thirds of this dose should be taken in the morning and one-third at night. Long-acting insulin is avoided in pregnancy to avoid hypoglycemia.

- Insulin is started in a dose of 2–4 units, 30 minutes before breakfast. Following this, two-hour PP levels are tested after two weeks. If the plasma glucose is within normal limits, i.e., within 120 mg/dL, the same dose of insulin is continued.
- If the values are higher, then the dosage is increased by 2–4 units (total dose taken 30 minutes before breakfast). At no point in time should the dosage be increased by more than 2–4 units. The dosage should be adjusted once in 15 days only after testing two-hour PP glucose levels. If the woman requires more than 16 units per day, then a split dose is given in the morning and in the evening. The measurement of HbA1C monthly is a useful indicator of diabetic control.
- If insulin is used throughout the day in women in whom fasting and postprandial hyperglycemia are present after most meals, a typical starting total dosage is 0.7–1 units/Kg daily; this dosage should be divided with a regimen of multiple injections using intermediate-acting insulin in combination with rapid-acting insulin.

Obstetric management

Antenatal care is important to diagnose complications and prevent macrosomia.

- In those diagnosed with GDM in the first trimester, thyroid function test and HbA1C are also carried out. An HbA1C level of 5–6% is desirable. The incidence of major congenital malformations is more if the values rise to 9.5% or more. HbA1C, though desirable, is not mandatory. In these women, retinal and renal assessments are also carried out at the first visit and again at 24–28 weeks of gestation.
- First-trimester aneuploidy screening is done at 11–14 weeks for nuchal translucency (NT) measurement.

- A detailed anomaly scan is done between 18 and 20 weeks of gestation.
- Fetal echo may be done at 24–26 weeks to detect any cardiac anomaly in the fetus if the woman is diagnosed with GDM at the first visit.
- Antenatal check-ups should be done once in 2 weeks until 32 weeks, and then weekly. At each visit, complications such as PIH, hydramnios and macrosomia and evidence of infections should be looked for.
- FBS and PPBS (2 hours) should be performed once a month in women with GDM who are on MNT and once in 2 weeks in women on insulin therapy when the sugar level is well controlled. If sugar is not under control, the tests should be repeated once in 3 days.
- From 28 weeks onwards, fetal growth and liquor volume should be monitored every 4 weeks.
- Hospitalisation should be advised whenever there is poor control of diabetes or if any complications develop.
- Antepartum surveillance in the form of a non-stress test, biophysical profile, etc. (described in Chapter 11, *Antepartum fetal surveillance*), should be started at around 32 weeks in gestational diabetes with any complications.
- Doppler studies may be indicated in cases complicated by pre-eclampsia.

Timing of delivery

The timing of delivery should be individualised depending on the presence and severity of various maternal and fetal risk factors and the degree of control of diabetes.

- If the woman has GDM that is well-controlled on diet and if there are no complications such as macrosomia or hydramnios and no other complications, pregnancy may be continued till near due date with fetal surveillance. In GDM pregnancies, there is a delay in the maturation of the fetal lung. For this reason, routine delivery prior to 39 weeks is not recommended.
- These women are not allowed to go beyond 40 weeks because of the risks such as macrosomia, shoulder dystocia and intrauterine death. Therefore, they are induced at 39–40 weeks of gestation.
- If GDM is being treated with insulin and the blood sugar levels are well-controlled, induction of labour should be scheduled at 39 weeks of pregnancy.
- Elective preterm delivery may be indicated if the diabetes is poorly controlled with hydramnios and macrosomia or associated pre-eclampsia/fetal

compromise. In these situations, steroid therapy is given to enhance the lung maturity of the fetus prior to the termination of pregnancy.

Management in labour

- If induction of labour is planned, a normal diet and the usual insulin regimen are given until the woman is in established labour.
- In established labour, the woman is kept NIL by mouth. An intravenous infusion is started with normal saline/dextrose saline.
- Blood sugar and urine acetone are checked hourly.
- Urea and electrolytes levels are checked on admission and thereafter, every 4 hours.
- In labour, blood sugar levels should be maintained between 90–120 mg/dL.
- When the blood sugar level exceeds 120 mg%, 4 units of insulin are added to 500 mL of NS/RL to run at a rate of 100 mL per hour. The insulin added to the infusion is gradually increased to 5 units, 6 units and so on, depending on the blood sugar levels. This is called the 'sliding scale'.
- Adequate pain relief is important in labour, as pain felt during labour contractions can release catecholamines which can induce hyperglycemia. Epidural analgesia is ideal for pain relief in labour.
- If oxytocin infusion is required for the augmentation of labour, normal saline should be used.
- Prophylactic antibiotics are started.
- The fetus is closely monitored to detect fetal distress early. As soon as the woman reaches the active stage of labour, the artificial rupture of membranes is performed to detect any meconium in the liquor.
- Labour progress should be carefully monitored.
- Cesarean section is performed if the baby is large or if there are other obstetrical indications such as fetal distress. In all cases of GDM, shoulder dystocia should be anticipated at the time of delivery.
- Neonatal monitoring should be carried out to look for hypoglycemia and other complications.

Mode of delivery

Elective cesarean is indicated when there is macrosomia, malpresentation, any other associated obstetrical factor or if shoulder dystocia is anticipated. When cesarean section is performed, prophylactic antibiotics should be given, the skin and uterine incision should be larger (to account for obesity and macrosomic baby), diabetic control should be by sliding scale (insulin dose adjusted to the blood sugar levels) and thromboprophylaxis should be mandatorily administered.

Management in the puerperium

- Antibiotics should be prescribed to prevent infection in the immediate puerperium.
- Women who have GDM often do not require any insulin after delivery.
- Breastfeeding may confer longer-term metabolic benefits on both the mother and offspring.

Postpartum care in women with GDM

Women who develop GDM during pregnancy have a 50% risk of developing overt diabetes within 20 years. Hence, women diagnosed with GDM in pregnancy should undergo 75 g OGTT to determine their glycemic status, ideally between 6–12 weeks postpartum (Table 31.3). The diagnostic criteria are similar to that laid out for non-pregnant adults.

Table 31.3 Normal and various glucose abnormality values for 75 g OGTT

Investigation	Values
Fasting plasma glucose (FPG)	<100 mg/dL (Normal)
2-hour 75 g glucose/postprandial plasma glucose (PPPG)	<140 mg/dL (Normal)
Impaired fasting glucose (IFG)	100–126 mg/dL
Impaired glucose tolerance (IGT)	140–199 mg/dL
Diabetes	>200 mg/dL

If fasting hyperglycemia develops during pregnancy, diabetes is more likely to persist postpartum. For those in whom the 75 g OGTT test is normal, a reassessment should be done at intervals of three years. Women with a history of gestational diabetes mellitus found to have pre-diabetes should receive intensive lifestyle interventions and/or metformin to prevent diabetes. Recurrence occurs in subsequent pregnancies in 50% of women. Therefore, such women should be advised to have preconception counselling prior to their next pregnancy. They also develop overt diabetes in 20 years.

Neonatal Problems

Infants of GDM mothers are more prone to certain neonatal problems, which are as follows:

- Respiratory distress may develop even in term babies.
- The neonate should be assessed for hypoglycemia 1–2 hours, 4–6 hours and 24–48 hours after birth. Hypoglycemia is defined as <40 mg/dL of glucose in term neonates. If hypoglycemia is diagnosed, IV glucose is given as per the newborn care protocols.
- Careful cardiac assessment is also important as there is a possibility of cardiac anomalies not picked by

antenatal USG. Cardiac septal hypertrophy can be seen.
- Hypocalcemia may be seen.
- There may be polycythemia due to chronic hypoxia. This may lead to renal vein thrombosis.
- Hyperbilirubinemia may be seen.

Late neonatal effects

- Macrosomic babies tend to become obese later in life.
- There is an increased incidence of diabetes mellitus developing in the offspring of women who had hyperglycemia in pregnancy.

Contraception

Low-dose combined hormonal contraceptives may be used safely in women with a history of gestational diabetes. Other options are IUCD and injectable progestogens.

PREGESTATIONAL OR OVERT DIABETES COMPLICATING PREGNANCY

Established diabetes complicates 4 of 1,000 pregnancies. Depending on the duration of diabetes, there could be endothelial damage involving the kidneys, eyes and cardiovascular system. Besides the diabetic status, the organ involvement also contributes to adverse maternal and fetal effects in overt diabetes.

Pregestational diabetes may be due to absolute insulin deficiency (type I) or defective insulin secretion or insulin resistance (type II). Type I is insulin-dependent diabetes, occurs in younger women and is difficult to control during pregnancy. These women are prone to recurrent attacks of ketoacidosis and complications related to organ damage.

Preconception Counselling

- In women with pre-existing diabetes, preconception counselling is important. Many of the complications of DM during pregnancy can be prevented with optimal medical care and patient education in the preconception period. The main aim of pre-pregnancy care is to reduce the incidence of congenital abnormality, to identify medical complications and to treat them appropriately and to identify women in whom pregnancy is contraindicated.
- Women with a previous history of gestational diabetes mellitus should also seek preconception screening

for diabetes and preconception care to identify and treat hyperglycemia and prevent congenital malformations.

In a woman with established pre-existing diabetes, pregnancy should be planned.

- Glycemic control is one of the most important aspects of preconception care. Ideally, HbA1C should be <6.5% to reduce the risk of congenital anomalies, pre-eclampsia, macrosomia and other complications.
- As the neural tube defects are increased, 5 mg tablet of folic acid supplementation should be given.
- Screening and treatment of diabetes complications should be carried out. Baseline glucose control and end-organ damage should be assessed, including renal function and retinopathy.
- In women who also suffer from hypertension, medications should be reviewed. ACE inhibitors are contraindicated. Cardiac assessment is very important in older women with long-standing diabetes.
- Those on oral hypoglycemic agents should be switched to insulin. Metformin use is safer in pregnancy.

Contraindications for Pregnancy

- In those with advanced diabetic nephropathy bordering on end-organ renal disease and those who have uncontrollable hypertension, pregnancy is contraindicated
- Women with microvascular heart disease should be discouraged from conceiving and continuing pregnancy.

Effect of Overt Diabetes on Pregnancy

In overt pregestational diabetes, the pregnancy outcome depends on the duration of diabetes and various vascular complications associated with diabetes. Women with White's class C (onset of diabetes between 10 and 19 years of age, duration of diabetes 10–19 years), class D (onset before the age of 10 and duration >20 years), class F diabetes (presence of nephropathy) and more have an increased risk of poor pregnancy outcomes. In women with classes A and B diabetes who receive good periconceptional, antenatal and intrapartum care, the incidence of congenital malformation is reduced, and the perinatal mortality can be reduced to levels similar to those in non-diabetic women.

- **Miscarriage:** There is an increased risk of miscarriages in women with uncontrolled diabetes in the first and early second trimesters.

- **Fetal malformations:** The incidence of major malformations is increased in overt diabetics. The incidence of major malformations in women with type I diabetes is 5%. Cardiac and neural tube defects are commonly seen. Heart anomalies include the transposition of the great vessels (most commonly, cardiac abnormality), ventricular septal defects (VSD) and atrial septal defects (ASD). Caudal regression is an anomaly specific to diabetes in a pregnancy where there is sacral agenesis with a short femur.
- **Preterm delivery:** Overt diabetes antedating pregnancy is a risk factor for preterm delivery. While attempting to prevent preterm labour in diabetic women, caution should be exercised in the control of glucose levels, as both beta-sympathomimetic drugs and glucocorticoids can increase the sugar levels. It is preferable to use calcium channel blockers such as nifedipine.
- **Pregnancy-induced hypertension and pre-eclampsia**: Diabetic women are more prone to develop PIH and pre-eclampsia; the risk is two-fold as compared to non-diabetic pregnant women. Therefore, a urine test for proteinuria, serum albumin and renal function tests are carried out at every antenatal visit. In women with pre-existing hypertension, worsening of hypertension may be seen.
- **Maternal infections:** A pregnant diabetic woman is more prone to urinary tract infections, especially pyelonephritis and monilial vulvovaginitis.
- **Other medical complications:** Deterioration of retinopathy leading to impaired vision. Therefore, regular retinal assessment is important. Other maternal complications include neuropathy and ischemic heart disease.
- **Hydramnios:** Hydramnios may be present if there is associated fetal malformation.
- **Placental insufficiency and IUGR:** In cases of overt diabetes, the blood supply may be impaired due to the vascular disease, leading to placental insufficiency and FGR. When there is no vascular involvement and no placental insufficiency and if the diabetes is uncontrolled, polyhydramnios can occur.
- **Unexplained fetal death:** Overt diabetes is associated with an increased risk of antenatal stillbirth—as high as a 5-fold increase. This may be due to compromised blood flow, maternal hyperglycemia/hypoglycemia or ketoacidosis. The main cause of unexplained stillbirth is maternal hyperglycemia in which the osmotically-induced villous edema leads to impaired fetal oxygen transport.

Effect of Pregnancy on Overt Diabetes

- Close monitoring of blood sugar is essential, and blood sugar needs to be estimated at two-weekly intervals as blood sugar control may be difficult during pregnancy. As early pregnancy is a time of enhanced insulin sensitivity and lowered glucose levels, many women with type 1 diabetes will have lower insulin requirements and an increased risk of hypoglycemia in early pregnancy. The situation rapidly reverses by approximately 16 weeks as insulin resistance increases exponentially during the second and early third trimesters to 2–3 times the preprandial requirement. The insulin requirement levels off toward the end of the third trimester with placental ageing. A rapid reduction in insulin requirements can indicate the development of placental insufficiency.

- Ketoacidosis is a serious complication that may occur in overt diabetes and can be precipitated by infections, hyperemesis in pregnancy and the use of tocolytics to prevent preterm labour. Therefore, ketone should be checked periodically, especially if the woman becomes hyperglycemic or unwell. These women may develop dehydration and metabolic acidosis, which should be corrected by fluid replacement and bicarbonate respectively. Women who are suspected of having diabetic ketoacidosis should be admitted immediately to a critical care unit. Maternal ketonemia is linked with impaired psychomotor development in the offspring.

- Retinal and renal changes if present, may be aggravated during pregnancy.

Investigations

The following investigations are carried out for women with overt diabetes.

- Thyroid function test and HbA1C should be performed at the booking visit. If glucose intolerance is detected in the early pregnancy, the HbA1C level will be helpful to differentiate between pregestational diabetes and GDM. If the HbA1C level is more than 6%, the woman is likely to have pregestational diabetes. The incidence of major congenital malformations is more if the values rise to 9.5% or more.

- Urine should be checked for microalbuminuria, and culture sensitivity should be carried out periodically every 4–6 weeks.

- Renal function test should be carried out every 4–6 weeks.

- ECG should also be performed at booking and whenever required.

Management of Pre-existing Diabetes in Pregnancy

Team care is important in the management of a diabetic pregnant woman. The team should be made up of a diabetologist, obstetrician, perinatologist and a dietician. In the presence of complications, other specialists such as a nephrologist and/or a cardiologist may have to be involved.

Medical management

- **Insulin management in diabetic pregnancies:** Insulin is the preferred agent for the management of both type 1 and type II diabetes in pregnancy. Those with type I diabetes who are already on insulin should be evaluated and their insulin dosage adjusted according to the sugar levels. If overt diabetes has been controlled on oral hypoglycemic agents prior to pregnancy, it is better to switch to insulin therapy once pregnancy is confirmed, since oral hypoglycemic agents may cause fetal defects. In cases of overt diabetes, it is always better to take the help of a physician as the sugar level becomes difficult to control, especially if the woman develops complications. These women should be carefully monitored for hyperglycemia/hypoglycemia and ketoacidosis; these complications may occur more commonly in early pregnancy due to vomiting or urinary tract infections. In the event of complications, the woman should be hospitalised. The insulin requirement increases after 24 weeks of gestation and hence, the dosage should be adjusted based on the blood sugar levels, which should be checked periodically.

- **Place of aspirin:** Women with type 1 or type 2 diabetes should be prescribed low-dose aspirin 60–150 mg/day (the usual dose is 81 mg/day) by the end of the first trimester in order to lower the risk of pre-eclampsia.

- **Blood pressure:** BP should be checked periodically to look for the development of hypertension/pre-eclampsia.

Assessment of medical complications

- Fundoscopy should be performed at the first visit and repeated at 24 weeks and 36 weeks. Retinopathy as such is not a contraindication for vaginal delivery.

- Renal function should be assessed every 4–6 weeks by checking 24-hour urinary protein, blood urea, serum creatinine and urine culture.

- In older women with long-standing diabetes, cardiac evaluation should also be done every 4–6 weeks.

- All diabetic women should be seen at least every 2 weeks until 34 weeks, and then weekly until delivery to ensure frequent alteration in insulin dosage, to provide dietary advice and to detect complications. If the control is poor, more frequent visits are required. At each visit, complications such as PIH, hydramnios, FGR and macrosomia should be looked for.
- Hospitalisation should be advised whenever there is poor control of diabetes, diabetic ketoacidosis or any other complications.
- Insulin resistance decreases dramatically immediately postpartum, and insulin requirements need to be evaluated and adjusted after delivery.

Fetal surveillance

The surveillance of fetal well-being involves the following investigations.

- Viability scan should be performed.
- Dating scan should be performed.
- NT scan—nuchal scan is carried out at 11–14 weeks.
- Down screening—the levels of alpha-fetoprotein and unconjugated estriol levels are low in diabetic pregnancies, and therefore, may lead to erroneous interpretation; amniocentesis and karyotyping are ideal to diagnose Down syndrome in such cases.
- Detailed anomaly scan at 18–20 weeks, in particular, to rule out renal and cardiac anomalies, sacral agenesis and short femur, should be carried out.
- If the facilities are available, maternal serum alpha-fetoprotein concentration is estimated at 16–20 weeks of gestation in an attempt to detect neural tube defects in the fetus.
- Fetal echo may be done at 24–26 weeks to detect any cardiac anomaly in the fetus.
- Assessment of fetal growth is important to diagnose growth restriction—head and abdominal circumferences are measured every 2–4 weeks from 24 weeks onwards for established diabetes complicating pregnancy.

Assessment of fetal well-being

Fetal well-being is assessed by performing a biophysical profile from 28 weeks onwards once in 2 weeks, and if necessary, more frequently. If there is fetal growth restriction, daily CTG, biophysical profile and Doppler studies are carried out (described in Chapter 10, *Imaging techniques*).

Timing of delivery

In overt diabetes complicating pregnancy, if the fetal and maternal well-being are normal, termination of pregnancy is considered after 38 weeks. Early delivery is indicated by maternal and fetal complications as indicated by fetal surveillance. Monitoring in labour is the same as that for GDM.

Post-delivery management

After delivery, in women with overt diabetes, there is a rapid decrease in the insulin requirement. Therefore, insulin dosage should be adjusted according to the blood sugar levels. Women with type II diabetes who were on metformin and glibenclamide prior to pregnancy can resume the same dosage as before.

Management in the puerperium

- Antibiotics are given to prevent infection in the immediate puerperium.
- Breastfeeding may confer longer-term metabolic benefits to both mother and offspring.

Contraception

Low-dose OC pills can be used following diabetic pregnancies if sugar is well under control. In diabetics with vascular disease, combined oral pills are contraindicated. Progestogen-only contraception may increase insulin resistance.

Neonatal Problems

Infants of diabetic mothers are more prone to certain neonatal problems.

- Respiratory distress may develop, even in term babies.
- The neonate should be assessed for hypoglycemia 1–2 hours, 4–6 hours and 24–48 hours after birth. Hypoglycemia is defined as <40 mg/dL of glucose in term neonates. If hypoglycemia is diagnosed, IV glucose is given as per the newborn care protocols.
- Careful cardiac assessment is also important as there is a possibility of cardiac anomalies not picked by antenatal USG. Cardiac septal hypertrophy may be seen.
- Hypocalcemia may develop.
- Hyperbilirubinemia could also develop.

KEY POINTS

✓ *In pregnancy, diabetes may antedate the pregnancy (overt diabetics) or may be detected during pregnancy (GDM).*

✓ *GDM is defined as carbohydrate intolerance resulting in hyperglycemia of variable severity with onset or first recognition during pregnancy.*

✓   *The incidence of GDM is 10–11-fold higher in Indians as compared to Caucasians.*

✓   *Pregnancy induces a diabetogenic state.*

✓   *The ideal time to perform the diagnostic test for GDM is at 12–16 weeks of gestation.*

✓   *The maternal and fetal effects of GDM include preterm labour, pre-eclampsia, infections, hydramnios and operative delivery, fetal loss, macrosomia, fetal death and hypertrophic cardiopathy.*

✓   *Established diabetes complicates 4 of 1,000 pregnancies.*

✓   *In women with established diabetes, the HbA1C should be <6.5% to reduce the risk of congenital anomalies, pre-eclampsia, macrosomia and other complications.*

✓   *Low-dose OC pills can be used following GDM or diabetic pregnancies if sugar is well under control.*

✓   *Proper control of blood sugar during pregnancy reduces perinatal morbidity/mortality.*

✓   *Prenatal counselling and proper guidance decrease the incidence of fetal malformations and fetal loss in women with established diabetes.*

Essay questions

1. Define gestational diabetes and discuss its management during pregnancy.
2. What are the effects of gestational diabetes on pregnancy?
3. What are the indications and methods of screening for diabetes during pregnancy?
4. A 33-year-old G2P1L1 presents at 14 weeks gestation with an OGCT value of 160 mg/dL. She had GDM in her previous pregnancy.
    a) What is the diagnosis in this case?
    b) What investigations should be carried out?
    c) What is the appropriate obstetric management?
    d) What is the appropriate medical management in this case? How should insulin be titrated optimally?
    e) Explain the management of labour and puerperium in this case.

Short answer questions

Write short notes on the following:

1. Fetal macrosomia
2. Diagnosis of diabetes in pregnancy
3. Medical nutrition therapy for a pregnant diabetic woman
4. Late sequelae of gestational diabetes on the mother and fetus

MCQs

1. The hormones responsible for the diabetogenic state of pregnancy include the following EXCEPT:
    a) Human placental lactogen
    b) Human chorionic gonadotrophin
    c) Progesterone
    d) Placental insulinase
2. What is carbohydrate intolerance diagnosed first during pregnancy called?
    a) Overt diabetes
    b) Insulin-resistant diabetes mellitus
    c) Insulin-deficient diabetes mellitus
    d) Gestational diabetes mellitus
3. GDM is associated with a significant increase in the risk of all of the following EXCEPT:
    a) Stillbirths
    b) Macrosomia-related morbidity
    c) Neonatal hypoglycemia
    d) Congenital malformations
4. For well-controlled diabetes in pregnancy, what should the 2 hours postprandial plasma glucose value be?
    a) <110 mg/dL
    b) <120 mg/dL
    c) <130 mg/dL
    d) <140 mg/dL
5. Which of the following is an anomaly specific to the infant of a diabetic mother?
    a) Down syndrome
    b) VSD
    c) Sacral caudal regression
    d) ASD
6. Which of these fetal complications is not more common in GDM pregnancy?
    a) Stillbirth
    b) Macrosomia
    c) FGR
    d) Hypoglycemia
7. What is the target postprandial blood glucose in the control of GDM pregnancy?
    a) <100 mg/dL
    b) 110–120 mg/dL
    c) 120–140 mg/dL
    d) 140–200 mg/dL
8. What is the preferred gestational age for delivery in a case of overt diabetes?
    a) 34 weeks
    b) 36–37 weeks
    c) 37–38 weeks
    d) 40 weeks
9. What is the incidence of malformations with type 1 DM?
    a) 1%
    b) 5%
    c) 10%
    d) 15%
10. Which of these changes is not associated with pregnancy?
    a) Increased insulin antagonising hormones
    b) Decreased insulin degradation
    c) Lowered renal threshold
    d) Aggravated retinal changes

Answers

1. (b), 2. (d), 3. (d), 4. (b), 5. (c), 6. (c), 7. (b), 8. (c), 9. (b), 10. (b)

Fill in the blanks

1. The desirable level of HbA1C in pregnancy is _____.
2. The level of HbA1C above which the incidence of major congenital malformation is markedly increased is _____.
3. The parameter used to estimate the control of sugar for the past 4–8 weeks is _____.

Answers

1. 5–6%, 2. 9.5% or more, 3. glycosylated hemoglobin

Case scenario-based discussion

1. A 28-year-old primigravida comes to the antenatal clinic at 10 weeks of gestation for an antenatal booking visit. She has had all the screening investigations for pregnancy including a single-step OGCT by the DIPSI method, in which her blood sugar level was 150 mg/dL. She does not have any significant medical history. On examination, she is obese, and her BMI is 31. In her past history, she was diagnosed with PCOS, for which she was treated for 2 years. Both her parents are diabetics. The USG shows a single intrauterine gestation corresponding to 10 weeks of gestation.

   a) How do you classify diabetes complicating pregnancy? What is the diagnosis in this case and what are the risk factors that could have contributed to this condition?

   b) What are the maternal and fetal complications you anticipate in this case?

   c) What is the medical management for GDM?

   d) How are maternal and fetal well-being monitored during such a pregnancy?

   e) What are the neonatal complications expected in this case?

   f) What are the long-term maternal and fetal effects of GDM?

Answers

a) Diabetes complicating pregnancy is classified into two types:

- Pregestational diabetes or overt diabetes—this is diabetes that is diagnosed before pregnancy. It is of two types: type I, which occurs due to absolute insulin deficiency, and type II, which occurs due to defective insulin secretion or insulin resistance.

- Gestational diabetes mellitus—it is defined as carbohydrate intolerance resulting in hyperglycemia of variable severity with its onset or first recognition during pregnancy.

The diagnosis in this case is gestational diabetes mellitus since the diabetes was diagnosed for the first time during this pregnancy. However, the possibility of unrecognised pregestational diabetes cannot be excluded. The risk factors for GDM in this case are obesity, family history of diabetes and pre-existing insulin resistance due to PCOS.

b) The woman may develop PIH/pre-eclampsia, recurrent urinary tract infections or hydramnios, and the chance of operative delivery is high. The fetal risks include macrosomia and intrauterine fetal death. In this case, since diabetes has been diagnosed in the first trimester, the possibility of unrecognised diabetes prior to pregnancy cannot be ruled out. Therefore, the risk of early fetal loss and congenital anomalies should also be kept in mind.

c) Once the diagnosis of GDM has been made, the woman should be given medical nutrition therapy for two weeks to keep the postprandial blood sugar <120 mg/dL and fasting <95 mg/dL. If this is achieved, the woman can continue with MNT with exercise and monthly checks of blood sugar levels. If the target values are not achieved in 15 days, the woman should be started on insulin therapy. Along with medical management, diet and exercise advice are also given.

d) Antenatal care is important to diagnose complications and to prevent macrosomia. In the first trimester, aneuploidy screening is done at 11–14 weeks for NT measurement, a detailed anomaly scan is performed at 18–20 weeks and a fetal echo is performed at 24–26 weeks to detect any cardiac anomaly. Antenatal check-ups should be done once in 2 weeks until 32 weeks, and then, weekly. At each visit, complications such as PIH, hydramnios, macrosomia and evidence of infections should be looked for. From 28 weeks onwards, fetal growth and liquor volume are monitored every 4 weeks. Antepartum surveillance in the form of a non-stress test and biophysical profile should be started at around 32 weeks. Doppler studies may be indicated in cases complicated by pre-eclampsia.

e) The neonatal problems seen in association with GDM are respiratory distress, hypoglycemia, hypocalcemia, polycythemia and hyperbilirubinemia.

f) Recurrence occurs in 50% of women in subsequent pregnancies. Approximately 50% of women with a past history of GDM develop type 2 DM later in life. As the vasculature in GDM is permanently altered, these women are also prone to cardiovascular disease (CVD) later in life. Infants born to GDM mothers tend to become obese later in life, and there is also an increased incidence of diabetes mellitus among such children.

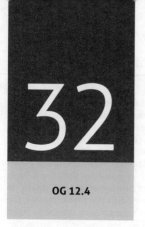

32

OG 12.4

Diseases of the Cardiovascular System

Learning Objectives

» To describe the physiological changes in the cardiovascular system during pregnancy and the symptoms produced by these changes

» To describe the etiology, classification and diagnosis of heart disease in pregnancy

» To discuss the adverse effects of heart disease on the mother and fetus

» To discuss the management of heart disease during pregnancy and labour

» To know the prenatal counselling given to women who have heart disease

» To know the indications for cardiac surgery during pregnancy

» To know the management of women who undergo valve replacement

■ INTRODUCTION

The incidence of heart disease varies in different parts of the world. In Western countries, rheumatic heart disease is now on the decline; on the other hand, there is a relative increase in congenital heart disease. The advances in investigative procedures and medical and surgical management have made it possible for women with congenital heart disease to have successful pregnancies. In India, **rheumatic heart disease** remains the major cause of heart disease encountered in pregnancy. Heart disease complicates about 1% of pregnancies and is one of the important indirect causes of maternal death in India.

■ CARDIOVASCULAR CHANGES DURING PREGNANCY

In pregnancy, the following changes occur in the cardiovascular system (Table 32.1).

Cardiac Output

- During pregnancy, the cardiac output is increased by as much as 30–50%—from about 4.5 L/minute before pregnancy to about 6–6.5 L/minute at term.
- This increase begins in early pregnancy, as early as 5 weeks, reaches a peak at 25–32 weeks of gestation and remains elevated for the remainder of the pregnancy.
- The increase in cardiac output is brought about by an increase in the heart rate and stroke volume.
- At the time of labour, the cardiac output further increases to 15% in the first stage of labour and 50% in the second stage of labour due to uterine

contractions, pain, anxiety and the autotransfusion of 500 mL of blood during each contraction.

- Immediately after delivery, due to the emptying of the uterine blood into the general circulation as well as the shifting of blood from the lower limbs (due to the sudden release of IVC compression), there is a marked increase in the intravascular volume, further increasing the cardiac output to as much as 60–80%.
- The stroke volume, heart rate and cardiac output remain elevated in the first two days postpartum. The cardiac output returns to normal 2 weeks after delivery.

Table 32.1 Changes in the cardiovascular system during pregnancy

Parameter	Changes during pregnancy
Cardiac output	Increases by 30–50%—from 4.5 L/minute to 6–6.5 L/minute
	Starts early in pregnancy, peaks at 25–30 weeks and remains so till the end of pregnancy
Heart rate	Increases by 10–15 bpm between 14 and 20 weeks and remains so till the end of pregnancy
Blood pressure	Systolic BP remains unchanged or slightly low till 20 weeks, after which it rises to pre-pregnancy levels
	Diastolic BP is slightly reduced
Femoral venous pressure	Rises from early pregnancy to term
Brachial venous pressure	Remains unchanged
Plasma volume	Rises between 12 and 32 weeks by 40–45%
RBC volume	Increases by 15–20%

Because of these changes, women with heart disease have the maximum risk of cardiac failure and pulmonary edema in the second stage of labour and the immediate post-delivery period.

Heart Rate

The heart rate increases by 10–15 beats per minute between 14 and 20 weeks, and this increase is maintained till term. In labour, the heart rate increases during contractions and returns to normal in-between contractions.

Blood Pressure

Despite the increase in the cardiac output, blood pressure does not rise in a normal pregnancy. This is because of the drop in the systemic vascular resistance caused by progesterone. Blood pressure normally varies from 110–120 mmHg systolic and 75–85 mmHg diastolic. There is a mid-trimester decrease in blood pressure and then a return to pre-pregnancy levels at term. In women predisposed to develop pre-eclampsia, this mid-trimester decrease in BP may not occur.

Venous Pressure

The femoral venous pressure rises steadily from early in pregnancy to term. This is more marked in the latter half of pregnancy because of the pressure exerted by the pregnant uterus on the IVC. This increase in the venous pressure in the lower limbs predisposes pregnant women to develop varicose veins, edema and hemorrhoids. Brachial venous pressure remains unchanged during pregnancy.

Plasma Volume

This increases by 40–45% between 12 and 32 weeks of gestation.

Red Cell Volume

The red cell volume increases by 15–20%.

Oxygen Consumption

Maternal oxygen consumption increases by 20–40% during pregnancy and further during the uterine contractions of labour.

Cardiac Signs

Due to the hyperdynamic circulation induced by the above changes, a benign ejection systolic murmur is heard in 96% of pregnant women.

These physiological CVS changes present as dyspnea, peripheral edema and palpitation, which are common complaints in pregnancy.

There is a significant overlap between the signs and symptoms of normal pregnancy and those of cardiac disease.

HEART DISEASE COMPLICATING PREGNANCY

Heart diseases are classified into acyanotic and cyanotic conditions.

Acyanotic Heart Diseases

- Congenital heart diseases—atrial septum defects (ASDs), ventricular septum defects (VSDs), patent ductus arteriosus (PDA) and coarctation of the aorta
- Acquired rheumatic diseases—valvular diseases namely mitral stenosis (MS), mitral regurgitation (MR), aortic stenosis (AS), aortic incompetence (AI) and pulmonary stenosis
- Acquired non-rheumatic diseases—peripartum cardiomyopathy, myocardial infarction and mitral valve prolapse

Cyanotic Heart Diseases

- Eisenmenger's complex
- Fallot tetralogy

Rheumatic Heart Disease

This is the most common type of heart disease encountered during pregnancy in India, contributing to 90–95% of cases. The most common lesion is **mitral stenosis**. Other lesions include mitral incompetence, aortic stenosis and aortic incompetence.

Congenital Heart Disease

These include atrial or ventricular septal defects and PDA. An atrial septal defect is the most common congenital heart disease.

These conditions are usually compatible with pregnancy as long as the left-to-right shunt is moderate. However, reversal of the shunt and cyanosis can occur with a sudden fall of BP with significant blood loss or at the time of induction of anesthesia. These conditions are amenable to surgical correction and should be undertaken prior to attempting pregnancy.

EFFECT OF PREGNANCY ON HEART DISEASE

Cardiac diseases are progressive conditions. Due to the profound hemodynamic changes taking place during pregnancy, there is further deterioration of cardiac status, which results in the risk of complications such as congestive cardiac failure (CCF), pulmonary edema, arrhythmias and infective endocarditis.

EFFECT OF HEART DISEASE ON PREGNANCY

Due to reduced oxygenation, preterm labour and FGR are more common in cases of tight mitral stenosis and cyanotic heart disease with a right-to-left shunt. There could also be fetal inheritance of the disease. In Marfan syndrome, there is a 50% chance of the child inheriting the condition. When the woman has a congenital heart disease such as ASD or VSD, the risk of inheritance ranges from 2–10%.

DIAGNOSIS OF HEART DISEASE

- Most cases of heart disease are diagnosed prior to pregnancy and such women are either on medical treatment or would have undergone surgical procedures such as ASD and VSD repair or valve replacement. In these women, the relevant details are available in the case records.
- Occasionally, the diagnosis of heart disease is made only during pregnancy as the physiological changes in pregnancy often unmask any underlying cardiac disease.
- The diagnosis of heart disease during pregnancy may be difficult as there is an overlap between the signs and symptoms of normal pregnancy and those of heart disease. However, it is crucial to identify an underlying heart disease as an undiagnosed condition may result in significant maternal morbidity and mortality.

Signs and Symptoms of Normal Pregnancy

The **signs and symptoms of normal pregnancy** are as follows:

- Fatigue
- Exertional dyspnea
- Palpitation (due to tachycardia or atrial and ventricular premature beats)
- Sinus tachycardia, 10–15% above normal heart rate
- Full volume pulse
- Third heart sound
- Systolic flow murmur
- Pedal edema

Signs and Symptoms That May Indicate an Underlying Heart Disease and Require Investigation

The following symptoms and signs may indicate an associated heart disease and require further investigations:

- Symptoms of progressive dyspnea, orthopnea, nocturnal cough, syncope, hemoptysis and chest pain and persistent edema of the face and feet
- Presence of diastolic murmur, pansystolic murmur radiating all over the pericardium, grade 3 or higher systolic murmur, increase in the intensity of the systolic murmur with advancing gestation
- Presence of thrill
- Presence of persistent arrhythmia like atrial flutter, fibrillation or ventricular tachycardia
- Systemic hypotension
- Sinus tachycardia >15% above the normal heart rate
- Presence of fourth heart sound
- Acute manifestation of pulmonary edema
- Features of heart failure such as increased jugular venous pressure
- Presence of clubbing or cyanosis indicating congenital heart disease

Investigations

The investigations that are generally carried out are X-ray chest, ECG and echocardiography.

X-ray chest

- In an X-ray chest with abdominal shielding, the mother is exposed to 0.1 rad and the fetus is exposed to 0.008 rad. Therefore, if necessary, an X-ray can be taken.
- X-ray changes that are seen in the normal pregnancy may mimic heart disease. There is mild enlargement in heart size, fullness of the left cardiac border and increased pulmonary vascular markings. Further, there may be a misdiagnosis of cardiomegaly due to the positional change of the heart.

ECG

- In a normal pregnancy, ECG may show sinus tachycardia, premature atrial and ventricular beats or right or left QRS deviation.
- ECG is more useful in diagnosing arrhythmias than in diagnosing structural abnormalities of the heart.

Echocardiography

- Echo is the diagnostic test of choice in pregnancy because it is non-invasive and does not expose the woman or the fetus to radiation.
- Echocardiography indicates the functional state of the heart as well as the structural abnormalities.
- Normal echocardiographic changes during pregnancy include the following:
  — Increase in heart size
  — Increase in left ventricular mass
  — Small pericardial effusion may be present
  — Mild valvular regurgitation may be present

■ MANAGEMENT

- The main aims of management are prevention, early diagnosis and prompt and efficient treatment of heart failure during pregnancy. The risk factors for heart failure should be identified and treated promptly.
- Heart diseases can be classified in terms of etiology, anatomical lesions and functional capacity of the heart. In the management of heart disease in pregnancy, it is important to assess the functional state of the heart and the severity of the disease.

Assessing the Severity of Heart Disease

The New York Heart Association's classification is used to assess the severity and the functional capacity of the heart (Table 32.2).

Table 32.2 The New York Heart Association classification

Class	Description
Class I	This is also known as the uncompromised state, wherein there is no limitation with regard to physical activity. There are no symptoms of cardiac insufficiency such as palpitation or dyspnea on ordinary physical activity.
Class II	This is a slightly compromised state, wherein patients with cardiac disease have a slight limitation of activity and are comfortable at rest. When ordinary physical activity is undertaken, discomfort results in the form of excessive fatigue, palpitation or dyspnea.
Class III	This is a markedly compromised state. Patients with cardiac disease have a marked limitation of physical activity. They are comfortable at rest, but even minimal activity causes discomfort and symptoms.
Class IV	The patient is in a severely compromised state, wherein the patient is unable to perform any physical activity without discomfort. Cardiac symptoms are present even at rest.

Antenatal Care

- Whenever heart disease is diagnosed during pregnancy, the woman should preferably be referred to a tertiary care centre or a centre where an experienced obstetrician and a cardiologist are available.
- Classes I and II cases could be treated as outpatients after the initial evaluation. Classes III and IV cases should be hospitalised.
- Women who have heart disease should be seen at least fortnightly until 30 weeks of gestation and then weekly until term. Even a woman with class I or II disease may be hospitalised near term for safe confinement if she lives in a remote area.

Identifying risk factors

Risk factors such as anemia, infection, hypertension and excessive physical activity, which increase the risk of CCF, should be avoided.

Anemia

As anemia increases the demand on the heart, prophylactic/therapeutic iron should be given to women. Besides correcting anemia, the woman's nutritional status should also be improved.

Infections

Infections are among the important risk factors that precipitate cardiac failure. Women who have heart disease must receive instructions to avoid contact with persons who have respiratory infections, including the common cold. Periodic screening for asymptomatic bacteriuria and dental infection is important. Prompt antibiotic therapy should be initiated in the presence of infection.

Relieving anxiety

Fear and worry increase the demand on the heart. All measures should be taken to allay fear and anxiety

Rest

Patients should be advised to limit physical activity and get adequate rest. They should also be advised to sleep or take rest in a semi-recumbent position.

Evaluation of medical risks

- Hypertension, pre-eclampsia, arrhythmia and multiple pregnancy are other conditions that can precipitate CCF.
- At each antenatal visit, the woman should be asked about her general well-being and whether there is an increase in breathlessness or limitation of

activity. Increasing dyspnea, orthopnea and signs of basal congestion in the lungs are indicative of the onset of cardiac failure. Such patients require hospitalisation.

USG assessment

At the time of the anomaly scan between 18 and 22 weeks, it is important to look for cardiac anomalies in the fetus, especially in those with cyanotic heart disease, ASD, VSD, PDA, etc. In those with cyanotic heart disease and severe heart disease, fetal growth monitoring should be performed to diagnose FGR.

Management of medical complications

CCF

The first warning signs of heart failure are persistent basal rales and nocturnal cough. The patient presents with tachycardia, edema and raised JVP. CCF during pregnancy and labour is treated with injection morphine 10 mg IM as a single dose; injection frusemide 40 mg IV, repeated if necessary or injection digoxin 0.5 mg IM as a single dose. A cardiologist should be involved in every stage of management.

Acute pulmonary edema

In the presence of tight mitral stenosis or precipitating factors such as atrial fibrillation or hypertension, the woman may develop pulmonary edema manifesting with acute-onset breathlessness, paroxysmal nocturnal dyspnea, cough with frothy sputum and hemoptysis. There will be evidence of rales on auscultation. These patients are made to sit in a propped-up position, oxygen is administered, and effective diuresis is carried out with large doses of intravenous frusemide. The precipitating cause should be treated. In those with recurrent and intractable pulmonary edema due to tight mitral stenosis, an emergency closed mitral valvotomy may be required.

Infective endocarditis

If the woman develops infective endocarditis during pregnancy, she may present with fever and other features such as hematuria. Infective endocarditis can occur in women on prosthetic valves and in those with congenital heart disease. It is caused by organisms such as *Streptococcus viridans*, *S. faecalis* and *S. aureus*. Echo may show vegetations. The mortality is high.

Infective endocarditis should be treated with appropriate antibiotics after blood culture studies. Beta-blockers such as metoprolol would be required to control the heart rate. In the presence of atrial fibrillation, digoxin may be useful for the control of ventricular rate.

Bacterial endocarditis prophylaxis

Antibiotic prophylaxis is given for indications such as dental extraction. Routine administration of antibiotics during pregnancy is not practised anymore. However, antibiotic prophylaxis is given during labour in certain groups of patients.

Management of Labour and Delivery

- Vaginal delivery is the safest for women with cardiac disease. Cesarean section should be avoided if possible.
- Spontaneous onset of labour is awaited, and the induction of labour is avoided as far as possible.
- Most labours progress rapidly, especially when the woman is on digoxin. Digoxin has a direct stimulatory effect on the myometrium. Moreover, due to water retention, the cervix dilates faster in valvular disease.

First stage of labour

- In the first stage of labour, the woman should be nursed in bed in a **semi-recumbent position.**
- Class III and IV patients are administered oxygen through a face mask. For others, oxygen should be readily available.
- **Vital signs** should be monitored every 30 minutes. Lung fields should be auscultated periodically. An increase in the pulse rate above 100 or a respiratory rate of more than 24, if associated with dyspnea, may indicate impending heart failure. Heart failure should be managed with oxygen inhalation, diuretics and digoxin.
- **Intravenous fluids should be restricted. If necessary, they should be administered through an infusion/syringe pump.** Women who have aortic stenosis may require adequate fluid because of fixed cardiac output.
- **Adequate analgesia** with injection pethidine/ epidural analgesia should be given since relief from pain and apprehension is very important. Epidural analgesia is the preferred method as it is well tolerated in the majority of women with adequate circulatory reserve. However, epidural should be avoided in those with restricted cardiac output such as in primary pulmonary hypertension and conditions with right-to-left shunt.
- **Bacterial endocarditis prophylaxis**—the current recommendation is to give antibiotic prophylaxis in labour for the following groups of patients:
  — Those with valvular heart disease
  — Those with prosthetic valves

— Those who have congenital heart diseases

— Those who have hypertrophic cardiomyopathy

— Those who have mitral valve prolapse with valvular regurgitation

Antibiotics are given at the onset of labour or when the membrane ruptures or at the time of the induction of anesthesia for cesarean section and continued for 6–8 hours after delivery. The drugs given are as follows:

— Injection amoxicillin 1 g IV 8th hourly and injection gentamycin 80 mg IV bd

— If allergic to penicillin, injection cephalexin 1 g IV is administered slowly along with gentamycin 80 mg IV twice daily

— Vancomycin can also be given

- Cardiac patients usually progress normally in spontaneous labour. If not, they should be augmented in the usual way with oxytocin administered through infusion or syringes pump. One should avoid administering too much fluid.
- Supine hypotension should be avoided in all stages.

Second stage of labour

- The second stage of labour should be shortened by using forceps or vacuum to prevent undue straining.
- If the woman is in cardiac failure, forceps should be used electively.

Third stage of labour

- In the third stage of labour, 10 units of oxytocin should be given IM and AMTSL should be followed. Ergometrine or syntometrine are absolutely contraindicated in heart disease complicating pregnancy. In patients with cardiac failure, oxytocics should be withheld as far as possible as they can worsen the condition.
- Following delivery, the woman should be closely observed in an ICU for 24–48 hours as cardiac failure can still occur.

Indications for cesarean section in heart disease (other than for obstetric indications)

- Coarctation of the aorta—when there is aortic root dilatation of >4 cm, cesarean section is indicated to prevent aortic dissection and rupture of the aneurysm
- Marfan syndrome with aortic diameter of >4 cm
- Severe aortic stenosis
- Occasionally, a woman in labour and presenting with CCF would benefit from CS under controlled anesthesia

Anesthesia

Though regional anesthesia can be used in cardiac diseases, it should be avoided in cases of aortic stenosis, coarctation of the aorta, pulmonary hypertension and hypertrophic cardiomyopathy. General anesthesia is recommended in these patients.

Management of the Puerperium

- Women who have shown little or no evidence of cardiac distress during pregnancy, labour or delivery may still decompensate after delivery. The first 48–72 hours are critical as the woman is prone to CCF during this time because of fluid shift.
- Meticulous care should be continued into the puerperium. Postpartum hemorrhage, anemia, infection and thromboembolism are much more serious complications of heart disease. One should be aware of pulmonary edema and thromboembolism in the postnatal period.
- Early ambulation is advised to prevent thromboembolic complications. Prophylactic anticoagulants may be required in some cases.
- Antibiotics should be continued for one week.
- The woman can be discharged after two weeks after being reviewed by the cardiologist.
- Contraceptive advice should be given before discharge.
- The newborn should be evaluated for cardiac disease.

■ CARDIAC SURGERY DURING PREGNANCY

Although careful medical therapy allows the successful completion of pregnancy in the great majority of women, repair or replacement of the valve during pregnancy may be required in select patients who remain symptomatic despite adequate medical therapy. In most cases, surgery is performed at the end of the second trimester or at the beginning of the third trimester.

Indications for Surgery in Mitral Stenosis

- Significant mitral stenosis with mitral valve area <1.5 cm² (normal mitral valve area is 4 cm²)
- More than functional class II despite aggressive medical therapy
- Presenting with intractable heart failure with recurrent hemoptysis
- Closed mitral valvotomy or percutaneous balloon mitral valvoplasty are usually carried out

MANAGEMENT OF WOMEN WITH PROSTHETIC VALVES

Pregnant women who have prosthetic valves are at the risk of the following:

- The woman may develop thromboembolism
- There may be an obstruction to flow due to fixed cardiac output
- The woman may develop hemolytic anemia due to the trauma caused to the red cells, which results in fragmented RBCs
- There may be valve regurgitation
- These women may develop arrhythmias

The fetus of a woman with a prosthetic valve may develop warfarin embryopathy.

The management of women who have mechanical heart valves is a major challenge. These patients are already on anticoagulants, which should be continued throughout pregnancy. As they are on warfarin, there is a risk of warfarin embryopathy in the first trimester, hemorrhagic complications in the mother and fetus and fetal loss throughout pregnancy. While choosing an anticoagulant during pregnancy, the benefits and the risks to the mother and fetus should be considered. In those who are on warfarin prior to pregnancy, the regimen should be modified during pregnancy as follows:

- Warfarin is discontinued at 6 weeks of conception.
- The woman is started on heparin until 14 weeks.
- Warfarin is restarted at 14 weeks and continued until 36 weeks.
- Aspirin may be started at a dose of 80–100 mg daily.
- Platelet count is checked periodically.
- The goal is to maintain INR at 2.5.
- At 36 weeks, unfractionated heparin or low-molecular-weight heparin (LMWH) is restarted.
- Heparin is stopped 6 hours before delivery and restarted 6 hours after vaginal delivery and 12 hours after CS to prevent PPH.
- Three days later, the woman is started back on warfarin.

- **Heparin** does not cross the placenta but is a less effective anticoagulant than warfarin; even if meticulously monitored, the mother is at risk of potentially fatal valve thrombosis.
- It is not advisable to prescribe LMWH throughout pregnancy because it is associated with an increased incidence of thrombosis.
- The fetal risk of warfarin is significantly reduced if the woman is adequately anticoagulated on ≤5 mg of warfarin.

If regional anesthesia is required, catheter placement for epidural anesthesia is not advisable within 10–12 hours of the last dose of heparin because of the longer half-life of LMWH.

PERIPARTUM CARDIOMYOPATHY

In this condition, the woman presents with **sudden-onset unexplained cardiac failure in the last weeks of pregnancy or in the postpartum period.** The diagnosis is made after excluding all known causes of cardiac failure. Some of the etiological factors proposed are genetic predisposition, an autoimmune process and viral infections. Peripartum cardiomyopathy is more common in obese multiparous women. The prognosis is poor due to grossly enlarged cardiac chambers and thromboembolic complications. Mortality is high, and if the woman survives, recurrence occurs in >85% of cases.

The criteria to diagnose the condition are as follows:

- The development of unexplained cardiac failure in the last month of pregnancy or within 5 months of delivery
- Absence of an identifiable cause of the cardiac failure
- Absence of pre-existing heart disease before the last month of pregnancy.
- LV systolic dysfunction as demonstrated by echo findings

CONTRACEPTION IN HEART DISEASE

There should be a discussion on contraception following delivery.

- As the functional state of the heart deteriorates as age advances, women diagnosed with cardiac disease should be advised to complete the family at the earliest.
- Contraception is required temporarily to facilitate corrective surgery before planning the next pregnancy.
- Combined oral contraceptive pills are best avoided as their use is associated with water and sodium retention, hyperlipidemia and a hypercoagulable state.
- Intrauterine contraceptive devices may be used, except in women on anticoagulants. At the time of inserting an IUCD, infective endocarditis prophylaxis should be administered.
- Progestogen-only contraception can be used with DMPA and progesterone-only pills. However, they can cause water retention.

- In women who have completed the family, tubal sterilisation can be undertaken but should be delayed for 6 weeks after delivery to ensure that the cardiac status is stable.

INDICATIONS FOR MEDICAL TERMINATION OF PREGNANCY IN HEART DISEASE

Therapeutic termination of pregnancy should be offered to all women who present early in pregnancy (before 12 weeks) and in whom there is significant risk of death should the pregnancy be allowed to continue.

The indications for therapeutic abortion include the following:

- **Class III or IV cardiac disease**—if such a patient is seen in the first trimester, it is better to treat the failure and then consider termination of pregnancy. However, if the woman is seen in the second trimester, it would seem advisable to continue treating the failure without interfering with the pregnancy.
- **Eisenmenger syndrome** is associated with a high maternal mortality, and hence, medical termination of pregnancy is advised if the patient is seen in the first trimester of pregnancy.
- **Primary pulmonary hypertension** is also an indication for medical termination of pregnancy.

PRECONCEPTIONAL COUNSELLING

In women with known cardiac disease, preconception counselling is mandatory to ensure that the woman is physically fit to go through pregnancy and labour. The goals of prenatal counselling are to find out whether there are any absolute contraindications for pregnancy, to assess the functional status of the heart and review the medications and to identify risk factors that can precipitate CCF in pregnancy and correct them appropriately. At the time of counselling, maternal and fetal risks associated with heart disease in pregnancy should be discussed. There should be a discussion on recommending corrective surgery for conditions that are suitable for surgery before embarking on pregnancy.

- Absolute contraindications for pregnancy:
  — Eisenmenger syndrome
  — Pulmonary hypertension (pulmonary pressure >40 mmHg)
  — Marfan syndrome with aortic root involvement (diameter >40 mm)
  — Previous peripartum cardiomyopathy

- Relative contraindications for pregnancy:
  — Coarctation of aorta
  — Prosthetic heart valve
  — Mitral stenosis with atrial fibrillation
  — Classes III and IV functional state of the disease
- Fetal inheritance of cardiac disease:
  — Marfan syndrome is inherited by the Mendelian mode of inheritance, wherein, there is a 50% chance of the child being affected; this should be explained to the parents
- Cardiac surgery prior to conception:
  — It is ideal to undertake corrective surgery for tight mitral stenosis, ASD, VSD and PDA before embarking on pregnancy
  — Surgically correctable cardiac conditions should be corrected prior to pregnancy
- Treating medical conditions:
  — It is important to diagnose and correct medical conditions such as anemia, UTI and dental infections, etc.
- Reviewing the medications:
  — Women who have a prosthetic valve and are on warfarin should be switched to heparin
- Assessment of functional state of the heart:
  — Echocardiography for the structural and functional state of the heart should be carried out
- Vaccination against viral infections:
  — All women with cardiac disease planning pregnancy should be vaccinated against viral infections

PROGNOSIS OF PREGNANCY WITH HEART DISEASE

Maternal Prognosis

Maternal prognosis depends upon the functional ability of the heart and the complications that develop during pregnancy. Many factors influence the prognosis of heart disease complicating pregnancy. Some of the important factors are listed below:

- **Age of the woman:** The older the woman (over 35), the less satisfactory will be the prognosis.
- **History of previous pregnancies:** If the woman has had no complications in her previous pregnancies and deliveries, the prognosis is satisfactory. However, she can still develop problems in a subsequent pregnancy.
- **Functional classification of the heart:** This is the most important factor. With rare exceptions, women who have class I disease and most of those with class II disease go through pregnancy without morbidity.

Women who have class III disease or more need intensive care and have higher morbidity.

- **Nature of the lesion:** Of the various lesions, **mitral stenosis** has a better prognosis, provided it is not severe mitral stenosis or associated with atrial fibrillation. **Eisenmenger syndrome** has the worst prognosis and a high maternal mortality rate. Though isolated mitral stenosis has a fair prognosis, it is the most common cause of cardiac death in pregnancy as it is the most common heart disease during pregnancy.

Risks associated with heart disease can be categorised in terms of mortality risk:

- High risk (mortality 25–50%; pregnancy contraindicated)
  1. Eisenmenger's complex
  2. Cyanotic heart disease (tetralogy of Fallot)
  3. Pulmonary hypertension
  4. Hypertrophic obstructive cardiomyopathy
  5. New York Heart Association classes III or IV with severe ventricular dysfunction

  6. Marfan syndrome with significant aortic root/ aortic valve involvement
  7. Acute myocardial infarction

- Moderate-to-high mortality (5–15%)
  1. Coarctation-uncomplicated
  2. Marfan syndrome with normal aortic root
  3. Mechanical prosthetic valves
  4. Valvular stenosis—classes III and IV

- Low risk (mortality <1%)
  1. Mild-to-moderate valvular regurgitation
  2. Mitral valve prolapse
  3. Small ASD, VSD, PDA
  4. Mitral stenosis—classes I and II

Fetal Prognosis

Besides prematurity and FGR, the incidence of congenital heart disease is high in infants born to women with heart diseases such as Marfan syndrome, aortic stenosis, ASD and VSD. The risk is highest with Marfan syndrome, in which 50% of infants are affected.

KEY POINTS

✓ The diagnosis of heart disease during pregnancy is difficult due to the physiological changes that occur in the cardiovascular and respiratory systems during pregnancy.

✓ Cardiac output increases by 40% from 6 weeks to peak at mid-pregnancy around 25–30 weeks; a further increase in cardiac output occurs at delivery.

✓ BP decreases in the second trimester.

✓ Types of heart diseases include rheumatic heart disease, congenital heart disease and other cardiac lesions. Rheumatic heart disease is the commonest type encountered during pregnancy in India.

✓ Echocardiography is the diagnostic test of choice in pregnancy to assess the functional state of the heart and to diagnose structural abnormalities.

✓ In the management of heart disease in pregnancy, it is important to assess the functional state of the heart and the severity of the disease.

✓ Complications during pregnancy and labour include CCF, pulmonary edema, arrhythmias and infective endocarditis. Fetal complications include prematurity, FGR and inheritance of cardiac condition.

✓ Risk factors for CCF include anemia, infection, hypertension and excessive physical activity.

✓ Severe mitral stenosis with mitral valve area <1.5 cm² may need cardiac surgery during pregnancy with a closed mitral valvotomy or percutaneous balloon mitral valvoplasty.

✓ Anticoagulant therapy is critical in the management of pregnant women with prosthetic valves.

✓ Peripartum cardiomyopathy is a condition in which there is an unexplained cardiac failure in the last month of pregnancy or within 5 months of delivery with significant LV systolic dysfunction.

✓ Preconceptional counselling is mandatory for women of reproductive age before planning pregnancy.

Essay question

1. Discuss the diagnosis, antenatal and intrapartum management and prognosis of rheumatic mitral stenosis of functional class II diagnosed at 14 weeks of gestation in a 27-year-old primigravida.

Short answer questions

Write short notes on the following:

1. Peripartum cardiomyopathy
2. Infective endocarditis prophylaxis
3. Contraceptive choices for women with heart disease
4. Functional classification of heart disease during pregnancy

MCQs

1. At what gestational age does cardiac output reach its peak?
   a) <6 weeks
   b) 6–12 weeks
   c) 12–28 weeks
   d) 28–32 weeks

2. Which of the following is the commonest heart disease complicating pregnancy?
   a) Mitral stenosis
   b) Mitral regurgitation
   c) Aortic stenosis
   d) Aortic regurgitation

3. The most common congenital heart disease encountered during pregnancy is:
   a) Atrial septal defect
   b) Ventricular septal defect
   c) Fallot tetralogy
   d) Eisenmenger syndrome

4. Which of the following cardiac conditions is best tolerated in pregnancy?
   a) Mitral stenosis
   b) Mitral incompetence
   c) Aortic stenosis
   d) Coarctation of the aorta

5. Pregnancy is contraindicated in the following heart diseases EXCEPT:
   a) Eisenmenger syndrome
   b) Severe aortic stenosis
   c) Marfan syndrome with significant aortic root/aortic valve involvement
   d) Mitral valve prolapse

6. Peripartum cardiomyopathy includes:
   a) The development of cardiac failure in the last month of pregnancy
   b) Absence of recognisable heart disease prior to the last month of pregnancy
   c) LV systolic dysfunction demonstrated by echo
   d) All of the above

7. As per the New York Heart Association Classification, uncompromised heart comes under which of the following classes?
   a) Class 1
   b) Class 2
   c) Class 3
   d) Class 4

8. High maternal mortality in heart disease during pregnancy is due to:
   a) Mitral stenosis
   b) Aortic stenosis
   c) Fallot teratology
   d) Eisenmerger syndrome

9. Which of the following drugs should be avoided in heart disease complicating pregnancy?
   a) Oxytocin
   b) Ergometrine
   c) Frusemide
   d) Morphine

10. Which of the following is used as an anticoagulant in the first trimester of pregnancy in women with mechanical prosthetic valves?
    a) Warfarin
    b) Heparin
    c) Both
    d) Neither

Answers
1. (d), 2. (a), 3. (a), 4. (b), 5. (d), 6. (d), 7. (a), 8. (d), 9. (b), 10. (b)

Fill in the blanks

1. The oxytocic drug of choice for the active management of the third stage of labour in a woman with heart disease is _____.

2. The mortality risk in a pregnant woman with Eisenmenger syndrome is _____.

3. The risk of the fetus inheriting the disease in Marfan syndrome is _____.

Answers
1. oxytocin, 2. 30–50%, 3. 50%

Case scenario-based discussion

1. A 28-year-old primigravida visits the antenatal clinic at 16 weeks gestation with complaints of palpitation and breathlessness, which she has been experiencing for a week. She is not able recall any illness in the past. On examination, she is not pale, there is no pedal edema, pulse rate is 88 bpm and the BP is 110/80 mmHg. On auscultation, a systolic murmur is heard.
   a) What are the possible diagnoses you will consider?
   b) What complications can occur during pregnancy in a woman with heart disease?
   c) What are the risk factors that can precipitate CCF in pregnancy?
   d) What are the absolute contraindications for pregnancy?

Answers
a) In this case, the possible diagnosis are as follows:
i) Normal physiological changes of pregnancy manifesting with breathlessness, palpitation and cardiac murmur
ii) Underlying heart disease, for which echo should be carried out
iii) Anemia should also be considered in the differential diagnosis and necessary investigations should be carried out
b) Such a patient is prone to medical complications such as CCF, pulmonary edema, thromboembolic complications and bacterial endocarditis. The baby may be growth-restricted, and the woman may go into preterm labour. There is also a possibility of the fetus inheriting the cardiac condition.
c) Anemia, hypertension, infections, increased physical activity, anxiety, multiple pregnancy and uterine contractions in labour are the risk factors that predispose to CCF.
d) The following are absolute contraindications for pregnancy:
— Eisenmenger syndrome
— Pulmonary hypertension (pulmonary pressure >40 mmHg)
— Marfan syndrome with aortic root involvement (diameter >40 mm)
— Previous peripartum cardiomyopathy

33 Liver and Gastrointestinal Disorders Complicating Pregnancy

OG 12.6

Learning Objectives

» To describe the physiological changes and the causes of liver disease in pregnancy
» To understand the management of a pregnant woman diagnosed with HBsAg-positive status
» To describe the clinical features, diagnosis and management of intrahepatic cholestasis of pregnancy
» To discuss the diagnosis and management of HELLP syndrome

■ INTRODUCTION

Liver disorders are important medical problems that can complicate pregnancy and are responsible for a considerable number of indirect causes of maternal deaths in India. Liver disorders in pregnancy can be grouped under three categories, which are as follows:

- Liver diseases peculiar to pregnancy
  — Hyperemesis gravidarum
  — Intrahepatic cholestasis of pregnancy
  — HELLP syndrome
  — Hepatic rupture
  — Acute fatty liver of pregnancy
- Liver diseases incidental to pregnancy
  — Viral hepatitis
  — Obstructive jaundice due to cholelithiasis
  — Jaundice due to hepatotoxic drugs such as paracetamol, chlorpromazine, INH, etc.
  — Hemolysis due to malaria, sickle cell disease, leptospirosis
- Liver diseases that may predate pregnancy
  — Familial haemolytic jaundice due to spherocytosis/elliptocytosis
  — Cirrhosis

▌ PHYSIOLOGICAL CHANGES IN PREGNANCY

In pregnancy, though the total blood volume is increased by 50%, the absolute hepatic flow does not increase significantly. In a healthy pregnancy, there is not much alteration in the metabolism and liver function. Therefore, any alteration in liver function suggests a hepatic complication. Some of the common biochemical changes of pregnancy are as follows:

- Serum levels of alkaline phosphatase increase by 2–4 times the upper limit of the normal and may remain elevated for 6 weeks postpartum.
- Due to hemodilution, the serum albumin levels decrease by up to 25%.
- Serum levels of aspartate aminotransferase (AST) and serum oxaloacetic transaminase (SGOT) rise during labour.
- Plasma cholesterol levels increase by 50% in the third trimester and triglycerides increase by 2–3 times the upper limit of normal.
- There may be delayed excretion of bilirubin in 15% of women, which may explain increased pruritus during pregnancy.
- Pregnancy is a procoagulant state, wherein clotting factors (I, II, V, VII, X, and XII) and fibrinogen are increased.
- The gallbladder empties slowly during pregnancy and may predispose to stone formation.
- Palmar erythema and spider naevi are common features of pregnancy and are seen in 70% of cases.

Elevation in transaminases, bilirubin or the prothrombin time during pregnancy is abnormal and indicate a pathological state which requires further assessment.

▌ LIVER DISEASES PECULIAR TO PREGNANCY

These are diseases induced by pregnancy that resolve after delivery.

Hyperemesis Gravidarum

Hyperemesis gravidarum complicates 0.3–2.0% of pregnancies. It is not a liver disease in the strict sense but leads to liver dysfunction in 50% of cases. Hyperemesis gravidarum is defined as **vomiting in pregnancy** that is severe enough to produce dehydration, weight loss, ketosis from starvation and warrants hospitalisation. The mechanism of liver involvement in hyperemesis is multifactorial and not well understood. There is mild to high (up to 20-fold) elevation in AST and ALT (ALT>AST) and rarely, mild hyperbilirubinemia. Liver function abnormalities and other biochemical abnormalities resolve upon the resolution of vomiting. Uncomplicated vomiting in pregnancy does not cause liver dysfunction. Viral hepatitis, hyperthyroidism and urinary tract infection must be excluded in women diagnosed with hyperemesis gravidarum.

The management of hyperemesis is supportive and includes intravenous rehydration with a short period of fasting followed by reintroduction of a diet rich in carbohydrates and low in fat. Antiemetics such as dopamine antagonists (metoclopramide and domperidone), phenothiazines (chlorpromazine and prochlorperazine) or antihistamine H1 receptor antagonists (cyclizine and promethazine) are used safely during pregnancy. Hospitalisation is necessary for rehydration, nutritional support and symptomatic measures with antiemetics. For more details, refer to Chapter 18, *Hyperemesis gravidarum*.

Intrahepatic Cholestasis of Pregnancy (ICP)

ICP is a pregnancy-related cholestatic disorder of uncertain etiology. It is an inheritable condition—50% of women who develop ICP may have a family history of jaundice. It is reported in nearly 2% of pregnant women. The incidence of ICP is high in South Asia.

The possible etiologies are genetic predisposition and increased susceptibility to sex steroids which induces abnormal biliary transport. ICP tends to recur in subsequent pregnancies, on account of which, it is also called 'recurrent jaundice of pregnancy' or 'icterus gravidarum'.

Pathophysiology

The serum levels of cholic acid and deoxycholic acid (bile acids) are elevated more than 10 times and are deposited in the skin, causing itching. The symptoms appear in the second half of pregnancy and are relieved within 48 hours of delivery. There is an increased risk of gallstones, and there may be associated gestational diabetes. ICP is more common in multiple pregnancy.

The major histological findings are dilated bile canaliculi with bile plugs in the centrilobular area. There is no change in the hepatocellular architecture and there are no inflammatory cells.

Clinical features

There is intense pruritus after 30 weeks of gestation, which progressively increases in severity and is relieved after delivery. Itching is most severe at night and over the trunk, palms and soles, with associated fatigue, anorexia, malaise and dark-coloured urine. There may be mild jaundice in 20–25% of women 2–4 weeks after the onset of pruritus, but this is not associated with rashes, fever, nausea and vomiting. Occasionally, cholestasis is complicated by diarrhea or steatorrhea.

Differential diagnosis

In pregnant women presenting with pruritus, viral hepatitis and gallstones should be ruled out by screening for viral markers and by USG.

Laboratory findings

- Fasting serum bile acid levels are >10 μmol/L, which is the key diagnostic test (may not be available in all healthcare settings).
- ALT and AST are usually raised 2–10 times the normal.
- The total plasma concentrations of bilirubin rarely exceed 4–5 mg/dL.
- The serum alkaline phosphatase is usually elevated to 5–10 times the normal.
- Cholesterol and triglycerides are markedly increased.
- Vitamin K, factor II, VII, IX and X are decreased, resulting in increased prothrombin time.

Effect on pregnancy

Common fetal risks include unexplained stillbirth, preterm delivery and meconium staining. Hence, antenatal surveillance is very important.

Management

- When pruritus is quite troublesome, orally administered antihistamines such as diphenhydramine may provide some relief.
- Phenobarbitone at night may help in inducing hepatic microsomal enzymes.
- Cholestyramine has also been shown to control pruritus by reducing the absorption of bile acids from the small intestine.
- Ursodeoxycholic acid (UCDA) at a dosage of 8–10 mg/Kg/day is an effective therapy for ICP. UDCA is superior to cholestyramine in relieving pruritus and

reducing serum aminotransferase. It is safe for both mother and fetus.

- Vitamin K (10 mg/day) should also be given from 36 weeks onwards.

Obstetric management

- Proper fetal surveillance (starting from 32 weeks) and timely intervention are required because cholestatic jaundice is known to be associated with adverse perinatal outcome, especially meconium-stained liquor and preterm delivery.
- Delivery should be considered at 37 weeks of gestation.
- Because of the reduced coagulation factors, one should be cautious about PPH.

Hepatic Disorders Associated with Pre-eclampsia/Eclampsia and HELLP Syndrome

In about 20% of women with severe pre-eclampsia or eclampsia, the liver may be involved. The pathological lesion is periportal hemorrhage, fibrin deposition and hepatocyte disruption with necrosis. Both the degree of dysfunction and the histological changes that develop can vary. HELLP syndrome (hemolysis, elevated liver aminotransferases and low platelet counts) is a variant of severe pre-eclampsia that occurs in up to 12% of patients with pre-eclampsia but can also occur in normotensive patients. Risk factors for HELLP are advanced maternal age and multiparity.

Pathophysiology

There is microvascular endothelial damage, which leads to the release of nitric oxide, prostaglandins and endothelin, which induces platelet activation and the release of thromboxane A2. These changes lead to vasospasm and hypertension. Hemolysis is due to the passage of red cells through damaged intima and fibrin mesh deposits. Liver dysfunction and hepatic necrosis are due to fibrin deposits in the sinusoids, resulting in sinusoidal obstruction, vasospasm of the liver vascular bed and liver ischemia. This may sometimes lead to large hematomas, capsular tears and intraperitoneal hemorrhage.

On HPE, there is diffuse petechial hemorrhage, hepatocellular necrosis in the periportal region and deposition of thrombi in the hepatic artery and portal vein.

Clinical features

Vague epigastric pain associated with nausea and vomiting and rarely, jaundice, hepatic tenderness with associated GI bleeding, hematuria and nephrogenic diabetes insipidus are the chief features.

Diagnostic criteria

In the Tennessee Classification System, the diagnostic criteria for HELLP comprise hemolysis with increased LDH (>600 IU/L), AST (≥70 IU/L) and platelets <100×10⁹/L. Depending on the severity of laboratory parameters, using the Mississippi classification, HELLP syndrome is further grouped as classes I, II and III (Table 33.1).

Table 33.1 Mississippi diagnostic criteria

Class	Criteria
Class I	Platelets ≤50×10⁹/L
	AST or ALT ≥70 IU/L
	LDH ≥600 IU/L
Class II	Platelets 50–100×10⁹/L
	AST or ALT ≥70 IU/L
	LDH ≥600 IU/L
Class III	Platelets ≤150×10⁹/L, ≥100×10⁹/L
	AST or ALT ≥40 IU/L
	LDH ≥600 IU/L

The acute fatty liver of pregnancy and pancreatitis may present with similar features. HELLP syndrome can recur in subsequent pregnancies.

Management

Management of women with pre-eclampsia and liver involvement usually involves prompt delivery (if it occurs after 34 weeks of gestation). Earlier delivery would be indicated if there is multiorgan dysfunction, disseminated intravascular coagulation (DIC), liver infarction or hemorrhage, renal failure, suspected abruption placentae or non-reassuring fetal status. The prognosis is better if pregnancy is terminated even before 34 weeks of gestation. Laboratory abnormalities peak by 24–48 hours postpartum and hepatic enzyme abnormalities and platelet counts begin to normalise within 2–3 days after delivery.

Hepatic Rupture

In cases complicated by HELLP syndrome, spontaneous rupture of the liver can occur due to necrosis and subcapsular hemorrhage. Hepatic rupture can be precipitated by vomiting, convulsions and trauma. It should be suspected when there is a triad of symptoms such as pre-eclampsia, right upper quadrant pain, referred pain to the right shoulder and shock. USG will show evidence of hemoperitoneum. Management is by laparotomy and packing/hepatic resection and immediate delivery. Embolization of the selective vessel also helps.

Acute Fatty Liver of Pregnancy (AFLP)

AFLP is an uncommon but potentially fatal complication that occurs in the third trimester of pregnancy or the early postpartum period. It is also called acute yellow atrophy. The etiology of this condition is unknown. However, current evidence suggests that recessively inherited mitochondrial abnormalities of fatty acid oxidation predispose a woman to fatty liver in pregnancy. It usually manifests in the third trimester and rarely in the immediate postpartum period. It is more common in primiparas, in multiple pregnancies and in women carrying a male fetus.

On histological examination of the liver, it is yellow and small, the hepatocytes are swollen and the cytoplasm is filled with microvesicular fat with central nuclei. There is evidence of intrahepatic cholestasis. These changes have a centrilobular distribution.

Clinical features

Patients often present with non-specific symptoms such as anorexia, nausea, vomiting, malaise, fatigue, headache and abdominal pain. On physical examination, the woman is usually febrile and >70% are jaundiced. Tenderness in the right upper quadrant or mid-epigastric area may be present. The liver is usually small and non-palpable. In severe cases, the woman may present with multisystem involvement including acute renal failure, encephalopathy, gastrointestinal bleeding, pancreatitis and coagulopathy. Marked hypoglycemia is common. Some women may have pre-eclampsia as well. AFLP also has a detrimental effect on the fetus. One of the complications of AFLP is maternal metabolic acidosis secondary to impaired clearance of serum lactate by damaged hepatocytes. Maternal metabolic acidosis directly affects the fetal acid–base status.

Laboratory findings

Laboratory investigations may show marked neutrophil leukocytosis, hypofibrinogenemia, abnormal clotting profile, hypoglycemia, hyperbilirubinemia, hemoconcentration and thrombocytopenia. The differential diagnosis includes viral hepatitis, drug-induced hepatotoxicity and HELLP syndrome.

Management

Early diagnosis, prompt delivery and intensive supportive care are the cornerstones of the management of AFLP. The most definitive test is liver biopsy, but this is often not done due to the presence of coagulopathy. Treatment with FFP, cryoprecipitate, platelets and whole blood/packed cells may be required. Management should aim at preventing hypoglycemic episodes. During the recovery period, acute pancreatitis can occur. In rare cases, patients progress to fulminant hepatic failure requiring liver transplantation. Maternal and fetal mortality are high. However, once recovery occurs, it is usually complete and does not recur in subsequent pregnancies.

LIVER DISEASES INCIDENTAL TO PREGNANCY

Viral Hepatitis

Viral hepatitis is the most common liver disease encountered in pregnant women. There are at least five distinct types of viral hepatitis—hepatitis A, B, C, D, E; hepatitis D is caused by the B-associated delta agent.

Clinical features

All forms of hepatitis are clinically similar in their acute phases. In many cases, infections are subclinical, but if clinically apparent, symptoms may precede jaundice by 1–2 weeks. Symptoms include nausea and vomiting, headache and malaise. Low-grade fever is more common with hepatitis A. When jaundice develops, symptoms usually improve, but there may be pain and tenderness over the liver. Diagnosis depends on the specific serological markers of acute and chronic infection.

Hepatitis A

Hepatitis A is caused by an RNA virus acquired by the ingestion of contaminated food and water. In developing countries, universal exposure occurs in infancy and childhood. The incubation period is 4 weeks.

Clinical features

Prodromal symptoms include nausea and vomiting, headache and malaise and a flu-like illness. In the cholestatic phase, jaundice develops with pale stools, dark urine and pruritus. Symptoms usually abate, but pain and tenderness over the liver may persist.

Diagnosis

Diagnosis is by the detection of IgM anti-hepatitis A antibodies in serum, which indicates acute infection. Presence of IgG antibody indicates immunity. Recovery is complete; there is no carrier state. There is no increased risk of spontaneous abortions, stillbirth, FGR or congenital anomalies. Infection with hepatitis A virus induces lifelong immunity against reinfection.

Immunoprophylaxis

- Pregnant women about to travel to high-prevalence areas should be considered for prophylaxis with immunoglobulins if they are already not immune to hepatitis A. An inactivated HAV vaccine is also safe to use in pregnancy.
- If a woman is exposed to HAV infection, immunoglobulins can be administered within 2 weeks; this ensures protection for 3 months.

Transmission to newborn

The neonate may contract the infection at the time of vaginal delivery by fecal contamination. Neonates born to mothers with HAV infection in the third trimester should be given immunoglobulin within 48 hours of birth. There is no contraindication to breastfeeding.

Hepatitis E

This is the commonest cause of epidemic viral hepatitis. The infection spreads through feco-oral contamination of drinking water. The disease course is severe and is associated with high maternal mortality. In the third trimester, it results in hepatic failure; it has a fulminant course and leads to stillbirth, premature delivery and PPH. Prevention is by using safe drinking water. Passive immunisation with IgG may be useful.

Hepatitis C

It occurs following blood transfusion, transfusion of clotting factors or organ transplantation. It is common in IV drug users, following multiple blood transfusions and in HIV seropositive cases. Following the acute infection, it develops into a chronic infection and results in cirrhosis. Perinatal transmission takes place if the infection occurs in the third trimester of pregnancy.

Hepatitis D

Hepatitis D is caused by the hepatitis delta virus (HDV). This is a defective virus with an incomplete RNA, which requires the assistance of hepatitis B surface antigen (HBsAg) to be infectious. Hepatitis D is mostly transmitted through the same route as the hepatitis B virus. The parenteral mode is the major mode of transmission, and vertical transmission during pregnancy is rare. Immunisation against hepatitis B infection also protects against HDV infection.

Hepatitis B

Formerly called 'serum hepatitis', hepatitis B infection (HBV) is a major cause of liver disease and hepatocellular carcinoma. The virus is made up of two components, namely:

1. The particulate form of the virus, which has an incomplete viral envelope containing the hepatitis B surface antigen–HBsAg
2. The Dane particle, which is a complete virion containing an envelope and the inner core; the core contains the hepatitis B core antigen, viral DNA and the hepatitis B e antigen—HBeAg; the presence of HBeAg is associated with infectivity and virion synthesis

Spread

- Perinatal transmission is the major route of spread.
- Parenteral transmission occurs through blood transfusion, needlestick injuries, drug use and occupational accidents.
- Sexual transmission occurs in both homo and heterosexuals through semen, vaginal secretions and saliva.

HBV infection in pregnancy

In India, 5% of pregnant mothers are positive for hepatitis B infection. Among them, nearly 12% are positive for HBeAg antigen. After acute hepatitis with HBV infection, 95% of patients recover completely, 5% become chronic carriers and 1% take a fulminant course.

Perinatal transmission

Vertical transmission to the fetus and neonate can occur from the mother if she is either a carrier or has an acute hepatitis B infection during the third trimester or in the early postpartum period. The degree of transmission depends on the maternal HBsAg and HBeAg levels, and HBV DNA positivity.

Routes of transmission

- Transplacental in utero transfer is rare.
- The chief mode of transmission is by the swallowing of infected amniotic fluid, infected blood, vaginal secretions, etc., at the time of delivery.
- Postnatally, the infection can be transmitted to the infant through a cracked nipple.

Risk of transmission of hepatitis B infection to the neonate

The chief risk factors for vertical transmission are the presence of HBe antigen and high maternal HBV DNA viral load.

- If the mother is HBsAg-positive and HBeAg-positive, the risk of transmission is >90%.
- If the mother is HBsAg-positive and HBeAg-negative, the risk of transmission is <30%.
- If the mother is anti-HBe-positive, the risk is further reduced to 1%.

The long-term risks of HBV infection in the newborn include chronic infection, development of cirrhosis and hepatocellular carcinoma.

Required investigations

In all pregnant women diagnosed with hepatitis B infection, the following investigations should be carried out:

- Tests for liver cell injury—ALT and AST
- Liver function test
- USG of the abdomen to diagnose chronic liver disease
- Tests for HBV antigens and antibodies:
  - Antigens detected in hepatitis B infection—HBsAg, HBcAg (core antigen) and HBeAg
  - Antibodies detected—anti-HBs, anti-HBc and anti-HBe
  - In acute infection, HBsAg is positive along with IgM anti-HBc (core antibody)
  - In chronic infection and carrier state, HBsAg is positive along with IgG anti-HBc for >6 months
  - The presence of HBeAg and HBV DNA indicates infectivity and viral replication
  - The presence of only hepatitis surface antibodies and the absence of antigen (HBsAg) indicates past infection
  - The mother should be carefully monitored with liver function tests every 3 months and 6 months after delivery as flares can occur intermittently
  - The need for antiviral therapy should be reviewed at 28 weeks by repeating the test for HBV DNA viral load and ALT levels

Prevention of neonatal transmission

- The screening of all pregnant women and selective immunisation of babies born to HBsAg-positive mothers are significant preventive measures.
- The newborn should be vaccinated within 24 hours with 10 micrograms of recombinant vaccine, and the vaccine should be repeated at 1, 2 and 12 months of age.
- HB immunoglobulin (250 micrograms) should be administered within 8–12 hours of birth. HBIG contains a high titre of anti-hepatitis B surface and core antigens. If HBIG is not available, gamma globulin can be used.
- The combined use of immunoglobulins and vaccination reduces the neonatal transmission risk by 80–85%.

Mode of delivery

Cesarean section is indicated only for obstetrical indications and breastfeeding is not contraindicated. At the time of delivery, universal precautions and biomedical waste management protocols should be followed.

Immunisation of pregnant woman

If the pregnant woman is not vaccinated and is at risk of acquiring the infection from her seropositive male partner, through her occupation or drug abuse, the vaccine can be safely given during pregnancy.

Place of antiviral therapy

Treatment with antivirals such as lamivudine is recommended in the third trimester if the HBV DNA viral load is >10,000 copies/mL in order to reduce the progression of the disease and the risk of mother-to-child transmission.

KEY POINTS

Intrahepatic cholestasis of pregnancy

- ✓ *ICP has a genetic preponderance and tends to run in families.*
- ✓ *There is increased susceptibility to sex steroids, which results in abnormal biliary transport.*
- ✓ *It recurs in subsequent pregnancies.*
- ✓ *Fasting serum bile acid levels are >10 μmol/L, which is the key diagnostic test.*
- ✓ *ICP is associated with adverse fetal outcomes such as unexplained stillbirth, preterm delivery and meconium-stained liquor.*

Hepatitis B virus infection in pregnancy

- ✓ *All pregnant women should be screened for hepatitis B infection by testing for HBsAg at the first antenatal visit.*
- ✓ *If positive, the HBeAg and HBV DNA status should be checked.*
- ✓ *The chief risk factors for vertical transmission are the presence of HBe antigen and a high maternal HBV DNA viral load.*
- ✓ *Perinatal transmission chiefly occurs at the time of delivery by the swallowing of infected amniotic fluid, infected blood, vaginal secretions, etc.*
- ✓ *Neonatal transmission is prevented by administering HB immunoglobulin and HBV vaccination at birth.*

Essay question

1. A 28-year-old G2P1 presents at 10 weeks of gestation for routine antenatal booking. On investigation, she is found to be hepatitis B-positive.
   a) What are the risks to the mother and the baby?
   b) What investigations should be carried out?
   c) How does perinatal transmission occur?
   d) How can neonatal infection be prevented?

Short answer questions

Write short notes on the following:
1. Acute fatty liver of pregnancy
2. HELLP syndrome

MCQs

1. What is the most common symptom of intrahepatic cholestasis of pregnancy?
   a) Pain in the right hypochondrium
   b) Yellowness of the eyes
   c) Pruritus
   d) Fatigue and malaise

2. Which of the following is true about acute fatty liver of pregnancy?
   a) Occurs mainly in a grand multipara
   b) Usually presents in the first trimester
   c) Is associated with DIVC
   d) Commonly leads to hyperglycemia

3. At what gestational age should delivery be considered in intrahepatic cholestasis?
   a) 34 weeks
   b) 37 weeks
   c) 38 weeks
   d) 40 weeks

4. At what period of gestation is pruritus most notable in intrahepatic cholestasis of pregnancy?
   a) Early pregnancy
   b) Late first trimester
   c) Second trimester
   d) Third trimester

5. Which of these is not associated with acute fatty liver of pregnancy?
   a) Hypoglycemia
   b) Coagulation failure
   c) Renal failure
   d) Macrosomia

6. Which type of hepatitis is associated with the maximum mortality?
   a) A
   b) B
   c) D
   d) E

7. How long after delivery do the laboratory abnormalities of HELLP syndrome normalise?
   a) 2–3 days
   b) 2–3 weeks
   c) 2–3 months
   d) 6 months

8. Which of these conditions can be caused by hyperemesis gravidarum?
   a) Acute fatty liver
   b) Hepatic dysfunction
   c) HELLP
   d) Cholestasis

Answers
1. (c), 2. (c), 3. (b), 4. (d), 5. (d), 6. (d), 7. (a), 8. (b)

Fill in the blanks

1. Liver disorders are _____ causes of maternal deaths.
2. Serum levels of alkaline phosphatase are _____ in pregnancy.
3. In idiopathic cholestasis of pregnancy, the level of _____ is increased.

Answers
1. indirect, 2. increased, 3. bile acid

Case scenario-based discussion

1. A 30-year-old G2P1 presents at 32 weeks of gestation with intense pruritus of one-week duration involving the body and the limbs. There is no history of fever or vomiting. She had a similar history at 34 weeks of gestation in her first pregnancy. On examination, she is not jaundiced and does not have any rashes. However, there are scratch marks on her body. Her uterus is enlarged corresponding to 34 weeks of gestation and the FH is 140 bpm.
   a) What is the most likely diagnosis?
   b) What investigations should be performed to confirm the diagnosis?
   c) The total bilirubin is 4 mg/dL, SGOT 100 U/L, SGPT 120 U/L. On USG, the gallbladder is normal and tests for viral markers are negative. Bile acid could not be checked. How would you manage this case?

Answers

a) The most likely diagnosis is intrahepatic cholestasis of pregnancy because this woman has had a similar problem in her first pregnancy and ICH has a tendency to recur in subsequent pregnancies. However, viral hepatitis should be ruled out. As there is no associated rash, pruritic urticarial papules of pregnancy can be ruled out.

b) LFT should be carried out to determine the levels of hepatic enzymes, as these are not markedly elevated in ICH. The levels of bile acids should be checked to confirm diagnosis. USG abdomen is required to rule out gallbladder disease. Tests for viral markers should be carried out to rule out viral hepatitis.

c) The woman should be treated with antihistamines and bile salt binders such as cholestyramine or ursodeoxycholic acid. Vitamin K supplements would also be required. As perinatal morbidity is increased in ICH with preterm birth and stillbirth, weekly biophysical profile is carried out, and the baby is delivered at 37 weeks of gestation.

Respiratory Diseases Complicating Pregnancy—Tuberculosis and Bronchial Asthma

---

Learning Objectives

» To understand the effect of tuberculosis on pregnancy
» To know the indications, dosages and side effects of first- and second-line anti-tuberculous drugs
» To understand congenital tuberculosis and its diagnosis
» To describe breastfeeding advice and the preventive measures to protect the newborn from tuberculosis
» To know the management of an HIV-infected pregnant woman with active tuberculosis
» To understand the management of chronic and acute bronchial asthma in pregnancy

---

TUBERCULOSIS COMPLICATING PREGNANCY

Despite the advances in the medical field, tuberculosis remains a major global health challenge. In 2013, 3.3 million tuberculosis cases and 5,10,000 tuberculosis deaths were reported to occur among women globally. More than 95% of new TB cases and deaths are reported from developing countries, with India and China sharing >40% of the global burden.

INCIDENCE

Tuberculosis may be encountered in 1–2% of pregnant women in India. The incidence may be higher among pregnant women who are HIV-positive. Pulmonary tuberculosis is the most common type of TB diagnosed during pregnancy. However, extrapulmonary lesions such as TB of the lymph nodes, bones and kidneys, abdominal tuberculosis and meningeal and miliary tuberculosis may be rarely encountered. Extrapulmonary TB is more common in HIV-positive women than in others.

EFFECT OF PREGNANCY ON PULMONARY TUBERCULOSIS

Though pregnancy was thought to aggravate pulmonary tuberculosis, it has been shown that the course of pulmonary tuberculosis is usually unaffected by pregnancy. Provided they are adequately treated, there is no difference in mortality between pregnant and non-pregnant women. Further, pregnancy does not increase the risk of relapse.

Women who are suffering from tuberculosis can get pregnant unless the disease is very advanced or is a multidrug-resistant tuberculosis, wherein pregnancy is contraindicated because some of the second-line drugs used in these situations are teratogenic.

> In women with multidrug-resistant TB (MDR-TB), one might need to consider therapeutic abortion, as some of the medications required to treat the disease may affect the fetus or may be teratogenic.

EFFECT OF TUBERCULOSIS ON PREGNANCY

- With timely diagnosis and initiation of effective anti-tubercular treatment (ATT), there are usually no adverse effects of TB on pregnancy.
- However, late diagnosis and inadequate treatment are associated with adverse obstetric outcomes such as miscarriages, FGR, intrauterine death, preterm labour and increased perinatal mortality. Tuberculosis is always associated with poor nutritional status, anemia, hypoproteinemia and malnutrition. These factors further contribute to maternal morbidity and mortality.

- Tuberculosis involving extrapulmonary sites (as in TB lymphadenitis) is not associated with adverse outcomes, whereas active pulmonary tuberculosis may even result in mortality.
- Tuberculosis rarely affects the fetus by transplacental passage. However, the newborn is at risk because of the close contact with the mother, if she has open tuberculosis.

DIAGNOSIS OF TUBERCULOSIS IN PREGNANCY

- In pregnancy, pulmonary tuberculosis may present with symptoms like cough, sputum, hemoptysis, fever or weight loss. Though the presentation in pregnancy is similar to that in non-pregnant women, there may be a delay in the diagnosis due to the non-specific nature of early symptoms. The physiological changes associated with pregnancy such as anemia, tachycardia and raised ESR may also confuse the clinical picture.
- There should be a high index of suspicion for tuberculosis in pregnant or puerperal women with unexplained cough and sputum. All pregnant and puerperal women with a history of contact with tuberculosis and those presenting with cough of more than 2 weeks' duration should be screened for tuberculosis.
- Occasionally, active tuberculosis may remain asymptomatic during pregnancy and manifest in the puerperal period when the diaphragm descends following delivery.

Investigations to Confirm Diagnosis

In all suspected cases of tuberculosis, the following investigations are carried out:

- Mantoux test with induration of >10 mm is considered positive.
- In clinically suspicious cases and in the presence of a positive tuberculin test, a single diagnostic X-ray can be taken, preferably after the first trimester. The abdomen can be shielded to protect the fetus from radiation effects.
- With a single diagnostic chest X-ray, there is <0.07 mrad radiation, which is not significant exposure to the embryo or to the fetus (adverse effects are produced when radiation exposure is >5 rad).
- Sputum must be checked for acid-fast bacilli at least twice. Under the Revised National TB Control Programme of India (RNTCP), at least one out of two sputum smears should be positive for acid-fast bacilli (AFB) to label the patient smear-positive.
- Even if the smear is negative, if there are radiological abnormalities on chest X-ray, the patient is diagnosed with pulmonary TB.
- For extrapulmonary tuberculosis, depending on the affected site, investigations are carried out such as FNAC/biopsy from lymph nodes, ascitic and pleural fluid aspiration and lumbar puncture for suspected TB meningitis.
- In selected cases, gastric washing and diagnostic bronchoscopy may be required.
- The samples are subjected to AFB smear, culture and rapid diagnostic methods using molecular studies. Currently available rapid diagnostic tests are PCR test for *Mycobacterium tuberculosis* (MTB) and cartridge-based nucleic acid amplification test (CBNAAT).
- All pregnant women diagnosed with tuberculosis should be counselled about getting HIV testing.

MANAGEMENT

Pregnant women who are diagnosed with active disease should be started on treatment as soon as TB is detected irrespective of the gestational age of the fetus. Before initiating treatment, the patient should be first categorised as per the WHO guidelines (Table 34.1).

The first-line drugs considered safe in pregnancy are ethambutol, pyrazinamide, isoniazid and rifampicin (Table 34.2). All the first-line drugs cross the placenta, but these drugs do not appear to have a harmful effect on the fetus except streptomycin, which should be avoided in pregnancy as it can cause ototoxicity to the fetus.

- In countries where compliance is not an issue, the treatment involves the 'standard recommended regimen' with daily dosing. However, for developing countries, the WHO recommends the DOTS regimen (directly observed treatment, short course) to prevent multidrug resistance.
- Due to the emergence of multidrug-resistant TB (MDR-TB), extremely drug-resistant TB (XDR-TB) and HIV co-infection, pregnant women may occasionally need second-line drugs, which include kanamycin, ofloxacin, ethionamide and cycloserine. The safety of these drugs in pregnancy is not known. These drugs are prescribed for 18–24 months. Because of the potential teratogenic effect of these drugs, therapeutic abortion may be considered in these women after adequate counselling.

Table 34.1   Categorisation of tuberculosis and its treatment regimen

Category	Criteria	Initial phase	Continuation phase
Category I	1. New smear-positive pulmonary TB 2. New smear-negative pulmonary TB with extensive parenchymal involvement 3. New cases of extrapulmonary tuberculosis	Isoniazid, rifampicin, pyrazinamide and ethambutol (HRZE) are given daily for 2 months (In the DOTS regimen, where every dose is directly observed, the above drugs can be given in three-weekly doses)	Isoniazid and rifampicin (HR) are given daily for 4 months
Category 2	1. Smear-positive relapse cases 2. Treatment failure 3. Treatment after interruption	Second-line drugs	

Table 34.2   First-line anti-tubercular drugs and the recommended schedule

Drug	Pregnancy category	Dose	Side effect	Special note
Isoniazid	Category A	5 mg/Kg or 300 mg	Peripheral neuropathy	Pyridoxine should be given during the entire period of therapy
Rifampicin	Category C	10 mg/Kg or 600 mg	Liver dysfunction	Check LFT once in 3 months during therapy
				Therapy should be discontinued if the elevation is five times the normal level
				Administer prophylactic vitamin K to the newborn
Ethambutol	Category A	15–20 mg/Kg	Retrobulbar neuritis	Ocular examination before and during treatment
				Patient is advised to report immediately if there are visual disturbances
Pyrazinamide	Category C	15–25 mg/Kg	Hepatitis	Inadequate data on teratogenicity
Streptomycin	Category D	–	Teratogenic	Contraindicated in pregnancy

Management of Pregnancy and Labour

The minimum duration of treatment is 6–9 months. Routine antenatal care should be continued, and attention should be paid to maternal nutrition and correction of anemia. More frequent bacteriological and laboratory investigations are required to detect improvement or deterioration of the respiratory condition. Any side effects of the chemotherapy should also be monitored. Fetal monitoring should be done to diagnose intrauterine growth restriction.

Obstetric management is generally no different than that of other pregnant women. Cesarean section is performed only for obstetric reasons.

ANTI-TUBERCULAR DRUGS AND TERATOGENICITY

Streptomycin has been proved to be potentially teratogenic and is contraindicated in pregnancy.

Though data regarding the use of pyrazinamide in pregnancy is limited, it has not been found to be associated with malformations.

CONGENITAL TUBERCULOSIS

Congenital tuberculosis is rare. The fetus may be affected through the hematogenous route, through the umbilical vein or by aspiration of infected amniotic fluid at delivery. The criteria for the diagnosis of congenital TB are as follows:

1. Lesions in the first week of life
2. Primary hepatic or caseating hepatic granulomas
3. Documented tuberculous infection of the placenta or endometrium

Congenital tuberculosis is usually seen in the first or second week of life with non-specific signs and symptoms presenting with poor feeding, respiratory distress, hepatosplenomegaly, fever, abdominal distension, lethargy or irritability. Failure to obtain a favourable response to broad-spectrum antibiotics should raise suspicion of congenital tuberculosis. Bronchoalveolar lavage is usually done to collect samples for testing for MTB. In women diagnosed with tuberculosis during pregnancy, the placenta may be sent for AFB and culture.

BREASTFEEDING IN WOMEN WITH TUBERCULOSIS

- Regardless of the TB status, the mother can breastfeed her baby. If she is sputum-positive, she should wear a face mask while breastfeeding.
- However, if the mother is diagnosed with MDR-TB or XDR-TB, the infant should be separated from the mother because of the risk of transmission and the lack of effective chemoprophylaxis.
- If the breastfeeding mother is on isoniazid, supplementary pyridoxine should be administered to the infant as pyridoxine deficiency may result in neonatal seizures.

NEONATAL RISKS AND MANAGEMENT

- A tuberculin-positive mother without active tuberculosis does not pose any risk to the neonate.
- If a pregnant woman with active tuberculosis is sputum-negative in the last three months of gestation, the risk to the infant is negligible.
- If the mother is sputum-positive, then the neonate needs to be evaluated for active tuberculosis with chest X-ray and gastric aspirate for AFB to rule out congenital TB.
- If there is no active tuberculosis in the neonate, it should receive isoniazid prophylaxis at (10 mg/Kg) for three months until the mother's sputum becomes negative.
- BCG vaccination is either postponed or given using isoniazid-resistant BCG vaccines.
- Supplemental pyridoxine should be administered to an infant who is on isoniazid or whose breastfeeding mother is on isoniazid as pyridoxine deficiency may cause seizures in the newborn.

TB AND CONTRACEPTION

As rifampicin is an enzyme inducer, it reduces the efficacy of contraceptive drugs. Therefore, either high-dose estrogen-containing OC pills or alternate methods should be used.

TUBERCULOSIS IN HIV-POSITIVE WOMEN

The risk of tuberculosis is 10 times higher in HIV-infected pregnant women; the perinatal and maternal morbidity and mortality are also significantly increased. Maternal tuberculosis also increases the risk of mother-to-child transmission of HIV infection. All HIV-infected women with active TB should be started on ART as early as possible irrespective of the CD4 count.

BRONCHIAL ASTHMA COMPLICATING PREGNANCY

Bronchial asthma is the most common respiratory disease in pregnancy and complicates 4% of pregnancies. It is a chronic inflammatory condition resulting in reversible airway obstruction, bronchial smooth muscle contraction, hypersecretion of mucus, hyper-responsiveness to various stimuli and increased secretion of cytokines. The common symptoms are cough, wheezing, shortness of breath and sputum production.

EFFECT OF PREGNANCY ON ASTHMA

One-third of pregnant women get better, one-third of women get worse and the remaining one-third experience no change. There may be exacerbation during labour and delivery.

EFFECT OF ASTHMA ON PREGNANCY

Asthma in pregnancy could be associated with an increased risk of preterm labour, low-birth-weight babies and increased perinatal mortality. In the presence of severe asthma with daily asthma symptoms, night awakening and limitation of daily activities, the woman may develop a pneumothorax, acute cor pulmonale and respiratory arrest.

INVESTIGATIONS

Pulmonary function tests are carried out to measure the forced expiratory volume and peak expiratory flow rate.

PREVENTION

Asthmatic pregnant women should avoid the following precipitating factors:
- All triggering factors such as exposure to pollen and animal hair

- Emotional disturbances
- Aspirin, beta-blockers
- Vigorous exercise and exposure to cold air
- They should be protected against viral infections—influenza vaccine is recommended for all patients with moderate and severe asthma and should be given every year

MANAGEMENT

Medical Management

The drugs used to manage asthma in pregnancy are presented in Table 34.3.

Table 34.3   Medications recommended during pregnancy

Class	Drugs	Dosage
Anti-inflammatory drugs	Cromolyn sodium	2 puffs/sprays × 4 times
	Beclomethasone	
	Prednisone	
Bronchodilators	Inhaled B2 agonist-salbutamol	Two puffs every 4 hours
	Theophylline	Oral
Antihistamine	Chlorpheniramine	4 mg orally 4 times a day
Decongestant	Pseudoephedrine	60 mg orally 4 times a day
Cough syrup	Dextromethorphan	
Antibiotics	Amoxicillin, erythromycin, cephalosporins	

Acute asthma is treated with IV methylprednisolone 1 mg/Kg every 6–8 hours, and then the drug is slowly tapered. SC terbutaline 0.25 mg is given if the patient does not respond to the above medications.

Obstetric Management

- If systemic steroids are used, pregnant mothers should be monitored for gestational diabetes and pre-eclampsia. Serial scans may be required to diagnose FGR.
- Use of theophylline may be limited as it causes tachycardia and nervousness.
- For labour induction, PGE_1 and PGE_2 are not contraindicated.
- During labour, the same medications are continued. In steroid-dependent patients, stress during labour is managed with IV hydrocortisone 100 mg 8-hourly until 24 hours after delivery.
- For labour analgesia, non-histamine narcotics such as fentanyl can be used. For cesarean section, conduction analgesia is preferable as tracheal intubation may trigger severe vasospasm.
- In refractory PPH, PGE_1 and other uterotonics such as oxytocin are used in place of PGF_2-alpha which can cause significant bronchospasm in asthmatics. Ergometrine can also cause bronchospasm.
- If oxygen saturation cannot be maintained, mechanical ventilation should be instituted.
- Breastfeeding is not contraindicated.

EFFECT ON THE CHILD

- The child may also develop an atopic disease.

KEY POINTS

✓ One should have a high index of suspicion to diagnose tuberculosis in pregnancy.

✓ Early diagnosis and adequate treatment will improve maternal and perinatal outcomes.

✓ First-line ATT is safe during pregnancy and can be given in the first trimester also.

✓ Streptomycin is contraindicated in pregnancy.

✓ Women with MDR-TB and XDR-TB need second-line drugs, which can be teratogenic. Therefore, women requiring these drugs should be counselled for therapeutic abortion.

✓ Breastfeeding should be encouraged except in MDR-TB and XDR-TB patients.

✓ Bronchial asthma in pregnancy can lead to preterm labour, low-birth-weight babies and limitation of daily activities.

✓ Acute asthma in pregnancy is treated with IV methylprednisolone.

✓ For cesarean section, conduction analgesia is preferable as tracheal intubation may trigger severe vasospasm.

✓ PGF_2-alpha can cause significant bronchospasm in asthmatics, and therefore, should be avoided for PPH management.

Essay question

1. Discuss the diagnosis and management of tuberculosis in pregnancy.

Short answer questions

1. What are the first-line anti-tuberculous drugs? Discuss the dosage and toxicity of these drugs.
2. What are the indications to use second-line anti-tuberculous drugs?
3. Discuss the drugs used for bronchial asthma in pregnancy.

MCQs

1. Which of the following is true regarding tuberculosis in pregnancy?
   a) There is no difference in TB-related mortality between pregnant and non-pregnant women if they are adequately treated.
   b) Pregnancy increases the risk of relapse.
   c) Pregnancy increases the risk of multidrug-resistant TB (MDR-TB).
   d) It is a frequent indication for therapeutic abortion.
2. If a woman is diagnosed with tuberculosis in the first trimester of pregnancy:
   a) Therapeutic abortion is advised.
   b) Anti-tubercular therapy should be instituted immediately.
   c) Anti-tubercular therapy should be instituted after the first trimester.
   d) Anti-tubercular therapy should be instituted after delivery.
3. Anti-tubercular drugs considered safe in pregnancy include the following EXCEPT:
   a) Ethambutol
   b) Isoniazid
   c) Rifampicin
   d) Streptomycin
4. Tuberculosis during pregnancy may lead to a slight increase in the incidence of all EXCEPT:
   a) Abortion
   b) Premature labour
   c) Intrauterine growth restriction
   d) Congenital malformations
5. Pyridoxine is used to treat neuropathy induced by which drug?
   a) Rifampicin
   b) Isoniazid
   c) Pyrazinamide
   d) Ethambutol
6. Pregnancy complicated by asthma is more likely to lead to:
   a) IUGR
   b) Congenital malformations

c) Prostaglandin E pessaries should be avoided
d) Pre-eclampsia is less common than in non-asthmatic women

7. Pregnant asthmatic women on synthetic steroids are at risk of:
   a) Diabetes mellitus
   b) Prolonged pregnancy
   c) Operative deliveries
   d) Abruption

Answers
1. (a), 2. (b), 3. (d), 4. (d), 5. (b), 6. (a), 7. (a)

Fill in the blanks

1. The dosage of isoniazid is _____.
2. Pyridoxine is given to reduce the risk of _____.
3. The dosage of rifampicin is _____.
4. The dosage of ethambutol is _____.
5. The dosage of pyrazinamide is _____.
6. The most common toxicity due to isoniazid is _____.

Answers
1. 5 mg/Kg daily, 2. isoniazid-induced neuropathy, 3. 10 mg/Kg daily, 4. 5–25 mg/Kg, 5. 15–25 mg/Kg, 6. hepatitis

Case scenario-based discussion

1. A 27-year-old G2P1, who had her last childbirth 2 years ago, presents with 8 weeks of amenorrhea and cough with low-grade fever of 3 weeks' duration. She was seen by her family physician and was prescribed antibiotics, but she was not getting better.
   a) How would you proceed to investigate this case?
   b) The woman's sputum is AFB-positive, there is >10 mm induration on the Mantoux test and the chest X-ray shows findings suggesting tuberculosis. How would you treat this woman?

Answers

a) Since the woman has had a cough of more than 2 weeks' duration and her symptoms are not relieved with antibiotics, one should suspect pulmonary tuberculosis. She should undergo a Mantoux test, her sputum should be sent for AFB smear twice, and a single X-ray chest should be taken.

b) This woman is a new case of smear-positive pulmonary tuberculosis and should be started on anti-tuberculous treatment without delay. First-line anti-tubercular drugs can be given safely in the first trimester since no teratogenic effect has been reported with these drugs. She should be started on isoniazid, rifampicin, pyrazinamide and ethambutol (HRZE), which should be given daily for 2 months followed by isoniazid and rifampicin (HR) given daily for 4 months. If the woman is non-compliant, she should be put on the DOTS regimen and be directly observed on three-weekly doses. Her anemia and hypoproteinemia should be corrected effectively. The woman should also be monitored for the development of side effects of anti-tuberculous drugs.

Maternal Infections During Pregnancy

Learning Objectives

» To describe the effect of TORCH infections on the fetus and the newborn

» To understand the principles of managing pregnant women exposed to rubella and chickenpox infections

» To describe the measures to prevent the transmission of HIV infection to the offspring from an HIV-infected mother

» To describe the management of malaria complicating pregnancy

» To describe the phases of dengue fever and its management in pregnancy

■ INTRODUCTION

The pregnant woman and her fetus are susceptible to many infections or infectious diseases caused by viruses, bacteria and protozoa. While some of these infections such as influenza, dengue and hepatitis may be quite dangerous to the mother, others such as rubella, CMV infection, toxoplasmosis, genital herpes, HPV infection and Zika virus infection may have adverse effects on the fetus and the newborn. The fetus may acquire the infection by hematogenous/transplacental passage or by ascending infection after the rupture of the membranes or it may be infected during birth. Breastfeeding and horizontal transmission are also modes by which the fetus may acquire an infection. In this chapter, the TORCH group of infections, sexually transmitted diseases and other important infections will be discussed.

TORCH INFECTIONS

TORCH infections include the following:
- Toxoplasmosis (TO)
- Rubella (R) infection
- Cytomegalovirus (C) infection
- Herpes simplex (H) infection

■ TOXOPLASMOSIS

Toxoplasma infection is caused by *Toxoplasma gondii,* which is an intracellular protozoan parasite. The infection is transmitted from cats, the definitive hosts, or through the consumption of raw meat. The parasite exists in several forms—primarily, as oocysts in cat feces or as cysts in infected meat. During acute infection, the cat excretes non-infectious oocysts in its feces. In favourable conditions such as warm and moist soil, the oocyst sporulates and becomes infectious. Toxoplasmosis is acquired by humans by the following routes:

- Eating raw or inadequately cooked meat (tissue cysts)
- Eating improperly washed fruits and vegetables which are contaminated with cat litter
- Hand-to-mouth transmission of oocysts after gardening or handling cat litter
- Vertical transmission from the mother to the fetus
- Through organ donation

Following the ingestion of oocysts, the infection spreads to various organs in the body through the intestinal epithelium. In healthy individuals, it remains asymptomatic or presents with mild flu-like symptoms with low-grade fever and myalgia. However, if acquired during pregnancy, it can lead to fetal infection resulting in miscarriage, intrauterine death, congenital infection, neurological manifestations, chorioretinitis, deafness and developmental delay.

Effect on Pregnancy

- In women who acquired the infection prior to pregnancy, antibodies are already produced; these protect against fetal infection in future pregnancies.
- For the fetus to be affected by toxoplasmosis, the mother should have acquired the infection during the current pregnancy.
- The risk of fetal infection is greater if the maternal infection occurs in the later weeks of pregnancy than in the early weeks. Fetal transmission is as high as 40–60% if the infection occurs in the third trimester

but is only 5–15% if the infection occurs in the first trimester. However, the risk to the fetus is more severe when the infection occurs in the first or early second trimester (40–50%) than in the latter half of pregnancy (10%). If the infection occurs in early pregnancy, it can result in miscarriage.

Effect on the Newborn

In untreated pregnant women with toxoplasmosis, the overall risk of congenital toxoplasmosis is 20–50%. Neonates born with congenital toxoplasmosis present with low birth weight, hepatosplenomegaly, jaundice and anemia. The nervous system manifestations include hydrocephaly, convulsions, microcephaly and mental retardation. Even if they are asymptomatic, they may develop chorioretinitis at a later age. Therefore, children known to have congenital toxoplasmosis should be kept under observation for months to years.

> **Features of congenital toxoplasmosis**
> - Low birth weight
> - Hepatosplenomegaly
> - Icterus
> - Anemia
> - Classical triad of hydrocephalus, chorioretinitis and intracranial calcifications (typical features)
> - Visual impairment, hearing loss, neurodevelopmental delay and seizures are other manifestations

Diagnosis

Universal screening for toxoplasmosis is not recommended. However, testing is carried out in the following situations:

- Possibility of exposure from pet cats at home or involvement in gardening
- Sudden intrauterine fetal death
- The presence of sonographic markers of fetal infection
- In HIV-infected women

Serological tests

Serology remains the mainstay of the diagnosis of *Toxoplasma* infection. Maternal serum is tested for *Toxoplasma*-specific IgM and IgG antibodies. Once infection has occurred, IgG remains positive throughout life and confers lifelong immunity.

- Positive IgG and negative IgM in the first and second trimesters indicate an old infection that could have occurred up to 6 months before, and, therefore,

does not pose a risk to the fetus. However, in the third trimester, the risk of fetal infection in early pregnancy cannot be ruled out.
- The presence of IgM antibodies with or without raised IgG suggests a recent infection.
- The most accurate confirmation of active infection is a four-fold increase in IgG titres in two samples taken at an interval of 3–4 weeks.
- The Sabin and Feldman cytoplasm-modifying (dye) test can also be used. Very high titres, greater than 1:512, are indicative of recent or current infection.
- IgG avidity test is performed to find out whether the presence of IgG antibody is due to recent infection or past infection. This test is based on the fact that antibodies bind less avidly to antigens in the active stage than in the chronic stage. Avidity of <30% indicates infection within the preceding 3 months, whereas avidity of >30% indicates that the infection happened more than 6 months ago. Therefore, high avidity in the first trimester may be reassuring.

Prenatal diagnosis

Prenatal diagnosis is required if a primary infection is suspected based on the following findings:

- IgM-positivity with low avidity
- Increasing titres of IgG
- Both IgG- and IgM-positivity with low avidity
- USG markers of fetal infection

Prenatal diagnosis includes amniocentesis and detection of *Toxoplasma* DNA by PCR testing in the amniotic fluid.

USG markers of toxoplasmosis of the fetus include the following:

- Hydrocephalus, calcifications and microcephaly
- Hepatosplenomegaly, enlarged placenta, liver calcification, ascites and early-onset IUGR

Management

- Treatment with spiramycin (1 g 8-hourly) reduces transmission and the incidence of fetal infection by 60% but does not modify its severity. Spiramycin is a macrolide antibiotic which does not cross the placenta.
- For the treatment of fetal infection, pyrimethamine (50 mg daily) plus sulphadiazine (1 g three times a day) is recommended. The treatment should be continued throughout pregnancy. This multidrug regimen is not recommended in the first trimester due to the possibility of teratogenicity with pyrimethamine, which is a folic acid antagonist.

- If primary toxoplasmosis infection is diagnosed in early pregnancy by a positive PCR and the presence of USG markers, because of the high likelihood of fetal damage, therapeutic termination of pregnancy may be considered.

RUBELLA INFECTION

Rubella (otherwise called German Measles) is caused by an enveloped RNA virus that causes an exanthematous infection commonly affecting children and young adolescents. Rubella is a vaccine-preventable disease and may be of minor importance in the non-pregnant state. However, if the infection is acquired during pregnancy, it is directly responsible for fetal wastage and major fetal malformations.

Clinical Features

The infection spreads through droplet infection from the upper respiratory tract. The incubation period is 14–21 days. Rubella infection presents with sore throat, low-grade fever, maculopapular rashes and cervical and occipital lymphadenopathy. Subclinical infections without rashes may go unnoticed. The course of the disease is the same as in the non-pregnant state. Though the disease course is very mild, occasionally, complications such as encephalitis and thrombocytopenia can occur. The clinical manifestations resolve in 3–5 days but the patient continues to be infective for a long period of time. During the period of viraemia, the virus spreads to the fetus through the placenta.

Effect on the Newborn

- Rubella acquired during pregnancy can lead to miscarriages, intrauterine death, preterm delivery and congenital rubella syndrome.
- The risk of fetal infection and its severity depends on the period of gestation at which infection occurs.
- The fetus is affected most severely if infection occurs in early pregnancy. If exposed during the first 11 weeks of gestation, >90% of fetuses are affected. If exposed between 13–16 weeks of gestation, nearly 35–40% of fetuses are affected. When infection occurs after 16 weeks of gestation, congenital malformations are uncommon, but extended rubella syndrome with panencephalitis, type I diabetes, hepatosplenomegaly, purpura, mental retardation and hearing loss can occur.
- Early-onset growth restriction is also a common feature of rubella, which can also occur in congenital CMV, herpes simplex virus and varicella infections.

Congenital Rubella Syndrome

- The characteristic triad—cataracts, sensorineural hearing loss and congenital heart disease
- Congenital heart diseases—patent ductus arteriosus (PDA) and pulmonary stenosis are common.; atrial septal defects (ASD) and ventricular septal defects (VSD) have also been reported; because congenital heart disease is present in more than 50% of children infected during the first two months of gestation, fetal echocardiography is recommended for women with known or suspected first-trimester rubella infection
- CNS defects, including meningoencephalitis
- Hepatitis
- Thrombocytopenia and anemia
- Rarely, myocarditis, microcephaly, microphthalmia and glaucoma are encountered

Diagnosis

Though universal screening for rubella is not recommended during pregnancy, screening may be indicated when there are USG features suggesting congenital rubella syndrome or in the presence of IUGR. In those who were exposed to rubella infection, serology testing should be done. Accurate diagnosis is made by serological testing for rubella-specific IgG and IgM antibodies.

- If a woman presents in the first trimester of pregnancy with a history of exposure to rubella from her children or other children or has developed a rash, she should be tested for rubella antibody status.
  — The presence of rubella-specific IgM antibodies is diagnostic of recent infection.
  — If rubella-specific IgG is >15 IU/mL, the woman is said to be immune and should be reassured. The presence of IgG antibodies signifies a past infection. Since the antibodies persist for a long time, they confer protection against rubella.
  — The absence of rubella IgG antibody indicates susceptibility to rubella infection. If the woman has no antibodies or if IgG is <15 IU/mL, the test should be repeated 1–2 weeks after the onset of the rash.
  — If seroconversion has occurred in the paired test, i.e., the rubella-specific IgG antibody titre has increased four-fold or specific IgM is detected, it is diagnostic of recent infection. Such a woman should be counselled about the risk of fetal damage, which is >90%, and termination of pregnancy is discussed.

- If the exposure occurs in the second or third trimester of pregnancy, fetal blood sampling (FBS) for IgM may be carried out.

Diagnosis of fetal infection

- Fetal infection can be diagnosed by performing PCR tests for rubella on chorion villus samples, amniotic fluid or fetal blood followed by cordocentesis.
- The presence of IgM also indicates infection.

Management

- Rubella is one of the most teratogenic agents known.
- Hence, if the fetus is likely to be affected, medical termination of pregnancy should be advised before 20 weeks of pregnancy.
- As the duration of pregnancy increases, fetal infections are less likely to cause congenital malformations.

Prevention

Vaccination

- As part of the national vaccination programme, the MMR vaccine is given to all children. If it is not given in infancy, girls should be given the rubella vaccination in their adolescent years before they enter the reproductive years.
- During the evaluation of an infertile couple, the woman should be encouraged to have her IgG antibody status checked and if not immune, she should be advised to have rubella vaccination before attempting pregnancy.
- Since the MMR vaccine is a live attenuated vaccine, there is a potential risk to the fetus. Therefore, women should be advised not to become pregnant for one month after immunisation.
- If the woman is inadvertently vaccinated during early pregnancy, there is no need to terminate the pregnancy as no congenital rubella syndrome has been reported in the offspring.
- The vaccine can be safely given to postpartum women who are breastfeeding.

■ CYTOMEGALOVIRUS INFECTION

Cytomegalovirus (CMV) belongs to the herpes group of viruses. The incidence of CMV infection in pregnancy is about 0.5–1%. It is the most common congenital infection to cause fetal damage. In pregnancy, this infection is transmitted to the fetus through the placental route. The primary infection is usually asymptomatic or produces only a mild non-specific glandular fever-like illness. Following primary infection, the virus becomes latent; there

is periodic reactivation with viral shedding despite the presence of serum antibodies. As there is relative depression of cell-mediated immunity in pregnancy, this places the fetus at high risk of the sequelae of these infections. Perinatal transmission can also occur through the aspiration of cervicovaginal secretions at delivery or through the ingestion of infected breast milk.

Congenital Infection

Since the primary infection in the mother is usually asymptomatic, the diagnosis is rarely made before birth. Following a primary infection in the mother, transmission from mother to fetus occurs in 50% of cases. Congenital infection causes cytomegalic inclusion disease only in 10% of cases. This is a syndrome that includes FGR, low birth weight, microcephaly, hydrocephalus, intracranial calcifications, chorioretinitis, mental and motor retardation, hepatosplenomegaly, jaundice, hemolytic anemia, thrombocytopenic purpura, hearing loss and pneumonitis. Cardiomegaly is the most frequently encountered cardiac manifestation of congenital infection with CMV.

Diagnosis

Serology

- The presence of specific IgM antibodies may indicate a recent infection.
- A paired test to check the IgG antibody levels may also be useful.
- IgG avidity test is also very useful. A low-avidity test prior to the 18th week of pregnancy indicates a high risk of congenital infection, whereas a high-avidity test in early pregnancy is a good indicator of past infection.

Diagnosis of fetal infection

Though USG markers may suggest CMV infection, they are not diagnostic as they can be seen in other infections also. Confirmation of fetal infection is by PCR testing of the amniotic fluid.

USG features of CMV infection
- Cerebral calcification
- Hydrocephalus
- Microcephaly
- Hepatosplenomegaly
- Ascites
- Hydrops
- Placental enlargement

Management

- There is no effective therapy for CMV infection but antiviral drugs like ganciclovir have been tried.
- Routine serological screening is not recommended in pregnancy. However, serological testing for CMV may be required if there are USG features suggesting CMV infection that cannot be explained by any other cause.
- No vaccine is available for prevention.

■ HERPES SIMPLEX VIRUS INFECTION

It is a sexually transmitted viral infection caused by a DNA virus. There are two types of herpes simplex virus (HSV) infections, namely HSV1 and HSV2.

- HSV1 causes oropharyngeal infections
- HSV2 causes genital infections

Effect on Pregnancy

During pregnancy, a woman may acquire HSV as a primary infection or as a recurrent infection. HSV infection presents with symptoms such as fever, myalgia, headache and the appearance of vesicles associated with pain. The woman also presents with dysuria, retention, perineal pain and discharge. Occasionally, it may present as a severe disseminating variety. The infection may also remain asymptomatic.

Infection acquired during pregnancy is transmitted to the fetus less commonly by intrauterine transmission and more commonly at the time of delivery through cervicovaginal secretions. Infection can spread from the lower genital tract into the uterine cavity with the rupture of membranes. The risk of transmission is greatest during primary infection than during a recurrence.

Untreated herpes infection may be associated with miscarriages, PROM and preterm labour and intrauterine death. Herpes infection before 20 weeks of gestation is associated with miscarriages and congenital malformations involving the CNS, eyes and skin. Infection after 20 weeks of gestation presents with FGR, PROM and preterm labour. In the severe form, the newborn may present with encephalitis and disseminated disease with increased perinatal morbidity and mortality. In immunocompromised women such as those who are HIV-infected, the course of the disease may be severe, leading to encephalitis and hepatitis.

USG features of congenital infection
- Hydrocephaly, microcephaly
- Non-immune fetal hydrops
- IUGR
- Skin scarring
- Calcification within the liver

Antenatal and Intrapartum Management

For pain relief, local lesions are treated with analgesics and topical anesthetic agents. Because of the pain, there may be retention of urine, which is treated by catheterisation. The specific treatment for HSV is with antiviral drugs such as acyclovir, valacyclovir, etc.— 200 mg of acyclovir five times a day can be prescribed for 5–7 days. In women who had recurrent herpetic lesions during pregnancy, acyclovir suppressive therapy is given, beginning at 36 weeks of pregnancy. The dosage for acyclovir is 400 mg three times a day for 7–14 days. Acyclovir is not shown to be associated with adverse fetal effects. It is a category C drug. In disseminated disease, parenteral therapy is given. Unless there is a lesion on the breast, breastfeeding is not contraindicated.

Mode of Delivery

- Cesarean delivery is recommended in women with an active genital lesion or prodromal symptoms such as vulvar pain as these may indicate an impending outbreak. Cesarean delivery should be performed even after the rupture of the membranes in women who have an active genital lesion.
- Cesarean is not recommended in women with non-genital lesions and in women with a history of HSV infection without active disease.

Neonatal Infection

Infection in the newborn may be disseminated, either with the involvement of the major viscera or localised with the involvement confined to the central nervous system, eyes, skin and mucosa. In some cases, the newborn may be asymptomatic.

OTHER VIRAL INFECTIONS IN PREGNANCY

■ INFLUENZA VIRUS INFECTION

Influenza viruses are a group of RNA viruses that are further classified into A, B and C groups. These viruses cause seasonal epidemics. Influenza is more likely to cause severe infection in pregnancy. The disease can progress from flu-like symptoms to tracheobronchitis and viral pneumonia. Though the symptoms are self-limiting and can be treated with rest and analgesics, antiviral medications such as oseltamivir may be required to reduce the severity and duration of the illness.

Prevention

The best way to prevent influenza is by administering inactivated influenza vaccination to pregnant women during the influenza season. The vaccination should be given before viral exposure occurs.

■ H1N1 INFECTION

H1N1 infection is a subtype of influenza A virus, which is a quadruple reassorted influenza virus (swine flu). This virus affects humans and contains segments of genes from pig, bird and human influenza viruses. It is transmitted by droplet inhalation, contact with infected objects and surfaces and direct contact with an infected person. The incubation period is 1–4 days.

In 2009, a pandemic influenza A H1N1 virus infection resulted in a widespread outbreak of respiratory infection across the world. The virus showed a predilection for the lower respiratory tract, producing acute respiratory distress. Data from past pandemics (1918–1919) and the 2009 outbreak have shown that pregnant women are at risk of complications from the infection. Besides the modification in the immune system to accommodate the developing fetus, the enlarging uterus produces mechanical effects, resulting in the elevation of the diaphragm, congestion and local edema, making pregnant women prone to complications such as pneumonia and ARDS.

Clinical Features

The typical symptoms of swine flu are a sudden fever of at least 38°C and a sudden cough with one or more symptoms such as chill, lethargy, headache, sore throat, running nose, muscle pain, diarrhea and vomiting. The signs and symptoms of severe disease include dyspnea, chest pain on breathing, purulent or bloodstained sputum, respiratory rate >30/minute, persistent tachycardia >100 beats per minute, hypoxia with SpO_2 <94%, shock and altered consciousness. Comorbidities such as asthma, chronic lung disease, heart disease, kidney, blood and liver disorders and metabolic and endocrine conditions weaken the immune system; marked obesity may increase the risk of influenza complications.

Effect on Pregnancy

Regarding the pregnancy outcome associated with H1N1 infection, a three-fold increase in preterm delivery and a five-fold increase in stillbirths have been reported. In early pregnancy, hyperthermia associated with H1N1 infection may lead to miscarriages and anomalies.

Diagnosis

RT-PCR test performed on throat swabs and nasopharyngeal swabs is diagnostic. It may be false-negative in nearly 30% of cases.

Management

- In pregnant women with suspected or confirmed H1N1 infection, irrespective of the RT-PCR results, antiviral treatment should be commenced as early as possible, particularly within the first 48 hours of the onset of symptoms. Antiviral drugs oseltamivir and zanamivir are used. Oseltamivir is given in a dose of 75 mg twice daily for 5 days. These are category C drugs with which no adverse fetal effects have been reported.
- Prophylactic antibiotics are given to prevent secondary bacterial infection.
- Supportive therapy with IV fluids, nutrition, oxygen and ventilatory support may be required.
- Aspirin is contraindicated in any virus infection.
- Breastfeeding is not contraindicated if the mother is using safety measures such as face masks.

Prevention

- All pregnant women should take preventive care to avoid contracting the infection.
- An inactivated monovalent vaccine, which is safe to use in pregnancy, is recommended for pregnant women.
- Personal protection equipment should be used by healthcare personnel.

■ ZIKA VIRUS INFECTION

Zika virus is an RNA virus transmitted by the bite of the female *Aedes* mosquito. The infection can spread by vertical transmission from the mother to the child. The incubation period is 3–14 days. It can remain asymptomatic or present with mild symptoms such as fever, malaise, headache and myalgia. Occasionally, it could have a severe course with neuropathy or myelitis.

Diagnosis

The diagnosis is made by real-time PCR (RT-PCR) test on blood, saliva or urine.

Effect on the Fetus

Zika virus infection in pregnancy can result in miscarriages, preterm labour, intrauterine death and FGR. The risk of congenital Zika virus syndrome is 10%. Fetal damage is greater if the infection occurs in early pregnancy. When the fetus is affected, the infection predominantly affects the neurological system, with major abnormalities such as microcephaly, cerebral calcifications, choroid plexus cyst and ventriculomegaly.

Antenatal Management

If Zika virus infection is confirmed in the mother by RT-PCR, a detailed anomaly scan should be performed every 4 weeks along with an MRI of the brain in selected cases. Fetal infection may be confirmed by an RT-PCR test on amniotic fluid. Termination may be considered if the fetal infection is confirmed in early pregnancy.

Management

There is no specific treatment for Zika virus infection; only supportive therapy is given. No preventive measures are available except for the prevention of mosquito bites.

■ COVID-19 VIRUS INFECTION

The World Health Organization (WHO) declared COVID-19 a global pandemic on March 11, 2020. COVID-19 is an infectious disease caused by a coronavirus. It is a respiratory virus transmitted from human to human. The spread occurs primarily through droplet infection, i.e., through droplets expelled when an infected person coughs or sneezes, from saliva or indirectly from fomites. The incubation period is 5–7 days. The virus enters the body through the oral and nasal mucous membranes, reaches the lung, proliferates rapidly in the lung parenchyma and manifests with a hyperinflammatory response.

Approximately 85% of infected persons suffer from mild symptoms with fever, myalgia, tiredness, sore throat and loss of taste and smell. Nearly 10–15% become seriously ill with a severe respiratory illness. Besides conditions such as diabetes, cardiac disease and cancer, pregnancy is also considered a risk factor for developing severe COVID disease because of the physiological changes occurring in the respiratory, reproductive, endocrine and immune systems during pregnancy. The effect of COVID-19 on the fetus is still not clear.

Diagnosis

Diagnosis is made by an RT-PCR test on swabs taken from the nasopharynx. There may be false-negative results in 20–30% of cases. X-ray chest/CT chest may be required to assess the severity of lung involvement in select cases after shielding the abdomen to protect the fetus.

Management

Antenatal management

- In pregnant women diagnosed with COVID-19, antenatal visits may be restricted, and protective measures should be taken at each visit. Until the end of the isolation period, routine medical visits may be delayed.
- 14 days after the resolution of symptoms, the woman should be referred for USG evaluation of the fetus.

Intrapartum management

- Extra vigilance is required in the management of pregnant women who have COVID infection.
- Induction of labour and cesarean section are carried out only for obstetrical indications.
- High rates of cesarean section have been reported, mainly for fetal distress.
- Continuous electronic fetal monitoring is recommended during labour for all cases of suspected or confirmed COVID-19.
- At the time of delivery, delayed cord clamping is not advocated.
- Healthcare providers should wear appropriate personal protective equipment when treating a patient with suspected or confirmed COVID-19.

Postpartum management

- Guidelines allow rooming-in of the baby for asymptomatic and mildly ill women. Separation of the baby is reserved for cases in which the mother has a severe or critical illness.
- The benefits of breastfeeding currently outweigh the risks of the transmission of the infection from the mother to the infant. Therefore, most organisations allow breastfeeding under specific hygiene conditions for COVID-19-suspected/-positive patients.
- In women presenting with severe respiratory disease, one should also consider pulmonary embolism as the differential diagnosis. As the risk of venous thromboembolism is increased in those infected with COVID-19 and since pregnancy is a hypercoagulable state, extra vigilance should be maintained.

- The mental health of the woman should also be addressed.

Medical Management

Medical management involves the use of various medications such as ivermectin, azithromycin and antiviral drugs such as remdesivir, oseltamivir, etc. These drugs can be safely given during pregnancy.

Prevention

Pregnant and breastfeeding women are advised to take the vaccine against COVID-19.

VARICELLA-ZOSTER (CHICKENPOX) INFECTION IN PREGNANCY

Varicella is a DNA virus of the herpes family which is highly contagious and transmitted through respiratory droplets and personal contact with vesical fluid and indirectly via fomites. The primary infection is characterised by fever, malaise and a pruritic rash, which develops as crops of maculopapules that become vesicular and form a crust before healing. The incubation period is 10–21 days. The disease is highly infectious 48 hours before the appearance of the rash and until the formation of crusts.

Most adults have a history of chickenpox during childhood and nearly 95% have serological evidence of immunity with IgG antibody. Following the primary infection, the virus remains latent in the dorsal root ganglia but can get reactivated to cause a vesicular rash known as herpes zoster or **shingles.** Shingles in pregnancy do not appear to cause fetal sequelae.

Effect on Pregnancy

Maternal effects

There is evidence that varicella infection can become severe during pregnancy. It can be associated with severe morbidity with complications such as pneumonia, hepatitis and encephalitis. Pneumonia develops in 10% of pregnant women.

Fetal and neonatal risks

- **Varicella infection before 20 weeks of gestation:** Fetal varicella syndrome occurs in 1–2% of cases where maternal varicella infection occurs before 20 weeks of gestation. This is characterised by skin scarring with dermatomal distribution, eye defects with microphthalmia, chorioretinitis, cataracts, hypoplasia of the limb and neurological abnormalities

such as microcephaly, cortical atrophy and mental retardation. Prenatal diagnosis is based on USG findings such as limb deformity, microcephaly, hydrocephaly, soft tissue calcification and IUGR. Varicella DNA can be detected by PCR in amniotic fluid.

- **Varicella infection after 20 weeks and before 36 weeks of gestation:** Maternal infection between 20 and 36 weeks of gestation does not appear to be associated with major adverse effects on the fetus.
- **After 36 weeks of gestation:** If maternal infection occurs 1–4 weeks before delivery, 50% of babies are affected and 1/4th develop clinical varicella (congenital varicella). Severe infection is likely to occur if the infant is born within 7 days of the onset of the rash.

Management

Management of a pregnant woman who has a history of contact with chickenpox

In the absence of a past history of chickenpox, VZV IgG levels are checked. If antibodies are detected within 10 days of contact, it is assumed that the woman must have acquired immunity in the past. If there are no antibodies and the woman is not immune to varicella virus and has had significant exposure (face-to-face exposure for 5 minutes or indoor contact for 1 hour), varicella-zoster immunoglobulin (VZIG) should be given as soon as possible; this can be done within up to 10 days of contact. Detailed USG is recommended between 18 and 20 weeks of gestation, and neonatal ophthalmological examination should be performed at delivery.

Management of a woman who develops chickenpox

- Personal hygiene and safety measures should be observed to prevent secondary bacterial infections.
- Oral acyclovir is started within 24 hours of the onset of rashes if the woman is at more than 20 weeks of gestation.
- These women are at a greater risk of developing pneumonitis. Delivery during the viremic period may be extremely dangerous. The maternal risks include bleeding, thrombocytopenia, DIVC and hepatitis. Besides supportive management, intravenous acyclovir is recommended.
- If maternal infection occurs at term, there is a significant risk of varicella of the newborn

(20–30%). If possible, delivery may be delayed for 5 days to allow the transfer of maternal antibodies to the fetus. However, if delivery occurs within 5 days of infection, the neonate should be given VZIG. If the neonate develops varicella infection, it should be treated with acyclovir.

Prevention

- Women seeking infertility treatment or preconceptional counselling should be screened for the presence of IgG antibodies. If seronegative, they should be offered vaccination.
- In women seeking antenatal care, at the initial visit, previous history of chickenpox should be elicited. If there is no such history, the woman should be advised to avoid contact with those who have chickenpox.

▌ DENGUE

Dengue fever is a viral disease caused by any of four closely related serotypes of flavivirus (RNA viruses) transmitted to humans by the bite of *Aedes* mosquitoes. Dengue is endemic in most tropical and subtropical countries. About half of the world's population is considered to be at risk. Most states in India are dengue-endemic.

Clinical Course

Nearly 80% of dengue infections remain asymptomatic, while the remaining 20% become symptomatic. In symptomatic cases, dengue fever occurs in three stages.

1. **Stage of acute febrile illness:** This stage lasts for 1–4 days, manifests with high-grade fever, myalgia, headache, facial flushing, conjunctival injection and retro-orbital eye pain. There may be anorexia, nausea and vomiting. General examination may be normal or there may be petechial and mucosal bleeding noted. The liver may be enlarged and tender after a few days of fever. The tourniquet test is positive (the BP cuff is inflated to the midpoint between SBP and DBP for 5 minutes; the test is positive when >10 petechial spots appear/square inch). The earliest abnormality in the FBC count is a progressive decrease in WBC, which should alert the physician to a high probability of dengue.

2. **Stage of critical illness:** This is a stage of capillary leak that manifests from day 3–8. During this stage, the fever starts subsiding. If not identified and treated effectively, one or more complications may arise, resulting in a fatality.

- There is significant plasma leakage from the intravascular compartment to the extravascular compartment, which results in shock. The woman presents with persistent vomiting and lethargy but remains mentally alert. There is an increase in liver size along with tenderness. There is a progressive decrease in WBC and platelets and a rise in the hematocrit levels (PCV).
- Hemorrhagic manifestations (dengue hemorrhagic fever)—overt bleeding can manifest as bleeding per vagina or hematemesis. However, significant bleeding could often be concealed. Such bleeding can occur into the GI tract (manifest later as melena), muscles, abdominal cavity or thoracic cavity and brain.
- Severe organ involvement may develop (hepatitis, encephalitis, myocarditis)—left unattended, it leads to compensated, and later uncompensated, shock and death.

3. **Phase of recovery:** After the patient survives the 48–72 hours of the critical phase, there is gradual absorption of fluid from the extravascular phase into the intravascular compartment. Hematocrit starts to fall, and the WBC and platelet counts start to increase. This phase lasts from 7–10 days. In this phase, one should be cautious about fluid overload. In pregnancy, the clinical manifestations and management are similar to that of non-pregnant individuals. Dengue may mimic some obstetrical conditions such as the HELLP syndrome.

Effect on Pregnancy

- Dengue fever does not warrant the termination of pregnancy. There is insufficient data on probable embryopathy in women who had DF in the first trimester of their pregnancy.
- The woman may go into preterm labour, and there is a risk of vertical transmission to the baby.
- Severe bleeding may complicate delivery and/or surgical procedures performed on pregnant women with dengue during the critical phase, i.e., the period coinciding with marked thrombocytopenia with or without plasma leak.

Diagnosis

- Rapid NS1 antigen—detected on day 3 of fever
- Dengue IgM—detected after day 5 of fever
- Full blood count as a baseline should be taken to monitor the progress of the disease

Management

Management in the antenatal period

Challenges in managing dengue in pregnancy
- Vomiting, which is one of the warning signs of dengue, may be mistaken as hyperemesis of pregnancy.
- There may be failure to recognise plasma leakage and shock early, which could lead to decompensated shock and multiorgan failure.
- When the woman goes into labour, bleeding complications can occur.

For the control of temperature, paracetamol can be used, and NSAIDs should be avoided. The woman should be carefully monitored for impending capillary leak presenting with lethargy, vomiting, rising hematocrit and falling platelet counts. Intense fluid resuscitation should be given without delay.

Labour management

- Labour management in the critical phase of dengue is vital. In the presence of warning signs, intense fluid resuscitation should be undertaken to prevent further complications. 0.9% normal saline is given in a bolus of 5–10 mL/Kg/hour for 2 hours followed by 3–5 mL/Kg/hour as maintenance.
- Neither planned induction nor surgical procedures should be taken up in the critical phase.
- Tocolytics may be considered to postpone delivery.
- If delivery is inevitable, bleeding should be anticipated and closely monitored. Blood and blood products should be cross-matched and kept ready in preparation for delivery. Trauma or injury should be kept to a minimum. There should be active management of the third stage of labour to prevent PPH. Even minimal blood loss should be replaced.
- Prophylactic platelet transfusion is not recommended unless delivery is inevitable (within 6 hours). Platelet count should be >50,000/cc for vaginal delivery and >75,000/cc for operative delivery.
- In the recovery phase of infection, one should be cautious about fluid overload.
- The newborn should be monitored for vertical transmission.
- Operative delivery should be attempted for obstetric indications only.

SEXUALLY TRANSMITTED INFECTIONS

Sexually transmitted infections can complicate pregnancy. During the booking visit, history suggesting syphilis, gonorrhea, chlamydia and human immunodeficiency virus (HIV) should be elicited discretely. In India, it is recommended to routinely screen for syphilis in the antenatal period, whereas investigations for other sexually transmitted infections are carried out if indicated and in high-risk populations.

■ SYPHILIS

Syphilis is a sexually transmitted disease caused by *Treponema pallidum*, a spirochete that crosses the placenta and infects the fetus from about 14 weeks of gestation and can result in major adverse effects on the offspring. If diagnosed and treated early in pregnancy, the adverse effects are minimised.

Effect of Pregnancy on Syphilis

In most cases, syphilis runs a mild course. However, some of the secondary manifestations such as condylomata and skin rashes may get aggravated because of the increased vascularity and immunosuppressive state of pregnancy.

Effect of Syphilis on Pregnancy

The effect of this disease on pregnancy and the fetus depends upon the period of gestation at which infection occurs. Miscarriages occur more commonly in the second trimester; first-trimester miscarriages are relatively uncommon. Other complications are preterm births, delivery of low-birth-weight infants and intrauterine fetal deaths.

Diagnosis

All pregnant women should be screened for syphilis. The VDRL (Venereal Disease Research Laboratory) test is routinely performed at the first antenatal visit. Occasionally, a VDRL test may be a false positive. In such a situation, its titres never rise above 1:8. The diagnosis can be confirmed by the fluorescent or treponemal antibody test, the *Treponema pallidum* immobilisation test or a PCR test for the *Treponema pallidum* DNA.

Management

Penicillin remains the treatment of choice. **Benzathine penicillin G**, 2.4 million units, is given intramuscularly as a single injection. Sometimes, a second dose is recommended one week after the initial dose, especially for those in the third trimester or those who contract secondary syphilis.

If penicillin cannot be used, erythromycin can be given in a dose of 500 mg orally once in 6 hours for a period of two weeks. The other option is injection ceftriaxone 1 g IM od for 10–14 days. These drugs may be curative for the mother but may not prevent congenital syphilis. Therefore, infants born to mothers treated with non-penicillin regimens should be re-treated.

Congenital Syphilis

Though fetal infection can occur at any stage of maternal syphilis, it is most common in women with primary or secondary syphilis. In a newborn delivered to a mother diagnosed with syphilis, the following **signs of congenital syphilis** should be looked for:

- Evidence of edema, ascites or hydropic features
- Large abdomen due to hepatosplenomegaly
- Jaundice with petechiae or purpuric skin lesions, lymphadenopathy, rhinitis (snuffles) or pneumonia
- Cutaneous lesions
- Saddle nose—the destruction of the nasal bone and cartilage
- Frontal bossing, perforated palate
- Interstitial keratitis
- Eighth nerve deafness
- Changes in permanent teeth—Hutchison's teeth, which develop later in life

> **Placental pathology**
> With syphilitic infection, the placenta becomes large, pale, bulky, greasy and heavier than usual. Spirochetes may be detected in the placenta.

Contact Tracing

In a woman diagnosed with syphilis, the sex partner should be screened and treated.

■ GONORRHEA

Nowadays, gonorrhea is very rarely encountered during pregnancy. In most pregnant women, gonococcal infection is limited to the lower genital tract, including the cervix, urethra and peri-urethral and vestibular glands.

Effect on Pregnancy

Gonorrhea exerts an adverse influence upon the pregnant woman and may cause abortion, premature labour, preterm premature rupture of membranes, chorioamnionitis and puerperal infection.

Management

Gonorrhea diagnosed during pregnancy is treated with injection ceftriaxone 250 mg IM or cefixime 400 mg given orally as a single dose. Other drugs that can be given are cefotaxime 500 mg IM, spectinomycin 2 g IM or 3 g amoxicillin plus 1 g probenecid orally.

Management of the neonate

Gonorrheal conjunctivitis is the chief danger since the eyes of the newborn get infected during its passage through the birth canal. Neonates born to untreated mothers are given ceftriaxone 25–50 mg/Kg.

■ CHLAMYDIAL INFECTIONS

Chlamydia trachomatis is an obligate intracellular bacterium that has several serotypes, including those that cause **lymphogranuloma venereum.** The most commonly encountered strains are those that cause **cervical infection**. Most pregnant women have a subclinical or asymptomatic infection.

Chlamydial Infection and Pregnancy Outcome

It has been observed that untreated maternal cervical chlamydial infection during pregnancy increases the risk of preterm delivery, preterm premature rupture of membranes and perinatal mortality.

Management

The first line of treatment is erythromycin base 500 mg orally four times a day for 7 days, or amoxicillin 500 mg orally three times a day for 7 days. Azithromycin is an alternative and is safe for use in pregnancy.

Neonatal Infections

Ophthalmic chlamydial infections are among the most common causes of preventable blindness. Inclusion conjunctivitis develops in as many as a third of neonates born to mothers with cervical infection.

HUMAN IMMUNODEFICIENCY VIRUS (HIV) INFECTION

Acquired immunodeficiency syndrome (AIDS) is caused by HIV (Fig. 35.1). This infection leads to a disorder of the immune system, which makes the individual susceptible to life-threatening infections. The prevalence of HIV infection among pregnant women is around 0.3%. Left untreated, the vertical transmission to the fetus occurs in around 30% of cases.

The following interventions reduce mother-to-child transmission from 25–30% to <2%:

- Antiretroviral therapy during the antenatal and intrapartum periods
- Antiretroviral therapy administered to the neonate for 4–6 weeks following delivery
- Delivery by elective cesarean section
- Avoidance of breastfeeding

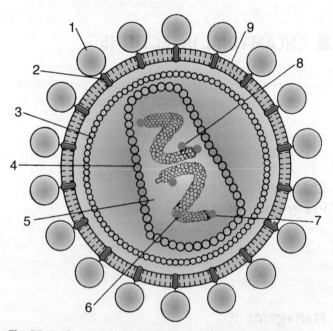

Fig. 35.1 Structure of HIV (diagrammatic representation): 1. Envelope glycoprotein spike (gp 120), 2. transmembrane pedicle glycoprotein (gp41), 3. outer icosahedral shell of nucleocapsid (p18), 4. cone-shaped core of the nucleocapsid (p24), 5. inner core, 6. viral proteins associated with RNA, 7. viral RNA, 8. reverse transcriptase and 9. envelope

Pathogenesis

HIV infection is caused by DNA retroviruses HIV 1 and HIV 2, the former being the most common infection. The infection is transmitted by the sexual route,

through blood transfusion/organ donation, through contaminated needles and through vertical transmission from the mother to the child in the antenatal, intrapartum and postpartum periods. Following the infection, predominantly T lymphocytes are affected, and there is severe immunosuppression which predisposes the individual to various opportunistic infections and neoplasms.

Clinical Features

The clinical manifestations occur in four stages—the incubation period, asymptomatic infection, symptomatic opportunistic infections and AIDS, which manifests with weight loss, chronic diarrhea and prolonged fever of >1 month. There may also be other manifestations such as persistent cough, generalised pruritus, recurrent herpes zoster, candidiasis, herpes simplex virus infection and generalised lymphadenopathy.

Routine antenatal screening

Infection with HIV is not a contraindication to pregnancy. With treatment, the risk of vertical transmission is <1%. However, without treatment, the risk is high at 15–45%. In India, the National AIDS Control Organisation (NACO) recommends that all pregnant women be counselled to undergo testing for HIV infection. The test is performed after getting the woman's informed consent. Women have the choice not to undergo HIV testing during routine antenatal care; such pregnant women should also be given the same antenatal care as others.

Diagnosis

The enzyme-linked immunosorbent assay (ELISA) is used as a screening test. If it is found to be positive, the Western blot test is carried out to confirm the diagnosis. The test becomes positive 3 months after viral transmission.

Effect on Pregnancy

The rate of fetal transmission is 25–30%, with nearly 20% occurring before 36 weeks of gestation, 50% near term and 30% due to breastfeeding if the mother is not on ART.

- During the antenatal period, the risk of mother-to-child transmission is increased due to malnutrition and invasive procedures such as amniocentesis and chorion villus sampling.
- In labour, the risk of transmission is high if the membrane is ruptured for >4 hours or if an

episiotomy is performed as this increases contact with the mother's infected blood and increases the risk of transmission. Transmission may occur at the time of vaginal delivery through exposure to cervicovaginal secretions.

- In the postnatal period, breastfeeding increases the risk of transmission.

Maternal complications

HIV infection in pregnancy can result in spontaneous abortions, ectopic pregnancies, preterm labour, PROM, abruptio placenta, genital infections with syphilis, gonorrhea, chlamydia, candida and trichomoniasis infection. Such women are also likely to suffer from recurrent urinary tract and respiratory infections. They may be malnourished and may present with anemia.

Fetal complications

Fetal complications include IUGR, low-birth-weight babies, intrauterine death and fetal infection, which may lead to fetal embryopathy presenting with microcephaly and craniofacial anomalies.

Management

Antenatal management

Besides the routine obstetrical history, history related to the involvement of the GI tract, respiratory system, genitourinary tract and nervous system and cutaneous manifestations should be elicited.

Investigations
- Complete blood count
- CD4 and CD8 count
- Viral load, LFT, RFT
- Serology for syphilis, toxoplasmosis, chlamydia, hepatitis C and B, CMV, rubella
- Urine analysis and culture
- Pap smear
- Mantoux test and screening for tuberculosis
- Stool analysis for ova and cyst
- CD4 count, as well as toxoplasmosis and syphilis serology, should be repeated periodically

- Iron, calcium, vitamin and nutritional supplements are essential to improve the general status of the individual.
- Vaccination against hepatitis should be given if HBsAg and HBC are negative.

- The HIV disease status needs to be evaluated based on the CD4 count.
- A woman who has a CD4 count of >350 will not need any therapy for herself but will need antiretroviral therapy for the prevention of perinatal transmission.
- A woman who has a CD4 count of <350 will need HAART (highly active antiretroviral therapy) for herself and to prevent perinatal transmission.

Antiretroviral drugs are classified as follows:
- Nucleoside reverse transcriptase inhibitors (NRTI): Lamivudine, zidovudine
- Non-nucleoside reverse transcriptase inhibitors (NNRTI): Nevirapine, efavirenz
- Protease inhibitors: Indinavir, lopinavir
  All of the above drugs have been found to be safe in pregnancy. However, nevirapine may cause liver toxicity.

PPTCT (prevention of parent-to-child transmission)

Under this scheme, antiretroviral therapy should be offered to all women.

Earlier regimen with zidovudine therapy

- Initiating the treatment at 28 weeks of pregnancy, in labour and to the neonate for 6 weeks reduces the risk to 6.5%.
- Initiating treatment at 36 weeks of gestation and in labour reduces the risk of transmission to 9%.
- When treatment is given in labour and to the neonate, this reduces the risk to 12%.

HAART therapy

NACO has revised their guidelines and the current technical guidelines recommend the following:
- Pregnant women with a CD4 count of <350 require HAART (highly active antiretroviral therapy).
- All HIV-infected pregnant/breastfeeding women should be initiated on lifelong ART (triple ART) at any CD4 count regardless of clinical staging. In this regimen, the WHO's three-drug regimen is recommended, wherein tenofovir (300 mg), lamivudine (300 mg) and efavirenz (600 mg) are used. This regimen should be continued lifelong for the mother.
- The neonate should be given nevirapine from birth until a minimum age of 6 weeks.

Management of labour in women living with HIV

- Antiretroviral (ARV) prophylaxis should be continued during labour.
- The number of vaginal examinations should be reduced.
- ARM should be avoided.
- Trauma during childbirth should be reduced by avoiding unnecessary episiotomy and instrumental deliveries.
- Invasive procedures on the fetus such as fetal blood sampling should be avoided.
- Active management of the third stage of labour should be practised to prevent PPH.
- Universal precautions should be strictly followed.

Cesarean section

- Elective cesarean section for obstetrical indications should be carried out preferably at 38 weeks of gestation. This reduces the risk of mother-to-child transmission.
- Cesarean section is not indicated for the prevention of mother-to-child transmission. The rate of transmission to the child is considerably low following vaginal delivery if the mother was on 3 drugs before delivery and her CD4 count was high.
- Hence, the decision for cesarean section is to be taken after deciding the benefits and risks.

Postpartum management

In the postpartum period, HIV-positive women are prone to develop puerperal sepsis and should be carefully followed up.

Breastfeeding

Nearly 30% of mother-to-child transmission takes place during breastfeeding. Though avoiding breastfeeding can reduce the risk of mother-to-child transmission, artificial feeding may be more harmful in certain socio-economic conditions wherein the family may not be able to afford to formula feed with a bottle; there is also a risk of the neonate dying of diarrhea. Therefore, the benefit of breastfeeding should be weighed against the risk of transmission of infection. There are two options:

- **Exclusive breastfeeding:** Women receiving ARV therapy can breastfeed the child; the newborn is given nevirapine prophylaxis.
- **Replacement feeding:** This completely eliminates mother-to-child transmission, especially when the neonate is receiving prophylaxis.

Contraception

Barrier methods, such as condoms, are the best methods of contraception for these women. PPIUCD can also be recommended.

Prophylaxis

Newborn prophylaxis

All babies born to HIV-positive women should be given a course of nevirapine for a period of 6 weeks, which should be started within 6–12 hours of birth. The newborn should be checked at birth, at 6 weeks, 12 and 18 months of age for HIV status.

Postexposure prophylaxis (PEP)—NACO guideline, 2014

All personnel who have had possible exposure to HIV should take medications to prevent getting infected with HIV. The medications should be taken within 3 days and preferably within 2 hours of exposure. The medications that are used are tenofovir 300 mg, lamivudine 300 mg and efavirenz 600 mg taken once daily for 28 days.

MALARIA COMPLICATING PREGNANCY

Malaria is caused by malarial parasites belonging to four species, namely *Plasmodium falciparum*, *P. vivax*, *P. ovale* and *P. malariae*. Malaria is transmitted by the bite of a sporozoite-bearing female anopheline mosquito. The parasite infects the red blood cells, causing hemolytic anemia. Compared to the general population, malaria is more common and severe among pregnant women. This is due to the immune-suppressive state of pregnancy and the availability of a new organ—the placenta—which allows the parasite to bypass the existing host immunity and multiply.

There are certain peculiarities of malaria in pregnancy—in 60–70% of cases, malaria occurs in primigravidae; the prevalence is higher in the second half of pregnancy, and two-thirds of malarial infections are caused by *P. falciparum*; these infections usually run a stormy course.

◼ SIGNS AND SYMPTOMS

- Symptoms of malaria are often non-specific.
- It can present with a flu-like illness, pyrexia, malaise, myalgia, chills, headache, diarrhea and

cough, sweating, pallor, splenomegaly, jaundice and respiratory distress.

- It can present with different patterns of fever—apyrexia, low-grade, continuous or hyperpyrexia. In the second half of pregnancy, there may be more paroxysms due to immunosuppression.
- Malaria may be associated with anemia and jaundice. Anemia may be the only presenting feature of malaria.
- In the evaluation of fever, travel-related infections such as malaria, typhoid, hepatitis, dengue, HIV, meningitis, encephalitis, SARS, avian influenza and viral hemorrhagic fever should be considered.
- Any pregnant woman presenting with pyrexia of unknown origin should be suspected of having malaria.

COMPLICATIONS

Pregnant women can develop severe complications due to *P. falciparum* infection.

- **Anemia:** Malaria can cause or aggravate anemia. This could be due to the hemolysis of red blood cells, increased demands of pregnancy or profound hemolysis, which can also cause folate deficiency. Anemia due to malaria is more common and severe between 16 and 29 weeks. It can develop suddenly due to high levels of parasitemia.
- **Acute pulmonary edema, respiratory distress and ARDS:** These can develop suddenly in the immediate postpartum period due to the autotransfusion of the peripheral blood with a high proportion of parasitised RBCs.
- **Hypoglycemia:** It is more common in pregnancy due to the increased demands of the hypercatabolic state and infecting parasites. In these women, the hypoglycemia may remain asymptomatic and consequently, go undetected; occasionally, there may be abnormal behaviour, convulsions, altered sensorium and sudden loss of consciousness. These symptoms of hypoglycemia may be easily confused with cerebral malaria. Therefore, in all women with falciparum malaria, blood sugar should be monitored every 4–6 hours.
- **Secondary infections:** As there is immunosuppression in all pregnancies, a woman who acquires malaria is prone to secondary infections such as UTI and pneumonia. Gram-negative septicemic shock can occur following secondary bacterial infection and is called 'algid malaria'.
- Pregnant women who have malaria can develop hyperpyrexia and acute renal failure.

EFFECT ON PREGNANCY

- Malaria in pregnancy is detrimental to the fetus. High-grade fever, placental insufficiency, hypoglycemia and anemia can adversely affect the fetus. Perinatal mortality ranges from 15–70%.
- Women may present with spontaneous miscarriage, premature birth, stillbirth, placental insufficiency and IUGR. Malaria may result in low-birth-weight babies, fetal distress and transplacental spread of infection to the fetus, leading to congenital malaria.
- Congenital malaria occurs in 5% of pregnancies complicated by malaria. All four species of *Plasmodium* can cause congenital malaria, but the chances are greatest with *P. malariae*. The newborn may present with fever, irritability, feeding problems and hepatosplenomegaly, anemia, jaundice, etc.

DIAGNOSIS OF MALARIA IN PREGNANCY

- The available methods for diagnosing malaria are the microscopic examination of thick and thin blood films for parasites and rapid diagnostic tests.
- Currently, microscopic examination remains the gold standard method for diagnosing malaria. It allows species identification and quantification of the number of infected red blood cells (parasitemia). It also helps to identify the stage of the parasite, namely trophozoite or schizont of *P. falciparum*.
- The rapid diagnostic test detects a specific parasite antigen or enzyme. This test should always be followed by microscopy to quantify parasitemia and to confirm the species and the stage of the parasite.
- In a febrile patient, three negative malaria smears 12–24 hours apart rule out the diagnosis of malaria.

In order to anticipate complications, the following investigations are done:
- Random blood sugar is checked every 4–6 hours
- Hemoglobin and parasite count should be performed every 12 hours
- Intake output chart
- Serum creatinine and serum bilirubin levels

Patients presenting with malaria can be broadly divided into two groups—those with uncomplicated malaria and those with severe and complicated malaria.

Uncomplicated Malaria

This is defined by the following features:

- The woman does not show signs and symptoms of severity
- There are no complications
- <2% of red cells are parasitised

Complicated Malaria

This is characterised by the following features:

- The signs, symptoms and laboratory test results indicate severity
- >2% of red cells are parasitised

The clinical manifestations of severe malaria include the following:

- Impaired consciousness
- Respiratory distress—ARDS, acidosis
- Pulmonary edema
- Convulsions
- Shock
- DIVC
- Jaundice
- Hemoglobinuria (without G6PD deficiency)

Laboratory tests that indicate severe disease are as follows:

- Severe anemia—Hb <8 g/dL
- Thrombocytopenia
- Hypoglycemia—<40 mg/dL
- Acidosis—pH <7.3
- Renal impairment—oliguria and raised creatinine levels
- Hyperlactatemia
- Hyper parasitemia—>2% of parasitised red blood cells
- Algid malaria—with superimposed gram-negative septicemia

■ MANAGEMENT

Malaria is a medical emergency, and women with suspected malaria should be evaluated immediately. The treatment of malaria in pregnancy should be energetic.

The management of malaria in pregnancy includes:

- Medical treatment of malaria
- Identification of complications and their management
- Management of labour

Medical Management of Malaria

The antimalarials commonly used in pregnancy are presented in Table 35.1.

Table 35.1 Antimalarials used to treat malaria in pregnancy

Trimester	Antimalarial drugs used
All trimesters	Chloroquine, quinine, artesunate (contraindicated in early pregnancy, but can be used in severe cases), artemether, arteether
2nd and 3rd trimesters	Mefloquine, pyremethamine, sulfadoxine

- Primaquine, tetracycline and doxycycline are contraindicated in pregnancy.
- **Management of non-falciparum malaria:**
  - The treatment of choice for non-falciparum malaria is a 3-day course of oral chloroquine. It is given in a dose of 600 mg followed by 300 mg 8 hours later and then 300 mg on day 2 and day 3.
  - Dormant parasites (hypnozoites) can persist in the liver after treatment. This can result in a relapse even after a year. In order to prevent relapses, the woman is treated with weekly chloroquine at a dose of 300–500 mg until delivery. Once lactation ceases, radical treatment with primaquine is instituted.
- **Treatment of uncomplicated falciparum malaria in pregnancy:**
  - Chloroquine should not be used for the treatment of falciparum malaria. Drugs that are used in uncomplicated falciparum malaria are quinine, mefloquine, proguanil and artesunates.
  - The WHO recommends an artemisinin-based combination therapy as the first-line treatment in the 2nd and 3rd trimesters of pregnancy.
  - Artemisinin is contraindicated in the first trimester due to embryo and fetal toxicity. However, it is a life-saving drug that can be used in the first trimester in a dose of 2 mg/Kg/day for 3 days **if other drugs are unsuitable**.
  - Sulphadoxine is contraindicated in the first trimester as it is a folic acid antagonist and can lead to NTD and cardiac anomalies.
- **Treatment of severe and complicated falciparum malaria in pregnancy:**
  - Parenteral therapy is used when the parasitic count is >2%.

Supportive Care in Malaria

- Monitor for hypoglycemia regularly
- Administer careful fluid therapy to prevent pulmonary edema
- Use antibiotics to prevent secondary infection

- Anemic patients are given packed cells/exchange transfusion
- Exchange transfusion is required when the parasite density is >10% or with complications such as cerebral malaria, ARDS or renal complications

Obstetric Management

- Falciparum infection can induce uterine contractions.
- The woman may present with preterm labour, IUGR or fetal heart rate abnormalities.
- Stillbirth and preterm labour can be prevented by effectively managing malaria.
- Uncomplicated malaria is not an indication for the induction of labour.
- In severe malaria, CTG abnormalities are very common with fetal tachycardia, bradycardia, late deceleration with uterine contractions due to high temperature and hypoglycemia. CTG changes will revert to normal with the control of temperature and correction of hypoglycemia.
- Standard obstetric principles apply. The life of the woman comes first in obstetric management.
- Tocolytic therapy and steroids can be given at the usual dose.

Management of labour

- In labour, careful fluid management is very important. Overloading and dehydration should be avoided as both are detrimental to the mother and fetus.
- The second stage should be shortened by forceps or ventouse if there is maternal or fetal distress.
- Acute malaria can cause thrombocytopenia and hence, the obstetrician should be cautious of PPH.
- In severe malaria, the role of cesarean section for a viable fetus is unproven.
- At delivery, placental and cord blood films should be prepared, and the placenta should be sent for HPE.
- If the parasitemia is very severe, exchange transfusion is required.

Antenatal care after recovery

This comprises the following measures:
- Periodical assessment of maternal hemogram
- Platelets and glucose
- Growth scans to diagnose FGR

CHEMOPROPHYLAXIS IN PREGNANCY

All pregnant women who live in malaria-endemic areas should be protected with chemoprophylaxis against malaria. Two strategies are followed:
1. Chemoprophylaxis with chloroquine
2. Intermittent preventive therapy

Choice of Drug for Chemoprophylaxis

- Chloroquine is the safest drug in pregnancy and should be the first choice. 500 mg chloroquine is administered every week during pregnancy and continued for one month after delivery.
- In women travelling to malaria-endemic areas, 300 mg of chloroquine is given orally every week and continued for a month after return.
- Because of poor compliance and drug resistance, intermittent preventive therapy with sulphadoxine and pyrimethamine can be used in the second trimester. Here, 2 doses of curative treatment are given 4 weeks apart in the 2nd and 3rd trimesters of pregnancy.

CONGENITAL MALARIA

Maternal malaria close to delivery can result in congenital malaria. Vertical transmission of malaria occurs when malarial parasites cross the placenta either during pregnancy or at birth, especially when the cord/placental bed is positive for malaria. It can occur in 5% of pregnancies. All four species of *Plasmodium* can cause congenital malaria, but the incidence is greatest with *P. malariae*. Congenital malaria can manifest in the first few weeks to months of delivery. The newborn may present with fever, irritability, feeding problems and hepatosplenomegaly, anemia, jaundice, etc. If the placenta is positive for parasites, weekly screening of the newborn for 28 days is useful for the early detection and treatment of congenital malaria The diagnosis can be confirmed by performing a smear test on cord blood or blood drawn from a heel prick to look for malarial parasites within a week of delivery. All neonates whose mothers developed malaria in pregnancy should be screened for malaria with standard microscopy of thick and thin films weekly for 28 days.

Prevention

Vaccines against malaria may be available in the near future.

KEY POINTS

Toxoplasmosis:

- ✓ The risk of fetal infection is highest in the third trimester, but if infection occurs, the severity is greatest in the first trimester.
- ✓ Diagnosis is based on serology showing positive IgM and low IgG avidity and the presence of increasing titres and seroconversion.
- ✓ Diagnosis of fetal infection is made by PCR test on amniotic fluid after 18 weeks of gestation.
- ✓ To reduce the risk of transmission to the fetus, spiramycin is used and should be continued throughout pregnancy.
- ✓ Fetal infection is treated with pyrimethamine and sulfadiazine, both of which cross the placenta.

Rubella:

- ✓ In cases where the rubella infection is acquired in the first trimester of pregnancy, >90% of the fetuses are affected. Therefore, the termination of pregnancy is recommended in such cases.
- ✓ If the infection is acquired in the second and third trimesters of pregnancy, the extended rubella syndrome can occur.
- ✓ The presence of rubella-specific IgG antibody >15 IU/mL indicates immunity against rubella.
- ✓ Rubella vaccination should not be given during pregnancy.

CMV infection:

- ✓ This is the commonest infection to cause fetal damage.
- ✓ Among pregnant women who are infected, 50% of the fetuses will be infected and 10% will suffer damage.

Herpes simplex virus infection:

- ✓ Cesarean delivery is recommended in women with an active genital lesion.
- ✓ The specific treatment for HSV is the use of antiviral drugs such as acyclovir, valacyclovir, etc. The dose is 200 mg of acyclovir five times a day for 5–7 days.

Zika virus infection:

- ✓ Zika virus infection is transmitted by the bites of **Aedes** mosquitoes.
- ✓ The risk of congenital Zika virus infection is 10%—the CNS is predominantly affected, and microcephaly is usually seen.

Chickenpox:

- ✓ A non-immune pregnant woman exposed to chickenpox should be given varicella-zoster immunoglobulin.
- ✓ Pregnant women suffering from chickenpox should be treated with acyclovir.

COVID-19:

- ✓ Induction of labour and cesarean section are carried out only for obstetrical indications.
- ✓ Pregnant and breastfeeding women are advised to take the vaccine against COVID.

Dengue:

- ✓ This is a common viral infection.
- ✓ If not managed properly, it has a potential to develop into life-threatening complications, more so in labour, during which period, complications may be easily missed.
- ✓ Dengue has a high mortality rate up of upto 20%.
- ✓ With prevention and early identification of complications and their treatment, mortality can be reduced to <1%.

HIV infection:

- ✓ Treating an HIV-positive pregnant woman reduces the transmission of the infection to the newborn significantly.
- ✓ Cesarean section is not indicated for the prevention of mother-to-child transmission.
- ✓ All HIV-infected pregnant/breastfeeding women should be initiated on lifelong ART (on triple ART) at any CD4 count regardless of clinical staging.

Malaria:

- ✓ Two-thirds of malarial infections are caused by P. falciparum. These infections can run a stormy course.
- ✓ Pregnant women can develop severe complications due to P. falciparum infection such as hypoglycemia, severe anemia and ARDS.
- ✓ Primaquine is contraindicated in pregnancy.
- ✓ Chloroquine is contraindicated in the management of falciparum malaria.

Essay questions

1. A 30-year-old primigravida presents at 8 weeks of gestation for routine antenatal care. She has had an HIV infection for the past one year.
   a) What are the antenatal complications she is expected to develop?
   b) What investigations need to be performed?
   c) What retroviral therapy should be given?
   d) What precautions should be taken in labour to prevent neonatal transmission?
2. Discuss the management of HIV during pregnancy.
3. Describe the diagnosis and management of malaria complicating pregnancy.

Short answer questions

Write notes on the following:
1. Congenital toxoplasmosis
2. Congenital syphilis
3. Fetal varicella syndrome
4. Congenital Zika virus syndrome
5. Management of H1N1 infection in pregnancy

MCQs

1. Which of the following is not included in TORCH infections?
   a) Toxoplasmosis
   b) Rubella
   c) Cytomegalovirus
   d) Herpes zoster
2. Which of the following is not a feature of congenital rubella syndrome?
   a) Cataract
   b) Heart disease
   c) Renal disease
   d) CNS defect
3. The classic triad of clinical manifestations of congenital toxoplasmosis constitutes the following EXCEPT:
   a) Hydrocephalus
   b) Chorioretinitis
   c) Intracranial calcifications
   d) Sensorineural deafness
4. Which of the following is not true for congenital toxoplasmosis?
   a) The mother must have acquired the infection during the current pregnancy.
   b) Fetal transmission is as high as 40–60% if the infection occurs in the third trimester.
   c) Fetal transmission is only 5–15% if the infection occurs in the first trimester.
   d) The risk to the fetus is more severe when the infection occurs in the latter half of pregnancy.
5. Which of the following drugs is not used for the treatment of toxoplasmosis during pregnancy?
   a) Spiramycin
   b) Pyrimethamine
   c) Metronidazole
   d) Sulphadiazine
6. The following are true of rubella antibody titres EXCEPT:
   a) The absence of rubella antibody indicates susceptibility.
   b) IgG antibodies to rubella can persist for a long time.

c) A non-immune person who acquires rubella viremia demonstrates peak antibody titres 4–6 weeks after the onset of the rash.
   d) The presence of rubella-specific IgM is diagnostic of a recent infection.
7. When should the screening for cytomegalovirus infection be done during pregnancy?
   a) First trimester
   b) Second trimester
   c) Third trimester
   d) Serological screening is not recommended
8. Which of the following is not a characteristic feature of the placenta in pregnancy complicated by syphilitic infection?
   a) Large
   b) Pale
   c) Greasy
   d) Calcified
9. A neonate born with congenital syphilis may have the following features EXCEPT:
   a) Hepatosplenomegaly
   b) Hydropic features
   c) Lymphadenopathy
   d) Chorioretinitis
10. Which of the following is not a risk associated with maternal chlamydial infection during pregnancy?
    a) Preterm labour
    b) Preterm premature rupture of membranes
    c) Intrauterine growth restriction
    d) Neonatal conjunctivitis
11. If a susceptible pregnant woman is exposed to chickenpox, the choice of treatment is:
    a) Termination of pregnancy
    b) Administration of varicella-zoster immunoglobulin
    c) Oral acyclovir
    d) Administration of varicella-zoster vaccine
12. The antimalarial contraindicated in pregnancy is:
    a) Chloroquine
    b) Primaquine
    c) Quinine
    d) Artesimine
13. Transplacental infection occurs in all the following except:
    a) Malaria
    b) Syphilis
    c) Gonorrhea
    d) Rubella

Answers
1. (d), 2. (c), 3. (d), 4. (d), 5. (c), 6. (c), 7. (d), 8. (d), 9. (d), 10. (c), 11. (b), 12, (b), 13. (c)

Fill in the blanks

1. Toxoplasmosis is caused by _____.
2. The drug of choice for herpes simplex infection during pregnancy is _____.
3. The mode of delivery in a woman with an active genital herpes lesion should be _____.
4. The drug of choice for the treatment of syphilis during pregnancy is _____.
5. The test used for the confirmation of the diagnosis of syphilis in pregnancy is _____.
6. The most common manifestation in a newborn of a woman suffering from gonorrhea is _____.

Answers

1. *Toxoplasma gondii*, 2. acyclovir, 3. cesarean section, 4. penicillin, 5. VDRL, 6. conjunctivitis

Case scenario-based discussion

1. A 9 weeks pregnant woman visits the clinic. She has an 8-year-old son who was diagnosed with rubella 10 days ago. On eliciting the history, she says that she has never suffered from rubella in the past and does not recall being immunised. What would your advice to her be?

Answers

- She should be told that she may still be immune to rubella.
- It should be explained to her that at her stage of pregnancy, almost all babies are affected if the mother is found to have recent or current infection. At gestational age <11 weeks, 100% defects can occur.
- Blood samples should be tested for IgM and IgG antibody titres.
- Termination of pregnancy should be recommended if the woman is IgM-positive.

36

OG 12.5

Diseases of the Urinary System Complicating Pregnancy

Learning Objectives

» To describe asymptomatic bacteriuria
» To discuss the predisposing factors for urinary tract infection in pregnancy
» To discuss the diagnosis and management of urinary tract infection in pregnancy
» To discuss the effect of urinary tract infection on pregnancy

---

■ INTRODUCTION

Though some urinary tract disorders may exist prior to pregnancy, the majority of urinary tract complications are encountered during pregnancy.

■ URINARY TRACT CHANGES DURING PREGNANCY

During pregnancy, a number of structural and functional changes take place in the urinary tract.

- Due to the smooth muscle relaxation caused by progesterone, there is dilatation of the renal calyces, pelvis and ureters.
- The pressure exerted by the enlarging uterus can also result in hydroureter and hydronephrosis.
- Effective renal plasma flow and glomerular filtration are increased, on average, by 40% and 65%, respectively. These changes have clinical relevance at the time of interpreting renal function tests. For example, serum concentrations of creatinine and urea are decreased in normal pregnancy.

■ FACTORS PREDISPOSING TO URINARY TRACT INFECTION IN PREGNANCY

Owing to the shortness of the urethra and its close proximity to the vagina, women are more prone to urinary tract infections than men, more so during pregnancy. A number of factors contribute to the increased prevalence of UTI in pregnancy. These are as follows:

- The apparent reduction in immunity of pregnant women along with stasis of urine appears to encourage the growth of both commensal and non-commensal microorganisms.
- The physiological increase in plasma volume and the resulting urine concentrations in pregnancy encourage bacterial growth in urine.
- Glycosuria and aminoaciduria, which develop during pregnancy, create an excellent culture medium for the growth of bacteria.
- Associated comorbid conditions like gestational diabetes mellitus also add to this burden.
- The stasis of urine due to dilated ureters along with the increased vesicoureteral reflux predisposes to upper urinary tract infections by facilitating the ascent of bacteria from the bladder to the kidney.
- Catheterisation in the intrapartum and postpartum periods are iatrogenic causes of UTI in pregnancy.

■ URINARY TRACT INFECTIONS

Urinary tract infections can manifest in three forms, which are as follows:

- Asymptomatic bacteriuria
- Cystitis
- Pyelonephritis

Asymptomatic Bacteriuria

Asymptomatic bacteriuria refers to the presence of more than $1,00,000$ colonies ($\geq 10^5$) of a single bacterial species per millilitre of urine, cultured from a midstream sample in the absence of symptoms. Asymptomatic bacteriuria occurs in 5–7% of pregnant women. Without treatment, 30–40% of pregnant women with asymptomatic bacteriuria will progress to symptomatic urinary tract infections such as cystitis and pyelonephritis.

Effect on maternal and fetal outcome

If asymptomatic bacteriuria is left untreated, it can lead to acute cystitis in 40% of cases and pyelonephritis in 20–30% of cases during the pregnancy. It can also lead to adverse obstetric events such as anemia, pre-eclampsia, abortions, preterm labour, IUGR and low-birth-weight infants and puerperal sepsis. Persistent anemia in spite of effective treatment should arouse the suspicion of asymptomatic bacteriuria which should be investigated and treated. Asymptomatic bacteriuria may recur or persist after delivery.

Effect of asymptomatic bacteriuria on pregnancy is associated with the following risks:
- Maternal anemia
- Maternal hypertension or pre-eclampsia
- Preterm delivery
- Intrauterine growth restriction
- Persistence of infection after delivery

The most common organisms that can cause asymptomatic bacteriuria are *Escherichia coli*, *Klebsiella*, *Proteus*, *Pseudomonas* and *Staphylococcus saprophyticus*. These organisms are mostly found in the periurethral and perianal areas. Among these, *E. coli* is the commonest organism, isolated in >90% of cases of asymptomatic bacteriuria.

Diagnosis

All pregnant women should be screened for asymptomatic bacteriuria during the first antenatal visit, before 14 weeks of gestation.

Urine culture is the gold standard method for the detection of bacteriuria in pregnancy. It is considered the most reliable method for the diagnosis of urinary tract infection. Though it is the definitive test to diagnose bacteriuria, universal screening with urine culture during pregnancy may not be feasible in low-resource settings, as the test is expensive, and the necessary laboratory support and staff may not be available at all centres. Therefore, in developing countries, simple methods such as pus cell count, nitrite test and leukocyte esterase test on dipsticks can be used. If these screening tests are positive, then urine culture should be carried out. The microscopic examination of the centrifuged urine in a wet film is used for the identification of pus cells. A pus cell count of more than 10/HPF indicates the presence of asymptomatic bacteriuria.

Frequent screening for asymptomatic bacteriuria every 4–6 weeks is recommended for the following groups of pregnant women:
- Previous h/o asymptomatic bacteriuria
- Pre-existing renal disease
- Renal calculi
- Structural and neuropathic abnormalities of renal tracts
- Pre-existing diabetes mellitus

Management

Women diagnosed with asymptomatic bacteriuria are treated as per the sensitivity pattern of the organism isolated. Commonly used drugs are ampicillin, amoxicillin and cephalosporins. The duration of treatment is 5–7 days. Nitrofurantoin is best avoided in the first trimester. In nearly 30% of cases, there is a risk of persistence of infection; therefore, urine culture should be repeated 7–10 days after the completion of the course of antibiotics.

Due to the risk of persistence and recurrence of infection, monthly urine cultures are preferred during the antenatal period.

Cystitis

Undiagnosed and untreated asymptomatic bacteriuria can progress to acute cystitis in 40% of cases presenting with dysuria, increased frequency, lower abdominal pain, fever, urgency, urge incontinence, suprapubic discomfort, offensive-smelling urine, strangury, nocturia and hematuria. In women presenting with urinary symptoms, urine culture and sensitivity tests are performed, and empirical antibiotic therapy is initiated while awaiting the culture results. Antibiotics are subsequently tailored according to the culture report. The duration of treatment and follow-up is similar to that of asymptomatic bacteriuria. When a woman presents with recurrent cystitis, she should be prescribed antibiotic prophylaxis throughout the duration of pregnancy with 100 mg nitrofurantoin or 500 mg of cephalexin daily. The woman should then be monitored for the development of pyelonephritis.

Acute Pyelonephritis

Acute pyelonephritis is a serious medical complication in pregnancy that can occur in 2% of patients. Renal infection is more common after mid-pregnancy. It is usually unilateral, with right-sided involvement seen more commonly. The infection is caused by bacteria that ascend from the lower urinary tract. Of the wide spectrum of microorganisms that cause acute pyelonephritis, the most common isolate (in 90% of cases) is *E. coli*.

Symptoms

Pyelonephritis usually has a sudden onset with symptoms of fever with chills, anorexia, nausea and vomiting, and pain in one or both lumbar regions. Symptoms of cystitis may be present.

Signs

The temperature is usually raised above 101°F. On palpation, tenderness is elicited in one or both costovertebral angles in the region of the kidney.

Complications

Complications include septic shock, ARDS and anemia. Women may go into acute renal failure due to suppurative pyelonephritis, and even maternal mortality can occur.

Differential diagnosis

In the acute stage of the disease, pyelonephritis may have to be differentiated from malaria, acute appendicitis, enteric fever and abruptio placentae. Fever with rigor may simulate an episode of malaria in areas where malaria is endemic. The examination of blood and urine aids in diagnosis. Enteric fever can be ruled out by blood culture in the early days and by Widal reaction later. The presence of pain and tenderness in the lower abdomen may be mistaken for an episode of acute appendicitis. Careful physical examination and the examination of the urine help in differentiation.

Investigations

- The examination of urine is the mainstay of the diagnosis of pyelonephritis. On microscopic examination, urine contains pus cells and, on staining the sediment, numerous bacilli can be demonstrated. In the early stages, renal function is not impaired. Urine culture and sensitivity will indicate the likely pathogen and its sensitivity pattern.
- A complete hemogram may be required to look for leukocytosis.
- Blood culture is performed in the presence of comorbidities such as diabetes or signs suggesting septicemia.
- Imaging studies with renal USG may be required for women with pyelonephritis who are severely ill, in those who present with symptoms of renal colic or a history

of renal stones, in diabetics or immunosuppressed patients or those who have urosepsis.

Management

- Patients with suspected or diagnosed pyelonephritis should be hospitalised.
- The treatment involves intravenous hydration and antimicrobial therapy. The choice of antimicrobial agent depends on the sensitivity of the organism. However, it may take 48 hours to get the sensitivity results. In the meantime, empirical treatment is initiated with ampicillin plus gentamicin, cefazolin or ceftriaxone. Patients usually respond well to cephalosporins, and the drug is effective in 95% of cases. As far as possible, aminoglycosides should be avoided in pregnancy because of the fetal risk. Once the culture report is available, the antibiotic therapy is changed accordingly. Intravenous antibiotics are given until the patient becomes asymptomatic and has no fever for 24–48 hours. After the parenteral therapy, oral medications are given for 10–14 days. Most urinary infections respond readily to adequate antimicrobial therapy.
- The physiological changes in the urinary tract due to pregnancy are unaltered by treatment. Hence, reinfection and recurrence of symptoms during pregnancy and puerperium are common. Pyelonephritis in pregnancy must not be considered as cured unless the urine remains sterile on repeated examination.

Effect on pregnancy outcome

Due to the hyperpyrexia of acute pyelonephritis, miscarriage, preterm labour and IUFD can occur.

■ CHRONIC RENAL DISEASE

Chronic kidney disease may be due to various causes such as chronic pyelonephritis, chronic glomerulonephritis, diabetic nephropathy, SLE, urolithiasis and renal artery disease or nephrotic syndrome. Nephrotic syndrome is characterised by the presence of proteinuria in excess of 3 g per day, hypoalbuminemia, hyperlipidemia and edema. Women who have chronic renal disease are at an increased risk of severe hypertension, superimposed pre-eclampsia, deterioration of renal function, episodes of acute pyelonephritis and resistant anemia due to erythropoietin deficiency. Fetal risks include FGR and preterm delivery. In chronic renal disease, the outcome of pregnancy will depend on the degree of renal functional impairment and the presence or absence of hypertension.

Preconceptional Care

Preconceptional care serves the following purposes:

- The severity of renal function can be assessed.
- When there is severe impairment of renal function as in end-stage disease, termination of pregnancy is recommended in early pregnancy.
- SLE patients should be in remission for at least for 6 months before attempting pregnancy.
- Hypertension should be under control; the medications reviewed as ACE inhibitors are contraindicated in pregnancy.

Antenatal Care

- A pregnant woman with chronic renal disease requires more frequent visits and frequent checking of BP and proteinuria.
- Renal function tests should be carried out periodically.
- Resistant anemia is treated with recombinant erythropoietin.
- Aspirin is started at a dosage 100–150 mg/day from the end of the first trimester as these patients are prone to pre-eclampsia, FGR and thrombotic complications.
- Uterine artery Doppler is carried out in early pregnancy to diagnose uterine artery resistance.
- Antepartum fetal surveillance should be carried out more frequently.
- Early delivery is indicated if there is deteriorating renal function, superimposed pre-eclampsia or severe FGR.

ACUTE RENAL FAILURE (ACUTE KIDNEY INJURY)

Acute renal failure is characterised by a decrease in the GFR, rise in creatinine levels and reduced urine output. In obstetrics, acute renal failure may be encountered in various complications of pregnancy. The important ones are as follows:

- Eclampsia, HELLP syndrome
- Severe grades of accidental hemorrhage, especially the concealed variety
- Severe postpartum hemorrhage
- Septic abortion
- Mismatched blood transfusion
- Hyperemesis gravidarum
- Sepsis

Pathology

Renal failure can occur in two forms—renal tubular necrosis and renal cortical necrosis.

- Tubular necrosis is the commonest type. Here, the renal tubules undergo ischemia and necrosis and are blocked with casts. The kidney lesion in acute tubular necrosis is focal. The most characteristic findings are dilatation and flattening of the epithelium of the distal convoluted tubules. There is slow regeneration of the tubular epithelium, and renal function tests return to normal in 1–2 weeks.
- In cortical necrosis, there is diffuse necrosis of the cortex due to the irreversible damage of the end arteries. There is thrombosis of the segments of the renal vascular system. The prognosis is poor in cortical necrosis as the pathological changes are irreversible and the mortality is high.

Clinical Features

Oliguria is an important sign of acutely impaired renal function. The woman may appear to be quite well despite reduced urinary output. The latter will be noticed only if a careful record of intake and output is maintained. These women are usually thirsty, warm to touch, gradually lethargic and irritable. The blood urea level is raised, and there is associated hyperkalemia, which gives rise to muscular changes and characteristic changes in electrocardiography. The dangers are hypertension, hyperkalemia and metabolic acidosis.

Management

Management involves the correction of the underlying cause, early termination of pregnancy, correction of sepsis and blood loss, supportive therapy and careful fluid management. Potassium-containing solutions and the use of nephrotoxic drugs should be avoided. A nephrologist should be involved at every stage of management. Occasionally, dialysis may be required. Early detection and prompt management of acute renal failure in pregnancy improve maternal outcome.

PREGNANCY IN WOMEN WITH RENAL TRANSPLANT

Women who have had renal transplants form a unique population. When such a woman wishes to get pregnant, she should ideally be advised to avoid pregnancy for about 1–2 years after transplantation—at least one year following a live donor transplant and two years following a cadaver transplant. Pregnancy within the first year is associated with a high risk of acute rejection, infection and fetal exposure to immunosuppressive drugs.

Preconceptional Counselling

At the time of counselling, information on optimal timing of pregnancy, expected maternal and fetal outcomes and the risks of immunosuppression on the fetus and deterioration of renal allograft function should be discussed. Such women should be given viral prophylaxis if this was not done earlier. Graft function should be adequate before conception with serum creatinine <1.5 mg/dL, protein excretion <50 mg/24 hours and normal USG of the allograft.

Management of Pregnancy

The maintenance of immunosuppression must be continued during pregnancy to prevent the rejection of the renal transplant. All immunosuppressive drugs cross the placenta and expose the fetus to potential risks. Maternal risks include worsening of hypertension, the development of pre-eclampsia, worsening or new-onset diabetes, resistant anemia and recurrent UTI. Graft function should be checked every 2–4 weeks.

KEY POINTS

✓ *Urinary tract infection is a common bacterial infection occurring during pregnancy.*

✓ *Urinary tract infections present as asymptomatic bacteriuria, cystitis or pyelonephritis.*

✓ *The most common cause of urinary tract infection is* E. coli.

✓ *Untreated pyelonephritis progresses to cystitis in 40% and acute pyelonephritis in 25% of cases.*

✓ *Acute pyelonephritis is an infection of the upper urinary tract involving the kidneys and presenting with fever, chills and loin pain. The management involves hospitalisation, parenteral antibiotics and adequate hydration.*

✓ *Women with chronic renal failure are at risk of developing severe hypertension, superadded pre-eclampsia, acute pyelonephritis and resistant anemia.*

✓ *The causes of acute renal failure in obstetrics include eclampsia, abruption, severe PPH and septic abortion.*

✓ *In women who have had a renal transplant, pregnancy should be avoided for 2 years. The woman should have stable graft and renal function before attempting pregnancy.*

Essay questions

1. A 27-year-old G3P1 attends the antenatal clinic at 14 weeks of gestation. Urine culture shows the presence *of E. coli*. She does not have any urinary symptoms.
   a) What are the various urinary tract infections a pregnant woman can develop?
   b) What is asymptomatic bacteriuria?
   c) What are the maternal and fetal effects of asymptomatic bacteriuria in pregnancy?
   d) How do you treat asymptomatic bacteriuria?

2. Discuss the clinical features, differential diagnosis and management of acute pyelonephritis during pregnancy.

Short answer questions

1. Discuss acute renal failure in obstetrics.
2. Describe the preconceptional counselling to be given to a woman who has a renal transplant.

MCQs

1. All the following renal changes occur during normal pregnancy EXCEPT:
   a) Dilatation of the renal calyces and pelvis
   b) Increase in plasma flow by 70%
   c) Increase in glomerular filtration rate by 65%
   d) Fall in serum concentrations of creatinine and urea

2. All the following complications in pregnancy can cause renal failure EXCEPT:
   a) Septic abortion
   b) Accidental hemorrhage
   c) Heart disease
   d) Eclampsia

3. A 24-year-old G2P1 comes for her first prenatal visit at 13 weeks of gestation. The urine culture showed >100,000 *E. coli* bacteria/mL of urine. The woman does not have any symptoms. Which of the following is the best course of action for this patient?
   a) Observation; no treatment required
   b) Initiate antibiotic therapy empirically
   c) Initiate antibiotic therapy based on the sensitivity
   d) Initiate treatment when the patient develops symptoms

4. Asymptomatic bacteriuria in pregnancy may be associated with an increased risk of the following EXCEPT:
   a) Maternal anemia
   b) Hypertension
   c) Low birth weight
   d) Renal failure

5. Acute renal failure may be encountered in the following complications of pregnancy EXCEPT:
   a) Eclampsia
   b) Gestational diabetes mellitus
   c) Severe postpartum hemorrhage
   d) Septic abortion

6. Nephrotic syndrome is characterised by the following EXCEPT:
   a) Proteinuria
   b) Hypoalbuminemia
   c) Hyperlipidemia
   d) Bacteriuria

Answers

1. (b), 2. (c), 3. (c), 4. (d), 5. (b), 6. (d)

Fill in the blanks

1. The most common organism causing urinary tract infection in pregnancy is _____.

2. Acute pyelonephritis is more common on the _____ side.

3. The duration of treatment in acute pyelonephritis during pregnancy should be at least _____.

4. Nephrotic syndrome is characterised by proteinuria in excess of _____ per day.

5. An important sign of acutely impaired renal function is _____.

Answers

1. *E. coli*,   2. right,   3. 10 days,   4. 3 g,   5. oliguria

Case scenario-based discussion

1. A 28-year-old primigravida attends the casualty at 34 weeks of gestation with high fever associated with chills and severe pain in the flanks. In her past history, she was diagnosed with asymptomatic bacteriuria at 14 weeks of gestation and was treated. Her temperature is 102°F, pulse is 100 bpm, tongue is dry, and BP is 100/70 mmHg. There is costovertebral tenderness. The uterus corresponds to 34 weeks of gestation, is well-relaxed and the FH is good.

   a) What is the most likely diagnosis and what investigation you will order?

   b) Which is the most commonly isolated microorganism in pyelonephritis?

   c) How would you treat this woman?

Answers

a) The most likely diagnosis is acute pyelonephritis. The chances of persistence or recurrent infection following treatment of asymptomatic bacteriuria is 30%. Following the treatment of asymptomatic bacteriuria in early pregnancy, the woman should have repeat urine cultures 10 days after the completion of the course of antibiotic therapy. Thereafter, the tests should be repeated once every month. Urine culture is the investigation to be ordered now.

b) The most commonly isolated organism in pyelonephritis is *E. coli*, which is the causative organism in 90% of cases. *Proteus* and *Klebsiella* can also cause pyelonephritis but are not the common causative organisms. *Candida* is not associated with urinary tract infection.

c) Acute pyelonephritis is a serious medical condition. Therefore, the woman should be hospitalised and treated with IV hydration and empirical antibiotic therapy until the culture results are available. Patients usually respond to parenteral cephalosporins/ampicillin and gentamycin combination. Once the patient is afebrile for 48 hours, oral medication is continued for 10–14 days. Urine culture is repeated once a month.

37 Epilepsy Complicating Pregnancy

Learning Objectives

» To know the pre-pregnancy counselling for epilepsy complicating pregnancy
» To know the effect of epilepsy on pregnancy and pregnancy on epilepsy
» To discuss the antenatal management of an epileptic woman

INTRODUCTION

Very often, epilepsy is diagnosed prior to pregnancy. However, if epilepsy manifests for the first time during pregnancy, other conditions causing seizures such as eclampsia, cortical vein thrombosis, brain tumours, and metabolic conditions such as hypoglycemia and hypocalcemia should be ruled out before making a diagnosis of epilepsy. These women need an MRI of the brain, EEG and other investigations to rule out other conditions.

PRE-PREGNANCY COUNSELLING

Women with epilepsy who intend to become pregnant should have pre-pregnancy counselling to discuss the following:

- All women should be counselled regarding the increased risks of fetal malformation and neurodevelopmental abnormalities and should be made aware of the dangers of stopping any medication during pregnancy unless indicated by a clinician.
- If the woman has been seizure-free for more than 2 years, withdrawal of anticonvulsant drugs may be considered because of the risk of teratogenesis.
- However, 20–50% of women will experience recurrence of convulsions when the anticonvulsant drugs are withdrawn.
- If the decision has been made to withdraw the drugs, this should be done gradually to reduce the risk of recurrence.
- The woman should not stop or reduce the medications on her own as doing so is associated with the risk of recurrence of seizures, which predisposes her to severe maternal risks including death.

EFFECT OF PREGNANCY ON EPILEPSY

In nearly 50% of women, there is no change in the frequency of seizures; in 37%, the frequency increases and in the remaining, which is a small proportion of women, the frequency of seizures reduces. Women who have been seizure-free in the previous year are likely to remain seizure-free during pregnancy. The increased frequency of seizures is usually due to non-compliance in taking the medication, sleep deprivation, stress, hormonal changes and altered concentration of the drug in the blood.

EFFECT OF EPILEPSY ON PREGNANCY

- Folic acid levels tend to decrease in those on antiepileptic drugs (AED), especially phenytoin and phenobarbitone. This predisposes women to folic acid deficiency anemia and neural tube defects in the fetus. Therefore, women should be given 5 mg folic acid supplement in the preconceptional period, which should be continued throughout pregnancy to prevent folic acid deficiency anemia.
- The chances of developing status epilepticus are high during pregnancy.
- Sudden unexplained death associated with epilepsy is twice more common during pregnancy. This is more common in patients taking lamotrigine because the serum levels of the drug tend to fall during pregnancy.
- In the postpartum period, there is a risk of accidents for both the mother and her offspring. In the interest of safety, the woman should be advised to have a companion with her at all times and to sleep on the floor.
- Because of the effect of the drug, the woman may suffer from irritability, depression and poor concentration.

EFFECT ON THE FETUS

- The incidence of fetal anomalies in the offspring of women on antiepileptic drugs is 4–6%, whereas, in the general population, it is 1–2%. This may be due to epilepsy itself, due to genetic predisposition, or in the majority of cases, due to antiepileptic medications.

- The incidence of fetal anomalies is increased in women taking more than one antiepileptic drug. Therefore, whenever possible, women of childbearing age should be maintained on single-agent therapy.

- Sodium valproate is considered to be the most teratogenic of all the AEDs and is associated with a lower IQ in offspring in addition to the autism spectrum disorders.

- Because of the high risk of fetal anomalies (>10%), sodium valproate is not used in pregnancy.

- The least risk is seen with the use of levetiracetam and lamotrigine.

- AEDs may increase the risk of hemorrhagic disease of the newborn.

- Lamotrigine and levetiracetam are the first-line therapy; however, the levels should be monitored periodically as the serum concentration can fall to >50–60% during pregnancy, predisposing to recurrence.

COMMON CONGENITAL ANOMALIES

Antiepileptic Drug Syndrome

- This was previously known as fetal hydantoin syndrome. The syndrome includes typical craniofacial abnormalities with epicanthic folds, hypertelorism, broad and flat nasal bridge, microcephaly, distal digital hypoplasia and nail hypoplasia.

- Spina bifida is associated with sodium valproate and carbamazepine use.

- Cleft lip and palate are seen with phenytoin and carbamazepine use.

- Due to genetic predisposition, the child can also develop epilepsy.

MANAGEMENT

Antenatal management

- In women who have been seizure-free for >2 years, the discontinuation of antiepileptic drugs during pregnancy may be considered. If discontinuation is not possible, monotherapy should be considered.

- Folic acid supplement should be continued throughout pregnancy.

- Women should be monitored for the development of anemia.

- A detailed USG scan is mandatory to diagnose anomalies.

- The risks of miscarriages, preterm delivery, IUGR and antepartum and postpartum hemorrhage are increased in women with epilepsy, and therefore, should be carefully monitored.

- Stress and insomnia should be avoided during pregnancy.

- Serial growth scans should be carried out from 28 weeks onwards to diagnose IUGR and fetal bradycardia.

- The serum concentration of antiepileptic drugs reduces during pregnancy due to volume expansion, increased hepatic and renal clearance and decreased intestinal absorption. Therefore, drug levels should be checked in each trimester.

- Antiepileptic drugs are enzyme inducers; further, they reduce the levels of vitamin K in the mother and the fetus. Consequently, offspring born to mothers on antiepileptic drugs are at risk of developing hemorrhagic manifestations. Therefore, vitamin K 10 mg tablets should be given to the mother from 36 weeks of gestation and the neonate should be given 1 mg IM after delivery.

Labour Management

Epilepsy is not an indication for cesarean delivery. Occasionally, women in status epilepticus may need cesarean section. Seizure may occur during labour, predisposing the mother to hypoxia and aspiration and the fetus to hypoxia. In such situations, the airway and oxygenation should be maintained and convulsions should be controlled with benzodiazepines or intravenous phenytoin. Occasionally, uterine hypertonus can occur, which can be relaxed by using tocolytic drugs. Obstetric analgesia, especially with epidural analgesia, is important to alleviate pain, which can precipitate seizures.

Postpartum Management and Breastfeeding

- The risk of seizures may be higher in the postpartum period.

- If the antiepileptic drug dose was increased during pregnancy, it should be gradually reduced to pre-pregnancy levels within a few weeks postpartum to reduce the toxicity of the drug.

- The risk of postpartum depression is also high and should be screened for.

- Though all anticonvulsant drugs are excreted in breast milk in small concentrations, breastfeeding is not contraindicated. However, the child may be irritable and may feed poorly due to the presence of small quantities of the drug in breast milk.

Contraception

As antiepileptic drugs are enzyme inducers, the use of combined oral contraceptive pills or progesterone-only pills may not be effective. Intrauterine contraceptive devices and injectable DMPA are the preferred choices.

KEY POINTS

✓ Epilepsy in pregnancy is associated with an increased incidence of congenital anomalies, mainly due to antiepileptic drugs.

✓ The chances of developing status epilepticus are high during pregnancy.

✓ Lamotrigine and levetiracetam are the first-line antiepileptic therapeutic agents.

✓ Sodium valproate is considered to be the most teratogenic of all the antiepileptic drugs, and therefore, should not be used in pregnancy.

✓ Folic acid supplement of 5 mg should be given preconceptionally and throughout pregnancy.

✓ Vitamin K supplement should be given to women on antiepileptic drugs from 36 weeks onwards and to the neonate after delivery.

✓ Seizures may occur during labour, predisposing the mother to hypoxia and aspiration and the fetus to hypoxia.

Essay question

1. Discuss the pre-pregnancy counselling and antenatal management of epilepsy complicating pregnancy.

Short answer questions

1. What is the effect of epilepsy on pregnancy?
2. What is the antiepileptic drug syndrome?

MCQs

1. All of the following antiepileptic drugs can be used in pregnancy EXCEPT:
   a) Phenytoin
   b) Carbamazepine
   c) Sodium valproate
   d) Lamotrigine

2. The first-line antiepileptic drug in pregnancy is:
   a) Phenytoin
   b) Lamotrigine
   c) Carbamazepine
   d) Diazepam

Answers
1. (c), 2. (b)

Fill in the blanks

1. The serum concentration of lamotrigine _____ during pregnancy.
2. The dosage of folic acid prescribed to women on antiepileptic drugs is _____.

Answers
1. decreases, 2. 5 mg

Case scenario-based discussion

1. A 26-year-old primigravida presents at 10 weeks of gestation for antenatal booking. She is a known case of epilepsy since the age of 13 and is being treated with phenytoin. She has been convulsion-free for the past 4 years.
   a) What is the counselling you would give her?
   b) What is the effect of epilepsy on the fetus?
   c) What is the antenatal management you will give this woman?

Answers

a) Since this woman has been seizure-free for more than 2 years, she may be advised on the withdrawal of anticonvulsant drugs because of the risk of teratogenesis. However, she should be made aware that 20–50% of patients experience recurrence of convulsions when the anticonvulsant drugs are withdrawn. There is also an increased risk of fetal malformation or neurodevelopmental abnormalities when pregnancy is complicated by epilepsy. The woman should be asked to increase the dose of folic acid to 5 mg.

b) The incidence of fetal anomalies in the offspring of women on antiepileptic drugs is 4–6% as compared to the rate of 1–2% in the general population. The common congenital anomalies noted are antiepileptic drug syndrome, where the neonate presents with typical craniofacial abnormalities with epicanthic folds, hypertelorism, a broad and flat nasal bridge, microcephaly, distal digital hypoplasia and nail hypoplasia. Spina bifida is associated with sodium valproate and carbamazepine use. Cleft lip and palate are seen with phenytoin and carbamazepine. Since antiepileptic drugs are enzyme inducers, they can reduce the levels of vitamin K, predisposing to hemorrhagic manifestations in the newborn.

c) The antenatal management for an epileptic pregnant woman is as follows:

- Folic acid supplement should be continued throughout pregnancy and women should be monitored for the development of anemia, especially the megaloblastic type. Detailed USG scan is mandatory to diagnose anomalies. The risk of miscarriages, preterm delivery, IUGR and antepartum and postpartum hemorrhage are increased in women with epilepsy. Stress and insomnia should be avoided during pregnancy.
- Serial growth scans are carried out from 28 weeks onwards to diagnose IUGR and fetal bradycardia.
- As antiepileptic drugs are enzyme inducers and since they reduce the levels of vitamin K in the mother and the fetus, therefore, offspring born to women on antiepileptic drugs are at risk of developing hemorrhagic manifestations. Therefore, vitamin K 10 mg tablet is given to the mother from 36 weeks of gestation, and the neonate is given 1 mg IM after delivery.

38 Tumours of the Uterus and Adnexae Complicating Pregnancy

OG 29.1

Learning Objectives

» To know the effects of fibroids on pregnancy
» To know the management of fibroids complicating pregnancy and labour
» To know the management of benign tumours of the ovary complicating pregnancy
» To understand the management of pre-invasive and invasive carcinoma of the cervix diagnosed in pregnancy

INTRODUCTION

Tumours of the uterus and adnexae, though rare, can complicate pregnancy. These tumours may be benign or malignant. In this chapter, fibroids, ovarian tumours and carcinoma of the cervix complicating pregnancy will be discussed.

FIBROIDS COMPLICATING PREGNANCY

Fibroids are the most frequently encountered tumours in pregnancy. Though they were originally believed to occur in 1–2% of pregnancies, with the increasing use of ultrasonography, more cases of fibroids in pregnancy are being diagnosed. Most often, they remain asymptomatic and do not have any adverse effect on the pregnancy. However, depending on the size and location, adverse effects can occur.

Effect of Fibroids on Pregnancy

Fibroids, especially the submucous variety, diminish the chances of conception. If pregnancy does occur, fibroids can lead to various obstetric complications.

- Abortion may occur due to the distortion of the uterine cavity and impaired blood supply to the implanted ovum. This is most commonly seen in submucous fibroids and large intramural fibroids.
- There may be retention of urine in the first trimester of pregnancy, especially with posterior and cervical fibroids.
- Posterior fibroids can get incarcerated in the pouch of Douglas.

- In cases of fibroids in the upper segment, the placenta implants in the lower segment, resulting in placenta previa.
- Malpresentations and malposition are common due to the distorted uterine cavity or due to the presence of a cervical fibroid or fibroids in the lower segment.
- Placental complications such as abruption placenta, placenta previa, adherent placenta and retained placenta have also been observed.
- Torsion of the uterus can be seen very rarely in subserous fundal myomas where there is torsion of the fibroid along with the uterus.
- Premature labour may occur.
- Labour may be prolonged due to uterine inertia.
- In cervical myoma or pedunculated subserous myoma impacted in the pelvis, the labour may become obstructed.
- Postpartum hemorrhage may occur due to interference with uterine contraction and retraction.
- Chances of puerperal sepsis are increased.
- Rarely, inversion of the uterus may occur in submucous fibroids.
- Subinvolution of the uterus may occur.

Effect of Pregnancy on Fibroids

During pregnancy, fibroids increase in size due to increased vascularity, edema and hypertrophy of the uterine musculature. There is also softening due to edema and vascularity. In pregnancy and the puerperium, fibroids are more likely to undergo degenerative changes, particularly red degeneration. Subserous fibroids may undergo torsion. Extrusion of submucous myoma may also rarely occur in the puerperium.

Diagnosis of Fibroids During Pregnancy

Most often, fibroids are asymptomatic and are diagnosed during USG assessment of early pregnancy. If fibroids are identified by USG, their number, size and location are noted. In cases of large fibroids complicating pregnancy, the size of the uterus is larger than the period of amenorrhea.

Management

Management in pregnancy

- In the majority of cases, no intervention is required during pregnancy. Subserous fibroids and intramural fibroids, even large ones, do not affect the pregnancy unless they involve the endometrium.
- If a miscarriage occurs, the chances of incomplete abortion and subsequent infection are high.
- Red degeneration of a fibroid is the most common type of degeneration that occurs in pregnancy and is reported in 8% of fibroids complicating pregnancy. This is due to the high levels of hormones in pregnancy. Usually, it occurs in the second trimester of pregnancy, when the rate of growth of the fibroid is more than the blood supply. There is arterial and venous thrombosis, leading to infarction and extensive necrosis. Histologically, the fibroid becomes soft and homogenous with necrosis in the centre. The cut section shows dark areas with a cut **'raw beef'** appearance and often contains cystic spaces. It appears red or salmon pink due to the hemolysis; there is thrombosis within the vessels. Clinically, it

presents with focal pain, tenderness over the area of the fibroid, slight abdominal distension, mild fever and vomiting. Moderate leukocytosis is common. The pain due to red degeneration may mimic acute appendicitis, abruption or pyelonephritis and other acute medical and surgical conditions. Red degeneration is managed with rest and analgesics. Antibiotics are given to prevent secondary infection. Reassurance is also important. With this conservative management, the symptoms subside within a few days, though the pain may recur at a later date. Laparotomy and myomectomy are not carried out in these patients as it results in torrential bleeding. MRI may be required to diagnose red degeneration.

- Torsion of a subserous fibroid may occur rarely, presenting with acute abdomen, which will require laparotomy and removal of the fibroid. This is the only indication for a myomectomy during pregnancy, as myomas with a discrete pedicle can be easily removed.

Management in labour

- Once fibroids have been diagnosed in pregnancy, their position and size are assessed to see whether they would interfere with pregnancy and labour (Fig. 38.1a and b). The possible complications that may arise during pregnancy should be discussed with patients. Nearing term, based on the location of the fibroid, a decision on the mode of delivery should be made. Obstructed labour and dysfunctional labour can occur in cases of fibroids complicating pregnancy. As pregnancy advances, most fibroids will ascend into the abdomen and will

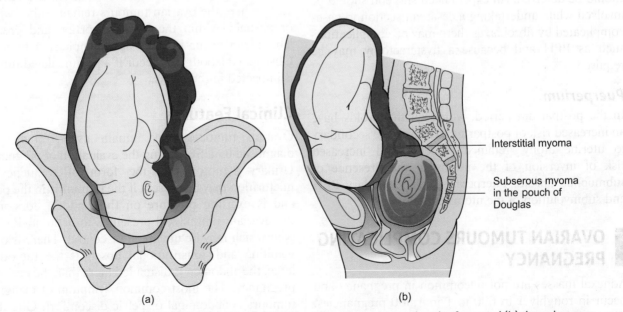

(a)   Interstitial myoma

Subserous myoma in the pouch of Douglas

(b)

Fig. 38.1 Multiple fibroids complicating pregnancy: (a) the fibroids are not obstructing the fetus and (b) the subserous myoma in the pouch of Douglas is obstructing the fetus

not complicate delivery. However, labour can be obstructed by cervical fibroids, posterior fibroids and broad ligament fibroids impacted in the POD. Dysfunctional labour can also occur due to inefficient uterine contractions.

- The presence of fibroids as such is not an indication for cesarean section. In cases where fibroids are situated above the pelvic brim, they are unlikely to obstruct the passage of the fetus and therefore, labour is allowed to proceed as for vaginal delivery. However, there are certain indications for cesarean section.

Indications for cesarean section

- Fibroids situated in the lower uterine segment that prevent the descent of the head
- Fibroids impacted in the pelvis
- Cervical fibroid, even if small, may cause problems
- Sometimes uterine inertia may occur due to the presence of fibroids
- Other obstetric complications such as oblique lie, transverse lie or other malpresentations

Technical aspects of cesarean section with fibroids

Fibroids should not be enucleated from the uterus at the time of cesarean section as this causes profuse bleeding, at times, requiring a hysterectomy. In recent years, there have been reports on enucleating fibroids that are situated on the incision site at the time of cesarean section. Typically, fibroids undergo remarkable involution after delivery. Therefore, myomectomy should be deferred. An experienced surgeon should be involved while undertaking a cesarean section in cases complicated by fibroids, as there may be complications such as PPH and because a hysterectomy may be required.

Puerperium

In the postpartum period, women with fibroids have an increased risk of postpartum hemorrhage secondary to uterine atony, retained placenta and increased risk of inversion of the uterus in the presence of submucous fibroid. Puerperal sepsis, secondary PPH and subinvolution of the uterus can also occur.

OVARIAN TUMOURS COMPLICATING PREGNANCY

Adnexal masses are not uncommon in pregnancy and occur in roughly 1 in 600 to 1 in 1,500 pregnancies. The majority of these are benign and only 1–3% may be malignant. The commonest benign tumours

encountered in pregnancy are mature cystic teratomas (dermoid cysts), followed by benign serous and mucinous cystadenomas. Physiological cysts such as corpus luteum cysts and theca luteal cysts are also encountered in pregnancy.

Effect of Pregnancy and Labour on Ovarian Tumours

Pregnancy does not have any particular effect on ovarian tumours. Torsion is the commonest complication, seen particularly in pedunculated tumours that lie above the pelvic brim. Due to the softening and edema of the pelvic tissues and the displacement of the ovary, there is also a predisposition to torsion. It is more common during the puerperium than pregnancy due to the lax abdominal wall; the large intra-abdominal space after birth allows free mobility of the tumour. Torsion can also occur in the first trimester of pregnancy. Hemorrhage and rupture are the other complications associated with ovarian cysts, especially in corpus luteal cysts. Infection is more likely to occur in the puerperium. Rarely, incarceration may occur with dermoid cysts, which have a tendency to remain in the pelvis.

Effect of Ovarian Tumours on Pregnancy

These depend on the size and location of the tumour. In the early weeks of pregnancy, ovarian tumours may give rise to pressure symptoms, particularly on the urinary bladder. In the later weeks of pregnancy, if the tumour is large, pressure symptoms such as difficulty in breathing can occur. Malpresentations are likely in cases where the ovarian tumours remain either wholly or partially within the pelvis. Abortion and preterm labour can occur in large and complicated tumours. Obstructed labour can occur if a pedunculated tumour is impacted in the pelvis.

Clinical Features

Ovarian tumours may remain asymptomatic and diagnosed by USG during the evaluation of pregnancy. Urinary symptoms in the form of frequency of micturition may be present if the tumour is in the pelvis and is exerting pressure on the bladder. Torsion of the ovarian tumour will present with acute abdominal pain which may be unilateral or central. There is often vomiting and constitutional upset. If the tumour is large, the abdomen is distended more than the period of pregnancy. The most common symptom of malignant tumours is abdominal or pelvic discomfort. One-third of ovarian cancers are diagnosed incidentally. The majority of tumours present as stage I tumours.

Diagnosis of Ovarian Tumours

Pelvic examination in early pregnancy may reveal the presence of a mass separate from the uterus. In some cases, a groove may be felt separating the tumour from the gravid uterus. When the tumour is large, there is overdistension of the abdomen. Confirmation of the presence of an ovarian tumour is by the USG of the abdomen and pelvis. Magnetic resonance imaging (MRI) is safe in all trimesters of pregnancy. It is the imaging technique of choice for diagnosing ovarian tumours complicating pregnancy. MRI (without contrast) is useful in assessing the extent of peritoneal disease and nodal metastases. Tumour markers are not useful as CA125, alpha-fetoprotein, and beta-hCG are otherwise also elevated in pregnancy.

Management

In the antenatal period

Management depends on the size and nature of the tumour and the period of gestation. The size of the tumour as well as its characteristics (cystic, solid, etc.) are determined by an ultrasound examination (Fig. 38.2a and b)/MRI, based on which, management is planned.

- In early pregnancy, the ovary may be enlarged, raising a suspicion of a neoplasm. Ovaries less than 6 cm in diameter are usually due to corpus luteum formation and do not need removal. Hence, the ultrasound is repeated in the second trimester. Removal of the ovarian cyst in the first trimester may lead to miscarriage, and therefore should be deferred.
- If an ovarian mass is 6 cm or larger and if it persists after 16 weeks of gestation, it may be better to

remove it surgically. Some clinicians manage cysts up to 10 cm conservatively, provided the cyst appears simple by USG. The removal of the cyst is carried out between 16 and 20 weeks of gestation as it may undergo torsion.
- At times, the ovarian cyst is diagnosed when the woman presents to the hospital with acute abdomen and the ultrasound reveals an extrauterine mass. Under these conditions, torsion of the ovarian cyst is suspected. In such cases, it is mandatory to perform a laparotomy and remove the cyst immediately.
- If an ovarian cyst is diagnosed in the third trimester of pregnancy and appears to be a simple cyst, surgery may be deferred until delivery.

> The chances of torsion are higher in the puerperium and hence it is better to electively remove the cyst at the earliest in the postpartum period.

Malignant ovarian tumours complicating pregnancy

Persistent simple cysts >10 cm after the first trimester should be evaluated for malignancy. Tumours that are solid with thick, irregular septae or solid and cystic areas/papillary excrescences are usually malignant. If malignancy is suspected, irrespective of the size of the cyst and duration of pregnancy, laparotomy and the appropriate surgical procedure must be performed.

During labour

- If the tumour lies above the pelvic brim and causes no obstruction, vaginal delivery is allowed, and the tumour is removed in the first week of the puerperium.

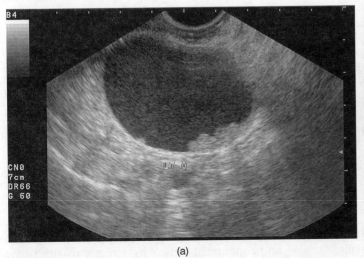
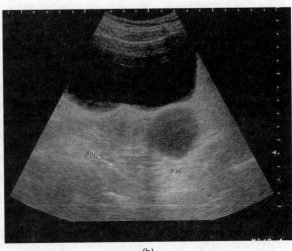

(a) (b)

Fig. 38.2 Ovarian cysts: (a) large cystic mass with a focal solid area and (b) a small, clear cyst

- If the tumour is impacted in the pelvis, causing obstruction, cesarean section with immediate removal of the tumour is performed.
- If a woman requires a cesarean section for any obstetric indication, and an ovarian cyst is identified, it can be removed concurrently following the delivery of the fetus.

During the puerperium

Tumours discovered for the first time should be removed immediately to avoid torsion.

CARCINOMA OF THE CERVIX COMPLICATING PREGNANCY

Nearly 3% of cervical cancers are diagnosed during pregnancy. The course of the disease and prognosis of cervical cancer in pregnant women are similar to those in non-pregnant women. The diagnosis and management of cervical cancer pose a number of problems in pregnancy.

- The diagnosis is usually made while evaluating abnormal cytology in pregnancy or when the woman presents with bleeding per vaginum. The abnormal vaginal bleeding or postcoital bleeding associated with carcinoma of the cervix can be easily mistaken for a miscarriage or antepartum hemorrhage. Therefore, all pregnant women presenting with bleeding should undergo a speculum examination as soon as the bleeding settles.
- On examination, the appearance of invasive cancer may be mistaken for pregnancy-induced cervical ectropion or cervical decidualization. Therefore, any suspicious lesion on the cervix should be biopsied; colposcopy carried out as it is easier to perform during pregnancy because of the physiological eversion of the cervix.

Effect of Invasive Carcinoma on Pregnancy and Labour

- Undiagnosed cervical carcinoma in labour can present with cervical dystocia, obstructed labour, cervical laceration, torrential bleeding and/or uterine rupture.
- Puerperal sepsis may occur.

Effect of Pregnancy and Labour on Invasive Carcinoma

- Due to the increased vascularity of pregnancy, there may be rapid growth of the tumour. This may result in rapid spread.

Management

The management of cervical carcinoma in pregnancy also poses a number of problems. The gestational age of the fetus should be taken into consideration while planning treatment. When radical hysterectomy is planned, excessive bleeding is a recognised complication. If cervical carcinoma is diagnosed in advanced pregnancy, vaginal delivery is contraindicated, and classical cesarean section is carried out to avoid excessive bleeding and dissemination.

Management of pre-invasive lesions of the cervix

The management of pre-invasive disease (CIN1 to CIN3) can be deferred until 6–8 weeks after delivery. However, it is recommended that a colposcopy be performed in each trimester to assess the lesion size and disease progression.

Management of invasive carcinoma of the cervix

The basic treatment is the same as that of non-pregnant women who have invasive carcinoma of the cervix. Management depends on the stage of the disease, gestational age at diagnosis and the woman's desire to continue pregnancy.

Management of advanced-stage disease (stages II–IV)

Treatment should be initiated promptly. In early pregnancy (first and second trimesters), external beam radiotherapy (EBRT) is given; spontaneous expulsion of the fetus occurs during pregnancy. If the fetus is sufficiently mature, treatment may be delayed for a maximum of 4 weeks and measures are taken to enhance lung maturity. Once this is achieved, pregnancy is terminated by classical cesarean section, followed by chemoradiation 2 weeks later.

Management of stage I disease

In most cases, cervical carcinoma is diagnosed in pregnancy in its early stage. In such cases, one of two alternatives are considered before planning management:

- If pregnancy is not desired:
  — If the gestational age is less than 20 weeks, in situ radical hysterectomy with pelvic lymphadenectomy is carried out.
  — When the gestational age is >20 weeks, pregnancy is terminated by a classical incision and concurrent radical hysterectomy with pelvic lymphadenectomy.

- If pregnancy is desired: Delivery can be delayed until fetal maturity. Then the baby is delivered by classical cesarean section with concurrent radical hysterectomy.

KEY POINTS

✓ Fibroids complicating pregnancy may result in an increased incidence of abortion, premature labour and postpartum hemorrhage.

✓ Red degeneration of fibroids seen in pregnancy is managed conservatively.

✓ Myomectomy is not attempted at the time of cesarean section unless the fibroid is subserous with a long pedicle.

✓ Ovarian cysts diagnosed during pregnancy are removed if the size is more than 6 cm or has features suggestive of malignancy. Benign cysts are removed between 16 and 20 weeks of pregnancy.

✓ Carcinoma of the cervix diagnosed during pregnancy is managed actively as in the non-pregnant state.

Essay questions

1. How will you manage a case of carcinoma cervix diagnosed during pregnancy?
2. Describe the management of a woman who was diagnosed with fibroids during pregnancy.

Short answer questions

1. What are the effects of fibroids on pregnancy?
2. Describe red degeneration of a fibroid.
3. What are the indications for cesarean section in a pregnancy complicated by fibroids?

MCQs

1. Which type of fibroid increases the risk of abortions?
   a) Submucous
   b) Intramural
   c) Subserous
   d) None

2. What is the common complication of fibroid associated with pregnancy?
   a) Hyaline
   b) Sarcomatous
   c) Red degeneration
   d) Cystic degeneration

3. Fibroids may lead to all of the following EXCEPT:
   a) Abortion
   b) Hydramnios
   c) Malpresentations of the fetus
   d) Premature labour

4. The management of red degeneration of fibroids in pregnancy may include all the following EXCEPT:
   a) Analgesics
   b) Sedation
   c) Antibiotics
   d) Myomectomy

5. The only indication for myomectomy during pregnancy is:
   a) Torsion of a subserous fibroid
   b) Red degeneration
   c) Malpresentation of fetus
   d) Preterm labour

6. A fibroid in pregnancy requires cesarean section for delivery in all EXCEPT:
   a) Lower segment fibroid
   b) Impacted fibroids
   c) Fundal fibroids
   d) Cervical fibroids

7. Which of these is not an indication for surgery for an ovarian cyst in pregnancy?
   a) Cyst <5 cm
   b) Persistent cyst >16 weeks
   c) Torsion of an ovarian cyst
   d) Simple cyst >10 cm

8. What is the best time to operate on an ovarian cyst diagnosed during pregnancy?
   a) As soon as the diagnosis is made
   b) First trimester
   c) Second trimester
   d) Third trimester

9. What is the best time to operate on an ovarian cyst when torsion is suspected?
   a) As soon as the diagnosis is made
   b) First trimester
   c) Second trimester
   d) Third trimester

10. What is the best time to operate if malignancy in an ovarian mass is suspected during pregnancy?
    a) As soon as the diagnosis is made
    b) First trimester
    c) Second trimester
    d) Third trimester

11. On examination of the cervix during pregnancy, an unhealthy area suspicious of malignancy is noted. A biopsy should be performed:
    a) At the earliest
    b) If the lesion becomes symptomatic
    c) After delivery
    d) After medical termination of pregnancy

Answers
1. (a), 2. (c), 3. (b), 4. (d), 5. (a), 6. (c), 7. (a), 8. (c), 9. (a), 10. (a), 11. (a)

Fill in the blanks

1. The most common type of degenerative change seen in pregnancy is _____.
2. The most common ovarian tumour complicating pregnancy is a _____.

Answers
1. red degeneration, 2. simple ovarian cyst

Case scenario-based discussion

1. A 25-year-old primigravida presents at 16 weeks of gestation with colicky pain of 6 hours duration which is localised to the right lower abdomen. She also has nausea

and vomiting with mild fever. She does not have any urinary or bowel symptoms. There is no previous history of surgery. Her scan at 10 weeks of gestation showed an ovarian cyst measuring 7 cm. She was reassured and advised to come for a repeat scan at 18 weeks to determine the size of the cyst. On examination, her temperature was 99°F, pulse was 100 bpm, and the BP was 100/70 mmHg. She is distressed and in pain. On abdominal examination, her uterus is enlarged to 16 weeks size; there is tenderness over the right lower quadrant with guarding. On vaginal examination, the cervix was closed, and the uterus corresponded to 16 weeks and no other details could be made out.

a) What is the most likely diagnosis?
b) What investigations will you order?
c) The USG shows an ovarian cyst measuring 8 cm in size with features suggesting a dermoid cyst. What is the further course of action?

Answers

a) The most likely diagnosis is torsion of the ovarian cyst, but the possibility of acute appendicitis should also be considered. The colicky pain is more suggestive of a torsion due to the ischemia of the ovarian vessel.

b) The woman needs an urgent USG of the abdomen and pelvis and a complete hemogram to look for leukocytosis.

c) As the findings are suggestive of torsion of an ovarian cyst, surgery should be the immediate treatment approach. Though the cyst can be taken out laparoscopically, this is best avoided during pregnancy. On opening the abdomen, the ovary should be examined for viability after untwisting it. If reperfusion takes place with viable ovarian tissue, ovarian cystectomy is carried out, preserving the normal ovarian tissue. If reperfusion does not occur and the ovary appears non-viable, an oophorectomy should be carried out. The appendix should also be inspected.

39

Surgical Emergencies Complicating Pregnancy

OG 9.3

Learning Objectives

» To know the surgical emergencies that may complicate pregnancy
» To know the diagnosis and management of acute appendicitis complicating pregnancy

INTRODUCTION

A pregnant woman may present with acute abdomen, which may be related to pregnancy or incidental to pregnancy (Tables 39.1 and 39.2). Some of the surgical conditions encountered in pregnancy are acute appendicitis, acute cholecystitis, renal colic, acute pancreatitis and intestinal obstruction. When a pregnant woman presents with acute abdomen, the changes in uterine activity, the position of the abdominal viscera and the response to peritoneal irritation pose challenges in the diagnosis of the underlying conditions.

ACUTE APPENDICITIS

Acute appendicitis can complicate 1 in 2,500 pregnancies. The woman usually presents with right-sided abdominal pain, nausea and vomiting. Depending upon the gestational age, the location of the pain and tenderness will vary. The pain is not typically in the right lower quadrant but is superior and lateral to the McBurney point. This is due to the enlarging uterus pushing the appendix upwards and laterally, occasionally mimicking pyelonephritis. In the first trimester of pregnancy, the pain is localised to the lower abdomen, gradually rising to the right hypochondrium in the third trimester of pregnancy. The diagnosis of acute appendicitis may be missed or delayed in pregnancy, especially in the third trimester due to various reasons, which are as follows:

• The pregnant uterus in front of the appendix may mask the tenderness and guarding; reflex uterine contractions occur frequently, confusing the diagnosis.

• Because of the upward displacement of the appendix, the pain may be felt at a higher level and is often mistaken for cholecystitis.

• Because of the displacement of the abdominal organs by the uterus, normal walling-off of the inflamed appendix does not occur; general peritonitis occurs more readily.

Table 39.1 Conditions incidental to pregnancy

Gastrointestinal	Genitourinary	Vascular	Respiratory	Others
• Acute appendicitis • Acute pancreatitis • Gastroenteritis • Bowel obstruction • Bowel perforation • Peptic ulcer	• Ureteric obstruction • Ureteric calculus • Ovarian cyst rupture • Rupture of the ovarian tumour	• Thrombosis • Splenic artery rupture • Ruptured visceral/ splenic artery aneurysm	• Pneumonia • Pulmonary embolism	• Intraperitoneal hemorrhage • Ruptured spleen • Abdominal trauma • Sickle cell disease

Table 39.2 Conditions associated with pregnancy

Pregnancy-associated conditions	Conditions resulting from pregnancy in the early weeks	Conditions resulting from pregnancy in the later weeks
• Acute pyelonephritis • Acute cholecystitis • Acute fatty liver of pregnancy • Acute cystitis	• Acute urinary retention • Septic abortion and peritonitis • Ruptured ectopic pregnancy	• Abruptio placentae • HELLP syndrome • Torsion of subserous myoma • Red degeneration

(Adapted from Taylor D, Perry RL. Acute Abdomen and Pregnancy. *Medscape Drugs & Diseases.* Updated March 28, 2014.)

- The WBC count is raised both in pregnancy and in appendicitis.

The woman may have an abortion or go into preterm labour if the diagnosis is delayed.

Management

If there is a suspicion of appendicitis, it is advisable to perform a laparotomy without any delay even if it is going to be negative. The incision is placed higher than usual depending on the site of maximum tenderness to allow adequate access.

INTESTINAL OBSTRUCTION

In a healthy pregnant woman, intestinal obstruction is rare. In some cases, however, it may occur due to bands and adhesions from a previous surgery. The presence of hernias, intussusception and volvulus can also lead to intestinal obstruction. The woman presents with acute abdominal pain, nausea, vomiting, constipation and distension of the abdomen, all occurring simultaneously.

Diagnosis

A plain X-ray abdomen will show distended loops of the bowel with fluid levels.

Management

If there are no signs of strangulation, conservative management with nasogastric aspiration and IV fluids may be attempted. If there is no improvement, laparotomy is mandatory. If pregnancy is advanced, cesarean section becomes necessary to facilitate the proper management of intestinal obstruction.

ACUTE CHOLECYSTITIS DURING PREGNANCY

Acute cholecystitis is usually associated with gallstones or biliary sludge during pregnancy and presents with acute upper abdominal pain, nausea and vomiting. Besides acute cholecystitis, the patient can also present with biliary colic and common bile duct obstruction. Symptomatic cholecystitis is initially managed conservatively, as it is for non-pregnant women—with antibiotics. However, it has been observed that there is a high recurrence rate as well as a possibility of pancreatitis if the condition is treated conservatively. Therefore, in the presence of cholecystitis or biliary obstruction, surgery should be the treatment of choice. Cholecystectomy appears to be a safe procedure in pregnancy. If cholecystitis recurs later in gestation, preterm labour is likely to occur.

ACUTE PANCREATITIS DURING PREGNANCY

It is a rare surgical complication of pregnancy that occurs in 1 in 4,000 pregnancies. The predisposing factors are increased lipid levels and biliary stasis in pregnancy, gallstones and alcohol intake. Women with pancreatitis present with nausea, vomiting and abdominal pain. The pain is upper and central, often radiating to the back. Occasionally, it can lead to shock. The diagnosis is made based on the detection of raised amylase levels (serum amylase may be mildly elevated in normal pregnancy). Management is mostly conservative with nasogastric aspiration and attention to electrolyte balance, glucose and calcium levels. Laparotomy should be avoided if possible.

HEARTBURN AND HIATUS HERNIA

As a result of the hormone-induced relaxation of the esophageal sphincter, there is a reflux of gastric acid from the stomach into the esophagus. This manifests as mild upper abdominal pain and burning sensation felt in the epigastrium, behind the sternum. Occasionally, hiatus hernia can manifest with vomiting and hemetemesis in the third trimester. It is treated like heartburn with antacids and metoclopramide. Occasionally, a large part of the intestine may herniate into the chest, presenting with acute abdominal pain, vomiting and shock. This condition mandates immediate surgical correction.

URETERIC COLIC

Pregnancy does not predispose to the formation of renal calculi. If there are pre-existing renal stones, due to the dilatation of the ureters, small ureteric calculi may be passed relatively painlessly. A large calculus may occasionally present with symptoms, usually, in the second or third trimester of pregnancy. Clinical features include acute flank pain which may radiate to the lower abdomen and is accompanied by hematuria. The diagnosis is confirmed by ultrasonography.

Renal colic in pregnancy is treated with antispasmodics and IV fluids to enhance the passage of the stone.

OTHER CONDITIONS

Other conditions such as sickle cell crisis, porphyria, drug abuse withdrawal and mesenteric vein thrombosis can present with acute abdomen complicating pregnancy.

INVESTIGATIONS FOR ACUTE ABDOMEN

When a pregnant woman presents with acute abdomen, the following investigations are carried out:

- USG abdomen and pelvis to diagnose gall bladder disease, renal calculi, ovarian cyst accidents, degenerating fibroids and rare intraabdominal tumours
- X-ray abdomen may be required in suspected cases of intestinal obstruction/perforation of peptic ulcer
- WBC to diagnose appendicitis
- Serum amylase to diagnose pancreatitis
- Urine microscopy and culture for pyelonephritis
- Hemoglobin and peripheral film for sickle disease
- LFT for biliary disease

KEY POINTS

✓ It is difficult to diagnose acute appendicitis during pregnancy. A delay in diagnosis leads to increased maternal morbidity.

✓ The risks of abortion and preterm labour are increased when acute appendicitis develops in pregnancy.

✓ In pregnancy, the appendix moves superiorly and laterally from the normal location.

✓ Intestinal obstruction is rare in pregnancy; early diagnosis and surgery reduce morbidity.

✓ Acute cholecystitis with lithiasis can recur during pregnancy. Therefore, surgical management is the preferred option.

✓ Pancreatitis with gallstones may occur and is managed conservatively.

Essay questions

1. Discuss the differential diagnosis, complications and treatment of acute appendicitis in pregnancy.
2. Discuss the differential diagnosis of acute abdominal pain in pregnancy.

Short answer question

1. Enumerate the investigations required for the evaluation of acute abdomen in pregnancy.

MCQs

1. Which of the following is not included in the management of acute appendicitis in pregnancy?
   a) Antibiotics
   b) Analgesics
   c) Appendicectomy
   d) Bowel resection
2. Which of the following is true about acute cholecystitis in pregnancy?
   a) Gallstones are less common during pregnancy
   b) Conservative management is the only form of treatment
   c) Can lead to increased mortality
   d) Surgery is preferred due to the risk of recurrence
3. What enzymes are used to detect pancreatitis in pregnancy?
   a) Amylase, lipase
   b) SGOT, SGPT
   c) Bilirubin values
   d) CA 125
4. Which of the following surgical emergencies can be managed without surgery?
   a) Acute appendicitis
   b) Torsion of an ovary
   c) Ruptured ectopic
   d) Gallstones

Answers
1. (d), 2. (d), 3. (a), 4. (d)

Fill in the blank

1. The most common cause of increased morbidity due to appendicitis in pregnancy is a _____.

Answers
1. delay in diagnosis

Case scenario-based discussion

1. A 30-year-old primigravida presents to the casualty at 28 weeks of gestation with complaints of anorexia of 2 days, fever, pain, nausea and vomiting since that morning. She does not have any urinary symptoms and the fetal movements are good. On examination she is febrile with a temperature of 102° F, her pulse rate is 106 bpm and BP is 100/60 mmHg. There is tenderness over the right lateral aspect of her abdomen at the level of the umbilicus. The uterus is well relaxed and the FH is good. On examination, there are no pus cells in the urine; the total count is 16,000/mm³.
   a) What is the most likely diagnosis?
   b) What further investigations will you order?
   c) The USG does not show cholecystitis. How would you manage this case?

Answers
a) When a pregnant woman presents with such findings, one should consider the possibility of pyelonephritis, appendicitis or cholecystitis. Abruption is ruled out as the uterus is well-relaxed with a good fetal heart. Pyelonephritis is also ruled out as there is no pyuria. The pain of cholecystitis is located in the right upper quadrant radiating to the right shoulder. Therefore, the most likely diagnosis is acute appendicitis.
b) In order to rule out cholecystitis and gallstones, USG of the abdomen should be carried out.
c) As acute appendicitis is the diagnosis, there should not be any delay in the management. A laparotomy and appendicectomy should be carried out immediately. Delay in diagnosis and management could lead to maternal morbidity and mortality.

Abnormal Fetal Position and Presentations (Occipitoposterior Position, Face and Brow Presentations)

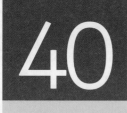

Learning Objectives

» To know the influence of the shape of the pelvis on the mechanism of engagement in labour

» To know the causes of malpositions and malpresentations

» To know the mechanism of labour in occipitoposterior position and face and brow presentations

» To know the indications and procedure of vacuum delivery in the occipitoposterior position

---

■ INTRODUCTION

At the onset of labour, the fetus enters the pelvis in the **cephalic presentation in 97% of the cases**. 3% of fetuses present as breech and 0.5% present as transverse or longitudinal lie.

■ SHAPE OF PELVIS AND MECHANISM OF ENGAGEMENT

In the cephalic presentation, engagement is the first step in the mechanism of labour. In this step, the head enters the pelvis in such a way that it adjusts according to the type of pelvic inlet. This, in turn, determines the position of the head during the further progress of labour. **Caldwell and Moloy** demonstrated the influence of the shape of the pelvis on the mechanism of engagement. During engagement, the long axis of the fetal head (the engaging diameter) adjusts itself to the longest inlet diameter of the pelvis. Accordingly, one of the following may happen:

- In the **anthropoid pelvis,** the anteroposterior diameter of the inlet is greater than the transverse, and therefore, the head enters the pelvis in an oblique manner.

- In the **flat or platypelloid** pelvis, the anteroposterior diameter is short, and the transverse diameter is wide. Therefore, engagement takes place in the transverse or occipitolateral position.

- In the **gynecoid** and **android** types of pelvises, the head enters in the transverse position in approximately 70% of cases and in the oblique position in the remaining. In the android type of pelvis, the occiput occupies posterior positions in the majority of cases.

■ MALPOSITIONS AND MALPRESENTATIONS

- The most common presentation of the fetus at term is **vertex**, where the occiput is the denominator and the vertex, which is bound anteriorly by the anterior fontanelle, posteriorly by the posterior fontanelle and laterally by parietal eminences, is felt by the vaginal examination. In nearly 70% of cases, the occiput occupies the left anterior quadrant. This is the normal position; in nearly 20–25% of cases, the occiput occupies the right posterior quadrant, which is a **malposition**.

- All other presentations other than vertex are called **malpresentations**—these include face, brow, breech and shoulder presentations.

Causes of Malpresentations and Malpositions

A number of factors may contribute to malpresentations and malpositions of the fetus; these are listed in the box that follows.

Defects in the powers
- Pendulous abdomen—laxity of the abdominal muscles
- The tight uterus and abdominal wall in a primigravida favour the occipitoposterior position as there is more room available for the back posteriorly
- Dextrorotation of the uterus—rotation of the uterus in the anti-clockwise direction favours the right occipitoposterior position

Defects in the passages
- Contracted pelvis, cephalopelvic disproportion (CPD)
- Android and anthropoid pelvis
- Pelvic tumours—uterine and adnexal tumours
- Uterine anomalies such as bicornuate, septate or fibroid uterus
- Placenta previa—anteriorly situated placenta

Defects in the passenger
- Macrosomia
- Prematurity
- Multiple pregnancy

■ OCCIPITOPOSTERIOR POSITION

Definition

It is a cephalic and vertex presentation in which the occiput is in the posterior quadrant of the pelvis. 20–25% of all vertex presentations engage in the posterior position—right or left (Fig. 40.1)—and a minority in the occipitosacral position. The right occipitoposterior position is more common for the following reasons:
- Greater space in the right oblique diameter
- Obliquity of the uterus to the right
- Sigmoid colon on the left reducing the space

Causes

Besides the causes of malpositions and malpresentations discussed earlier, transverse narrowing of the midpelvis, as seen in an android pelvis is a major contributing factor for the occipitoposterior position. During the course of labour, more than 80% of occipitoposterior positions rotate to the anterior position.

Diagnosis

On abdominal examination

An occipitoposterior position is usually diagnosed by abdominal palpation if the uterus and abdominal walls are not too tense.

- Inspection shows flattening below the umbilicus known as subumbilical flattening.
- The head is high or mobile at term. Occipitoposterior position is the commonest cause for a mobile head at term, especially in a primigravida.
- As the right occipitoposterior position is more common, the back is felt on the right side. Because the back is towards the flank, there is difficulty in identifying the same.
- The fetal limbs are more easily felt than usual and lie nearer to the midline of the body.
- There is a delay in the engagement of the head. The anterior shoulder is usually at a higher level and farther out from the midline than in the anterior position.
- In the second pelvic grip, the occiput and the sinciput are at the same level. The fetal heart sounds are heard best in the flanks.

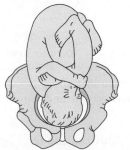 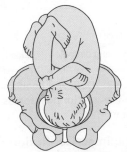

Right occipitoposterior positions   Left occipitoposterior positions

Fig. 40.1 Right and left occipitoposterior positions

Vaginal examination

- Vaginal findings are appreciated only in labour. When the cervix is sufficiently dilated, the sagittal suture is felt in the right oblique diameter.
- The large anterior fontanelle of the fetus is well-appreciated in the anterior quadrant of the pelvis and the small posterior fontanelle can also be reached. As the head is deflexed, both the fontanelles are felt.
- There may be early rupture of membranes, or the membrane may be hanging loose; the latter is called a **'sausage-shaped membrane'**.

Mechanism of Labour in the Occipitoposterior Position (OP Position)

- The engaging diameter in the OP position is either suboccipitofrontal or occipitofrontal and measures 11 cm.
- The engaging diameter occupies the right oblique diameter of the pelvis.
- The occiput is opposite the right sacroiliac joint and the brow is opposite the left obturator foramen.

- The attitude of the fetus is normal—the head is flexed, but the degree of flexion is lesser than the occipitoanterior position. This is because the fetus lies with its spine against the mother's spine. As a result, the natural convexity of the fetal spine is undone and is replaced by straightening, which results in a certain amount of deflexion (Fig. 40.2).

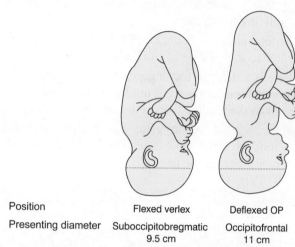

Position	Flexed vertex	Deflexed OP
Presenting diameter	Suboccipitobregmatic 9.5 cm	Occipitofrontal 11 cm

Fig. 40.2 Deflexed head and straightened spine in occipitoposterior position as compared to flexed vertex position

The imperfect flexion (deflexion) of the fetal head in the OP position is due to the following reasons:

- The pelvic floor may be weakened by previous deliveries, and thus, may offer no resistance. Consequently, it may fail to produce full flexion.
- The military attitude of the child contributes to imperfect flexion.

The attitude of the child is not the universal 'round shouldered' one but a military one.

- An important factor is the relation of the fetal head to the brim of the pelvis. In the occipitoanterior position, the biparietal diameter lies approximately in a line passing from one of the sacroiliac joints to the symphysis pubis and measures more than 9.4 cm. Therefore, the head is able to maintain flexion and descend. In contrast, in the occipitoposterior position, the biparietal diameter occupies the sacrocotyloid diameter, which runs from the sacral promontory to the iliopectineal eminence on the same side (9–9.2 cm), which is smaller than the biparietal diameter (9.4 cm). As a result, the narrow sinciput descends first in advance to the occiput, thus undoing the flexion and leading to deflexion.

Normal mechanism

Given enough time, with a good uterine contraction and a favourable pelvic shape, long anterior rotation takes place and delivery occurs as in normal labour in 90% of cases. Factors that favour anterior rotation are gynecoid pelvis, average-sized head, good uterine action, rupture of the membranes after full cervical dilatation and good tone of the pelvic floor.

The following are the cardinal movements of labour:

- After descent with flexion, the occiput becomes the leading part. It meets the resistance of the pelvic floor and rotates to the front.
- There is a long internal rotation to 3/8th of a circle.
- The occiput rotates under the symphysis pubis.
- Extension, restitution and external rotation take place as in the occipitoanterior position.

Abnormal mechanism

The most common cause for prolonged labour in a vertex presentation is the occipitoposterior position.

- Approximately 10% of OP positions fail to go through the normal mechanism, and there is a failure of anterior rotation. Factors that hinder forward rotation include an android pelvis or a pelvis with a straight sacrum and converging side walls, a large baby weighing over 3.5 Kg, premature rupture of the membranes, weak uterine action and poor tone of the pelvic floor.
- Occipitoposterior position may persist, with the head either persisting in the right posterior quadrant or rotating (Fig. 40.3) into the hollow of the sacrum (direct occipitoposterior).
- Alternatively, the head may get arrested during the long internal rotation. The arrest can occur at any level. If it occurs at the level of ischial spines with the cervix fully dilated, it is called deep transverse arrest.

Deep transverse arrest is a condition in which the fetal head is at the level of the ischial spines with the sagittal suture in the transverse diameter of the midpelvis, but no further descent occurs despite full cervical dilatation and good uterine contractions for more than one hour. Deep transverse arrest is common in android and anthropoid pelvises.

Management of Labour

During labour, adequate fluid balance should be maintained. Pain relief is mandatory with analgesics or epidural analgesia. One should try to keep the membranes intact as long as possible as the intact membrane acts as a cervical dilator and stimulates uterine contractions.

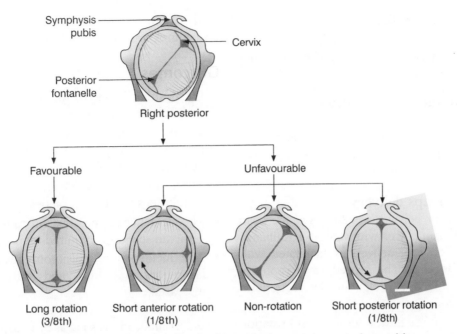

Fig. 40.3 Favourable and unfavourable rotation of the fetal head in the occipitoposterior position

The progress of labour should be carefully monitored with a partogram to identify slow progress or arrest of labour. If the labour is slow, the pelvis should be carefully assessed to rule out cephalopelvic disproportion. After ruling out CPD, if the uterine contractions are weak, labour can be augmented with oxytocin infusion to facilitate anterior rotation.

> Pain relief is mandatory with analgesics or epidural analgesia.

Modes of Delivery in the Occipitoposterior Position

Spontaneous vaginal delivery

With adequate pelvis and good uterine contractions, labour may progress normally, sometimes, with a slight delay due to the long internal rotation. Spontaneous vaginal delivery may take place as in the occipitoanterior position.

Delivery as direct occipitoposterior position (face-to-pubis delivery)

Here, the occiput passes under the hollow of the sacrum by reversely rotating by 1/8th of a circle while the sinciput rotates anteriorly to the front. This mechanism of labour occurs in the anthropoid type of pelvis since the AP diameters of the pelvis are longer at all levels. There is extreme flexion of the head followed by extreme extension. With flexion, the brow or part of the head in front of the bregma is fixed under the

pubic arch. With marked flexion, the vertex and the occiput sweep over the perineum. Then by extreme extension, the nose, mouth and chin are delivered. The face then slips behind the symphysis pubis. This mechanism may overdistend the perineum, resulting in a complete perineal tear. This is also called 'face-to-pubis delivery'. It is followed by restitution and external rotation of the occiput to the right. Here, the vulva is distended by the occipitofrontal diameter (11.5 cm); the bulky occiput distends the perineum. Hence, in all cases of face-to-pubis delivery (Fig. 40.4), a very liberal episiotomy is mandatory, and perineal lacerations should be anticipated and managed. At this stage, assistance may be required with a ventouse or forceps.

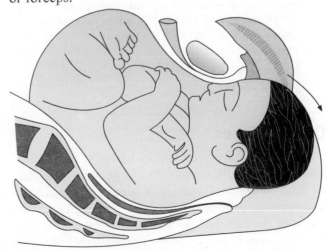

Fig. 40.4 Face-to-pubis delivery

Failure of anterior rotation

During the internal rotation of the occiput, there may be a failure of anterior rotation, or the occiput may remain in the OP position.

Management of failure of rotation

- If the arrest occurs at or above the levels of the ischial spines, cesarean section should be undertaken.
- Nowadays, a fetal head at the +1 level is also delivered by cesarean section.

Ventouse and forceps delivery

- If the head is at or below the +2 station, the head can be rotated manually or with ventouse/Keillands forceps. After rotation, delivery is facilitated with a ventouse or forceps. The procedure of ventouse delivery is discussed in detail in the section on operative deliveries.
- Ventouse assists in the flexion, descent and rotation of the head.
- Quite often, even when the head is not engaged, the scalp may be visible at the introitus due to severe moulding and caput formation, giving the false impression of the head being low in the pelvis. For this reason, before applying forceps or a ventouse for assisted delivery, it is important to check for the fetal poles per abdomen. Cesarean section should be performed without attempting vaginal delivery if any fetal pole is palpable per abdomen.

> **Indications for cesarean section in the occipitoposterior positions**
> - Deep transverse arrest
> - Failure of rotation with persistent occipito-posterior position/occipitosacral position or failure to rotate and the head persisting at or above the level of the +1 station
> - CPD
> - Failed ventouse delivery
> - Fetal distress

Delayed Cases

Often, women are seen late in labour with the fetal head jammed in the cavity with a large caput obscuring all landmarks, thus making it almost impossible to ascertain the position of the head. In such cases, the pinna of the ears will point to the occiput. The fetus in these cases is usually in a moribund condition with a very faint fetal heart and is often dead. Even in such cases, a cesarean section is preferable in the interest of the mother rather than attempting any destructive procedures or instrumental vaginal delivery.

Outcomes

- OP position is one of the most common causes of mobile head in primigravidae and prolonged labour.
- When compared to the occipitoanterior position, the first and second stages of labour are prolonged in the occipitoposterior position.
- There are increased chances of early rupture of membranes and cord prolapse.
- The incidence of operative intervention is higher and cesarean section is required more often.
- The incidence of episiotomy extension, perineal lacerations and third- and fourth-degree tears is increased.

> Fetal complications such as birth asphyxia and birth trauma due to operative interventions are more common in OP presentation.

- Head moulding—in the persistent occipitoposterior position, the head is shortened along the occipitofrontal diameter, and there is a compensatory increase in the suboccipitobregmatic diameter.

> The caput succedaneum is situated over the anterior fontanelle, and the head appears square. The 'jam pot' type of moulding is characteristic of persistent OP position.

Fig. 40.5 summarises the normal and abnormal mechanisms of labour in the occipitoposterior position.

■ OCCIPITOTRANSVERSE POSITION

The occipitotransverse position is usually transient as the occiput eventually rotates to the anterior position. However, this position may persist in the presence of pelvic architectural abnormality or hypotonic uterine action. The diagnosis of occipitotransverse position is made by vaginal examination. When the head is below the +1 station without caput or moulding, ventouse delivery can be attempted. Otherwise, it is safer to perform a cesarean section.

■ FACE AND BROW PRESENTATIONS

These two malpresentations are considered together because of their common etiology. Both presentations commonly arise from an occipitoposterior position

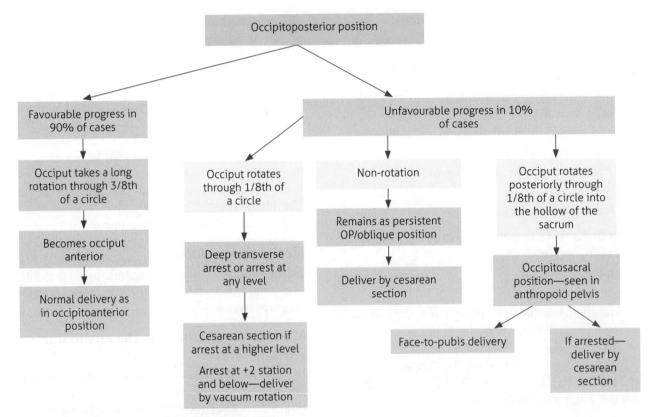

Fig. 40.5 Mechanisms and management of OP position

in which there is deflexion of the head. Any pressure along the fetal spine will cause the extension of the head. If this extension is partial, brow presentation results. If complete, face presentation occurs. This is why secondary face and brow presentations are more common than the primary. Secondary face presentation occurs in cases of CPD and abnormal pelvis.

Face Presentation

Definition

It is a cephalic presentation with the fetal head in complete extension. It occurs in 1 in 500 cases. The part of the cephalic pole that lies between the chin and the frontal eminence tries to engage in the pelvis. The engaging diameter is the submentobregmatic (9.4 cm) with the chin as the denominator. In the face presentation, the normal attitude of flexion is undone, and the head is hyperextended so that the occiput is in contact with the fetal back. Four positions (Fig. 40.6) are possible with the chin as denominator; these are as follows:

- Right mentoposterior (RMP)
- Left mentoposterior (LMP)
- Right mentoanterior (RMA)
- Left mentoanterior (LMA)—more than 75% of cases

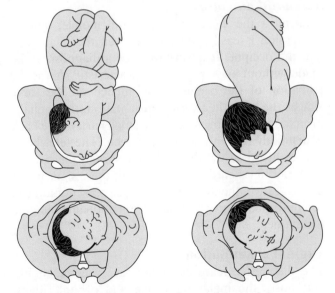

Fig. 40.6 Anterior and posterior positions of the chin

Causes

The factors responsible for primary face presentation are those that favour extension or prevent head flexion. The varieties of face presentations are primary and secondary face presentations.

Fetal causes (primary face presentation):

- Anencephaly—because of the absence of the cranium, the face is palpable easily
- Prematurity
- Multiple pregnancy
- Large fetus
- Cord around the neck, tumours and goitre
- Arms folded under the chin
- Spasm of the extensor muscles of the neck
- Large thorax
- Dolichocephalic head

Maternal causes (secondary face presentation):

- Contracted pelvis
- Platypelloid pelvis
- Uterine obliquity
- Multiparity with a lax abdomen which allows the fetus to extend the cervical and thoracic spine
- Pelvic tumours

These factors act by causing the occiput to hitch onto the brim of the pelvis when labour begins and when the head is attempting to engage.

Diagnosis

Abdominal palpation

Antenatal diagnosis

Clinically, the head is high and mobile, and a depression is easily palpable between the fetal spine and the occiput. It is very rare for a diagnosis to be made without an X-ray. The characteristic sign is the palpation of the cephalic prominence on the same side as the back (in a vertex presentation, the cephalic prominence is on the side of the small parts). The back is distinctly felt only near the breech. The fetal heart is best heard below the umbilicus; when the back is posterior, it is heard distinctly. While these signs might be suggestive, the diagnosis of a face presentation can be confirmed only by vaginal examination and imaging techniques.

Vaginal examination

The distinctive features of the face are the mouth and nose, the malar eminence and orbital ridges. At times, a breech may be mistaken for a face when the anus is mistaken for the mouth. In breech presentation, the ischial tuberosities are always in line with the anus, whereas, in the face presentation, the mouth and malar eminences form a triangle. These findings help in avoiding the mistake of confusing a face presentation for a breech. The anus can be differentiated from the mouth based on whether or not it admits a finger—the former, due to the sphincter tone, does not allow the introduction of a finger, whereas the latter easily allows this. It is not uncommon to come across the sucking response from the fetus when the finger in introduced into its mouth. Before the availability of USG, plain X-ray abdomen was used for diagnosis and would reveal a hyperextended head with facial bones at or below the pelvic inlet. Nowadays, ultrasound has replaced X-ray as the diagnostic imaging modality of choice. The characteristic hyperextended head of the fetus can be clearly seen on ultrasound.

Mechanism of labour

The mentum is the denominator in the face presentation. The fetal face may present as **mentoanterior** or **mentoposterior.**

Mechanism of labour in the mentoanterior position

In the face presentation, the chin simulates the part played by the occiput in a vertex presentation (Fig. 40.7). The movements that help to deliver the face are descent with increased extension, internal rotation of the chin, flexion, restitution and external rotation.

- At the beginning of labour, the head is fairly high and may not always be in an attitude of complete extension.
- When labour starts and descent begins, an exaggeration of extension takes place. The chin becomes the most dependent part, and the face engages by its submentobregmatic diameter (9.5 cm) in one of the oblique diameters of the pelvis.
- As the head descends further, the chin meets the pelvic floor first, and anterior rotation of the chin takes place through one-eighth of a circle to bring it underneath the symphysis pubis. After the head is fixed there, flexion occurs. As a result of this, the mouth, nose, forehead and sinciput escape, sweeping over the perineum.

As soon as the head is delivered, restitution takes place, as in a vertex presentation. Simultaneously, there is external rotation of the head corresponding to the movement of internal rotation of the shoulders. The rest of the body is delivered after this.

Mechanism of labour in the mentoposterior position

With the fetus in the mentoposterior position, delivery by the vaginal route is impossible. In this position,

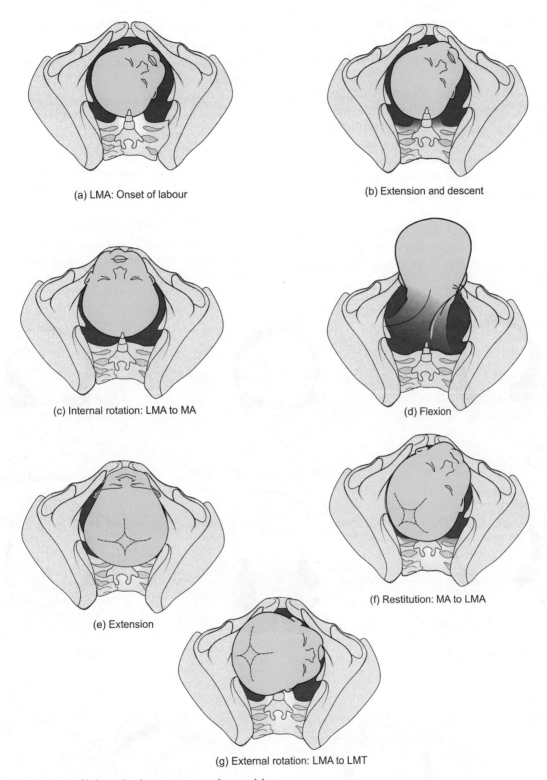

(a) LMA: Onset of labour

(b) Extension and descent

(c) Internal rotation: LMA to MA

(d) Flexion

(e) Extension

(f) Restitution: MA to LMA

(g) External rotation: LMA to LMT

Fig. 40.7   Mechanism of labour in the mentoanterior position

with each uterine contraction, along with the head, the neck and a portion of the body are also pushed down, thereby increasing the diameter of the presenting part. This causes impaction of the fetus in the pelvis and

may result in fetal death and uterine rupture. If vaginal delivery is to take place, the chin must rotate anteriorly. Occasionally, if the size of the fetus is small, the chin may rotate through the larger arc of 3/8th of a circle

(135°) to become mentoanterior (Fig. 40.8). During the process of internal rotation, the chin may not rotate at all or it may be arrested at any stage in the course of internal rotation.

- When the chin remains posterior, further efforts at delivery only impact the face more tightly (Fig. 40.9). This is because each attempt pushes the head down; a portion of the neck and the body of the fetus are also pushed down simultaneously so that the diameter of the engaging part increases to accommodate the thickness of the chest of the fetus.

- While occipitoposterior delivery is possible, delivery as mentoposterior is impossible in face presentations. A cesarean section has to be performed to deliver the baby.

Causes of prolonged labour in face presentation

Labour is prolonged in face presentation for the following reasons:

- The membrane is sausage-shaped and therefore, is not a good dilator; as a result, it ruptures easily.
- The face is not a good dilator of the cervix.
- The facial bones do not mould, but get altered in shape. The submentobregmatic diameter is reduced, and there is a compensatory increase in the occipitofrontal diameter.
- There is long internal rotation.
- The uterine force is not transmitted to the head in the correct axis due to the angulation between the head and neck.

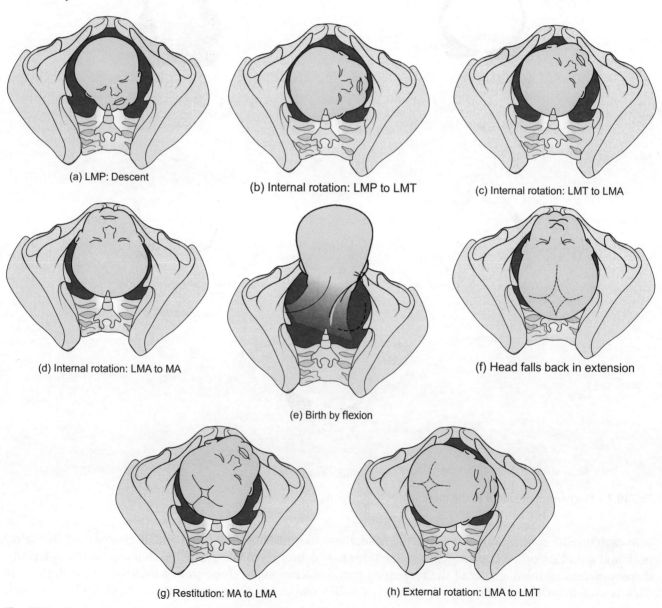

(a) LMP: Descent

(b) Internal rotation: LMP to LMT

(c) Internal rotation: LMT to LMA

(d) Internal rotation: LMA to MA

(e) Birth by flexion

(f) Head falls back in extension

(g) Restitution: MA to LMA

(h) External rotation: LMA to LMT

Fig. 40.8 Mechanism of labour in the left mentoposterior position

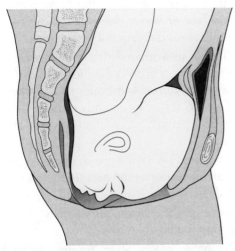

Fig. 40.9 Impacted face in a persistent mentoposterior position

- In mentoposterior position, long rotation has to take place.

Prognosis

For the mother
- There is prolonged labour, increased necessity for obstetric interventions and risk of rupture in the mentoposterior position.

For the baby
- Asphyxia and birth injury
- There is a risk of cord prolapse
- Caput succedaneum is well-marked with swollen and discoloured lips and eyelids with conjunctival hemorrhages
- The baby will show facial edema and bruising; these may lead to problems in resuscitation and feeding
- Laryngeal and tracheal edema may occur after 24 hours of birth and may require nasotracheal intubation; therefore, the baby should be carefully monitored
- Breastfeeding may become difficult as the baby is unable to suck the breast

Management (Fig. 40.10)

Management of mentoanterior position
- If the diagnosis is made during the antenatal period, a decision has to be made regarding the mode of delivery. In those with suspected or evident cephalopelvic disproportion or the presence of a low-lying placenta or a large baby, cesarean section should be resorted to. At the time of cesarean section, the incision should be carefully made on the lower uterine segment to avoid injuring the fetal face.

- Mentoanterior presentations may be allowed to deliver vaginally. However, the face has to be protected. Episiotomy is essential. If required, forceps can be applied; however, ventose is contraindicated.
- If allowed for vaginal delivery, spontaneous labour should be allowed as far as possible, and the membranes should be left intact to prevent cord prolapse.
- In labour, when a face presentation is diagnosed, a careful study of the pelvis should be made to rule out a pelvic contraction at all levels as the cause of the face presentation. If no such cause is found, and the fetus is not unduly large, management will depend upon the position of the chin. If the chin is anterior, the delivery can be dealt with as in vertex presentations.
- No attempt should be made to convert a mentoanterior into a vertex because the resulting position is occipitoposterior, which is less favourable.
- There is a high likelihood of premature rupture of the membranes and delayed engagement of the presenting part. With increasing uterine contractions, the face descends to the pelvic floor and is usually delivered spontaneously. Adequate episiotomy should be given in all cases of face presentations.
- During cesarean section, care should be taken to gently flex the fetal head to avoid nerve damage.
- Fetal mortality is not usually higher than in vertex presentations.

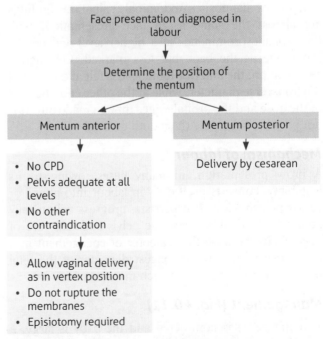

Fig. 40.10 Management of face presentation

Management of the mentoposterior position

- When the chin is posterior, cesarean section is the treatment of choice in the interest of the fetus.
- Cesarean section may have to be undertaken even if the fetus is dead.

Brow Presentation

This is the most unfavourable of all cephalic presentations. There is partial extension of the head, midway between complete flexion and complete extension. With the onset of labour, the brow may be converted to vertex by complete flexion or to face by complete extension. Here, the portion of the fetal head between the anterior fontanelle and the glabella (root of the nose) forms the presenting part. The incidence is 1 in 1,000 to 1 in 1,500 deliveries. Verticomental is the engaging diameter, measuring 13.5 cm; it is the largest. During moulding, the verticomental diameter is decreased and occipitofrontal diameter is increased.

Causes

Transitory presentation of the brow in the beginning of labour is occasionally observed. When labour is established, it might correct itself into a face or vertex presentation. The causes of a brow presentation are practically identical to those giving rise to a face presentation and depend on factors that interfere with flexion or promote the extension of the head.

Diagnosis

Brow presentation is rarely diagnosed by abdominal examination. Vaginal examination is necessary for a definite diagnosis. Abdominal palpation findings are almost the same as in face presentation, with the cephalic prominence at a higher level and on the same side as the back but less marked. On vaginal examination, the anterior fontanelle is felt at one end of the transverse diameter, while at the other end, the root of the nose and the orbital ridges may be made out. It is not possible to palpate the mouth or chin.

Mechanism of labour

A brow presentation, in many cases, owing to its instability, converts itself early in labour into a face or vertex presentation. If it persists, progress will usually be arrested in cases where the pelvis and fetus are of normal size because the diameter of engagement in a brow presentation is the longest diameter of the fetal head—the mentovertical, which measures 13.5 cm.

Management (Fig. 40.11)

- If the pelvis is contracted and the baby is large, a cesarean section should be performed early in labour.

- In about 30–40% of cases, the brow may convert itself into face or vertex presentation during labour, and spontaneous delivery may take place.
- In a multiparous woman with a good-sized pelvis and an average fetus, if brow is diagnosed in early labour, one may observe for 4–6 hours to see whether the head flexes to vertex or extends to face. If the brow presentation persists, a cesarean section should be performed.
- Brow presentation is a very dangerous condition, and cesarean section is the best treatment even if the fetus is dead.
- Except in cases of extreme prematurity, delivery as a brow is impossible.
- When a brow presentation progresses to labour, the membranes rupture early, and there is delay in the first and second stages of labour. Eventually, obstructed labour develops with large caput and moulding. If assistance is not given at this stage, rupture uterus results.

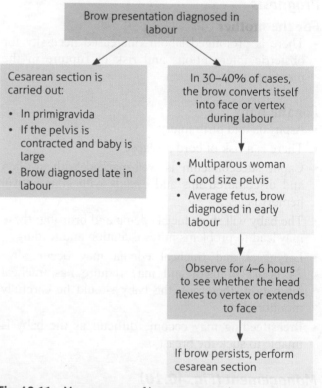

Fig. 40.11 Management of brow presentation

Management of Occipitoposterior, Face and Brow Presentations in a Primary Care Settings

If an occipitoposterior position is diagnosed and the mother is not in labour, it is best to refer her to a higher facility. However, if delivery is imminent, then delivery should be conducted with liberal episiotomy, and the woman should be carefully observed for postpartum hemorrhage. All cases of face and brow should be immediately referred to a higher facility for delivery.

KEY POINTS

✓ *Android pelvis predisposes to occipitoposterior position.*

✓ *The labour in occipitoposterior position is usually more prolonged than that in the occipitoanterior position.*

✓ *90% of occipitoposterior positions have a long anterior rotation and deliver normally.*

✓ *In the anthropoid pelvis, the occiput can rotate to the occipitosacral position and deliver as face-to-pubis, which is associated with extensive perineal tears.*

✓ *If the vertex is below the +2 station, instrumental delivery can be undertaken with ventouse.*

✓ *Cesarean section is performed in cases where the head is arrested at the brim and remains high in the cavity or when there is a failure of rotation.*

✓ *Face and brow presentations occur due to causes that favour the extension of the fetal head or prevent flexion.*

✓ *Vaginal delivery is not possible in persistent mentoposterior and brow presentations and cesarean section is indicated.*

Essay questions

1. Describe the mechanism and conduct of labour in an occipitoposterior position.
2. Describe the mechanism of labour in a face presentation.

Short answer questions

1. Describe the face-to-pubis delivery.
2. What are the findings on abdominal and pelvic examination if the fetus is in the occipitoposterior position?
3. What are the abdominal and pelvic findings in a face presentation?
4. How is the diagnosis of brow presentation made?

MCQs

1. What is the commonest cause of occipitoposterior position of the fetal head during labour?
   a) Maternal obesity
   b) Android pelvis
   c) Multiparity
   d) Multiple pregnancy
2. What is the engaging diameter in the occipitoposterior position?
   a) Suboccipitobregmatic
   b) Occipitofrontal
   c) Submentobregmatic
   d) Biparietal diameter
3. Which of the following is the most unfavourable cephalic presentation?
   a) Brow presentation
   b) Face presentation
   c) Occipitoanterior
   d) Occipitoposterior
4. In the majority of cases, the occipitoposterior positions at the onset of labour:
   a) Spontaneously rotate anteriorly
   b) Become direct occipitoposterior
   c) Become occipitotransverse
   d) Remain as occipitoposterior
5. Factors that hinder the forward rotation of an occipitoposterior position include all the following EXCEPT:
   a) Android pelvis
   b) Oxytocin augmentation

   c) Poor pelvic muscle tone
   d) Premature rupture of membranes
6. The best option for delivery if the head is arrested at the pelvic brim in the transverse position in a viable fetus is:
   a) Cesarean section
   b) Ventouse delivery
   c) Forceps rotation of the occiput to anterior position and delivery
   d) Forceps delivery with occiput directly posterior
7. All the following conditions predispose to face presentations EXCEPT:
   a) Anencephaly
   b) Hydrocephalus
   c) Tumours of the neck
   d) Cephalopelvic disproportion
8. What is the treatment of choice in a live fetus in the mentoposterior position?
   a) Rotation to mentoanterior
   b) Rotation to occipitoanterior
   c) Cesarean section
   d) Forceps delivery
9. What is the engaging diameter in a brow presentation?
   a) 9.4 cm
   b) 11 cm
   c) 12.5 cm
   d) 13.5 cm
10. Which of these is not true in occipitoposterior presentation?
    a) Common in android pelvis
    b) Presents with subumbilical flattening
    c) Fetal heart sounds are best heard near the flanks
    d) 50% spontaneously rotate anterior at the onset of labour

Answers

1. (b), 2. (b), 3. (a), 4. (a), 5. (b), 6. (a), 7. (b), 8. (c), 9. (d), 10. (d)

Fill in the blanks

1. The incidence of transverse lie is about _____.
2. The denominator in the face presentation is the _____.
3. When the portion of the fetal head between the anterior fontanelle and the glabella forms the presenting part, the presentation is known as _____.

4. The diameter of the engagement in a brow presentation is _____.

Answers

1. 0.5%, 2. chin, 3. brow presentation, 4. verticomental

Case scenario-based discussion

1. A 21-year-old primigravida is admitted at 39 weeks of gestation with labour pains for the previous 6 hours and leaking fluid for the last two 2 hours. She does not have any antenatal risk factors. Her general examination findings are normal. On abdominal examination, the uterus is at term and the fetus is in a cephalic presentation with its back on the right side and the head 3/5th palpable with a good fetal heart. The uterus is contracting once in three minutes, each contraction lasting for 45 seconds. On vaginal examination, the cervix is 4 cm dilated, the membrane is absent, the head is felt at the −2 station with the sagittal suture in the transverse diameter of the pelvis; the anterior fontanelle is easily palpated on the left side. The pelvis is adequate.

a) What is the probable diagnosis? What complications do you expect?

b) After 4 hours, the cervix is fully dilated, the occiput has rotated to the right anterior quadrant and the head is at the +2 station. The woman has been in the second stage of labour for one hour; she is exhausted and the CTG showed bradycardia. How would you deliver her?

Answers

a) The woman is in active labour with the fetus in the occipitoposterior position. The complications that may occur in this position are prolonged labour, deep transverse arrest or arrest of anterior rotation at any level.

b) As there is maternal exhaustion and fetal bradycardia, the baby should be delivered immediately either by vacuum application or forceps delivery.

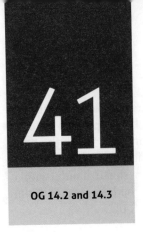

41

OG 14.2 and 14.3

Transverse Lie/Oblique Lie/Unstable Lie

Learning Objectives

» To know the etiology and diagnosis of transverse lie
» To discuss the complications of transverse lie and neglected shoulder presentation
» To describe the antenatal management of transverse and oblique lie

---

■ DEFINITIONS

- **Transverse lie**: When the long axis of the fetus is at a right angle to the long axis of the uterus, it is called a transverse lie.
- **Oblique lie**: When the fetal long axis crosses the maternal long axis obliquely at an angle other than a right angle, it is called an oblique lie. An oblique lie is only temporary or short-lived because with the onset of labour, it becomes either a longitudinal or a transverse lie.
- **Unstable lie**: When the fetal lie changes repeatedly after 37 weeks of gestation, it is known as an unstable lie.

■ TRANSVERSE LIE

Transverse lie is otherwise known as shoulder presentation because the shoulder of the fetus lies over the pelvic brim with the cephalic pole at one of the iliac fossae; the breech is felt at the opposite iliac fossa. The incidence of transverse lie at term is 0.3%. The acromion process is the denominator in shoulder presentation. There are four variants of the transverse lie, which are as follows:

- Dorso anterior is the commonest, seen in 60% of cases
- Dorso posterior
- Dorso superior
- Dorso inferior

Etiology

The causes of transverse lie are generally the same as the ones that favour a malpresentation. These are listed in the box that follows.

Maternal factors
- Contracted pelvis
- Uterine anomalies

- Unusual relaxation of the abdominal wall resulting from high parity
- Tumours complicating pregnancy
- Congenital uterine malformations
- In a primigravida with an oblique or transverse lie or in a woman with recurrent transverse lie, uterine malformation should be ruled out as the cause of malpresentation

Pregnancy factors
- Placental abnormalities (placenta previa or fundal implantation of the placenta)
- Hydramnios
- Prematurity

Fetal factors
- Multiple pregnancy (more common in the second of twins)
- Fetal anomalies such as hydrocephalus, tumours of the neck and sacrococcygeal teratoma

Diagnosis

Abdominal examination

- On inspection, the uterus appears broader, asymmetrical and not pyriform as it does in a longitudinal lie.
- On palpation, the fundal height is lesser than the period of amenorrhea.
- With **fundal grip**, neither the cephalic nor the podalic pole is palpable. On **lateral grip,** the head is felt in the iliac fossa on one side and the soft podalic pole is felt on the other side. Sometimes, the head may be felt at a higher level near the fundus. In dorsoposterior positions, where the spine is posterior, the limb buds are easily palpable. When the back is anterior, a hard resistance is felt across the abdomen (Fig. 41.1a and b). On **pelvic grip,** the lower pole is empty.

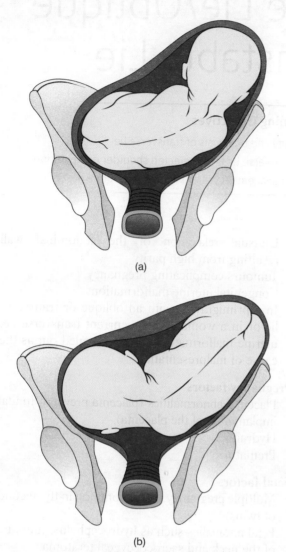

Fig. 41.1 Types of oblique lie: (a) Breech on iliac fossa and (b) head in the iliac fossa

- The **fetal heart** is generally heard at the level of the umbilicus. In vertex presentations, it is heard well below the umbilicus, and in breech, well above the umbilicus.
- USG should be carried out in all cases to rule out fetal anomalies, uterine tumours and placenta previa.

Vaginal examination

Vaginal examination should not be carried out without ruling out placenta previa by USG. When the woman is in labour and the cervix is dilated, the membrane will be hanging loose, and through it, the fetal parts can be felt. But most often, the membranes are ruptured and the fetal hand, elbow the shoulder can be felt; if the fingers are passed up further, the side of the chest may be palpable. The shoulder can be recognised by palpating the acromion process, the scapula, the clavicle and

axilla. On palpating further, the chest of the fetus can be felt by noting the ribs, which run parallel to each other and have a typical 'grid iron feel'. When the hand is prolapsed in the vagina, the side to which it belongs can be determined by trying to shake hands with it (Fig. 41.2). Occasionally, when the hand is still within the vagina, it is mistaken for the foot.

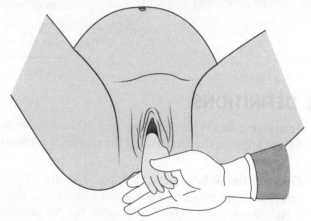

Fig. 41.2 Oblique presentation with one hand prolapsed; method of recognising the side to which the hand belongs by shaking hands—the doctor's right hand shakes the baby's right hand

Course of Labour in Transverse Lie

In the presence of a normal pelvis and a normally developed fetus at term presenting by the shoulder, there is no mechanism of labour. Spontaneous termination of pregnancy is impossible without serious risks to the mother and the child.

Sequence of events if an oblique lie/transverse lie is neglected in labour (Fig. 41.3a–c)

Under normal circumstances, transverse lie at term should be delivered only by **cesarean section**. In the past, due to the lack of information and inadequate transport facilities, women used to reach the health facility many hours after the onset of labour, presenting with neglected shoulder presentation. With improvement in the healthcare system, such catastrophic events are rarely seen nowadays. If the woman is unattended for long hours during labour, the following sequence of events is likely to occur:

1. When the woman goes into labour, the membranes rupture prematurely and there could be cord or hand prolapse.
2. With each uterine contraction, the fetal hand descends more and more into the vagina and may present at the vulva as a hand prolapse. Sometimes, even the shoulder may be impacted in the vagina.

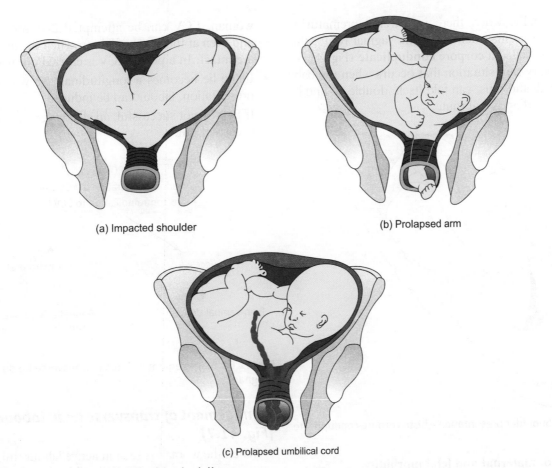

(a) Impacted shoulder

(b) Prolapsed arm

(c) Prolapsed umbilical cord

Fig. 41.3(a–c) Oblique lie and difficulties in delivery

3. The hand becomes swollen, edematous and bluish.

4. Continued uterine action forces the fetus to descend into the distended lower uterine segment. The lower uterine segment is thus stretched to accommodate the fetus.

5. As a result of the contraction of the upper segment and dilatation of the lower segment, a line of demarcation between the two uterine segments becomes demonstrable. This demarcation is known as the **Bandl's ring** or retraction ring. It gradually rises higher and higher as the obstructed labour progresses. The ring may even rise to the level of the umbilicus (Fig. 41.4a and b).

6. The height at which this ring is noted indicates the extent to which the stretching of the lower uterine segment has taken place and, thereby, the degree of thinning of its wall. This situation is referred to as a **neglected transverse lie** leading to obstructed labour.

7. Finally, a stage is reached when the lower uterine segment can stretch no more and the **uterus ruptures**.

8. When rupture takes place, the woman feels a momentary relief as uterine contractions cease.

Normal shape of the abdomen

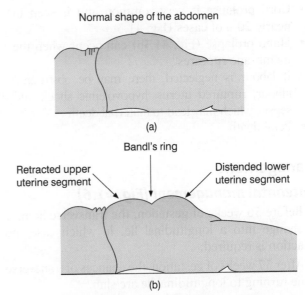

(a)

Bandl's ring

Retracted upper uterine segment

Distended lower uterine segment

(b)

Fig. 41.4 (a) Normal abdomen and (b) line of demarcation demonstrable between the two uterine segments

However, as a result of the rupture, the fetus and placenta escape partially or wholly into the abdominal cavity. Because of the intraperitoneal bleeding, the woman goes into shock and collapses. If assistance is not available, fetal and/or maternal death occurs.

Occasionally, when there is extreme prematurity, a transverse lie may deliver by the vaginal route; this condition is called a **corpore conduplicate** (Fig. 41.5). This is a very rare situation that occurs when the baby is very small and thus, can fold itself, double up and be delivered by the vaginal route.

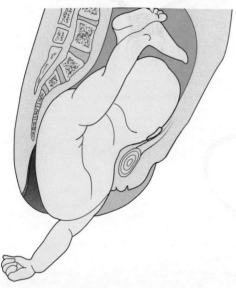

Fig. 41.5 Shoulder presentation—birth corpore conduplicate

Causes of maternal and fetal morbidity associated with shoulder presentation
- Cord prolapse is very common and is seen in nearly 20% of cases (Fig. 41.3c)
- Hand prolapse (Fig. 41.3b) can occur when the membrane ruptures
- If labour is neglected, there may be obstructed labour, ruptured uterus, hypovolemic shock and sepsis, which may lead to maternal death
- Fetal death

Management

Antenatal management (Fig. 41.6)
- Before 36 weeks of gestation, the transverse lie may change into a longitudinal lie, in which case, no action is required.
- After 37 weeks of gestation, the chances of transverse lie turning to longitudinal lie are slim.
- All women with transverse lie after 36 weeks should be hospitalised to avoid the risk of membrane rupture and cord prolapse.
- If there are no contraindications, the woman should be offered external cephalic version (ECV) so that cesarean section can be avoided. In a multiparous

woman, ECV can be attempted 2–3 times a week and even at the onset of labour when the membranes are intact. In a primi, ECV is carried out weekly.
- If the lie becomes a longitudinal one with cephalic presentation, labour can be induced.
- If ECV is not successful, an elective cesarean section is carried out.

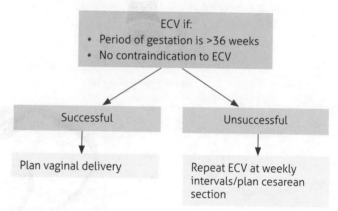

Fig. 41.6 Management of fetus in transverse lie during pregnancy

Management of transverse lie in labour (Fig. 41.7)
- When the woman is seen in active labour, this would present with an impacted shoulder; the folded fetus would have been driven to a varying amount down the pelvis.
- In such cases, an immediate cesarean section should be performed even if the fetus is dead because of the risk of uterine rupture.

Cesarean section in transverse lie
- The lower segment may be thick and narrow as there is no fetal part occupying the lower pole. The incision may have to be converted to a J-shaped or inverted T-shaped incision to deliver the baby. Occasionally, a classical incision may be required.

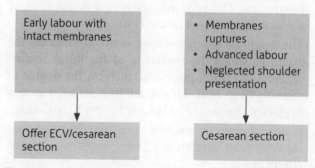

Fig. 41.7 Management of fetus in transverse lie at the time of labour

- If the membrane has ruptured and the liquor has drained, there will be difficulty in delivering the fetus. Due to the tonic uterine contractions and absence of liquor, the uterus will be closely applied to the fetus and it would be difficult to insinuate the hand into the uterus to reach the foot and deliver as breech.
- In the dorsoanterior position, accessing the fetal legs may be difficult.
- The uterine incision may extend laterally into the broad ligament or in the downward direction behind the bladder.
- It is important that an adequate incision is made on the anterior abdominal wall and the uterus. Occasionally, uterine relaxation may have to be provided by the anesthetist if difficulty is encountered in delivering the baby.
- The position of the fetus and the side on which the legs are present should always be confirmed by USG prior to the cesarean section. The baby should be delivered by grasping the feet and not the arms.

UNSTABLE LIE

When the fetal lie changes repeatedly after 37 weeks of gestation, it is known as an unstable lie.

Management

Antenatal management of unstable lie

Women diagnosed with unstable lie should be hospitalised because of the risk of hemorrhage from placenta previa, prolapse of the umbilical cord and obstructed labour. The following steps should be taken upon admission:

- The bladder and bowel should be emptied as this may stabilise the lie of the fetus
- CPD and fetal anomalies should be ruled out
- USG should be performed to locate the placental site
- Vaginal examination should be performed to rule out pelvic tumours

In the majority of cases, no cause will be found. In such cases, the woman is usually multiparous and has a lax uterus or abdominal wall. In these women, external cephalic version can be attempted if there are no contraindications.

Management during labour

- Blood is cross-matched and kept ready, as the chance of CS is high.
- In a primigravida, cesarean section is carried out at 38 weeks.
- In a multigravid woman, in the presence of CPD or other risk factors, a cesarean section is carried out.
- In the absence of any such risk factors, the spontaneous onset of labour should be awaited. Once labour begins, the lie is corrected to vertex and is held there until the head is stable. If the membranes ruptures, cord prolapse should be looked for. Occasionally, controlled ARM can be undertaken. Initially, the hindwaters are ruptured, and once the head stabilises in the pelvis, the forewater can be ruptured. This should preferably be done in the theatre.

KEY POINTS

✓ *Transverse lie is a presentation in which the long axis of the fetus lies at a right angle to that of the uterus.*

✓ *With a normal pelvis and a normally developed fetus at term presenting by the shoulder, spontaneous termination of labour is impossible without serious risks to the mother and the child.*

✓ *When an oblique lie/transverse lie is recognised in the later weeks of pregnancy, efforts should be made to correct it into a vertex presentation by external version if there are no contraindications.*

✓ *If a woman is seen in active labour with a transverse lie, a cesarean section should be performed.*

✓ *If the unstable lie persists, external cephalic version can be performed at 38–39 weeks followed by stabilising induction.*

Essay questions

1. How would you manage a primigravida at 36 weeks of gestation with transverse lie?
2. Discuss the management of unstable lie of the fetus after the 36th week of pregnancy.

Short answer questions

1. How is the diagnosis of transverse lie made?
2. What are the complications of transverse lie?

3. Describe the role of external cephalic version in correcting the lie of the fetus.

MCQs

1. Which of the following is not among the etiologies of malpresentations?
   a) Contracted pelvis
   b) Small baby
   c) Polyhydramnios
   d) Abruptio placenta

2. The complications of transverse and unstable lie are all except:
   a) Cord or hand prolapse
   b) Obstructed labour
   c) Shoulder dystocia
   d) Uterine rupture

3. Which of the following is the most common cause of compound presentation?
   a) Pelvic tumours
   b) Multiple pregnancy
   c) Prematurity
   d) Rupture of the membranes

4. Which of the following is the management of transverse lie with hand prolapse?
   a) External cephalic version
   b) Internal podalic version
   c) Cesarean delivery
   d) Evisceration

5. The causes of transverse lie include all the following EXCEPT:
   a) Contracted pelvis
   b) Placenta previa
   c) Multiple pregnancy
   d) Oligohydramnios

6. The pathological retraction ring of Bandl is associated with:
   a) Preterm labour
   b) Obstructed labour
   c) Abruptio placenta
   d) Chorio amnionitis

7. What is the preferred mode of delivery for an intrauterine dead fetus with hand prolapse?
   a) Decapitation
   b) Craniotomy
   c) Internal podalic version
   d) Cesarean section

8. What is the incidence of cord prolapse in transverse lie?
   a) 10%
   b) 20%
   c) 30%
   d) 40%

9. What is the most common cause of recurrent transverse lie?
   a) Contracted pelvis
   b) Uterine anomaly
   c) Multiple pregnancy
   d) Polyhydramnios

10. What is the denominator in transverse lie?
    a) Mentum
    b) Occiput
    c) Acromion
    d) Sacrum

Answers

1. (d), 2. (c), 3. (c), 4. (c), 5. (d), 6. (b), 7. (d), 8. (b), 9. (b), 10. (c)

Fill in the blanks

1. When the long axis of the fetus lies at a right angle to that of the uterus, it is called a _____.
2. The denominator in a transverse lie is the _____.
3. The condition in which a very premature baby in transverse lie is delivered by folding on itself is called _____.

Answers

1. transverse lie,   2. acromion,   3. corpore conduplicate

Case scenario-based discussion

1. A 30-year-old gravida 3, para 2, with a history of two normal deliveries presents at 37 weeks of gestation with a diagnosis of transverse lie. She is not in labour.
   a) How would you proceed with managing this case?
   b) If the ECV is unsuccessful, what is the further course of action?
   c) If the woman goes into labour, what are the complications expected?

Answers

a) The woman should be hospitalised to avoid the risk of membrane rupture and cord prolapse when she goes into labour. If there are no contraindications, ECV may be offered.

b) If the ECV is unsuccessful, it can be repeated weekly; alternatively, an elective cesarean can be performed after 38 completed weeks of gestation.

c) Cord prolapse, arm prolapse, obstructed labour and rupture of uterus, PPH and sepsis are the complications that can be expected.

42
OG 15.1 and 15.2

Breech Presentation and Compound Presentation

Learning Objectives

» To discuss the definition, causes and types of breech presentation
» To be able to make the antenatal diagnosis of breech presentation
» To describe the mechanism of labour in breech presentation
» To know the steps and conduct of assisted breech delivery
» To know the difference between assisted breech delivery and breech extraction
» To discuss the maternal, fetal and neonatal complications in breech presentation
» To know the risks associated with a compound presentation

■ BREECH PRESENTATION

Breech presentation is defined as a fetus in a longitudinal lie, wherein the buttocks or the feet (the podalic pole) of the fetus occupy the lower segment of the uterus.

Types of Breech Presentation (Fig. 42.1)

The types of breech presentation are the following:

1. Flexed or complete breech
2. Extended or frank breech
3. Incomplete breech

- **Complete breech presentation:** Here, the fetus maintains an attitude of universal flexion with the thighs flexed at the hips and the legs at the knees ('tailor sitting' or squatting position) (Fig. 42.1a). This type of breech is seen in 5–10% of all cases. It is more commonly seen in multiparous women.

- **Frank breech or extended breech:** Here, both the thighs are flexed against the abdomen but the legs are extended at the knee sothat the lower limbs lie along the ventral surface of the baby's trunk (Fig. 42.1b). It is the commonest and most favourable type of breech presentation, accounting for nearly 70% of cases. It is more common in nulliparous women.

- **Incomplete breech presentation:** This includes knee and footling presentations. In the knee presentation, the thigh is extended at the hip, but the leg is flexed at the knee. In the footling presentation, the thigh is extended at the hip and the leg at the knee (Fig. 42.1c). In knee and footling presentations, one or both the legs may be involved. This type of breech is associated with a high risk of cord prolapse and therefore, is an indication for cesarean section.

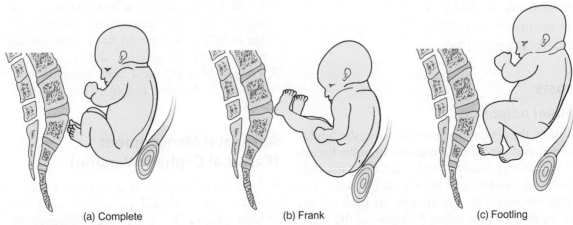

(a) Complete   (b) Frank   (c) Footling

Fig. 42.1(a–c) Types of breech

Incidence

The frequency of breech presentation depends upon the period of gestation. Breech presentation accounts for nearly 3% of all deliveries and is more common in preterm fetuses. At 28 weeks of gestation, the incidence could be as high as 25%. The incidence of breech presentations at term at the Govt. Hospital for Women and Children, Chennai, Tamil Nadu, in 2011 was 1.9%.

Etiology

Anything that interferes with the movement of the fetus can predispose to breech presentation. In 40–50% of cases, no underlying cause may be found. The common etiological factors are as follows:
- Prematurity
- Conditions that interfere with the kicking movement of the fetus, e.g., extended legs, oligohydramnios, multiple pregnancy
- Uterine anomalies
- Congenital malformations of the fetus—hydrocephalus, fetal ascites, spina bifida
- Placenta previa, cornuofundal implantation of the placenta
- Contracted pelvis, pelvic tumours
- Fetuses with skeletal or neuromuscular malformations—inability to move
- Maternal alcohol abuse, use of anticonvulsants due to decreased tone
- Previous breech presentation

Positions

In a breech presentation, the sacrum is the denominator. Four such positions have been described:
1. Left sacroanterior (LSA), which is the most common
2. Right sacroanterior (RSA)
3. Right sacroposterior (RSP)
4. Left sacroposterior (LSP)

Diagnosis

Abdominal palpation

On palpation, the cephalic pole will be felt at the fundus of the uterus and can be differentiated from the breech because the head is smaller, harder and more movable and ballots independently of the rest of the body. The lateral grip will reveal the presence of the back on one side and the limbs on the other. By means of the pelvic grip, the large breech is felt at the lower pole; it is broader, bulkier and softer and moves with the rest of the body.

Auscultation

The fetal heart will be heard above the level of the umbilicus, either to its right or left, depending upon the position of the back. It is heard closer to the midline when the back is anterior, and further out when the back is posterior.

Vaginal examination

A breech presentation is detected on vaginal examination by the palpation of the ischial tuberosities on either side, with the anus in the middle and the sacrum behind. In a complete breech, the feet can be felt beside the buttocks, whereas in an extended breech, the feet are not felt. In the footling presentation, one or both feet may be felt hanging in the vagina. Sometimes, the external genitalia may be felt. The anus may sometimes be mistaken for the mouth and the ischial tuberosities for malar eminences, leading to a diagnosis of face presentation. These errors can usually be avoided by performing a careful examination. When a finger is introduced into the anus, the grip of the sphincter is usually felt; there may also be staining with meconium. The anus and the ischial tuberosities form a straight line, distinguishing the breech from the face. The heel helps to differentiate between the foot and the hand.

Imaging techniques

All women presenting with breech or suspected of having breech after 36 weeks of gestation should undergo USG of the abdomen to confirm the presentation, classify the type of breech, assess the estimated fetal weight, rule out the presence of congenital anomalies and ascertain the location of the placenta. USG also helps in the diagnosis of a hyperextended (star gazing attitude—the angle between the thoracic and cervical spine is >90°) or deflexed head, which might lead to cervical extension injuries during vaginal delivery. Adequacy of liquor and cord presentation can also be assessed. Routine use of X-ray pelvimetry is not advisable.

Antenatal Management (External Cephalic Version)

If breech presentation is diagnosed in the antenatal period, women should be offered external cephalic version (ECV) to lower the incidence of breech presentations in labour. External cephalic version is a method of converting a breech presentation into a cephalic presentation by external manipulation. The advantages of ECV are that it is safe, non-invasive, relatively easy to perform and relatively painless for the mother. Further, it may reduce the need for a cesarean section. However, there are certain contraindications for the procedure (see box below).

Contraindications for external cephalic version
- Absolute contraindications
  — Multiple pregnancy
  — APH, placenta previa
  — Ruptured membranes
  — Significant fetal abnormalities
  — When there is a need for CS for other indications
  — Known uterine anomalies
- Relative contraindications
  — Scarred uterus
  — IUGR
  — Severe pre-eclampsia
  — Rh-isoimmunisation

ECV is performed starting from 36 weeks in a nullipara and 37 weeks in a multiparous woman. If it is performed earlier, the chances of reverting to breech are higher. Moreover, if the baby has to be delivered on account of complications arising during ECV, the chances of prematurity are minimal after 36 weeks. The procedure is successful in nearly 60% of cases. If ECV is successful, vaginal delivery should be allowed. If ECV was not successful, it can be repeated at weekly intervals. Though ECV can be performed even in early labour with intact membranes, there may be difficulties in converting breech to cephalic because of the advanced gestation and reduced liquor. If ECV is repeatedly unsuccessful, the woman can be offered an elective cesarean section or assisted vaginal breech delivery at the onset of labour. Anti-D immunoglobulin must be given if the mother is Rh-negative. Version can be complicated by abruption, preterm labour, preterm premature rupture of membranes, fetal distress and cord entanglement.

Indications for Elective Cesarean Section

There are certain indications for elective cesarean section that is carried out as a planned procedure after 38 weeks of gestation.

- Breech with other obstetrical problems or previous cesarean section
- Severe IUGR, oligohydramnios
- Fetal weight >3.5 Kg
- Inadequate pelvis
- Hyperextended head as shown by imaging studies
- Footling /knee presentation
- An obstetrician inexperienced in conducting an assisted vaginal breech delivery

Mechanism of Labour

Compared to the vertex presentation, labour in breech presentation is more complicated because progressively larger and less compressible parts of the fetus are delivered. The labour is usually prolonged because the engagement of the breech occurs only with the onset of labour. Moreover, breech—especially the flexed breech—is a poor cervical dilator as it does not fit snugly in the lower segment. The chances of cord prolapse and premature rupture of membranes are also high.

Labour in breech presentation consists of three stages—delivery of the breech, delivery of the shoulders and delivery of the head.

Delivery of the breech

Engagement
In breech, the denominator is the sacrum, and the engaging diameter is the bitrochanteric diameter, which is 9.5 cm. When the position is left sacroanterior (LSA), the breech enters the brim with the bitrochanteric diameter occupying the left oblique diameter of the pelvis.

Descent with compaction
When labour begins, the first movement is descent with compaction. Compaction means that every part of the fetal body becomes a little more flexed; this movement is akin to the flexion noted in vertex presentation.

Internal rotation
This descent with compaction drives the breech down through the pelvis until the anterior buttock reaches the floor of the pelvis. Then, the second movement takes place, namely, internal rotation. It always results in the anterior buttock moving towards the symphysis pubis through one-eighth of a circle, regardless of whether the sacrum is in the anterior or posterior position (there is always one buttock positioned anteriorly, which can move through one-eighth of a circle and thus, bring the buttock to the symphysis pubis).

Lateral flexion

After internal rotation has taken place, the next movement is lateral flexion. This movement is, in fact, the counterpart of the movement of extension in a vertex presentation and flexion in a face presentation. It is only by lateral flexion that the breech is able to pass through the cavity and present at the outlet. The breech then distends the perineum, after which, the body and limbs are born (Fig. 42.2).

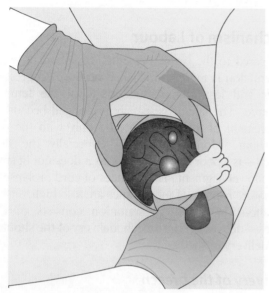

Fig. 42.2 Breech distending the perineum

Delivery of the shoulders

Once the breech has been delivered outside the vagina, the body slips out; the engaging diameter at the shoulder is the bisacromial diameter, which is 12 cm. It engages in the same left oblique diameter as the breech, and by the movement of internal rotation by one-eighth of a circle, the shoulder becomes anteroposterior and the anterior shoulder hitches against the symphysis pubis; by lateral flexion, the posterior shoulder sweeps over the perineum and is born first, the anterior shoulder following later.

Delivery of the head

After the shoulders have descended, the head engages in the opposite oblique diameter; if the breech has passed through the left oblique diameter, the head will engage with suboccipitofrontal diameter (10.5 cm), occupying the right oblique diameter. There is further descent of the head with increasing flexion. Now, rotation takes place, bringing the occiput underneath the symphysis pubis. Then, by a movement of flexion, the head is born.

Conduct of Vaginal Breech Delivery

In the conduct of vaginal breech delivery, case selection is very important. The clinician should be experienced in conducting assisted breech delivery, and there should be careful intrapartum management. As operative interventions and perinatal complications are more common with vaginal breech delivery than with vertex, informed consent must be taken from the mother. Besides a skilled obstetrician, vaginal breech delivery also requires facilities for emergency cesarean section and an anesthetist and pediatrician.

Vaginal delivery may be undertaken in women with an adequate pelvis, an average-sized baby (<3.5 Kg—fetal weight should be assessed by USG), extended/flexed breech (preferably extended breech), well-flexed head and spontaneous onset of labour. There should not be any other indications for cesarean section. Footling and knee presentations are contraindications for vaginal delivery. In women with breech presentation, to identify those who will be most suitable for vaginal delivery, a scoring system (Zatuchini–Andros scoring system) is available. In this system, scores are assigned based on parity, gestational age, estimated fetal weight, previous breech delivery, dilatation and station of the breech at presentation.

Vaginal delivery is accomplished by the following methods:

1. Spontaneous breech delivery—the infant is expelled spontaneously without any assistance or manipulation. Spontaneous delivery is possible only in extremely preterm babies.

2. Assisted breech delivery—all breech deliveries at term require assistance in the delivery of the head, and some, in the delivery of the shoulders. In assisted breech delivery, the fetus is delivered spontaneously up to the umbilicus; the rest of the baby is delivered by various manoeuvres.

3. Total breech extraction—a routine breech extraction is not favoured and is recommended only when there is a definite indication. This will be discussed later.

Management of the first stage of labour

- To avoid the risk of cord prolapse at the time of the rupture of membranes, it is advisable to nurse the woman in bed.

- As operative interventions and anesthesia may be required, the woman should be prepared as for a cesarean section. Intravenous fluid should be given for nutritional support.

- Because of the risk of cord compression and cord prolapse, it is important to observe the fetal heart rate every 15 minutes, especially after the rupture of the membranes. Continuous electronic monitoring of the fetal heart is preferable as it can pick up cord compression and occult cord prolapse early. This is mandatory in the second stage of labour.

- Good progress in labour is the best indicator of fetopelvic adequacy. Therefore, as in the vertex presentation, labour progress should be monitored using a partograph.

- Amniotomy should be avoided. If there is spontaneous rupture of membranes, vaginal examination should be performed to rule out cord prolapse. CTG changes should be carefully looked for. Cervical dilatation and the type and position of the breech should also be noted.

- With increasing uterine contractions, the breech begins to descend. With an extended breech, engagement and progress occurs earlier than with a fully flexed breech. With good progress in labour and no cord complications, the labour is allowed to progress. If there are weak uterine contractions and inadequate labour progress, it is preferable to opt for a cesarean section rather than augmentation with oxytocin infusion as there may be subtle fetopelvic disproportion.

- Pain relief is important, preferably with epidural analgesia as it avoids premature pushing through an undilated cervix. Also, if the woman was on epidural analgesia, she can be taken up for CS or breech extraction if necessary.

Management of the second stage of labour

- Assessing full cervical dilatation is difficult in breech. In cephalic presentation, the cervix disappears behind the cephalic crown. In breech, the cervix remains palpable as the fetal trunk descends. It requires experience to diagnose full cervical dilatation.

- In the early second stage, the breech descends well into the pelvis. Once the breech reaches below the ischial spine, active pushing begins.

- At this stage, the availability of a skilled obstetrician, neonatologist and immediate theatre facility is essential.

- Conducting an assisted breech delivery requires proper planning. All arrangements must be made to treat neonatal asphyxia. Each step of the assistance should be planned, purposeful and deliberate and not haphazard in any way. There should be no panic, especially in the delivery of the arms and the head. There is no need to hurry and complete the delivery (five to seven minutes is not a long interval and will not adversely affect a well-oxygenated baby). The umbilical cord pulsation will provide an indication of the baby's well-being.

Assisted breech delivery (Fig. 42.3a–f)

- With the descent of the breech to the pelvic floor, the pain increases in intensity and frequency and the breech appears at the vulval outlet. At this stage, the woman should be brought to the edge of the board and kept in the lithotomy position.

- If the woman is not on epidural, pudendal block anesthesia is given, and the bladder is catheterised.

- When the baby's anus is visible at the vulval outlet between contractions—otherwise called 'breech climbing the perineum'—a liberal mediolateral episiotomy is performed. The timing of the episiotomy is important. It should not be performed too early. It is best done when, between contractions, the baby's anus is visible at the vulval outlet. Episiotomy should always be performed for a primigravida; often, it is required in a multipara as well. Failure to do so might occasionally give rise to difficulty in the delivery of the aftercoming head.

- At this stage, the 'hands-off approach' should be practiced until the baby is delivered to the level of umbilicus. With increasing uterine contractions, the breech emerges out of the vulval outlet. With a fully flexed breech, a foot may sometimes be caught in the vagina; it should be released by hooking it out with a finger. With further contractions and straining by the woman, the baby is born as far as the umbilicus spontaneously. At this stage, there should not be any attempt to apply traction on the fetus. The obstetrician must ensure that the baby's back is facing him. No attempt should be made to draw down a loop of the cord; rather, it should be kept to one side to prevent it from being compressed. The baby should be covered in a warm towel to avoid early breathing attempts and aspiration of the amniotic fluid. The body of the baby should be steadied around the pelvic girdle with a femoropelvic grip (Fig. 42.3a)—the fingers are kept on the anterior superior iliac crest and the thumbs on the sacrum to avoid injury to the abdominal organs and prevent femoral fracture.

- With further effort on the part of the woman, the axillary folds of the baby come into view under the

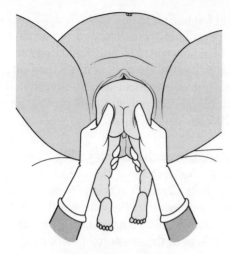

(a) Femoropelvic grip

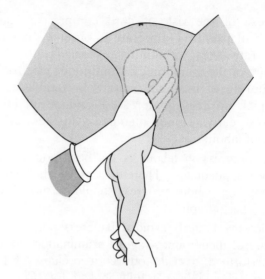

(d) Extended arms: Subsequently bringing down
the anterior right arm without rotating the fetus

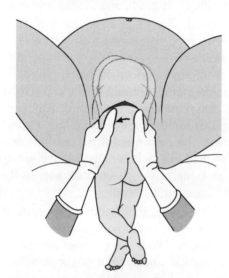

(b) Rotate the fetal shoulders
(in direction of arrow)
to bring the arm posterior

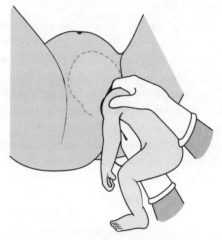

(e) Jaw and shoulder traction: First stage of traction

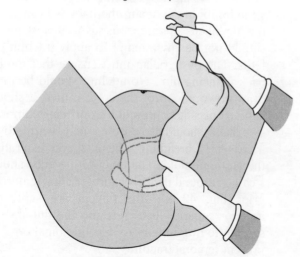

(c) Extended arms: Bringing down the
posterior left arm

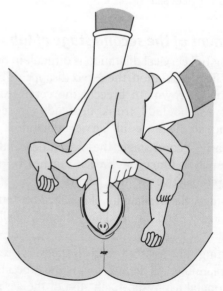

(f) Jaw and shoulder traction: Second stage of traction

Fig. 42.3 Assisted breech

symphysis. There should not be any attempt to deliver the shoulder until the scapula and one axilla are visible. Heavy sedation and dense epidural should be avoided to maximise expulsive effort. Ordinarily, since the arm is flexed at the elbow, the shoulders deliver without much difficulty. The posterior arm is usually born first, followed by the anterior arm. If the arm is not flexed, and if there is delay, the Lovset manoeuvre is used to deliver the arms.

Lovset manoeuvre

The baby is held by the femoropelvic grip and rotated with gentle traction until the posterior shoulder becomes anterior and comes under the symphysis pubis. As soon as the shoulder is seen under the symphysis, a finger is passed along the arm down to the elbow, which is then flexed. As a result, the hand drops down. The baby is then rotated again so that the other shoulder comes under the symphysis and the same manoeuvre is repeated. This is based on the principle that the posterior shoulder is always at a lower level and below the brim. The Lovset manoeuvre is resorted to only when the normal mechanism fails. After both the arms are delivered, the child hangs from the vulval outlet with its back directly facing the obstetrician. Allowing the child to hang down from the vulval outlet for a few minutes is believed to facilitate the entry of the head into the pelvis by flexion and the action of gravity. Should further assistance be required, it is provided by moderate suprapubic pressure on the head to promote flexion and descent.

Delivery of the head (Fig. 42.4a–d)

Once the hairline is seen under the symphysis, with the assistant applying suprapubic pressure to maintain flexion, the obstetrician, with steady traction on the feet, swings the fetus in an arc over the mother's abdomen. This manoeuvre must be carefully executed; care must be taken to see that the head does not suddenly come out of the vagina. This manoeuvre has the potential to make the head hyperextended and cause injury to the cervical vertebra and the spinal cord. The episiotomy already performed provides enough room for the safe passage of the head, which can be controlled. This method of delivery of the head is known as the **Marshall–Burns technique**. The head can also be kept flexed by jaw flexion and shoulder traction—the Mauriceau–Smellie–Veit manoeuvre, which is described later in this chapter.

Delivery of the after-coming head by forceps

Some obstetricians, at this stage, prefer to deliver the after-coming head by forceps. Either a pair of straight

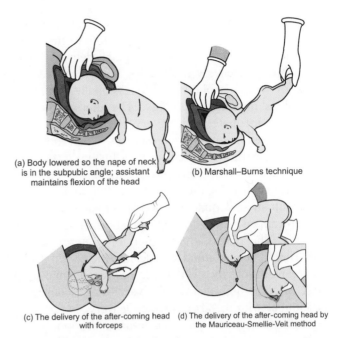

(a) Body lowered so the nape of neck is in the subpubic angle; assistant maintains flexion of the head

(b) Marshall–Burns technique

(c) The delivery of the after-coming head with forceps

(d) The delivery of the after-coming head by the Mauriceau-Smellie-Veit method

Fig. 42.4   Delivery of the head

forceps or Piper's forceps with their long and parallel shanks can be used. Before applying the forceps, an assistant holds the body of the child straight using a towel and lifts it up to make sure that the body remains parallel to the floor. Then, the operator introduces the blades of the forceps from below, placing one on either side of the head, and applies steady traction. The advantages of using forceps are that the delivery of the head can be controlled and the sudden exit of the head can be avoided. The traction on the head promotes flexion and prevents traction and injury to the neck and cervical vertebra. Further, the space created by the forceps allows the baby to breathe.

Management of the third stage of labour

The third stage of labour is managed on the usual lines. Prophylactic use of oxytocics prior to the completion of the delivery is not recommended.

Indications for Cesarean Section in Labour

During the course of assisted breech delivery, the baby may have to be delivered by emergency cesarean section for various indications, which are as follows:

- Cord prolapse in first and early second stages of labour
- Fetal distress
- Failure to progress in the first and second stages of labour
- High breech and failure to descend
- Impacted breech

At the time of cesarean section, the delivery of the breech, shoulders and head should follow the same sequence as that in assisted vaginal delivery. Very often, hurried delivery of the baby at cesarean section leads to fetal morbidity and occasionally, mortality as well as maternal morbidity. The uterine incision should be adequate; if necessary, it can be converted to an inverted T- or J-shaped incision. When the lower uterine segment is not well-formed, further difficulties will be encountered. Uterine relaxants may be required just before delivering the baby. Struggling to deliver the head with an inadequate incision is as bad as delivering an entrapped after-coming head during vaginal delivery. The risk is even higher for preterm babies. One should bear in mind that despite the liberal use of cesarean section, the overall risk for breech babies is at least twice as high as others. Every obstetrician must be familiar with the art of breech delivery, as the same versatility is required even in a cesarean section.

Complications Encountered During Breech Delivery

Many complications may occur during a breech delivery, some of which may result in fetal death and maternal trauma.

Premature rupture of the membranes

This is a very common feature in breech deliveries and is relatively more common in complete breech and footling presentations due to the presenting part imperfectly fitting into the lower uterine segment. It cannot be prevented, and to some extent, affects the fetal prognosis adversely since labour may be prolonged, and intrapartum infection is likely to occur. With the premature rupture of the membranes and a partially dilated cervix, the foot sometimes slips into the vagina in a flexed breech presentation. No attempt should be made to extract the breech when the cervix is not fully dilated. Such attempts often end in cervical tears and difficulties in delivering the arms and head, ending most often in stillbirth. It is far better to deliver the baby by cesarean section.

Head entrapment

Here, through an incompletely dilated cervix, the soft breech and shoulder are delivered, and the head gets trapped by the undilated cervix. It commonly occurs with preterm breech vaginal delivery. In these cases, the cord also gets compressed between the tight cervix and the fetal head. In these situations, the delivery of the baby should be brought about rapidly. If the cervix is rigid and unyielding, a Dührssen's incision is made at the 4 o'clock and 7 o'clock positions so that the cervix opens sufficiently to allow the delivery of the head.

Prolapse of the umbilical cord

The incidence of cord prolapse is 0.5–1% in frank breech (which is almost similar to that of cephalic [0.5%]), 4–5% in complete breech and nearly 10% in knee and footling presentations. Prolapse of the cord is an indication for immediate delivery of the baby if it is viable. When the cord prolapse occurs in the first or second stage of labour and the fetus is not well in the pelvis, cesarean section should be undertaken. If the breech is imminent to deliver in the second stage of labour, breech extraction can be performed to save the child.

Extended arms

Ordinarily, the arms are well-flexed and easily delivered during an assisted breech delivery. However, at times, one or both arms may be extended. Extension of the arms can also be produced by unnecessary traction of the fetus from below. When such difficulty is encountered, it can most often be dealt with by performing the Lovset manoeuvre already described in assisted breech delivery. Should this manoeuvre fail, an attempt should be made to deliver the posterior arm first. In this manoeuvre, the baby is held up to one side by its feet while a hand passed into the vagina. This hand is passed into the hollow of the sacrum and along the side of the baby's arm until the elbow is reached. The arm is then flexed and brought down in front of the baby's body. It should never be brought across the back as doing so will certainly fracture the humerus. Once the posterior arm is delivered, the anterior one can be delivered as in the Lovset manoeuvre. If there is any difficulty, the baby can be rotated so that the anterior arm is made posterior, and the delivery can be completed by the technique mentioned. Particular care should be taken to see that all movements are gentle and deliberate.

Nuchal position of the arms

This is not a common complication. This term is applied to denote that the hand is behind the occiput. One or both arms may be in the nuchal position. The diagnosis is made when the obstetrician notices that the medial border of the scapula is not parallel to the spine. In such a situation, the direction in which the fingers are pointing should be ascertained and the baby should then be rotated in that direction. With this manoeuvre, the arms drop down.

Difficulty in delivering the after-coming head

The most difficult step in the conduct of assisted breech delivery is the delivery of the after-coming head. This is because the bitrochanteric diameter is less than the biparietal diameter—9.25 cm vs. 9.4 cm. Therefore, even if the breech passes through the pelvis, it may not be adequate for the after-coming head. Further, the after-coming head does not have time for moulding. In vaginal breech delivery, successively larger and less compressible parts of the fetus pass through the pelvis. Therefore, the most common difficulty encountered in breech delivery is the delivery of the after-coming head.

The hyperextended fetal head, undiagnosed disproportion between the head and the pelvic brim and delivery through an undilated cervix are the other factors that result in difficulties in delivering the after-coming head. In premature babies, the head may be trapped by an undilated cervix. The Marshall–Burns technique is often successful (Fig. 42.4b) if the flexion of the head is maintained by an assistant applying gentle suprapubic pressure during the process of delivery. Forceps application to deliver the after-coming head is also effective (Fig. 42.4c).

Another method to deliver the head is the **Mauriceau–Smellie–Veit method** (Fig. 42.4d). In this method, the fetus is supported astride the left forearm, and the index and middle fingers are applied over the maxilla to flex the head. The index or middle finger of the right hand is then slipped over the clavicles from behind. Downward traction is applied until the nape of the neck appears. At this time, the direction of the traction is changed, and the fetus is swung up over the mother's abdomen. Suprapubic pressure over the head is combined with the manoeuvre. Occasionally, the back and the occiput may be directed posteriorly; such a complication should not happen. If it happens, attempts at delivery may be made by gripping the shoulders with two fingers of one hand and by first pulling the baby backwards, so that the forehead is fixed against the posterior surface of the symphysis pubis, and then carrying the trunk upwards onto the mother's abdomen. If there is still a difficulty in the delivery, forceps may be applied. Deep tears of the perineum are inevitable, and it is preferable to perform a prophylactic episiotomy in such cases.

Extended legs

In an extended breech, there may be difficulty in delivering the extended leg. In these cases, the Pinard's manoeuvre is performed. The gloved hand is introduced into the vagina and the fingers are guided along the posterior aspect of the thigh to reach the knee. Gentle pressure is then exerted in the popliteal space. This will cause the leg to flex at the knee when the fingers are passed along the shin until they reach the foot. The foot is then grasped and brought down to the vulva. Under no circumstances should the breech be extracted if cervical dilatation is not complete.

Impacted breech

Impaction of the breech can occur when the breech is extended. The most common cause of impaction is a disproportion between the size of the breech and the pelvis. If this is present at the brim or in the cavity, the breech will not descend into the cavity and should be delivered by cesarean section. If within 30 minutes of full cervical dilatation, descent has not occurred to the outlet, cesarean section should be performed. Such impaction may also occur at the outlet. It is very important that the adequacy of the pelvis be confirmed prior to allowing vaginal delivery for a breech. Impaction at the outlet is dealt with by episiotomy and traction with a finger in the groin. Traction can also be applied to both sides of the groin by the fingers of the two hands; this is often successful.

Fig. 42.5 is an algorithm for the management of breech presentation.

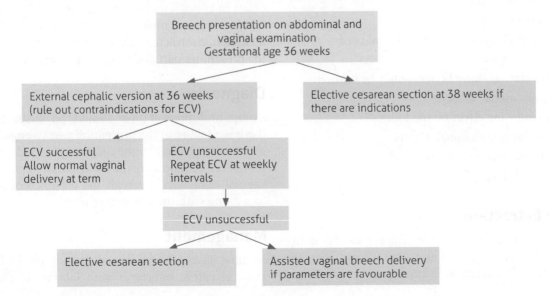

Fig. 42.5 An algorithm for the management of breech presentation

Prognosis

For the mother

Maternal morbidity is slightly higher than in vertex presentations because of the increased operative interventions.

For the baby

Breech presentations are divided into complicated breech and uncomplicated breech.

- Complicated breech is associated with factors that are pre-existing and detrimental to the fetus namely, prematurity, pre-eclampsia/eclampsia, antepartum hemorrhage, fetal abnormalities, contracted pelvis and maternal diseases like hypertension, cardiac disease and so on.
- In an uncomplicated breech, there are no pre-existing adverse factors, but complications can occur during the delivery.

Causes of Increased Perinatal Loss in Breech Presentations

In breech presentation, the perinatal mortality is four times that of cephalic presentation. Preterm delivery, congenital anomalies and the effect of pre-existing adverse factors contribute to the perinatal loss in breech presentation. In an uncomplicated breech, the major complications are cord prolapse leading to birth asphyxia and birth trauma. Birth injuries are seen in 6–7% of vaginal breech deliveries. The following birth injuries are noted in breech presentations:

- Cephalohematoma
- Intracranial hemorrhage with rapid and uncontrolled delivery of the head
- Medullary coning
- Injury to the brachial plexus or spinal cord
- Facial nerve paralysis
- Fracture clavicle, long bones, femur or humerus
- Tearing of lumbar muscles
- Crush syndrome effect on the kidney
- Injury to intra-abdominal organs
- Injury to the sternomastoid muscle
- Soft tissue injury

Breech Extraction

Breech extraction involves the delivery of the entire fetus by the clinician without any effort from the woman. Breech extraction is carried out rarely, when urgent delivery is needed in the second stage of labour. The following are the indications for breech extraction:

- Fetal distress/cord prolapse in the second stage of labour or when there is maternal distress
- The main indication is when the second of twins is presenting as transverse lie; in this situation, under general anesthesia, internal podalic version with breech extraction is carried out

Breech Presentation in Twin Pregnancy

- When the first twin is breech, cesarean section is performed.
- If the second twin is a breech, vaginal breech delivery is conducted.

■ COMPOUND PRESENTATION

Compound presentation is a condition in which more than one part of the fetus presents at the brim of the pelvis (Fig. 42.6) when the woman goes into labour. Usually, a hand, arm or foot prolapses alongside the head or breech. There could also be a cord prolapse.

Incidence and Types

Compound presentation is seen in almost 1 in 1,000 deliveries and the head and hand are the most common forms.

Etiology

Most often, there is no demonstrable cause for compound presentation. However, conditions that prevent complete filling and occlusion of the pelvic inlet by the presenting part can predispose to compound presentation. It can occur in conditions like prematurity, premature rupture of membranes, multiparity, high head, laxity of the abdomen, contracted pelvis or pelvic tumours displacing the presenting part and multiple pregnancy.

Diagnosis

Compound presentation should be suspected when there is a failure of the presenting part to engage during active labour. Mostly, the diagnosis is made in the late first stage of labour or in the second stage, when the vaginal examination reveals the presence of a hand or foot along with the presenting part.

Management

In most cases, the prolapsed part should be left alone since it rarely interferes with labour. If the arm is prolapsed alongside the head, the condition should be observed closely to see if the arm rises out of the way with the progress of labour. If the arm does not retract, it can be pushed gently upward. Cesarean section is the method of delivery when compound presentation is associated with cord prolapse, non-reassuring fetal status or arrest of labour or when a non-vertex compound presentation is seen in a term fetus.

KEY POINTS

✓ Breech presentation is associated with increased perinatal loss due to prematurity, congenital anomalies and birth trauma.

✓ Prematurity is the most common cause of breech presentation.

✓ The fetal prognosis depends upon the weight of the baby, the type of breech, the pelvic configuration, the presence of any maternal complication and the skill of the obstetrician.

✓ The chances of cord prolapse are less with frank breech.

✓ If there are no contraindications to external cephalic version, it should be attempted in all breech presentations.

✓ External cephalic version is performed after 36 weeks of gestation.

✓ If suitable for vaginal delivery, the mode of delivery is an assisted breech delivery.

✓ The indications for elective cesarean section in breech presentation are in the presence of other associated obstetrical problems such as a previous cesarean section, severe FGR, fetal weight >3.5 Kg, inadequate pelvis, hyperextended head and footling/knee presentation.

✓ Emergency cesarean section would be required in the presence of cord prolapse, failure to progress in labour and impacted breech.

✓ Compound presentation usually does not interfere with the progress of labour.

✓ Cesarean section is the method of delivery when compound presentation is associated with cord prolapse, non-reassuring fetal status or arrest of labour.

Essay questions

1. Describe the mechanism of labour in the breech presentation.
2. Outline the management of a second gravida with a previous normal delivery at 36 weeks of gestation during which there was breech presentation in labour.

Short answer questions

1. What are the types of breech presentation?
2. What are the indications for cesarean delivery in a breech presentation?
3. List the complications of breech delivery.
4. Discuss perinatal loss in breech presentations.

MCQs

1. What is the most common cause of breech presentation?
   a) Contracted pelvis
   b) Prematurity
   c) Placenta previa
   d) Oligohydramnios
2. The Marshall–Burns method is used in the delivery of the:
   a) After-coming head
   b) Shoulder
   c) Nuchal arm
   d) Leg
3. Which of the following is not a method used in breech delivery?
   a) Marshall–Burns
   b) Piper's forceps
   c) Pinard's manoeuvre
   d) Brandt Andrew's technique

4. The following are methods of delivering the after-coming head of a breech EXCEPT:
   a) Lovset manoeuvre
   b) Marshall–Burns technique
   c) Piper's forceps
   d) Mauriceau-Smellie-Viet manoeuvre
5. What is the process of labour in breech where every part of the body becomes a little more flexed called?
   a) Engagement
   b) Universal flexion
   c) Compaction
   d) Internal rotation
6. Spontaneous correction of breech to vertex is significantly less after how many weeks of gestation?
   a) 30 weeks
   b) 32 weeks
   c) 34 weeks
   d) 36 weeks
7. Which of these manoeuvres is used to deliver the arms in breech delivery?
   a) Lovset
   b) Mauriceau–Smellie–Viet
   c) Pinard
   d) Marshall–Burns
8. In which of the following is recurrent breech presentation seen?
   a) Congenital uterine anomalies
   b) Multiparity
   c) Prematurity
   d) Placenta previa

Answers

1. (b), 2. (a), 3. (d), 4. (a), 5. (c), 6. (d), 7. (a), 8. (a)

Fill in the blanks

1. The denominator in a breech presentation is the _____.
2. The diameter of engagement in a breech presentation is the _____.
3. The condition in which more than one part of the fetus presents at the pelvic brim is called_____.

Answers

1. sacrum, 2. bitrochanteric diameter, 3. compound presentation

Case scenario-based discussion

1. A 27-year-old gravida 2, para 1 presents at 38 weeks of gestation with labour pains for the past 8 hours and ruptured membranes 2 hours ago. In her previous obstetric history, she previously had a vaginal breech delivery at 39 weeks and the birth weight of the baby was 2.7 Kg. On examination, the fetus is in a longitudinal lie with a breech presentation and the uterus is contracting once in 3 minutes. The fetal heart is 110 bpm, and during contractions, there are decelerations to 90 bpm. On vaginal examination, the cervix is fully dilated, the membrane is absent and the buttocks and feet are felt at the +2 station. There is a loop of cord by the side of the foot, and pulsations are felt.
   a) What is the diagnosis?
   b) What is the management?

Answers

a) This is a case of breech presentation in the second stage of labour with flexed breech and cord prolapse.

b) In view of the cord prolapse, the baby should be delivered immediately by breech extraction under anesthesia.

Shoulder Dystocia and Umbilical Cord Prolapse

OG 14.3

Learning Objectives

» To know the clinical presentation and risk factors for shoulder dystocia

» To discuss the management of shoulder dystocia

» To describe the complications of shoulder dystocia

» To know the risk factors and management of cord prolapse

■ SHOULDER DYSTOCIA

Shoulder dystocia is an uncommon but unpredictable obstetric emergency. It is defined as the arrest of the delivery of the shoulders after the fetal head has been born. It is arbitrarily taken as a head-to-shoulder delivery interval exceeding 60 seconds. It occurs in <1% of all deliveries.

Diagnosis

Clinically, shoulder dystocia is diagnosed after the delivery of the head, when there is a failure to deliver the anterior shoulder with the standard manoeuvre of downward traction on the fetal head. In such cases, additional obstetric manoeuvres are required to deliver the shoulders. The fetal head remains tightly applied to the vulva and the chin retracts and depresses the perineum. The head protrudes with maternal effort and then retracts. This is called the 'turtle' sign (Fig. 43.1).

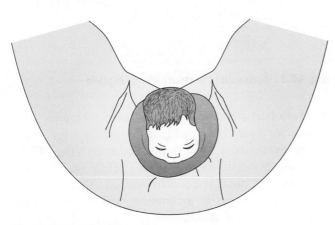

Fig. 43.1 Turtle sign

Risk Factors (Table 43.1)

Most cases of shoulder dystocia cannot be predicted.

Antenatal risk factors

Certain antenatal risk factors may indicate the possibility of shoulder dystocia—a history of shoulder dystocia in a prior vaginal delivery (10% risk), fetal macrosomia, diabetes/impaired glucose tolerance (the upper part of the baby's body is larger in the presence of maternal diabetes), obesity, postdated pregnancy and excessive weight gain during pregnancy. Increased birth weight is the most common single risk factor for shoulder dystocia; it may be caused by maternal obesity, diabetes or multiparity.

Intrapartum risk factors

Intrapartum factors that can predict the risk of shoulder dystocia are a precipitous second stage (<20 minutes), operative vaginal delivery—forceps/ventouse, slow progress in the first stage of labour and prolonged second stage of labour.

Table 43.1 Risk factors for shoulder dystocia

Antenatal risk factors	Intrapartum risk factors
• Previous history of shoulder dystocia	• Precipitous second stage (<20 min)
• Fetal macrosomia	• Operative vaginal delivery
• Diabetes/impaired glucose tolerance	• Slow progress in the first stage of labour
• Obesity	• Prolonged second stage of labour
• Postdated pregnancy	
• Excessive weight gain during pregnancy	

Complications of Shoulder Dystocia

Even with appropriate action and intervention, there is an increased incidence of maternal and perinatal complications.

Fetal complications

Fetal complications occur in nearly 20% of cases.

- Brachial plexus injury—In ERB–Duchenne palsy, C5 and C6 nerve roots are affected; the arm is adducted and internally rotated at the shoulder and pronated at the elbow
- Klumpke paralysis—C8 and T1 nerve roots are affected, and the child presents with a claw hand deformity
- Facial nerve paralysis
- Clavicular fracture and humeral fracture
- Birth asphyxia
- Fetal and neonatal death

Maternal complications

- Postpartum hemorrhage due to vaginal or cervical lacerations or uterine atony
- Third- and fourth-degree perineal lacerations
- Rupture uterus
- Symphyseal separation
- Lateral femoral cutaneous neuropathy

Prevention

Based on epidemiological data, it is reasonable to offer a prophylactic cesarean section for an estimated fetal weight (EFW) of >4.5 Kg for women with diabetes mellitus and for an EFW of 5 Kg for women who do not have diabetes mellitus. However, there is no evidence to support this.

Management

In all vaginal deliveries, shoulder dystocia should be anticipated. Shoulder dystocia can occur without any warning signs, and the diagnosis is made only after the delivery of the head. The aim is to deliver the baby with the minimum possible head-to-body delivery interval.

- As soon as shoulder dystocia is recognised, one should call for help and should not panic.
- A generous episiotomy should be given.
- Pulling the baby damages the brachial plexus and pressing either suprapubically or fundally wedges the shoulder further. Pivoting on the neck damages the structures in the area.

- Fundal pressure should not be applied as it can result in further impaction of the shoulder and rupture uterus.
- The bladder should be drained.

Executing Manoeuvres

It should be borne in mind that no fundal pressure should be applied; neither should there be any pulling or pushing of the baby.

If the shoulder remains undelivered, the following steps should be followed. The aim is to release the anterior shoulder from behind the pubic symphysis.

- **Applying suprapubic pressure (Fig. 43.2):** The assistant applies direct posterior or oblique suprapubic pressure on the anterior shoulder in an attempt to dislodge the shoulder from behind the symphysis pubis. At the same time, the obstetrician applies gentle downward traction on the fetal head.

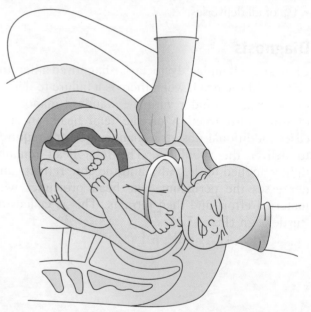

Fig. 43.2 Suprapubic pressure being applied

- **McRobert's manoeuvre:** In this technique, the woman's legs are forcibly abducted, and the thighs are hyperflexed against the abdomen (Fig. 43.3). In this position, the sacrum is straightened, and the symphysis pubis is caudally rotated. This decreases the angle of pelvic inclination, which helps in the delivery of the anterior shoulder from behind the symphysis pubis.

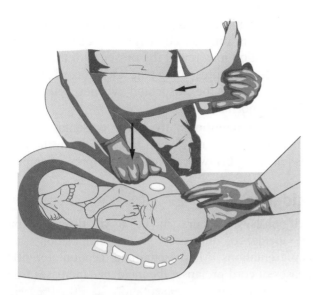

Fig. 43.3 McRobert's manoeuvre

- **Rubin's manoeuvre (Fig. 43.4):** The operator applies pressure on the posterior surface of the most accessible shoulder and exerts pressure towards the fetal chest, thereby causing shoulder adduction. This moves the fetus into an oblique position and reduces the bisacromial diameter.

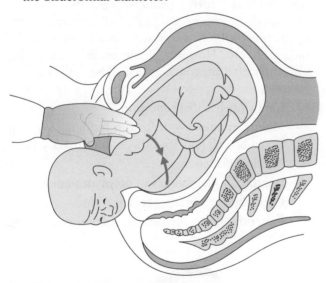

Fig. 43.4 Rubin's manoeuvre

- **Wood's corkscrew manoeuvre (Fig. 43.5):** In this manoeuvre, continuous pressure is applied to the anterior surface of the posterior shoulder to push it posteriorly towards the fetal back. This results in progressive rotation of the shoulder girdle in a corkscrew fashion—the shoulder rotates to an oblique plane, releasing the impacted anterior shoulder from behind the symphysis pubis (posterior shoulder moves to the anterior position).

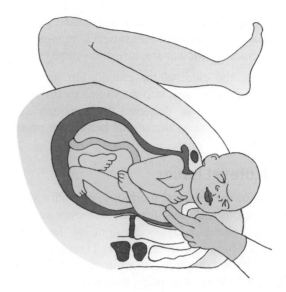

Fig. 43.5 Wood's corkscrew manoeuvre

- **Delivery of the posterior arm—Barnum's manoeuvre (Fig. 43.6):** Another method of tackling shoulder dystocia is by delivering the posterior arm. To perform this manoeuvre, the hand is inserted posteriorly in the vagina along the curve of the sacrum. The posterior arm of the fetus is identified, and pressure is applied at the antecubital fossa to flex the fetal forearm. Then, the arm is swept across the fetal chest and is delivered at the perineum. Once the arm is delivered, there is a 20% reduction in the shoulder diameter.

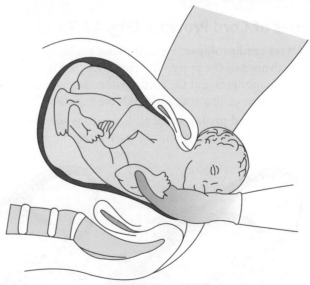

Fig. 43.6 Delivery of the posterior arm—Barnum's manoeuvre

- **Zavanelli's manoeuvre:** When shoulder dystocia seems intractable and vaginal delivery does not seem possible, one may need to consider performing cephalic replacement (Zavanelli's manoeuvre) or intentional clavicular fracture and symphysiotomy.

Here the cardinal movements are reversed, the head is pushed back into the vagina by firm pressure and the baby is delivered by cesarean section. Tocolytics to relax the uterus before the procedure may be considered.

Medicolegal Issues

Because of the neonatal morbidity, mortality, maternal complications and long-term neurological sequelae in the child, shoulder dystocia is one of the important causes for litigation in obstetrics. Therefore, accurate documentation of events is very important. This should include the mode of delivery, time interval between the delivery of the head and the body, the sequence of the manoeuvres performed, neonatal status at birth and neonatal and maternal complications. It is also very important to explain these details to the woman and her family and document that this has been done.

UMBILICAL CORD PROLAPSE AND PRESENTATION

Cord prolapse is a condition in which the umbilical cord comes out through the cervical os, either in advance or along with the presenting part. The fetal outcome is poor as the cord is compressed between the fetus and the maternal bony pelvis.

Types of Cord Prolapse (Fig. 43.7a–c)

* **Overt cord prolapse:** Here, the cord prolapse occurs in advance of the presenting part after the rupture of the membranes and the cord is either palpable within the vagina or protrudes through the vagina.
* **Occult cord prolapse**: Here, the cord is seen by the side of the fetal presenting part after the rupture

of the membranes but not below it. Occult cord prolapse is difficult to diagnose. Careful vaginal examination may reveal the presence of the cord by the side of the presenting part. Occult cord prolapse should always be suspected whenever there are CTG abnormalities.
* **Cord presentation:** In cord presentation, the membranes are intact, and through them, the cord is felt either below or along with the presenting part.

Incidence

Cord prolapse occurs in 0.5% of deliveries but the incidence increases with malposition and malpresentations. Malpresentations account for 50% of cases of cord prolapse; the incidence increases from 2.5–3% with breech presentation to 20–30% with compound presentations.

Etiology

Several risk factors have been identified that are associated with umbilical cord prolapse. It can occur spontaneously or due to obstetric interventions.

* **Spontaneous cord prolapse** occurs due to inadequate or improper filling of the maternal pelvis by the presenting part or due to abnormalities of the umbilical cord. However, it can occur in otherwise uncomplicated pregnancies also. The causes are as follows:
    — Cephalopelvic disproportion
    — Malpresentations—10% with footling, 5% with flexed breech and 15–20% with transverse lie
    — Multiple gestation
    — Rupture of membranes in polyhydramnios
    — Cord abnormalities—very long cord
    — Preterm delivery/growth restriction due to low birth weight

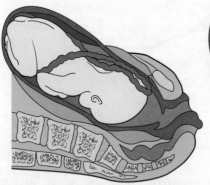

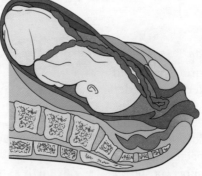

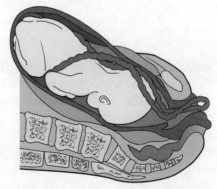

(a) Cord prolapsed at the inlet   (b) Cord prolapsed into the vagina   (c) Cord prolapsed through the introitus

Fig. 43.7(a–c)   Types of cord prolapse

— Spontaneous rupture membrane is a risk factor, as is preterm PROM

- **Iatrogenic cord prolapse** can occur due to various obstetric interventions. Nearly 50% of cases of cord prolapse are attributed to iatrogenic factors such as the following:
  — Amniotomy, especially when the fetal presenting part is not engaged
  — ECV
  — During amnioinfusion or amnioreduction
  — While applying forceps or vacuum

Diagnosis

Overt cord prolapse is easier to diagnose than occult cord prolapse. The cord may be palpable within the vagina or may be visible outside the introitus. It is often accompanied by severe, sudden fetal heart rate decelerations, prolonged bradycardia and variable decelerations. Occult cord prolapses may often go undiagnosed. Most often, this leads to cesarean section for unexplained fetal bradycardia. Other palpable soft masses in the vagina such as the fetal limb, caput or fetal intestines may be confused with the umbilical cord.

Prevention

- When there is a possibility of cord prolapse, as in malpresentations, women with transverse and oblique lie may be hospitalised by 37 weeks.
- A woman who has a high risk of cord prolapse should be counselled and advised to report immediately if the membrane ruptures or there is reduced fetal movement so that immediate action can be taken.
- In women with known risk factors for cord prolapse, continuous CTG monitoring is important in labour. Intermittent auscultation is contraindicated.
- Following the rupture of membranes in labour, immediate vaginal examination should be performed to rule out cord prolapse, and CTG monitoring should be carried out to pick up fetal heart abnormalities.
- Whenever there is unexplained fetal distress in labour, cord prolapse should be looked for.

There are also other conditions with rapid fetal heart rate decelerations such as vasa previa, placental abruption, uterine rupture and maternal hypotension due to any reason.

- If the head is well-applied and within the pelvis, amniotomy may be undertaken. If the head is not engaged but amniotomy has to be undertaken, then a controlled rupture of the membrane is performed, which should allow a slow release of fluid rather than sudden decompression. Instead of using ARM forceps or an amniotomy hook, a thin hypodermic needle should be used so that fluid can be released very slowly.
- While performing procedures such as catheter placement or scalp electrode placement, care should be taken not to elevate the fetal head.
- Cervical balloon catheters elevate the fetal head out of the pelvis, as a result of which, there is a risk of cord prolapse. However, the use of balloon catheters can be avoided when the membranes have already ruptured.

Management (Fig. 43.8)

Umbilical cord prolapse with a live fetus is an obstetric emergency. One should act very quickly, otherwise, it can lead to fetal death or long-term disability. Delivery should be accomplished as quickly as possible. The decision-making-to-delivery interval should be <20–30 minutes. The absence of pulsation does not necessarily indicate fetal death. Auscultation of the fetal heart by USG and CTG is mandatory before declaring fetal death.

- Women in the first stage or early second stage are delivered by cesarean section.
- In women who are imminent to deliver, vaginal delivery is undertaken, and the decision on spontaneous/operative vaginal delivery is taken based on the fetal heart tracing. Breech in the late second stage of labour with cord prolapse can be delivered by breech extraction.
- Until the baby can be delivered, the pressure on the umbilical cord by the presenting part should be relieved. This is called **funic decompression** and can be achieved by adopting various measures, which are as follows:
  — The woman is advised not to push.
  — Oxygen is administered to the woman.
  — In order to avoid the drying and vasospasm of the cord, it is important to keep the cord in the vagina and wrap it with a moist pad or sterile linen soaked in warm saline.
  — The woman is positioned in such a way so as to allow gravity to help in the decompression. This can be achieved either by the deep Trendelenburg position or knee–chest position, which moves the presenting part away from the pelvis.
  — Bladder filling by Vago's method—a distended bladder exerts upward pressure on the fetal presenting part. Filling the bladder with

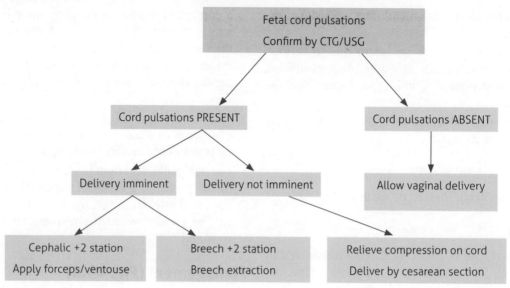

Fig. 43.8 Management of cord prolapse

500–750 mL of normal saline through a Foley's catheter helps to lift the presenting part above the pelvis. This is especially useful when the anticipated diagnosis-to-delivery interval is likely to be prolonged.

— Manual elevation of the fetal head—with two fingers or the entire hand inserted into the woman's vagina, the presenting part is gently elevated. During the procedure, care should be taken to avoid exerting pressure on or touching the cord as this could lead to vasospasm. Continuous elevation of the presenting part is difficult for both the woman and the clinician.

— Tocolytics can be used as an adjunct to elevation as they reduce the uterine tone and contraction, thereby reducing the pressure on the cord. The use of tocolytics may be helpful when delay in delivery is anticipated.

— In rural settings where facilities for cesarean are not available, besides decompression, funic reduction can be attempted along with the use tocolytics.

• In situations where there is a lethal fetal anomaly or fetal demise, the woman is allowed spontaneous delivery. No intervention is required is such cases.

• The overall prognosis is good if the baby is delivered within 30 minutes. If the woman is already in the hospital for immediate intervention, the prognosis for the baby is good.

• Proper documentation should be maintained. There should also be effective communication with the woman and her relatives.

Occult Cord Prolapse

In a woman in labour, if the FHR is abnormal after the rupture of membranes, the presence of occult cord prolapse should be looked for. The woman may also feel excessive fetal movements. In these cases, the maternal position should be changed to look for FHR improvement. If the FH changes persist, it necessitates immediate delivery. When in doubt, Doppler may be carried out to determine the position of the umbilical cord.

Funic Presentation (Cord Presentation)

Here, the cord is felt below the presenting part through the intact membranes. If necessary, the presence of cord presentation can be confirmed by Doppler. Once a diagnosis of cord presentation is made, the baby is delivered by cesarean section.

KEY POINTS

✓ *Shoulder dystocia is the failure of the shoulder to deliver following the delivery of the head.*

✓ *Risk factors for shoulder dystocia include fetal macrosomia, diabetes, postmature baby, prolonged labour and instrumental delivery.*

✓ *Fetal complications occur in nearly 20% of cases of shoulder dystocia.*

✓ Factors such as contracted pelvis, malpresentations, placenta previa and small fetus prevent the proper fitting of the presenting part at the pelvic brim, thus causing compound presentation and cord prolapse.

✓ In women with predisposing factors such as malpresentations, prematurity or polyhydramnios, per vaginal examination should be performed to exclude cord prolapse.

✓ Prolapse of the umbilical cord with a live fetus is an obstetric emergency and warrants immediate delivery of the fetus.

✓ While preparing for delivery, pressure on the prolapsed umbilical cord should be minimised by putting the woman in the Trendelenburg position, filling the bladder and preventing uterine contractions using tocolytic drugs.

Essay questions

1. How is shoulder dystocia diagnosed and what are the manoeuvres to deliver the baby?
2. How would you manage a case of cord prolapse with a live and viable fetus?

Short answer questions

1. What is the etiology of cord prolapse?
2. What are the risk factors for shoulder dystocia?
3. Describe the McRoberts manoeuvre.
4. What is cord presentation and its management?

MCQs

1. The complication of artificial rupture of membranes when presenting part is high is:
    a) Cord prolapse
    b) Abruption placentae
    c) Chorioamnionitis
    d) Non-progress of labour
2. A 28-year-old primigravida at 35 weeks of gestation presents to the labour ward with complaints of watery discharge. On examination, she is found to have a pulsating cord below the presenting part, the vertex. All of the following should be done EXCEPT:
    a) The woman should be placed in the head–knee position.
    b) She should be prepared for immediate delivery.
    c) A Foley's catheter should be inserted to empty the bladder.
    d) A tocolytic should be given to inhibit uterine contractions.
3. Umbilical cord prolapse is associated with all the following, EXCEPT:
    a) Postmaturity
    b) Cephalopelvic disproportion
    c) Multiparity
    d) Footling breech presentation
4. A primigravida at term is seen in active labour. After the delivery of the head, the neck does not descend, and the chin is retracting against the perineum. What is the most likely diagnosis?
    a) Uterine rupture
    b) Uterine inversion
    c) Placenta previa
    d) Shoulder dystocia
5. Which of the following manoeuvres is NOT used for the management of shoulder dystocia?
    a) McRobert's manoeuvre
    b) Suprapubic pressure
    c) Wood's corkscrew manoeuvre
    d) Mauriceau–Smellie–Veit manoeuvre

6. A 34-year-old gravida 2, para 1 presents in labour at 36 weeks of gestation. Her membranes ruptured 20 minutes earlier. CTG shows bradycardia. On vaginal examination, the cervix is 3 cm dilated and there is cord prolapse. What is the mode of delivery?
    a) Continue with labour
    b) Forceps delivery
    c) Ventouse delivery
    d) Emergency cesarean section

Answers

1. (a), 2. (c), 3. (a), 4. (d), 5. (d), 6. (d)

Fill in the blanks

1. The presence of the umbilical cord between the fetal presenting part and the cervix with an intact membrane is called _____.
2. The most common cause of cord prolapse is _____.
3. Retraction of the fetal chin onto the maternal perineum upon the delivery of the head is a sign of shoulder dystocia known as the _____.

Answers

1. cord presentation, 2. malpresentation, 3. turtle sign

Case scenario-based discussion

1. A 26-year-old primigravida is admitted at 39 weeks of gestation with labour pains for the last 8 hours and draining for the last 2 hours. She was diagnosed with gestational diabetes at 32 weeks and is on insulin. The estimated fetal weight determined one week earlier was 3.7 Kg. On examination, a cephalic presentation is noted with the head 2/5th palpable, the FH was good. Uterine contractions are occurring at a frequency of 1 in 7 minutes and are weak. On vaginal examination, the cervix is 8 cm dilated, the membrane is absent, the head is LOA at 0 station. Since the contractions are weak, oxytocin infusion is stated. After 2 hours, the baby is delivered up to the neck, but the shoulder cannot be delivered.
    a) What is the diagnosis and what are the risk factors in this case?
    b) How would you proceed to manage this case?
    c) What complications are expected in this case?

Answers

a) The diagnosis is shoulder dystocia and the risk factors in this case are diabetes, large (3.7 Kg) baby and oxytocin augmentation.

b) The immediate response is to call for help. The woman should be asked not to push. No fundal pressure should be applied. The bladder should be catheterised, the woman should be brought to the edge of the table, placed in lithotomy position and given a liberal episiotomy. All the manoeuvres for shoulder dystocia should be performed.

c) Maternal complications are perineal, vaginal and cervical tears and PPH. Fetal complications are Erb's palsy, clavicle fracture, birth asphyxia and death.

Abnormal Labour and Dystocia Due to Anomalies of the Expulsive Force

---

Learning Objectives

» To discuss the causes and risk factors associated with abnormal labour
» To describe the uterine activity in normal labour
» To describe dystocia due to hypotonic and hypertonic uterine actions and their management
» To discuss protracted dilatation in the active phase of labour, its causes and management
» To discuss protracted descent, its causes and management
» To diagnose abnormal labour on partograph
» To describe precipitate labour
» To understand cervical dystocia

■ NORMAL LABOUR

Labour has been traditionally divided into three stages, which are as follows:

First stage of labour

- It begins with regular uterine contractions and ends with complete cervical dilatation at 10 cm.
- It is divided into a latent phase and an active phase
- The latent phase begins with mild, irregular uterine contractions that soften and shorten the cervix; simultaneously, progressive cervical dilatation takes place.
- The latent phase begins with the onset of true labour pains and ends when the cervix is 4 cm dilated.
- The active phase of labour extends from 4 cm dilatation to full cervical dilatation, during which period, the contractions become progressively more rhythmic and stronger.

Second stage of labour

It begins with full cervical dilatation and ends with the delivery of the baby.

Third stage of labour

This stage extends from the delivery of the baby to the delivery of the placenta.

Factors Influencing Normal Labour

- In the first stage of labour, progress depends on the uterine contractions, the resistance offered by the cervix (when the presenting part is well-applied to the cervix, it dilates faster) and the forward pressure exerted by the fetal head.
- In the second stage of labour, besides the above factors, the mechanical relationship between the fetal head (size and position) and the pelvic capacity is important (fetopelvic relationship).

Normal Uterine Activity

- From early pregnancy, contractions known as Braxton Hicks contractions occur, which are painless, irregular and intermittent contractions that occur at long intervals, last for a short period of time and are not associated with the dilatation of the cervix or descent of the presenting part. Nearer to term, these contractions become more frequent, regular and coordinated; they last longer and are converted into true labour pains by the time labour sets in.
- True labour pains are painful, more frequent and last longer. They are associated with the dilatation of the cervix and the descent of the fetus.
- Cervical dilatation is the result of a gradient of diminishing physiological activity from the fundus to the lower uterine segments. There is a balanced action between the upper and the lower segments known as polarity, whereby, when the upper segment contracts, the lower segment dilates.
- The uterus has a baseline intrauterine pressure of 5–10 mmHg in early labour. Any pressure exceeding this will be felt as a contraction on abdominal

palpation. Pain is felt by the woman when the intrauterine pressure exceeds 15 mmHg.

- In early labour, contractions occur approximately every 3–5 minutes with a pressure build-up of 20–30 mmHg above resting tone. In active labour, contractions usually occur every 2–4 minutes with a pressure that is 30–50 mmHg above the resting tone. Between contractions, the pressure comes back to the normal base-level tone. With pushing, the pressure may rise to 100–150 mmHg.

- In addition to increased frequency and tone, the duration of contractions lengthens from 30–60 seconds in early labour and to 60–90 seconds at the end of the first stage and in the second stage of labour.

- The contractions are also coordinated with fundal dominance; the upper segment contracts while the lower segment dilates to receive the presenting part.

- In normal progressive labour, the contractions of the fundus rise quickly to a maximum and are strong and sustained. The middle zone of the uterus contracts simultaneously, but less intensely and for a shorter time, while the lower segment remains inactive and its tone is low.

Recording uterine activity

- The frequency and duration of contractions can be recorded using a cardiotocography (CTG) machine.

- Intrauterine pressure can be recorded using internal tocography, which involves placing a sensor-tipped catheter inside the uterus. This is not routinely carried out as it is an invasive procedure.

- The uterine contractions are expressed in Montevideo (MVU) units. A uterine contraction is considered adequate when it exceeds 200 MVU for a 10-minute contraction.

Partograph

- A partograph is a graphical representation of the progress of labour based on the rate of cervical dilatation and descent of the presenting part. It is a simple and inexpensive tool to monitor labour in a cost-effective manner. Any deviation from the normal progress is considered abnormal labour. It provides an early warning system and assists in making an early decision on transfer, augmentation and termination of labour. Early detection of abnormal progress and prevention of prolonged labour significantly reduce the risk of maternal and perinatal morbidity and mortality.

- The original partograph was designed by Friedman and has gone through various revisions. The one currently in use is the modified WHO partograph. Further changes were made in 2018 which may come into practice and will be discussed later.

— The WHO partograph is recorded from the time when the woman goes into active labour, i.e., at a cervical dilatation of 4 cm.

— The time at which a woman is seen with 4 cm dilatation is recorded as the 0 hour. The actual time at 0 hour is noted in the time column.

— Cervical dilatation is marked with an X.

— Vaginal examination is performed every 2–4 hours, and the cervical dilatation is noted.

— In order to identify abnormal labour in the active phase, two lines are drawn—the alert line and the action line (Fig. 44.1).

— In the active phase, labour is expected to progress at a rate of 1 cm cervical dilatation per hour, which corresponds to the alert line. This means that the alert line starts at 4 cm of cervical dilatation, showing the cervix dilating at 1 cm per hour up to 10 cm. This is the normal expected cervical dilatation in any labour.

— The action line is drawn 4 hours to the right and parallel to the alert line.

— The progress of labour is considered normal when the labour curve of the woman falls to the left of the alert line (Fig. 44.2). The partograph is described in detail in Chapter 14, *Conduct of normal labour.*

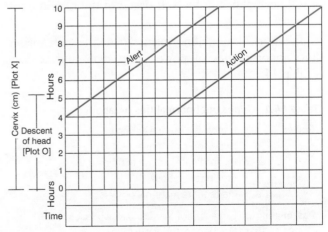

Fig. 44.1 Alert and action lines on a partograph

■ ABNORMAL LABOUR

Abnormal labour is otherwise known as dysfunctional labour or labour dystocia. It refers to the abnormally slow progress of labour. The process of labour involves two mechanisms, namely progressive cervical dilatation and

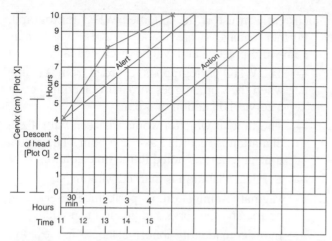

Fig. 44.2 A partograph showing the normal progress of labour with the woman's labour curve to the left of the alert line

descent of the fetal head. If either of these does not occur as expected, the labour is considered to be abnormal.

Etiology

Labour dystocia arises due to the following four abnormalities, which can exist either alone or in combination:

1. Abnormality of the uterine contractions and maternal expulsive efforts
2. Abnormalities of the presentation and position or weight of the fetus
3. Abnormalities of the maternal pelvis (contracted pelvis)
4. Abnormalities of the soft tissue of the reproductive tract

In short, these abnormalities can be categorised into abnormalities of power, passenger and passage (Table 44.1).

Table 44.1 Types of abnormalities of labour

Power	• Hypotonic uterine action • Hypertonic uterine action • Incoordinate uterine action • Precipitate labour • Inadequate maternal powers
Passenger	• Large size of the fetus, which leads to CPD • Occipitoposterior position • Malpresentations with face, brow and shoulder • Fetal anomalies such as hydrocephalus, fetal ascites, etc.
Passage	• Contracted pelvis • CPD • Abnormalities of the soft parts interfering with the labour progress

Risk Factors Associated With Labour Dystocia

- Advanced maternal age
- Nulliparity
- Short maternal stature
- Obesity
- Contracted pelvis/CPD/obstructed labour
- Malposition and malpresentations
- Macrosomia
- Post-term pregnancy (>41 weeks)
- Uterine overdistension (multiple pregnancy, polyhydramnios)
- Injudicious use of oxytocic agents, induction of labour
- Medications
- Chorioamnionitis
- Prelabour rupture of membranes
- Psychological factors
- Maternal exhaustion or motor blockage from epidural analgesia resulting in ineffective maternal expulsive efforts in the second stage

Complications of Labour Dystocia

Maternal complications:
- Obstructed labour
- Maternal exhaustion and dehydration
- Genital tract injuries/rupture
- Increased risk of both instrumental and operative deliveries
- Atonic postpartum hemorrhage
- Increased risk of chorioamnionitis and postpartum endometritis
- Pelvic injuries (especially from a prolonged second stage)

Neonatal complications:
- Risk of meconium-stained fluid
- Increased risk of neonatal infection
- Increased risk for birth asphyxia
- Low APGAR scores
- Admission to NICU

Delayed complications:
- Pelvic floor dysfunction
- Vesiscovaginal fistula (VVF)

Diagnosis and Management of Abnormal Labour

- Abnormal labour is identified by using a partograph in which the cervical dilatation and the descent of the fetal head are plotted against time.
- When there is a delay in the progress of labour for any reason, the labour curve will cross the alert line to the right.
- Abnormal labour patterns (Table 44.2) are seen in both the first and second stages of labour.

Disorders of the first stage of labour

Prolonged latent phase

The latent phase extends from the onset of true labour pains until the active phase of cervical dilatation is reached (i.e., when the cervix is 4 cm dilated). Prolonged latent phase was defined by Friedman and Sachtleben (1963) as one exceeding 20 hours in the nullipara and 14 hours in the multipara.

> A diagnosis of labour dystocia should not be made before the onset of the active phase when the cervix is less than 4 cm dilated.

Risk factors for prolonged latent phase include the following:

- An unripe cervix at the onset of labour
- Abnormal position of the fetus (occipitotransverse or posterior positions)
- Cephalopelvic disproportion
- Weak uterine contractions
- Induction of labour
- Prelabour rupture of amniotic membranes

- Early administration of regional anesthetic with heavy motor block
- Heavy sedation

Management

- A prolonged latent phase is not an indication for cesarean delivery.
- After excluding CPD, malposition and malpresentation, expectant management is recommended.
- The maternal and fetal parameters should be checked to ensure that they are normal.
- The presence of a supportive partner, regular attention to the bladder, maintaining the fluid balance and relieving the woman's fear and anxiety are measures that aid the progress of labour.
- Occasionally, false labour pain may be diagnosed as a prolonged latent phase. With expectant management, false labour pain will disappear.

> False labour pains may be mistaken for prolonged latent phase.

- The supine position should be avoided as it may result in supine hypotension and compromise the blood flow to the fetus. As a result of supine hypotension, CTG abnormalities may be noted.
- Therapeutic rest involves providing pain relief through effective support and analgesia. Excessive pain or anxiety during labour can lead to an increased production of catecholamines, which have a direct inhibitory effect on uterine contractility.
- Ambulation should be encouraged.
- With these measures, in more than 80% of women, regular contractions will begin. If the latent phase is

Table 44.2 Abnormal labour patterns and management

Labour patterns	Diagnostic criteria		Treatment	Exceptional treatment
	Nullipara	Multipara		
Prolongation disorder				
Prolonged latent phase	>20 hr	>14 hr	Bed rest	Oxytocin
Protraction disorders				
Protracted active phase dilatation	<1.2 cm/hr	<1.5 cm/hr	Expectant management	Cesarean delivery—CPD
Protracted descent	<1 cm/hr	<2 cm/hr		
Arrest disorders				
Secondary arrest of dilatation	>2 hr	>2 hr	Rule out CPD, malposition	Cesarean section
				Oxytocin augmentation if CPD is ruled out
Arrest of descent	>2 hr	>1 hr		Head below +2 station—instrumental delivery

prolonged, labour can be augmented with oxytocin infusion.

- Amniotomy should be avoided in the latent phase of labour.

Active-phase disorders

In the active phase, the labour disorders are divided into **protraction disorders** and **arrest disorders**.

- A protraction disorder is one where the labour progresses slowly (slow dilatation of the cervix).

- An arrest disorder is one where there is complete cessation of progress, and labour comes to a stop (cervical dilatation stops).

Protracted active phase (Fig. 44.3)

According to Friedman's data, a rate of cervical dilatation at less than 1.2 cm/hour in nulliparas and less than 1.5 cm/hour in multiparas is evidence of some abnormality. According to the WHO partograph, cervical dilatation of <1 cm/hour for a minimum of four hours is considered protracted labour.

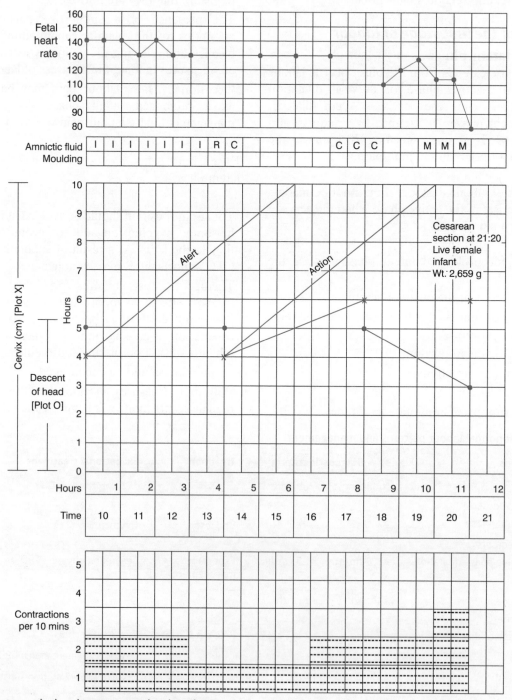

Fig. 44.3 Partograph showing protracted active phase

Management

- Mechanical factors such as cephalopelvic disproportion and malpositions should be ruled out. If there is cephalopelvic disproportion, cesarean section is indicated.
- Fluid balance should be maintained, and pain relief provided.
- Amniotomy—in prolonged labour, in the active phase, amniotomy is recommended in all women with intact membranes. Amniotomy increases local prostaglandin levels, which, in turn, increase the strength and frequency of uterine contractions. This has been shown to shorten the duration of the first stage of labour. Moreover, the colour of the liquor can be noted.
- Oxytocin—for hypotonic uterine contractions, medical management is carried out as long as the fetus and mother are in good condition. When artificial rupture of membranes (ARM) has failed to stimulate more effective contractions, it is recommended that labour augmentation be started with oxytocin infusion to achieve 3–4 strong contractions every 10 minutes. If there is a failure to progress despite oxytocin augmentation, a cesarean section should be performed.

Arrest of dilatation (Fig. 44.4)

According to the WHO partograph, arrest of dilatation is defined as complete cessation of cervical dilatation for >2 hours with good uterine contraction (equivalent to 200 Montevideo units) in the active phase of labour.

Management

- When the arrest of dilatation is diagnosed, it is important to rule out mechanical factors such as CPD, malposition and malpresentations.
- Occasionally, there may be associated inefficient uterine contractions, which may be due to mechanical factors rather than primary uterine dysfunction. Therefore, caution should be taken before augmenting labour with oxytocin infusion. Most such cases require a cesarean section.

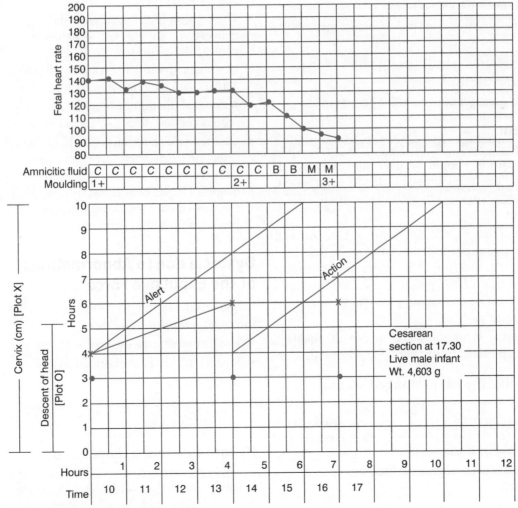

Fig. 44.4 Partograph showing arrest of dilatation

Disorders of the second stage of labour

- Many of the cardinal movements necessary for the fetus to negotiate the birth canal occur during the second stage. Accordingly, cephalopelvic disproportion frequently becomes apparent during this stage. The second stage of labour lasts for two hours in a nullipara and one hour in a multipara. In women on regional analgesia, this time frame may increase by one more hour.
- The labour disorders noted in the second stage of labour are protracted descent and arrest of descent.
  — In protracted descent, the descent of the presenting part is <1 cm/hour in a nullipara and <2 cm/hour in a multipara.
  — In the arrest of descent, there is no progress in descent for >2 hours in a nullipara and for >1 hour in a multipara.

The causes of a prolonged second stage of labour include the following:

- Cephalopelvic disproportion
- Malpresentation and malposition
- Primary inefficient uterine contractions, myometrial fatigue
- Maternal exhaustion and poor expulsive efforts
- Regional anesthesia
- Soft tissue dystocia due to a rigid perineum

Management

- In all women with second-stage disorders, CPD and malposition should be carefully excluded. If the delay is due to insufficient uterine contraction, labour can be augmented with oxytocin once CPD is ruled out.
- If the presenting part is below the +2 station and there is no disproportion, the baby can be delivered by forceps or vacuum. It is important to ensure that the station of the presenting part is correctly assessed as caput or moulding can be mistaken for the presenting part.
- If the woman is in the active phase of pushing, maternal expulsive efforts should be encouraged.

Risks associated with prolonged second stage

A prolonged second stage is associated with increased maternal risks including chorioamnionitis, postpartum hemorrhage, operative vaginal delivery and third- and fourth-degree perineal lacerations and fetal asphyxia.

Recent revisions made to the criteria for the diagnosis of abnormal labour by partograph (WHO, 2018):

- The latent phase of labour lasts up to 5 cm dilatation.
- Earlier, the active phase of labour was thought to begin at 4 cm; now, as per the 2018 WHO guidelines, the active phase of labour is said to start at 6 cm dilatation and hence, the partograph should be plotted from 6 cm dilatation.
- Arrest of labour in the first stage should be defined as more ≥6 cm dilatation with ruptured membranes and one of the following—4 hours or more of adequate contractions (>200 MVU) or 6 hours or more of inadequate contractions and no cervical change.

Recommendations of the Obstetric Care Consensus Committee (2016)

- A prolonged latent phase is not an indication for cesarean delivery.
- The committee recommends against cesarean delivery if labour is progressive but slow—a protraction disorder. Such labour should typically be managed with observation, assessment of uterine activity and stimulation of contractions as required.
- A cervical dilation of 6 cm and not 4 cm is now the recommended threshold for active labour.
- Cesarean delivery for active-phase arrest 'should be reserved for women at or beyond 6 cm of dilation with ruptured membranes who fail to progress despite 4 hours of adequate uterine activity or at least 6 hours of oxytocin administration with inadequate contractions and no cervical change'.

Dystocia due to Abnormalities of the Expulsive Force

Labour dystocia due to abnormalities of the expulsive forces are grouped as follows:

- Hypotonic uterine dysfunction
- Hypertonic uterine dysfunction
- Incoordinate uterine action
- Tonic uterine contraction
- Constriction ring

Hypotonic uterine dysfunction

- This type of dysfunction can occur at any stage of labour and is characterised by low or no basal tone, the interval between the contractions is long and the contractions are weak, lasting for <40 seconds each. On palpation of the uterus, even at the height of a contraction, the uterus rarely hardens under the palpating hand. The uterine contractions have a normal gradient pattern, but the pressure during a contraction is insufficient to dilate the cervix. As the cervical dilatation is slow, it leads to prolonged labour which can be easily identified on a partograph.

- Besides the causes discussed earlier, some of the medications given during labour may alter uterine contractility. The latent phase of labour is particularly sensitive to narcotics. Nifedipine and magnesium sulphate used in the management of hypertensive disorders can cause hypotonic uterine action. Similarly, nitroglycerine infusion or patches used in the treatment of hypertension can also relax the uterus. Epidural anesthesia may cause a transient decrease in uterine contractility; it also prolongs the second stage of labour.

Management

Whenever there is hypotonic uterine action, it is imperative to rule out CPD, malposition and malpresentations. Whenever an obstruction is encountered, in an effort to protect the uterus, the uterus goes into inertia, especially in a primigravida. Once CPD, malposition and malpresentations are ruled out, labour can be augmented with ARM and oxytocin infusion. Careful monitoring should be continued.

Hypertonic uterine dysfunction

- Hypertonic uterine contractions are characterised by elevated resting pressure, frequent contractions that last for a longer time and a delay in return to baseline uterine tone. The pressure gradient may be distorted.
- One of the commonest causes of uterine hypertonicity is the use of oxytocic drugs such as oxytocin or prostaglandins, especially misoprostol. These medications can result in tachysystole, wherein there are >5 contractions in 10 minutes.
- Hypertonic uterine action can also be encountered when there is obstructed labour, especially in a multigravida. To overcome the obstruction, the uterine contractions become frequent and stronger, and unless appropriate action is taken, this leads to rupture uterus.

Management

If the woman is on oxytocin infusion, it should be stopped immediately, and the woman should be turned to the left lateral position and be given oxygen through a face mask. 0.25 mg of terbutaline injection should be given subcutaneously to relax the uterus. If there is persistent hypertonus of the uterus or evidence of fetal hypoxia, a cesarean section should be performed immediately. CS should also be undertaken if the hypertonicity is due to obstructed labour.

Incoordinate uterine action

- Incoordinate uterine action is a type of hypertonic dysfunction, wherein the frequency of the contraction increases, but there is no coordination. The basal tone is increased, the gradient of uterine contraction is altered and the frequency, duration and intensity of contractions are irregular. There may be more forceful contraction of the midsegment of the uterus than the fundus. Despite strong contractions, cervical dilatation proceeds slowly.
- The woman is usually anxious and distressed, which makes the incoordination worse. Labour is prolonged, and all the complications of prolonged labour follow.
- Management involves adequate analgesia and fluid balance. Stimulation of the uterus by oxytocin is best avoided in these cases. If the membranes have ruptured prematurely, prophylactic antibiotic therapy should be instituted.
- With these measures, normal uterine action may be established and labour may progress normally. Sometimes, despite analgesia and sedatives, the incoordination persists, and labour fails to progress; a cesarean section should be performed in such cases. Conditions such as elderly primiparity and disproportion or malpresentation, when found in association with incoordinate uterine action, also necessitate immediate cesarean section.

Tonic uterine contraction

- Occasionally, the uterus goes into tetanic contractions, wherein there is no relaxation, and the contractions last for 2–3 minutes.
- Tetanic contractions are highly dangerous and lead to fetal death, abruption and rupture. The uterus should be relaxed using uterine relaxants, and an immediate cesarean section carried out.

Irregular contractions of the uterus

Contraction ring and hourglass contraction

'Contraction ring' refers to an area of tetanic contraction confined to a segment of circular muscle fibres in the uterus. It is also called a 'constriction ring'.

The contraction ring is distinct from the retraction ring or the Bandl's ring.

- A retraction ring is a physiological phenomenon. It is the demarcation between the upper and lower uterine segments. It becomes more prominent in the second stage of labour. In obstructed labour, it develops into a pathological ring, which is prominent enough to be seen and palpated (Bandl's ring) above the level of the symphysis pubis.

- A contraction ring, on the other hand, is not physiological. The contraction ring may develop around a part—often a small part—of the fetus such as the neck or the breech or occasionally, a limb. Alternatively, it may be entirely dissociated from any portion of the fetus and may occur below the level of the fetus instead. A contraction ring could also develop after the delivery of the first twin. Occasionally, it can form an hourglass contraction with a retained placenta. The diagnosis of contraction ring can usually be made only at the time of cesarean section performed for prolonged labour. At the time of cesarean section, the ring may not relax and may have to be cut to deliver the baby. Differences between the pathological ring and constriction ring are presented in Table 44.3.

Other Abnormal Labours

Precipitate labour

Precipitate labour, otherwise called rapid labour, is defined as the expulsion of the fetus in less than three hours of the onset of labour.

Table 44.3 Differences between a pathological ring and a constriction ring

Pathological ring	Constriction ring
Occurs in prolonged second stage	Occurs in prolonged first, second or third stage
Always between upper and lower uterine segments	Could develop at any level of the uterus
Uterus rises	The position of the uterus does not change
Felt and seen abdominally	Diagnosis is usually made at the time of cesarean section
Uterus is tonically retracted and tender; fetal parts cannot be felt	The uterus is not tonically retracted; fetal parts can be felt
Maternal and fetal distress and fetal death may occur	Maternal and fetal distress may not be present
Relieved only by delivery of the fetus	May be relieved by anesthetics and antispasmodics

Etiology

- A multipara with abnormally low resistance and relaxed pelvic or perineal floor muscles may have an extremely short duration of labour.
- Precipitate labour may also occur in a multipara with spontaneous, unusually strong and forceful contractions. Two to three powerful contractions may cause the baby to appear with considerable rapidity.
- Hypertonic uterine contractions following induction or augmentation with oxytocic agents could result in precipitate labour.
- A previous history of precipitate labour is a predisposing factor.

Complications

Maternal complications
- Lacerations of the cervix, vaginal walls and perineum due to the rapid stretching of tissues
- Uterine rupture
- Uterine atony due to muscular exhaustion after unusually strong and rapid labour; may result in PPH
- There may be infection as a result of unsterile delivery
- In some cases, inversion of the uterus may take place

Fetal complications
- Fetal asphyxia
- Due to the rapid expulsion, the baby may sustain intracranial hemorrhage
- Occasionally, the baby may be delivered while the woman is standing; if it drops to the floor unattended, the baby may sustain serious injuries
- The cord may snap, leading to severe hemorrhage before assistance is available

Management

As precipitate labour is very rapid, it is most often recognised only after it has occurred. However, in cases with a previous history, precautions can be taken to see that the woman is kept in bed and that assistance is available as soon as the first signs of labour appear. The use of tocolytics or general anesthesia to impair uterine contractility has been attempted. If oxytocic agents are being administered, they should be discontinued immediately. After delivery, the woman should be carefully examined for any tears; If found, they should be sutured with due antiseptic precautions. The third stage of labour must be carefully conducted.

Cervical Dystocia

Cervical dystocia is one of the manifestations of abnormal labour. When the cervix fails to dilate even in the presence of good, regular uterine contractions, it is called cervical dystocia. There are two types of cervical dystocia—primary and secondary cervical dystocia.

Primary cervical dystocia

Primary dystocia is commonly seen in primigravidae. Here, the external os of the cervix fails to dilate and remains rigid despite efficient uterine contractions. This may be due to the lack of softening of the cervix during pregnancy or cervical spasm as a result of overactive sympathetic tone or excessive fibrous tissue. Cervical dystocia may also be associated with malposition and malpresentations.

Secondary cervical dystocia

Secondary cervical dystocia is usually due to excess scarring or rigidity of the cervix due to the effect of a previous operation or disease of the cervix such as amputation of the cervix, cone biopsy, extensive cauterisation or previous tears of the cervix and cervical cancer.

Management

The general condition of the woman is monitored based on maternal pulse and blood pressure; hydration and ketoacidosis are monitored and corrected as required.

Careful monitoring of the fetal heart is important. Malposition and malpresentations should be ruled out. The labour should be monitored using a partograph. Cervical dystocia usually manifests as protraction or arrest disorder in the first stage of labour.

KEY POINTS

✓ The first stage of labour has two phases—the latent phase and the active phase of labour.

✓ The latent phase extends from the onset of true labour pains to 4 cm cervical dilatation.

✓ Prolonged latent phase is not an indication for cesarean section.

✓ Labour progress is assessed by using a partograph.

✓ A partograph is a simple, inexpensive tool to monitor the progress of labour.

✓ The recording of a partograph should be started in the active phase of labour at 4 cm of cervical dilatation.

✓ Abnormal labour is defined as slow progress in labour.

✓ In all cases of abnormal labour, CPD, malposition and malpresentations should be ruled out.

✓ The use of a partograph significantly reduces maternal and perinatal morbidity and mortality.

✓ First-stage labour disorders are protracted dilatation of the cervix and arrest of dilatation.

✓ Abnormal labour can occur with hypotonic and hypertonic uterine action.

✓ In precipitate labour, the total duration of labour is <3 hours.

✓ Bandl's ring, otherwise known as the retraction ring, is seen in obstructed labour.

Essay questions

1. Define abnormal labour. What are the causes and consequences of abnormal labour?
2. How do you diagnose abnormal labour? Discuss the management of protracted active phase dilatation.

Short answer questions

1. What are the various types of uterine dysfunction?
2. How is a case of hypotonic inertia managed?
3. Write a short note on the partograph and its uses.
4. Enumerate the complications of precipitate labour.
5. What are the causes of hypertonic uterine activity?
6. What are the signs and symptoms of hypertonic uterine action?
7. Differentiate between Braxton Hicks contractions and true labour pains.
8. Differentiate between the contraction ring and the retraction ring.

MCQs

1. The following are true of Braxton Hicks contractions EXCEPT that they:
   a) Are painful
   b) Occur at long intervals and last for a short time
   c) Are not accompanied by dilatation of the cervix
   d) Are not accompanied by descent of the presenting part

2. During labour, a uterine contraction is considered adequate when it exceeds:
   a) 50 MVU
   b) 100 MVU
   c) 150 MVU
   d) 200 MVU

3. In the modified WHO partograph, cervical dilatation is plotted from:
    a) 2 cm
    b) 3 cm
    c) 4 cm
    d) 5 cm

4. Which of the following is true for a partograph?
    a) Started in the latent phase of labour
    b) Used to assess the progress of labour
    c) Not used in low-risk pregnancies
    d) It is used by the patient

5. Which of the following is a partograph is used for?
    a) To assess neonatal condition
    b) To assess the well-being of the fetus in utero
    c) To assess the progress of labour
    d) To assess maternal well-being

6. The second stage of labour is prolonged in a multipara if it is more than:
    a) 30 minutes
    b) One hour
    c) Two hours
    d) Four hours

7. A partograph includes all the following except:
    a) Fetal heart rate
    b) Colour of liquor
    c) CTG
    d) Uterine contractions

8. Hypertonic uterine contractions are characterised by:
    a) Increased frequency of contractions
    b) Proper coordination
    c) Reduced resting pressure
    d) Immediate return to baseline

9. Hypotonic uterine contraction can be managed by:
    a) Prostaglandin gel
    b) Oxytocin
    c) Betamimetics
    d) Immediate cesarean section

Answers
1. (a), 2. (d), 3. (c), 4. (b), 5. (c), 6. (b), 7. (c), 8. (a), 9. (b)

Fill in the blanks

1. The strength of uterine contractions is expressed in _____.

2. With hypertonic uterine contractions, a demarcation between the upper and lower uterine segments becomes very prominent and is known as _____.

3. A localised area of tetanic contraction confined to a segment of circular muscle fibres in the uterus due to hypertonic uterine action is called a _____.

Answers
1. Montevideo units (MVU),   2. Bandl's ring,   3. constriction ring

Case scenario-based discussion

1. A 30-year-old primigravida reports at 39 weeks of gestation with labour pains. On examination, her vitals are normal, and her uterus is contracting once in 6 minutes, with each contraction lasting for 30 seconds. The head is 3/5th palpable and the fetal heart rate is good. On pelvic examination, the cervix is 5 cm dilated, and the vertex is at the −2 station. The pelvis appears adequate.
    a) How would you manage this woman?
    b) When the woman is reviewed after 4 hours, her contractions are still 1 every 6 minutes and are weak. The head is 3/5th palpable and the cervical dilatation remains at 6 cm. What is the interpretation on partograph?
    c) What is the management recommended for this diagnosis?

Answers

a) The maternal and fetal condition should be monitored periodically, and the labour progress should be documented on the partograph.

b) As there is no cervical dilatation for 4 hours, this is a case of arrest of dilatation.

c) The case should be very carefully assessed to rule out CPD, malposition and malpresentation such as brow. After ruling out these factors, augmentation with oxytocin may be attempted to treat hypotonic uterine action. If the labour progress resumes, vaginal delivery should be allowed. Otherwise, a cesarean section should be performed.

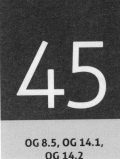

45

OG 8.5, OG 14.1, OG 14.2

Cephalopelvic Disproportion (CPD) and Obstructed Labour

Learning Objectives

» To describe pelvic assessment

» To describe and demonstrate cephalopelvic disproportion (CPD) in a model

» To discuss the causes of CPD

» To diagnose CPD

» To understand the trial of labour

» To discuss the causes and management of obstructed labour

▌ CEPHALOPELVIC DISPROPORTION (CPD)

It is important to understand the difference between cephalopelvic disproportion (CPD) and contracted pelvis.

Cephalopelvic Disproportion

Cephalopelvic disproportion refers to the anatomical/ mechanical disproportion between the fetal head and the maternal pelvis for that particular pregnancy. CPD may be due to either diminished pelvic capacity or abnormal fetal size. It does not necessarily recur in subsequent pregnancies.

Contracted Pelvis

- A contracted pelvis refers to a permanent deformity of the pelvis in which one or more diameters of the pelvis are reduced. This can affect the normal mechanism of labour and could be a recurrent cause of dystocia in subsequent labours.
- Though a contracted pelvis could be a cause of CPD, not all cases of CPD are due to a contracted pelvis.
- There are many types of contracted pelvises.
- In a contracted pelvis, one or more diameters in one or more of the planes of the pelvis may be shorter than normal. The contraction may occur at the brim of the pelvis, cavity or outlet or it may be present at all three levels. If contraction occurs at all levels, it is called a generally contracted pelvis. The contraction may affect the anteroposterior diameter or the transverse diameter or both. A contraction in one diameter may be compensated for by an increase in the other diameters.

Therefore, in assessing the possibilities of vaginal delivery, the obstetrician should take into consideration the capacity of the pelvis as a whole at all levels.

- The pelvic contraction may be symmetrical or asymmetrical, thus causing several varieties of deformities. Lower limb shortening or deformities caused by the fracture of the pelvis/lower limbs, poliomyelitis and tuberculosis of hip joints can result in asymmetrical pelvic contractions affecting the pelvic diameters on one side of the pelvis. Similarly, kyphosis and scoliosis affecting the lumbar region can also result in asymmetrical pelvic contractions. Congenital dislocation of the hip can also result in a contracted pelvis.
- Rickets and osteomalacia are rare causes of a contracted pelvis. Rickets results in a triradiate pelvis; the pelvic inlet is kidney-shaped (reniform).
- Naegele's pelvis and Robert's pelvis (see Chapter 1, *The pelvis*) are congenital causes of a contracted pelvis. These are rarely encountered and occur due to the defective development of one or both sacral alae.

Contracted Inlet

As the fetal biparietal diameter is approximately 9.5 cm, for the head to pass through a pelvic inlet, the available anteroposterior diameter should be >10 cm. The anteroposterior diameter of the inlet, which is the obstetrical conjugate, cannot be manually measured. Instead, it is calculated by measuring the diagonal conjugate (Fig. 45.1) and subtracting 1.5–2 cm from it (refer to Chapter 1 for measurement). Therefore, inlet contraction is usually defined as a diagonal conjugate of <11.5 cm or a calculated obstetric conjugate of <10 cm.

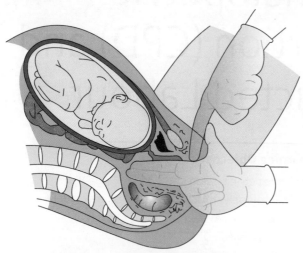

Fig. 45.1 Measurement of diagonal conjugate

Effects of inlet contraction

- A contracted inlet can result in abnormal presentations. In nulliparas with normal pelvic capacity, at term, the head commonly descends into the pelvic cavity before the onset of labour. When the inlet is contracted, the descent of the head does not take place. Cephalic presentations still predominate, but the head floats freely or rests more laterally in one of the iliac fossae (oblique lie) presenting with cephalopelvic disproportion. Inlet contraction can also result in malposition and malpresentations such as deflexed head, face or brow presentation or transverse lie.

- When the inlet is contracted, there may be premature rupture of membranes or spontaneous rupture of the membranes early in labour. As the head is unable to descend into the pelvis, the force of the uterine contractions is directly borne by the membranes, causing them to rupture early.

Contracted Midpelvis

- The average midpelvis measurements are as follows:
  - The transverse or interischial spinous diameter—10 cm
  - The anteroposterior diameter from the lower border of the symphysis pubis to the junction of S4–5—11.5 cm
  - The posterior sagittal diameter is a part of the AP diameter, which lies posterior to the interspinous diameter—6 cm
- The distance between the two ischial spines (the interspinous diameter) is assessed by measuring the distance between the stretched index and middle fingers trying to touch the ischial spines. Midpelvic

contraction is suspected whenever the interspinous diameter is <10 cm. When it measures <8 cm, the midpelvis is definitely contracted.

- There is no precise manual method to measure the midpelvic dimensions. However, mid-cavity assessment can be carried out by palpating the pelvic architecture. In a mid-cavity contraction, the ischial spines are prominent, the interspinous diameter is <10 cm, the sacrum is flat and not curved and the side walls of the pelvis are converging. The sacrosciatic notch does not allow two fingers; the sub-pubic arch is also narrow and does not admit two fingers either. Narrowing of the interspinous diameter can be anticipated when the intertuberous diameter at the outlet is narrow.

Effects of midpelvic contraction

Midpelvis contraction causes the transverse arrest of the fetal head and prolonged labour and obstructed labour, resulting in cesarean delivery.

Contracted Outlet

- If the outlet is normal, it should be possible to place four knuckles of the closed fist in-between the ischial tuberosities (Fig. 45.2) and the subpubic arch should admit two fingers.

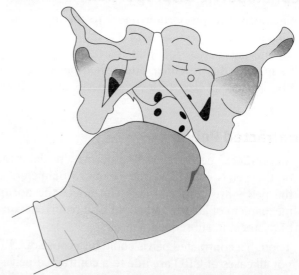

Fig. 45.2 Assessment of the intertuberous diameter

- A contracted outlet is defined as an interischiotuberous diameter of 8 cm or less and is usually associated with narrow a subpubic arch. Decreased intertuberous diameter with consequent narrowing of the anterior triangle inevitably forces the fetal head posteriorly. Outlet contraction occurring alone is rare and is almost always associated with concomitant mid-cavity contraction. Although the disproportion between the fetal head and the pelvic outlet may not give rise to severe dystocia, it may cause third- and fourth-degree perineal tears.

Diagnosis of CPD

Though the diagnosis of CPD is made by history, clinical examination and clinical pelvimetry, the progress of labour is the best determinant to assess CPD in labour.

History

Previous obstetric performance

- In a multiparous woman, previous obstetric performance provides important information about the possibility of a contracted pelvis and CPD.
- Safe vaginal delivery of average-size, live babies at term without fetal compromise or fetal morbidity usually denotes a pelvis of normal capacity.
- On the other hand, a history of prolonged labour, difficult vaginal delivery (forceps), cesarean section, fetal asphyxia or stillbirth or neonatal death, in the absence of other etiological factors, would strongly suggest the possibility of a contracted pelvis or cephalopelvic disproportion. The delivery of a macrosomic baby with morbidity may also suggest CPD.

Past history

History of post-polio residual paralysis, fractures affecting the lower limbs or pelvis and tuberculosis affecting the pelvic joints point to the possibility of an obliquely contracted pelvis.

Examination

- Short-statured women (<145 cm) tend to have a small, gynecoid pelvis in which all the diameters are reduced. In women who are of less than average height, labour should be carefully monitored for abnormal labour patterns and pelvic dystocia.
- Dystocia dystrophia syndrome—women who are short, obese and stocky may have abnormal labour on account of an android pelvis.
- A pendulous abdomen, deformities of the spine, especially those involving the lower lumbar region, shortening of a lower limb, tilting of the pelvis and a waddling gait may predict an abnormal pelvis/cephalopelvic disproportion.
- An unengaged or floating head in a primigravida at term should always alert the obstetrician to the possibility of cephalopelvic disproportion. It is also important to remember that the deflexed head may

simulate or exaggerate disproportion. The causes of a floating head in a primigravida are presented in the box below.

- In the presence of CPD, malpresentations such as face, breech and transverse lie are common.

Causes of a floating head in a primigravida
- Full bladder
- CPD
- Malposition and malpresentations such as occipitoposterior position or face or brow presentations
- Placenta previa
- Tumours occupying the lower segment such as fibroids and ovarian tumours
- Cord around the neck
- Fetal anomalies such as hydrocephalus or tumours in the region of the fetal neck
- Polyhydramnios
- Multiple pregnancy
- Wrong dates

After taking the woman's history and performing thorough general and abdominal examinations, all primigravidae and multigravidae with previous history suggesting CPD should be assessed for the presence of a contracted pelvis as well as cephalopelvic disproportion. The assessment should be carried out at or after 38 weeks of gestation.

Assessment of the pelvis (clinical pelvimetry)

The clinical assessment of the pelvis provides information on the type of pelvis. It also helps to determine whether there is any reduction in the measurable diameters such as the diagonal conjugate and the interischial and intertuberous diameters.

Procedure of clinical pelvimetry

The bladder should be emptied prior to the assessment. After explaining the procedure to the woman, she is placed in the dorsal position. With sterile precautions, the middle and index fingers of the right hand are introduced into the vagina, and a systematic assessment of the pelvis is carried out.

The inlet

Diagonal conjugate—attempts should be made to palpate the sacral promontory and to measure the diagonal conjugate. Normally, the diagonal conjugate is 12.5 cm and the sacral promontory cannot be reached. If the sacral promontory of the pelvis is reached, the pelvis is considered contracted. The obstetric conjugate can be calculated by subtracting 1.5 cm from the diagonal conjugate.

The cavity

- Shape and inclination of the sacrum: The sacral concavity, which extends from the promontory to the sacral tip, should be well-developed so that at the midpelvic and higher level, the bone can be reached only with difficulty. Flattening of the sacrum is an unfavourable sign, which may produce 'transverse arrest'.

- Side walls: To determine whether the side wall is straight, convergent or divergent, palpation is performed starting from the pelvic brim down to the base of ischial spines in the direction of the base of the ischial tuberosity.

- Ischial spines: The ischial spines are palpated to see whether they are blunt (difficult to identify at all), prominent (easily felt but not large) or very prominent (large and encroaching on the mid-plane).

- Interspinous diameter: Using the two examining fingers, if both spines can be touched simultaneously, the interspinous diameter is <9.5 cm, which is inadequate for an average-sized baby.

- Sacrosciatic notch: If the sacrospinous ligament admits two and a half fingers, the sacrosciatic notch is considered adequate.

The outlet

- The subpubic angle should normally admit two fingers.

- The intertuberous diameter—the distance between the two ischial tuberosities—should normally admit the closed fist of a hand (four knuckles).

Assessment of cephalopelvic disproportion

CPD is assessed by abdominal and abdominopelvic methods. Normally, assessment for CPD is carried out at 38 weeks of gestation. However, the adequacy of the pelvis for the particular fetus is best assessed in labour.

Abdominal methods

In these methods, per abdomen, an attempt is made to push the head down the pelvic brim to look for CPD.

Head fitting test

- The bladder should be emptied prior to the procedure.

- The woman is placed in a semi-sitting position with her legs semi-flexed at the thighs and knees so that the fetal axis is perpendicular to the brim.

- Standing to the right of the woman, the obstetrician uses the left hand to push the fetal head downwards and backwards into the pelvis while the fingers of the right hand are placed over the symphysis pubis to detect disproportion (Fig. 45.3). If the head descends into the pelvis, there is no CPD. If the fetal head is flushed or if it overhangs the symphysis pubis, CPD is inferred.

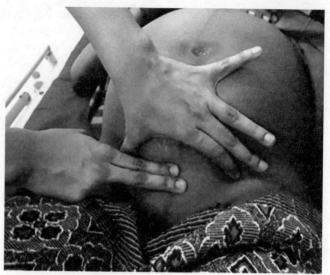

Fig. 45.3   Head fitting test

Donald's method

In this method, the woman lies on her back with semi-flexion of the thighs and knees and the legs separated. The clinician stands on the right side of the woman, and using the third, fourth and fifth fingers of both hands, holds the fetal head at the sinciput and the occiput (Fig. 45.4). The index fingers of both hands palpate the symphysis pubis while the thumbs exert downward and backward pressure on the parietal eminence of the fetal head. An assistant may exert downward pressure on the breech at the fundus at the same time. The index fingers on the symphysis pubis are used to assess whether the fetal head can descend into the pelvis or if there is over-riding of the fetal head.

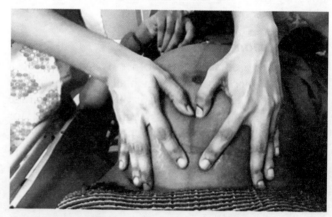

Fig. 45.4   Donald's method of assessing CPD

Abdominopelvic method—the Munro–Kerr–Müller method

By this method, the adequacy of the maternal pelvis in relation to the size of the fetal head is assessed.

- Before starting the assessment, the procedure is explained to the woman, and she is asked to empty her bladder.

- The woman is placed in the dorsal lithotomy position and the obstetrician stands at her side facing her.
- Under aseptic conditions, the obstetrician passes two fingers into the vagina and positions them at the level of the ischial spines.
- With the other hand on the abdomen, the obstetrician grasps the fetal head and presses it into the pelvic brim (Fig. 45.5).
- The thumb of the vaginal hand is used to palpate the head over the symphysis.
- From the extent of the descent of the head into the maternal pelvis or the degree of over-riding of the head over the symphysis, the severity of CPD can be assessed as given below:
  a) If the head can be pushed down to the level of the ischial spines, there is no CPD.
  b) If the head can be pushed down a little but not to the level of the ischial spines, there is a minor degree of CPD. In this condition, the head will be in line with the thumb placed at the level of the symphysis pubis.
  c) When the head cannot be pushed into the pelvic cavity and there is marked over-riding of the head on the thumb, it is known as a major degree CPD.

Limitations of this procedure
- The important limitation of this procedure is that if it is performed prior to labour, a deflexed head may simulate disproportion, which may result in an incorrect diagnosis. Prior to labour, mild disproportion can be exaggerated by deflexion, which is usually corrected during active labour pains.
- This method helps in diagnosing disproportion at the brim level but is not useful to assess CPD at the cavity or at the outlet.

Imaging studies in the diagnosis of CPD
Imaging studies by X-ray pelvis, MRI and USG are not very helpful in the diagnosis of CPD, and therefore, are not routinely used.

Complications of CPD
- Floating head
- Malpositions and malpresentations such as occipitoposterior position, brow, face, breech, transverse and oblique lie
- Premature rupture of membranes
- Prolonged labour
- Obstructed labour and rupture uterus

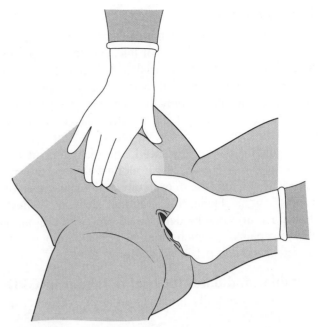

Fig. 45.5 Munro–Kerr–Müller method of estimating disproportion

- Cord prolapse, fetal distress, stillbirth
- Increased operative deliveries

Management of CPD
- Major degrees of CPD and obliquely contracted pelvis are diagnosed in the antenatal period without difficulty. Minor degrees of CPD are also suspected or diagnosed during the antenatal period. In many cases, the diagnosis of CPD is made during labour or in retrospect due to prolonged labour, non-descent of the fetal head or excessive caput or moulding.
- When CPD occurs in a nulliparous woman, the uterus goes into uterine inertia following good uterine contractions. On the other hand, in a multiparous woman, the uterus contracts vigorously to overcome the obstruction; this may result in rupture uterus.
- If disproportion is diagnosed during the antenatal period, the case is managed either by elective cesarean section or trial of labour. The management depends on the degree of disproportion and the associated risk factors.

Indications for elective cesarean section
- In those diagnosed with a major degree of CPD or in the presence of an obliquely contracted pelvis due to deformities of the lower limbs or the spines, a cesarean section is performed as a planned procedure.
- In those diagnosed with minor disproportion, in the presence of associated malpresentations or associated high-risk pregnancies, elective cesarean section should be undertaken.

Trial of labour

In women diagnosed with minor disproportion, trial of labour can be undertaken. If it fails, a cesarean section is carried out. The aim of trial of labour is to reduce cesarean section rates. The basis of trial of labour is that during normal labour, the diameters of the pelvis increase to some extent due to the relaxation of the pelvic joints and soft tissue. At the same time, due to the moulding of the fetal head, the diameters of the fetal skull also decrease. These, along with good uterine contractions, may help overcome minor degrees of disproportion, facilitating vaginal delivery. These clinical features can be determined only with the onset of labour pains, at which time, the adjustment between the fetal head and pelvis will favour progress.

Suitable candidates for trial of labour in CPD

- Minor degree CPD (contraction in one diameter in one plane)
- The most favourable outcome is with the platypelloid pelvis since only the AP diameter at the pelvic brim is reduced
- Primigravida without comorbidities
- Vertex presentation
- No mid-cavity or outlet contractions
- Average-sized baby

Contraindications for trial of labour in CPD

- Major degree of CPD
- Associated malpresentations
- Associated obstetrical risk factors such as elderly primi, GDM, hypertension and postdated pregnancy

The procedure of trial of labour in CPD

- Trial of labour should be carried out in a hospital where facilities for cesarean section are readily available.
- Spontaneous onset of labour is preferable.
- The procedure should be carried out in a dual setting, wherein the woman is prepared and prepped for both vaginal delivery and cesarean section.
- The woman must be psychologically prepared for trial of labour, and her consent should be taken beforehand.
- Once labour begins, its progress should be monitored by abdominal palpation as well as vaginal examination. Labour progress should be documented using a partograph.
- The maternal condition should be carefully monitored and should include a pulse chart, temperature, BP estimation and fluid balance.
- When the membrane ruptures, cord prolapse should be ruled out.

- The fetal condition should be monitored by continuous CTG.
- The woman should be kept on nil per oral as she may require a cesarean section.
- Pain relief should be given—epidural analgesia is preferable.

The **good prognostic signs** of trial of labour
- Presence of good uterine action
- Early engagement of the head
- The cervix is thinned out, dilating progressively and well-applied to the vertex
- Occipitoanterior position

The **bad prognostic signs** of trial of labour
- Weak uterine contractions
- Slow descent of the head
- Rupture of the membranes with an uneffaced and partially dilated cervix
- Slow dilatation of the cervix
- Occipitoposterior position of the head

Termination of trial of labour

If the progress of labour is unsatisfactory despite good uterine action, with poor cervical dilatation, slow descent of head or evidence of obstruction with excessive caput and moulding, labour should be terminated with a lower segment cesarean section. Maternal and fetal distress are also indications for the immediate termination of trial of labour. A trial of labour is considered successful if vaginal delivery results in a healthy baby and mother. The vaginal delivery may be either spontaneous or assisted by forceps/vacuum. The trial of labour is considered failed if it results in a cesarean delivery or perinatal complications/death.

■ OBSTRUCTED LABOUR

Obstructed labour should not occur in modern obstetric practice. With the use of a partograph, prolonged labour should be identified early, and necessary action should be taken before obstruction develops. Labour is considered obstructed if it does not progress due to anatomical/mechanical factors causing obstruction to delivery.

Etiology of Obstructed Labour

- CPD (due to a contracted pelvis or a large baby)
- Persistent occipitoposterior position and deep transverse arrest
- Fetal anomalies such as hydrocephalus, fetal ascites and conjoined twins

- Malpresentations such as brow presentation, mento posterior, shoulder presentation or compound presentation
- Pregnancy complicated by tumours such as fibroids and ovarian tumours
- Uterine anomalies

Diagnosis of Obstructed Labour

Obstructed labour that is not diagnosed and treated could lead to rupture uterus and maternal and fetal deaths. Therefore, the diagnosis should be made without delay.

- In women presenting with obstructed labour, there will be a history of prolonged labour, prolonged rupture of membranes, loss of fetal movements and use of oxytocic drugs. The woman will also complain of severe and continuous abdominal pain. There may be a history of delivery attempted elsewhere.
- On examination, the woman may be cold and clammy, anxious, restless, exhausted or in agony. She will be febrile, dehydrated and pale, and her tongue will be dry. The pulse will be rapid with tachycardia; there may be laboured respiration.
- On abdominal examination, the uterus is hard and tender and tonically contracted on the baby, making palpation difficult. The uterus is in a state of continuous contraction and retraction so that there is no relaxation between contractions. The major portion of the fetal head is palpable per abdomen. The round ligaments are prominent.
- Pathologic retraction ring or Bandl's ring— Normally, during labour, under the influence of uterine contractions, the uterus gradually becomes differentiated into two distinct portions. The upper segment is thicker and more active and becomes progressively thicker as labour advances. The lower portion, i.e., the lower segment with the cervix, is passive and becomes thinner and more stretched out to receive the descending fetus as labour advances. The junction between the upper and lower segments is characterised by a ring of circular muscle fibres— the physiological retraction ring. Above this level is the contracting thick upper segment, and below is the dilatating and stretching lower segment and cervix. This ring becomes prominent in obstructed labour and is termed the pathologic retraction ring or Bandl's ring (Fig. 45.6a and b), which can be made out by abdominal palpation.
- The Bandl's ring may run obliquely or transversely across the uterus, showing the demarcation between the lower and upper uterine segments. Depending on the duration of the obstruction, the retraction

ring of Bandl is felt at a higher level. At times, the round ligaments may stand out as tense cords on either side. If assistance is not rendered in time, the uterus ruptures.

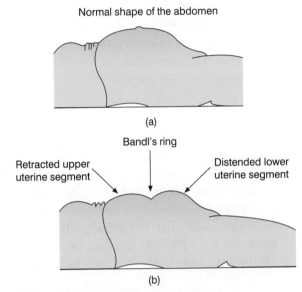

Fig. 45.6 Uterus showing Bandl's ring

- There may be difficulty in identifying the fetal heart sounds, which may not be heard distinctly on auscultation. CTG and USG may be useful in identifying fetal heart sounds. Most often, the fetus is in distress or the fetal heart is absent as the child is dead.
- There may be distended bowel loops due to sepsis or ileus.
- On vaginal examination, the vagina is hot and dry, the perineum, vagina, cervix, urethra and bladder may be lacerated due to attempts at vaginal delivery. There may be an offensive vaginal discharge. A large caput may be visible on the presenting part. In many cases, though a large caput is visible at the introitus, 3/5th or more of the fetal head is still palpable per abdomen. The head may be high despite full cervical dilatation. The large caput may obscure the landmarks on the presenting part; marked, irreducible moulding may be present. The cervix may be hanging loose and edematous, and there may be edema of the vagina and perineum. In cases of neglected shoulder presentation, the edematous arm can be seen protruding through the vagina.
- If a partograph was maintained, it will show slow progress in the first stage of labour/arrest of labour in the second stage.
- Threatened rupture—at this stage, the patient is in a state of threatened rupture, and if the uterus is not emptied, rupture uterus will result. It is important

to rule out rupture uterus in these cases, as such women need a laparotomy. The woman's consent should be taken for a hysterectomy if it is required. The necessary appropriate preparations are required to manage rupture uterus.

- Once the uterus ruptures:
  - The woman shows signs of shock.
  - Uterine contractions cease.
  - Fetal parts are easily palpable.
  - There may be vaginal bleeding.
  - Fetal heart is absent.
  - The presenting part recedes from the pelvis.
  - The bladder may be distended with retained urine, which may be concentrated or bloodstained due to the pressure on the bladder by the fetal head and symphysis pubis.
  - In some cases, the tamponade effect of an impacted head prevents bleeding as in the case of rupture uterus. If the head is dislodged, bleeding will be obvious.

Management

Once obstructed labour is diagnosed, the following measures should be instituted immediately:

- The woman should be resuscitated with NS or Ringer's lactate solution.
- Blood should be grouped, cross-matched and kept available.
- Dehydration, acidosis and hypovolemia should be corrected.
- Hemoglobin, renal function and electrolytes should be checked.
- The bladder should be catheterised and continuous bladder drainage carried out.
- Antibiotics should be given by the parenteral route to cover aerobic and anaerobic organisms.
- The stomach should be emptied by nasogastric aspiration to prevent aspiration pneumonitis.
- Immediate steps should be taken to empty the uterus. If facilities are not available, the woman should be shifted to the nearest higher centre. Before shifting, IV fluid should be started, sedation should be given and the uterus should be relaxed with subcutaneous terbutaline.

Obstetric management

- Even if the fetus is dead, cesarean section must be undertaken without delay in the interests of the mother. In modern obstetric practice, destructive operations are not undertaken as most clinicians do not have the necessary skills to perform them.

- At the time of cesarean section, care should be taken while opening the abdomen as the bladder may be drawn up and may be injured. To avoid this, the uterovesical fold of the peritoneum should be opened at a higher level.
- There may be difficulty in the delivery of the fetal head, which is impacted in the pelvis. The head may have to be disimpacted by the vaginal route by an assistant.
- Injury to the bladder may occur and should be carefully looked for.
- The uterus should be delivered outside the abdominal incision and carefully evaluated for rupture in the posterior surface, the presence of broad ligament hematoma and downward and lateral extension of the uterine incision.
- Atonic/traumatic PPH should be anticipated, and necessary preventive measures should be taken to avoid such an occurrence.
- Following cesarean section, it is important to leave the catheter for 10–14 days in order to prevent avascular necrosis of the bladder and vesicovaginal fistulae.

Complications of Obstructed Labour

The complications of obstructed labour include the following:

- Rupture of the uterus may occur.
- There is a risk of atonic/traumatic postpartum hemorrhage.
- Trauma to the perineum and vagina may occur.
- Puerperal infection and septicemia may develop.
- Due to prolonged pressure exerted by the fetal head on the vagina and surrounding structures such as the bladder and rectum, pressure necrosis may occur, resulting in a vesicovaginal fistula (VVF) or rectovaginal fistula (RVF).
- Prolonged pressure on the sciatic nerve and nerve roots results in neurological complications affecting the lower limbs; foot-drop is not uncommon.
- With strong expulsive efforts, the fetal head may be forced through the pelvis, resulting in rupture or subluxation of the symphysis pubis. The sacroiliac joints may also be involved in the subluxation. Fracture or fracture–dislocation of the coccyx and sacrococcygeal joint is likely to occur.

- With prolonged obstructed labour, there could be stillbirth or severe trauma to the baby, resulting in neonatal death. Trauma to the fetal scalp may result in cephalhematoma. Extreme moulding of the fetal head may result in intracranial hemorrhage and neonatal asphyxia.
- The mother may die from rupture uterus and the fetus from asphyxia.

Complications of obstructed labour
- Rupture uterus
- Postpartum hemorrhage
- Puerperal sepsis
- Perineal and vaginal tears
- VVF and RVF
- Foot-drop
- Subluxation of the symphysis pubis/sacroiliac joints
- Maternal, fetal and neonatal death

KEY POINTS

✓ *In a contracted pelvis, one or more diameters in one or more planes are shorter than normal and this affects the normal mechanism of labour.*

✓ *In cephalopelvic disproportion, there is an anatomical disproportion between the fetal head and the maternal pelvis for that particular pregnancy. CPD may occur due to either diminished pelvic capacity or abnormal fetal size.*

✓ *The management options for CPD include elective cesarean section and trial of labour.*

✓ *Trial of labour is allowed only in minor CPD. The most favourable type of pelvis is one in which there is contraction at one diameter in one plane only. The presentation should be vertex, and labour should be preferably spontaneous in onset. Labour should be monitored with a partograph and continuous CTG.*

✓ *The causes of obstructed labour include CPD, malpresentations, fetal anomalies such as hydrocephalus and tumours complicating pregnancy.*

✓ *Obstructed labour is managed by a cesarean section.*

Essay question

1. What is cephalopelvic disproportion? How do you diagnose CPD? Discuss the conduct of trial of labour in CPD.

Short answer questions

Write short notes on:

1. Diagonal conjugate
2. Assessment of mid-cavity contraction
3. Munro–Kerr–Müller method for assessment of CPD
4. Causes of obstructed labour
5. Bandl's ring
6. Complications of obstructed labour

MCQs

1. In which of the following conditions is trial of labour not allowed?
   a) Minor degree of CPD
   b) Small gynaecoid pelvis
   c) Platypelloid pelvis
   d) Postdated pregnancy

2. In trial of labour, the following are the good signs of progress except:
   a) Progressive dilatation of the cervix
   b) Progressive descent of the fetal head
   c) Cervix well-applied to the fetal head
   d) Early rupture of membranes in labour

3. In a primigravida, the pelvic assessment is carried out at:
   a) 32 weeks
   b) 34 weeks
   c) 36 weeks
   d) 38 weeks

4. Obstructed labour occurs due to all of the following except:
   a) Hydrocephalus
   b) Transverse lie
   c) Obliquely contracted pelvis
   d) Congenital talipes

5. The Munro–Kerr–Müller method is used to diagnose:
   a) Contraction at the inlet
   b) Contraction at the cavity
   c) Contraction at the outlet
   d) Asymmetric pelvic contraction

6. What is the ideal pelvis for a trial of labour?
   a) Gynaecoid pelvis
   b) Android pelvis
   c) Anthropoid pelvis
   d) Platypelloid pelvis

7. Absence of one sacral ala is seen in:
   a) Rachitic pelvis
   b) Osteomalacic pelvis
   c) Robert's pelvis
   d) Naegele's pelvis

8. Which of the following is true about Robert's pelvis?
   a) Both pelvic alae are absent
   b) Single pelvic ala is absent
   c) It is a triradiate pelvis
   d) It is a flat pelvis

9. Triradiate pelvis is seen in:
   a) Kyphosis
   b) Scoliosis

c) Rickets

d) Robert's pelvis

10. Which of the following methods is NOT used to assess cephalopelvic disproportion?

a) Mariceau–Smillie–Viet method

b) Head fitting test

c) Donald's method

d) Munro–Kerr-Müller method

Answers

1. (d), 2. (d), 3. (d), 4. (d), 5. (a), 6. (d), 7. (d), 8. (a), 9. (c), 10. (a)

Fill in the blanks

1. With hypertonic uterine contractions, a demarcation between the upper and lower uterine segments becomes very prominent. This is known as _____.

2. Triradiate pelvis occurs in _____.

Answers

1. Bandl's ring,   2. rickets

Case scenario-based discussion

1. A 21-year-old primigravida at 40 weeks of gestation presents with labour pains of 12 hours' duration and leaking per vaginum of 24 hours' duration. She was seen and managed by a *dai* at home for 10 hours. She reports that she has not been able to feel the fetal movements for nearly 6 hours.

   She is a short-statured woman, is distressed with pain and on examination, is found to be febrile, exhausted and pale. Her tongue is dry, pulse is 100 bpm and BP is 100/80 mmHg. On abdominal examination, the uterus is tonically contracted and tender on palpation; the head is 4/5th palpable and the FH is not heard. The lower segment is stretched and a Bandl's ring is seen. On vaginal examination, the vagina is warm, the cervix is 8 cm dilated and edematous, the membrane is absent, and a large caput is felt at the +1 station.

   a) What is the diagnosis?

   b) What immediate measures should be taken?

   c) What is the management of obstructed labour and what precautions should be taken in such cases?

   d) What are the complications of obstructed labour?

   e) How can obstructed labour be prevented?

Answers

a) The diagnosis is primigravida at term pregnancy in obstructed labour with IUFD.

b) The woman should be resuscitated immediately with crystalloids; dehydration, acidosis and hypovolemia should be corrected, electrolytes should be administered, and blood samples should be taken for grouping and cross-matching and for checking hemoglobin levels. Renal function test should be performed. Blood should be made available. The bladder should be catheterised, and continuous bladder drainage should be carried out. Antibiotics should be given by the parenteral route to cover aerobic and anaerobic organisms. The stomach should be emptied by nasogastric aspiration and immediate steps should be taken to empty the uterus.

c) The woman should be delivered by immediate cesarean section by a senior obstetrician. Before this, it is important to rule out rupture uterus. At the time of cesarean section, care should be taken while opening the abdomen as the bladder may be drawn up and may get injured. There may be difficulty in the delivery of the fetal head which is impacted in the pelvis. PPH should be anticipated, and preventive measures should be taken. Downward and lateral extension of the uterine incision, broad ligament hematoma and rupture of the posterior surface of the uterus may occur and hence, should be carefully looked for and managed. Postoperatively, there should be continuous bladder drainage to prevent bladder fistulae.

d) The complications of obstructed labour include rupture of the uterus, atonic and traumatic postpartum hemorrhage, trauma to the perineum and vagina and puerperal infection. Delayed complications include vesicovaginal and rectovaginal fistulae. There may be stillbirth, neonatal death and trauma to the fetus with cephalhematoma and intracranial haemorrhage.

e) The following measures help prevent obstructed labour:

- All women, both primigravidae and multigravidae, with a previous mishap suggesting CPD should be assessed for CPD at 38 weeks of gestation. In cases diagnosed with a major degree of disproportion and malpresentation, an elective cesarean section should be performed at the appropriate time.

- When such women go into labour, the progress of labour should be carefully monitored using a partograph to look for abnormal labour patterns. If the labour is prolonged and the labour curve crosses the alert line, the woman should be carefully evaluated for the presence of CPD and malpresentations. If present, necessary action should be taken. In centres where facilities for cesarean section are not available, once the labour curve crosses the alert line, the woman should be referred without delay to the nearest centre where facilities are available.

Abnormalities of the Reproductive Tract

Learning Objectives

» To know the pregnancy complications encountered in women with congenital uterine anomalies
» To manage a case of uterine prolapse complicating pregnancy
» To know the manifestations of retroverted gravid uterus and the management of urinary retention
» To know about genital mutilation and its obstetric complications

A number of pregnancy complications and abnormalities of labour can be caused by abnormalities of maternal soft parts. These abnormalities could be either congenital or acquired.

ABNORMALITIES OF THE VULVA

Vulval Atresia

The vulva and the vaginal introitus may be occluded completely or partially due to adhesions and scar formation following injury or infection. Pregnancy cannot occur when there is complete atresia of the vulva. However, when there is incomplete occlusion, which is common, pregnancy is possible.

At the time of vaginal delivery, in order to avoid extensive perineal tears involving the rectum, an adequate episiotomy may need to be performed.

Rigid Perineum

This is often seen in elderly primigravidae and in multiparous women who have had previous perineal lacerations repaired. For these women, adequate episiotomy should be given at the time of delivery.

Edema of the Vulva

In pregnancy, edema of the vulva can occur as a result of pre-eclampsia, anemia or cardiac disease. Being a dependent area, the vulva can easily be affected as a part of generalised edema. Treating the underlying cause can relieve this problem. However, if the edema is intractable and painful, dressing with magnesium sulphate and glycerine over the edematous area provides relief.

Healed Scars

Scarring can occur from lymphogranuloma venereum, which produces severe cicatrisation resulting in a narrow vulval outlet. In such cases, the difficulties at the time of vaginal delivery may be prevented by performing an episiotomy; if severe, a cesarean section may be required.

Bartholin Abscess

A Bartholin abscess may be encountered occasionally in pregnancy. This abscess is situated in the lateral lower one-third of the vagina. It should be drained, either under local or general anesthesia. After drainage, the cavity is left open with the help of a gauge drain until granulation is complete. A broad-spectrum antibiotic is administered. Excision of the cyst wall during pregnancy is difficult and not advised because of increased vascularity and longer operating time.

Bartholin Cyst

If asymptomatic, the treatment should be delayed until after delivery. If it causes obstruction during vaginal delivery, needle aspiration can offer a temporary solution.

Female Genital Mutilation

Female genital mutilation (FGM) involves the partial or total removal of external female genitalia for non-medical reasons. It is practised in some African and Middle-Eastern countries. Several obstetric complications may arise due to the obstruction of the birth canal by scar tissue. FGM is associated with an increased risk of cesarean section, postpartum hemorrhage, recourse to episiotomy, difficult labour, obstetric tears/lacerations, instrumental delivery, prolonged labour and extended maternal hospital stay. Because of prolonged labour, the bladder could be compressed between the fetal head and the symphysis pubis, which could lead to an obstetric fistula. These obstetric complications can result in a higher incidence of infant resuscitation at delivery and intrapartum stillbirth and neonatal death.

Vulval Warts

Genital warts known as condyloma accuminata are caused by human papillomavirus (HPV) infection. They present as small, skin-coloured/brown/grey, painless growths around the vulva, vagina, anus or upper thighs and can grow into large cauliflower-like lesions They can manifest for the first time in pregnancy or small lesions may become very large and make vaginal delivery difficult. Large warts on the vulva or in the vagina can bleed when stretched during delivery. Neonates may become infected during passage through an infected birth canal. The incidence of perinatal transmission to the infant's pharynx may be as high as 50%. Routine treatment of external genital warts in pregnant women is not required unless they are very large and cause discomfort. In such cases, the warts can be removed using cryotherapy. These warts usually regress following delivery. Unless there are large lesions in the vagina that can bleed or obstruct labour, a cesarean section is not indicated.

■ ABNORMALITIES OF THE VAGINA

Vaginal Atresia

Congenital atresia, most common in the upper one-third of the vagina, is associated with Müllerian duct anomalies. Acquired atresia is secondary to inflammatory lesions, trauma or cicatrisation following vaginal operations. In all cases where there is marked obstruction due to cicatrisation or atresia, a cesarean section would be indicated.

Septate Vagina or Double Vagina

If the septum is vertical and complete and involves the cervical canal and uterus, labour usually progresses normally with one portion of the vagina dilating and the other getting compressed by the passage of the fetus. However, when the septum is transverse, it may form a definite band in front of the presenting part and thus cause obstruction. Delivery is by cesarean section if the septum is thick and high up. Often, a thin septum may be identified in the lower part of the vagina and can be excised easily.

Vaginal Wall Cyst (Gartner Duct Cyst)

A Gartner duct cyst is usually small. In labour, it easily slips above the presenting part and does not cause obstruction.

■ ABNORMALITIES OF THE CERVIX

Cervical Stenosis

This may be due to inflammatory lesions of the cervix or trauma following childbirth, leading to irregular cicatrix formation. Operations on the cervix such as amputation of the cervix also cause the cervix to become rigid. In these cases, if given sufficient time, the cervix dilates normally in labour. Most often, a cervix that was considered hard and rigid becomes soft and dilates easily to reach full dilatation. If cervical dilatation does not occur as expected despite good uterine contractions, a cesarean section should be carried out.

Hypertrophic Elongation of the Cervix

In this condition, there is congenital elongation of the cervix where by the infravaginal portion of the cervix is long and has more muscle tissue. As a result, the cervix is further away from the seminal pool, and conception may be difficult. When conception occurs, management of pregnancy and labour are as usual. However, due to the excessive muscular tissue, the cervix may not dilate; as a result, there may be cervical dystocia.

■ ABNORMALITIES OF THE UTERUS

These include uterine malformations and displacement of the body of the uterus.

Malformations of the Uterus

The female genital tract develops from two Müllerian ducts on either side. Initially, there is fusion of the two Müllerian ducts, which is followed by canaliasation at a later date. Defects in the fusion or subsequent canalisation result in uterine deformities, the severity of which depends on the extent of the defect.

While most congenital uterine anomalies are asymptomatic and associated with normal reproductive outcomes, some may be associated with adverse reproductive outcomes such as recurrent pregnancy loss (RPL), first- and second-trimester pregnancy loss, intrauterine growth restriction, preterm labour and delivery, cervical insufficiency, placental abruption, retained placenta, malpresentation and intrauterine fetal demise. The overall prevalence of congenital uterine anomaly is 5.5% in an unselected population, 8.0% in infertile women and 13.3% in those with a history of miscarriage. The most common uterine malformations are presented in Fig. 46.1.

The American Society of Reproductive Medicine (ASRM) classifies Müllerian anomalies as follows:

• Hypoplasia/agenesis of the uterus

• Unicornuate uterus

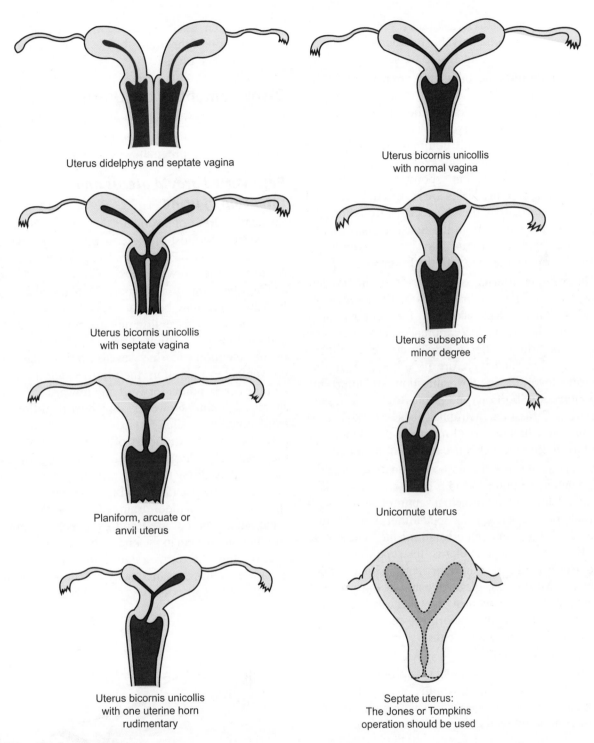

Uterus didelphys and septate vagina

Uterus bicornis unicollis
with normal vagina

Uterus bicornis unicollis
with septate vagina

Uterus subseptus of
minor degree

Planiform, arcuate or
anvil uterus

Unicornute uterus

Uterus bicornis unicollis
with one uterine horn
rudimentary

Septate uterus:
The Jones or Tompkins
operation should be used

Fig. 46.1 Uterine anomalies

- Uterine didelphys
- Bicornuate uterus
- Septate uterus
- Arcuate uterus
- In **hypoplasia/agenesis**, there is no development of the Müllerian ducts.
- The **unicornuate uterus** accounts for approximately 20% of Müllerian duct anomalies. In this type of

malformation, the main body of the uterus and cervix develop from one Müllerian duct only. It is usually associated with varying degrees of a rudimentary uterine horn from the other Müllerian duct. Common obstetric complications include abnormal fetal lie, fetal growth restriction and spontaneous abortions. The cause for spontaneous abortions may be inadequate vascularisation and compromised uteroplacental blood flow to the unicornuate uterus. Occasionally, pregnancy may occur in the rudimentary horn; this is dangerous when it ruptures around 16–20 weeks of gestation.

- **Uterus didelphys** accounts for approximately 5% of Müllerian duct anomalies. It results from nearly complete failure of fusion of the Müllerian ducts. Each Müllerian duct develops into a distinct body and cervix. There is no communication between the duplicated endometrial cavities. Pregnancy may take a normal course but, spontaneous abortions, IUGR and premature births are reported. In some of these cases, menstruation may occur throughout the course of pregnancy from the non-pregnant uterus. The non-pregnant uterus may be mistaken for a tumour or may interfere with the progress of labour.

- A **bicornuate uterus** is the result of incomplete fusion of the uterovaginal horns at the level of the fundus. This defect accounts for approximately 10% of Müllerian duct anomalies. Women who have a bicornuate uterus usually conceive without treatment provided there are no other extrauterine factors involved in the causation of infertility. Spontaneous abortions and premature deliveries are reported. Strassman metroplasty has been advocated in women with a history of recurrent pregnancy loss and in whom no other cause has been identified.

- The **septate uterus** is the most common Müllerian duct anomaly, accounting for 55% of all such anomalies. In this defect, the uterovaginal septum fails to resorb partially or completely. In the septate uterus, the septum extends through the entire length of the endometrial cavity; in the subseptate uterus, the septum is partial and usually confined to the upper portion for a variable distance. Most often, pregnancy and labour progress normally. In some women, however, the condition manifests with recurrent abortions, recurrent breech or retained or adherent placenta.

- In an **arcuate uterus**, the cavity of the uterus is normal, except for a slight depression in the midline over the fundus. This gives the uterus a saddle-shaped or arcuate appearance. The arcuate uterus is most commonly seen in breech presentations.

Surgical interventions for uterine malformations

- In women with uterine didelphys or a unicornuate or bicornuate uterus, there could be associated cervical incompetence. In these women, cervical cerclage is indicated if there is recurrent pregnancy loss due to an incompetent cervix.

- If the recurrent pregnancy loss is due to uterine anomalies, necessary surgical procedures may be

undertaken such as excision of the septum and unification of the uterus by the Strassman surgery in a bicornuate uterus.

Displacement of the Uterus

Retroverted uterus, anterior displacement of the uterus and prolapse of uterus are conditions that can cause problems during pregnancy and labour.

Retroverted gravid uterus and retention of urine

In nearly 20% of women, the uterus is normally retroverted. In most of these women, retroversion gets corrected by the 12th week of pregnancy (Fig. 46.2). As the uterus grows, the cervix is pushed forward against the symphysis, compressing the bladder neck. Initially, there may be frequency of micturition; later, the woman may have difficulty in emptying the bladder and eventually, retention of urine can occur. As a result of the retention of urine, severe cystitis may develop. On vaginal examination, the uterus is felt in the POD, and the cervix points forward and upwards towards the symphysis pubis. However, this must be differentiated from conditions such as extrauterine gestation with pelvic hematocele, tumours of the ovary or a fibroid in the posterior wall of the uterus. The diagnosis can be confirmed by USG. The management involves emptying the bladder by a catheter with all aseptic precautions and continuous bladder drainage for 24–48 hours. The urine should be cultured and examined for pus cells. Nursing the woman in the knee–chest position may help in correcting the retroversion. If retroversion persists, it can be corrected manually or under anesthesia. Insertion of a soft pessary is also helpful.

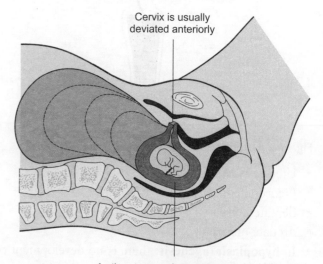

Cervix is usually deviated anteriorly

As the uterus enlarges, a posterior sacculation remains

Fig. 46.2 Retroverted gravid uterus

Sacculation

On very rare occasions, a retroverted gravid uterus may become incarcerated in the hollow of the sacrum. The possible risk factors for this incarceration include uterine fibroids, uterine malformation and pelvic adhesions caused by abdominal surgery or endometriosis. As the uterus is retroverted, the cervix becomes displaced above the symphysis pubis. As the fundus of the uterus is incarcerated, it cannot enlarge further. Therefore, in order to accommodate the growing fetus, the lower part of the anterior uterine wall begins to thin out, and balloons into the upper abdomen. This is called sacculation. Along with the anterior wall of the uterus, both the bladder and the cervix are also pulled up into the abdominal cavity toward the umbilicus. Uterine sacculation can be asymptomatic. It is difficult to diagnose sacculation antenatally owing to its rarity and non-specific symptoms such as abdominal pain, constipation, urgency and urinary retention. Complications associated with sacculation include intrauterine death, uterine rupture, adherent retained placenta and postpartum hemorrhage. Pregnancy may proceed to term, and if the sacculation is marked, vaginal delivery is not possible. When labour begins, the contractions of the uterus do not result in the dilatation of the cervix. As a result, labour is prolonged and can result in rupture uterus.

Anterior (forward) displacement of the gravid uterus

Very rarely, when the uterus is enlarging in size, the anteversion becomes extreme and the uterus is displaced forward, through the abdominal wall, resulting in a pendulous abdomen. This is seen in multiparous women who have a weak abdominal wall. The displacement may also be encountered in women who have a contracted pelvis, particularly in those with kyphosis, lordosis or spondylolisthesis. With repeated pregnancies, the abdominal wall becomes flaccid, and the muscles atrophy, facilitating the anteversion of the uterus. Divarication of the recti may also contribute to the forward displacement of the uterus.

Common symptoms include an abnormal sensation of heaviness and general abdominal discomfort. Pressure and pulling on the bladder may result in frequent micturition. There may also be dragging pains in the loins and difficulty in movements. During labour, severe dystocia may arise. The forward displacement results in the cervix being pushed back towards the hollow of the sacrum; occasionally, it may even be above the level of the sacral promontory. In such cases, the force of the uterine contractions is directed posteriorly and not along the axis of the birth canal. The presenting part is displaced posteriorly, and engagement of the head in the brim of the pelvis does not occur. Malpresentations are therefore frequent. Labour is usually prolonged. During labour, the woman should be kept in the recumbent dorsal posture. Once the head engages in the brim of the pelvis, labour pains usually proceed in a more orderly manner.

Downward displacement (prolapse) of the gravid uterus

- When prolapse of the first- or second-degree complicate pregnancy, spontaneous rectification usually occurs as the uterus rises above the pelvic brim, dragging the prolapsed hypertrophied cervix with it. In the majority of cases, pregnancy and labour proceed normally and complications are uncommon.

- When the prolapse is of a major degree (third-degree or procidentia), urinary complications like frequency, urinary infection and retention are common because of the cystocele. As the pregnancy continues, the prolapsed cervix may recede to a certain extent into the vagina. In some, it remains outside the vulval outlet and becomes ulcerated and infected. When this happens, the woman should be advised bed rest with the foot end of the bed raised. The infected cervix should be kept in position by a sterile vaginal pack which should be changed twice a day. No attempt at replacement of the cervix should be made if there is gross edema and infection. Once the edema subsides and the infection clears, the cervix should be replaced in the vagina with a ring pessary. As pregnancy advances, the enlarged uterus enters the abdominal cavity, and the prolapsed cervix gradually recedes into the vagina. If a pessary is inserted, it should be removed around 36 weeks of gestation. The size of the pessary may vary as the pregnancy progresses.

- During labour, the woman should be confined to bed and if the prolapse is outside the vagina, it should be covered with gauze soaked in glycerine–magnesium sulphate. Adequate time should be given for the dilatation of the cervix. In rare cases, a cesarean section may become necessary if the cervix is edematous and does not dilate. More often, the woman is able to deliver vaginally.

- In women who have undergone a Fothergill operation for a prolapsed uterus, due to the scarring of the cervix, there may be failure to dilate or slow dilatation; cervical tears may occur during delivery. If this complication is anticipated, it is better to resort to cesarean section. If labour is progressing well, second-stage straining should be avoided to prevent recurrent prolapse. Unyielding perineum following perineorrhaphy can be dealt with by performing an episiotomy.

- An isolated cystocele or rectocele may be seen in multiparous women. These women may present with recurrent urinary infection or difficulty in emptying the bladder during the antenatal period. During labour, a large cystocele or rectocele may sometimes cause dystocia. In the second stage of labour, the cystocele may have to be lifted to allow the descent of the head. If forceps application is required, care should be taken to protect the bladder.

Torsion of the Gravid Uterus

This is a dangerous (but fortunately rare) complication. The signs and symptoms are the same as those of acute abdomen—the woman presents with shock, intense pain and tenderness over the uterus. The fetal heart is most often absent, depending upon the degree of torsion. It is difficult to differentiate this condition from concealed accidental hemorrhage. The diagnosis is made only at laparotomy. If there is complete torsion, the diagnosis is very often made only after delivering the baby, at which time, the obstetrician will be surprised to see the incision on the posterior wall of the uterus. Antepartum diagnosis may be improved by MRI—the vagina, which is normally seen as an H-shaped structure, appears X-shaped because of torsion. After delivering the baby, the torsion of the uterus is corrected. If there is significant damage to the uterus and adnexa, a hysterectomy may have to be performed, with or without the removal of the adnexa.

KEY POINTS

✓ A number of soft tissue abnormalities of the genital tract could lead to difficulties during pregnancy and labour.

✓ Female genital mutilation can result in adverse obstetric outcomes.

✓ The commonest congenital malformation of the uterus is a septate uterus.

✓ A retroverted uterus can lead to retention of urine and incarceration of the uterus leading to sacculation.

✓ There is no indication for cesarean section unless genital warts are large and likely to bleed and obstruct labour.

✓ Major degrees of prolapse complicating pregnancy are treated with a pessary.

✓ Torsion of the gravid uterus is an acute emergency.

Essay questions

1. Describe the different uterine anomalies and enumerate the pregnancy complications that may be encountered in women with these anomalies.
2. Discuss female genital mutilation and its obstetric complications.
3. What are the clinical manifestations of a retroverted gravid uterus and how are they managed?
4. How will you manage a case of uterine prolapse complicating pregnancy?

Short answer questions

1. What is a bicornuate uterus?
2. Describe incarceration of the uterus.
3. Write a short note on torsion of the gravid uterus.

MCQs

1. What is the most common uterine anomaly associated with recurrent breech presentation?
   a) Uterus didelphys
   b) Septate uterus
   c) Uterus bicornis unicollis
   d) Uterus bicornis bicollis
2. Septate uterus may be associated with all the following complications in pregnancy EXCEPT:
   a) Recurrent abortions
   b) Malpresentations
   c) Retained placenta
   d) Abruption of the placenta
3. A retroverted gravid uterus usually undergoes spontaneous correction by:
   a) 12 weeks
   b) 20 weeks
   c) 28 weeks
   d) 32 weeks
4. The malformation in which there are two separate uterine cavities, each communicating with its own cervical and vaginal canal is known as:
   a) Uterus didelphys
   b) Arcuate uterus
   c) Bicornuate uterus
   d) Septate uterus
5. What is the most common malformation of the female genital tract?
   a) Cervical stenosis
   b) Imperforate hymen
   c) Vaginal atresia
   d) Septate uterus
6. Which of the following complications is not associated with Müllerian anomalies?
   a) Malpresentation
   b) Abortion
   c) Postpartum hemorrhage
   d) Polyhydramnios

7.   In which of the following conditions are recurrent abortions common?
  a)   Cervical atresia
  b)   Arcuate uterus
  c)   Bicornuate uterus
  d)   Vaginal atresia

8.   In which of the following conditions is cervical cerclage not indicated?
  a)   Uterine didelphys
  b)   Arcuate uterus
  c)   Unicornuate uterus
  d)   Bicornuate uterus

9.   Metroplasty performed on an anomalous uterus to improve pregnancy outcomes is called:
  a)   Shirodkar procedure
  b)   McDonald procedure
  c)   Strassman procedure
  d)   Vechietti procedure

Answers
1. (b),   2. (d),   3. (a),   4. (a),   5. (d),   6. (d),   7. (c),   8. (b),   9. (c)

Fill in the blanks

1.   A condition in which there are two complete uteri, each with a distinct body and cervix is known as _____.

2.   A common complication of a retroverted gravid uterus is _____.

Answers
1. uterus didelphys,   2. retention of urine

Case scenario-based discussion

1.   A 22-year-old primigravida is admitted at 10 weeks of gestation with acute retention of urine.
  a)   What is the immediate management?
  b)   What is the further course of management if retroversion is diagnosed?
  c)   What investigations should be ordered?
  d)   What risks are expected if the uterus remains in the pelvis at 14 weeks of gestation?

Answers
a) The bladder should be catheterised and vaginal examination should be performed to diagnose a retroverted uterus.
b) Continuous bladder drainage should be done for 24–48 hours, the woman should be nursed in the knee–chest position and retroversion should be corrected either manually or with a pessary.
c) A urine sample should be collected for culture and USG pelvis should be carried out to diagnose posterior fibroids/endometriomas.
d) Sacculation of the uterus may occur if the uterus remains in the pelvis at 14 weeks of gestation.

Complications of the Third Stage of Labour

Learning Objectives

» To know the causes of postpartum hemorrhage (PPH) and its prevention
» To discuss the diagnosis and management of atonic PPH
» To know the resuscitative measures and use of blood and blood products in PPH
» To know the causes of secondary postpartum hemorrhage
» To discuss the management of retained placenta
» To understand the causes, prevention and management of acute inversion of the uterus
» To know the causes of postpartum collapse

The complications encountered in the third stage of labour are as follows:

1. Postpartum hemorrhage
2. Retained placenta
3. Uterine inversion
4. Postpartum collapse

POSTPARTUM HEMORRHAGE

DEFINITION

- Postpartum hemorrhage (PPH) is defined as blood loss of more than 500 mL after vaginal delivery and more than 1000 mL after cesarean section (WHO).
- A 10% decrease in hematocrit level as compared to the prelabour values is also defined as PPH (ACOG). This is a retrospective definition and is useful for research purposes.
- A small blood loss that makes the woman hemodynamically unstable is also termed PPH because women who have anemia, cardiac disease or contracted blood volume states such as pre-eclampsia or dehydration do not tolerate even a minimal blood loss.

INCIDENCE

- Every year, about 14 million women around the world suffer from PPH; 25% of all maternal deaths are due to PPH (WHO).
- In India, PPH accounts for 38% of all maternal deaths (Sample Registration Scheme [SRS], 2001–2003). PPH occurs in 2–4% of mothers after vaginal delivery and 6% after cesarean section.

CLASSIFICATION OF PPH

PPH can be classified according to the time of its occurrence and the amount of blood loss.

- According to the time of occurrence, PPH is classified into:
  — **Primary PPH**, in which PPH occurs within 24 hours of the delivery of the baby
  — **Secondary PPH**, wherein hemorrhage occurs 24 hours after delivery, but within 6 weeks postpartum
- According to the amount of blood loss, PPH is classified as presented in Table 47.1.

Table 47.1 Categorisation of PPH based on the amount of blood loss

Severity	Volume of blood loss (mL)
Minor	500–1,000
Moderate	1,000–2,000
Severe	>2,000
Life-threatening	>2,500
Major PPH: Blood loss >1,000 mL and/or blood loss in an unstable patient irrespective of the amount of blood loss	

Though PPH can be classified based on the amount of blood loss, it is very difficult to accurately estimate blood loss as it is subjective. Most often, the blood loss is underestimated as the hemorrhage may be concealed within the uterine cavity or as a hematoma. A persistent small trickle of blood loss may also go unnoticed.

ETIOLOGY OF PPH

The chief causes of primary postpartum hemorrhage are grouped as follows and can be represented as the 4 'T's as presented in Table 47.2:

1. Uterine atony (tone)—accounts for >70% of cases
2. Genital tract trauma (trauma)
3. Retained placental fragments (tissue)
4. Coagulation disorders (thrombus)

Table 47.2   Causes of primary postpartum hemorrhage

Mechanism of blood loss	Causes
Tone	Atonicity of the uterus due to: • Overdistension of the uterus as in multiple pregnancy, polyhydramnios or due to a large baby • Uterine exhaustion due to high parity, prolonged labour, chorioamnionitis, abruption placenta, fibroid complicating pregnancy or the use of anesthetic agents • Previous PPH
Trauma	Due to scar rupture following previous cesarean section, uterine rupture following obstructed labour, cervical and vaginal tears following instrumental delivery, extension of episiotomy and hematoma, broad ligament hematoma or forniceal tear (colporrhexis)
Tissue	Retained placental tissue and membranes
Thrombus	Coagulation failure following APH, pre-eclampsia, IUFD, amniotic fluid embolism

ATONIC POSTPARTUM HEMORRHAGE

During the normal process of the third stage of labour, the separation, descent and expulsion of the placenta are not associated with heavy bleeding. This is because the contraction and retraction of the uterus result in the shortening of the myometrial fibres and occlusion of the vessels, thereby minimising blood loss. This is known as the **'living ligature'** of the uterus.

Atonic hemorrhage is a placental site hemorrhage caused by any factor that prevents proper contraction and retraction of the uterus. The factors that predispose to atonic hemorrhage are as follows:

• Multiparity
• Overdistension of the uterus in polyhydramnios, macrosomia and multiple pregnancy
• Injudicious induction and augmentation of labour, especially with oxytocin
• Fibroids of the uterus that interfere with proper contraction and retraction of the uterus
• Anemia
• Antepartum hemorrhage
• Prolonged labour leading to uterine exhaustion
• Precipitate labour
• Use of halogenated anesthetics like isoflurane or enflurane or heavy sedation in labour which interferes with proper contraction and retraction of the uterus
• Use of agents that inhibit calcium entry into the cells like magnesium sulphate and nifedipine, which are used in hypertensive disorders of pregnancy
• Previous history of PPH

> Though there are a number of predisposing factors for atonic PPH, it occurs most often in low-risk deliveries.

Causes of atonic PPH
• *Maternal factors*
  — Multiparity
  — Previous history of PPH
  — Fibroids complicating pregnancy
  — Maternal anemia
• *Pregnancy complications*
  — Antepartum hemorrhage
  — Overdistension of the uterus as in multiple pregnancy, hydramnios or macrosomia
• *Labour complications*
  — Prolonged labour
  — Induction of labour
  — Precipitate labour
• *Effect of drugs*
  — Anesthetic drugs
  — Magnesium sulphate
  — Nifedipine

Prevention of PPH

Every attempt must be made to prevent postpartum hemorrhage. Good antenatal and intranatal care help to reduce the incidence of postpartum hemorrhage considerably. This includes the following measures:

• In the antenatal period, the woman's general nutrition should be improved, and any persisting anemia should be properly treated.

- All pregnant women must have their blood group determined. For those in whom PPH is anticipated, compatible blood should be made available at the time of delivery.
- Whenever risk factors for PPH are identified, the woman should be advised to have the delivery in a hospital where facilities for blood transfusion and specialists are available.
- Active management of the third stage of labour (AMTSL) should be practised (WHO, 2012). This comprises the following:
  — Administration of inj. oxytocin 10 units IM immediately after the delivery of the baby (within 1 minute)
  — Delay clamping the cord for at least 1–3 minutes to reduce the risk of infant anemia (early cord clamping is no longer recommended)
  — Controlled cord traction by Brandt–Andrews technique
  — Postpartum vigilance—the uterine tone should be immediately assessed to ensure a contracted uterus; thereafter, it should be checked every 15 minutes for 2 hours; if there is uterine atony, a fundal massage should be performed, and the woman should be monitored more frequently

It has been estimated that routine use of AMTSL reduces the chances of PPH by nearly 60%.

Third stage management is discussed in detail in Chapter 14, *Conduct of normal labour*.

Clinical Features

Depending on the woman's general condition and the amount of blood loss, the clinical features of PPH vary. The amount of bleeding may range from a slow trickle to heavy bleeding. Occasionally, bleeding may not be evident externally and may collect inside the uterus instead. The earliest clinical signs of blood loss are increased pulse rate, dizziness and evidence of pallor followed by a drop in blood pressure. If the bleeding continues, the woman usually becomes restless, anxious, complains of thirst; there is sweating, air hunger and shallow respiration and death may supervene if timely and appropriate intervention is not provided (Table 47.3). Along with these features, the uterus will be flabby, soft and enlarged, often reaching above the umbilicus.

Table 47.3 Clinical findings in relation to the amount of blood loss

Class	Amount of blood loss (mL)	Percentage of blood loss	Clinical picture
I	500–1,000	15%	There are no signs and symptoms; occasionally, there may be dizziness The woman is in a compensated state
II—mild	1,000–1,500	20–25%	The woman presents with tachycardia, hypotension and increased respiratory rate
III—moderate	1,500–2,000	25–35%	There is overt hypotension, severe tachycardia, tachypnea with cold, clammy skin, restlessness and oliguria
IV—severe	>2,000	40%	The patient is in profound shock with ↑ pulse, ↓ B.P, air hunger, renal failure. This is a massive obstetric hemorrhage requiring urgent volume replacement

(*Source: Benedetti's classification of acute blood loss according to volume deficit*)

Occult shock can be diagnosed using the shock index (SI), which is calculated by the following equation.

$$SI = \text{Heart rate} \div \text{Systolic BP (mmHg)}$$

The normal shock index is 0.5–0.7. Higher values are more sensitive in the detection of occult shock than either vital sign in isolation.

Diagnosis of PPH

In the management of PPH, it is necessary to differentiate atonic postpartum hemorrhage from traumatic PPH (Table 47.4).

- In atonic PPH, the uterus is flabby and large. It may be felt above the level of the umbilicus. On examination, there may not be any evidence of injury.

- In traumatic PPH, the uterus is well-contracted and hard in consistency. There is fresh bleeding from the genital tract and evidence of genital tract injuries.

Table 47.4 Differences between atonic and traumatic PPH

Atonic PPH	Traumatic PPH
Uterus is flabby and large	Uterus is contracted and appropriate for postpartum stage
Blood is dark	Fresh and bright red blood
No lacerations or injuries can be found	Speculum examination will reveal lacerations, tears or other injuries to the genital tract

At times, atonic and traumatic PPH may co-exist.

Management of PPH

The objectives of treatment are to:

1. Correct hypovolemia and maintain circulatory volume by timely replacement of IV fluids, blood and components
2. Correct atonicity and control the bleeding either by medical or surgical methods

In the management of PPH, resuscitation, stabilisation and identification of a potential cause and its treatment should take place simultaneously. The '**golden hour**' should be kept in mind during management—if the woman is not effectively resuscitated and treated in the first hour, the chance of survival decreases. While resuscitating, the principles of basic and advanced life support should be followed. Senior staff and multi-disciplinary teams should be involved in the management. One should call for help as the management of PPH requires more assistance.

Resuscitation

- At least two large-bore intravenous cannulae, preferably 16 gauge, should be inserted.
- Blood should be drawn for cross-matching and the estimation of hemoglobin, packed cell volume, coagulation profile, baseline urea and electrolytes.
- Fluid replacement should be commenced immediately. Crystalloid solutions such as 0.9% saline should be infused rapidly at the rate of 500 mL in 15 minutes to restore systolic blood pressure.
- The bladder should be catheterised, and a strict input–output record should be maintained.
- Pulse, BP, respiration and other vitals should be checked.
- The woman should be kept warm.
- Oxygen should be administered by a face mask at the rate of 8–10 litres/minute.

- Even if the woman is not in shock, her condition may worsen rapidly.
- Blood transfusion should be started as soon as possible, ideally within 30 minutes. Adequate quantities of blood should be replaced (the blood loss should not be underestimated). Most cases require 1–2 units of red blood cells initially, which will increase the hematocrit by 3–4 % for each unit transfused. Further transfusion may be required if there is ongoing bleeding or if the initial loss is heavy. Fresh frozen plasma (FFP) is indicated to correct clotting deficiencies related to a large amount of hemorrhage or a large amount of transfusion. Cryoprecipitate can be given when the fibrinogen levels are very low and when there is active oozing. This is particularly useful when volume overload is the concern.

Identifying the potential causes

- The uterus should be palpated for tone. The position of the uterus should be determined, and the woman should be examined to look for cervical and vaginal tears.
- A flabby, enlarged uterus is indicative of atonic PPH.
- If the fundus is not palpable per abdomen or the shock is disproportionate to the blood loss, inversion should be suspected.
- If the uterus is not in the midline and displaced to one side, broad ligament hematoma should be suspected.

Control of bleeding

Medical methods

Oxytocic drugs (Table 47.5) are given in a stepwise and quick progression.

- When the uterus is atonic, 20 units of inj. oxytocin in 500 mL of NS or RL should be started and run at the rate of 60 drops per minute (dpm), titrated according to the response (first-line management). Infusion pumps are the preferred method of delivery.
- Care should be taken to avoid fluid overload as oxytocin can cause water retention.
- If bleeding is controlled, oxytocin infusion with 10 units in 500 mL of fluid at a rate of 20 dpm should be maintained.
- Uterine massage should be performed to expel blood and blood clots from the uterus.
- The placenta should be re-examined to confirm whether all the placental lobes and membranes have been expelled.
- If there is no response to oxytocin infusion or if oxytocin is not available, inj. methylergometrine

0.2 mg can be given intravenously. This drug should be avoided in cases of maternal heart disease or hypertension. In other cases, this drug can be repeated for up to four doses (second-line management).

- If bleeding continues, inj. prostaglandin PGF$_2\alpha$ can be given in a dose of 250 µg IM and can be repeated for up to eight doses (third-line management). Prostaglandin should be used with caution in asthmatic patients. Its side effects include vomiting, diarrhea, fever and tachycardia.

- If oxytocin, ergometrine and prostaglandins are not available, then 600–800 µg of misoprostol can be given rectally.

- Oxytocin stimulates the upper segment of the myometrium to contract rhythmically.
- Methyl ergometrine is an ergot alkaloid that causes generalised smooth muscle contraction in the upper and lower segments of the uterus.
- Prostaglandin enhances uterine contractility and causes vasoconstriction.

Table 47.5 Oxytocic drugs used in PPH

Drugs	Oxytocin	Methylergometrine	PGF$_2\alpha$
Dose	20 units of inj. oxytocin in 500 mL of NS or RL run at 60 dpm minute	0.2 mg given intravenously (should be avoided in hypertensive and cardiac patients)	250 µg IM
Maintenance dose	10 units in 500 mL of NS run at 20 dpm	If necessary, it can be repeated every 4 hours IM or IV	Can be repeated every 15 minutes
Maximum dose		4 doses	8 doses

Intravenous tranexamic acid

In recent years, tranexamic acid has been recommended by slow IV bolus of 1 g, followed by another 1 g four hours later (WHO).

Uterine and aortic compression

While oxytocic medications are being used, other measures such as bimanual compression of the uterus and compression of the abdominal aorta should also be undertaken to reduce blood loss. Bimanual compression of the uterus has been a very successful life-saving technique to reduce the amount of bleeding.

Bimanual compression of the uterus (Fig. 47.1)

- After donning sterile gloves, a hand is inserted into the vagina to remove any blood clots from the lower part of the uterus or cervix.
- The hand is closed into a fist and inserted into the anterior fornix. The fist is then used to apply pressure on the anterior wall of the uterus.
- The other hand is used to press deeply into the abdomen behind the uterus and apply pressure against the posterior wall of the uterus.
- Compression should be maintained until bleeding is controlled and the uterus contracts and becomes hard.
- Care must be taken to avoid aggressive massage as this can injure the large vessels of the broad ligament.

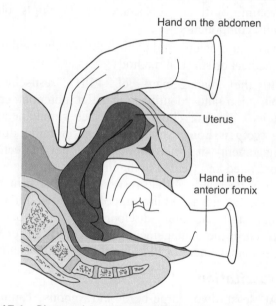

Hand on the abdomen

Uterus

Hand in the anterior fornix

Fig. 47.1 Bimanual compression of the uterus

Manual aortic compression

- Another method that has been used in emergencies for the control of PPH is the compression of the abdominal aorta.
- Direct pressure is applied to the aorta with the fist just above and to the left of the umbilicus (Fig. 47.2). The abdominal aorta is compressed against the vertebrae a few centimetres superior to the sacral promontory. The bifurcation into the common iliac arteries is just distal to this point.
- The femoral pulse is palpated. Successful aortic compression is defined as the absence of a femoral pulse and unrecordable blood pressure in a lower limb.
- An external aortic compression device is also available.

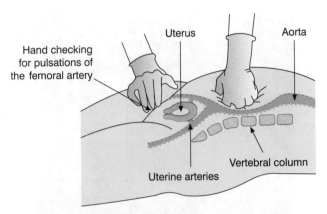

Fig. 47.2   Manual aortic compression

Persistence of bleeding despite medical measures

If bleeding persists despite medical measures, the diagnosis should be reviewed.

- The placenta should be examined again. Even if it appears appropriate, an ultrasound of the uterus can be performed to ensure that no placental tissue is retained in the uterus and causing bleeding.
- If the bleeding persists, trauma to the genital tract should be ruled out. To do this, the woman should be examined under good light and under anesthesia. If tears of the cervix or vagina are found, they must be sutured.
- The coagulation profile should also be reviewed.

If bleeding persists due to an atonic uterus after the above conditions are ruled out, the management options are as presented in the box below.

Management options for unresponsive hemorrhage due to atonic PPH

Conservative
- Tamponade techniques—gauze, balloons, condom, gloves

Conservative surgical techniques
- Vessel ligation—uterine, ovarian, internal iliac
- Uterine vertical full-thickness sutures
  — Compression suture (B-Lynch, 1997)
  — Modified B-Lynch (Hayman, 2002)
- Uterine horizontal full-thickness sutures
  — Square suture
  — Figure-of-eight stitch
  — Combination of sutures
  — Uterine artery embolisation
  — Hysterectomy

Tamponade techniques

Various techniques are used to compress the bleeding vessels and occlude the bleeding surface of the uterus:

- Sengstaken–Blakemore tube
- A large Foley's catheter
- Rüsch urologic hydrostatic balloon
- SOS Bakri tamponade balloon
- Condom

The most commonly used of these are the Foley's catheter (Fig. 47.3) and condoms.

- 2–3 Foley's catheters are inserted into the uterine cavity, and the individual Foley's bulbs are distended with 60–80 mL of saline. Depending on the response, these can be left in situ for up to 24 hours.
- A saline drip is connected to a condom and is inserted into the uterine cavity. The condom is distended with 100 mL of saline and kept distended.
- Whenever a tamponade technique is used, there should be counterpressure from the uterus. This is achieved by starting a 20-unit oxytocin drip and running it at a speed that is enough to establish effective uterine contractions.

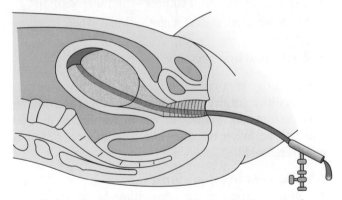

Fig. 47.3   Use of Foley's catheter for uterine tamponade

Tamponade with uterine packing
- Under anesthesia, a long, sterile roll of gauze tape is used to pack the uterus tightly from the fundus downwards.
- The end of the tape is brought out through the vagina and left there for 24 hours.
- This method may be useful in cases where laparotomy cannot be performed, in cases of PPH in jaundice and DIVC.

Uterine vacuum retraction system

It is a relatively new method that works on the principle that by creating a vacuum, the uterine walls can be brought closer to each other. This assists in the natural process of contraction and retraction of the uterus, and thereby, the closing of the vessels. A uterine vacuum retraction cannula is inserted into the uterine cavity to create negative pressure (Fig. 47.4).

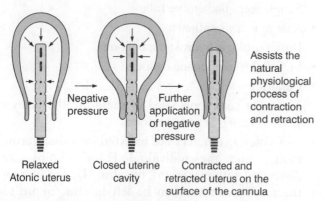

Fig. 47.4 Uterine vacuum cannula

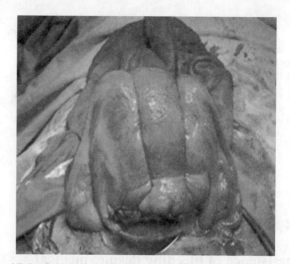

Fig. 47.5 B-Lynch brace suture on the uterus

If bleeding does not stop despite treatment using uterotonics and other available conservative interventions (e.g., uterine massage, balloon tamponade), the use of surgical interventions is recommended.

Surgical methods
- Uterine compression sutures—first intervention
- Stepwise uterine devascularisation—when bleeding continues
- Peripartum hysterectomy

Conservative surgical techniques
Conservative surgical procedures are aimed at avoiding hysterectomy in women in whom fertility is desired and can be taken up when the woman's condition is relatively stable.

Uterine compression sutures
- The objective of this procedure is to effectively compress the myometrium to reduce the bleeding.
- The B-Lynch brace suture (Fig. 47.5) was the earliest method devised to achieve this.
- Currently, a number of techniques such as the Cho suture (multiple, square sutures) are available.
- These procedures result in good hemostasis without grave complications and also preserve future fertility in most women.
- Delayed complications such as uterine necrosis, pyometra and uterine synechiae can occur, more often with Cho sutures.

Stepwise devascularisation of the uterus
- Stepwise devascularisation of the uterus is a procedure in which the vessels supplying the uterus are ligated step-by-step to reduce the blood flow to the uterus.

- In this technique, the uterine artery, uterine–ovarian anastomosis and descending cervical branch of the uterine artery are ligated successively on one side and then on the other. If there is no response, internal iliac artery ligation can be done on one or both sides. This results in an 85% reduction in the pulse pressure and promotes hemostasis and clot formation.

Uterine artery embolisation
- Angiographic embolisation is sometimes carried out.
- However, in the face of acute hemorrhage it is logistically challenging and not always possible or available in most places.
- The anterior division of the internal iliac artery is accessed via a femoral artery approach and gelatin particles are injected into the vessels to occlude them.
- Resuscitative endovascular balloon occlusion of the aorta (REBOA) has recently been attempted to temporarily occlude the aorta.

Hysterectomy
- Hysterectomy is the definitive treatment. It should be performed when bleeding is not controlled quickly with other measures and if the blood loss is >2,000 mL.
- Peripartum hysterectomy is indicated in persistent atonic PPH, rupture uterus, when repair is not possible, and when there is abnormal placentation with placenta increta, accreta or percreta.
- Subtotal hysterectomy is the procedure of choice unless there is trauma to the cervix or lower uterine segment or PPH in cases of placenta previa.
- It is a life-saving measure and should be performed without hesitation irrespective of parity. It should not be put off until the woman is moribund.

PPH with placenta in situ

If the bleeding starts with the placenta in utero, the fundus of the uterus must be grasped and massaged to make it contract. If the placenta shows signs of separation, it must be expressed by the commonly used **Brandt–Andrews technique**. When there is no evidence of placental separation, it should be considered to be a retained placenta and should be removed as explained in the section on retained and adherent placenta.

PPH during cesarean delivery

If hemorrhage is experienced during cesarean delivery, the uterus is compressed and uterotonic agents are administered. If bleeding persists after these measures, the uterus is taken out, compressed manually and flexed caudally; if the bleeding stops, there is a good chance of controlling the bleeding with uterine sutures (compression test). The angles should be identified, and hemostasis should be achieved as soon as possible. If the bleeding is still persistent, the other manoeuvres explained earlier should be attempted. It is always tempting for the obstetrician to proceed to a hysterectomy as the abdomen is already opened. It is important for the obstetrician to weigh the benefits against the possible risks quickly as decision-making has to be swift in cases of PPH.

Assessment of blood loss

Though the assessment of blood loss is mostly visual and not accurate, there are certain simple techniques that can be used for assessing blood loss. One such method is the use of a blood drape, which consists of a conical plastic sheath sutured over another broad plastic sheath (Fig. 47.6). This drape is placed under the woman's

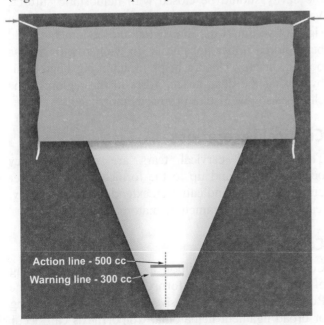

Action line - 500 cc
Warning line - 300 cc

Fig. 47.6   Blood drape

buttocks after the placenta is delivered. The blood lost from the uterine cavity collects in the conical bag. The markings in the bag indicate the volume of blood loss. One should remember that the necessity for adequate and timely blood transfusion is most important.

Transporting the patient

If the woman needs to be transported to another centre, to combat shock, a non-pneumatic anti-shock garment (NASG) can be used (Fig. 47.7). It should, however, be clearly understood that NASG is only a temporary method to prevent shock and is not a treatment for PPH. The NASG acts by shunting the blood accumulating in the lower extremities back to the vital organs including the brain, heart and lungs.

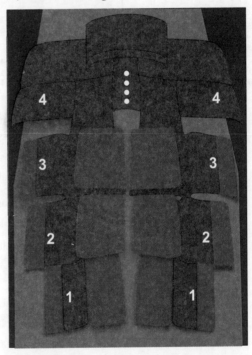

Fig. 47.7   NASG—the compression bands should be applied from below upwards in the order shown in the figure

Monitoring of the Patient Following PPH

- Continue monitoring.
- Review fluid balance, electrolytes and coagulation status.
- Continue oxytocin infusion for another 12 hours.
- Administer antibiotics.
- Check hematocrit after 24 hours.
- Administer hematinics at discharge.
- Advise woman to report if there is further bleeding.
- Secondary PPH can also occur in these women and should be looked for.

Fig. 47.8 is an algorithm for the management of PPH.

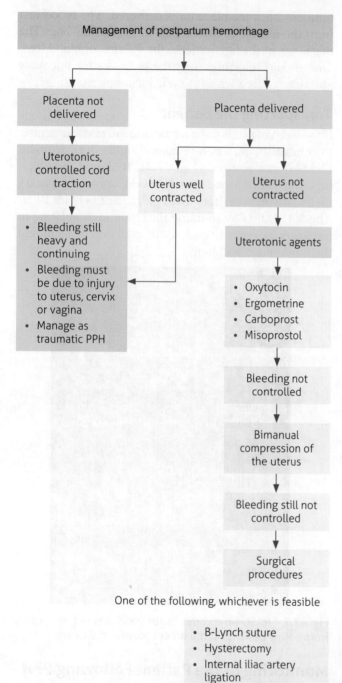

Fig. 47.8 Management of PPH

Complications of PPH

- Hypovolemic shock and renal failure
- Multiorgan failure
- Infections
- Venous thromboembolism
- Occult myocardial ischemia
- Transfusion-related problems
- Dilutional coagulopathy
- Anemia, fatigue, orthostatic hypotension
- Postpartum anemia, which increases the risk of postpartum depression
- Postpartum pituitary necrosis (Sheehan's syndrome)
- Maternal death

▌ TRAUMATIC POSTPARTUM HEMORRHAGE

(All the conditions listed here are discussed in detail in Chapter 48, *Injury to the Parturient Canal*.)

In the event of brisk hemorrhage following an operative delivery or continued bleeding despite the uterus being contracted, genital tract injuries should be suspected. It is critical to recognise these injuries early as they are usually associated with brisk bleeding, which can quickly lead to decompensation and shock.

Vaginal Hematomas

Vaginal lacerations, extension of episiotomies, and forceps application can lead to vaginal hematomas due to injury to the vaginal and pudendal arteries. Small hematomas usually do not expand and often result in tamponade. Large and enlarging hematomas, on the other hand, should be explored and the bleeding vessel should be identified. If the vessel cannot be identified, the cavity should be closed with hemostatic sutures. Vaginal packing is mandatory. When there are persistent signs of volume loss, the vagina and abdomen should be explored under anesthesia. In women with diffuse oozing, layered closure helps in achieving hemostasis by closing the dead space. Tears in the region of the clitoris also give rise to profuse hemorrhage.

Cervical Lacerations

Though small cervical tears are common, they occasionally extend up to the fornices and the lower uterine segment and can even extend retroperitoneally, leading to broad ligament hematoma.

Colporrhexis

Colporrhexis is a condition in which there is tearing of the posterior vaginal fornix which extends into the POD. It can cause extensive intraperitoneal bleeding or broad ligament hematoma. Colporrhexis can occur spontaneously or as an extension of a cervical tear. The tear cannot be repaired from below and usually requires a hysterectomy with subsequent vaginal repair of the tear.

Uterine Rupture

Uterine rupture is rare in an unscarred uterus. However, significant uterine rupture occurs following vaginal delivery in women who have had a previous cesarean section—it occurs in 0.6–0.7% of cases of low transverse incision. The risk increases significantly following a classical cesarean section, uterine surgeries or multiple cesarean deliveries. Compared to spontaneous labour, induction or augmentation will increase the risk of traumatic PPH. Misoprostol should not be used for cervical ripening when attempting vaginal birth after a previous cesarean delivery. Before delivery, the primary sign of uterine rupture is fetal bradycardia. Fetal tachycardia and decelerations may also indicate uterine rupture. Other signs are vaginal bleeding, abdominal tenderness, maternal tachycardia and circulatory collapse.

■ PPH DUE TO COAGULATION FAILURE

Coagulation disorders are rare causes of PPH. Such cases do not respond to conventional management. Most coagulopathies are identified before delivery. DIVC can develop following severe pre-eclampsia, eclampsia, amniotic fluid embolism (AFE), abruption, prolonged fetal demise or HELLP syndrome. A coagulation defect should be suspected in women who have not responded to the usual measures used for treating PPH, those who are not forming clots and those who are oozing from puncture sites. Rapid infusion of fluids can also result in dilutional coagulopathy. In the event of a massive transfusion, if the components are not replaced adequately, clotting failure can occur. Conditions such as von Willebrand disease and idiopathic thrombocytopenic purpura can also present with PPH.

■ SECONDARY POSTPARTUM HEMORRHAGE

Definition

Any heavy bleeding from the genital tract occurring from 24 hours after delivery to 6 weeks postpartum is defined as secondary postpartum hemorrhage.

Etiology

Secondary PPH usually occurs due to the retention of portions of the placenta or membranes, which may be infected. Rarely, submucous fibroids and choriocarcinoma can present with secondary PPH. Following a cesarean section, when there is brisk, fresh bleeding around the 7–10th day, scar dehiscence following infection should be suspected. Infection can also erode the vessels to cause life-threatening hemorrhage. Women who have von Willebrand disease or idiopathic thrombocytopenic purpura can also present with secondary PPH. With increasing cesarean section rates, the incidence of arteriovenous malformations of the uterus is on the rise. In such cases, the artery opens directly into the venous system without an intervening capillary network. In this situation, if the venous pressure exceeds certain limits, it ruptures, resulting in life-threatening hemorrhage.

> **Causes of secondary postpartum hemorrhage**
> - Retained placental bits and membranes
> - Infected retained tissue
> - Infection and scar dehiscence following cesarean section
> - Submucous fibroids
> - Von Willebrand disease
> - Idiopathic thrombocytopenic purpura
> - Choriocarcinoma
> - AV malformation

Clinical Features

The bleeding may be continuous or very heavy, leading to hemodynamic instability. The general condition of the woman will depend upon the amount of blood loss. The bleeding may be preceded by persistent, foul-smelling lochia, subinvolution of the uterus and fever.

Diagnosis

A high vaginal swab should be taken for culture in all cases. An ultrasound scan would reveal the presence or absence of retained products. If the bleeding follows a cesarean section or if an AV malformation is suspected, Doppler and MRI studies should be performed. In women with suspected bleeding disorders, hematological investigations should be carried out.

Management

- Broad-spectrum antibiotics should be started if the ultrasound scan reveals retained products. The uterus should be evacuated under anesthesia by an experienced obstetrician as there is a high risk of perforation.
- Manual vacuum aspiration of the retained products of conception is a safe technique which should

replace the conventional D&C. The tissues obtained should be sent for culture and histopathological examination.

- If there is clinical evidence of sepsis, the evacuation of retained products should be delayed for 12–24 hours and the woman should be put on broad-spectrum intravenous antibiotics. This reduces the risk of septicemia following evacuation.
- As retained products following cesarean section are rare, in the presence of heavy bleeding, scar dehiscence should be the first diagnosis rather than that of retained products.
- Occasionally, bleeding may be very severe, and it may become necessary to undertake uterine artery ligation, embolisation or hysterectomy.
- Oxytocic drugs are rarely effective in the management of secondary PPH.

RETAINED PLACENTA

The placenta separates from the uterine cavity within a few minutes of the birth of the child and is expelled within 15–20 minutes or even much earlier.

■ DEFINITION

A placenta is said to be retained when it is not separated and expelled within half to one hour after the delivery of the baby.

■ PATHOGENESIS

The causes of retained placenta can be grouped under three headings—trapped placenta, atonic non-detached placenta and adherent placenta.

- **Trapped placenta:** Here, the placenta is separated but does not get expelled from the uterus due to inefficient uterine contractions or as a result of the formation of a constriction ring.
- **Atonic non-detached placenta or placenta adherens:** Here, the placenta does not get separated from the uterus due to inefficient uterine contractions and atony of the uterus. Uterine anomalies and submucous fibroids can also result in the non-detachment of the placenta.
- **Adherent placenta:** It is an invasive placenta with abnormal placentation such that the placenta invades the myometrium to varying depths due to the complete or partial absence of the decidua basalis, especially the spongiosa layer.

■ MANAGEMENT

When a placenta is not expelled within 15–20 minutes of delivery, bleeding does not occur and the signs of placental separation and descent are not evident, the woman should be prepared for manual removal of placenta. The first step is to catheterise the bladder, which will very often result in the placenta being delivered. During the preparation stage, the woman should be kept under careful observation. Her pulse and blood pressure should be recorded. Oxytocin infusion should be started to promote uterine contractions. A hand may be placed on the abdomen behind the fundus of the uterus to check for uterine retraction. In the meantime, adequate blood and components should be kept ready.

Manual Removal of the Placenta

- Manual removal should be performed in the operation theatre under general anesthesia using aseptic techniques and under antibiotic cover.
- The woman is first placed in the lithotomy position.
- One hand is placed on the abdomen. The fingers of the second hand placed in the vagina follow the umbilical cord into the uterine cavity. The lower end of the placenta is located by this hand and the fingers are inserted into the placental bed (Fig. 47.9). With sweeping movements, the placenta is stripped from the uterine wall (akin to turning the pages of a book).
- The abdominal hand is used to exert counterpressure.

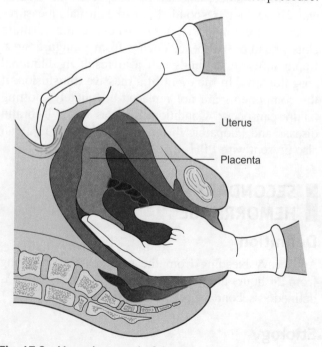

Fig. 47.9 Manual removal of the placenta

- When there is total separation of the placenta, intravenous oxytocics are administered to promote uterine contraction and expulsion.
- Following manual removal, the birth canal is checked for tears, and the placenta is checked to see if it is complete.
- Blood transfusion, if necessary, should be started without delay.
- Even after manual removal, it is advisable to continue oxytocin infusion to prevent uterine atony.
- Likewise, continuous bladder drainage should also be maintained.

> At the time of the manual removal of the placenta, if the tissue plane between the uterine wall and the placenta cannot be developed through blunt dissection with the edge of a gloved hand, an invasive placenta should be considered.

ADHERENT PLACENTA

An adherent placenta can be life-threatening. The incidence of this complication has increased due to the increase in cesarean section rates.

Definition

Adherent placenta has been defined as abnormal adherence of the placenta—either in whole or in part—to the underlying uterine wall. Pathologically, there may be a complete or partial absence of the decidua basalis, especially the spongiosa, thus placing the trophoblast in direct contact with the myometrium.

Types of Adherent Placenta

Depending on the area of involvement, an adherent placenta may be **total** (involving the entire placenta), **partial** (involving one or more cotyledons) or **focal** (involving a part of a single cotyledon). Depending on the depth of invasion, adherent placenta is classified as follows:

- **Placenta accreta**, in which the placental villi are attached to the myometrium
- **Placenta increta**, in which the trophoblast has invaded the myometrium
- **Placenta percreta**, in which the villi have penetrated the myometrium to reach or cross the serosa

Risk Factors

The basic cause of adherent placenta is decidual deficiency. The risk factors include advanced maternal age, high parity, previous cesarean delivery, placenta previa and previous adherent placenta.

- Women who have had previous cesarean sections and subsequent pregnancy with placenta previa are at the highest risk of adherent placenta. The risk is 3.3% following the first and 11% following the second cesarean section.
- Previous cesarean section alone without placenta previa is also an independent risk factor for adherent placenta, the risk increasing with the number of cesarean sections.
- Placenta previa alone without previous uterine surgery is also associated with an increased risk of adherent placenta.
- Advanced maternal age, myomectomy, endometrial ablation and dilatation and curettage, submucous fibroids, Asherman syndrome and uterine artery embolisation are other risk factors.

Diagnosis

Antenatal diagnosis

- Antenatal diagnosis is vital to optimise patient outcomes. All women with previous cesarean section and those diagnosed with placenta previa should be evaluated for adherent placenta.
- Greyscale USG predicts abnormal placentation with a sensitivity of 77–86% and a specificity of 63–88%.
- MRI should only be used in ambiguous cases or to assess organ involvement.

Ultrasonic findings suggestive of adherent placenta

- The presence of multiple placental lacunae gives the placenta a 'moth-eaten' or 'swiss cheese appearance'
- Turbulent blood flow through the placenta lacunae on Doppler
- Obliteration of clear space between the placenta and the uterus
- Hypervascularity of the adjacent bladder wall
- Thinning of the myometrium overlying the placenta; myometrial thickness <1 mm
- Vessels extending into the myometrium and bladder

Diagnosis in labour

A partially adherent placenta is often associated with partial separation and hence presents with bleeding in the third stage of labour. A completely adherent placenta does not give rise to bleeding and should be suspected when there is a well-contracted uterus with a non-separated, retained placenta without bleeding.

Management

If diagnosed postpartum

- Placenta accreta is usually diagnosed only when attempts at manual removal are made. These efforts result in a failure to find the place of cleavage in a totally adherent placenta.

- If a single cotyledon is involved, it may be removed from the uterine wall. Excessive bleeding may be controlled with oxytocics. Follow-up is essential as there is an increased risk of secondary PPH and placental polyp formation. If there is evidence of retained bits that are vascular on Doppler, they can be medically managed with methotrexate under antibiotic cover.

- When the entire placenta or a large part of the placental bed is involved, the safest treatment is prompt hysterectomy under antibiotic cover. Leaving the placenta in situ can lead to severe infection and hemorrhage.

- However, if the woman is keen to preserve her fertility, and if there is no bleeding and the entire placenta is adherent, the placenta may be left in situ after counselling the woman and explaining to her the possible risk of bleeding/infection and the possible need for an emergency hysterectomy. In such cases, the woman can be treated with methotrexate therapy. While on methotrexate, the woman should be monitored with weekly USG for the size of the placenta, Doppler of the placental site for vascularity, serial β-hCG measurements, investigations for evidence of infection and hematological parameters for evidence of methotrexate toxicity.

If diagnosed in the antenatal period

- The management of adherent placenta should be in a tertiary care centre and should have a multidisciplinary approach involving the urology and vascular surgery departments.

- Experienced senior obstetric and anesthetic staff should be available for the management of this life-threatening condition.

- A blood bank should be able to support massive transfusion.

- The pre-delivery hematocrit should be raised to 30 by oral or parenteral iron or, if necessary, erythropoietin.

- When placenta accreta is suspected or present, serial USG should be done every 3–4 weeks to know the depth of placental invasion.

- Planned surgery should be the goal. Delivery timing should be individualised, usually between 34–35 weeks in adherent placenta and 36–37 weeks in uncomplicated placenta previa. As these patients need delivery early, steroids can be given to the woman to promote fetal lung maturity.

- The woman and her family should be counselled regarding the high potential for hysterectomy, profuse hemorrhage, transfusion, increased complications and maternal death.

- General anesthesia is commonly recommended. Alternatively, a continuous epidural can be given. Surgical technique—a midline incision is preferable to allow better access to the fundus. A classical incision is made on the upper segment, away from the placenta. After the delivery, the cord is ligated and cut as close to the placenta as possible. Then, the vertical incision is quickly approximated with mass sutures to reduce the bleeding. Oxytocics are given. No attempt should be made to remove the placenta. A cesarean hysterectomy (Fig. 47.10) should be carried out with the placenta.

Conservative methods

Conservative therapy is associated with serious and genuine risks such as severe sepsis and torrential hemorrhage.

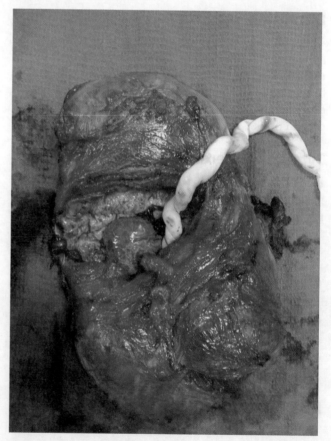

Fig. 47.10   Hysterectomy specimen with adherent placenta in situ

- When there is a strong fertility desire, interventional radiology and uterine artery embolisation can be carried out. Pre-operative catheterisation and balloon occlusion can prevent massive blood losses. These measures are helpful when a conservative approach is planned.
- Arterial ligation to reduce the blood flow to the placental site can also be undertaken.
- Systemic/intraumbilical administration of methotrexate can be used.
- All women managed conservatively should be carefully monitored for regression and autolysis of the placenta and evidence of impending sepsis. All preparations should be available for an emergency hysterectomy.

SEQUELAE OF ADHERENT OR RETAINED PLACENTA

If adherent placental bits are left behind, the woman can develop the following complication:
- Puerperal infection
- Subinvolution of the uterus
- Secondary postpartum hemorrhage
- The formation of placental polyps

PUERPERAL INVERSION OF THE UTERUS

Inversion of the uterus refers to the uterus being turned inside out. This may occur immediately after delivery. Inversion is caused either by pressure on the uterus from above or by traction on the umbilical cord from below in the presence of an atonic uterus and a soft, dilated cervical os. Uterine inversion is rare—it occurs 1 in 2,000 deliveries—and is a life-threatening emergency.

ETIOLOGY

- Injudicious attempts at the removal of the placenta
- Excessive cord traction with an unseparated placenta
- Fundal pressure and squeezing the placenta down
- Placenta accreta
- Fundal implantation of the placenta
- Short umbilical cord
- When the woman is on tocolysis and the uterus is relaxed
  — Manual removal of the placenta
  — Uterine malformations
  — Prolonged labour

— Uterus overdistended due to macrosomia, multiple pregnancy, etc., wherein the uterus has a tendency to relax

DEGREES OF INVERSION

Depending on the level to which the fundus has descended through the cervix, inversion can be graded (Fig. 47.11).

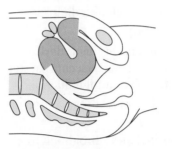

1st Degree
Inverted fundus up to the cervix

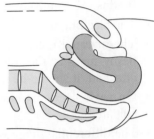

2nd Degree
Body of the uterus protrudes through the cervix into the vagina

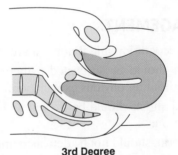

3rd Degree
Prolapse of inverted uterus outside the vulva

Fig. 47.11   Degrees of inversion of the uterus

- First degree—inverted fundus is at the level of the cervix
- Second degree—the body of the uterus protrudes through the cervix into the vagina
- Third degree—prolapse of the inverted uterus outside the vulva

Inversion can present as acute inversion within 24 hours of delivery or in the puerperal period as chronic inversion.

CLINICAL FEATURES

- Acute puerperal inversion of the uterus is one of the most serious obstetric complications. It presents with pain, hemorrhage or sudden collapse. The cause of the shock may be hemorrhagic or neurogenic due to the stretching of the infundibulopelvic ligaments and the compression of the ovaries.
- Because of the vasovagal effect, the degree of shock would be disproportionate to the amount of blood loss.

- Uterine inversion should be suspected whenever a woman develops unexplained shock following delivery.
- If the placenta is still attached to the inverted fundus and appears at the vulval introitus, it can be easily mistaken for retained placenta; in such cases, inversion will be missed.
- Per abdomen, one may not be able to feel the uterine fundus. Alternatively, it may be felt as a dimple.
- The bleeding may be very heavy.
- The inverted uterus usually appears as a dark red, fleshy mass at the introitus. If the placenta is still attached, it should be left in place until reduction.
- On vaginal examination, the cervical os cannot be palpated.
- The differential diagnosis includes fibroid polyps or prolapse of the uterus with atonic hemorrhage.
- When in doubt, emergency USG can be performed to locate the fundus of the uterus.

■ MANAGEMENT

- Prompt recognition and treatment are crucial.
- Inversion should be suspected if there is profound shock without an obvious explanation.
- Vasovagal shock should be treated with the ABC of resuscitation.
- The placenta should not be detached until the uterus is replaced and contracted.
- The uterus should be replaced immediately under anesthesia and tocolytics to relax the constriction ring.

Replacing the Uterus

- Manual replacement
- Hydrostatic replacement
- Surgical replacement

Manual replacement

- The principle of manually replacing an inverted uterus is that the portion that comes down last should be replaced first.
- Generally, a portion of the cervical canal is the last to come down and should be replaced first; the fundal portion should be replaced last.
- The protruding fundus is held with the palm of the hand and the fingers are directed towards the posterior fornix; then, steady upward pressure is applied.
- In the majority of cases, during the replacement of an inverted uterus, the fundal portion flops back into position once the greater part of the inverted uterus has been replaced.

- The other hand should be placed on the abdomen to support the uterus as it is being replaced (Fig. 47.12a, b and c).
- Tocolytic agents such as ritodrine, magnesium sulphate or terbutaline can be used to relax the uterus during manual repositioning. Once the correction is achieved, oxytocic drugs are given to assist uterine contraction and to prevent recurrence.

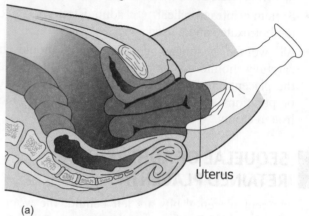

(a)

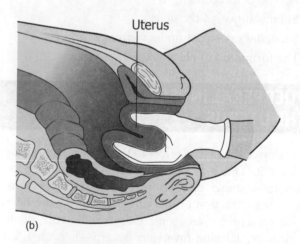

(b)

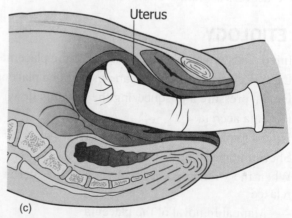

(c)

Fig. 47.12 Manual repositioning of the uterus: (a) Fundus of the uterus held in the palm, (b) steady pressure being applied to the fornix and (c) the uterus after repositioning

- If the placenta is attached to the fundus, it is removed after repositioning the inverted uterus. If removed prior to repositioning, major hemorrhage can occur, which may not be controllable.

If the initial methods fail or if a cervical contraction ring is formed, other methods should be attempted.

O'Sullivan's hydrostatic replacement

- The woman is placed in the Trendelenburg position (her head lowered about 0.5 meters below the level of the perineum).
- A sterile douche system is prepared using warmed normal saline and an ordinary IV administration set.
- The posterior fornix is identified easily in partial inversion when the inverted uterus is still in the vagina. In other cases, the posterior fornix is recognised by where the rugose vagina becomes the smooth vagina.
- The nozzle of the douche is placed in the posterior fornix.
- At the same time, the labia are sealed over the nozzle with the other hand.
- An assistant is asked to turn on the douche with full pressure (the water reservoir is raised to at least 2 meters).
- In this method, water distends the posterior fornix of the vagina gradually so that it stretches. This causes the circumference of the orifice to increase, relieves cervical constriction and results in the correction of the inversion.

Surgical replacement of the uterus

In surgical methods, either the constriction ring is stretched, or the posterior part of the ring is divided, and then the fundus is pulled up. This requires an abdominal approach.

- **Huntington's method:** A pair of Allis forceps are placed at the dimple of the inverted fundus and gentle upward traction is applied (47.13a). The forceps are further advanced until the fundus is repositioned.
- **Haultain's technique** (Fig. 47.13b): If the constriction ring still prohibits repositioning, it is incised posteriorly with a longitudinal incision. The fundus is then pulled up, and the uterus is repaired in two layers. After repositioning, the fundus should be massaged carefully, uterine contractions should be promoted, and the woman should be treated for shock and collapse. Appropriate antibiotics should be given.

■ PREVENTION

One should wait for signs of placental separation before attempting placental removal by controlled cord traction. Fundal pressure should not be applied.

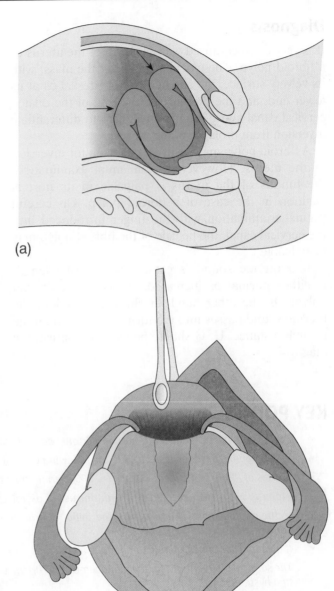

(a)

(b)

Fig. 47.13a and b Surgical replacement of the uterus—(a) Huntington's method where the inverted uterus is pulled up and (b) the pulling up of the fundus and incised constriction ring posteriorly

■ CHRONIC PUERPERAL INVERSION

In some cases, inversion may not be recognised at the time of its occurrence and the diagnosis is made at a later date. In such cases, the woman suffers repeated hemorrhage and a slight rise in temperature. The exposed endometrium has a granular, shaggy appearance due to chronic congestion and infection, particularly over the placental site. Vaginal examination reveals the presence of a globular swelling, with the soft, thickened endometrium presenting a hyperemic appearance.

Diagnosis

It is very often confused with prolapse of the uterus or a fibroid polyp. The globular nature of the mass, with its velvety surface, the absence of the external os at its lower end, and the presence of the ring of the dilated cervical canal above the mass will help to differentiate inversion from prolapse of the uterus.

A fibroid polyp may easily be mistaken for inversion of the uterus. However, on bimanual examination, the fundus of the uterus is palpable in its normal position in the case of a fibroid polyp. On careful vaginal examination with the finger introduced into the cervical canal, the pedicle of the fibroid polyp may be palpable.

If a uterine sound is passed, the uterine length is either normal or increased in cases of a fibroid polyp. On the other hand, in chronic inversion, the uterine sound passes into the fornices to less than the normal distance. USG should be used to confirm the diagnosis.

Management

The immediate treatment is to combat infection with antibiotics. Later, an attempt may be made under an anesthetic to replace the inverted uterus. If this proves unsuccessful, an operation for the replacement of the inverted uterus either by the vaginal route (Spinelli's) or by the abdominal route (Haultain's) may be performed.

NON-HEMORRHAGIC POSTPARTUM COLLAPSE

Besides PPH, the following conditions can cause postpartum collapse:
- Amniotic fluid embolism
- Cerebrovascular accidents in eclampsia
- Anesthesia complications
- Pulmonary embolism
- Drug toxicity and anaphylaxis
- Hypoglycemia and ketoacidosis in diabetes

KEY POINTS

✓ Postpartum hemorrhage (PPH) is an important cause of maternal mortality.

✓ PPH is defined as blood loss of >500 mL following vaginal delivery and >1,000 mL following cesarean section.

✓ Causes of PPH include uterine atony (>70%), genital tract trauma and coagulopathy.

✓ Atonic PPH can be prevented by the routine use of oxytocics and controlled cord traction in the third stage of labour.

✓ In the management of atonic PPH, the initial approach is resuscitation, the use of oxytocic drugs and bimanual uterine compression.

✓ If bleeding continues, uterine tamponade techniques should be attempted.

✓ The surgical interventions for the management of PPH include compression sutures on the uterus, stepwise devascularisation and hysterectomy.

✓ Early and adequate replacement of blood is important for a favourable maternal outcome.

✓ The assessment of blood loss is important so that adequate blood transfusion can be given.

✓ Inversion of the uterus refers to the uterus being turned inside out, which may occur immediately after delivery. It is a life-threatening emergency presenting with hemorrhagic and neurogenic shock. Prevention is by awaiting signs of placental separation before attempting placental removal by controlled cord traction. Fundal pressure should not be applied.

Essay questions

1. What do you understand by postpartum hemorrhage? Enumerate the causes of primary postpartum hemorrhage.
2. What is a retained placenta? How would you manage a woman with a retained placenta?

Short answer questions

1. Outline the steps in the management of PPH.
2. Elaborate on stepwise devascularisation.
3. What are the predisposing factors for PPH?
4. Describe the active management of the third stage of labour (AMSTL).

5. Describe the antepartum diagnosis of adherent placenta.
6. What is acute inversion of the uterus?

MCQs

1. The definition of PPH is blood loss more than _____ after vaginal delivery:
   a) 250 mL
   b) 500 mL
   c) 1,000 mL
   d) 1,500 mL

2. The most common cause of secondary PPH is:
   a) Uterine atony
   b) Ruptured uterus

c)   Retained placental bits
d)   Vaginal lacerations

3.   The options for the treatment of total placenta percreta include all of the following EXCEPT:
a)   Manual removal of placenta
b)   Hysterectomy
c)   Leave the placenta in situ
d)   Leave the placenta in situ and administer methotrexate

4.   Factors favouring uterine inversion include all of the following EXCEPT:
a)   Hypertonic uterus
b)   Traction on the umbilical cord
c)   Fundal implantation of the placenta
d)   Improper pressure over the fundus

5.   The treatment of uterine inversion does not include:
a)   Manual reposition
b)   Oxytocin infusion
c)   Applying hydrostatic pressure
d)   Surgical correction

6.   The following is not included in the active management of the third stage of labour:
a)   Controlled cord traction
b)   Administration of oxytocin
c)   Uterine massage
d)   Prophylactic misoprostol

7.   The most common cause of primary PPH is:
a)   Atony
b)   Trauma
c)   Retained placenta
d)   Coagulation disorders

8.   The dose of injection prostaglandin $PGF_2\alpha$ for the management of PPH is:
a)   100 μg
b)   150 μg
c)   200 μg
d)   250 μg

9.   The ideal treatment for placenta accreta is:
a)   Cesarean hysterectomy with the placenta in situ
b)   Vaginal delivery followed by manual removal of placenta
c)   Cesarean with manual removal of placenta
d)   Cesarean and leaving the placenta in situ

10.   B-Lynch suture is applied on the uterus for the treatment of:
a)   Incompetent os
b)   Atonic PPH
c)   Rupture uterus
d)   Bleeding from the placental bed of placenta previa

11.   All the following are used in PPH except:
a)   Ergometrine
b)   Carboprost

c)   Misoprostol
d)   Mifepristone

Answers

1. (b), 2. (c), 3. (a), 4. (a), 5. (b), 6. (d), 7. (a), 8. (d),
9. (a), 10. (b), 11. (d)

Fill in the blanks

1.   The abnormal placental adherence in which the villi penetrate through the myometrium is known as _____.

2.   If the trophoblast invades into the myometrium, it is called _____.

3.   The oxytocic drug contraindicated in the management of atonic PPH in a hypertensive patient is _____.

Answers

1. placenta percreta,   2. placenta increta,   3. methylergometrine

Case scenario-based discussion

1.   A 32-year-old para 3 had a spontaneous vaginal delivery at a nearby PHC 30 minutes ago. Following the delivery of the placenta, she had profuse vaginal bleeding. On admission to the hospital, she looks pale, her pulse is 110 bpm and BP is 100/70 mmHg.
a)   What is the possible cause of bleeding?
b)   What measures should be taken?
c)   If the woman continues to bleed despite these measures, how would you manage her?
d)   If the bleeding continues due to an atonic uterus and there is a further decrease in BP, what is the further course of action?

Answers

a) The possible cause of bleeding could be atonic PPH. However, traumatic causes should be ruled out before making a diagnosis.

b) Resuscitative measures, investigations to identify the cause and the treatment of PPH should be carried out simultaneously. Two IV lines should be started with wide-bore needles, blood samples should be collected for investigations, IV fluid with normal saline should be started, oxygen should be administered by a face mask, the bladder should be catheterised, the uterus should be palpated to ascertain its tonicity and oxytocin should be started as an infusion with 20 units in 500 mL NS to run at a rate of 40 dpm. The uterus should be massaged to expel blood clots. Bimanual uterine compression should be performed. Blood should be transfused as soon as possible.

c) Second- and third-line oxytocic drugs such as ergometrine and prostaglandin should be given in a stepwise manner. The placenta should be checked again, the clotting profile should be reviewed, and traumatic causes should be ruled out.

d) Adequate blood should be transfused, and the woman should be taken for surgery. While shifting her to the theatre, condom tamponade should be undertaken to reduce the bleeding. Being a multipara, this woman would benefit from a quick hysterectomy rather than conservative procedures.

48

OG 14.2 and 14.3

Injuries to the Parturient Canal

Learning Objectives

» To discuss the management of vulval and vaginal hematomas
» To know the etiology, classification, prevention and repair of perineal tears
» To discuss the causes, diagnosis and management of rupture uterus
» To identify the symptoms and signs of uterine rupture

Injuries to the genital tract are common, both in spontaneous and operative deliveries. Genital tract injuries account for nearly 10% of all PPH cases. Besides genital tract injuries, musculoskeletal injuries can also occur following delivery.

INJURY TO THE BONY PARTS

INJURY TO THE SYMPHYSIS PUBIS (DIASTASIS OF THE SYMPHYSIS PUBIS)

Relaxin and progesterone hormones secreted by the placenta cause the relaxation of pelvic ligaments and contribute to the softening of the cartilage of the pubic symphysis, leading to increased joint mobility. This is more common in the third trimester of pregnancy. This increased joint mobility results in the widening of the pubic symphysis during childbirth, which is physiological and helpful in increasing the pelvic diameters to some extent; this is called the '**give of the pelvis**'. However, excessive widening of the pubic symphysis can occur due to various reasons. A separation of more than 1 cm of the symphysis pubis is considered to be pathological.

The risk factors for postpartum pubic symphysis diastasis are multiparity, delivery of a macrosomic baby, forcible extraction of the fetal head in forceps or breech delivery and McRoberts manoeuvres used for shoulder dystocia. It can also occur spontaneously.

The symptoms include the following:

• Suprapubic pain, sharp pain in the pubic area and pain that worsens with walking, climbing stairs and getting out of bed
• Difficulty in walking

• The woman can present with bladder dysfunction such as urinary incontinence or occasionally, retention of urine

Signs

A distinct gap can be felt between the pubic bones. The gap between the pubic bones, the tenderness on pressure and pain felt more particularly with the movement of the limbs suggest the diagnosis. X-ray and ultrasonography are useful to confirm the diagnosis. Occasionally, MRI may be required.

Treatment

Treatment consists of keeping the woman at rest on a firm bed with strips of adhesive plaster applied tightly around the entire pelvis to immobilise the joint. A firm binder around the pelvis may also be applied. This gives the woman a feeling of security and comfort. Mild analgesics and walking devices may be used. Strengthening and stabilisation exercises for the pelvic girdle also help.

FRACTURE AND DISLOCATION OF THE COCCYX

This injury generally occurs during delivery when the head is at the outlet. It is more likely to occur in cases where the subpubic angle is so narrow that the head has to emerge more posteriorly at the outlet. The injury may not be recognised until some months after delivery, at which time the woman may complain of pain in the lower part of the sacrum, particularly in the sitting posture. On palpation, the coccyx will be unduly mobile or displaced and tender. Occasionally, persistent neuralgia is present and is known as **coccydynia**. Management is usually symptomatic. Mild analgesics can be given. The woman should be advised to avoid direct pressure over the coccygeal region. Constipation should be avoided as it puts pressure on the coccyx. If the pain is very severe, the woman will need a referral to an orthopedic specialist who may treat her by injecting lidocaine or steroids into the sacrococcygeal joint.

■ INJURIES TO THE SACROILIAC JOINT

Pain in the sacroiliac joints can start early in pregnancy due to the effect of relaxin. The sacroiliac joint, which normally resists the forward flexion of the sacral ala, becomes lax. This gives rise to pain. The iliac bones flare out and the ligaments of the joints are stretched. This results in the hypermobility of the joints.

Symptoms include backache, sharp pain in the pelvic region and numbness in the legs. The pain may originate at the joint and spread to the thighs, groin, buttocks and upper part of the back. The main aims of treatment are to decrease stress on the joint and to strengthen the muscles surrounding the joint to provide greater pelvic stability. Bed rest with proper support to the pelvis with the help of strapping relieves the pain. Specific exercises may help in alleviating the pain.

INJURIES TO THE GENITAL TRACT

Genital tract injuries occur following spontaneous and assisted deliveries. They are more common than injuries to the bony parts and tend to be more severe with instrumental deliveries, operative procedures and manipulations (Table 48.1).

Table 48.1   Causes of genital tract injuries

Spontaneous	• Precipitate labour • Obstructed labour • Grand multipara • Drug-induced—oxytocin, misoprostol • Previous uterine surgery
Iatrogenic	• Instrumental delivery (forceps or vacuum) • Manipulations—external version, internal version, breech extraction, shoulder dystocia • Manual removal of the placenta • Extension of cesarean section incision into the broad ligament, vagina, bladder
Physical trauma	• Fall or accident

Injuries may occur in the upper genital tract or in the lower genital tract.

• Upper genital tract injuries:
— Uterine rupture
— Cervical tear or lacerations
— Vaginal vault rupture (colporrhexis)
• Lower genital tract injuries:
— Vulval injuries include clitoral tears, paraurethral tears, vestibular injury, avulsion of the urethra and perineal tears
— Vaginal tears and hematoma

■ INJURIES TO THE VULVA

Small lacerations of the labia minora, the fourchette, vestibule, perineal body and superficial vagina are frequently seen following vaginal delivery. Small lacerations that do not bleed may not require any treatment. However, deep lacerations may involve the large vessels, and if not repaired, could cause serious hematomas.

Vulvar hematomas are infralevator in location. Their extension is limited superiorly by the levator ani muscle. However, they can dissect below the levator muscle to cause vulval or vulvovaginal hematomas involving the lower part of the vagina. If large, they can dissect into the ischiorectal fossa. The vessels that are injured in vulvar hematomas are branches of the pudendal artery—the inferior rectal, transverse perineal, posterior labial and anteriorly clitoral arteries.

> • Injury to the pudendal artery is responsible for the majority of vulvar hematomas.
> • Injury to the descending branch of the uterine artery accounts for the majority of vaginal hematomas.

Vulval Hematoma

The collection of blood in the vulvar region is known as a vulval hematoma. This can occur following a spontaneous vaginal delivery and more often, following instrumental vaginal delivery or an episiotomy that is not sutured properly. Clotting abnormalities and injuries to the pudendal vessels at the time of a pudendal block can also present with vulvovaginal hematoma. This complication usually occurs after delivery and rarely, in the second stage of labour. In the second stage of labour, when an instrumental delivery is carried out, excessive stretching of the vulval tissues may result in the spontaneous rupture of the blood vessels. The risk is greater when there are engorged veins in the vulva or vulval varicosities. Usually, the pressure exerted by the head reduces the bleeding before delivery, and the hematoma becomes apparent only once the baby is delivered. The blood extravasates into the soft, loose areolar tissue of the labium, producing a large hematoma. A large vulvar/vaginal hematoma can also occur if the episiotomy or perineal tears are not sutured properly.

Clinical features of vulval hematoma

Symptoms

* A steadily increasing swelling is usually present on one side of the vulval region.
* The swelling is very often extremely painful and tender; there may be rectal pain if there is extension into the ischiorectal fossa.
* There might be difficulty in passing urine, which may result in the retention of urine.

> * In the immediate postpartum period, whenever a woman complains of severe pain in the vulval region, it should raise the suspicion of vulval/vaginal hematoma.
> * Very often, the pain is wrongly interpreted as episiotomy-related pain; vulval hematoma can be easily missed.

Signs

* The swelling may appear bluish or purplish due to the blood collected inside the vulval tissue (Fig. 48.1).

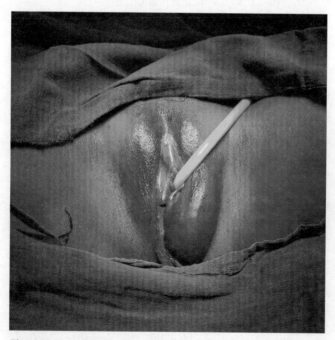

Fig. 48.1 Vulvar hematoma

* Depending on the severity of bleeding, the woman may go into hemorrhagic shock requiring blood transfusion and effective resuscitation.
* The woman should be examined in the lithotomy position with good light. Vaginal and rectal examinations should be carried out to know the extension into the vagina and the pararectal space.

Treatment

* Any hematoma that is sufficient to cause symptoms requires incision, drainage and suturing. Unrecognised bleeding from vulval and vaginal tears may be severe enough to necessitate a blood transfusion.
* The hematoma must be incised under general anesthesia, and the clots removed. If possible, bleeding vessels should be identified and ligated. If this is not possible, the cavity should be closed from the base with multiple mattress sutures to secure hemostasis. The cavity may be closed with a drain in situ. Most obstetricians prefer to use a running–locking suture because it is more hemostatic. A large, round-bodied needle with 00 chromic sutures may be used.
* If the lacerations are close to the urethra as in clitoral and para-urethral tears, it is important to insert a Foley's catheter which will facilitate the repair without compromising the urethra. The catheter also helps to overcome the postoperative voiding difficulty that may be encountered by the woman. These tears should be repaired with very fine 000 or 0000 chromic catgut, Dexon or Vicryl.
* Tight packing of the vagina is important. If there is rectal extension, rectal packing for a short period of time may also help.
* Blood transfusion is given depending on the size of the hematoma and the woman's condition.

VAGINAL LACERATIONS AND HEMATOMAS

Lacerations of the vagina are not uncommon and generally occur in forceps deliveries and breech extractions. They are more frequent in cases where the head has to be rotated, and are severe if the forceps slip upon traction. When the tear involves the fornices, it may extend to the pelvic cellular space. Extension of episiotomies and tears following forceps application can lead to vaginal hematomas due to injury to the vaginal and pudendal arteries. Some deep lacerations involve the descending branch of the uterine artery. Vaginal hematomas are more concerning because they can extend into the paravaginal and ischiorectal fossae without any changes in the external genitalia. Moreover, if a vessel is injured high in the vagina, it can retract into the retroperitoneum and become a supralevator hematoma. It may then extend into the broad ligament and cause retroperitoneal hematoma, which can extend as high as the kidneys. The diagnosis of these injuries can be easily missed until hypotension sets in and the patient becomes hemodynamically unstable. Since this is a life-threatening situation, it is imperative that the diagnosis is not missed.

Diagnosis

Following all difficult or instrumental deliveries, vaginal and rectal examinations should be performed to diagnose vaginal hematoma. While suturing perineal tears and episiotomies, the apex of the tear should be secured properly. Vaginal packing is important following suturing. When there is a suspicion of extension into the retroperitoneal space, USG should be carried out.

Treatment

Small hematomas usually do not expand and generally result in tamponade. On the other hand, large and enlarging hematomas should be explored, and the bleeding vessel identified. If the vessel cannot be identified, the cavity should be closed with hemostatic sutures. Vaginal packing is mandatory. In women who have diffuse oozing, layered closure helps in achieving hemostasis by closing the dead space. In the event of supralevator hematomas, abdominal exploration is mandatory, and may require internal iliac artery ligation.

PERINEAL TEARS

The perineum is the most common location for a tear during labour. The extent of the tear often depends upon the care taken and skill displayed during the delivery of the head.

■ ETIOLOGY

Perineal tears occur both in spontaneous and assisted deliveries. There are many etiological factors for these tears, which are as follows:

- More common in nulliparous women, especially in elderly primigravidae, as the perineum is rigid
- Rapid delivery of the head or shoulders
- Birth weight over 4 Kg
- Persistent occipitoposterior position
- Shoulder dystocia
- Instrumental delivery

- Face-to-pubis delivery
- Prolonged second stage
- Perineal cicatrisation due to previous injury or surgery

■ DEGREES OF PERINEAL LACERATION

Four degrees of perineal lacerations have been described (Fig. 48.2).

- **First degree:** Injury to perineal skin and/or vaginal mucosa only
- **Second degree:** Injury to the perineum involving perineal muscles but not involving the anal sphincter
- **Third degree:** Injury to the perineum involving the anal sphincter complex
  — **3a:** Less than 50% of the external anal sphincter thickness is torn
  — **3b:** More than 50% of the external anal sphincter thickness is torn
  — **3c:** Both the external and internal anal sphincters are torn
- **Fourth degree:** Injury to the perineum involving the anal sphincter complex (external and internal anal sphincters) and anal epithelium

(Adapted from RCOG Green-top Guidelines No. 29. Classification by Sultan.)

1st Degree
(Just the skin)

2nd Degree
(Skin and muscle)

3rd Degree
(Skin, muscle, and anal sphincter)

4th Degree
(Skin, muscle, anal sphincter, and the rectum)

Fig. 48.2 Degrees of perineal tears

■ PRINCIPLES IN THE MANAGEMENT OF PERINEAL INJURY

The management of perineal injury involves the following steps:

1. The first step is the recognition of the injury and its severity (type of perineal tear).

2. The woman should be examined in lithotomy position under good lighting.

3. The woman should be asked to contract the anal sphincter to look for puckering around the anal orifice.

4. A combined vaginal and rectal examination is important to exclude associated anal sphincter injuries.

5. Immediate repair of the perineal injury is preferred over delayed repair as it will reduce the bleeding and pain associated with the injury. This may, in turn, affect early breastfeeding and bonding. Immediate repair also prevents the development of edema and fibrosis, which may affect the subsequent recognition of structures involved and also reduce the possibility of infection.

6. If there is any doubt about the extent of the injury, a second opinion must be sought. The presence of an experienced person at the time of assessment and treatment of perineal injury improves the outcome.

7. A successful first repair offers the best cure rate.

8. The labia, clitoris and urethra should also be examined.

■ REPAIR

- All tears of the perineum must be carefully sutured. This must be taken as a surgical emergency.

- Though first-degree tears can be sutured in the labour room, all third- and fourth-degree tears should be sutured only in the operation theatre under regional or general anesthesia. Second-degree tears are also best sutured in the operation theatre.

- For suturing first-degree tears, the woman is brought to the edge of the bed and placed in the lithotomy position. The area is cleaned and exposed to light. After thoroughly cleaning the wound and the adjoining surfaces, the area may be kept fairly dry by inserting a large sterile sponge into the vagina to prevent the flow of blood.

Suturing of First- and Second-Degree Tears

The extent of the vaginal tear and its apex should be identified. The suture materials used are 2-0 chromic catgut and delayed absorbable sutures such as polyglactin (Vicryl). The vaginal mucosa is sutured with continuous sutures, the perineal muscles are approximated by interrupted sutures and then the skin is sutured.

Suturing of Third- and Fourth-Degree Tears

Third- and fourth-degree tears (Fig. 48.3) require much more thorough repair.

- The rectal mucosa is first identified and repaired with fine 3–0 suture such as polyglactin (Vicryl). Either continuous or interrupted sutures are made without tension.

- Next, the retracted ends of the internal anal sphincters are identified (pale pink in appearance) and approximated with interrupted or mattress sutures using 2–0 Vicryl.

- The external sphincters are identified and approximated using 2–0 Vicryl.

- This is followed by the approximation of the vaginal mucosa, perineal muscles and the skin.

Postoperative Care

For proper union, the postoperative care of the woman is very important. Broad-spectrum antibiotics should be used for 5–7 days. The site should be kept clean and dry. It is better in cases of perineal tears to prescribe stool softeners in the postoperative period. Particular care should be taken to see that after each evacuation, the perineum is thoroughly cleaned and dried; a mild antiseptic should also be applied. For bowel rest, the woman should be kept on a liquid diet for two days; a soft diet should be followed for the next three days and then a normal diet can be resumed. After 6–12 weeks, the woman should be offered physiotherapy and instructed on pelvic floor exercises. Laxatives should be given for two weeks and bulking agents should be avoided.

Follow-up and Management in Subsequent Pregnancy

Following the repair of third- and fourth-degree perineal tears, the woman should be assessed at 6–12 weeks postpartum. History related to bowel symptoms should be elicited. The healing of the perineal wound and sphincter tone may be checked. Endoanal sonography may be useful to assess the integrity of the repair. If necessary, manometry may be used.

- In asymptomatic women with low squeeze pressures and a defect of greater than one quadrant by anal USG, the option of cesarean section should be offered in subsequent pregnancies.

- Women who are asymptomatic and have no clinical evidence of a deficient perineum or low anal sphincter tone may be allowed vaginal delivery with detailed counselling.

- Symptomatic women with severe injuries should be offered secondary sphincter repair and subsequent pregnancies should be delivered by cesarean section.

Complications of perineal tear repair include repair failure and rectovaginal fistula.

LACERATIONS OF THE CERVIX

After parturition, the cervix is never the same as before. Minor lacerations occur in practically all cases. The causes of cervical lacerations include the following:

- Rapid delivery of the fetus as in precipitate labour
- Following an instrumental delivery
- Delivery through an undilated cervix—e.g., injury due to the application of forceps before full cervical dilatation or the extraction of a breech when the cervix is not adequately dilated
- Delivery through a scarred cervix, which occurs following Fothergill's surgery, amputation of the cervix or conisation
- Occasionally, a circular tear or 'avulsion of the cervix' may occur—this may be due to the faulty application of a vacuum cup (more so with metal cups), wherein the cervix is caught between the cup and the head, so that when traction is applied, a whole ring of the cervical tissue tears off; in some cases, it may occur spontaneously when the uterus suddenly forces the head down

■ CLINICAL FEATURES

Most times, small tears do not bleed and hence, go unrecognised. Larger tears present as traumatic PPH. If the cervical tear is extensive and extends into the fornix, causing colporrhexis, the woman presents with hemodynamic instability.

■ MANAGEMENT

- Following all difficult and instrumental deliveries, the cervix should be visualised to diagnose cervical tears.
- In all cases of atonic PPH, if the bleeding is not controlled with adequate medical methods, vaginal and cervical injuries should be looked for.
- The vulva, vagina and cervix should be routinely inspected following any delivery.
- Whenever a cervical tear is suspected, the woman should be examined in the lithotomy position under good light.
- A broad Sims speculum/right-angled retractor is inserted into the vagina anteriorly and posteriorly to expose the cervix. The anterior lip of the cervix is held

with a pair of sponge-holding forceps. Keeping this as an identification point, another pair of sponge-holding forceps is applied to the lateral side, and the cervix is examined.

- Then, keeping the lateral wall sponge-holding forceps in situ, the first pair of forceps is removed and applied to the posterior lip of the cervix. This pair of forceps is then kept in situ, and the lateral wall forceps are removed and applied to the other lateral wall of the cervix.
- This technique is called '**walking round the cervix**' and is very useful in identifying cervical tears.
- Applying suprapubic pressure will help in visualising the entire circumference of the cervix. Most often, cervical lacerations are noted at the 3 o'clock and 9 o'clock positions.
- Upon the identification of a cervical tear that is bleeding and needs suturing, the cervix is held by a couple of sponge-holding forceps, and the two torn edges are brought into close apposition by means of interrupted catgut sutures. The first suture should be applied beyond the upper angle of the tear for satisfactory hemostasis (Fig. 48.3).
- Small tears of the cervix that are not bleeding do not require suturing. However, during the healing process, the cervix may get everted, leading to ectropion and persistent cervicitis.

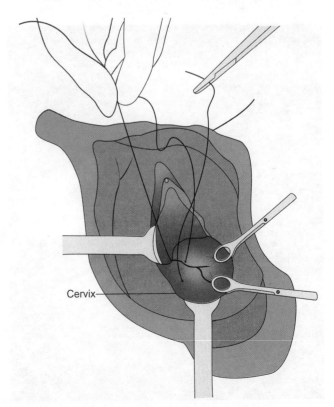

Cervix

Fig. 48.3 Repair of a cervical tear

RUPTURE OF THE UTERUS

This is one of the most serious complications that may occur during pregnancy or in labour (Fig. 48.4).

TYPES OF UTERINE RUPTURE

Two types of uterine rupture are described—complete and incomplete.

- In a complete rupture, all the layers of the uterus including the peritoneum are torn. As a result, the fetus and the placenta escape into the peritoneal cavity. There is fetal death, and the mother presents with hemodynamic instability.

- In an incomplete rupture, otherwise called scar dehiscence, the visceral peritoneum remains intact. Therefore, the fetus does not enter the peritoneal cavity and may be alive occasionally.

ETIOLOGY

- **Rupture uterus following previous surgery on the uterus:** The most common causes of rupture uterus are surgical procedures on the uterus.
  - Cesarean section
  - Myomectomy
  - Metroplasty

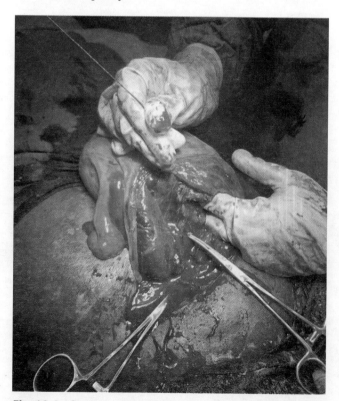

Fig. 48.4 Rupture of the right lateral wall of the uterus

  - Cornual resection of the fallopian tube for cornual ectopic pregnancy
  - Previous injury to the uterus—perforation during suction evacuation
- **Traumatic rupture:** Rupture uterus can occur following various operative procedures and manipulations such as:
  - Internal podalic version
  - Instrumental delivery
  - Breech extraction
  - Shoulder dystocia
  - Manual removal of the placenta
  - Destructive operation
- **Spontaneous rupture:** Spontaneous rupture can also occur in an unscarred uterus in the following scenarios:
  - Obstructed labour
  - Grand multiparity
  - Misuse of oxytocic drugs
  - Pregnancy in a rudimentary uterine horn
  - Placenta percreta

Most cases of rupture uterus occur during labour. However, in certain situations, rupture can occur during the antenatal period, e.g., when there has been a previous classical cesarean section or in cases of placenta percreta, pregnancy in a rudimentary horn or trauma to the uterus following road traffic accidents.

CLINICAL FEATURES

The clinical manifestations vary depending on the cause of rupture.

- Ruptures occurring during the antenatal period are difficult to diagnose. Rupture during the antenatal period can occur in cases of previous classical cesarean section, pregnancy in a rudimentary horn, in cases of placenta percreta and following accidents or trauma.
- There should be a high index of suspicion in the presence of risk factors such as classical cesarean section.
- The usual presentation is unexplained collapse in the antenatal period. If there is a small trickle of blood as in cases of placenta percreta, the woman may present with recurrent fainting episodes prior to the rupture. There is also diminution or loss of fetal movements in these cases.
- Classical cesarean section scar rupture is seen in 4–8% of cases. The rupture usually occurs around 34–36 weeks of gestation when the uterus starts to enlarge in the transverse direction. Therefore, women who have

had a classical cesarean section should be hospitalised early—at around 32 weeks—and an elective cesarean should be carried out at 36 weeks of gestation.

In women presenting with unexplained collapse during the antenatal period, besides rupture, conditions such as abruptio placenta and amniotic fluid embolism should also be suspected.

- Following difficult instrumental delivery or manipulations such as breech extraction, there will be evidence of traumatic PPH with a well-contracted uterus. There is hemodynamic instability, and the uterus is not felt in its normal position in the suprapubic region. Either the uterus is high up or pushed to one side due to broad-ligament hematoma.
- Spontaneous rupture due to obstructed labour caused by CPD and malpresentations used to be more common in the past. With the advent of improved healthcare systems and the routine use of partographs, rupture uterus due to obstructed labour is rarely seen nowadays.
- The typical presentation consists of prolonged labour, protracted first and second stages, maternal exhaustion and evidence of fetal heart rate changes. On abdominal palpation, the uterus is tonically contracted, not relaxing between contractions, and a distinction between the upper and the lower segments is clearly made out (Bandl's ring). On vaginal examination, the head is obstructed in the pelvis with a big caput and marked moulding. At this stage, it is called threatened rupture. If left unattended, the uterus ruptures during a contraction. For a short while, the woman is relieved of pain as the uterine contractions cease. Soon after, the rupture manifests with hemorrhagic shock. On abdominal examination, the fetal parts are easily palpable, FH is absent and the contracted uterus is felt separately on one side; there are no uterine contractions. Fluid in the peritoneal cavity may be demonstrated. On vaginal examination, there is bleeding per vaginum, the presenting part appears to have receded and the cervix hangs loose. If the bladder is involved, there is hematuria.

Occasionally, the woman may complain of pain at her shoulder tip, which is caused by the hemoperitoneum irritating the diaphragm.

Rupture of Cesarean Section Scar in Labour

Rupture of the uterus can occur in 0.5% of lower segment cesarean section scars in labour. Women who are taken for VBAC should be carefully monitored for the possible occurrence of rupture uterus. When there is scar dehiscence with an intact peritoneum, the symptoms are not acute. The earliest indications of possible dehiscence are fetal tachycardia and maternal tachycardia. Therefore, there should be continuous CTG monitoring, and a pulse chart should be prepared every 15 minutes for the mother. Suprapubic pain, swelling, bleeding per vaginum and hematuria are late manifestations in labour.

▌ MANAGEMENT

Treatment consists of immediate laparotomy with simultaneous treatment of shock by rapid and sufficient blood transfusion. The following resuscitative measures should be undertaken:

- Two large-bore cannulae should be instituted with NS or RL and compatible blood on flow
- 8–10 litres/minute of oxygen should be administered by a face mask
- Continuous bladder drainage
- Continuous monitoring of pulse, BP and respiration
- Adequate amount of blood and components should be ordered and kept ready
- Written consent should be obtained for hysterectomy

At laparotomy, the fetus and placenta, which are often lying free in the peritoneal cavity, are removed. Broad-spectrum antibiotic therapy is essential to control postoperative peritonitis. The choices at laparotomy are hysterectomy or conservative surgery.

Hysterectomy

Hysterectomy is indicated in the following situations:
- In a multiparous woman who has completed her family
- If the uterus is damaged beyond repair
- Rupture uterus with sepsis

It is preferable to undertake subtotal hysterectomy rather than total hysterectomy as it is difficult to differentiate the cervix from the vagina owing to the complete distortion of the anatomy by lacerations and hematoma formation. Sometimes, the bladder is involved; such lacerations must be recognised and repaired. When there is associated broad-ligament hematoma, it is important to ligate the bleeding vessel or carry out internal iliac artery ligation. Extension behind the bladder into the vagina should be identified and sutured. In all cases with rupture uterus, the integrity of the bladder should be checked by distending the bladder with sterile methylene blue. If rupture occurs following obstructed labour, the bladder should be catheterised for 7–10 days to prevent ischemic necrosis of the bladder.

Conservative Surgery

Conservative surgery involves repairing the rent in the uterus. It can be undertaken only in certain situations and may be considered if preserving fertility is a major concern. Before undertaking the procedure, one should ensure that the general condition of the woman is stable, the bleeding is controlled, and the uterine wound is clean without sepsis. Conservative surgery should be avoided if there is extension of tears into the upper segment, laterally into the broad ligament or downwards into the vagina.

Dehiscence of a cesarean section scar is ideally suited for rent repair. This procedure should be combined with tubal ligation if the woman has completed her family. If only rent repair is to be undertaken in women who have not completed their family, it is important to counsel them regarding the recurrent risk of rupture in future pregnancies, which could be as high as 10%. The woman should be advised to stay in the hospital from the early third trimester onwards, and an elective cesarean section should be carried out at 36 weeks.

■ COLPORRHEXIS

This is a rupture of the vaginal vault that can occur after normal labour in a multiparous woman due to the weakening of the posterior fornix. Extension of cervical lacerations into the fornix and instrumental deliveries can also lead to vault rupture. Clinical presentation and management are the same as those of rupture uterus. In these cases, a total hysterectomy should be carried out to occlude the descending cervical artery and the vaginal artery. Care should be taken to avoid including the ureters in the clamps.

■ PROPHYLAXIS

- Early diagnosis and proper management of cephalopelvic disproportion, malpresentation and other factors giving rise to obstruction will prevent the rupture of the uterus.
- Extreme care should be taken in the selection of cases for vaginal delivery after a previous cesarean section; careful monitoring of labour is important.
- All precautions should be taken at the time of instrumental delivery.
- If threatened rupture is diagnosed, immediate cesarean section should be performed even if the fetus is dead.

KEY POINTS

✓ *The injuries to the parturient canal can occur following instrumental as well as spontaneous delivery.*

✓ *Trauma to the genital tract should be suspected whenever there is excessive bleeding after delivery with a well-contracted uterus.*

✓ *All the tears of the perineum must be carefully sutured.*

✓ *Injury to the pudendal vessels leads to vulval hematoma.*

✓ *Vaginal hematomas, especially at a higher level, can be easily missed as they can dissect the pararectal and paravaginal tissue easily and extend into the retroperitoneal area.*

✓ *In vaginal hematoma, besides the pudendal vessels, the descending branch from the uterine artery can also be injured.*

✓ *Vulval hematoma should be drained under anesthesia, and the cavity obliterated by mattress sutures.*

✓ *Uterine rupture is one of the most serious complications of labour and is associated with significant maternal morbidity and fetal mortality.*

✓ *Treatment of ruptured uterus consists of resuscitation and immediate laparotomy.*

Essay questions

1. Describe the management of third-degree perineal tears.
2. Discuss the causes, diagnosis and management of rupture uterus.

Short answer questions

1. What is the cause of symphysis pubis diastasis?
2. How is a vulval hematoma managed?
3. What are the vessels injured in vaginal hematoma?
4. Describe the diagnosis and management of cervical tears.
5. What are the presenting features of ruptured uterus?
6. What are the causes of rupture uterus in the antenatal period?
7. What are the causes of perineal tears?

MCQs

1. A second-degree perineal tear involves all the following EXCEPT
   a) Skin
   b) Vaginal mucosa
   c) Anal sphincter
   d) Perineal muscles

2. What is the characteristic sign of injury to the symphysis pubis?
   a) Suprapubic pain with difficulty in walking
   b) Hematoma
   c) Numbness
   d) Loss of consciousness

3. A woman complaining of giddiness and tender vulval swelling after an instrumental delivery should be managed with:
   a) Reassurance
   b) Immediate exploration of hematoma in the labour room
   c) Vaginal packing
   d) Exploration of hematoma under anesthesia

4. When more than 50% of the external anal sphincter is involved, the perineal tear is classified as:
   a) 3a degree
   b) 3b degree
   c) 3c degree
   d) Fourth degree

5. Which of the following is not a risk factor for fourth-degree perineal tears?
   a) Baby weight >4 Kg
   b) Shoulder dystocia
   c) Mediolateral episiotomy with perineal support
   d) Forceps delivery

6. Which of the following is not a risk factor for uterine rupture during labour?
   a) Previous myomectomy
   b) Previous cesarean
   c) Prematurity
   d) Obstructed labour

7. Cervical lacerations result in all except:
   a) Hemorrhage
   b) Abortions
   c) Amenorrhea
   d) Cervicitis

8. Which of the following is not a characteristic sign of uterine rupture?
   a) Maternal tachycardia
   b) Fetal heart rate abnormality

c) Hematuria
d) Hypertension

Answers

1. (c), 2. (a), 3. (d), 4. (b), 5. (c), 6. (c), 7. (c), 8. (d)

Fill in the blanks

1. The treatment for symphyseal separation is _____.
2. _____-degree perineal tears involve both external and internal anal sphincters and the anal mucosa.

Answers

1. immobilising the joints, 2. Fourth

Case scenario-based discussion

1. A 24-year-old para 1 delivered two hours ago. The labour was assisted by an episiotomy and ventouse because of occipitoposterior presentation. The baby weighed 3.6 Kg. The estimated blood loss was 350 mL. The episiotomy wound was sutured. Two hours later, the woman complains of perineal and rectal pain and feels dizzy while getting out of bed. Her pulse is 100 bpm and her BP is 90/70. The uterus is well-contracted.
   a) What is the next step in evaluating this woman?
   b) On examination, the labia majora on the right side is swollen, and there is a hematoma measuring 8 cm involving the labia and lower part of the vagina. What is your diagnosis and how would you manage this case?

Answers

a) Resuscitative measures should be undertaken for possible blood loss. As the uterus is well-contracted and since the woman has had an instrumental delivery, traumatic PPH should be considered. Immediate vaginal and rectal examination should be carried out.

b) The diagnosis is vulvovaginal hematoma. As this is a big hematoma, it should be explored under anesthesia. If the bleeding vessel is identified, it should be ligated. If the bleeding vessel is not identified after evacuating the blood clots, the space should be sutured with continuous locking sutures. Rectal examination should also be carried out to rule out extension into the ischiorectal space. Following the suturing, the vagina should be tightly packed.

Puerperal Infection and Other Postpartum Complications

Learning Objectives

» To discuss the causes of puerperal pyrexia and the evaluation and management of puerperal sepsis
» To know the management of postpartum breast complications
» To know the risk factors and preventive measures for deep vein thrombosis and pulmonary embolism
» To understand the psychological morbidity related to pregnancy

■ PUERPERAL PYREXIA

According to the International Classification of Diseases, puerperal pyrexia or postpartum fever is defined as a rise of temperature greater than 38°C (100.4°F) on any two occasions in the first 10 days following childbirth, miscarriage or termination of pregnancy excluding the first 24 hours. The most common cause of puerperal fever is puerperal sepsis, which complicates 5–7% of all deliveries. According to the WHO's estimates, puerperal sepsis accounts for 15% of the gross maternal mortality and causes at least 75,000 maternal deaths every year, mostly in developing countries.

Etiology

There are a number of causes of puerperal infection leading to puerperal pyrexia. Among these, infection of the genital tract after childbirth (puerperal sepsis) is the commonest cause of puerperal pyrexia.

Causes of fever that affect the general population such as viral fevers, malaria, tuberculosis, and respiratory infections could also cause puerperal pyrexia.

Causes of puerperal pyrexia
- Puerperal sepsis
- Infection of episiotomy wound, vagina or perineum
- Abdominal wound infection following cesarean section
- Urinary tract infection
- Mastitis, breast abscess
- Septic thrombophlebitis
- Respiratory complications such as pneumonia, atelectasis
- Meningitis following regional anesthesia

■ PUERPERAL SEPSIS

Puerperal sepsis refers to uterine infection following childbirth (puerperal infection). There are a number of risk factors that predispose a woman to puerperal sepsis. These factors may exist before delivery or may be related to labour and delivery (Table 49.1).

Table 49.1   Risk factors for puerperal sepsis

Pre-existing factors	• Low socio-economic status • Anemia, malnutrition • Diabetes, immune compromised state • Pre-existing genital infections—bacterial vaginosis, sexually transmitted infection, Group B *Streptococcus* infection • Poor hygiene • BMI >30
Risk factors related to labour and delivery	• Home birth in unhygienic conditions • Prolonged labour • Prolonged rupture of membranes • Multiple vaginal examinations • Operative vaginal delivery • Trauma to the genital tract • Cesarean section • PPH, manual removal of placenta • Retained placenta and membranes • Use of fetal scalp electrode • Droplet infection from caregivers and attendants

Infecting Organisms

The organisms responsible for puerperal infection are typically those that colonise the cervix, vagina and perineum. The trauma of labour allows these bacteria to multiply and cause clinical infection. The following organisms are most commonly implicated in puerperal sepsis:

- *Streptococcus* (groups A, B and D)

- *Staphylococcus aureus*
- Gram-negative bacteria like *Escherichia coli*, *Klebsiella* species and *Proteus* species
- *Peptococcus* and *Peptostreptococcus* species
- *Clostridium* species
- *Gardnerella vaginalis*
- *Chlamydia*

Pathogenesis

Devitalised tissue, trauma and the alkaline nature of lochia predispose to uterine infection, which starts as endometritis. The common routes of spread are the following:

- Direct spread along the endometrial surface
- Spread along the veins into the pelvic venous channels
- Spread along the lymphatics into the parametrial tissue
- Bloodborne transmission, leading to septicemia

The infection from the endometrium spreads along the lymphatics to the pelvic cellular tissue, resulting in parametritis. The infection can also spread to the tubes and ovaries, forming tubo-ovarian masses and abscesses. Pus may collect in the pouch of Douglas (POD)—this is known as a pelvic abscess. Untreated puerperal sepsis progresses to pelvic and generalised peritonitis. There may also be involvement of the veins, resulting in septic pelvic thrombophlebitis. When the infection spreads to the bloodstream, septicemia results, leading to endotoxic shock.

Grades of Puerperal Sepsis

- Grade I: Infection involving the lower genital tract and the uterus
- Grade II: Besides the uterus, the adnexa are also involved
- Grade III: Spread to the entire pelvic structures with pelvic peritonitis
- Grade IV: Spread to the upper abdomen (general peritonitis) and septicemia

Complications

Complications of puerperal sepsis include peritonitis, abscess formation, adnexal infection, the formation of tubo-ovarian masses (T–O mass), septic pelvic thrombophlebitis, septicemia and endotoxic shock.

- The spread of infection to the tubes and ovaries results in **salpingo-oophoritis** and **pelvic cellulitis**. This presents as severe abdominal pain, persistent or increasing temperature and a bilateral, or occasionally, unilateral mass palpable in the fornices.
- When pus collects in the POD, **pelvic abscess** results. If not drained, it may burst into the rectum, and the infection may spread to the inguinal region or retroperitoneally to the perinephric region. If the abscess bursts into the peritoneal cavity, it will result in generalised peritonitis.
- **Septicemia** develops due to gram-negative organisms such as *E. coli*, *Klebsiella*, *Proteus* and *Pseudomonas* releasing endotoxins from their cell walls. The released endotoxins and inflammatory mediators result in multi-organ failure and disseminated intravascular coagulation.
- **Septic pelvic thrombophlebitis** occurs very rarely following puerperal infection. This is a manifestation of severe infection with thrombi in the veins. In a woman who is being treated for puerperal sepsis, if the temperature does not decrease in response to effective antibiotic therapy, CT or MRI may be required to diagnose the involvement of the veins.
- Delayed complications are chronic pelvic infection, chronic pelvic pain and infertility.

Signs and Symptoms (Fig. 49.1)

- Whenever a woman presents with puerperal pyrexia, uterine infection should be suspected. The first indication of infection is a rise in temperature, usually on the third or fourth day after delivery. In the early stages of endometritis, there is low-grade fever, abdominal pain and uterine tenderness, and the lochia is unhealthy. Alteration in the nature of lochia is an indicator of sepsis; it can be easily seen on the sanitary pad and subsequently becomes foul-smelling.

While healthy lochia stains dark in the centre of the pad and lightly at the periphery, the reverse occurs with unhealthy lochia, i.e., there is dark staining at the periphery of the pad and light staining at the centre.

- With deeper and more widespread infection, there is high-grade fever, rigor and malaise. The uterus is tender. There will be tenderness in the iliac fossae if the adnexae are involved. The lochia is foul-smelling.
- In the event of the development of peritonitis or pelvic abscess formation, the woman looks toxic and besides fever and rigor, she has abdominal pain and bloating, often associated with diarrhea.
- Persistent fever with rigor indicates that the infection has spread into the systemic circulation. With the development of septicemia, the temperature is

initially high; there is tachycardia, the pulse is over 110, repeated rigor is present, and the woman looks toxic. With the release of endotoxin from the gram-negative organism, the temperature becomes subnormal, and there is hypotension. The woman then goes into endotoxic shock. A positive blood culture will confirm the diagnosis.

Examination

- The breast should be examined for engorgement and abscess.
- The neck should be examined for rigidity to rule out meningitis following regional anesthesia.
- The throat and chest should be examined for infections, especially following general anesthesia.
- The lower limbs should be examined for thrombophlebitis and deep vein thrombosis.
- Suprapubic and renal angle tenderness should be looked for to rule out urinary tract infection.
- On abdominal examination, for women who have undergone cesarean section, signs of wound infection should be looked for. The abdomen should be palpated for the presence of organomegaly. In the presence of peritonitis, there would be abdominal distension, guarding and rigidity.
- On local examination, there may be purulent vaginal discharge with infected lacerations in the perineum; the episiotomy wound may show wound breakdown with necrotic edges.
- A pelvic examination is carried out to look for infected vaginal and perineal tears, to note the colour of the lochia and to look for subinvolution and tenderness of the uterus. With the involvement of the adnexa, forniceal tenderness may be present. In such cases, the movement of the cervix will be painful due to parametritis. There may be bilateral adnexal masses.
- When there is a pelvic abscess formation, a boggy swelling can be felt through the posterior fornix, which is well appreciated by rectal examination.

Laboratory Investigations

Evaluation of puerperal pyrexia
- Complete blood count for total count and ESR
- High vaginal swab for culture
- Blood culture (in cases of suspected septicemia)
- Urine analysis for pus cells, culture and antibiotic sensitivity
- Wound cultures (in case of wound sepsis)
- Renal function test, serum electrolytes
- Coagulation studies

- In areas where typhoid, malaria and other fevers are prevalent, investigations to rule out these may have to be carried out
- USG would be required to diagnose retained placental bits, adnexal masses and pelvic abscess
- Venous Doppler, CT and MRI are indicated if deep vein thrombosis and pelvic vein thrombosis are suspected

Management

General measures

- General measures include bed rest, adequate fluid intake and control of temperature with antipyretics and tepid sponging. The woman should be given supportive therapy and her urine output should be monitored.
- When the infection is severe or if there is evidence of peritonitis, intravenous fluid resuscitation is required.
- Local wound cleaning should be done.

Antibiotic therapy

Antibiotics should be started immediately after collecting the necessary swabs for culture. A broad-spectrum antibiotic is given to cover both aerobic and anaerobic organisms.

- When there is a mild infection following a vaginal delivery, amoxicillin with clavulanic acid and metronidazole are used by the oral or parenteral route. Alternatively, cephalosporins such as cefotaxime can be used.
- When the infection is moderate to severe following a vaginal delivery or in case of any infection following cesarean section, it is important to give parenteral therapy with higher antibiotics such as a combination of piperacillin and tazobactam. In MRSA-positive cases, vancomycin may be given. The combination of clindamycin and gentamicin plus ampicillin is another commonly used regimen for patients with severe infection or infection following cesarean section.
- Antibiotics are continued for 7–10 days in cases of mild infection. For moderate to severe infection, parenteral therapy should be continued at least for another 48 hours after the temperature has become normal. When the blood culture is positive, parenteral therapy should be continued for two weeks.

Other measures

- Retained products should be removed 24 hours after antibiotic cover has been instituted.
- Pelvic abscess is drained by colpotomy.

- Infected perineal wounds should be treated, the sutures should be removed, and the infected wound opened and drained.
- Heparin is required if the diagnosis is septic thrombophlebitis.

Improvement is usually seen within 48–72 hours of initiating antibiotic therapy. If fever persists despite antibiotic therapy, the woman should be evaluated for other sources of infection such as pelvic abscess, infected hematomas, septic thrombophlebitis and other non-pelvic causes of fever.

> In any woman with postpartum fever, puerperal sepsis should be the primary diagnosis unless proved otherwise.

Prevention

- Prophylactic antibiotics should be given to all women undergoing a cesarean section.
- Aseptic precautions should be observed with adequate hand washing, restricting the number of vaginal examinations and minimising tissue trauma.
- Post-delivery cleanliness is very important.

An algorithm for the evaluation of puerperal pyrexia is presented in Fig. 49.1.

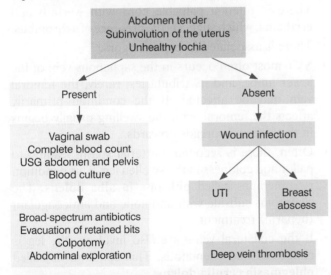

Fig. 49.1 Evaluation of puerperal pyrexia

OTHER POSTPARTUM COMPLICATIONS

■ MASTITIS AND BREAST ABSCESS

Mastitis

Mastitis is an inflammatory condition of the breast that usually occurs during the first six weeks postpartum but can occur at any time during lactation. Risk factors for mastitis include maternal age above 30 years, sore and cracked nipples and a history of mastitis in the previous pregnancy. Breast engorgement, blocked lactiferous ducts and milk stasis also contribute to the development of mastitis.

Etiology

- The most common causative microorganism is *Staphylococcus aureus*; infections caused by methicillin-resistant *Staphylococcus aureus* (MRSA) are on the rise.
- Rarely, other organisms such as *Escherichia coli* and *Haemophilus influenzae* are also implicated.
- The organism is transmitted to the mother's breast from the child's nasopharynx through the milk ducts or from the mother's skin, from where they gain entry through cracked or fissured nipples.

Clinical features

- Puerperal mastitis presents with acute-onset maternal fever (100.4°F or higher), chills, myalgia, malaise and breast tenderness with associated erythema.
- Mastitis is most commonly unilateral. On examination of the breast, the erythema is segmental, usually in the upper, outer quadrant, with variable degrees of induration and tenderness.
- If a palpable, fluctuant mass is felt, breast abscess should be suspected and confirmed by ultrasound.
- Culture of the breast milk is not carried out routinely. It may be indicated when there is recurrent mastitis.

Treatment

- The treatment of breastfeeding women with mastitis includes early antibiotic therapy, regular emptying of the breasts and local comfort measures. As the majority of *S. aureus* are penicillin-resistant, penicillinase-resistant penicillin antimicrobial agents such as dicloxacillin, amoxicillin or first-generation cephalosporins can be used. Erythromycin and vancomycin are appropriate choices for women who have a penicillin allergy. Antibiotic therapy should be continued for 10–14 days to avoid the development of resistant organisms.
- Women who have mastitis should be instructed to continue breastfeeding; consideration should be given either to increasing the frequency of feeds or manually emptying the breast between feeds. Continued breastfeeding is not harmful to the infant. In fact, women who wean or decrease feeding during an episode of mastitis have a higher risk of developing a breast abscess.

- Analgesics such as ibuprofen or acetaminophen may be taken for symptomatic relief. Increased fluid intake and adequate nutrition should be encouraged. Either cold or warm compresses may be used for pain relief.

Breast Abscess

- Breast abscess can develop when there is a delay in initiating antibiotic treatment or inadequate emptying of the breast in the presence of mastitis.
- Once breast abscess is suspected, one should not wait for the appearance of fluctuation before opening it as delay may cause the destruction of breast tissue.
- When in doubt, USG of the breast can be taken.
- During incision and drainage, all loculations should be opened, and biopsy of the abscess wall should be considered to rule out rare cases of carcinoma. The pus should be sent for culture and sensitivity.
- Antibiotic therapy should be continued.
- In abscesses involving the parenchyma, there is segmental involvement. Therefore, the incisions should radiate outwards from the nipple so as to open up any pockets or lobules that are distended with the suppurating material.
- The resulting cavity should be loosely packed with gauze, which should be removed after 24 hours.
- Efficient drainage should be ensured after evacuation.
- If there is an abscess behind the areola, it is best opened towards the lower and outer quadrant and also at any spot where the pus points.

▌ VENOUS COMPLICATIONS IN THE PUERPERIUM

Venous complications in the puerperium comprise thrombophlebitis, deep vein thrombosis and pulmonary embolism.

Thrombophelebitis

Inflammation and infection may involve the venous channels of the pelvis or the lower limbs, leading to thrombus formation.

- **Septic pelvic thrombophlebitis:** Bacterial infection usually begins at the placental site, causing myometrial venous thrombosis before spreading to the ovarian veins. The clot may extend to the inferior vena cava or the left renal vein. The clinical manifestation includes persistent high fever with chills despite antibiotic therapy and abdominal pain. The diagnosis may be confirmed by either CT or MRI imaging. The addition of heparin to the antimicrobial therapy may improve the outcome.

- **Superficial vein thrombophlebitis of the lower limb:** Superficial vein thrombophlebitis (SVT, also known as superficial venous thrombosis) refers to thrombus formation in a superficial vein of the leg and inflammation in the tissue surrounding the vein. It is infective in origin.

Etiology

- The primary source of infection is the uterus.
- Anaerobic streptococci are commonly involved.
- The risk factors include anemia, varicose veins and thrombophilic disorders.
- The infection occurs by direct spread from adjacent cellulitis or by retrograde spread from pelvic thrombophlebitis.
- Embolism is uncommon in this condition because the thrombi are adherent to the vein walls as a result of infection.

Clinical features

- Superficial thrombophlebitis is characterised by pain, tenderness, induration and/or erythema in a superficial vein.
- There is often a palpable cord with warmth and erythema, which suggests the presence of a thrombus.
- There is associated fever with rigors.
- SVT most often occurs in the saphenous vein of the lower limbs, and its tributaries; rarely, the femoral vein may be affected. If the condition primarily affects the femoral vein, the swelling usually begins in the foot and spreads upwards.
- Often, there is secondary arterial spasm leading to pallor and coldness in the swollen leg. This condition is sometimes called **phlegmasia alba dolens**. The symptoms subside with antibiotic and anticoagulant (heparin) treatment.
- If the collateral veins are also involved, the leg is congested and edematous. This condition is called **phlegmasia cerulia dolens**.

Venous Thromboembolism (VTE) in Pregnancy and the Puerperium

Venous thromboembolism (VTE) includes deep vein thrombosis (DVT) and pulmonary embolism (PE). During pregnancy and the puerperium, women are at an increased risk of venous thromboembolism (VTE). During normal pregnancy, the concentrations of the clotting factors fibrinogen VII and VIII and von Willebrand IX, X and XII are all increased, resulting in a hypercoagulable state, which exposes pregnant women to an increased risk of thrombosis. Moreover, the mechanical obstruction produced by the growing uterus compromises venous outflow and subsequently increases the susceptibility of pregnant and postpartum women to developing thromboembolisms. Pregnant women are at an approximately 5-fold increased risk of VTE compared to non-pregnant women. The risk of VTE increases further (to ≥20-fold) in the puerperium and remains high until approximately 12 weeks postpartum. Pregnancy-related VTE is a major cause of maternal mortality in developed countries and accounts for about 10% of maternal deaths in the developed world. It is being reported more commonly in developing countries also.

The risk factors for VTE in pregnancy and the puerperium are presented in Table 49.2.

Table 49.2 Risk factors for VTE

Pre-existing	New onset
• Previous VTE • Congenital thrombophilia with antithrombin deficiency, protein C or protein S deficiency, factor V Leiden mutation • Acquired thrombophilia—APLA • Age >35 years • BMI >30 • Gross varicose veins • Anemia • Paraplegia • Sickle cell disease, polycythemia or nephrotic syndrome	• Hyperemesis, dehydration • Severe infection—puerperal sepsis, pyelonephritis • Prolonged immobility after delivery • Pre-eclampsia • Prolonged labour • Postpartum hemorrhage

Prevention

Since the mortality associated with VTE is very high, it is important to take preventive measures as soon as possible after delivery in the following situations:

- In the absence of previous VTE or thrombophilia, if two or more of the risk factors mentioned in Table 49.2 are present, the woman should be given low-molecular-weight heparin (LMWH) for 3–5 days postpartum.
- Women who have inherited thrombophilia or previous VTE should be given LMWH for 6 weeks postpartum.
- In women with acquired thrombophilia, LMWH may be offered for 3–5 days postpartum.

Currently, LMWH is recommended for prophylaxis as well as for the treatment of DVT and PE. The commonly used drugs are:
- Inj. enoxaparin 40–60 mg daily depending on the woman's weight
- Inj. dalteparin (Fragmin) 5,000–6,000 units daily depending on the woman's weight

Other preventive measures

- Other preventive measures are the correction of anemia and sepsis; the prevention of dehydration and early mobility.
- When there is previous history of VTE/thrombophilia, graduated elastic compression stockings should be used throughout pregnancy and for 6–12 weeks after delivery.
- While travelling by air, pregnant women should be advised to maintain adequate hydration. There may be a place for low-dose aspirin for the duration of travel.
- Prophylactic anticoagulant should be given when there is prolonged immobilisation.

Deep Vein Thrombosis (DVT)

DVT begins in the deep veins of the calf or soles of the feet and extends upwards. In the early stages, DVT can be easily missed. If it remains undiagnosed and untreated, 15–24% of these patients will develop pulmonary embolism, which is fatal.

Clinical features

- The symptoms and signs of DVT include leg pain and swelling (usually unilateral), tenderness on palpation and lower abdominal pain (reflecting extension of thrombus into the pelvic vessels and/or development of collateral circulation), often on the left side.
- Sharp dorsiflexion of the foot elicits pain in the calf. This is termed the **Homans' sign**. However, it may not be demonstrated in all cases.
- There may be a slight rise in temperature and pulse rate, with no obvious cause, usually on the 7–10th day of the puerperium.
- These early signs are very often missed. The condition may first manifest when pulmonary embolism occurs or when generalised edema of the leg sets in.

Diagnosis

- Compression duplex ultrasound is the primary diagnostic test for DVT.

- When iliac vein thrombosis is suspected (back and buttock pain and swelling of the entire limb), Doppler ultrasound of the iliac vein and magnetic resonance venography should be carried out.

Pulmonary Embolism (PE)

Symptoms

The symptoms of PE include dyspnea, chest pain, hemoptysis, cough, pink and frothy sputum and collapse. In massive embolisms, death occurs within a few minutes.

> In any woman presenting with unexplained collapse or respiratory distress in the puerperal period, pulmonary embolism should be suspected.

Laboratory investigations

- In women presenting with symptoms and signs of an acute PE, an electrocardiogram (ECG) and a chest X-ray (CXR) should be performed.
- In women with suspected PE without symptoms and signs of DVT, a ventilation/perfusion (V/Q) lung scan or a computerised tomography pulmonary angiogram (CTPA) should be performed.
- Blood gas analysis and echocardiogram are other helpful investigations.

Management

- The initial management of DVT consists of elevating the leg and using a graduated elastic compression stocking to reduce the edema. Mobilisation with graduated elastic compression stockings should be encouraged. Antibiotics should be prescribed to prevent infection.
- Consideration should be given to the use of a temporary inferior vena cava filter in the peripartum period for women with iliac vein VTE to reduce the risk of PE.
- Anticoagulant therapy is the mainstay of management in VTE.

In the management of DVT, therapeutic doses of subcutaneous LMWH should be employed during the remainder of the pregnancy and for at least 6 weeks postnatally. These drugs can be used by breastfeeding women. In the management of pulmonary embolism, intravenous unfractionated heparin is the preferred initial treatment with a loading dose of 80 units/Kg, followed by a continuous intravenous infusion of 18 units/Kg/hour. The activated partial thromboplastin time (APTT) is measured periodically to maintain the APTT level at 1.5–2.5 times the average laboratory control value.

PUERPERAL PSYCHIATRIC MORBIDITY

During the puerperal period, postpartum mothers are vulnerable to psychological disturbances. Nearly 85% of women experience some type of mood disturbance. For most of these women, the symptoms are mild and short-lived. However, 10–15% of women develop more significant symptoms of depression or anxiety. Postpartum psychiatric illness is typically divided into three classes, which are as follows:

A. Postpartum blues
B. Postpartum depression
C. Postpartum psychosis

The mood changes and psychiatric morbidity following delivery have been attributed to abrupt changes in cortisol, oxytocin, endorphins, thyroxine, progesterone and estrogen levels. It has been suggested that the sudden decrease in estrogen in the postpartum period triggers a hypersensitivity of certain dopamine receptors, which may be responsible for the severe mood disturbance in the postpartum period. Fatigue after labour and delivery, caring for a newborn that requires 24/7 attention, sleep deprivation, the lack of support from family and friends, financial stress, marital/relationship strain and caring for premature or sick infants may be contributory factors.

Postpartum Blues

Postpartum blues is a very common but self-limiting condition that begins shortly after childbirth and lasts up to two weeks in duration. The symptoms include tearfulness or crying 'for no reason', mood swings, irritability, anxiety, loss of appetite and sleep and fatigue. The symptoms are mild and do not affect daily activities. Treatment is supportive, including ensuring adequate sleep and emotional support. If symptoms are severe enough to affect daily functioning or last longer than two weeks, the individual should be evaluated for postpartum depression.

Postpartum Depression

Between 10 and 15% of women suffer from some form of depression in the first year after the delivery of their baby. The recurrence rate of postnatal depression in subsequent pregnancies could be as high as 50%. Symptoms of severe postnatal depressive disorder include early morning wakening, poor appetite, low energy and libido, loss of enjoyment, lack of interest, impaired concentration, tearfulness, feelings of guilt and failure, thoughts of self-harm/suicide and thoughts of harming the baby. The Edinburgh Postnatal Depression Scale (EPDS) is available to screen for postnatal depression. The adverse sequelae of postnatal depressive illness are suicide/infanticide, prolonged psychiatric morbidity, psychiatric morbidity in the child and marital breakdown. Tricyclic antidepressants or selective serotonin reuptake inhibitors (SSRIs) are appropriate for treatment. A psychiatrist should be involved in every stage of management.

Puerperal Psychosis

This is a severe and acute mental disorder that develops in the early postnatal period. It affects between 1:500 and 1:1,000 women. It manifests between the 5th day and 4 weeks postpartum with an abrupt onset. The symptoms include restlessness, agitation, crying spells, fear, suspicion, delusions and hallucinations and thoughts of self-harm. The sequelae are suicide, infanticide, homicidal thoughts and marital/family problems. Puerperal psychosis should be treated as a medical emergency and an urgent referral to a psychiatrist should be made. Usually, such patients require admission to a psychiatric unit. They are treated with antipsychotics such as chlorpromazine or haloperidol and mood stabilisers such as lithium carbonate. Breastfeeding is contraindicated in a case of puerperal psychosis, especially during lithium treatment.

CEREBRAL VENOUS AND SINUS THROMBOSIS (CVT)

Pregnancy and the immediate postpartum period are associated with a significant increase in the risk of cerebral venous thrombosis due to the hypercoagulable state of pregnancy. Contributing factors for the occurrence of CVT are infection, cesarean section, obesity, prolonged bed rest, anemia, pre-eclampsia/eclampsia and dehydration in the postpartum period. Most commonly, the superior sagittal and transverse sinuses are affected. This condition is associated with headache, seizures, visual disturbances, altered consciousness and focal neurological findings such as hemiparesis or aphasia. The majority of cases manifest in the second postpartum week. CT scan remains the first imaging modality. CVT is treated with anticonvulsants, anti-edema measures and anticoagulants.

POSTPARTUM PITUITARY NECROSIS OR SHEEHAN SYNDROME

This is a rare condition in which there is necrosis of the anterior pituitary following hemorrhagic shock due to PPH/APH. The degree of ischemic necrosis is proportional to the amount of blood loss, sludging and thrombosis of the vessels supplying the anterior pituitary. The presence of 15–20% of pituitary tissue is compatible with normal endocrine function. When the anterior pituitary is destroyed more than this, severe clinical symptoms of panhypopituitarism results, which manifests as decreased gonadotrophic activity, decreased corticotrophic activity, decreased thyrotrophic activity and decreased somatotrophic hormones.

Clinical Features

- The first symptom is failure to lactate. The patient is apathetic with prominent asthenia and lethargy; hypothyroidism, decreased insulin tolerance and frequent attacks of hypoglycemia develop.
- Adrenal cortical failure is indicated by the loss of pubic and axillary hair, decrease in skin pigmentation and decreased sweating.
- The woman becomes anemic due to the deficiency of pituitary erythropoietin; there is weight loss and atrophy of breast and genital organs. This presentation is collectively called '**pituitary cachexia**'. If not recognised, even death can occur due to severe hypotension and hypoglycemia.
- Whenever there is a failure of lactation, the evaluation of thyroid and adrenal function is of paramount importance. Serum gonadotropin and gonadal steroid levels are typically low in hypopituitarism.

Management

- The woman should be treated with a maintenance dose of thyroxine, corticosteroids and HRT.
- These women need exogenous pulsatile GnRH if pregnancy is desired.
- The individual should be provided with a medical alert bracelet to alert physicians as to the need for additional corticosteroids at times of stress.

KEY POINTS

✓ Puerperal sepsis is defined as a postpartum infection of the genital tract.

✓ The causes of puerperal fever include genital tract infection, breast engorgement, mastitis, urinary tract infection, thrombophlebitis and other intercurrent infections.

✓ The organisms responsible for puerperal infection are usually the normal inhabitants of the vagina, which become pathogenic in the presence of damaged tissues.

✓ The complications of puerperal sepsis include salphingo-oophoritis, pelvic abscess, peritonitis, septic pelvic thrombophlebitis and septicemia.

✓ The commonest organism responsible for breast abscess is Staphylococcus aureus.

✓ In women with past history of VTE or thrombophilia, thromboprophylaxis should be given for 6 weeks postpartum.

✓ Postpartum blues are mild and short-lived and usually disappear in two weeks.

✓ The first symptom of postpartum pituitary necrosis is a failure of lactation.

Essay questions

1. Discuss are the causes of puerperal fever. How would you manage a case of puerperal sepsis?
2. Discuss the prevention and management of deep vein thrombosis.

Short answer questions

1. Define puerperal sepsis.
2. What are the risk factors for deep vein thrombosis?
3. Describe Homans' sign.
4. What is Sheehan syndrome?
5. Write a short note on breast abscess.
6. What are the predisposing factors for puerperal sepsis?
7. What is phlegmasia alba dolens?
8. Describe postpartum blues.

MCQs

1. Which of the following is the most common causative organism of acute mastitis?
   a) *Staphylococcus aureus*
   b) *Escherichia coli*
   c) *Streptococcus*
   d) *Proteus*

2. Puerperal infection can be caused by:
   a) Unclean delivery
   b) Prolonged rupture of the membranes
   c) Multiple digital vaginal examinations
   d) All of the above

3. Which of the following is the mode of treatment of breast abscesses?
   a) Incision and drainage at the earliest
   b) Incision and drainage after the appearance of fluctuation
   c) Cessation of breastfeeding
   d) Antibiotics

4. The first symptom of Sheehan syndrome is:
   a) Failure of lactation
   b) Subinvolution of the uterus
   c) Loss of axillary and pubic hair
   d) Cold intolerance

5. Which of these is not a recognised complication of puerperal infection?
   a) Endotoxic shock
   b) Future infertility

   c) Neonatal sepsis
   d) Increased BP

6. The most common organism causing thrombophlebitis following puerperal infection is:
   a) Anerobic *Streptococcus*
   b) *Escherichia coli*
   c) *Chlamydia trachomatis*
   d) *Gardnerella vaginalis*

7. Which is not true of cerebral venous thrombosis?
   a) Affects lateral or superior sagittal sinus
   b) Presents as headache and fits
   c) Seen after 30 days of delivery
   d) Anticonvulsants, antimicrobials and anticoagulants are required

8. Sheehan syndrome is characterised by all except:
   a) Failure of lactation
   b) Amenorrhea
   c) Hypertension
   d) Genital atrophy

Answers
1. (a), 2. (d), 3. (a), 4. (a), 5. (d), 6. (a), 7. (c), 8. (c)

Fill in the blanks

1. Cerebral venous thrombosis usually involves the _____.
2. Ischemic necrosis of the anterior lobe of the pituitary is called _____.

Answers
1. lateral or superior sagittal sinus, 2. Sheehan syndrome

Case scenario-based discussion

1. A 27-year-old para 1 had a vaginal delivery at home 4 days ago. The delivery was conducted by a *dai*. The baby cried after stimulation. The woman had leakage per vaginum for 2 days prior to the onset of labour pains. Now she complains of high-grade fever for two days with foul-smelling discharge from the vagina. Her temperature is 102ºF.
   a) What is the diagnosis?
   b) How is puerperal sepsis diagnosed?
   c) What is the further course of action?
   d) If, on examination, there is only uterine tenderness and no forniceal masses, how would you treat this woman?

Answers
a) This is a case of puerperal pyrexia, probably due to puerperal sepsis.
b) Given that the woman was leaking PV for 2 days prior to delivery and that the delivery was conducted at home by a *dai*, there is a strong

possibility of infection. Moreover, besides fever, the woman is also complaining of foul-smelling vaginal discharge. All these indicate puerperal sepsis.

c) A detailed examination should be carried out—systemic examination to rule out other causes of pyrexia, abdominal examination for tenderness, guarding and rigidity and pelvic examination for tears, subinvolution of uterus and uterine and forniceal tenderness and rectal examination for the presence of pelvic abscess. Swabs should be collected for culture and sensitivity; urine analysis and complete hemogram should be ordered.

The woman also needs a USG pelvis to rule out retained placenta, pelvic abscess and adnexal masses.

d) The woman's temperature should be controlled with antipyretics. Fluid balance should be maintained. Antibiotics should be started immediately without waiting for the results. The prescribed antibiotic should cover both aerobic and anerobic organisms. The preferred antibiotic would be amoxicillin with clavulanic acid and metronidazole and should be given for 7–10 days.

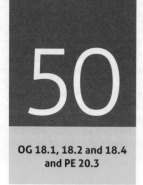

50

OG 18.1, 18.2 and 18.4 and PE 20.3

Resuscitation and Examination of the Newborn

Learning Objectives

» To be able to identify babies needing resuscitation
» To perform resuscitation in the appropriate sequence
» To know how to provide essential newborn care at birth

RESUSCITATION

The most important event after birth is to establish spontaneous respiration. In utero, the placenta supplies the necessary nutrients and oxygen to the fetus and removes fetal waste products. Soon after birth, when the baby is separated from the mother, the baby must breathe on its own to supply adequate oxygen to the vital organs of the body.

Failure to breathe at birth occurs due to perinatal events. If this is prolonged, it leads to hypoxic damage to the brain. Perinatal asphyxia is one of the most important causes of death within the first seven days of life. Significant asphyxia also leads to long-term neurodevelopmental abnormalities like cerebral palsy and global developmental delays. Hence, all deliveries should be treated as medical emergencies, and trained personnel should be available for all high-risk deliveries.

Though most babies establish spontaneous respiration at birth, approximately 3–10% of babies need some help (resuscitation) at birth.

It is advisable to start resuscitation as per the algorithm presented in Fig. 50.2 soon after birth in any apneic baby. Apgar scores are not useful in the context of resuscitation, as these measures should be started at birth without waiting to assign an Apgar score.

Delivery Room Preparation

The minimum preparation for any delivery should include the following:

- A resuscitation kit should be kept ready.
- All equipment should be checked and prepared for use; a suitable team should be organised.
- Additional help should be called for if necessary.
- A pre-resuscitation checklist should be referred to.
- The delivery room should be clean and warm (26–28°C).

- Resuscitation equipment should be checked during every shift.
- Fans should be switched off to avoid cold draughts.
- All members of staff should wash their hands with soap and water before entering the labour room or nursery and before making any attempt at resuscitation.
- Universal precautions for asepsis should be taken for all deliveries.

Apart from these measures, the maternal, obstetric and family history should be reviewed by the attending doctor to anticipate complications. The following details should be determined:

- Outcome of previous pregnancies
- Gestational age and fetal assessment
- Results of fetal growth monitoring and fetal size
- Evidence of fetal maturity and any malformations
- Current status of maternal complications and details of fetal intrapartum monitoring

All deliveries should be attended by healthcare personnel trained in resuscitation; this includes the knowledge of how to provide intermittent positive pressure ventilation (IPPV) and the indications and procedure for intubation, chest compression and administration of drugs. In uncomplicated preterm birth, delayed cord clamping (DCC) should be attempted for a minimum of 60 seconds after delivery. DCC must be done even if the mother has an HIV infection.

Steps Involved in Resuscitation

Maintenance of temperature

Immediately after delivery, the baby should be placed on the mother's abdomen, dried thoroughly with a prewarmed towel, covered with another dry, prewarmed towel and then moved up so that it lies on the mother's chest, between her breasts. A wet baby loses heat rapidly. Drying with prewarmed towels reduces this evaporative heat loss. It is recommended that the baby be received under a preheated radiant warmer only if resuscitation is necessary.

Suctioning

If the baby is a 'vigorous baby' (one with strong respiratory efforts, heart rate >100 bpm and a good muscle tone), no suctioning of the oropharynx or the trachea is required. Non-vigorous and apneic babies require resuscitation and hence, should be moved and placed under a preheated radiant warmer.

> In vigorous babies, routine suctioning should not be done even if the liquor is meconium-stained.

- The baby is placed in a supine position with its neck slightly extended by placing a shoulder roll under the shoulders to ensure a straight airway.
- Secretions may be removed from the airway by wiping the nose and mouth with a towel or by suctioning with a mucus extractor or suction catheter.
- In all non-vigorous babies, oropharyngeal suctioning should be done to ensure a clear airway before applying positive pressure ventilation.
- If suctioning is done, the mouth should be suctioned before the nose to avoid any aspiration of the contents in case the baby gasps while the nose is being suctioned. The neonate's mouth may be suctioned gently to remove excess mucus or blood (Fig. 50.1).
- Vigorous suctioning of the posterior pharynx is harmful, produces significant reflex bradycardia and may damage the oral mucosa, which may result in difficulty in sucking later. Care must be taken to ensure that the suction pressure does not exceed 100 mmHg.

Ventilation

The normal newborn breathes within seconds of delivery and establishes regular respiration within a minute of delivery. The baby needs positive pressure ventilation in the following scenarios:

- The baby is apneic or gasping
- The fetal heart rate is less than 100

Before applying positive pressure ventilation, the airway should be cleared, and the head should be placed in a sniffing position with the help of a shoulder roll. IPPV is performed using an appropriately-sized Ambu bag and face mask. The face mask should cover the chin, mouth and nose and should be sealed tightly over the baby's using the 'C' grip with the thumb and index finger of the left hand. Most babies respond to bag-and-mask ventilation, though it may be difficult sometimes in premature babies with non-compliant lungs. Initial

lung inflation may require 30–40 cm H_2O with room air and subsequent breaths may need 15–20 cm H_2O given at the rate of 40–60 per minute.

Indications for intubation

- Antenatally diagnosed congenital diaphragmatic hernia
- Depressed newborn with a history of meconium-stained liquor
- For the administration of drugs through endotracheal (ET) tube
- Prolonged bag-and-mask ventilation or ineffective ventilation with bag and mask

Chest compression

- If the heart rate does not increase to more than 60 per minute after effective ventilation for 30 seconds, chest compression is required along with positive pressure ventilation at the rate of 90 compressions and 30 ventilations (3:1).
- The chest is compressed on the lower third of the sternum to a depth of one-third of the chest diameter. If there is no response after 30 seconds despite this, drug therapy should be initiated.
- It is important to have two persons attending to chest compression as compression should be simultaneously assisted with bag-and-mask ventilation. The person performing the chest compression should have uninterrupted access to the chest to place her fingers over the chest correctly for efficient compression. The person providing ventilatory support should be positioned at the head end.
- There are two techniques for performing chest compression. The most common one is the '**thumb technique**', where both the thumbs are used to depress the sternum, while the hands encircle the torso and the fingers support the spine. The other is the **two-finger technique**.

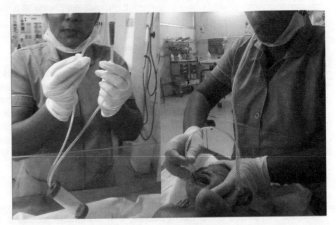

Fig. 50.1 Dee Lee mucus extractor

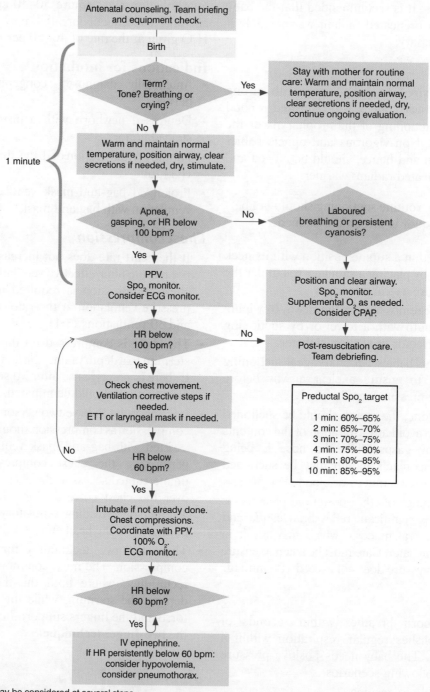

Fig. 50.2 Neonatal resuscitation flowchart, 2020 update (NRP India Guidelines, Ministry of Health and Family Welfare)

A few salient changes that have been incorporated in the Neonatal Resuscitation guidelines by AAP/AHA in 2015, 2017 and 2021 are as follows:

— The colour and meconium staining of liquor have been removed from the initial assessment.

— Routine suctioning of the oropharynx and airway is not recommended soon after birth in vigorous babies even if it is meconium-stained.

— Routine intubation for tracheal suctioning is not recommended when there is meconium-stained liquor.

— Rubbing the newborn's back, trunk or extremities is preferred over flicking the soles of the feet for stimulation.

— When IPPV is required, room air with 21% oxygen is preferred over 100% oxygen to initiate IPPV; oxygen delivery is subsequently increased based on the baby's response and pulse oximeter reading.

— When IPPV is needed in preterm babies, oxygen is delivered starting with 21–30% and gradually increased based on targeted preductal oxygen saturation.

— Whenever chest compression is performed, the recommendation is to use 100% oxygen.

— If IPPV is needed for preterm babies, it is preferable to use a device that can provide positive-end expiratory pressure (PEEP). This is done using the T-piece resuscitator device.

— For chest compressions, the two-thumb technique is preferred over the two-finger technique.

ASSESSMENT OF NEWBORN AT BIRTH

After initial resuscitation and stabilisation (Fig. 50.2), the baby should be examined thoroughly to determine the level of care required for any systemic abnormality, congenital malformations, weight and gestational age.

The routine examination of newborns includes the following:
- General physical examination, which includes a head-to-toe examination
- Recording of vital parameters (heart rate, respiratory rate, colour, temperature, oxygen saturation)
- Gestational age assessment
- Any kind of malformation
- Signs of respiratory distress, presence of any murmur, any stigmata of intrauterine infection, hepatosplenomegaly

Apgar Score

Though the Apgar score has lost its importance as 'the measure' to assess neonatal condition, it is still a useful tool to make a rapid assessment of the condition of the newborn, particularly in places where access to qualified/trained staff and facilities is not always available. For this reason, the Apgar score is recorded for every baby, at one and five minutes after birth. Scores of 0–2 are assigned each of the following parameters—heart rate, respiration, muscle tone, reflex response and colour. The Apgar scoring system is presented in Table 50.1.

- The Apgar score is useful for describing the status of the neonate at birth and his subsequent adaptation to the extrauterine environment. It should be recorded 1 and 5 minutes after birth. If the score is less than 7, scores should be assigned every 5 minutes for up to 20 minutes (extended Apgar scoring).

Though there is no uniform definition of asphyxia, a score of less than 6 at 1 minute suggests asphyxia of some degree.

- The WHO defines asphyxia as a failure to initiate and sustain breathing at birth. The National Neonatology Forum of India (NNF) uses a score of 4–6 with slow gasping breathing to define moderate asphyxia and a score of 0–3 with no respiratory efforts to define severe asphyxia.

Table 50.1 Apgar scoring system

Sign	0	1	2
Heart rate	Absent	Below 100 beats/min	Over 100 beats/min
Respiration	Absent	Slow/gasping	Good cry
Muscle tone	Flaccid	Some flexion	Active motion of the extremities; Grimace and withdraw
Colour	Blue or pale	Body is pink, extremities are blue	Completely pink

- In compromised clinical situations, the time taken for the successful establishment of respiration and/or colour should be noted. If more than 5 minutes are required to establish spontaneous breathing, it should be labelled as severe asphyxia; if the time taken is less than 5 minutes, it is considered to be moderate asphyxia.
- ACOG and the American Academy of Pediatrics have proposed that the term perinatal asphyxia be reserved for an infant who manifests all of the following:
  — Umbilical cord artery pH of <7.0 with a base deficit of >12 mEq/L
  — Apgar score <3 at 5 minutes
  — Neonatal neurological manifestations suggestive of hypoxic–ischemic encephalopathy (HIE)
  — Evidence of multi-organ dysfunction (e.g., cardiovascular, gastrointestinal, hematological, pulmonary or renal system)

Meconium-staining of liquor, non-reassuring fetal heart rate patterns, low 1-minute Apgar score and prolonged labour in the absence of encephalopathy and seizures have no predictive value for long-term injury or cerebral palsy.

Babies Who Need Special Care

- Babies <35–37 weeks old
- Babies who weigh <1.8–2 Kg
- Babies who have perinatal asphyxia or respiratory distress
- Small-for-gestational-age (SGA) babies <2 SD
- Babies born to diabetic mothers
- Babies who have hypoglycemia
- Babies who have suspected sepsis/meningitis
- Babies who have seizures
- Babies who have major congenital malformations

Assessment of Gestational Age

The correct gestational age should be assigned to every newborn; it is important to counsel the parents for the following reasons:

- Neurological examination depends on gestational age
- Complications depend on gestational age

There are various methods available for the accurate assessment of gestational age. The **New Ballard Score** (NBS) is a widely accepted method of assessing gestation. This score is dependent on two major criteria—physical parameters and neurological parameters. The major advantages of the NBS are that this score can be used for extremely preterm babies as the lowest score denotes 20 weeks of gestation. Moreover, this score can be applied to sick and even ventilated neonates as none of the parameters require any gross movement of the baby.

Classification of Newborns as per Gestational Age

- Early preterm: Less than 34 weeks (237 days)
- Preterm: Less than 37 weeks, that is, birth occurs at the end of the last day of the 37th week (259 days)
- Term: 37–41 weeks (259–293 days)
  - Early term: Born between 37 0/7 and 38 6/7 weeks (259–272 days)
  - Full term: Born between 39 0/7 and 40 6/7 weeks
  - Late term: Born between 41 0/7 and 41 6/7 weeks
- Post-term: Born after 42 weeks or more

■ ESSENTIAL NEWBORN CARE

Babies who are stable and do not require shifting to any special care area should be given to the mother so that she can provide skin-to-skin care. This maintains the infant's temperature better and improves successful breastfeeding rates.

Breastfeeding

- The baby should be put directly to the breast and fed within half an hour of birth.
- The mother should be counselled about the advantages of breastfeeding in the antenatal period (optimal nutrition, growth and developmental advantages, protective role against infection, etc.).

- Early initiation and exclusive breastfeeding comprise the rule and are most advantageous for the baby and the mother.
- No prelacteal feeds in the form of honey, glucose, water or tea should be given to the infant.
- Colostrum must never be discarded; all babies should receive it because it is rich in protein, protective antibodies and cellular elements.
- The physiological inadequacy of lactation during the first three days of nursing does not impose any hazard to healthy newborns. No supplemental feeding is required in such cases.
- In the subsequent postnatal days, if the baby sleeps well for 2 hours following a feed, voids 5–6 times/day, passes 1–2 soft stools and gains 20–30 g/day, breastfeeding is considered adequate.

Thermal Protection

The body temperature of newborns is unstable and hence, they are prone to cold stress and hypothermia. Hypothermia can be prevented by ensuring skin-to-skin contact with the mother, keeping the room temperature at 25–28°C and not allowing cold draughts.

Indications for Urgent Referral from PHC to a Neonatal Specialist

- Feeding difficulties: Not suckling/choking on feeds/not feeding well
- Lethargy
- Cyanosis, grunting, severe chest in-drawing
- Hypothermia (axillary temperature <35.5°C) or hyperthermia (temperature ≥38°C)
- Jaundice within 24 hours or yellow staining of palms and soles
- Convulsions
- Excessive vomiting
- Weak or absent cry

Newer Strategies for Improving Clinical Outcomes of Preterm Delivery

- Antenatal magnesium sulfate ($MgSO_4$) can be administered for neuroprotection.
- It is indicated for pregnant women <31 weeks of gestation in whom preterm birth is imminent (active labour with >4 cm of cervical dilatation with or without PPROM and planned preterm deliveries for fetal or maternal indications).

- The drug is administered as 4 g IV loading dose administered over 30 minutes followed by 1 g/hour maintenance infusion until birth. Therapy should be discontinued if delivery does not occur or after a maximum infusion period of 24 hours. This therapy is safe for neonates without an increased need for resuscitation at birth.
- Preterm neonates have surfactant deficiency, poor respiratory drive, weak and compliant chest wall,

fragile capillary network in the brain and higher sensitivity to oxygen-induced free radical damage. Hence, specific interventions at birth should focus on the following:
- Delayed cord clamping
- Thermoregulation
- Gentle respiratory support
- Avoidance of hyperoxia

KEY POINTS

✓ *Asphyxia is defined as the failure to establish sufficient breathing at one minute after birth.*

✓ *Perinatal asphyxia is one of the most important causes of perinatal morbidity and mortality.*

✓ *The steps involved in resuscitation include suctioning, ventilation and maintenance of temperature.*

✓ *Apgar score is useful for describing the status of the neonate at birth.*

✓ *Early, exclusive and frequent breastfeeding is the rule, and the mother should be informed about its advantages.*

✓ *Classification of babies at birth according to gestational age and weight helps in management according to expected complications.*

Essay questions

1. Discuss the steps of resuscitating a newborn.
2. What are the indications for urgent referral to a neonatal specialist?

Short answer questions

1. Enumerate the indications for the intubation of a neonate.
2. Write a short note on Apgar score.
3. Define perinatal asphyxia.
4. Define prematurity and list the complications encountered in preterm babies.

MCQs

1. The diagnosis of perinatal asphyxia is made when:
   a) Umbilical artery pH at birth is 7.3
   b) Apgar score at 5 minutes is 4
   c) There is transient tachypnea
   d) Clinical features suggestive of HIE

2. The Apgar score of a pale newborn with a heart rate of 90 and slow respiration and some flexion of extremities will be:
   a) 1
   b) 2
   c) 3
   d) 4

Answers

1. (d), 2. (c)

Fill in the blanks

1. One of the criteria for defining perinatal asphyxia is an Apgar score of _____.
2. One of the widely accepted methods of assessment of gestation of the newborn is the _____.

Answers

1. <3 at 5 minutes,   2. New Ballard Score (NBS)

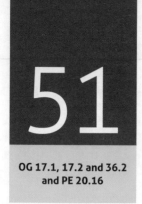

51 Feeding of the Newborn and Immunisation

OG 17.1, 17.2 and 36.2 and PE 20.16

Learning Objectives

» To understand the nutritional requirements of a preterm baby and how these requirements should be met

» To know the National Immunisation Schedule

Breast milk (Table 51.1) is the ideal food for all newborns. In term babies, breastfeeding should be initiated soon after birth and should preferably be continued until six months of age. The mother should be guided to help place the newborn properly at the breast and to ensure that the baby is well-attached/latched onto the breast.

Table 51.1 Comparison of the composition of breast milk, baby milk powder, cow milk and buffalo milk

Per 100 mL	Breast milk	Baby milk powder	Cow milk	Buffalo milk
Calories (Kcal/dL)	67	67	67	117
Proteins (g/dL)	1.1	1.7	3.2	4.3
Fats (g/dL)	4.5	3.3	4.1	6.5
Carbohydrates (g/dL)	7.1	7.5	4.4	5.1
Calcium (mg/dL)	33	62	120	210
Phosphorus (mg/dL)	15	47	90	–
Iron	0.03	0.8	0.2	0.2
Vitamin A (IU/dL)	250	200	–	–
Vitamin D (IU/dL)	2.2	40	–	–
Sodium (mEq/dL)	0.8	1.3	–	–

▮ FEEDING PREMATURE BABIES

Nutrition is one of the most important aspects of the management of preterm babies. The goal of the nutrition of preterm babies is to achieve accretion of nutrients at the same rate as in utero. The expected weight gain is approximately 15–20 g/Kg birth weight per day after an initial period of weight loss.

Feeding premature babies is slightly different from feeding term babies because of their anatomical and physiological immaturity—sucking and swallowing are not coordinated; they have a small stomach and low capacity, poor gastric emptying and immature digestive enzymes. In extreme preterm and extreme low-birth-weight babies, the current practice is to start total parenteral nutrition on the first day of life as soon as the baby is stabilised. Enteral feeding is initiated in this group of preterms as **colostrum swabbing**. The practice of colostrum swabbing in the first few days of birth promotes early gut maturity, reduces the risk of neonatal necrotising enterocolitis (NNEC) and helps to achieve a quick transition to full enteral feeds. Gavage feeding in the form of minimal enteral feeds (MEN) using orogastric or nasogastric tubes is started early to augment parenteral nutrition; following this, enteral nutrition is gradually advanced to achieve full enteral feeds.

Expressed human breast milk is the first choice for enteral feeding. Progressively, as the baby stabilises and attains oromotor maturity, direct breastfeeding in the form of non-nutritive sucking is started and slowly progressed to full direct breastfeeds. Preterm babies aged 34 weeks and more are started on direct breastfeeds soon after birth. VLBW and early preterm babies aged less than 34 weeks are started on gavage feeds through orogastric or nasogastric tubes, advanced to *palladai* feeds and finally, progressed to direct breastfeeds.

▮ RECOMMENDATIONS FOR WATER INTAKE

- Preterms have higher insensible water loss (40–100 mL/Kg); hence, water intake must be adequate to replace the losses through the skin, renal system and GI tract and sufficient to excrete the metabolic wastes and provide for growth requirements.

- Excess water intake in preterm babies is also associated with higher incidence of patent ductus arteriosus, chronic lung disease and necrotising enterocolitis, whereas dehydration can lead to metabolic acidosis.

- The approximate fluid requirements for term and preterm babies in mL/Kg/day are presented in Table 51.2. Fluid intake should be titrated based on accurate recording.

Table 51.2 Approximate fluid requirements for term and preterm babies (in mL/Kg/day)

	Day 1	Day 2	Day 3	Day 4	Day 5 and beyond
Term	60–80	80–100	100–120	120–140	150
Preterm	80–100	100–120	120–140	150	Up to 180

RECOMMENDATIONS FOR NUTRIENT INTAKE

- An intake–output chart (e.g., the volume of blood given, drugs used, losses from gastric aspirates) should be maintained.
- Weight should be recorded twice a day for sick babies and once a day for stable babies.
- The natural course of weight loss—in the postnatal period, term babies lose approximately 5–10% of birth weight by 5–7 days and regain birth weight in 7–10 days; preterms may lose weight of upto 10–15% for up to 10–15 days (with the use of early parenteral nutrition, the maximal weight loss over the first few days of life can be restricted to 5–7%) and gain as much as 10–15%.
- Serum sodium and potassium values must be checked, and the prescribed levels must be maintained.

- Urine osmolality or specific gravity should be checked, especially in more mature babies (>34 weeks).

Table 51.3 presents the nutritional requirements of term and preterm babies.

IMMUNISATION SCHEDULE

The suggested National Immunisation Schedule (NIS) is presented in Table 51.4. Under the Universal Immunisation Programme (UIP), the Government of India provides vaccinations to prevent seven vaccine-preventable diseases—diphtheria, pertussis, tetanus, polio, measles, hepatitis B and tuberculosis.

In addition, Japanese encephalitis vaccination is provided in 113 districts; an additional 62 Japanese encephalitis-endemic districts have recently been identified. The second dose of Japanese encephalitis vaccination was introduced under UIP in these endemic districts in April 2013. A pentavalent vaccine has been introduced in eight states—Tamil Nadu, Kerala, Haryana, Jammu and Kashmir, Gujarat, Karnataka, Goa and Puducherry.

The injectable polio vaccine (IPV) has been introduced into the National Immunisation Schedule. Recently, the pneumococcal vaccine has been introduced in Tamil Nadu and a few other states under UIP.

Table 51.3 Nutritional requirements of term and preterm babies

Nutrients	Requirements		Comments
	Term babies	**Preterm babies**	
Energy	90–100 Kcal/Kg/day	120–130 Kcal/Kg/day	
Proteins	1.5–2 g/Kg/day	3–4 g/Kg/day	Should be 10–15% of the total calories.
Fats	3–4 g/Kg/day		Should be 40–60% of the energy intake.
Carbohydrates	10–12 g/Kg/day		Should be 35–40% of the energy intake.
Calcium	75–150 mg/Kg/day	150–240 mg/Kg/day	Higher requirements cannot be met by the preterm mother's milk or formula alone. Supplements are required in such cases. The calcium:phosphorus ratio of the supplement must be 1.6:2.
Sodium	2–3 mEq/Kg/day	3–4 mEq/Kg/day	
Iron	Term babies need iron supplementation from 5–6 months of life till at least 1 year of age or until fully weaned	The stores of iron are very low in preterm babies, but RBC synthesis being low, the requirements are minimal in the first 5–7 weeks of life. Babies who weigh <1,000 g should be given 3–4 mg/Kg. Babies who weigh >1,000 g should be given 2–3 mg/Kg/day of iron starting at 6–8 weeks till one year of age	If the baby had frequent phlebotomies (blood sampling), iron should be started at 4 weeks of life. Iron supplementation prevents late anemia of infancy.

Table 51.4 National Immunisation Schedule (India)

Vaccine and its presentation	Protection against	Route	Number of doses	Vaccination schedule
BCG (Bacillus–Calmette–Guérin)—lyophilised vaccine	Tuberculosis	Intradermal	1	At birth (up to 1 year, if not given earlier)
OPV (oral polio vaccine)—liquid vaccine	Poliomyelitis	Oral	5	Birth dose for institutional deliveries; primary—three doses at 6, 10 and 14 weeks and one booster dose at 16–24 months of age
Hepatitis B—liquid vaccine	Hepatitis B infection	Intramuscular	4	Birth dose (within 24 hours) for institutional deliveries; primary—three doses at 6, 10 and 14 weeks
DPT (diphtheria, pertussis and tetanus toxoid)—liquid vaccine	Diphtheria, pertussis and tetanus	Intramuscular	5	Three doses at 6, 10 and 14 weeks and two booster doses at 16–24 months and 5–6 years of age
Measles—lyophilised vaccine	Measles	Subcutaneous	2	First dose at 9–12 months of age and second dose at 16–24 months
Td (tetanus toxoid with low-dose diphtheria)—liquid vaccine	Tetanus	Intramuscular	2	Two does at 10 years and 16 years of age; for pregnant woman, two doses are to be given (one dose if previously vaccinated within 3 years)
Japanese encephalitis (JE)—lyophilised vaccine (in selected high disease burden districts)	Japanese encephalitis (brain fever)	Subcutaneous	2	First dose at 9–12 months of age and second dose at 16–24 months (6 months after vaccination drive)
Hib (given as a pentavalent containing Hib [*Haemophilus influenzae* type B]+ DPT+ hep B [hepatitis B])—liquid vaccine (in 8 states)	Hib pneumonia and Hib meningitis	Intramuscular	3	6, 10 and 14 weeks of age
IPV is given in a few states including Tamil Nadu	Poliomyelitis	Intradermal/ Intramuscular	2	Two doses at 6 weeks and 14 weeks in the dose of 0.1 mL; in a few states, it is given at 14 weeks as a single dose intramuscularly
PCV—pneumococcal conjugate vaccine	Pneumonia and invasive pneumococcal disease	Intramuscular	2	6 weeks and 14 weeks

KEY POINTS

✓ *Breastfeeding must be initiated soon after birth.*
✓ *Enteral feeding should be initiated early in preterm babies.*
✓ *Preterm babies require additional nutrition and hence may have to be referred to a specialist for care.*
✓ *An extremely premature baby would need parenteral nutrition support.*
✓ *The immunisation schedule should be explained to the mother at the time of discharge from the hospital.*

Essay question

1. Describe the immunisation schedule, starting from birth to two years of age.

Short answer question

1. Write a short note on the nutritional requirements of a neonate.

MCQs

1. What is the energy requirement for term babies?
   a) 70–80 Kcal/Kg/day
   b) 90–100 Kcal/Kg/day
   c) 80–90 Kcal/Kg/day
   d) 120–130 Kcal/Kg/day

2. What are the energy requirements for a preterm baby?
   a) 70–80 Kcal/Kg/day
   b) 120–130 Kcal/Kg/day
   c) 90 –100 Kcal/Kg/day
   d) 150–160 Kcal/Kg/day
3. What is the approximate weight loss in term babies in the first few days?
   a) 20%
   b) 30%
   c) 1%
   d) 5–10%
4. What is the anticipated weight loss in preterm babies in the first few days?
   a) 5%
   b) 1%

c) 10–15%
d) 30%

Answers

1. (b), 2. (b), 3. (d), 4. (c)

Fill in the blank

1. The expected weight gain after an initial period of weight loss in a preterm neonate is approximately _____.

Answer

1. 15–20 g/Kg

52 Respiratory Distress and Neonatal Sepsis

OG 18.1 and PE 20.8 and 20.16

Learning Objectives

» To know the causes of respiratory distress in the newborn
» To be able to diagnose respiratory distress and assess its severity
» To identify airway anomalies that may require surgery
» To know the causes, clinical features, required investigations and management of neonatal sepsis

RESPIRATORY DISTRESS

DEFINITION

Respiratory distress in a newborn is defined as the presence of at least two of the three clinical features mentioned below.

- Tachypnea (respiratory rate >60/min)
- Retractions
- Grunting

Etiology

The common causes of respiratory distress in preterm and term babies are outlined below.

Preterm
- Hyaline membrane disease
- Pneumonia
- Delayed clearance of lung fluid
- Air leaks
- Metabolic causes—acidosis, hypoglycemia, polycythemia, anemia
- Hypovolemia

Term
- Delayed clearance of lung fluid
- Aspiration of liquor, meconium or blood
- Air leaks
- Pneumonia

Preterm and term
- Surgical causes—choanal atresia, tracheo-esophageal fistula, diaphragmatic hernia
- Congestive cardiac failure
- Intracranial bleed

HISTORY

A detailed relevant antenatal and perinatal history should be taken based on the following:

- Gestational age at birth
- Maternal complications such as diabetes and antepartum hemorrhage
- Previous preterm babies with respiratory distress
- Antenatal corticosteroid prophylaxis in the present pregnancy, if delivered preterm
- Premature or prolonged rupture membranes
- Maternal fever
- Unclean vaginal examination
- Foul-smelling liquor, chorioamnionitis
- Fetal bradycardia
- Meconium-stained liquor—history of aspiration of meconium from the trachea at birth
- Traumatic delivery
- Birth asphyxia
- Intermittent positive pressure ventilation (IPPV)

DETAILED EXAMINATION

The neonate should be examined in detail to look for the following:

- Tachycardia, weak pulse, low BP, prolonged capillary filling time
- Hyperinflated chest
- Meconium-staining of cord and nails (MAS)
- Scaphoid abdomen
- Location of heart sounds
- Congenital diaphragmatic hernia (CDH)—equality of air entry on two sides
- Transillumination (to look for air leaks)

- Evidence of congenital heart failure (CHF)—hepatomegaly, tachycardia, murmur, cyanosis
- Evidence of intracranial bleeds—bulging anterior fontanelle, pallor, hypotonia, pupillary size and reactions, neurological obtundation

The neonate should be checked for **choanal atresia** and **esophageal atresia** by passing a size 10 Fr stiff rubber catheter.

The severity of respiratory distress can be assessed by using the **Downe score** (Table 52.1), wherein a score of 6 indicates severe respiratory distress. In such cases, the newborn should be referred to a special care unit.

Table 52.1 Downe score

Downe score	0	1	2
Respiratory rate	<60	60–80	>80 or apneic
Cyanosis	None	In room air	In 40% FiO$_2$
Grunt	None	Audible with stethoscope	Audible to the naked ear
Retractions	None	Mild	Moderate–severe

MANAGEMENT

- The goal of respiratory treatment is to provide **adequate tissue oxygen** and **carbon dioxide removal**.
- Oxygen should be administered only when needed and based on pulse oximeter reading. Excessive oxygen administration to preterm babies is associated with toxic injury to the retina, brain and other tissues.
- Supplemental oxygen is administered through a hood (headbox) or nasal cannula only to babies who have established spontaneous respiration. For babies with apnea or inadequate respiratory efforts, respiratory support is provided using mechanical ventilators and appropriate FiO$_2$.
- Oxygen is always administered only after appropriate humidification.
- Gentle ventilation is the rule of thumb for preterm babies who need respiratory support. It is provided using a CPAP machine, ideally, the bubble CPAP.
- Most babies who have spontaneous respiration but respiratory distress and inability to maintain tissue oxygen saturation improve with CPAP ventilation.

NEONATAL SEPSIS

DEFINITION

Neonatal sepsis is defined as an **invasive infection**, usually bacterial in nature, occurring in the neonatal period. Depending upon the time of occurrence, neonatal sepsis is categorized as:

- **Early**—within 3 days of birth
- **Late**—after 3 days of birth

Probable sepsis/clinical sepsis is defined as the presence of clinical features along with a positive septic screen in the absence of positive blood culture.

INCIDENCE

Sepsis is a major cause of morbidity and mortality among neonates. The **incidence** of neonatal sepsis varies between 10 and 45 per 1,000 live births in India, depending upon the type of service provided and the number of premature and sick babies cared for. The incidence among very-low-birth-weight (VLBW) babies is likely to be many times more.

The **common organisms responsible for sepsis** comprise chiefly gram-negative bacteria such as *E. coli*, *Klebsiella pneumoniae*, *Pseudomonas* and *Acinetobacter* and less frequently, gram-positive bacteria like *Staphylococcus aureus*.

DIAGNOSIS

Diagnosis is based on the following:

- Clinical features
- Sepsis screen
- Blood culture
- CSF examination

Clinical Features

Neonatal sepsis can present with very non-specific signs and symptoms and clinical manifestations such as the following:

- Poor feeding
- Diminished spontaneous activity
- Lethargy
- Bradycardia
- Temperature instability
- Respiratory distress

- Apnea
- Vomiting
- Diarrhea
- Abdominal distention
- Shock
- Jaundice
- Convulsions

> It is important to remember the following:
> - These clinical signs also indicate the presence of many **non-septic conditions** like hypoglycemia, hypothermia, electrolyte disturbances, inborn errors of metabolism, etc.
> - On the other hand, neonates, especially premature ones, may have very subtle features or even no features; if these are not identified and managed promptly, they can lead to rapid deterioration.

Sepsis Screen

The sepsis screen has **five components** and is considered positive if two or more parameters are positive.

1. **Total leukocyte count** (TLC): The normal total leukocyte count ranges from 7,000–14,000. A count of less than 5,000 or more than 15,000 should raise suspicion of sepsis.

2. **Micro-ESR:** Blood is collected in a standard pre-heparinised microhematocrit tube (75 mm length, internal diameter of 1.1 mm and outer diameter of 1.5 mm) so that the tube is completely filled; the tube is then kept upright. The drop in the erythrocyte column is read after one hour. A value of >10 mm is suggestive of infection.

3. **Absolute neutrophil count (ANC):** After performing a total leukocyte count, a differential count is performed on a peripheral smear. ANC is considered low if it is below the normal for the age, according to the nomogram of Monro for term babies and the nomogram of Zipursky for preterm babies.

> ANC = Total leukocyte count (TLC) × percentage of polymorphs

4. **C-reactive protein (CRP):** CRP is a rapidly responsive acute phase reactant synthesised by the liver within 6–8 hours of an inflammatory stimulus. CRP is estimated by the latex agglutination test. A positive CRP latex agglutination test on an undiluted sample corresponds to a plasma CRP concentration of 0.6–0.8 mg/dL. Normalisation of CRP elevation appears to be a helpful tool in determining response to antimicrobial therapy.

5. **Band cell count (I/T ratio):** The ratio of immature to total neutrophils (I/T ratio) is 0.16 at birth and declines to 0.12 after 72 hours of birth. An I/T ratio of >0.20 is suggestive of infection. A band cell count is also done whenever the WBC count is performed as part of the sepsis screen in neonates.

> $$\text{I/T ratio} = \frac{\text{Immature neutrophils (bands/myelocytes/metamyelocytes/promyelocytes)}}{\text{Total neutrophils (mature + immature cells)}}$$

Procalcitonin: This is an acute inflammatory marker specific for infection. Its estimation in blood is slowly becoming popular and is widely used. This is a recent addition, which is being used in several centres for screening.

Blood Culture

Blood culture must be obtained using two culture media. At least 1 mL of blood must be collected in each bottle. If this amount of blood is not available, 0.5 mL of blood may be used in bile broth media. Blood culture is the gold standard for the diagnosis of septicemia.

Cerebrospinal Fluid (CSF) Examination

CSF examination must be performed in all babies with suspected or proven sepsis, preferably before starting antibiotics. However, it should be borne in mind that there is a risk of hypoxia in already hypoxemic babies; sometimes, oxygen supplementation may be required. CSF examination may not be performed in asymptomatic babies who are born with adverse perinatal factors.

Abnormal CSF

- More than 25 WBC per cubic millimetre
- More than 60% of the WBC are polymorphs
- CSF glucose—blood glucose ratio less than 50%
- Protein concentration greater than 170 mg/dL
- Positive Gram stain/presence of microorganisms in CSF culture

Note: Blood for glucose estimation should be taken just prior to the lumbar puncture.

EARLY-ONSET SEPSIS

Early-onset (within 48–72 hours) infections are associated with certain high-risk obstetric factors. These risk factors have been given a relative score as presented in Table 52.2. However, the perinatal risk score is just a guideline, to which there may be exceptions. Thus, management should be individualised. If the cause of prematurity is an elective cesarean section, prematurity should not be considered while calculating the perinatal score.

Table 52.2 Perinatal risk score

Perinatal risk	Score
Birth asphyxia (Apgar <6 at 5 min)	2
Unclean vaginal examination	2
Foul-smelling liquor	2
Duration of labour >24 hours	2
Gestation <37 weeks	3
Duration of rupture of membranes >24 hours	2
Maternal pyrexia >38°C	1

Actions based on score:
- Score 0–3: Observe clinically
- Score ≥4: Refer to a special care unit

LATE-ONSET SEPSIS OR NOSOCOMIAL SEPSIS

The **risk factors** for late-onset sepsis (after 72 hours of life) include prolonged intravenous administration, central line, ventilation or any other invasive procedures.

During hospital stay, if the baby shows clinical features suggestive of sepsis, a complete septic workup with lumbar puncture should be performed, as the incidence of meningitis is significantly higher in this type of sepsis than in perinatally acquired early-onset sepsis.

MANAGEMENT OF NEONATAL SEPSIS

Antibiotics

Prophylactic antibiotics have no role and should not be used as they favour the development of drug-resistant bacteria. The antibiotics should have good broad-spectrum cover against gram-negative organisms and *Staphylococcus aureus*. A combination of two antibiotics should be used to provide good broad-spectrum cover and minimise the emergence of drug resistance.

The choice of antibiotics changes with time on the basis of the prevalent organisms and the sensitivity pattern. After the initiation of antibiotics, they must be reviewed periodically depending upon the organisms grown (Table 52.3).

Early-onset sepsis

Antibiotics are decided upon based on one of the following two factors:

1. On the basis of the bacteria isolated from the mother (e.g., urine culture, high vaginal/cervical swab culture)
2. According to the existing unit policy

Late-onset/Hospital-acquired sepsis

Antibiotics are decided upon based on one of the following three factors:

1. On the basis of the pathogen isolated from surface swabs (e.g., tracheal aspirate)
2. On the basis of the currently prevalent organism in the nursery
3. According to the existing unit policy

Table 52.3 Type of sepsis and duration of antibiotic therapy

Type of sepsis	Duration
Suspected sepsis (rapid diagnostic test [RDT] positive)	7 days
Proven sepsis (blood culture positive)	14 days
Gram-positive meningitis	14 days
Gram-negative meningitis and culture-negative meningitis	21 days
Septic arthritis/osteomyelitis/necrotising pneumonia, emphysema, ventriculitis	4–6 weeks

Adjunctive Modalities

These include the use of immunoglobulin, exchange transfusion and cytokines. These are administered only by a specialist.

KEY POINTS

✓ *Respiratory distress syndrome is seen commonly in preterm babies.*

✓ *A newborn with severe distress needs special care in a neonatal unit.*

✓ *Early-onset sepsis is treated based on the perinatal risk score.*

✓ *Late-onset sepsis is usually hospital-acquired and needs broad-spectrum antibiotic therapy.*

Essay questions

1. Discuss the diagnosis of neonatal sepsis.
2. How do you approach a case of respiratory distress in a newborn?

Short answer question

1. Define respiratory distress in a newborn and list the causes of respiratory distress in preterm and term babies.

MCQs

1. The Downe score for the assessment of respiratory distress includes the following EXCEPT:
   a) Respiratory rate
   b) Cyanosis
   c) Grunt
   d) Oxygen saturation
2. The components of a sepsis screen in a neonate include the following EXCEPT:
   a) Band cell count
   b) Fever
   c) Micro-ESR
   d) C-reactive protein (CRP)
3. The following are the criteria for abnormal CSF EXCEPT:
   a) >25 WBC per cubic millimetre
   b) >60% of the WBC being polymorphs
   c) CSF glucose—blood glucose ratio >50%
   d) Protein concentration greater than 170 mg/dL

Answers

1. (d), 2. (a), 3. (c)

Fill in the blanks

1. Respiratory distress in a newborn is defined as the presence of tachypnea or a respiratory rate of _____.
2. The severity of respiratory distress can be assessed by the _____ score.
3. Downe score of _____ indicates severe respiratory distress.
4. Early-onset neonatal sepsis is defined as sepsis occurring within _____ of birth.
5. A value of _____ of micro-ESR is suggestive of infection.

Answers

1. >60/minute, 2. Downe score, 3. 6, 4. 48–72 hours, 5. >10 mm

Neonatal Jaundice

Learning Objectives

» To be able to differentiate physiological jaundice from pathological causes
» To know the causes of neonatal jaundice and its evaluation
» To know the management of neonatal jaundice

PHYSIOLOGICAL JAUNDICE

About 97% of healthy full-term infants have bilirubin values of >2 mg/dL during the first week of life; 65% are clinically jaundiced. This is termed physiological jaundice.

However, jaundice in the newborn might signal a serious, potentially treatable illness which may cause neurological damage if the bilirubin level is sufficiently elevated.

PATHOLOGIC OR NON-PHYSIOLOGICAL JAUNDICE

This is clinical jaundice that develops in the first 24 hours of life and is defined by the following:

- Total serum bilirubin (TSB) increasing by >5 mg/dL/day
- TSB >12 mg/dL in full-term infants and >10–12 mg/dL in preterm infants
- Conjugated serum bilirubin >2 mg/dL
- Clinical jaundice persisting for >2 weeks in full-term and >3 weeks in preterm infants
- Elevation of TSB that requires phototherapy
- A rise of TSB or transcutaneous bilirubin (TCB) by more than 0.2 mg/dL/hour

The terms 'physiologic' and 'non-physiological' jaundice in low-birth-weight infants are no longer relevant. Hyperbilirubinemia in these infants is invariably treated at levels far below those previously defined as non-physiological.

Etiology of Neonatal Jaundice

- Physiological causes
  - Prematurity
  - Rh-incompatibility and ABO-incompatibility
  - Glucose-6-phosphate dehydrogenase (G6PD) deficiency
- Intrauterine infections
- Asphyxia
- Use of oxytocics during labour
- Congenital causes

Evaluation of a Jaundiced Neonate

Severity of jaundice

When a neonate is clinically jaundiced, the TSB is usually 5–7 mg/dL. Jaundice in newborns progresses in a cephalocaudal direction, and thus, the extent of yellowness of the skin is useful to assess the level of bilirubin clinically. With experience, one can reliably assess jaundice clinically (Table 53.1).

Table 53.1 Clinical assessment of neonatal jaundice

Area of the body	Bilirubin level
Face	5–7 mg/dL
Chest and upper abdomen	7–10 mg/dL
Lower abdomen/thigh	10–15 mg/dL
Arms and lower legs	15–18 mg/dL
Soles/palms	>18 mg/dL

For a baby who has significant jaundice or is receiving phototherapy, clinical assessment may be fallacious. Hence, serum/plasma bilirubin must be checked for appropriate management.

Complications of Jaundice

Bilirubin-induced neurological damage (BIND) is the most important complication of neonatal jaundice. After assessing the degree of jaundice, a complete neurological examination should be performed to look for evidence of bilirubin encephalopathy. This depends on the tone, cry, neonatal reflexes, eye movements and general activity of the infant.

Stages of bilirubin encephalopathy (for term babies)

- Stage 1: Poor Moro reflex, decreased tone, lethargy, poor feeding, vomiting and high-pitched cry
- Stage 2: Opisthotonus, seizures, fever, rigidity, oculogyric crisis and paralysis of upward gaze
- Stage 3: Spasticity is decreased
- Stage 4: Late sequelae including spasticity, athetosis, deafness, mental retardation, paralysis of the upward gaze and dental dysplasia

Preterm babies do not show the above-mentioned temporal evolution of bilirubin encephalopathy.

Investigations

A blood sample is collected for all neonates with significant jaundice. The following investigations are performed:

- Blood grouping
- Rh type of baby and mother
- Screening for G6PD deficiency
- Hemogram to check for evidence of hemolysis (elevated reticulocyte count, fall in packed cell volume [PCV] or hemoglobin)
- Peripheral smear to look for microspherocytes, nucleated RBCs, anisopoikilocytosis and polychromasia
- Conjugated bilirubin fraction should be estimated at least once and when cholestasis is suspected

Monitoring

Total serum bilirubin (TSB) should be estimated when pathological jaundice is suspected; the test should be repeated every 6–8 hours. More frequent assessment of jaundice is done when hemolysis is suspected/proven. In Rh-isoimmunised mothers, cord blood is screened for TSB, PCV, blood grouping and direct Coombs test (DCT).

Management

Babies with neonatal jaundice should be treated to decrease their bilirubin levels and thereby prevent bilirubin encephalopathy. The various treatment modalities include the following:

- Phototherapy
- Exchange transfusion
- Immunoglobulins

- Oral phenobarbitone
- Metalloporphyrins

The decision to treat depends on the severity and cause of jaundice. The American Academy of Pediatrics has published guidelines for the management of non-hemolytic neonatal jaundice in term and near-term babies. For premature babies, Cockington charts are the most commonly used guidelines for treating neonatal jaundice.

Phototherapy

- Phototherapy is given to a baby when the TSB is higher than normal and likely to rise but has not yet reached the exchange level. As a rough guideline, phototherapy needs to be given when TSB reaches half the exchange value. Once, TSB is in the exchange zone, exchange transfusion must be done.
- Phototherapy is not a substitute for exchange transfusion. It is most effective with a combination of blue and green lights and with a minimum irradiance of 30 $\mu W/cm^2/nm$. The higher the irradiance, the better the effect, but care must be taken not to overheat the body.
- While under phototherapy, the baby's eyes should be covered with an opaque mask without applying undue pressure on the face and nose.
- The mother should be encouraged to remove the baby from under the lights, uncover its eyes and breastfeed it every 2–3 hours.
- The baby should be alternated between the prone and supine positions.
- Hydration, fluid and electrolyte status should be monitored.

Effects of phototherapy

Babies under phototherapy may develop hypothermia or hyperthermia. Hence, temperature should be monitored diligently. Some degree of loose green stools is fairly common during phototherapy. Sometimes, a rash may develop on the skin. The mother should be reassured about the transient and benign nature of these conditions.

Clinical assessment of jaundice in babies under phototherapy may be fallacious. Hence, they need to be monitored by 8-hourly TSB estimation. Before stopping phototherapy, there should be consecutive TSB values below the phototherapy zone for a period of 24 hours. After stopping phototherapy, one should check for a rebound rise in TSB after 12 hours. Phototherapy is not recommended for babies who have conjugated hyperbilirubinemia. It may cause a bronze discolouration of skin in these babies.

Exchange transfusion

Indications for exchange transfusion at or soon after birth in a baby born to an Rh-isoimmunised mother are as follows:

- Hydrops (if the baby cannot tolerate double-volume exchange, partial exchange may be given initially to increase hematocrit)
- A history of elder siblings requiring exchange because of Rh-isoimmunisation in a baby born with pallor, hepatosplenomegaly and positive DCT
- Cord Hb <11 g/dL
- Cord TSB >5 mg/dL
- Rate of rise of TSB >1 mg/dL/hour despite phototherapy if Hb is 11–13 g/dL
- Any TSB >12 mg/dL in the first 24 hours
- Any TSB >20 mg/dL in the neonatal period

Total serum bilirubin is taken as the marker to make a decision regarding exchange transfusion. The conjugated fraction is to be subtracted from the total value only when it is >5 mg/dL.

Albumin, which was used as an adjunct before ET, is no longer recommended.

In cases of Rh-isoimmunisation, the first choice is Rh-negative blood of the baby's ABO blood group. If this is not available, O-negative blood may be used. If the baby has undergone intrauterine or exchange transfusion with O-negative blood, then O-negative blood must be used for the next exchange as well. In case of ABO incompatibility, the first choice is a suspension of O-group cells in AB plasma. If this is not available, O-group blood is to be used. For other babies, the baby's blood group should be used.

IV immunoglobulins

The role of IV immunoglobulins (in a dose of 0.5–1 g/kg) used to prevent repeated ET in jaundiced babies has become limited to settings where ET is not possible.

The following drugs should be avoided in hyperbilirubinemia caused by G6PD deficiency:

- Acetanilide
- Niridazole
- Doxorubicin
- Nitrofurantoin
- Furazolidone
- Methylene blue
- Primaquine
- Nalidixic acid
- Sulphamethoxazole
- Phenazopyridine

PROLONGED UNCONJUGATED HYPERBILIRUBINEMIA

Clinical jaundice persisting beyond two weeks in term and three weeks in preterm babies is termed prolonged jaundice. Yellow stools and the absence of diaper staining should be confirmed before labelling the jaundice as unconjugated. A conjugated bilirubin fraction should be obtained for confirmation.

Etiology

- Hemolytic diseases—blood group incompatibility, hereditary spherocytosis and G6PD deficiency
- Hypothyroidism
- Breast milk jaundice
- Pyloric stenosis/intestinal obstruction
- Concealed hemorrhage
- Malaria
- Urinary tract infection (UTI)

Investigations

- Blood grouping, DCT, reticulocyte count, peripheral smear and smear for malarial parasite in endemic areas
- Suprapubic urine culture
- X-ray knee joints for bone age; T3, T4, TSH and LFT if jaundice persists for more than 2 weeks of life

Management

Management depends on the cause of the hyperbilirubinemia. Breastfeeding should not be stopped even if breast milk jaundice is suspected. If the workup shows negative results but jaundice continues (TSB >15 mg/dL), phenobarbitone should be given for a week at a dosage of 3–5 mg/Kg/day, and the child should be re-evaluated after a week.

Fig. 53.1 presents an algorithm for the management of neonatal jaundice.

HEMOLYTIC DISEASE OF THE NEWBORN

Hemolytic disease or erythroblastosis fetalis is caused by incompatibility between the blood groups of the mother and the fetus. The characteristic clinical features are edema, jaundice and anemia. These infants require special antenatal, intranatal and neonatal care. Hence, whenever a diagnosis of Rh-isoimmunisation is made, the patient should be referred to a high-risk obstetric unit.

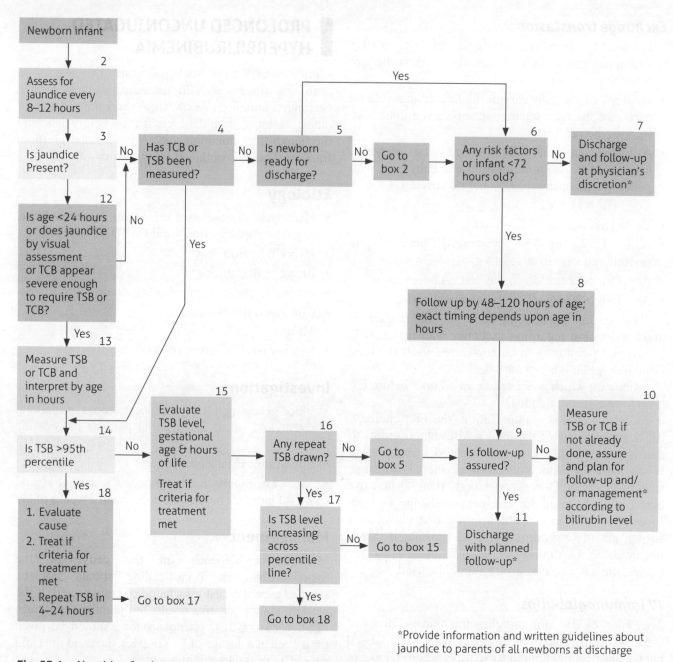

Fig. 53.1 Algorithm for the management of jaundice in the newborn

ABO Incompatibility

Hemolysis due to ABO incompatibility may be associated with the following features:

- The mother's blood group is O with anti-A and anti-B in her serum, while the fetus is group A, B or AB.
- There is onset of jaundice within 24 hours.

- In 5% of babies, the incompatibility develops into hemolysis. The process is less severe than Rh-hemolysis. ABO incompatibility is the common cause of hemolytic anemia in the newborn. The newborn develops jaundice within 24 hours, and the first baby is affected more often. Jaundice is mild and disappears in a week. ABO incompatibility provides protection against Rh-hemolytic disease.

KEY POINTS

✓   *Jaundice in the newborn may signal a serious, potentially treatable illness.*

✓   *Bilirubin encephalopathy is the most important complication of neonatal jaundice.*

✓   *Causes of jaundice include ABO incompatibility and Rh-incompatibility, G6PD deficiency, prematurity, asphyxia and so on.*

✓   *The main line of treatment of jaundice is phototherapy along with exchange transfusion if required.*

Essay questions

1.   Discuss the causes of neonatal jaundice and its complications.
2.   Discuss the available treatment modalities for neonatal jaundice.
3.   What are the causes and management of prolonged unconjugated hyperbilirubinemia?

Short answer questions

1.   Write a short note on phototherapy.
2.   What are the indications for exchange transfusion at or soon after birth in a baby born to an Rh-isoimmunised mother?
3.   Write a short note on hemolytic disease of the newborn.

MCQs

1.   If jaundice is clinically detected at the neonate's chest, the likely TSB is:
     a)   5 mg/dL
     b)   10 mg/dL
     c)   15 mg/dL
     d)   20 mg/dL
2.   If the neonate shows opisthotonus, seizures and oculogyric crisis, the bilirubin encephalopathy is at which stage?
     a)   1
     b)   2
     c)   3
     d)   4

3.   Neonatal jaundice is considered as non-physiological or pathological if:
     a)   It appears at 36 hours
     b)   Total serum bilirubin increases by 3 mg/dL/day
     c)   Conjugated bilirubin is more than 2 mg/dL
     d)   Clinical jaundice persists for more than one week in preterm babies

Answer

1. (b),   2. (b),   3. (c)

Fill in the blanks

1.   The most important complication of neonatal jaundice is _____.

2.   Clinical jaundice persisting beyond _____ in term and _____. in preterm babies is termed prolonged jaundice.

Answers

1. bilirubin-induced neurological damage (BIND),   2. two weeks, three weeks

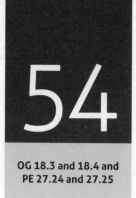

54 Neonatal Problems and Their Management

OG 18.3 and 18.4 and
PE 27.24 and 27.25

Learning Objectives

» To be able to diagnose neonatal hypoglycemia and know its causes and management
» To know about the adverse effects of neonatal hypoglycemia
» To know the risk factors for birth trauma and measures that should be taken to prevent neonatal injury

■ HYPOGLYCEMIA

Neonatal hypoglycemia is defined as a condition that occurs whenever the blood glucose level falls below **45 mg/dL** in the first 48 hours of life and that is less than **50 mg/dL** thereafter.

Etiology

The three most common associations of hypoglycemia are as follows:

- Prematurity
- Intrauterine growth restriction (IUGR)
- Infants of diabetic mothers (IDM)

Additional Risk Factors

- Small-for-gestational-age (SGA) babies
- Preterm with IUGR
- Rh-isoimmunised babies
- Babies who have asphyxia, hypothermia, polycythemia, septicemia or any sickness
- Any baby on IV fluids or total parenteral nutrition (TPN)

Monitoring of Blood Glucose

Blood glucose should ideally be monitored in a proper laboratory setting. However, it may become necessary in emergency situations to monitor blood glucose with bedside capillary blood glucose monitors.

Blood glucose estimation is done using bedside point-of-care capillary blood glucose estimation with a glucometer or glucostix.

Symptoms of Hypoglycemia

On the first or second day of life, hypoglycemic infants may be asymptomatic or have life-threatening CNS and cardiopulmonary disturbances.

Symptoms of hypoglycemia
- Poor feeding
- Jitteriness, tremors
- Seizures
- Hypothermia
- Hypotonia
- Lethargy, apathy
- Cyanosis
- Apnea

Prevention

Early feeding started before one hour of age should be ensured in IDMs and SGAs. In IDMs, the first three feeds should be given at intervals of one hour as 5 mL/Kg per feed. If the blood glucose remains normal, the interval can be increased to two-hourly. Only breast milk or formula feeds should be given.

Once transferred to the mother, breastfeeding should be carefully supervised in IDMs and SGAs to ensure adequate intake. In babies on IV fluids, dextrose should be administered continuously.

Management

- Asymptomatic and symptomatic cases should be managed similarly. While treatment for hypoglycemia is instituted, it is important to remember to identify and correct the secondary causes of hypoglycemia, e.g., polycythemia and sepsis.
- Minibolus—200 mg/Kg glucose should be given with 2 mL/Kg of 10% dextrose over one minute.

- Immediately following that, an infusion of 10% dextrose should be started at the rate of 6 mg/Kg/min (3.6 mL/Kg/hour of 10% dextrose).
- Blood glucose should be checked after 15 minutes. If normal, the same infusion should be continued. If low, the glucose infusion rate should be increased by 2 mg/Kg/min. If blood glucose is consistently low, the infusion rate should be increased by 2 mg/Kg/min every 15 minutes to a maximum of 12–14 mg/Kg/min. The maximum concentration of dextrose that can be used by the peripheral vein is 12.5%. While increasing the glucose infusion rate, care should be taken to ensure that the baby does not suffer from fluid overload.
- Infusion pumps should be used to ensure continuous and smooth delivery of glucose. When large amounts of glucose have to be infused, two IV lines should be used.
- Once the blood glucose is normal, it should be rechecked two more times, 15 minutes apart. If normal, it should subsequently be checked twice at one-hour intervals, then after two hours and then four-hourly.
- If there is no other contraindication, tube feeds should be started with expressed breast milk (EBM) or formula simultaneously. This will help prevent drastic fluctuations in blood glucose.
- Dextrose infusion should be tapered.
- When blood glucose has remained normal for 6–12 hours or if blood glucose exceeds 100 mg/dL, the infusion should be decreased by 2 mg/Kg/min every 6 hours while checking blood glucose.
- Once the infusion rate has been brought down to 4 mg/Kg/min, the feeds can be increased and IV fluids can be tapered off.
- If hypoglycemia persists despite treatment, the newborn should be referred to a special care unit.

THERMOREGULATION IN THE NEWBORN

The newborn baby is homeothermic, but its ability to stay warm may be easily overwhelmed by extremes of temperatures. Neonatal hypothermia is an important cause of neonatal morbidity and mortality.

Mechanisms of Heat Production

Non-shivering thermogenesis

This is the main mechanism of heat production in the newborn. Term neonates have brown fat that forms 4–7% of their body weight. This is located in the neck, interscapular region, groin, axillae and around the kidneys. This fat is highly vascularised and innervated by sympathetic neurons. When the infant faces cold stress, there is increased production of norepinephrine, which acts locally in the brown fat to stimulate lipolysis and release free fatty acids, which are oxidised or re-esterified to produce heat.

Problems in Thermoregulation

Premature infants have specific problems that place them at a disadvantage in terms of temperature maintenance.

- The skin surface area is disproportionately large for the weight of the infant.
- There is decreased subcutaneous fat, and thus, less insulation.
- There are fewer well-developed brown fat stores.
- The premature infant is unable to take in enough calories to provide nutrients for thermogenesis.
- Oxygen consumption is limited in some premature babies because of pulmonary problems.

Measurement of Temperature

Axillary temperature

For routine use, the measurement of axillary temperature is adequate. The bulb of the clinical thermometer is held firmly against the roof of the axilla, free from moisture, with the baby's arm pressed against the side of the chest. The reading is taken after three minutes of placing the thermometer. The normal range of temperature is 36.5–37.5°C. The exact reading is recorded.

Skin temperature

This is to be monitored continuously in babies kept in incubators and radiant warmers by lightly taping a thermistor probe to the skin over the upper abdomen. The aim is to maintain skin temperature at 36.5°C.

Rectal temperature

This method is not used for routine monitoring. However, it is the best way to measure core temperature in hypothermic neonates. Temperature is recorded by inserting the bulb of the thermometer into the rectum to a depth of 3 cm in a term baby and 2 cm in a preterm baby. The thermometer is kept in place for at least two minutes. The normal range is 36.6–37.2°C.

Interpretation of temperature by touch

The baby's temperature can be assessed with reasonable precision by human touch, the reliability of which can be enhanced by training. Abdominal temperature is representative of the core temperature and is reliable in the diagnosis of hypothermia. Warm and pink feet indicate that the baby is in thermal comfort. But when the feet are cold and the abdomen is warm, it indicates that the baby is in cold stress. In hypothermia, both feet are cold to touch.

Environmental Temperature Control

The temperature at which neonates are nursed has a measurable effect on their mortality and morbidity. Neutral thermal environments are associated with the lowest mortality rates.

Thermoneutral zone

The thermoneutral zone is defined for each infant as the range of ambient temperature within which body temperature is normal, metabolic rate is minimal and temperature regulation can be achieved by non-evaporative physical processes alone.

Incubators

The incubator works on the principle of forced convection. The incubator is a closed system with a heating element underneath and a transparent canopy around the baby tray. Air is sucked in through a microfilter over the heating element and circulated by a fan to attain a uniform temperature.

Modes of control

- **Air temperature servo-control:** The air temperature is set to the desired level and the air is heated to the preset level by a servo loop. The control is proportional, that is, the heater output is proportional to the difference between the set temperature and the actual temperature. If the incubator air temperature is just below the set temperature, the heater output will be low; if it is substantially below the set temperature, the heater will be on full power.
- **Skin (patient) temperature servo-control:** The baby's temperature is recorded, and the output of the heater is set to the desired level. A thermistor or thermocouple is taped to the baby's skin, preferably on the upper abdomen, and the heater output is servo-controlled to keep the skin temperature constant. In practice, air temperature fluctuations are greater in skin mode than in air mode, especially when the infant is handled. For this reason, the air mode is preferred for routine care.

Indications for use of incubators

- For neonates weighing less than 1,800 g

- For isolating an infected baby
- When the ambient temperature is extremely low (<20°C)
- For transporting babies (transport incubator)

Radiant warmer (open care system)

Radiant warmers provide an intense source of radiation energy. Here, an overhead quartz rod produces heat. This heat is reflected by a parabolic reflector onto the bassinet and thereby, the baby.

Modes of control

- **Skin temperature (patient) servo-control:** The desired skin temperature is set, and the baby's skin temperature is recorded by a skin temperature probe and continuously displayed. The heater output is servo-controlled to maintain the baby's skin temperature at a set level. This is the preferred mode of caring for babies in open care.
- **Manual mode:** This mode is used to preheat the open care unit. Here, the heater output is set at a desired level (25–100%) and kept constant. As a protective mechanism, this heater output level is reset from time to time (usually 30 minutes); after this time, the heater output switches off and the system sounds a continuous alarm till it is reset.

Tips for using warmers

- The warmer should not be used in a cold room; it works best when the ambient temperature is above 20°C.
- Air currents reduce the efficacy of the warmer and increase transepidermal water loss. Hence, the warmer should be kept away from such drafts.
- The warmer must be prewarmed before placing the baby inside.
- While using the manual mode in a warmer without a temperature display, the baby's temperature should be measured hourly and the heater output should be adjusted accordingly.
- Open care increases transepidermal water loss; hence, 20 mL/Kg/day of fluid in excess of daily maintenance requirements should be given and the fluid status should be monitored carefully.
- The use of clear plastic tenting and plastic wrap (cling film) decreases both convective heat loss and transepidermal water loss.
- Clothing babies who do not need frequent observation decreases heat loss and transepidermal water loss. The head and lower extremities must be covered.

Hazards of temperature control methods

- Hyperthermia
- Servo-controlled warmers can generate excess heat and cause severe hyperthermia if the probes become detached from the infant's skin (Tables 54.1 and 54.2)
- Undetected infection
- Servo-control may mask hypothermia and hyperthermia seen with infection
- Dehydration
- Radiant heaters cause increased insensible water loss; if the fluid is not adequately replaced, this can result in dehydration

Table 54.1 Abdominal skin temperature setting for infants nursed under radiant warmers or in skin mode in incubators

Weight (Kg)	Abdominal skin temperature (°C)
<1.0	36.9
1.0–1.5	36.7
1.5–2.0	36.5
2.0–2.5	36.3
>2.5	36.0

Table 54.2 Average incubator air temperature to provide thermoneutral environment for a naked healthy infant

Birth weight (Kg)	35°C	34°C	33°C	32°C
1.0–1.5	For 10 days	After 10 days	After 3 weeks	After 5 weeks
1.5–2.0		For 10 days	After 10 days	After 4 weeks
2.0–2.5		For 2 days	After 2 days	After 3 weeks
>2.5				After 2 days

Hypothermia

When the axillary temperature is **less than 36.5°C**, it is known as hypothermia. When the temperature is less than 32°C, it is called severe hypothermia (Table 54.3).

Table 54.3 Axillary temperature in the newborn infant

Temperature range (°C)	Category
36.5–37.5	Normal range
36.5–36	Cold stress
36–32.0	Moderate hypothermia
32.0	Severe hypothermia

Risk

- Preterm babies
- Small-for-gestational-age (SGA) babies
- Babies requiring frequent manipulation and intervention
- Low environmental temperature (winter)
- Unattended delivery

Signs and symptoms

- Peripheral vasoconstriction
- CNS depression
- Increased metabolism
- Increased pulmonary activity
- Tachypnea, respiratory distress, shock
- Acrocyanosis, cold extremities, decreased peripheral perfusion
- Lethargy, poor feeding, apnea, bradycardia
- Hypoglycemia, hypoxia, metabolic acidosis

Prevention

In the delivery room

- The baby should be dried properly and wet linen should be removed. A fresh warm towel should be used to wrap the baby.
- Normal term babies should be transferred to the mother's side as soon as possible after being clothed appropriately.

In the nursery

- The nursery should be kept warm, and room temperature should be maintained at 28–30°C.
- The doors and windows of the nursery should be kept closed to avoid cold draughts.
- The baby should be received in warm linen under a preheated radiant warmer.
- The temperature of babies kept in the nursery for observation should be monitored every two hours and the results must be recorded.
- Avoiding hyperthermia—the baby should not be kept under the radiant warmer for prolonged periods without monitoring its temperature. Babies in warmers can also get overheated, and hence, should be monitored closely.
- Babies should not be bathed in the nursery.

By the mother's side

- The baby should be clothed adequately (usually one layer of clothing more than that worn by adults) with the head and extremities sufficiently covered.

- In cold weather, the baby should be wrapped in multiple layers of clothes; in hot weather, loose and light clothes should be used.
- The mother should be taught how to assess the baby's temperature, either with a thermometer or by touch.

Kangaroo mother care

This method helps to prevent hypothermia in newborns, especially in cold climates and can also be used while transferring newborns to special care centres wherever incubators for transfer are not available (Fig. 54.1).

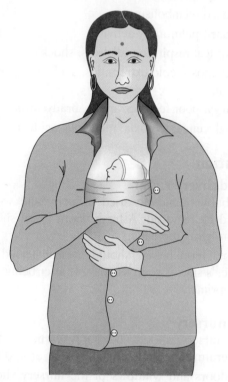

Fig. 54.1 Kangaroo mother care

- The baby is clothed in a prewarmed shirt that is open at the front, a napkin and socks.
- The baby is placed in an upright position directly against the mother's skin.
- The baby is secured in skin-to-skin contact as mentioned above.
- The baby's hips and elbows should be flexed in a frog-like position and the baby's head and chest should be on the mother's chest with the head in a slightly extended position.
- The baby should be placed directly on the mother's chest under her clothes and should be covered with a prewarmed blanket.
- A soft piece of fabric (about 1 square metre) should be folded diagonally, wrapped over the

baby and secured with a knot at the mother's back. The knot should be tight enough to prevent the baby from sliding out if the mother stands up, but not so tight that it obstructs the baby's breathing movements.
- After positioning the baby, the mother should be allowed to rest with the baby and should be encouraged to move around when she is ready.

During procedures

- **Exchange transfusion:** The procedure should be performed under a functioning radiant warmer. The blood to be used for exchange transfusion should be brought to room temperature before use and a blood warmer should be used during transfusion. The baby's temperature should be monitored continuously during the procedure with a skin probe (placed on the chest or upper arm).
- **Minor procedures:** For babies cared for in an incubator, the door of the incubator should not be opened wide for minor procedures like peripheral venous cannulation, lumbar puncture, suction and so on. If the door of the incubator needs to be kept open, the incubator should be put on air mode and the set limit should be raised appropriately. If the procedure gets unduly prolonged, the general condition of the baby, including temperature, should be closely monitored. In case of fluctuations, the procedure should be stopped and the temperature should be normalised before attempting the procedure again.

During transport

- The baby's temperature should be allowed to stabilise before transport.
- The baby's temperature should be recorded before transport and documented.
- The transport incubator should be prewarmed to 37°C before transport and the baby should be moved into it only just before the transfer.
- The baby should be wrapped well if close observation is not required. The head and extremities should be covered in all babies.
- The receiving ward should be informed about the transport immediately before starting.
- In the receiving ward, the incubator or open care should be prepared for receiving the baby.
- Immediately on arrival, the temperature and other vital signs should be checked.
- If the incubator or open care is still not ready, the transport incubator should be plugged into an electrical source while awaiting transfer.

Management

Neonates with hypothermia are managed by rewarming them in the incubator or by providing open care as follows.

- The baby is kept in the incubator naked and the incubator is set to air control mode. The control temperature is set to 1.5–2°C more than the baby's temperature (not more than 36.5°C). This set temperature is increased as the baby's skin temperature improves so as to reach normal temperature.
- The baby's body should not be covered with cotton or clothes during rewarming as this will delay the process. After rewarming to normal temperature, the baby can be appropriately clothed.
- Setting the open care to manual mode and keeping the heater output to the maximum helps to rewarm the baby in an open care setting. Alternatively, the open care unit can also be kept in the skin control mode.
- The control temperature is set at 1°C above the baby's skin temperature; the set limit is raised gradually as the baby's temperature increases so as to reach normal temperature.
- The baby's skin temperature is monitored continuously while rewarming; the axillary temperature is also checked with a thermometer every 15–30 minutes.
- Hyperthermia should be avoided during rewarming.
- In babies with severe hypothermia (32°C), during rewarming, the following should be done:
  - IV drip of 10% dextrose should be started.
  - Blood sugar should be monitored with a glucostix every 30 minutes.
  - Oxygen saturation should be monitored, and supplemental oxygen should be given if necessary.
  - Vitamin K should be given if the baby has not received it in the first seven days.

Cold Stress

A neonate is said to be in cold stress if the axillary temperature is 36.0–36.5°C and the baby has cold extremities. A baby is usually able to maintain the core temperature by increasing its metabolism. In the process, nutrients that would have otherwise been used for tissue building are burnt to maintain body temperature. Cold stress is an important cause of poor weight gain in growing preterm babies. Babies with cold stress need appropriate modification of environmental temperature control (warming the environment with room heaters or blowers) and appropriate clothing.

Hyperthermia

Hyperthermia is defined as an axillary temperature above 37.5°C.

Etiology

- High environmental temperature
- Sepsis
- Iatrogenic
  - Use of extra heat source
  - Excessive clothing
  - Phototherapy
- Dehydration
- CNS damage with injury to the hypothalamic centres

Clinical features

These include lethargy, irritability, increased/decreased activity, poor feeding, hypotonia and weak/absent cry.

Management

- The external heat source is removed, the amount of clothing is reduced and the environmental temperature is brought down.
- Tepid sponging is done only if the temperature is more than 39°C.
- The cause of the hyperthermia should be evaluated and treated. The baby should be referred to a specialist if the condition does not settle.

■ NEUROLOGICAL DISORDERS

If a neurological disorder is suspected, the newborn should be referred to a special care unit. A seizure may occur, indicating an alteration in neurological function; such a development needs to be investigated.

Etiology

Common causes of neonatal seizures are as follows:

- Birth trauma
- Intracranial bleed
- Hypoglycemia and hypocalcemia

These account for the majority of cases of neonatal seizures in the first three days of life. After the third day of life, meningitis is the most important cause, but it should be considered strongly in seizures at any age. Hyponatremia and hypernatremia may also occur at any age. Seizures due to structural malformations of the CNS and drug withdrawal can occur at any time. Rare causes include inborn errors of metabolism and storage disorders.

■ RETINOPATHY OF PREMATURITY

Retinopathy of prematurity (ROP) is a vasoproliferative disorder of the retina and vitreous in preterm infants. ROP manifests clinically by the abnormal growth of developing retinal vessels. An indirect ophthalmoscopic examination of the retina is required for the early detection of this disorder. ROP is an important cause of visual impairment in preterm infants. Early screening, appropriate treatment and follow-up can improve the outcome.

Risk Factors

Many factors have been associated with ROP. A consistent association has been with low gestational age, low birth weight, and duration of mechanical ventilation. Other factors implicated in the pathogenesis of ROP include hyperoxia, hypoxia, hypocarbia, acidosis, alkalosis, vitamin E deficiency, bright-light exposure, respiratory distress syndrome, intraventricular hemorrhage, bronchopulmonary dysplasia, patent ductus arteriosus, sepsis, candidiasis and multiple blood transfusions.

Incidence

Nearly 50% of very-low-birth-weight (VLBW) babies develop some degree of ROP, while 10% develop severe ROP (stage 3 or more). If this condition is suspected on examining the retina, the newborn should be referred to a special care unit.

Screening

The aim is to identify the following:
- ROP that has the potential to reach stage 3
- Severe (stage 3) ROP that may require treatment

Whom to screen
- Gestational age ≤32 weeks
- Birth weight ≤1,700 g
- Neonates who have received prolonged oxygen administration irrespective of gestation and birth weight

When to screen
The first ophthalmological examination should be conducted in all infants at 4–6 weeks postnatal age.

■ BIRTH TRAUMA

Birth trauma is defined as injuries sustained during the process of labour and delivery. Birth trauma frequently accompanies birth asphyxia, both being the result of difficult and prolonged deliveries. Sometimes, trauma may occur despite skilled and competent obstetric care. Intrauterine invasive procedures like amniocentesis, intrauterine transfusions and neonatal injuries after resuscitation are not considered birth injuries.

The importance of the recognition of birth trauma is that even an apparently minor injury can have long-term sequelae or lead to an acute catastrophic outcome. The injuries may be mild to severe and may need care ranging from simple observation to aggressive management.

Predisposing factors for birth trauma

Maternal
- Primigravida
- Small maternal stature, pelvic anomalies contributing to CPD

Pregnancy, labour and complications at delivery
- Oligohydramnios
- Abnormal presentations like breech
- Deep transverse arrest
- Use of mid-cavity forceps or vacuum extraction
- Internal podalic version and extraction

Fetal factors
- Fetal macrosomia
- Large fetal head
- VLBW babies and extreme prematurity
- Fetal anomalies

Though mortality related to birth trauma has significantly decreased, this continues to be a major cause of morbidity. The spectrum of birth injury ranges from minor skin injury to devastating intracranial hemorrhage and spinal cord injuries. Broad groups of injuries associated with birth trauma are those involving:
- The head, neck and face
- The nerves
- The spine, viscera and bones
- The soft tissues

Head Injuries

Injuries to the head and neck include intra- and extracranial injuries. Three major extracranial injuries are caput succedaneum, cephalohematoma and subgaleal hemorrhage. These lesions occur in different planes between the skin and the cranial bones.

Caput succedaneum

It is an area of edema over the presenting part, which is present at birth and resolves spontaneously within the next few days (Fig. 54.2).

Cephalohematoma

It represents a subperiosteal collection of blood overlying a cranial bone and limited by suture lines (Fig. 54.2). There are several clinical features that differentiate cephalohematoma from subgaleal hemorrhage and caput succedaneum; these are as follows:

- Cephalohematoma usually resolves within one to two months.
- Significant hyperbilirubinemia can result from a big cephalohematoma.
- Common associated complications include skull fractures and intracranial bleeds.

Subgaleal hemorrhage

It is a collection of blood in the soft tissue space between the galea aponeurotica and the periosteum of the skull. This usually results from forceps delivery or vacuum extraction. This is a serious and life-threatening complication which is sometimes associated with systemic signs and symptoms of blood loss. Mortality may be as high as 25%.

Intracranial bleed

Intracranial hemorrhage is a life-threatening complication. The hemorrhage may be subdural, intraparenchymal or intraventricular. Intracranial hemorrhages are often associated with significant mortality and morbidity.

Neck Injuries

Neck injuries include shoulder dislocation, clavicular fracture and muscle injury.

Clavicular fracture

Fracture to the clavicle occurs during a difficult delivery of the shoulder in vertex presentation and extended arms in breech delivery. Immobilisation of the arm and pain relief are important in the first one to two weeks; these measures are well-associated with recovery.

Sternocleidomastoid muscle injury

Injury to the sternocleidomastoid muscle may present as congenital torticollis or swelling over the sternocleidomastoid muscle (SM), which is usually detected two to three weeks after birth. This may result from abnormal intrauterine pressure or injury at birth. Physiotherapy of the neck improves the condition in two to three months. For persistent deformity, surgical intervention may be required before the age of one year.

Facial Injuries

Facial injuries include bruising of the face, fracture and dislocation of the facial bones and injuries to the eyes and ears. These injuries have variable prognosis depending on the type and site of injury.

Nerve Injuries

Though various nerves can be injured during delivery, brachial plexus injury is the most common. Other nerves injured are the phrenic nerve, facial nerve and peroneal nerve.

Brachial plexus injury

Brachial palsy occurs due to trauma to the spinal roots of the C5 vertebra through the first thoracic nerves.

The three main presentations are:

- Erb's upper arm palsy (C5, C6, C7)
- Klumpke's lower arm paralysis (C8, T1)
- Paralysis of the entire arm

Most cases follow a prolonged and difficult delivery leading to avulsion of the nerve root and tearing of the

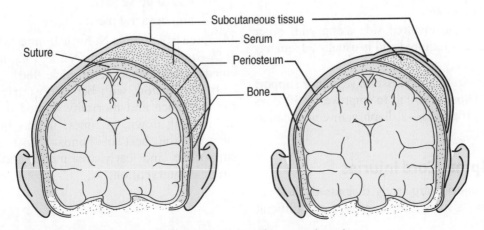

Fig. 54.2 Caput succedaneum (left) and cephalohematoma (right)—coronal section

nerve sheath; as a result, nerve fibres are compressed due to hemorrhage and edema. The clinical features are classical.

- In upper arm paralysis, the arm is adducted and internally rotated. There is extension at the elbow, pronated forearm and flexion of the wrist.
- It may be associated with ipsilateral phrenic nerve injury.
- In lower arm paralysis, the hand is paralysed and grasp is absent. It may be associated with an ipsilateral Horner syndrome due to concurrent injury to the sympathetic fibres of T1.
- When total paralysis occurs, the entire arm is motionless and flaccid with all reflexes absent and there is sensory deficit.
- However, arm palsy should be differentiated from cerebral injury leading to arm paralysis and shoulder injury. A CT scan or USG can detect shoulder dislocation, which may be difficult to pick up on plain X-ray. Treatment is primarily conservative with periodic reevaluation.
- Those who fail to improve in three months may need exploration of the brachial plexus. About 95% of patients improve with conservative therapy. For the rest, long-term sequelae are expected. Early surgical intervention may improve the outcome significantly.

Phrenic nerve palsy

This results in diaphragmatic paralysis and is more often associated with brachial plexus injury than an isolated manifestation.

- Lateral hyperextension of the neck during breech delivery leads to the avulsion of C3, C4 and C5 roots which supply the phrenic nerve.
- Irregular and laboured breathing points towards the diagnosis.
- Real-time ultrasound can pick up abnormal motion of the hemidiaphragm.
- Positioning on the involved side along with other supportive care is required and is usually adequately supported.
- For severe respiratory depression, ventilator support is required. Those who fail to improve by 30 days have a poor prognosis—a diaphragm complication is a probability.

Spine and Spinal Cord Injuries

Though spinal injuries are rarely diagnosed, they are not uncommon. Usually, they result from difficult breech deliveries.

Visceral Injuries

Though visceral injuries are relatively uncommon, they are fatal when they do occur.

Bone Injuries

The various bones and related structures injured during delivery are the humerus and the femur; there could also be dislocation of the hip and knee and epiphyseal separation. Skull fractures include linear fracture, depressed fracture and occipital osteodiastasis.

In addition to the injuries described above, intrapartum fetal monitoring can lead to injuries due to fetal scalp electrode application and fetal blood sampling.

Prognosis

- Skull injuries with a favourable long-term prognosis include the following:
  — Caput succedaneum
  — Cephalohematoma
  — Linear fractures
- Facial injuries with a favourable long-term prognosis include the following:
  — Subconjunctival hemorrhage
  — Retinal hemorrhage
- Musculoskeletal injuries with a favourable long-term prognosis include the following:
  — Clavicular fracture
  — Fractures of the long bones
  — SM injuries
- Peripheral nerve injuries with a favourable long-term prognosis include the following:
  — Facial palsy
  — Unilateral cord paralysis
  — Radial nerve palsy
  — Lumbosacral plexus injury

(Adapted from Laroia N. Birth Trauma. *Medscape Drugs & Diseases*. Updated February 2, 2015. Available at http://emedicine.medscape. com/article/980112-overview.)

In conclusion, with better obstetric care, though the incidence and mortality related to birth trauma are coming down, at times, it may be unavoidable even in the best of hands. Most injuries need supportive and early treatment, and only rarely, surgical intervention.

KEY POINTS

✓ *Neonatal hypoglycemia is defined as blood glucose <40 mg/dL irrespective of gestation and day of life. This is commonly seen in infants of diabetic mothers, IUGR infants and premature infants.*

✓ *Neonatal hypothermia is an important cause of neonatal morbidity and mortality. Hypothermia should be prevented or detected early and corrected.*

✓ *Hyperthermia is defined as axillary temperature above 37.5°C.*

✓ *Common causes of neonatal seizures include birth asphyxia, birth trauma, intracranial bleed, hypoglycemia and hypocalcemia.*

✓ *Retinopathy of prematurity is a vasoproliferative disorder of the retina and vitreous in preterm infants.*

✓ *Birth trauma is defined as injuries sustained during the process of labour and delivery.*

Essay questions

1. Define neonatal hypoglycemia. List its causes and principles of management.
2. List the causes of neonatal hypothermia and the measures that can be adopted to prevent this complication.

Short answer questions

1. What are the indications for the use of incubators?
2. Write a short note on 'kangaroo mother care'.
3. Enumerate the common causes of neonatal seizures.
4. Write a short note on retinopathy of prematurity.
5. Write a short note on brachial plexus injury.
6. Define the following:
   a) Caput succedaneum
   b) Subgaleal hemorrhage
   c) Cephalohematoma

MCQs

1. The following are true of cephalohematoma EXCEPT:
   a) It is a subperiosteal collection of blood
   b) It is limited by suture lines
   c) It usually resolves within one to two days
   d) It may be associated with significant hyperbilirubinemia

2. The nerve roots involved in Klumpke's paralysis are:
   a) C5, C6
   b) C6, C7
   c) C8, T1
   d) C5, C6, C7

Answers

1. (c), 2. (c)

Fill in blanks

1. Neonatal hypoglycemia is defined as a condition that occurs whenever the blood glucose level falls below_____ in the first 48 hours of life and less than _____ thereafter.
2. When the axillary temperature is less than _____ it is known as hypothermia, and when the temperature is less than _____ it is called severe hypothermia.

Answers

1. 45 mg/dL, 50 mg/dL, 2. 36.5°C, 32°C

55

The Forceps and the Vacuum Extractor

OG 15.1 and 15.2

Learning Objectives

» To know the indications for vacuum and forceps deliveries
» To know the prerequisites for the application of vacuum
» To know the prerequisites for the application of outlet forceps
» To know the complications of vacuum and forceps delivery

■ FORCEPS DELIVERY

The obstetric forceps are an integral part of obstetric management and were widely used until the last decade. However, in recent years, with the increasing incidence of cesarean sections, the incidence of instrumental vaginal deliveries has come down.

Forceps and vacuum application are two essential components of obstetric care, the knowledge of which is essential for all medical professionals. With proper case selection and proper application, cesarean section rate can be reduced, while at the same time, keeping maternal and neonatal morbidity low.

Types of Forceps

Forceps are broadly classified into three categories, which are as follows:
• Traction forceps
   — Short, straight forceps such as Wrigley's forceps (Fig. 55.1)
   — Long, straight forceps such as Simpson's forceps
   — Axis traction forceps (Fig. 55.1) such as Milne Murray's forceps

   The straight Wrigley's forceps and Simpson's forceps are used in outlet forceps delivery. Axis traction forceps are used in cases of low mid-cavity delivery.
• Rotational forceps
   — Kielland's forceps (Fig. 55.1) are rotational forceps that are used in the occipitoposterior position to facilitate rotation.
• Special forceps
   — Piper forceps are special forceps used in the delivery of the after-coming head of the fetus

Parts of the Forceps

All obstetric forceps consist of the following four parts (Fig. 55.2) with minor variations to suit their particular

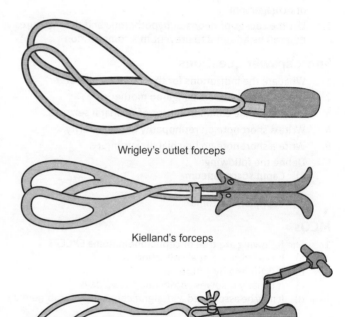

Wrigley's outlet forceps

Kielland's forceps

Axis traction forceps

Fig. 55.1 Types of forceps

indication or preference—the blade, the shank, the lock and the application handle. In addition, some types of forceps also have a traction handle and traction rods.

The blades

The obstetric forceps consist of two blades that cross each other. These are called the left or lower blade and the right or upper blade, according to the side of the pelvis to which they are applied.

The fenestrated blade

Each fenestrated blade possesses two curves—a cephalic curve, which enables the blade to be applied closely to the cephalic pole of the fetus and a pelvic curve (Fig. 55.2), which enables it to be introduced so as to lie more or less in the axis of the parturient canal (curve of Carus).

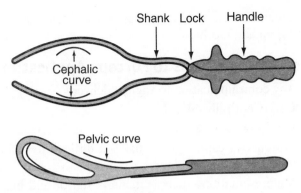

Fig. 55.2   Components of forceps

The shank

The shank connects the blades to the handle and gives the instrument its length. The shank is parallel in straight forceps (e.g., Simpson's forceps) or crossed over (e.g., Tucker–McLean's forceps).

The lock

The two blades articulate at the lock, which may be of the English type or the French type. The English type is the simpler and more efficient of the two and allows the shank of one blade to slip into the socket of the other. In the French lock, there is a pivot located in the shank of the left blade and a notch in the right blade into which the pivot can be aligned; the screw is tightened after locking the blades.

The handle

Finger grips or lateral flanges on the handle help in getting a secure grip.

Axis traction

Axis traction was devised by Tarnier in 1877. With straight forceps, traction becomes difficult when the head is in the mid-cavity. The addition of traction rods, which enables traction to be applied in the axis of the pelvic cavity, helps overcome this difficulty.

The common forms of axis traction forceps currently in use are the improved Tarnier's forceps, Milne Murray's axis traction forceps and Neville's axis traction forceps. The Milne Murray's axis traction forceps is preferred, as it is suitable for all types of forceps delivery

Types of Forceps Delivery

Depending on the station of the fetal head in relation to the ischial spines and the rotation of the fetal skull, forceps application is classified into three types (Table 55.1)—outlet forceps, low forceps and mid forceps application. In modern obstetric practice, only outlet forceps and low forceps applications are in use. Low forceps application helps in gaining traction to bring the fetal head to the pelvic floor. Outlet forceps application helps in the extension of the fetal head.

Table 55.1   Types of forceps delivery

Forceps delivery	Criteria for application
Outlet forceps	• Fetal head is at or on the perineum, +3 station • The scalp is visible at the introitus without separating the labia • The fetal skull has reached the pelvic floor • The sagittal suture is in the anteroposterior diameter or the rotation is not >45°
Low forceps	• The leading point of fetal skull at ≥+2 cm station or below, but not on the pelvic floor • Rotation ≥45° or ≤45° in the occipitoanterior or occipitoposterior position
Mid forceps	• Head is engaged, not palpable per abdomen or 1/5th palpable • The leading point of the fetal skull is above 2 cm but below the ischial spines • Rotation is <45° or >45°

Indications for Forceps Application

Forceps application is indicated in any condition that threatens the well-being of the mother or the fetus in the second stage of labour and is likely to be relieved with safe vaginal delivery. Forceps may be applied prophylactically or when there are definite indications.

Maternal indications

• Conditions where prolonged expulsive efforts should be avoided as in anemia/cardiac disease, in failure, eclampsia, pulmonary compromise, etc.

• Prolonged second stage of labour can occur due to maternal exhaustion, failure of secondary powers or weakness of muscles associated with neurological conditions such as myasthenia gravis.

• Prolonged second stage can also occur following epidural analgesia. In a woman on epidural, if the second stage of labour is prolonged for more than 3 hours in a nulliparous woman and more than 2 hours in a multiparous woman and if the criteria for instrumental delivery are fulfilled, forceps application is carried out.

Fetal indications

When there is fetal distress in the second stage of labour due to cord prolapse, abruptio placenta or any other reason, the baby is quickly delivered by forceps application.

Types of Forceps Application

Prophylactic forceps

The term 'prophylactic forceps' has been used to indicate delivery by forceps in cases where there is no definite indication for forceps delivery. Instead, the forceps are applied to reduce the stress on the mother and damage to the baby. The indications for prophylactic forceps are as follows:

- In medical conditions such as pre-eclampsia, cardiac disease or severe anemia, prophylactic forceps are applied to prevent the woman from straining in the second stage of labour, which may worsen her condition.
- While conducting vaginal birth after cesarean section, prophylactic forceps may be applied to prevent scar dehiscence/rupture at the time of pushing in the second stage of labour, if it is prolonged.
- For controlled delivery of the head in a preterm baby and to avoid prolonged pressure on the baby's head from being left on the perineum for a long time, prophylactic forceps may be required.

Indicated forceps

The term 'indicated forceps' is used when forceps are applied when there are maternal or fetal indications for their use.

Trial of forceps

When the operator anticipates the possibility of failure and makes advance preparations for cesarean delivery, and attempts forceps application, it is known as a trial of forceps.

> Trial of forceps is attempted only in an operating room that is both equipped and staffed for immediate cesarean delivery. The procedure is abandoned if the forceps cannot be applied satisfactorily or if there is no descent with one single downward pull along with uterine contraction. In such cases, the delivery is accomplished by cesarean section.

Failed forceps

The term failed forceps refers to an error of judgement. It refers to cases in which forceps are applied under conditions that are not favourable for their application. The main causes of failed forceps are undiagnosed CPD, malpositions, high head or incorrect application. In these circumstances, the team is not prepared for the emergency cesarean section, and the delivery is usually attempted in surroundings not suitable for immediate cesarean delivery. Failed forceps demands immediate cesarean section and is associated with high maternal and perinatal morbidity.

Contraindications to Forceps Application

- Any contraindication to vaginal delivery
- Cervix not fully dilated
- Unengaged head
- Presence of caput, which makes it difficult to define the position and station
- Malpresentations such as mentoposterior and brow presentations
- Even a minor degree of CPD
- A mother infected with HIV is a relative contraindication as forceps may be associated with scalp trauma
- Bleeding disorders in the fetus

Prerequisites for Forceps Application

- There should be a clear indication for forceps application.
- The cervix must be fully dilated.
- The membranes must be recently ruptured.
- The presentation should be vertex (occipitoanterior or occipitoposterior) or the after-coming head in a breech presentation.
- There should not be any cephalopelvic disproportion; all the diameters of the pelvis should be adequate.
- The head should be engaged (the greatest transverse diameter of the head should have passed through the brim of the pelvis).
- No part of the fetal head should be palpable per abdomen.
- The head should be well rotated.
- The position of the head should be ascertained by palpating the fontanelles and sagittal suture.
- Analgesia should be satisfactory.
- The uterus should be contracting and relaxing.
- The bladder should be empty.
- Informed consent should be obtained from the woman and her family.

Methods of Application

The fundamental principle involved in the application of forceps is to complete delivery with minimum trauma to the mother and the child. Faulty technique can result in failure to extract the head, damage to the fetal head, lacerations of the maternal soft parts and the increased incidence of morbidity in the puerperium.

Forceps application is best performed under pudendal block anesthesia; regional or general anesthesia may be necessary on occasion. The woman is brought to the edge of the bed and made to lie in the dorsal posture with her legs supported mechanically or by assistants. The operative field is then covered with sterile towels or sheets.

There are two ways of applying the forceps: the cephalic method and the pelvic method.

Cephalic method

In the cephalic method, the blades are applied at either end of the biparietal diameter so that each ear is at the centre of each fenestra of the forceps (Fig. 55.3). When the blades are locked, there is compression in the biparietal diameter, where it does least harm. Since the blades are well-applied to the sides of fetal head, this does not allow the head to slip. Irrespective of its position in relation to the maternal pelvis, the blades are applied to the sides of the fetal head.

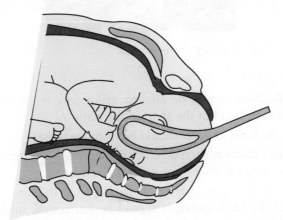

Fig. 55.3   The ideal position of the blades relative to the fetal head

Pelvic method

This method is rarely practiced now.

Low Forceps Delivery—Occipitoanterior Position (Fig. 55.4a–e)

The most commonly used forceps is the axis traction Milne Murray forceps.

Identification of position

The exact position of the fetal head is determined by examining the sagittal sutures and the fontanelles. The head should have completely rotated into the occipitoanterior position with the sagittal suture lying in the AP diameter of the outlet.

Assembly of blades (Fig. 55.4a)

The blades are assembled carefully. The left blade is that which is applied on the left side of the mother's pelvis. The handle is held in the operator's left hand.

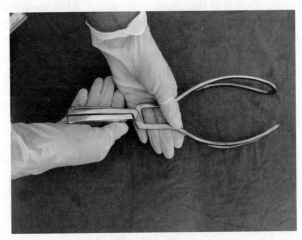

Fig. 55.4a   Assembly of the blades

Introduction of the blades

- The patient is anesthetised, and the perineum is carefully prepared. The operator sits on a stool of convenient height.
- After emptying the bladder by passing a catheter, the operator selects and picks ups the left blade in her left hand.
- She introduces two fingers of her gloved right hand into the vaginal cavity (Fig. 55.4b) on the left and posterior quadrant of the pelvis so that the palmar surface of the fingers faces upwards and to the right. The left blade is lightly held with the handle parallel to the right inguinal ligament as one would hold a spoon.

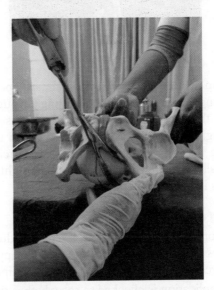

Fig. 55.4b   Introduction of the left blade

- The tip of the blade is held at right angles to the palmar surface of the fingers in the vagina and gently slipped along the fingers into the vaginal cavity.

- The blade thus introduced is gently rotated laterally to position it at the appropriate place. That the lower blade has been correctly applied can be verified by pressing the handle well against the perineum. If the handle is seen to be perfectly straight without any tilting to one side or the other, it can be presumed to have been properly applied. If the lower blade has been applied properly, it will rest there and will not tend to slip out. An assistant may, if necessary, lightly steady the handle in this position.

- The operator then removes her right hand and introduces two fingers of the left hand—this time, above and to the right, so that the palmar aspect of the two fingers is facing downwards and towards the left (Fig. 55.4c). The right blade is taken in the right hand by gripping the handle. The blade is now held parallel to the mother's left inguinal ligament.

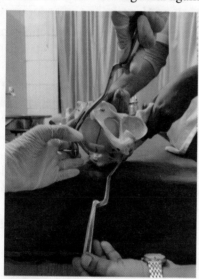

Fig. 55.4c Introduction of the right blade

- The tip is pressed against the palmar aspect of the two fingers, and by gently rotating through half a circle, the cephalic portion is gradually inserted into the vagina to lie in close apposition with the head. As the blade passes through half the circle, it will generally, be found that it slips into the right side and adapts itself to the cephalic pole.

Locking of the forceps (Fig. 55.4d)

- As soon as the blades have been introduced, the forceps should be locked. With proper application, the forceps lock easily or with minor manipulation.

- The application is checked to see whether the blades are equidistant from the sagittal suture.

- If the blades do not lock easily, undue manipulation should not be applied. In such cases, it is advisable to remove the forceps and reassess the situation.

- The obstetrician should proceed with traction only after reassuring the woman that the forceps have been applied properly and locked.

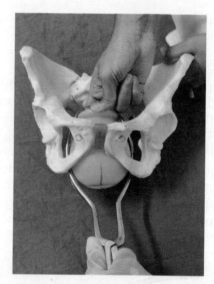

Fig. 55.4d Locking of the forceps

Traction

- Traction should be applied using only the traction handle and not the shaft of the blade.

- The force exerted should be from the wrist.

- The traction should be applied during a contraction so that minimal force needs to be exerted.

- The direction of traction should be in the direction of the birth canal. It should be horizontal, initially downwards and backwards, and once the fetal head distends the perineum, the direction should be changed to upward and forward (Fig. 55.4e).

- As the vulva is distended by the occiput, an episiotomy may be given.

- If the traction is applied properly and there is descent of the head, the head will automatically move upwards so that there is no need for the operator to try to extend the head for delivering the same.

- When the occiput has emerged from under the symphysis, the blades may be removed, and the delivery completed in the manner described in Chapter 14, *The conduct of normal labour*.

- While removing the blades, the right blade is removed first followed by the left blade.

- Some obstetricians prefer to complete the delivery with the forceps in situ as this gives a greater degree of control over the advance of the head. After the delivery of the head, the shoulders are delivered, following which, the rest of the body slips out.

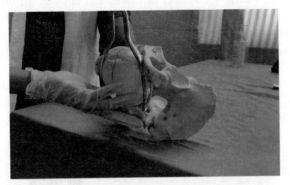

Fig. 55.4e   Traction and extension of the fetal head

Outlet Forceps Delivery

For outlet forceps delivery, Wrigley's outlet forceps are used. It is used only to facilitate the extension of the head and should not be used for traction. Traction with outlet forceps may lead to extensive lacerations and trauma.

Procedure

- The woman is placed in the lithotomy position and brought to the edge of the table.
- Local analgesia with perineal infiltration is administered with about 10–12 mL of 1% xylocaine.
- Local preparations and draping are done to ensure strict asepsis.
- Vaginal examination is done to confirm that the head lies in the pelvic outlet, with the parietal eminences lying below the ischial spines and the fetal head at or on the perineum at the +3 station.
- The scalp should be visible during contractions without separating the labia.
- The internal rotation should be complete, and the sagittal suture should be felt in the anteroposterior diameter of the outlet.
- The introduction of the blades is as described in low forceps application.
- The locking of the blades is usually easy. If there is any difficulty, the handle should be brought down, pressing over the perineum. Otherwise, the blades are removed, and vaginal examination is repeated to confirm the full rotation of the head. This should be corrected, and the blades reinserted. There is no fixation screw, and the operation is easy. The handles of the forceps are held with the operator's right hand and extension of the head is facilitated during a uterine contraction. During the procedure, an episiotomy is given when the head is crowning and the perineum is thinned out.

- With outlet forceps application, trauma to the fetus and the maternal soft parts is minimal.
- After any instrumental delivery, the cervix, vagina and perineum should be examined for injuries.

Forceps in Malpositions/ Malpresentations

Direct occipitoposterior position

In the direct occipitoposterior position, when the head is on the perineum, the blades are applied correctly as described earlier and a generous episiotomy is given. Horizontal traction is applied until the base of the nose is under the symphysis pubis. The handle should then be elevated till the occiput emerges over the anterior margin of the perineum. Then, with a downward motion of the instrument, the nose, face and chin emerge from the vulva (face-to-pubis delivery). In direct occipitoposterior delivery, whether spontaneous or assisted by forceps, there is a greater risk of severe lacerations of the perineum and complete perineal tears.

Keilland's forceps

It is one of the rotational forceps. Kielland's forceps were used in the past in the delivery of occipitoposterior position. Because it has a sliding lock, it permits satisfactory cephalic application even if there is asynclitism. It also facilitates rotation because it has minimal pelvic curvature. The use of this type of forceps requires special training. In inappropriate and unskilled hands, Kielland's forceps are technically difficult to operate. Improper use of the instrument may lead to spiral vaginal tears. In modern obstetrics, Kielland's forceps are rarely used having been largely replaced by vacuum delivery/cesarean section depending on the situation.

Forceps application for the after-coming head of the breech

Forceps application is one of the methods used to deliver the after-coming head of the breech. Some clinicians use it routinely while others use it when they encounter difficulty in delivering the after-coming head. Either straight forceps or Piper's forceps with their long and parallel shanks can be used. To apply the forceps, an assistant holds the baby's body straight using a towel and lifts it so that the body remains parallel to the floor. The operator then introduces the blades from below, one on either side of the head, and applies steady traction. The advantages of using forceps are that the delivery of the head can be controlled, the sudden exit of the head can be avoided and the traction is on the head, promoting flexion; this avoids traction injury to the neck and cervical vertebra. The space created by the forceps also allows the baby to breathe.

Forceps in face presentation

In the mentoanterior position, outlet forceps may be applied. It is contraindicated in the mentoposterior position.

Complications of Forceps Application

If cases are properly selected, the risks to the mother and child are negligible. However, maternal and fetal complications can develop due to the faulty and injudicious use of the instrument.

Maternal complications

- Extension of episiotomy
- Vaginal lacerations and cervical tears
- Perineal lacerations including third- and fourth-degree tears
- Extension of vaginal tears to the fornices, resulting in colporrhexis
- Occasionally, rupture uterus can result
- Broad-ligament hematoma
- Postpartum hemorrhage
- Bladder injury, which may later lead to vesicovaginal fistulae and rectal injury
- Puerperal sepsis

Fetal complications

- Intracranial hemorrhage
- Skull fractures
- Cephalohematoma
- Facial nerve palsy
- Facial injuries
- Birth asphyxia

Slipping of the forceps

Sometimes, the forceps may slip when traction is applied. This may be due to faulty application, occipitoposterior position, a small head or a macerated fetus.

■ VACUUM EXTRACTOR

The vacuum extractor, like the obstetric forceps, is a method of delivering the fetal head from the birth canal. It was in 1956 that Malmström published a monograph in which he justified and showed that, on mechanical grounds, the vacuum extractor is less dangerous than forceps when used under given clinical conditions.

Parts of a Vacuum Extractor

The instrument consists of extraction cups of different sizes—30, 40, 50 and 60 mm in diameter, a vacuum generator apparatus consisting of a vacuum bottle and gauge and the connecting tubing (Fig. 55.5). Attached to the metal cup is a traction chain with a handle. Metal cups were widely used in the past, but with the advent of soft silastic cups, metal cups are slowly being replaced by soft cups which are less traumatic.

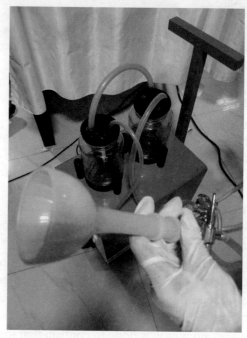

Fig. 55.5 Vacuum generator apparatus and silastic cup

Indications and Prerequisites

The indications and prerequisites for the use of a vacuum extractor for delivery are the same as for forceps delivery. There should not be any CPD, it should be a vertex presentation and the head should be engaged. The bladder should be empty, and the cervix should be fully dilated—at least >8 cm dilated. The indications are maternal/fetal distress in the second stage of labour and prolonged second stage. The vacuum extractor is very useful in the occipitoposterior position as it also helps in the rotation of the head.

Contraindications

- Brow, face or other non-vertex presentations
- Prematurity (gestation <34 weeks)
- Fetal coagulopathies
- Recent scalp blood sampling
- Presence of significant degree of caput, which may preclude the correct placement of the cup and indicate cephalopelvic disproportion

Technique

Application of the cup

- If the woman is on epidural labour analgesia, the same is continued. Otherwise, a pudendal block is given with perineal infiltration for an episiotomy.
- The woman is placed in the dorsal position at the edge of the table. Her flexed lower limbs are supported on the supporting rods on either side. Under aseptic precautions, the bladder is emptied before the procedure.
- A suitable cup is selected and introduced into the vagina sideways and then turned for proper placement. With the present-day silastic or soft cups, the rim of the cup can be pressed together for proper placement.
- Under the control of two fingers, the cup is pushed towards the head and placed in direct contact with it at its most inferior and/or posterior parts. Determining the flexion point is important so as to keep the head flexed; this helps in successful delivery.
- In an average-term infant, the flexion point is located along the sagittal suture, 3 cm anterior to the posterior fontanelle (and thus, 6 cm posterior to the anterior fontanelle). This is known as the 'application distance'.
- The centre of the cup should be placed directly over this point. Failure to adequately position the cup can lead to a progressive deflexion of the fetal head during traction and result in an increased risk of detachment due to obliquely diverted traction.
- Creating negative pressure—the dome is held in place manually at the chosen site, while the assistant creates a vacuum at the rate of 0.2 Kg/cm².
- At the same time, taking advantage of the few minutes required for the formation of the chignon within the cup, the operator carefully verifies, with the forefinger moved around the brim of the cup, that it is directly applied to the head without the inclusion of maternal tissue such as portions of the vaginal wall or cervix; this is especially important in a multipara.
- The vacuum is gradually increased every two to three minutes until the pressure gauge shows a reading of 0.8 Kg/cm². This will allow a traction force of 20–22 Kg.
- Traction should not be initiated without pausing for the above-mentioned time intervals. This is important. The quality of the chignon or artificial caput, which is the most important factor in good adhesion, depends essentially on the time allowed for its formation.
- With silastic cups, there is no need to wait for chignon formation. Full vacuum can be applied directly.

Correct application of silastic vacuum cup

The centre of the cup should be over the sagittal suture and about 3 cm (1.2 inches) in front of the posterior fontanelle (Fig. 55.6). The cup is generally placed as far posteriorly as possible (American Academy of Family Physicians, www.aafp.org).

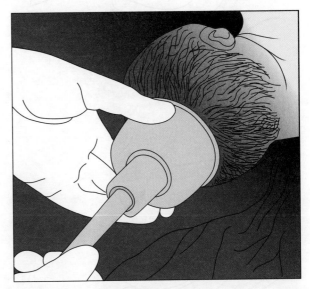

Fig. 55.6 Application of silastic vacuum cup

Traction

Traction should be applied so as to coincide with spontaneous uterine contractions. It must be exerted at right angles to the cup; otherwise, one edge will be lifted off and the vacuum will be broken (Fig. 55.7a–c).

Since general anesthesia is not employed, it is possible to coordinate traction with spontaneous uterine contractions. Traction also stimulates uterine contractions in a hypotonic uterus. When traction is being applied, it is important that the mother be encouraged to use all her effort to push down. It takes 8–10 minutes to build the vacuum slowly to the required level (0.8 Kg/cm²), so that the chignon may fill the cup. Traction must be applied intermittently along with the uterine contractions and maternal bearing down efforts. The duration of delivery should not exceed 20 minutes, as a longer duration produces severe trauma to the fetal scalp, causing hematoma formation and sloughing.

When the vacuum is applied at a higher level, similar to applying an axis traction forceps, the direction of traction should follow the curve of the pelvis, with initial downward and backward traction followed by downward and horizontal traction, and finally, upwards traction.

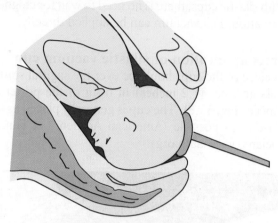

(a) Traction downwards and posteriorly

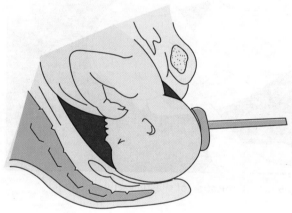

(b) Traction downwards and horizontally

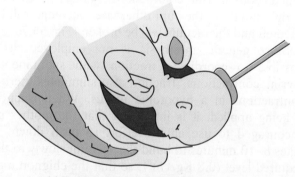

(c) Traction upwards and anteriorly

Fig. 55.7 Traction applied with a vacuum extractor

As mentioned earlier, with the present-day silastic cups, vacuum can be created without the conventional 'waiting time' and this reduces the overall procedure time.

After the delivery, the mother and baby should be examined for the presence of any soft tissue injury.

Attempts at vacuum extraction should be abandoned when there is no evidence of progressive descent with each pull or when delivery is not imminent following three pulls of a correctly applied instrument by an experienced operator.

Advantages of Vacuum Extractors

One of the main advantages of the vacuum extractor is that it causes minimum trauma to the mother and the child. The artificial caput formed disappears within 24–48 hours. However, when it is used to deliver a head at high level, intracranial injury can occur; when it is applied over a cervix that is incompletely dilated, avulsion of the cervix can occur. A vacuum extractor requires maternal effort, and therefore, may not be ideal in cases of heart disease complicating pregnancy.

Table 55.2 lists the advantages and disadvantages of vacuum extractors.

Table 55.2 Advantages and disadvantages of the vacuum extractor

Advantages	Disadvantages
• It occupies less space and does not add to disproportion • It allows the fetal head to follow its own path of descent and rotation • Only a little extra pain relief is required • It can be used when the exact position of the fetal head cannot be ascertained • It does not require a high level of skill to operate • It is less likely to be associated with significant maternal perineal and vaginal trauma	• The equipment is more complex and requires more maintenance • The equipment is less portable than forceps • It is more likely to fail at achieving vaginal delivery • The time taken for delivery is a minimum of 10–15 minutes after the application of the cup when the head is at the outlet; hence, if there is an urgency to deliver the child because of distress, forceps would be the better option • The incidence of neonatal jaundice and fetal hematoma is relatively higher with vacuum than with forceps • It is likely to be associated with cephalohematoma • It is more likely to be associated with retinal hemorrhage

Complications

- Circular avulsion of the cervix may occur if a rim of the cervix gets caught inside the cup
- Spiral vaginal tears
- Postpartum hemorrhage
- Fetal complications include scalp injury, subgaleal bleed, cephalohematoma, intracranial bleeds,

subconjunctival hemorrhage, neonatal jaundice and birth asphyxia

The Kiwi Omni Cup

This is a new-generation 'hand-held' vacuum extractor which does not require a cumbersome external suction source. It is designed for use in all fetal head positions—occiput anterior (OA), occiput posterior (OP) and occiput transverse (OT)—and during cesarean section. Its flexible stem and low-profile cup (Fig. 55.8) enable placement over the flexion point, 3 cm forward of the posterior fontanelle along the sagittal suture, so that the smallest diameter of the fetal head is presented into the birth canal. The traction force indicator located on the device measures the force exerted during traction.

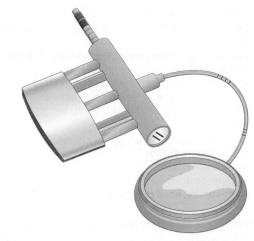

Fig. 55.8   The Kiwi OmniCup

KEY POINTS

✓   *The obstetric forceps and vacuum extractor are instruments designed for the extraction of the fetal head.*

✓   *Their use is indicated when a quick delivery is likely to be beneficial to the mother or the baby and vaginal delivery is expected to be safe.*

✓   *The fundamental principle involved in the application of the forceps or vacuum is to complete delivery with minimum trauma to the mother and the child. If the cases are properly selected, the risk to the mother and the child is minimum.*

✓   *Forceps and ventouse applications offer many advantages in carefully selected cases. Every obstetrician should learn the skills related to applying these.*

✓   *When the leading point of the fetal skull is at station +2 cm and not on the pelvic floor, a low forceps application is performed.*

✓   *When the operator anticipates the possibility of failure and makes advance preparations for cesarean delivery, the forceps application is known as trial of forceps.*

✓   *The artificial caput that is formed due to the application of a vacuum cup is called a chignon.*

Essay questions

1.   What are the indications and contraindications for forceps application?
2.   What are the prerequisites for forceps application? Describe outlet forceps application.
3.   What are the contraindications for vacuum delivery? Describe the technique of vacuum delivery.
4.   Compare the advantages and disadvantages of forceps and vacuum extractors in an assisted vaginal delivery.
5.   A 25-year-old primigravida is admitted at 39 weeks of gestation in active labour. The first stage of labour progressed normally, and she has been in the second stage of labour for one hour and 20 minutes. On examination, she looks exhausted and is unable to push during contractions. The baseline fetal heart rate is 120 per minute and decelerating to 80 beats per minute during contractions for the past 5 minutes. On vaginal examination, the cervix is fully dilated, there is no caput or moulding and the vertex is felt below the +2 station.
   a)   What should be the mode of delivery in this woman?
   b)   What are the indications to resort to operative vaginal delivery?

c)   What criteria should be fulfilled before resorting to operative vaginal delivery?
d)   What are the complications associated with forceps/vacuum delivery?

Short answer questions

1.   Describe the parts of an obstetric forceps.
2.   What do you understand by the term prophylactic forceps?
3.   What is a failed forceps delivery?
4.   Enumerate the complications that may occur due to forceps application.
5.   What are the advantages of vacuum extraction over forceps?

MCQs

1.   If the blades of the forceps do not lock easily, the next step is:
   a)   They should be locked by applying force
   b)   Removal of forceps and reassessment
   c)   The obstetrician should proceed with traction
   d)   Forceps application should be abandoned

2.   The criteria for outlet forceps include all EXCEPT:
   a)   The leading part of the fetal head is at the +2 station
   b)   The sagittal suture is in the anteroposterior diameter

c) Rotation does not exceed 45°
d) The scalp is visible at the introitus without separating the labia

3. Prerequisites for forceps application include all EXCEPT:
a) The membranes must be ruptured
b) The uterus must be contracting and relaxing
c) The cervix must be at least 8 cm dilated
d) No part of the fetal head must be palpable per abdomen

4. The forceps may be applied on all of the following presenting parts EXCEPT:
a) Occipitoanterior
b) Occipitoposterior
c) After-coming head of a breech
d) Brow

5. Contraindications for vacuum application include all EXCEPT:
a) Brow presentation
b) Occipitotransverse
c) Fetal coagulopathy
d) Extreme prematurity

6. Which of the following is not a contraindication for vacuum delivery?
a) Brow presentation
b) Fetal distress
c) Fetal coagulopathy
d) Recent fetal scalp blood sampling

7. In which of these conditions is forceps delivery not recommended?
a) Maternal heart disease
b) Prolonged second stage of labour
c) Hand prolapse
d) Non-reassuring CTG

8. After how many pulls should one abandon vacuum delivery if there is no descent of the head?
a) 1 pull
b) 2 pulls
c) 3 pulls
d) 4 pulls

9. Which of the following is not an axis traction forceps?
a) Wrigley's forceps
b) Milne Murray's forceps
c) Tarnier's forceps
d) Neville's forceps

10. Which is the flexion point in vacuum application?
a) 6 cm anterior to anterior fontanelle
b) 6 cm posterior to posterior fontanelle
c) 3 cm posterior to anterior fontanelle
d) 3 cm anterior to posterior fontanelle

11. What is the negative pressure required in vacuum delivery?
a) 0.2 Kg/sq. cm
b) 0.4 Kg/sq. cm
c) 0.6 Kg/sq. cm
d) 0.8 Kg/sq. cm

12. A primigravida is in the second stage of labour for the past two hours. The fetal head is at the +2 station. Despite effective uterine contractions, she is unable to push as she is exhausted. What will be the next step in management?
a) Wait for 1 more hour
b) Sedate the mother
c) Emergency cesarean section
d) Instrumental delivery

Answers

1. (b), 2. (a), 3. (c), 4. (d), 5. (b), 6. (b), 7. (c) 8. (c), 9. (a), 10. (d), 11. (d), 12. (d)

Fill in the blanks

1. When the leading part of the fetal skull is at the +2 station and not on the pelvic floor, the forceps application that should be used is _____.
2. The artificial caput that is formed due to the application of a vacuum cup is called a _____.
3. When the operator anticipates the possibility of failure and makes advance preparations for cesarean delivery, the forceps application is known as a _____.

Answers

1. low forceps, 2. chignon, 3. trial of forceps

56

OG 15.1

Version and Destructive Operations

Learning Objectives

» To know the indications, contraindications, procedure and complications of external cephalic version

» To know the indications for internal podalic version

■ INTRODUCTION

The cesarean section rates and morbidity associated with cesarean section are on the rise. One of the measures adopted to reduce the cesarean section rates is to reduce the incidence of breech presentations in labour. This can be achieved by external cephalic version, wherein a breech is converted into a cephalic presentation with the help of external manipulations.

■ VERSION

Version is a procedure in which the presentation of the fetus is altered, either by substituting one pole of a longitudinal presentation for the other or by converting an oblique or transverse lie into a longitudinal lie.

- External cephalic version is one in which by external manipulations, a breech or a transverse lie is converted into a cephalic presentation.
- External podalic version is one in which by external manipulations, the transverse lie of the second of twins is converted to a breech.
- Internal podalic version is one in which by internal manipulations, an oblique or transverse lie in the second of twins is converted to a breech presentation.

External Cephalic Version (ECV)

External cephalic version is a method of converting a breech presentation or a transverse lie into a cephalic presentation by external manipulation. If breech presentation is diagnosed in the antenatal period, women should be offered external cephalic version to lower the incidence of breech presentations in labour and thereby reduce the cesarean section rates. The advantages of ECV are that it is safe, non-invasive, relatively easy to perform and generally painless and that it may reduce the need for a cesarean section. However, there are certain contraindications for the procedure.

Contraindications

Absolute contraindications

- Multiple pregnancy
- Antepartum hemorrhage
- Ruptured membranes
- Significant fetal abnormalities
- Known uterine anomalies
- When there is a need for CS for other indications such as a contracted pelvis, severe IUGR with non-reassuring fetal status, severe pre-eclampsia or previous classical cesarean section scar
- High-risk pregnancies such as elderly primigravida, bad obstetric history and a large baby, which may lead to CPD

Relative contraindications

- Maternal obesity
- Rh-isoimmunisation
- Previous lower segment cesarean section scar

Timing of external cephalic version

ECV is performed at 36 weeks in a nullipara and at 37 weeks in a multipara. If done earlier, the chances of reverting to breech are higher. Moreover, if the baby has to be delivered due to complications during ECV, the chances of prematurity are minimal after 36 weeks.

The procedure is successful in nearly 60% of cases. If ECV is successful, vaginal delivery should be allowed. If ECV was not successful, it can be repeated at weekly intervals. Though ECV can be performed even in early labour when the membranes are intact, there may be difficulties in converting breech to cephalic because of the increasing size of the fetus and the diminishing liquor amnii.

Factors associated with successful version

The average success rate of external cephalic version for breech is 60% and that for transverse lie is 80%.

The factors associated with successful version include the following:

- Multiparity
- Complete breech
- Adequate liquor
- Woman not obese

The procedure (Fig. 56.1a–c and 56.2)

Version should be performed in a facility where an emergency cesarean section can be performed readily if needed. The procedure, its benefits and the probable complications should be explained to the woman and her consent should be taken. If the pregnant woman wishes to have an elective cesarean section, then this procedure should not be attempted. The woman should be prepared and ready for a cesarean section if required.

- An ultrasound is carried out to confirm breech presentation and the type of breech, to check for adequacy of amniotic fluid, to estimate fetal weight, to rule out congenital anomalies of the fetus and to identify the placental location.

- A non-stress test or modified biophysical profile is carried out to confirm the well-being of the fetus prior to the procedure; continuous CTG monitoring is carried out throughout the procedure.

- There is no need for anesthesia; however, if the mother is already in labour and has been given analgesia with epidural, it can be continued.

- Tocolysis with 0.25 mg terbutaline may be given subcutaneously before the procedure so that the uterus is well relaxed.

- The woman is positioned in the supine position with a slight left lateral tilt and the Trendelenburg position. The knees are slightly flexed.

- The presentation and position of the fetus are carefully ascertained, and the fetal poles are grasped with each hand. The breech is gently elevated out of the maternal pelvis and pushed laterally. Meanwhile, with the other hand, the cephalic pole is gently manipulated towards the pelvis. By a series of gentle stroking and pushing movements, the head is brought over the pelvic brim and the breech is moved to the fundus. While manipulating the fetus, two thirds of the force is on the breech and one third on the head to keep it flexed. A 'forward roll' of the fetus is gently attempted first. If it is unsuccessful, the 'back flip' technique is attempted.

- The attitude of flexion must be maintained throughout the procedure.

- After the completion of the procedure, CTG is continued for 10 minutes to ensure that there are no abnormal fetal heart rate changes.

- A binder may also be placed on the abdomen to hold the fetus in place.

- During the manipulations, any significant alterations in the fetal heart rate should be taken as a warning, and the version should be discontinued immediately.

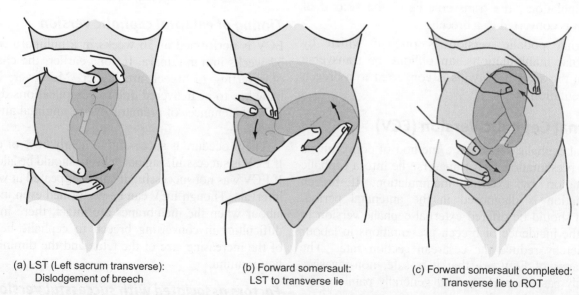

(a) LST (Left sacrum transverse): Dislodgement of breech

(b) Forward somersault: LST to transverse lie

(c) Forward somersault completed: Transverse lie to ROT

Fig. 56.1 External version in breech: (a) LST (left sacrum transverse)—dislodgement of breech, (b) forward somersault—LST to transverse lie and (c) forward somersault complete—transverse lie to right occipitotransverse (ROT)

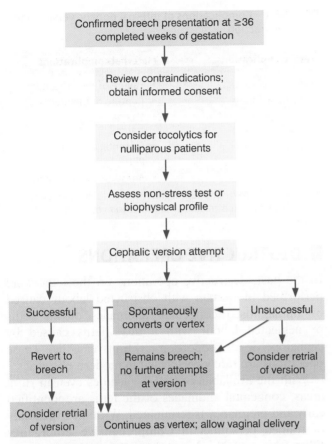

Fig. 56.2 Algorithm for ECV

- The procedure should also be discontinued if there is excessive maternal discomfort or a persistent abnormal fetal heart rate.
- Anti-D immunoglobulin is given to RhD-negative unsensitised women.
- If the presentation reverts to breech, version can be re-attempted even in early labour.

Complications

Version can be complicated by abruption, preterm labour, preterm premature rupture of membranes, fetal distress, cord entanglement, fetomaternal hemorrhage and rarely, fetal death and rupture uterus. These complications result from injudicious manoeuvres.

Internal Podalic Version

Internal version is always podalic. By intrauterine manipulations, one or both feet of the fetus are caught and drawn out through the cervix while transabdominally pushing the upper portion of the fetal body in the opposite direction. In modern obstetrics, the only indication for internal podalic version is the delivery of a second twin in transverse lie where the baby has to be delivered immediately because of fetal

distress, cord prolapse or abruption. Internal podalic version is always followed by breech extraction.

Prerequisites for internal version

There must be plenty of liquor amnii in the uterus, as this permits easy movement. Hence, the membranes must be intact or very recently ruptured with enough liquor still left. Internal podalic version should not be carried out when all the liquor has drained away and the uterus is tonically contracted as this may result in rupture of the uterus. The cervix should be fully dilated.

Contraindications

- When all the liquor has drained out
- When the woman is in obstructed labour
- When fetopelvic disproportion is anticipated, and vaginal delivery is not possible
- In the presence of a scarred uterus

The procedure

Before attempting internal podalic version for the second of twins in a transverse lie, after the delivery of the first twin, all efforts must be made to convert the second twin into a cephalic presentation by external cephalic version. Only when ECV fails should the woman be offered the option of internal podalic version. Before starting the procedure, the woman should be prepared as for a major obstetric operation, and her informed written consent should be obtained.

- For good relaxation of the uterus, deep general anesthesia is important. After being anesthetised, the woman is brought to the edge of the bed and made to lie in the lithotomy position.
- The bladder should be emptied under all sterile precautions.
- The clinician's right hand is introduced into the uterus to identify the baby's knee.
- The hand is then passed along the shin, and the foot is gripped along with the heel (Fig. 56.3a and b).
- An episiotomy should be performed at this stage.
- By gentle traction, the foot is brought out of the cervical canal and the vagina. Unless there are complications, gentle traction on one foot is usually sufficient to allow the breech and the other foot to be born. The other hand is kept on the fundus to provide assistance from above.
- Once both the feet are brought down, the breech is delivered by breech extraction as explained in Chapter 42, *Breech presentation and compound presentation*. One should ensure that the back of the fetus is anterior throughout the procedure.

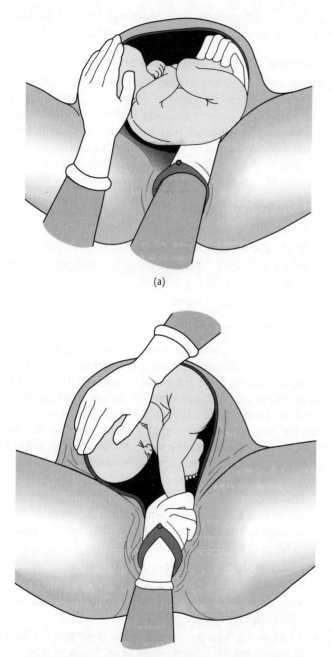

Fig. 56.3 (a and b) Internal podalic version in transverse/oblique lie

- At this stage, the uterus-relaxing anesthetic agent is discontinued, and the placenta is delivered or manually removed. Uterine exploration is performed, and oxytocin is administered by intravenous infusion. Fundal massage or bimanual compression is done to hasten myometrial contraction. The lower genital tract is explored to identify any lacerations, which are then sutured along with the episiotomy.
- Internal podalic version may be associated with the complications listed in Table 56.1.

Table 56.1 Complications of internal podalic version and breech extraction

Fetal complications	Maternal complications
• Cord prolapse • Visceral injury • Skeletal injury—femur • Neural injury • Fetal demise	• Failure of the procedure • Rupture of the uterus • Vaginal and perineal trauma • Placental abruption • PPH • Anesthetic complications

(Modified from Webster SNE, Loughney AD. 2011. Internal podalic version with breech extraction. *The Obstetrician & Gynecologists.* 13:7–14)

DESTRUCTIVE OPERATIONS

In the past, destructive operations on the fetus were performed in women with obstructed labour caused by undiagnosed congenital anomalies of the fetus or neglected labour with a dead fetus caused by cephalopelvic disproportion or transverse lie. These operations are rarely performed in modern obstetrics.

With the availability of USG facilities even in rural areas, congenital anomalies of the fetus are identified early and pregnancy is terminated. With the availability of trained personnel in **Comprehensive Emergency Obstetrics and Newborn Care** (CEmONC) centres, transfusion facilities and provision for early referral of cases to higher centres, the occurrence of obstructed and neglected labour has come down tremendously. Even if a pregnant woman is received with obstructed labour with a dead fetus, the antibiotic usage, anesthesia and blood transfusion facilities have made cesarean sections safer than before. Therefore, more often, cesarean section is carried out in the event of obstructed labour with a dead fetus. Hence an obstetrician practicing in a developing country is rarely faced with the need to perform a destructive operation, but should, nevertheless, be familiar with the procedures.

Contraindications to Destructive Operations

- When the uterus is threatening to rupture
- In the presence of a live fetus
- Any obstruction in the lower segment such as a tumour

The destructive operations performed on the fetus are elaborated below.

1. Craniotomy

It consists of perforating the skull, evacuating the cranial contents and extracting the fetus. It is indicated for the delivery of a dead fetus when labour is neglected and obstructed in a cephalic presentation. Usually, it is indicated when the head has become impacted in the pelvis. If the head is > 3/5th palpable per abdomen, craniotomy becomes difficult and dangerous, and it is wiser to deliver the baby by cesarean section.

2. Cephalocentesis

It is one of the most common destructive operations performed in modern obstetrics. It is indicated in fetal hydrocephalus if associated with lethal anomalies such as holoprosencephaly and Dandy–Walker malformation. In these conditions, the cerebrospinal fluid (CSF) is drained using a needle, which results in the decompression of the fetal head, permitting vaginal delivery.

Technique

- In cases of cephalic presentation, the hydrocephalic head can be decompressed transabdominally under USG guidance using a spinal needle. A collapsed head is easily delivered once the cervix is fully dilated. If the woman presents in labour, when the cervix is sufficiently dilated, a spinal needle can be passed through the fontanelle or through the thinned-out skull bone.
- In cases of breech presentation, a cephalocentesis can be performed by perforating the base of the occiput after the delivery of the body of the baby using an 18G spinal needle. The drainage of CSF is continued until the biparietal diameter is decreased sufficiently to allow vaginal delivery. When there is hydrocephalus with spina bifida presenting as breech, CSF can be drained by passing a catheter into the spinal canal up to the cranium.

3. Decapitation

It is indicated in obstructed labour with a dead fetus due to neglected shoulder presentation. In this operation, the head is separated from the trunk by cutting through the neck with a special decapitating hook, or a knife, or a pair of scissors. After decapitation, traction is applied on the arm, and the trunk is delivered, followed by the head.

4. Cleidotomy

This procedure consists of cutting through the clavicle so as to reduce the bisacromial diameter, which facilitates delivery. It may be indicated in shoulder dystocia with a dead fetus, shoulder dystocia in an anencephalic fetus or impacted shoulders in breech presentation. In shoulder dystocia, cleidotomy can be performed even in a live fetus if all methods to deliver the baby fail.

5. Embryotomy

It is indicated for an abdominal tumour or a very large fetus following craniotomy. An incision is made in the thorax or abdomen, the visceral contents are evacuated manually, and the fetus is extracted. It is easy to perform embryotomy if the fetus is presenting as breech.

6. Symphysiotomy

It is an operative method employed to enlarge the pelvic cavity. In cases of obstructed labour due to borderline disproportion and a dead fetus, in order to facilitate vaginal delivery, symphysiotomy used to be combined with destructive procedures. In modern obstetric practice, these procedures are not carried out. However, it may have a place in the management of shoulder dystocia, as a last resort.

Technique

- The woman's legs are supported in the lithotomy position at an angle of 80°.
- A 14 Fr Foley's catheter is placed in the urethra and the bladder is emptied.
- A half-an-inch long incision is made on the symphysis pubis and the blade of the knife passed through this incised wound until it gradually cuts through the symphysis pubis. With a finger inserted into the vagina, the knife is controlled so that only the joint and the subpubic ligament are divided.
- Before the final separation of the symphysis pubis, care must be taken to see that the assistant on either side holds the hips pressed inwards, thereby preventing the sudden flaring out of the iliac bones as the two pelvic bones spring apart.
- If the cervix is fully dilated at the time of symphysiotomy, the delivery can be completed by vacuum extraction or forceps under pudendal block anesthesia and episiotomy. Spontaneous delivery may also be awaited.
- After completion of delivery, the legs should be kept strapped together for 24 hours. The bladder should be kept continuously drained for three to four days. A broad belt may help ambulation, which begins on the fifth to seventh day in uncomplicated cases.
- Complications include hematoma, sepsis, stress incontinence, injuries to the urethra and the bladder, pelvic pain and backache.

Complications Associated with Destructive Procedures

- Rupture uterus
- PPH

- Vesicovaginal fistula (VVF) due to avascular necrosis caused by the spicule of a bone or an instrument
- Injury to the rectum
- Infection

Postoperative Care

- The genital tract should be carefully evaluated for any injury.
- Precautions should be taken to prevent PPH.
- A catheter should be left in place for 5–7 days to prevent VVF.
- Antibiotics should be given to prevent sepsis.

KEY POINTS

✓ *External cephalic version is indicated in breech or transverse lie after 36 weeks of gestation. Internal version is used mainly for the delivery of the second of twins in a transverse lie.*

✓ *The main indication for procedures such as version, destructive operations or symphysiotomy is to avoid a cesarean section.*

✓ *Destructive operations are performed on the dead fetus with a view to diminish its bulk so as to facilitate vaginal delivery. These operations include craniotomy, decapitation, cleidotomy and evisceration.*

✓ *With the availability of a safe alternative (cesarean section), there is hardly any place for these procedures in modern obstetrics.*

Essay questions

1. Discuss the indications, contraindications and the procedure of external cephalic version.
2. A 27-year-old G2P1 who had a previous full-term normal vaginal delivery presents at 36 weeks of gestation with a scan report showing breech presentation. The placenta is located in the upper segment and the liquor is adequate. On examination, it is a complete breech above the brim.
   a) What is the course of management in this patient?
   b) What are the contraindications to external cephalic version?
   c) Describe the technique of ECV.
   d) What are the complications and success rate of ECV?
3. A 29-year-old G2P1L1 had a previous normal vaginal delivery. In the current pregnancy, the USG at 28 weeks of gestation showed a breech presentation. She wants a normal delivery.
   a) What counselling would you offer this woman?
   b) If breech persists, at what gestational age will you attempt the procedure?
   c) Define the procedure.
   d) What are the prerequisites for the procedure?
   e) What are the contraindications?
   f) Explain the technique of the procedure.

Short answer questions

Write short notes on the following:
1. External cephalic version
2. Craniotomy
3. Decapitation
4. Internal podalic version
5. Cephalocentesis
6. Definition, indication, technique, complications of internal podalic version

MCQs

1. When a baby in breech presentation is manipulated abdominally into a cephalic presentation, the procedure is called:
   a) External cephalic version
   b) External podalic version
   c) Internal cephalic version
   d) Internal podalic version
2. The contraindications for external cephalic version include all EXCEPT:
   a) Contracted pelvis
   b) Antepartum hemorrhage
   c) Previous classical cesarean section
   d) Multiparity
3. ECV is contraindicated in all except:
   a) IUGR with Doppler changes
   b) Rh-negative isoimmunised pregnancy
   c) IUI pregnancy
   d) Placenta previa
4. What is the success rate of ECV?
   a) 40%
   b) 50%
   c) 60%
   d) 70%
5. Which of these does not favour a successful ECV?
   a) Multiparity
   b) Unengaged breech
   c) Oligohydramnios
   d) Complete breech
6. Which of the following is a drug used for tocolysis prior to ECV?
   a) Salbutamol
   b) Terbutaline
   c) Nifedipine
   d) Atosiban
7. Internal podalic version is recommended in:
   a) Delivery of the second twin in a transverse lie
   b) Cord prolapse in early labour
   c) Transverse lie not in labour
   d) Oblique lie after 24 hours of membrane rupture
8. Which of these complications is not associated with internal podalic version?
   a) Cord prolapse
   b) Rupture uterus
   c) Placental abruption
   d) Preterm labour

9. Which of these destructive procedures can be attempted in incompatible fetal hydrocephalus to permit vaginal delivery?
    a) Cephalocentesis
    b) Cleidotomy
    c) Evisceration
    d) Spondylotomy
10. The procedure of cutting the pubic bone to enlarge the pelvis is called:
    a) Cleidotomy
    b) Spondylotomy
    c) Symphysiotomy
    d) Craniotomy

Answers
1. (a), 2. (d), 3. (c), 4. (c), 5. (c), 6. (b), 7. (a), 8. (d), 9. (a), 10. (c)

Fill in the blanks

1. The procedure of perforating the skull, evacuating the cranial contents and extracting the fetus is known as _____.
2. The process of cutting through the clavicles so as to reduce the bisacromial diameter is called _____.
3. The removal of the viscera from the abdominal or thoracic cavity after opening the abdominal or the thoracic wall is known as _____.

Answers
1. craniotomy, 2. cleidotomy, 3. embryotomy

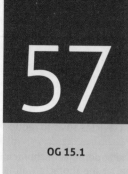

57

OG 15.1

Cesarean Section

Learning Objectives

» To know the types of cesarean section
» To know the indications for cesarean section
» To know the procedure of cesarean section
» To know the complications associated with cesarean section
» To know how to reduce cesarean section rates
» To understand VBAC

■ INTRODUCTION

Cesarean section is defined as the delivery of a viable fetus through an incision in the abdominal wall and the uterine wall. The term does not include the removal of a fetus from the abdomen following uterine rupture or cases of abdominal pregnancy. Cesarean section is indicated when vaginal delivery might pose a risk to the mother or the baby.

■ INCIDENCE

Rates of cesarean birth are rising throughout the world. The WHO recommends an ideal cesarean rate of 15–20%. However, in most countries, it is >30%. The NFHS-4 (2014–2015) report from India shows that 7 states in India have CS rates >30% with Telangana at 58%, Andhra Pradesh at 40.1%, Kerala at 35.8% and Tamil Nadu at 34.1%.

Though cesarean sections are effective, considered relatively safe and potentially life-saving for the fetus, the mother or both in certain cases, it is still a major surgery with its own risks and associated complications, which are more than those associated with vaginal birth. The increasing cesarean section rates pose an increased risk of maternal morbidity and mortality and have an implication for future pregnancies.

The two major contributors to the increase in cesarean section rates are the increase in primary cesarean sections and the decrease in vaginal birth after cesarean (VBAC).

The common indications for primary cesarean sections are as follows:

- Failure to progress in labour
- Non-reassuring fetal heart rate tracing
- Failed induction of labour
- Fetal malpresentations

- Multiple gestation, especially following IVF
- Suspected fetal macrosomia
- Maternal request for cesarean section without medical and obstetric indications
- Maternal medical complications such as pre-eclampsia/diabetes
- Fetal indications such as IUGR, macrosomia, severe oligohydramnios
- Clinician concerned about litigation and resorting to defensive practice

The VBAC rates in the developed world are 60–70%, whereas, in India, almost 80–90% of previous cesarean sections are delivered by repeat cesarean sections. The practice of 'cesarean always by cesarean' needs to be changed. Complications related to VBAC can be reduced with proper selection of cases, preparedness for adverse events, one-to-one care, intensive monitoring and continued psychological support throughout labour. The couple should be counselled adequately, and their informed consent should be taken beforehand.

■ MEASURES TO REDUCE PRIMARY CS RATES

- **Correct diagnosis and management of labour using partograph**:
  — Prolonged latent phase should not be taken as an indication for cesarean delivery; instead, it should be considered an indication for augmenting labour.
  — The threshold to diagnose arrest and performing a cesarean section.
  — In the active phase of labour, arrest should be diagnosed if there is a failure of dilatation for more than 4 hours after 6 cm dilatation of the cervix with good uterine contractions.

- **Resorting to operative vaginal delivery**: If all criteria are met for operative vaginal delivery, forceps/ventouse should be attempted instead of cesarean section. This needs the presence of experienced clinicians on site.
- **Proper interpretation of CTG:**
  — Absent fetal heart rate variability with recurrent late decelerations, recurrent variable decelerations or bradycardia or a sinusoidal rhythm are indications for immediate delivery. Recurrent variable decelerations alone may indicate cord compression, which requires evaluation, continued surveillance and initiation of appropriate corrective measures before deciding on cesarean section.
  — In cases of meconium-stained liquor, intrauterine resuscitation may be carried out by supplementing oxygen, intravenous fluid bolus, tocolytic agents to relax the uterus and amnioinfusion to dilute the meconium.
- **ECV for singleton breech presentations**: In cases of breech presentations, ECV should be offered after 36 weeks of gestations.
- **Labour induction:** Unwarranted induction of labour should be avoided. Before 41 weeks of gestation, induction of labour is generally performed for maternal and fetal medical indications. In cases of postdated pregnancy, labour induction is carried out at 41 weeks.
- **Maternal request:** Women may request cesarean section without maternal or fetal indications due to various reasons such as fear of pain, pelvic floor injury, sexual dysfunction, fear of harm to the baby, previous unpleasant experience and a desire to give birth on a designated day and time. In such situations, the woman should be counselled and alerted about the true risks of major abdominal (C section) surgery, compared to normal vaginal deliveries; this counselling should be documented. A defensive cesarean section should be avoided. The woman should be advised in honesty about the likelihood of achieving positive outcomes with different birth plans.
- **Support during labour**: A pregnant woman needs continuous physical and emotional support throughout labour and birth. Encouraging a birth companion and providing one-to-one care for the woman helps in reducing the cesarean section rates. Attention should be paid to nutrition in labour, as good hydration will help in good uterine contractions and provide energy in the second stage of labour for maternal pushing. Effective pain management also helps to reduce cesarean section rates.
- **Audits:** The Robson Ten Group Classification System is based on the indications for cesarean section. Periodic auditing should be carried out using this classification to identify cases in which cesarean section could have been avoided.

INDICATIONS FOR CESAREAN SECTION

There are many indications for cesarean section, which can be divided into three groups as follows:

1. Fetomaternal indications—when both maternal and fetal indications coexist.
2. Fetal indications—when prompt delivery is needed for fetal well-being or when labour and vaginal delivery have to be avoided for the sake of the fetus.
3. Maternal indications—when safe vaginal delivery is unlikely, or labour is contraindicated, or prompt delivery is needed to safeguard the woman's health.

More than 75% of cesareans are performed due to prior cesarean delivery, dystocia, fetal distress or breech presentation.

Cephalopelvic Disproportion and Contracted Pelvis

When the pelvis is contracted or there is a major degree of cephalopelvic disproportion and the delivery of the baby per vaginum is not possible, elective cesarean section is the treatment of choice. In a borderline pelvis and with minor degrees of disproportion, a trial of labour may be opted for. When trial of labour fails, cesarean section becomes necessary to deliver a live child. Cesarean section is also indicated when there is a contracted pelvis due to kyphoscoliosis, pelvic deformities, polio or a fracture affecting the pelvic dimensions.

Malpresentations and Malpositions

The common malpresentations necessitating cesarean section are transverse lie, mentoposterior position, brow presentation, breech presentation and deep transverse arrest in the occipitoposterior position.

Multiple Pregnancy

When the first of twins is in a presentation other than cephalic presentation, cesarean section is undertaken. Cesarean section is also indicated in the presence of discordant fetal growth, monochorionic twins, conjoined twins and higher-order multiple pregnancies.

Previous Cesarean Section

Cesarean section is recommended in the following scenarios:

- Previous classical cesarean section: A classical cesarean section should be followed by repeat cesarean section in the subsequent pregnancies. The CS should be performed before the onset of labour because of the high risk of uterine scar rupture.
- Previous two cesarean sections should be followed by a cesarean section.
- Previous lower-segment cesarean section: A repeat cesarean section may be indicated in a pregnancy subsequent to a lower-segment cesarean section if the chance of successful vaginal delivery is assessed and found to be low and the likelihood of scar dehiscence is high.

Antepartum Hemorrhage

- Placenta previa: It is almost always a rule to perform a cesarean section in all cases of major placenta previa. In minor types of placenta previa, cesarean section is carried out if the labour does not progress or if bleeding is not controlled by the artificial rupture of the membranes and oxytocin infusion.
- Abruptio placenta: Cesarean section is indicated in cases of Couvelaire uterus or in cases in which there is a failure to progress in labour or maternal and fetal deterioration.

Eclampsia or Pre-eclampsia

In a woman with eclampsia/imminent eclampsia or deteriorating severe pre-eclampsia, cesarean section may be required unless rapid vaginal delivery is feasible.

Gestational Diabetes Mellitus (GDM)

In cases of GDM, if the baby develops macrosomia which leads to CPD or when shoulder dystocia is anticipated, cesarean section may be indicated.

Bad Obstetric History and Habitual Intrauterine Death of the Fetus

Women who have had recurrent miscarriages and a history of unexplained perinatal deaths may be delivered by cesarean section in a subsequent pregnancy.

Maternal Infections

- When there is maternal HIV infection, cesarean section reduces maternofetal transmission, particularly in women with high viral load and low CD4 counts.

Therefore, it may be indicated in selected cases. In women who are treated with multiple antiretroviral agents and in those with low viral load and high CD4 counts, vaginal delivery can be allowed.

- Cesarean section is also indicated in women with active herpes infection diagnosed in the third trimester of pregnancy.

Pregnancy Following Previous Surgical Procedures

In cases of pregnancy following VVF repair, third- or fourth-degree perineal tear or stress incontinence repair, cesarean section would be indicated.

Fetal Indications

In severe IUGR or severe oligohydramnios with Doppler changes diagnosed during the antenatal period, the fetus will not be able to withstand the stress of labour. Therefore, cesarean section is performed in such cases.

Miscellaneous Indications

- In the presence of cord presentation or vasa previa
- Carcinoma cervix complicating pregnancy
- Aortic aneurysm with root dilatation in Marfan syndrome
- Maternal request

Indications for Cesarean Section in Labour

- Obstructed labour due to CPD, transverse lie or obstruction caused by ovarian or uterine tumours
- Deep transverse arrest in the occipitoposterior position
- Failure to progress in labour due to inadequate uterine contractions, malpositions or malpresentations such as brow presentation
- Failed induction of labour
- Fetal distress—non-reassuring fetal heart rate patterns and the passage of meconium are indicators of fetal hypoxia and are indications for cesarean section if prompt delivery by the vaginal route is not imminent
- When there is prolapse of the umbilical cord and the cord is pulsatile indicating a live fetus, but delivery is not imminent
- Failed forceps/ventouse in the second stage of labour
- The second of twins is larger than the first twin
- Impending uterine rupture or scar dehiscence in labour in a woman who has had a previous cesarean section

Elective and Emergency Cesarean Section

Cesarean section may be performed as an elective planned procedure for various indications or as an emergency procedure due to complications arising during labour or conditions necessitating urgent delivery. Elective cesarean sections are usually planned after 39 weeks of pregnancy to reduce **respiratory distress** in the neonate, which is known as **transient tachypnea of the newborn**.

■ OPERATIVE PROCEDURE

Preparation for Surgery

The preparation for surgery depends on whether it is an elective or emergency cesarean section.

Preparation for elective cesarean section

In an elective cesarean section, the woman is usually advised 12-hour fasting. Some basic investigations like urine for albumin and sugar and complete blood count (CBC) are repeated prior to surgery. Blood is grouped and typed and adequate blood is reserved beforehand. An IV line with RL is started and an indwelling urinary catheter is inserted. Depending on the policy of the hospital, an intravenous prophylactic antibiotic is given 60 minutes prior to skin incision or after cord clamping following the delivery of the baby. Anti-thromboembolic stockings with or without low-molecular-weight heparin should be prescribed as required.

Preparation for emergency cesarean section

Pregnant women lying flat for a cesarean section are at risk of Mendelson's syndrome (aspiration of gastric contents into the lung), leading to chemical pneumonitis. This is because of the pressure exerted by the gravid uterus on the stomach. Moreover, in an emergency cesarean section, since the woman may not be fasting, an H2-receptor antagonist like ranitidine +/- metoclopramide (an anti-emetic that increases gastric emptying) is given preoperatively to reduce the risk of aspiration of acid and gastric contents. The rest of the procedures are similar to those described under the elective cesarean section. Pubic hair encroaching on the proposed line of incision is clipped. Shaving should be discouraged as it causes abrasions which may promote infection. The woman is preferably placed in a moderate Trendelenburg position with 15° left lateral tilt while carrying out the operation to avoid vena caval compression.

Anesthesia

The anesthesiologist monitors the pulse, BP and other vitals. The preferred anesthesia is regional—either spinal or epidural anesthesia. However, general anesthesia may be required if there are contraindications to regional anesthesia or when there is a need to expedite delivery as in cases of fetal distress or in cases of failure of regional anesthesia.

Incision
Abdominal incisions (Fig. 57.1)

- **Transverse incision:** The low transverse incision (Pfannenstiel) incision is commonly performed because the chances of wound dehiscence and incisional hernia are low and it is more comfortable for the woman, with lesser postoperative pain. Besides having a good cosmetic result, it also allows easy palpation of the uterine fundus in subsequent pregnancies. In this incision, a transverse curvilinear incision is made above the pubic hair line.

- **Midline vertical incision:** The abdomen may have to be opened by a vertical incision when a classical cesarean section is contemplated or when procedures need to be carried out in the upper abdomen. Gaining entry into the abdomen is much faster with a vertical incision as compared to a transverse incision. However, the incidences of incisional hernia, wound dehiscence or postoperative pain are higher with a vertical incision.

- **Joel–Cohen incision:** It is a modification of the transverse incision, wherein a transverse incision is made 3 cm below the line joining the anterior superior iliac spines on either side. This incision is higher than the Pfannenstiel incision.

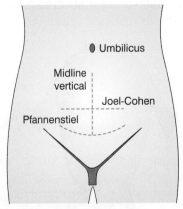

Fig. 57.1 Types of abdominal incisions

Opening the abdomen

- Following the skin incision, the subcutaneous tissue is incised either by using a scalpel or by stretching the incision bluntly with the fingers from the medial to the lateral side (both superficial fatty layers, the Camper's fascia, the deeper membranous layer and the Scarpas' fascia are incised). Then, the rectus sheath is incised transversely with a scalpel and extended with scissors. Once the rectus sheath is dissected off the rectus muscle, the two recti muscles are separated in the midline. Occasionally, cutting of the rectus sheath may be required to achieve more space if difficulty is anticipated in the delivery of the fetus as in breech delivery. This is followed by the opening of the peritoneum well above the bladder. At this stage, blunt and sharp dissections are required, and care should be taken to prevent injury to the bladder and the underlying organs. Identification of the ligamentum teres prevents injury to the bladder.

Uterine Incision

Lower segment incision

- The lower segment uterine incision or Munro–Kerr incision (a transverse curvilinear incision made 1 cm below the reflection of the peritoneum over the bladder) is the preferred incision. The advantages of the lower segment uterine incision are as follows:
  — As the lower segment is thin and stretched out, the approximation of the edges of the uterine wound is easy; this helps in achieving good hemostasis and strength.
  — There is lesser bleeding when the incision is in the lower segment.
  — Since the lower segment is comparatively quiescent in the puerperium, it allows better healing. Hence, rupture in a subsequent pregnancy is much less frequent.
  — The convalescence is also much smoother than that after the classical operation.

- The uterus is exposed. Any rotation of the uterus, which is commonly to the right, is corrected. This is important, as otherwise, there is a fair chance of injuring the uterine blood vessels. Once dextrorotation is corrected, it becomes possible to view both the round ligaments simultaneously.

- The peritoneum on the anterior wall of the uterus just above its reflection over the bladder is then held loosely by dissecting forceps, and a transverse incision made over the peritoneal attachment at this level, extending from one side of the anterior uterine surface to the other (Fig. 57.2a).

- The peritoneum with the bladder in front is separated from the uterine wall and pushed down; the separation should be adequate to expose the lower segment of the uterus. The bladder should be retracted using a Doyen's retractor to expose the lower segment.

- At this stage, a curvilinear transverse incision is made in the musculature of the lower uterine segment, about 1–2 cm below the junction with the upper segment. The incision is deepened until the uterine cavity is opened. At this point, the shiny fetal membrane should be visible, bulging through the uterine incision. The incision is extended laterally with upward curvature using curved scissors or with the two index fingers introduced at either side and moving the fingers in opposite directions. The length of the incision should be at least 10 cm in size so as to allow the hand to pass and to deliver the head in a term fetus.

Classical uterine incision

In certain situations (see box below), a vertical incision is required in the upper segment, starting from above the reflection of the uterovesical fold of the peritoneum and extended upwards in the midline as far as required. The incision should not extend beyond the take-off of

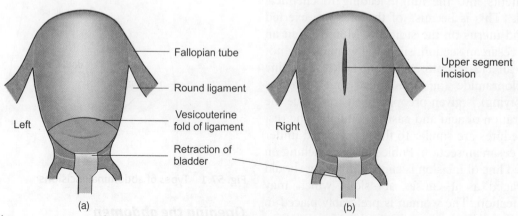

Fig. 57.2   (a) Lower segment cesarean section incision and (b) upper segment or classical cesarean section

the round ligaments (Fig. 57.2b). Difficulty in entering the uterine cavity and excessive bleeding should be anticipated because of the thick uterine musculature in the upper segment.

The baby is grasped by the foot and delivered as a breech. The uterine wound is then closed in three layers. The risks associated with a classical scar are delayed healing, resulting in a weak scar and subacute intestinal obstruction (due to the intestine adhering to the uterine inscision). In subsequent pregnancies, the risk of scar rupture is high, especially in a late pregnancy presenting as a silent rupture. If the placenta implants in the anterior wall of the uterus, it can perforate through the scar, presenting as placenta percreta.

Indications for classical cesarean section
- Carcinoma of the cervix complicating pregnancy
- Inability to approach the lower uterine segment due to maternal skeletal abnormalities such as kyphoscoliosis or extensive adhesions due to previous surgery, a large fibroid in the lower uterine segment
- Conjoined twins
- Adherent placenta in the lower segment
- Central/anterior placenta previa with large tortuous vessels in the lower segment
- Impacted shoulder presentation

Lower segment vertical incision (De Lee's incision)

In cases where the lower segment is not formed, as in transverse lie, an incision can be made vertically in the lower segment. However, the risk associated with this incision is that it can extend vertically down into the cervix, vagina and bladder.

Delivery of the Head

After opening into the uterus, the membrane is ruptured, the hand is passed into the uterine incision and the palm of the hand is used to lift the head out while an assistant helps with fundal pressure. The head is brought up to the level of the uterine incision, and then the occiput is rotated anteriorly before the head is delivered through the uterine incision (Fig. 57.3). Occasionally, one blade of the forceps or the soft vacuum extractor cup may be used for this purpose, especially if the head is floating. Care should be taken before the delivery of the head to see that the incision is sufficiently large to allow the head to be delivered without tearing the lateral ends of the wound in an irregular manner. Once the head of the child has been delivered, the rest of the body follows

easily. If there is difficulty in delivering the head, an inverted T-shaped incision or a J-shaped incision may be required (Fig. 57.4).

In cases of breech presentation or transverse lie, the hand is passed into the uterine cavity and the foot of the fetus is grasped and brought out through the incision and delivered as in vaginal breech delivery.

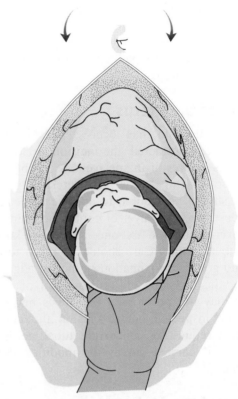

Fig. 57.3 As the fetal head is lifted through the incision, pressure is usually applied to the uterine fundus through the abdominal wall to help expel the fetus

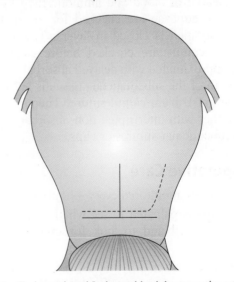

Fig. 57.4 T-shaped and J-shaped incisions on the uterus

Delivery of the Placenta

After the delivery of the anterior shoulder, oxytocin infusion is administered. Most often, it will be found that the placenta has separated by the time the child is extracted. The third stage can then be completed easily by pulling on the cord. While the placenta separates, the angles of the uterine incision, the midpoint of the lower uterine incision and any actively bleeding points of the uterine incision are secured with broad hemostatic Green–Armytage forceps to reduce the blood loss. If the placenta does not separate by cord traction, it may be manually removed.

Closure of the Uterus

Once the placenta has been removed and the uterus is well contracted, the incision is closed with continuous sutures, using delayed absorbable sutures such as polyglactin (Vicryl). The lateral angle of the incision should be secured to achieve hemostasis at the angles. A second layer of continuous sutures are made, overlapping the first one. This is also known as the Lembert suture. Care should be taken to obtain close and good approximation of the cut edges when suturing the incision. The uterovesical peritoneum may or may not be closed. The tubes and ovaries should be inspected before closing the abdomen. In women requesting concurrent tubal sterilisation, tubectomy is carried out by the modified Pomeroy technique.

Closure of the Abdomen

The abdominal cavity, paracolic gutters and cul-de-sac are cleared of blood and amniotic fluid by gentle suction; the adnexae are checked for any pathology and the abdomen is closed in layers. The swab and instrument counts are checked before closure. The fascia is approximated with delayed absorbable sutures. If the depth of the subcutaneous tissue is ≥2 cm, it is closed with 1-0 plain catgut suture. Then, the skin is closed, either with interrupted non-absorbable sutures or with subcuticular sutures or clips.

Postoperative Care

- The vitals are monitored every 4 hours for 24 hours.
- The uterus is palpated to see whether the uterus is well-contracted and to look for excessive vaginal bleeding.
- IV fluids are given for first 24 hours. If there are no contraindications, oral fluids can be started in 6 hours. Soft solid diet is started after 48 hours.
- The bladder is continuously drained for 24 hours, and then the catheter is removed.
- Adequate pain relief is given.
- Antibiotics may be continued for 24 hours to 3 days.
- Leg movement, early ambulation and breathing exercises are encouraged to prevent thromboembolic complications.
- Breastfeeding is initiated within 4 hours.
- The wound dressing is removed after 48 hours and observed for infection.
- A laxative may be required on the third day if the bowel was not opened.

COMMON DIFFICULTIES ENCOUNTERED DURING CESAREAN SECTION

Delivery of the Head

The most common difficulty encountered is in delivering the head through the incision in the lower segment.

1. Floating head

In a fetus with a floating head, the delivery of the head may be difficult. This difficulty is exaggerated if the woman is in the Trendelenburg position. In such situations, making the incision at a higher level in the lower segment may help. By gentle manipulation, the head is made to engage in the incision and fixed in that position by the left hand or by the assistant; meanwhile, with the right hand, the head can be lifted out. Gentle fundal pressure may also help. The single blade of a pair of forceps or a vacuum extractor can also be used to deliver the floating head. With this technique, the chance of uncontrolled extension of the uterine wound is reduced and delivery of the head is brought about slowly and carefully. Occasionally, internal podalic version and extraction through the incision may be required, but this can result in lateral extension of the uterine incision, resulting in excessive bleeding.

2. Deeply engaged head

Greater difficulty may be experienced when a lower segment cesarean section is undertaken in the second stage of labour when there is obstructed labour or when there is deep transverse arrest of the head in the cavity. When the head is deeply wedged in the cavity, it can be delivered by passing a hand through the incision and well behind the head and levering it out. The Trendelenburg position may help in dislodging the head from the pelvis. The head may also be disimpacted from the vagina by pushing it up (this can be done by an assistant).

Another technique that has been described and found to be useful for delivering a deeply engaged head is Patwardhan's technique, which is performed as follows:

- In cases of occipitotransverse or occipitoanterior positions of the vertex, when a transverse incision is made in the lower uterine segment, most often, it is found to be at the level of the shoulder; the anterior shoulder usually, fairly 'pops' out of the incision line. If it does not, it is delivered out of the incision line.
- Next, the posterior shoulder is also delivered out of the incision line. Then, the surgeon hooks her fingers under both the axillae and with gentle traction aided by fundal pressure by the assistant, brings the body of the fetus out of the uterus.
- At the end of the above step, the baby's head is still wedged in the pelvis and is gently delivered by lifting the baby.
- When the back is posterior after delivering the anterior shoulder, a hand is introduced into the uterus to reach for a foot. By applying traction on the foot coupled with fundal pressure, the breech is delivered, followed by the trunk. The head is delivered by applying traction on the legs. This technique needs practice and experience; it is not advisable for the inexperienced surgeon to attempt it without being assisted by a senior consultant.

Impacted Shoulder Presentation

In impacted shoulder presentation and arm prolapse, lower segment cesarean section offers considerable difficulty in delivering the child. With the lower uterine segment thinned out, the delivery of the child by version may give rise to the extension of the incision laterally. Often, it may be difficult to get a grip on the foot. Under these circumstances, a vertical incision may need to be made, extending into the upper segment (inverted T incision; Fig. 57.4).

Dilated Blood Vessels in the Lower Segment

At times, especially in the case of anterior placenta previa, some large blood vessels are seen coursing over the lower segment. These can be ligated above and below and cut in-between before proceeding with the operation; failure to do so may result in profuse bleeding. Excessive bleeding can occur due to large sinuses in the myometrium, extension of the uterine incision laterally into the uterine arteries or the involvement of the broad ligament.

If the head is too large for the incision or the lower segment itself is not broad enough for the size of the head, lateral extension of the incision may occur. It is necessary to avoid this. To do so, the incision must be made as long as possible, and the head should be delivered slowly. At the time of delivery of the head, the lateral angles of the incision should be watched carefully. Treatment involves the placement of sutures lateral to the edge of the lower segment incision and securing the bleeding vessels. The uterus may have to be exteriorised outside the abdominal incision, which helps in the proper suturing of the angles.

▌ COMPLICATIONS OF CESAREAN SECTION

A primary cesarean section carries a lower risk of perineal trauma and pain, urinary and anal incontinence, uterovaginal prolapse, late stillbirth and early neonatal infections than vaginal birth. However, it is associated with immediate, intermediate and late complications, which are listed below.

- **Anesthetic complications**: General anesthesia may cause the aspiration of gastric contents resulting in ARDS.
- **Hemorrhage:** The risk factors for hemorrhage include cesarean section for placenta previa, placental abruption, uterine atony in multiple pregnancy and multiparity, and prolonged labour. The hemorrhage may be primary or secondary. Primary hemorrhage may arise from the placental bed due to atony or from the uterine vessels due to the extension of the incision. Secondary hemorrhage and secondary PPH may occur due to infection or scar dehiscence, which usually manifests 7–10 days after cesarean section. The risk of PPH is four times higher with emergency cesarean section and twice as high following elective cesarean section compared to vaginal delivery.
- **Endomyometritis:** The risk of endometritis is increased with prolonged labour, premature rupture of membranes and a number of vaginal examinations performed in labour. The common causative organisms are *E coli*., beta *Streptococcus* and anaerobic organisms. Endometritis is 10–20 times higher following cesarean section than vaginal delivery.
- **Wound infection:** Women who have had a cesarean in labour after prolonged rupture of membranes are

more prone to infection. Infection may involve the uterine wound or abdominal wall incision and is treated with antibiotics. Infection is more common in obese women. The reported incidence of wound sepsis is 1–9%.

- **Urinary complications:** The risk of bladder injury or ureteric injury with cesarean section is <1%. Injury is more common with repeat cesarean sections. Ureteric injury can occur if the uterine incision extends laterally and blind suturing is done; it can include the ureter. Pressure necrosis of the bladder can occur in obstructed labour. Urinary tract infection is a common complication following cesarean delivery. The urinary tract infection is chiefly due to urinary catheterisation and is higher with a longer duration of catheter use and in diabetic patients. Proper asepsis during catheterisations prevents such an infection, which is treated by antibiotics.

- **Bowel complications:** Paralytic ileus can occur following cesarean for obstructed labour and is treated by gastric suction and parenteral fluids until the bowel sounds are heard. Subacute intestinal obstruction is a delayed complication that may occur due to adhesions. Though rare at cesarean section, bowel injury may occur during a repeat procedure if the bowel is adherent to the abdominal scar.

- **Thromboembolism:** The risk of developing thromboembolic complications is much higher following cesarean section compared to vaginal delivery. Early mobilisation and the use of heparin in indicated cases such as obesity will reduce the incidence of thromboembolism.

- **Chest infection:** In women who are obese and those who have a pre-existing upper respiratory tract infection, there may be segmental atelectasis after cesarean section. Postoperative pain may cause the woman to reduce the efforts at breathing, further aggravating the condition.

- **Injury to the baby:** Occasionally, the baby may be injured while making the incision on the lower uterine segment.

- **Re-laparotomy:** Re-laparotomy may be required if there are complications such as atonic PPH, secondary PPH or intraperitoneal bleeding due to the extension of the angles or severe endomyometritis.

Late Sequelae of Cesarean Section

- Delayed effects of a cesarean section include scar site endometriosis, endometriosis of the bladder, incisional hernia, AV malformation and subacute intestinal obstruction.

- The subsequent pregnancy may be affected.
- Future pregnancies may be complicated by uterine scar ectopic pregnancy, placenta previa, adherent placenta and uterine rupture in labour. The incidence of rupture with lower segment cesarean section is 0.5–2%, whereas it is 9% with classical cesarean section.

Maternal Mortality

The relative risk for maternal mortality is 4–7 times higher in a cesarean section than in vaginal delivery due to infection, hemorrhage and thromboembolism. However, most deaths are associated with complicated emergency procedures than with elective cesarean sections.

▋ WOUND HEALING FOLLOWING CESAREAN SECTION

Following a cesarean section, wound healing occurs by the approximation of the connective tissue and muscle fibres between the upper and the lower edges of the cesarean wound. The integrity of the resultant scar depends on the proper approximation of the edges without a gutter underneath. The following conditions can interfere with the wound healing and the integrity of the scar:

- At the time of the previous cesarean section
  — Improper approximation of the uterine wound
  — Intrapartum sepsis
  — Uterine wound hematoma
  — Malnutrition or anemia
  — Previous indication for cesarean section such as placenta previa, prolonged labour, obstructed labour
  — Intrapartum complications such as lateral extension or vertical extension of the wound
- Current pregnancy
  — Current pregnancy occurring within a short interval of less than one year
  — Stretching of the scar due to polyhydramnios, multiple pregnancy
  — Placenta previa in the current pregnancy

▋ PREGNANCY FOLLOWING CESAREAN SECTION

In a woman who had a previous cesarean section, the decision to allow vaginal delivery in the subsequent pregnancies depends on the following factors:

- The risk of rupture of the cesarean section scar in pregnancy and labour
- The chances of a successful vaginal delivery

Rupture of Uterine Scar

A pregnancy following a cesarean section is considered a high-risk pregnancy because it carries a risk of rupture of the cesarean section scar during pregnancy or labour. The uterine rupture may be dangerous for the mother as well as the baby. Therefore, vaginal birth after cesarean section (VBAC) should be allowed only in institutions equipped to provide emergency care. Before proceeding further, it is essential to understand the terms scar rupture and scar dehiscence.

- **Rupture of the uterine scar** is said to have occurred when all the layers of the uterus including the serosa give way; the fetus may be found in the peritoneal cavity.
- In **scar dehiscence**, the visceral peritoneum (serosal layer) is intact and the fetus, cord and placenta are still within the uterine cavity. Bleeding is also comparatively less with scar dehiscence.

The integrity of a uterine scar and the risk of scar rupture depend upon the type of previous cesarean section, number of cesarean sections, the postoperative period, wound healing in the previous pregnancy and the interval between pregnancies.

The integrity of the cesarean section scar can be assessed during the antenatal period using transabdominal USG. It has been shown that a scar thickness of >4 mm indicates a good scar, whereas, a scar thickness of <2 mm is associated with a high risk of rupture.

- **Type of previous uterine incision:** The estimated incidence of the rupture of the scar is 0.5–2% for a lower segment cesarean section and up to 9% for a classical cesarean section. Moreover, the classical scar tends to rupture during the antenatal period and presents as a silent rupture. The incidence of the rupture of a previous inverted T-shaped scar is similar to that of a classical cesarean section. Women who have sustained scar dehiscence or rupture in the previous pregnancy are also at a high risk of subsequent rupture.
- **Number of previous cesarean sections**: The rate of scar rupture increases as the number of previous cesarean sections increases.
- **Indication for previous cesarean section:** If the previous cesarean section was performed for obstructed labour or when there was associated intrapartum sepsis, the wound healing may be poor, leading to a weak scar.
- **Birth interval:** Pregnancy within one year of a previous cesarean section may predispose to scar rupture in labour due to poor healing.

- **Puerperal sepsis with endomyometritis:** This also leads to a weak scar, which can rupture in subsequent pregnancies.

MODE OF DELIVERY FOLLOWING A PREVIOUS CESAREAN SECTION

In a woman who had a previous cesarean delivery, in subsequent pregnancies, there are two management options at the time of delivery:
- Repeat cesarean delivery
- Allowing vaginal delivery (vaginal birth after cesarean section [VBAC]); currently, it is also called trial of labour after cesarean section (TOLAC)

Indications for Repeat Cesarean Section

In the following situations, an elective repeat cesarean section is carried out:
- When there is a recurrent indication such as absolute CPD with an obliquely contracted pelvis caused by polio, kyphosis, tuberculosis of the pelvic joint or accidents causing the shortening of the lower limbs; a repeat cesarean is also carried out even in a gynecoid pelvis when there is minor CPD
- When the woman has had more than two cesarean sections
- When the previous cesarean involved a classical incision, low vertical (De Lee or modified classical) incision or inverted T or J incisions
- When the type of cesarean section is not known
- When the previous cesarean section was carried out for failed instrumental delivery
- When the cesarean section was done for obstructed labour or threatened rupture
- When the woman had intrapartum or postpartum complications such as the extension of the uterine incision or postoperative puerperal sepsis following the cesarean section
- When the current pregnancy is complicated by malpresentations, placenta previa or any other obstetric factors such as advanced maternal age or conception following a long period of infertility
- When there are associated medical disorders such as pre-eclampsia, diabetes, etc.
- When the woman desires to have a repeat cesarean section
- When facilities for emergency cesarean section are not available

Vaginal Birth After Cesarean Section (VBAC)

Nearly 70% of women with a previous cesarean section are suitable for a trial of vaginal delivery; about 80% of these trials are successful. The success of VBAC depends on the selection of cases for trial of scar and the careful monitoring of labour.

Criteria to allow VBAC

- A detailed history and review of the woman's records with regards to previous obstetric history is important before selecting cases for VBAC. The conditions mentioned under indications for repeat cesarean section are contraindications to VBAC; if these are ruled out, the woman may be considered for VBAC.
- The success rate may be as high as 90% if the previous section was performed for a non-recurring indication such as breech presentation, non-reassuring fetal heart rate pattern and conditions such as placenta previa or abruption. It is as low as 60% when it was done for failure to progress in labour.
- Previous vaginal delivery either before or after the cesarean section significantly improves the successful vaginal delivery.
- In the current pregnancy, the fetal weight should be assessed carefully to rule out CPD. In a floating head at term, VBAC should be avoided.
- Malpresentation and placenta previa should be ruled out.
- In a woman selected for VBAC, the pregnancy should not be allowed to go beyond the EDD as the fetal size increases, BPD increases and moulding reduces. Spontaneous onset of labour is associated with successful VBAC. If induction of labour is required, the mechanical method with Foley's catheter is advised. There is no place for induction with misoprostol. Dinoprostone gel can be used with caution.
- An interdelivery interval of less than 18 months is associated with a three-fold increase in uterine rupture as compared to an interval of >18 months.

Selection criteria for VBAC
- One previous lower segment cesarean section
- Non-recurrent indication
- No CPD
- Scar integrity considered adequate based on the previous history and intraoperative findings
- Personnel and infrastructure facilities available for continuous monitoring and emergency cesarean section
- Informed consent obtained from the patient

Conduct of Labour in VBAC

- The woman should be counselled adequately regarding the success of VBAC and the potential risks (need for emergency cesarean section, fetal distress and scar rupture). All discussions should be documented. After the woman fully understands the implications, her written informed consent should be obtained.
- VBAC should be under a double set-up and conducted only in a centre where facilities for urgent cesarean are available round the clock.
- The theatre personnel, anesthesiologist, pediatrician and blood bank personnel should be informed in advance about the trial.
- The woman should be prepared as for cesarean section. She should be kept nil per oral; nutrition should be provided by intravenous fluids, medications given for gastric emptying, parts prepared for anesthesia and surgery and blood grouped and reserved.
- The woman should be attended to at all times.
- The maternal condition should be monitored by automatic monitoring of pulse and BP every 15 minutes. A rising pulse rate is one of the earliest indicators of impending rupture.
- For pain relief, epidural analgesia is safe for both the mother and fetus. Regional analgesia is easier and safer and can be continued if cesarean section or instrumental delivery is required.
- The fetus should be monitored by continuous CTG throughout labour. Fetal tachycardia is another early indicator of impending rupture.
- Labour progress should be monitored by partograph. When there is a failure to progress, there should be a low threshold for CS. When required to augment labour, oxytocin can be judiciously administered by infusion pump with utmost care and at the lowest dose.
- Suprapubic pain and tenderness may indicate a weak scar that may rupture and are late signs.

Signs of uterine rupture
- A sudden abnormality in fetal heart rate pattern such as fetal tachycardia, prolonged bradycardia, severe and prolonged variable deceleration
- Maternal tachycardia, hypotension
- Cessation of uterine contractions
- The presence of a suprapubic bulge indicates that there is a hematoma underneath
- Hematuria
- Vaginal bleeding

- The presenting part receding from the pelvis and fetal parts being superficial and easily palpable per abdomen
- Following delivery, when there is fresh bleeding, PPH or postpartum collapse or if the uterus is pushed to one side, uterine rupture should be suspected

- Scar dehiscence and rupture occur more commonly in the second stage of labour when the woman is pushing. These can be avoided by applying outlet forceps prophylactically when the head is distending the perineum.
- If the placenta is expelled easily, there is no extra blood loss and the woman's condition as judged by blood pressure and pulse rate is satisfactory, the uterine cavity, particularly the lower segment, need not be explored. However, if there is a delay in the separation of the placenta or there has been fairly heavy blood loss and the woman shows evidence of it, the uterus should be explored in the theatre for any evidence of rupture.

Indications for Cesarean Section During Trial of Labour

- Failure to progress in labour
- Fetal distress
- Maternal distress
- Impending rupture

Successful VBAC

VBAC is considered successful if it results in a vaginal delivery spontaneously or with the assistance of instruments without any morbidity and mortality to the mother and the fetus.

▌ PERIPARTUM HYSTERECTOMY

Occasionally, a hysterectomy may be indicated as a life-saving measure following a vaginal or cesarean delivery. Usually, only a sub-total hysterectomy is possible as it is difficult to locate the cervix. The indications for hysterectomy following delivery are the following:

- Rupture of the uterus—whether the rupture of the uterus is spontaneous, traumatic or due to the rupture of a previous cesarean section scar, it is most often treated by hysterectomy, except when the rent is clean and found to be repairable; tubal ligation may be done along with the repair of the rent
- Postpartum hemorrhage—PPH may be due to intractable uterine atony, lower segment bleeding because of placenta previa or the laceration of major uterine vessels; in these situations, a hysterectomy may be necessary to save the mother from hemorrhage
- Placenta accreta is often associated with repeat cesarean delivery and is one of the commonest indications for peripartum hysterectomy
- Co-existing cervical fibroid, cervical carcinoma
- Severe intrauterine sepsis

▌ PERIMORTEM/POSTMORTEM CESAREAN SECTION

Occasionally, when the mother is in a critical condition with a cardiac arrest, the quick delivery of the fetus may relieve the aorto-caval compression and improve the chances of survival. This is called a perimortem cesarean section. The procedure is also called resuscitative hysterotomy as it can be performed even before the period of viability.

In cases of maternal death with a viable fetus, in order to save the child, a cesarean section may be indicated. This should be carried out within four minutes of the maternal cardiac arrest. As the timeline is critical, a classical section is carried out following a midline incision on the abdomen. This is called a postmortem cesarean section.

KEY POINTS

✓ Cesarean section is the delivery of the baby per abdomen when vaginal delivery may be harmful to the mother or the baby. Cesarean delivery rates have increased worldwide over the last 20 years.
✓ The lower segment uterine incision is preferred over the upper segment because the healing of the lower segment incision is better and risk of rupture in a subsequent pregnancy is low.
✓ Maternal morbidity is higher after cesarean section than after vaginal delivery.
✓ A pregnancy following cesarean section is a high-risk pregnancy because it carries the risk of rupture of the cesarean section scar during labour.

Essay questions

1. What are the indications for cesarean section?
2. What are the possible complications of cesarean section?
3. What are the indications of peripartum hysterectomy?

Short answer questions

1. Compare and contrast transverse and vertical abdominal incisions.
2. Why is the LSCS scar stronger than the classical section scar?

MCQs

1. Which of the following refers to cesarean delivery?
   a) Removal of the baby with an incision on the abdominal and uterine walls
   b) Removal of the baby after the rupture of the uterus
   c) Removal of the baby in an abdominal pregnancy
   d) All of the above

2. The advantages of a transverse abdominal incision over vertical incision include all EXCEPT:
   a) It is more comfortable postoperatively
   b) There is less chance of incisional hernia
   c) Gives good cosmetic results
   d) Is less liable to hematoma formation

3. Which of these is not an indication for cesarean delivery?
   a) Fetal distress
   b) Contracted pelvis
   c) Cord around the neck
   d) Cord prolapse

4. What is the name of the incision made on the lower uterine segment, 1 cm below the reflection of the peritoneum over the bladder to deliver the baby by cesarean section?
   a) Pfannenstiel
   b) Munro–Kerr
   c) Cherney
   d) Lembert

5. Which of the following techniques can be employed to deliver a deeply impacted head in a cesarean?
   a) Deliver by force
   b) Extension of incision
   c) Use vacuum forceps
   d) Patwardhan technique

6. What of the following is an absolute indication for classical cesarean section?
   a) Carcinoma cervix
   b) Obstructed labour
   c) Severe bradycardia of fetus
   d) Low lying placenta

7. What is the name of the hemostatic forceps used to secure bleeding points in a uterine incision?
   a) Green Armytage
   b) Babcock
   c) Allis
   d) Kocher

8. The estimated incidence of the rupture of the scar for a classical cesarean section is:
   a) 1–2%
   b) 3–5%
   c) 6–7%
   d) 8–9%

9. What is the incidence of scar rupture after a classical cesarean?
   a) 0.3%
   b) 2%
   c) 5%
   d) 9%

10. Which of the following is NOT a sign of rupture uterus?
    a) Hematuria
    b) Sudden cessation of pain
    c) Fetal heart rate 130 bpm with accelerations
    d) Easily palpable fetal parts

11. Indications of peripartum hysterectomy include all of the following EXCEPT:
    a) Atonic PPH
    b) Previous classical cesarean section
    c) Placenta accreta
    d) Uterine rupture

12. A cesarean section should be done in all of the following cases EXCEPT:
    a) Previous classical cesarean section
    b) Carcinoma cervix
    c) Abruptio placentae
    d) Major degree placenta previa

13. The incidence of rupture of a previous lower segment cesarean scar is approximately:
    a) 0.3–2%
    b) 2–4%
    c) 4–6%
    d) 6–8%

14. All the following signs may be seen in ruptured uterus EXCEPT:
    a) Hematuria
    b) Bleeding per vaginum
    c) Easily palpable fetal parts
    d) FHR 140 per minute

Answers

1. (a), 2. (d), 3. (c), 4. (b), 5. (d), 6. (a), 7. (a), 8. (d), 9. (d), 10. (c), 11. (b), 12. (c), 13. (a), 14. (d)

Fill in the blanks

1. Women with carcinoma cervix should be delivered by _____ cesarean section (classical).
2. Elective repeat cesarean section is done in case of gestational age of at least _____ weeks.

Answers

1. upper segment, 2. 39

Case scenario-based discussion

1. A 30-year-old G3P2L2 presents to the clinic. Her first baby was delivered by the vaginal route and second baby was delivered by LSCS—the indication being breech presentation; the LCB was 3 years ago. She did not have any postoperative complications. She is at 38 weeks of gestation and the baby is in a cephalic presentation and 2/5th palpable. There are no other complications. On assessment, there is no CPD. She enquires about VBAC.
   a) Will you recommend VBAC for her? If so, why?
   b) What are the factors determining the success of VBAC?
   c) What is the management protocol for VBAC?
   d) What is the most important complication to be monitored during VBAC? How is it monitored?
   e) What is a successful VBAC?

Answers

a) This woman's previous cesarean section was for a non-recurrent indication and was done by LSCS 3 years ago. Her postoperative period was uneventful and she has also had a prior normal delivery. In the current pregnancy, there are no contraindications for VBAC. Therefore, VBAC is recommended in this woman.

b) The factors determining the success of VBAC are an average-size baby, a good pelvis, spontaneous onset of labour and a prior normal delivery.

c) The woman should be counselled regarding the benefits and risks of VBAC, and her informed consent should be taken. VBAC should be carried out in a centre where facilities for an emergency cesarean section are available. The woman should be prepared as for a cesarean section, which may become necessary. The fetal and maternal conditions and the progress of labour should be carefully monitored.

d) Scar rupture is the most important complication to be monitored for. Maternal tachycardia and fetal tachycardia are important indicators of impending rupture.

e) Successful VBAC is one in which the woman delivers vaginally either spontaneously or assisted by instruments without any morbidity and mortality to the mother or the fetus.

58

OG 1.1, CM 10.1 and
FM 3.28

Maternal Mortality

Learning Objectives

» To know the definition of maternal death and maternal mortality ratio (MMR)
» To know the classification, causes and factors influencing maternal deaths
» To know the strategies for the prevention of maternal mortality
» To know the national health strategies to reduce maternal mortality

■ INTRODUCTION

The maternal mortality ratio (MMR) is a very sensitive index of maternal and child health (MCH) care available in a community. It also reflects the socio-economic status of a country and the facilities available in the health system in terms of infrastructure, trained personnel and other facilities. Maternal mortality is an avoidable tragedy since the majority of the direct causes of maternal deaths are preventable and treatable.

■ MATERNAL DEATH

According to the WHO, maternal death is defined as the 'death of a woman while pregnant or within 42 days of the termination of pregnancy, irrespective of the duration and site of pregnancy, from any cause related to or aggravated by the pregnancy or its management, but not from accidental or incidental causes'.

Registration of Maternal Death

In India, though it is mandatory to have all births and deaths registered within a specified period of time, the implementation of this act is not effective, resulting in a paucity of exact data on maternal deaths. Therefore, improving the surveillance and reporting of maternal deaths is crucial.

Maternal Death Surveillance and Response (MDSR)

The MDSR system is a continuous cycle of identification, notification and reviewing of maternal deaths followed by actions to improve the quality of care and prevent future deaths. The Maternal Death Review (MDR) process initiated by the Government of India in 2010 attempted to improve the quality of obstetric care and reduce maternal mortality and morbidity by exploring the pregnancy- and childbirth-related lacunae in the healthcare system. The aim of the MDR process is to identify the factors contributing to maternal deaths at various levels—the community, facility, district, regional and national levels—so that preventive action can be taken. The first and foremost step of the Maternal Death Review process is preparing a line list of all the maternal deaths in the area, followed by facility and/or district-based maternal death reviews.

Classification of Maternal Deaths

The causes of maternal deaths are broadly classified as follows:

1. **Direct maternal death:** This is a death resulting from obstetric complications of the pregnant state (pregnancy, labour, and the puerperium), from interventions, omissions or incorrect treatment, or from a chain of events resulting from any of the above (includes deaths related to hemorrhage, hypertensive disorders of pregnancy, sepsis, abortions, amniotic fluid embolism and deaths due to interventions).

2. **Indirect maternal death:** This refers to maternal death resulting from a pre-existing disease or a disease that developed during pregnancy and that was not directly due to obstetric causes but was aggravated by the physiological effects of pregnancy (includes deaths related to medical conditions such as anemia, cardiac disease, viral infections, malaria, HIV, etc.).

3. **Non-obstetrical maternal death:** This refers to the death of a pregnant woman resulting from incidental causes (e.g., accident, assault, suicide, snake bite, burns, etc.).

4. **Late maternal death:** This refers to the death of a woman from direct or indirect obstetric causes more than 42 days but less than one year after the termination of pregnancy.

ICD-10 classification of maternal deaths

It is recommended that maternal deaths be classified on the basis of ICD-10, according to which, the following nine categories for the classification of maternal deaths have been included in the MDSR formats:

- M01—Pregnancies with an abortive outcome (maternal death: direct)
- M02—Hypertensive disorders in pregnancy, childbirth and puerperium (maternal death: direct)
- M03—Obstetric hemorrhage (maternal death: direct)
- M04—Pregnancy-related infections (maternal death: direct)
- M05—Other obstetric complications (maternal death: direct)
- M06—Unanticipated complications of management (maternal death: direct)
- M07—Non-obstetric complications (maternal death: indirect)
- M08—Unknown/undetermined (maternal death: unspecified)
- M09—Co-incidental causes (death during pregnancy, childbirth and the puerperium)

MATERNAL MORTALITY RATIO (MMR)

MMR is defined as the number of maternal deaths per 100,000 live births occurring during the same period of time. This ratio is used as a measure of the quality of healthcare available in a country. The denominator is live births rather than all pregnancies because of the difficulty in ascertaining the number of abortions in the population.

Trends in Maternal Mortality Across the World and in India

There are large disparities in MMR between countries and also within countries; maternal deaths are more common in low-income groups and rural areas as compared to high-income groups and urban areas.

The incidence of maternal death has dropped significantly since the adoption of the Millennium Development Goals (MDGs) in 2000. The MDG-5 goal was to reduce the MMR by three quarters between 1990 and 2015 and to achieve universal access to reproductive health by 2015. In 2015, the era of MDG ended. In 2016, the Sustainable Development Goals (SDGs) were initiated, and new targets were fixed to further reduce maternal mortality. The global target is to reduce the MMR to less than 70/100,000 live births. As per the recent UN target for Sustainable Development Goals, India is committed to reducing its MMR to less than 70/100,000 live births by 2030. As per the National Health Policy (NHP), 2017, the target for MMR is 100/1,00,000 live births by 2020.

In 2017, the global MMR was 211/100,000—highest in African countries at 525/100,000 and lowest in Europe at 13/100,000 live births (Table 58.1).

India's Maternal Mortality Ratio (MMR) has seen a decline from 130 per 1 lakh live births in 2014–2016 to 122 per 1 lakh live births in 2015–2017. Maternal mortality in India has a wide regional variation; it is highest in northern Indian states like Assam and lowest in southern Indian states like Kerala. Mortality depends on many factors including social and economic factors, literacy rate and the availability of healthcare facilities. From 2016 to 2018, the north-eastern state of Assam in India had the highest maternal mortality ratio at 215 deaths per 100,000 live births, whereas Kerala had

Table 58.1   MMR trends in various WHO regions (2000–2017)

WHO region	2000	2005	2010	2015	2017	Overall reduction in MMR in 2000–2017 (%)
Africa	857	735	615	548	525	38.7
America	73	68	64	60	59	21.2
South-East Asia	355	280	214	165	152	57.3
Europe	27	22	17	14	13	52.8
Eastern Mediterranean	330	275	220	175	164	50.3
Western Pacific	75	61	51	43	41	45.8
World	342	296	248	219	211	38.4

(*Source*: World Health Organization, UNICEF, United Nations Population Fund and The World Bank, Trends in Maternal Mortality: 2000 to 2017 WHO, Geneva, 2019)

the lowest mortality ratio with 43/100,000 live births (Fig. 58.1).

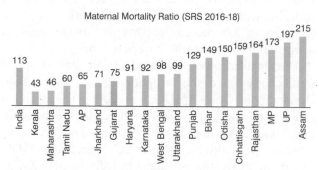

Maternal Mortality Ratio (SRS 2016-18)

Fig. 58.1   Graph showing MMR in various states of India

FACTORS INFLUENCING MATERNAL MORTALITY

Maternal Factors

Age

Maternal mortality is higher in pregnancies occurring at the extremes of age. When pregnancies occur in the adolescent age, there is malnutrition, anemia and cephalopelvic disproportion, leading to a greater number of operative deliveries with associated maternal morbidity and mortality. Hypertensive disorders such as pre-eclampsia are more common in teenage pregnancies. In pregnancies occurring at advanced maternal ages, mortality is increased not only due to obstetric factors but also due to the increase in age-related medical disorders such as hypertension, diabetes and renal and vascular diseases.

Parity

Mortality is lowest in second and third deliveries and shows a significant rise after the fourth delivery.

Socio-economic Issues

In developing countries, poor socio-economic status, inadequate transport facilities, the unavailability of timely transport and communication, delay in making the decision to shift the patient to a higher centre, poor nutrition, anemia and infectious diseases contribute to the increase in maternal mortality.

Gender discrimination, illiteracy, preference for a male child over a female and the related sex-selective feticide and domestic violence are the other social issues that have bearing on maternal mortality.

Medical Issues

The majority of complications leading to maternal death can be avoided with effective antenatal care, skilled monitoring in labour and the availability of emergency obstetric care measures. The lack of blood and blood products and essential drugs such as oxytocic agents and magnesium sulphate are significant contributing factors for maternal deaths. Maternal death reviews have shown that junior staff members dealing with high-risk cases without supervision significantly contributes to maternal death. There may be a delay in diagnosis/incorrect diagnosis. The place of delivery and the presence of a skilled birth attendant is also important. According to National Family Health Survey (NFHS)-3, in 2005–2006, only 43% of deliveries were attended by a skilled birth attendant. This had risen to around 52% by 2010–2012. In developing countries, inadequate transport facilities and delay in transporting the patient are a major issue contributing to maternal deaths.

Well-trained doctors, nurses and midwives form the backbone of any efficient obstetric service, and the availability of infrastructure facilities along with the awareness to utilise such services can significantly reduce the maternal mortality rate.

CAUSES OF MATERNAL DEATHS

A WHO systematic analysis looking into the global causes of maternal deaths in 2014 showed that between 2003 and 2009, 73% of all maternal deaths were due to direct obstetric causes and 27% were due to indirect causes. Hemorrhage accounted for 27.5% of maternal deaths, hypertensive disorders to 14% and sepsis to 10.7%. 8% of deaths were due to abortions, chiefly unsafe abortions. 52% of all maternal deaths are attributable to three leading preventable causes namely hemorrhage, sepsis and hypertensive disorders (Table 58.2).

Table 58.2   Causes of maternal deaths

Cause of death	%
Hemorrhage	27.5%
Hypertensive disorders	14%
Sepsis	10.7%
Unsafe abortions	8%

(*Source*: Say L et al., 'Global causes of maternal death: A WHO systematic analysis', *Lancet Global Health*. 2014)

Direct Causes

Hemorrhage

Hemorrhage accounts for >25% of all maternal deaths. The hemorrhagic causes of maternal deaths include antepartum hemorrhage, postpartum hemorrhage and bleeding associated with abortions and trophoblastic diseases. The most common cause of maternal mortality due to hemorrhage is postpartum hemorrhage. Antepartum hemorrhage (APH) accounts for less than 5% of maternal deaths. This is mainly because the number of women seeking early institutional care when there is bleeding in the antepartum period has increased; further, improved blood transfusion facilities have improved the outcome in APH. On the other hand, mortality due to postpartum hemorrhage (PPH), both atonic and traumatic, including cases in which the retained placenta does not come down to the expected level, continues to be a major cause of maternal deaths. In recent years, due to the increase in cesarean section rates, the incidence of adherent placenta is on the rise. This is one of the significant causes of maternal deaths due to PPH.

The strategies to reduce maternal deaths due to PPH are as follows:

- Providing quality antenatal care with the aim to increase the hemoglobin level
- Monitoring in labour using a partograph to diagnose abnormal labour early and employing measures to prevent obstructed labour
- Skilled care at birth
- Antenatal diagnosis and appropriate interventions to manage adherent placenta performed by senior personnel
- Practising active management of the third stage of labour
- The availability of high-quality emergency obstetric care (with trained medical personnel and adequate infrastructure) and improved access to these services
- Promoting institutional deliveries

Hypertension

Hypertensive disorders of pregnancy, particularly pre-eclampsia and eclampsia, account for nearly 12–14% of all maternal deaths. The main causes of death are neurological complications, especially cerebral hemorrhage, followed by pulmonary edema.

Some strategies to prevent maternal deaths due to pre-eclampsia/eclampsia are as follows:

- Early detection of pre-eclampsia and appropriate management before the onset of convulsions (eclampsia) and other life-threatening complications
- Creating awareness among the public to seek early medical attention
- Educating healthcare professionals and paramedical staff about timely identification and the treatment of pre-eclampsia by careful and periodical monitoring of blood pressure and detection of albuminuria during pregnancy
- Effective use of antihypertensives as and when necessary to prevent cerebrovascular accidents
- Timely use of magnesium sulphate to prevent and treat convulsions—wherever indicated, the medical officers at primary health centres (PHC) and auxiliary nurse midwives (ANMs) should be empowered to start a magnesium sulphate regimen before transferring the woman to a higher institution; this system has been established in states like Tamil Nadu, where the staff nurse in the PHC is also empowered to start magnesium sulphate regimen before transferring the patient to a higher facility
- Careful fluid management to prevent pulmonary edema
- Careful monitoring and management of a pregnant woman from the antenatal period through labour and the postpartum period

Puerperal sepsis

Puerperal infections, often the consequence of poor hygiene during delivery, account for about 15% of maternal mortality. Severe intrapartum infection can result from prolonged labour, home births in unhygienic conditions, prolonged rupture of membranes, multiple vaginal examinations, operative vaginal delivery, trauma to the genital tract, PPH, manual removal of placenta, retained placenta and membranes and droplet infection from caregivers. Following simple practices like proper hand washing before and after examining the patient, the use of separate linen and footwear for the labour room, restricting the number of vaginal examinations to the minimum, the use of prophylactic antibiotics for cesarean section and post-delivery cleanliness can help reduce the incidence of sepsis. The use of disposable /sterile delivery kits for deliveries and meticulously following the 'five cleans' of delivery will reduce the mortality due to sepsis to a great extent.

The five 'cleans' of delivery
1. Clean hands
2. Clean surface
3. Clean blade
4. Clean cord
5. Clean cord tie

Abortion

To avoid maternal deaths due to abortions, it is also vital to prevent unwanted pregnancies. All women, including adolescents, need access to contraception, safe abortion services to the full extent of the law, and quality post-abortion care. Introducing comprehensive abortion care practices at all first referral units (FRUs) is one of the key interventions to decrease criminal abortions by unqualified persons. Similarly, the Medical Termination of Pregnancy Act (MTP Act) has also been amended to include medical abortion in routine practice. Moreover, the upper limit for termination has been increased from 20 to 24 weeks for certain categories of women.

Rupture uterus

Rupture uterus can occur in a scarred uterus following cesarean section; it can occur spontaneously following obstructed labour or occur due to grand multiparity and injudicious use of oxytocics and due to traumatic causes following difficult instrumental deliveries. If not properly managed, it can lead to maternal deaths. All post-cesarean pregnancies should be carefully monitored in the antenatal period, and there should be proper selection of cases for vaginal birth after cesarean section. In the event of scar dehiscence/rupture it should be managed appropriately. With the availability of improved healthcare systems and the routine use of partographs, rupture uterus due to obstructed labour has become a rarity. Effective counselling during antenatal visits on the use of contraception also reduces the incidence of grand multiparity, and thereby, rupture uterus.

Other direct causes

Other direct causes include ectopic pregnancies, embolism and death due to interventions.

Indirect Causes

Around 20% of maternal deaths in India are due to indirect causes, as a result of pre-existing diseases or a disease that developed during pregnancy. A number of medical conditions such as anemia, cardiac diseases, tuberculosis, infective hepatitis, viral infections such as COVID, swine flu and dengue, malaria, gastrointestinal diseases and malnutrition can complicate pregnancy. These conditions can deteriorate during pregnancy or predispose to obstetrical complications.

Anemia in pregnancy accounts for 11.5% of all maternal deaths. The World Health Organization (WHO)/World Health Statistics data show that in 2016, 40.1% of pregnant women worldwide were anemic. The condition is prominent in South-East Asian countries. India contributes to about 80% of maternal deaths due to anemia in South Asia. Anemia among pregnant women is often due to nutritional causes and worm infestations; most women are anemic at the commencement of pregnancy. Even with the prophylactic administration of oral iron, women continue to be anemic as most iron preparations are not easily tolerated. To combat the high prevalence of iron deficiency anemia (IDA), several Government programmes and state-level schemes were rolled out in various states of India. The National Nutritional Anemia Prophylaxis Programme 1970, National Anemia Control Programme 1991 and the 12/12 Initiative 2007, are some of the nationwide initiatives to reduce the incidence of anemia. The National Health Policy 2017 also addressed malnutrition and micronutrient deficiencies interventions. With the introduction of parenteral iron preparations like iron sucrose, there is likely to be a decrease in the prevalence of anemia.

Heart disease in pregnancy accounts for 8.2% of all deaths. Infective hepatitis, especially when it occurs in epidemics, is also associated with high mortality.

■ STRATEGIES FOR THE PREVENTION OF MATERNAL MORTALITY

In order to reduce maternal mortality, the health status of women should be addressed before pregnancy and during pregnancy, childbirth and the postpartum period and effective contraception should be provided in the postpartum period to prevent unwanted pregnancies and promote birth spacing.

Health Education

- Age at marriage—pregnancy in young women may be associated with increased morbidity and maternal mortality due to anemia and hypertensive disorders; currently, the minimum legal age of marriage for girls is 18 years and there is a proposal to increase it to 21 years
- Utilisation of RCH services
- Awareness of antenatal care
- Use of prophylactic iron and deworming
- Raising awareness of danger signs during pregnancy
- Nutritional education
- Importance of immunisation
- Spacing/limitation of births

Safe Abortion Services

Preventing unwanted births and reducing unsafe abortions by:
- Sex education and contraception (adolescent clinics)
- MTP Act

Improving Healthcare Infrastructure

- Provision of RCH services in remote rural areas/urban slums
- Improved staffing
- Skilled intrapartum care
- Facilities for essential/emergency obstetric care
- All births attended by skilled health professionals
- Training of traditional birth attendants (TBAs) in remote and inaccessible areas
- Training of medical and paramedical personnel through CMEs, workshops and drills on the management of emergencies
- Conducting periodic audits
- Developing first referral units (FRU) where emergency obstetric care and anesthesia can be provided by trained doctors who can provide effective support to qualified obstetricians and anesthesiologists
- Strengthening of transport facilities

Anemia Prevention

- Through iron supplementation and deworming, it should be ensured that all adolescent girls have a hemoglobin level of >12 g%

- Hemoglobin level should be checked at each antenatal visit
- During pregnancy, all antenatal women should receive at least 100 tablets of iron
- Oral iron tablets should be continued during lactation

Addressing the Causes of Maternal Deaths and Taking Preventive Action

- Addressing deaths related to hemorrhage, hypertensive disorders, sepsis, anemia, unsafe abortions, etc.
- Addressing certain diseases like malaria, TB, RTI/STI, HIV/AIDS and hepatitis
- Implementing government policies and programmes to reduce maternal mortality (also refer to Chapter 66, *Maternal and newborn health: Initiatives and programmes by the Government of India*)

NATIONAL HEALTH STRATEGIES TO REDUCE MATERNAL MORTALITY (Table 58.3)

Table 58.3 National health policies and programmes to reduce maternal mortality

Health programmes	Year	Goals
Child Survival and Safe Motherhood Programme (CSSM) Sponsored by the central govt.	1992	To improve child and maternal mortality and morbidity rates
Reproductive, Maternal, Newborn, Child plus Adolescent Health (RMNCH + A) Sponsored by the central govt.	1997 2013	Maternal and reproductive health—covers facilities for the antenatal period, delivery, postnatal period, birth spacing counselling and provisions for MTP Child health—skilled care at birth, breastfeeding, neonatal and childhood illness, vitamin A, iron and folic acid prophylaxis Adolescent health—nutrition, iron and FA supplementation, sexual health and mental health services BEmOC—basic emergency obstetric care CEmOC—comprehensive emergency obstetric care
Janani Suraksha Yojna Sponsored by the central govt.	2005	Cash incentives to reduce maternal and neonatal mortality by promoting institutional deliveries among poor pregnant women
Janani Shishu Suraksha Karyakram Sponsored by the central govt.	2011	Expenses related to delivery in public institutions borne by the govt.
Pradhan Mantri Matritva Vandhana Yojna Sponsored by the central govt.	2017	Promoting appropriate practice, care and institutional service utilisation during pregnancy, delivery and lactation All pregnant women given financial benefit of Rs 5,000
Pradhan Mantri Surakshit Matritva Abhiyan (PMSMA) Sponsored by the central govt.	2016	Quality maternal care, free of cost to all pregnant women on the 9th of every month

(Continued)

Table 58.3 (*Continued*) National health policies and programmes to reduce maternal mortality

Health programmes	Year	Goals
Dr. Muthulakshmi Reddy Maternity Benefit Scheme Sponsored by the state govt.	1987	Rs 18,000 given in seven instalments for the first two deliveries of pregnant women above 19 years of age
Mother And Child Tracking System (MCTS)	2009	Web-based programme introduced by the Ministry of Health and Family Welfare to facilitate timely delivery of antenatal and postnatal care services and immunisation to all children
Comprehensive Abortion Care Services (under RMNCH +A) Sponsored by the central govt.	2013	To provide quality MTP services Supply of NISCHAY kits Mala N, Mala D, CHHAYA (centchroman) IUCDs– CuT 380A, 375 Emergency pills Permanent methods
LAQSHYA Launched by the Ministry of Health and Family Welfare on 11 December 2017	2017	It is a labour ward quality improvement initiative to reduce preventable maternal and newborn mortality, morbidity and stillbirths by ensuring care in the labour room and maternity theatres
Manyata programme Launched by FOGSI	2017	A nationwide initiative to improve the quality of maternal and neonatal care in the private sector in India
SUMAN—Surakshit Matritva Aashwasan National Programme	2019	Assuring free medicines to pregnant women and mothers upto 6 months after delivery Sick newborns also receive free health benefits

KEY POINTS

✓ *More than 75% of maternal deaths are due to direct causes.*

✓ *Important causes of direct maternal deaths include hemorrhage, hypertension, sepsis and unsafe abortions.*

✓ *The indirect causes of maternal deaths include anemia, cardiac disease, infective hepatitis and viral infections complicating pregnancy.*

✓ *Proper antenatal care, intrapartum care by a skilled birth attendant, and proper referral to the appropriate centre when required can help in reducing the maternal mortality in India.*

Essay questions

1. Define maternal death and maternal mortality ratio and list the causes of maternal deaths.
2. What are the factors that influence maternal mortality?
3. Discuss the strategies to reduce maternal mortality.
4. Discuss the Government Policies and Programmes to reduce maternal mortality in India.

Short answer question

1. Discuss the strategies to reduce maternal deaths due to PPH.

MCQs

1. The WHO definition of maternal mortality extends to how many days after delivery?
   a) 7 days
   b) 21 days
   c) 42 days
   d) 6 months

2. What formula is used to calculate the maternal mortality ratio?
   a) Number of maternal deaths/100,000 women of reproductive age
   b) Number of maternal deaths/1,000 women of reproductive age
   c) Number of maternal deaths/100,000 live births
   d) Number of maternal deaths/1,000 live births

3. What was the target of MDG-5?
   a) To reduce maternal mortality ratio by 1/4 between 1990 and 2015
   b) To reduce maternal mortality ratio by 1/2 between 1990 and 2015
   c) To reduce maternal mortality ratio by 3/4 between 1990 and 2015
   d) To reduce maternal mortality ratio by 4/5 between 1990 and 2015

4. What is the most common indirect cause of maternal death?
   a) Anemia
   b) Hypertension
   c) Heart disease
   d) Renal disease

5. Which of these measures is not beneficial in reducing maternal mortality?
   a) Active management of the third stage of labour
   b) Presence of a trained birth attendant
   c) Strengthening first referral units
   d) Providing emergency obstetric care only at tertiary care centres
6. The states with low MMR include the following EXCEPT:
   a) Kerala
   b) Maharashtra
   c) Rajasthan
   d) Tamil Nadu

Answers
1. (c), 2. (c), 3. (c), 4. (a), 5. (d), 6. (c)

Fill in the blanks

1. Maternal death is defined as the death of a woman while pregnant or within _____ of the termination of pregnancy.
2. The target for MDG-5 was to reduce the maternal mortality ratio by _____ between 1990 and 2015.
3. The most common cause of maternal mortality in India is _____.
4. The most commonly used measure of maternal mortality is the _____.

Answers
1. 42 days, 2. three-quarters, 3. postpartum hemorrhage,
4. maternal mortality ratio

Perinatal Mortality

Learning Objectives

» To know about the perinatal period and perinatal and neonatal mortality rates
» To know the causes of and factors influencing perinatal deaths
» To know the causes of perinatal asphyxia and birth injuries
» To know the strategies to prevent perinatal deaths

■ INTRODUCTION

Perinatal mortality in any community/country is dependent on the status of maternal health and the quality of the available obstetric and pediatric services. The major causes of stillbirths and neonatal deaths can be classified into avoidable and unavoidable causes. The avoidable causes are poor maternal health, inadequate care during pregnancy, inappropriate management of complications occurring during pregnancy and delivery, lack of infection control measures at birth and non-availability of efficient newborn care. The unavoidable causes are congenital malformations and chromosomal disorders.

The following are some important definitions in this context:

*   **The perinatal period:** It commences at 22 completed weeks (154 days) of gestation and ends at seven completed days after birth.
*   **The fetal period:** The period extending from 22 completed weeks of gestation until birth is known as the fetal period. This is further classified into intermediate and late fetal periods.
    — Fetal deaths occurring between 22 and 27 weeks of gestation are known as **intermediate fetal deaths.**
    — Deaths occurring after 28 weeks of gestation are known as **late fetal deaths**.
*   **Neonatal period:** The first 28 days of postnatal life is called the neonatal period. It is subdivided into the immediate (first 24 hours), early (first 7 days) and late (8–28 days) neonatal periods.
*   **Stillbirth:** According to the WHO, stillbirth is the birth of a baby with a birth weight of 500 g or more at 22 or more completed weeks of gestation or with a body length of 25 cm or more, who died before or during labour and birth. For international comparisons, the WHO recommends reporting stillbirths with a birth weight of **1,000 g or more, 28 weeks' gestation or more or a body length of 35 cm or more**.

The WHO recommends that for the uniformity of international statistics, a weight of 1,000 g (or when weight is unknown, a gestational age of 28 weeks and crown–heel length of 35 cm) be used to determine these rates.

*   **Neonatal mortality:** This term refers to neonatal death. It is the death of a newborn within the first 28 days of life. Neonatal deaths may be subdivided into early neonatal deaths, occurring during the first seven days of life, and late neonatal deaths, occurring after the seventh day but before the 28th day of life.
*   **Perinatal mortality:** This refers to the death of a fetus between the age of viability and the 7th day of life. It equals the sum of stillbirths and early neonatal deaths.
*   **Perinatal mortality rate (PNMR):** For defining the PNMR, the lower limit of the perinatal period varies between and within countries based on the available newborn care and the fetal viability of a particular unit. This period ranges from 22–28 weeks.

    Perinatal mortality rate is defined as the number of perinatal deaths (late fetal deaths + early neonatal deaths)/1,000 total births (live births and stillbirths).

$$\text{PNMR} = \frac{\text{Late fetal deaths} + \text{early neonatal deaths}}{1,000 \text{ total births}}$$

*   **Neonatal mortality rate (NMR):** This is defined as the number of neonatal deaths from birth to 28 days of life per 1,000 live births during the same period.
*   **Stillbirth rate:** This is the number of fetal losses prior to or during labour, i.e., babies born dead divided by the total number of births in a given period. It is expressed as stillbirths per thousand births.

PREVALENCE

Perinatal mortality accounts for about 90% of all fetal and infant mortality. In India, stillbirths are seldom registered. Hence, most studies on perinatal mortality are hospital-based. According to the SRS 2014 report, the national PMR was 28/1,000 (stillbirths were 5/1,000 and early neonatal deaths were 23/1,000). The report also showed marked interstate variability (e.g., Kerala 10/1,000 and Odisha 37/1,000). The Sample Registration System's estimate of perinatal mortality for the year 2016 was 23/1,000 live births + stillbirths with about 26 in rural and 14 in urban areas. The neonatal mortality rate (NMR) declined from 52 per 1,000 live births in 1990 to 28 per 1,000 live births in 2013 and 22 per 1,000 live births in 2019 (WHO, UNICEF).

The maternal factors resulting in increased perinatal loss include adolescent pregnancies, maternal undernutrition, low socio-economic status, iron deficiency anemia and other micronutrient deficiencies, interpregnancy intervals of <12 months or >60 months, lack of antenatal care, maternal infections, pre-eclampsia and type 2 diabetes. The three major causes of neonatal deaths are complications from preterm birth (35%), infections (33%) and intrapartum-related conditions or birth asphyxia (20%). It is estimated that around 40% of all stillbirths and neonatal deaths take place during labour and the day of birth, i.e., approximately within 48 hours. About three-fourths of the total number of neonatal deaths occur in the first week of life.

ETIOLOGY OF PERINATAL DEATHS (Fig. 59.1)

General Causes

- Pregnancy during adolescence or at an advanced age
- Increasing parity
- Low socio-economic status
- Inadequate antenatal care
- Poor nutritional status (malnutrition and anemia)
- Low rates of literacy
- Large numbers of deliveries by untrained personnel

Maternal Causes

Antenatal causes

- Maternal diseases such as hypertension, diabetes, anemia, SLE, renal disease, cholestasis of pregnancy, liver disease and APLA, which can lead to placental insufficiency

- Anatomical defects of the uterus such as uterine anomalies and cervical incompetence may result in preterm delivery and neonatal death
- Antepartum hemorrhage—perinatal mortality is increased in both major degree placenta previa and abruptio placentae
- Rh-incompatibility may lead to the formation of a hydropic fetus, resulting in stillbirth or neonatal death
- Chorioamnionitis and other infections
- Malaria and viral infections
- Maternal infections such as syphilis or group B streptococci or parvovirus infections, which are transmitted to the fetus
- Smoking and drug abuse

Intrapartum causes

- Birth injuries
- Birth asphyxia
- Prolonged/obstructed labour
- Intrauterine infection
- Placental abruption

Fetal Causes

- Malpresentations
- Multiple pregnancy
- Genetic abnormalities
- Prematurity, FGR (SGA)
- Congenital anomalies (such as anencephaly) that are incompatible with life; cardiac anomalies, renal anomalies or other anomalies of the central nervous system may lead to early neonatal death
- Hypoxia due to cord accidents, birth trauma

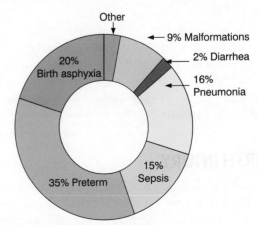

Fig. 59.1 Causes of perinatal deaths (*Source:* Liu et al., Statistical Report, *Lancet*, 2012)

Postnatal Causes

- Neonatal deaths account for about 40% of all child deaths worldwide; 99% of these deaths occur in developing countries.
- The highest NMR is in Sub-Saharan Africa (over 45 deaths per 1,000 live births).
- The main causes of neonatal death are prematurity, neonatal infections, aspiration pneumonitis, respiratory distress syndrome, low birth weight, perinatal hypoxic insult and asphyxia.

■ PERINATAL HYPOXIA

Hypoxia is the result of interference with the transport of oxygen from the maternal blood to the fetal blood in the placenta or obstruction of blood flowing through the umbilical cord.

Etiology

There are many causes of hypoxia during pregnancy, labour and delivery. These include the following:

- Hypertension or renal disease may affect the vessels in the placental site and, consequently, prevent proper placental oxygenation
- Premature separation of the placenta, placenta previa, vasa previa
- Prolapse of the cord and cord compression
- Obstructed labour
- Prolonged labour, especially a prolonged second stage
- Difficult instrumental delivery
- Malpresentations like breech or conditions like unexpected shoulder dystocia
- Sudden lowering of maternal blood pressure, as in maternal shock
- The injudicious use of analgesic drugs, which may interfere with the establishment of normal breathing in the baby by depressing the respiratory centre
- Placental changes that occur in postmaturity, resulting in hypoxia

■ BIRTH INJURY

- Intracranial injury and hemorrhage result from any condition that causes excessive stress during labour, such as cephalopelvic disproportion, difficult forceps delivery, precipitate labour and very rapid delivery of the after-coming head in breech. The premature fetus is more vulnerable to birth injury; it is not uncommon to see such injuries even after a normal spontaneous labour. While the most common type of birth injury is subdural hemorrhage resulting from the rupture of the vein of Galen, any of the cerebral veins may rupture. Congestion and edema of the brain and meninges may also result from the prolonged compression of the head. Extradural subarachnoid and intraventricular hemorrhage may also be found occasionally.
- Injuries to the spine are occasionally encountered in cases of breech delivery and impacted shoulders.
- Rarely, injury to the viscera is seen.

Though neonatal death may occur following severe birth trauma, with subtle injuries, neurological manifestations and cognitive function defects may be noted only as the child grows.

■ FETAL MALFORMATION

The prevalence of birth defects among live-born infants is 2–4%. Risk factors for congenital malformations include family history, maternal age, illness, drug use, exposure to infectious or environmental agents and the intrauterine environment.

Etiology

In 65–75% of cases, the etiology of fetal malformation is multifactorial.

- Genetic factors: These include single gene disorders or chromosomal abnormalities. The abnormalities associated with death are aneuploidies like trisomies 18, 13 and 21, sex chromosome aneuploidy and unbalanced translocations.
- Maternal medical conditions
  — Substance abuse, including smoking and the consumption of alcohol
  — Diabetes mellitus
  — Infections—viral infections like rubella have been shown to result in abnormalities of the fetus
  — Medications such as thalidomide, warfarin and phenytoin
  — Exposure to radiation and hyperthermia
  — Mechanical constraints on fetal development (10%) as in severe oligohydramnios and multifetal pregnancy

Strategies to reduce perinatal mortality
- Preconception counselling
- Proper antenatal care
- Good maternal hygiene and control of genital infections
- Early recognition and effective treatment of high-risk maternal factors
- Prevention of preterm labour
- Timely delivery of prolonged pregnancy, diabetes, GDM, pre-eclampsia, FGR, oligohydramnios, PROM
- Hygienic labour room practices
- Prompt management of non-reassuring CTG
- Avoiding traumatic delivery
- Avoiding prolonged labour by maintaining a partograph
- Proper resuscitation and suction of the newborn
- Prevention of hypothermia and neonatal infections
- Emphasis on breastfeeding and education of proper feeding techniques

GOVERNMENT PROGRAMMES AND POLICIES TO REDUCE PNMR

- The Every Newborn Action Plan (ENAP), which was launched in June 2014 by the WHO and endorsed by the World Health Assembly calls for a national SBR of ≤12/1,000 births by 2030 and a further reduction to 10/1,000 births by 2035.
- The India Newborn Action Plan (INAP) being launched by the Government of India incorporates the same principles. The goals of the INAP are as follows:
  1. Eliminating preventable stillbirths to achieve "single digit SBR" by 2030, with all states required to individually achieve this target by 2035. The INAP targets are to achieve a stillbirth rate of <10 by 2030.
  2. Eliminating preventable newborn deaths to achieve "single digit NMR" by 2030, with all states required to individually achieve this target by 2035.

  In order to achieve these goals, the INAP interventions focus on the following areas:
  — Preconception and antenatal care
  — Care during labour and childbirth
  — Immediate newborn care
  — Care of small and sick newborns
  — Care of healthy newborns

KEY POINTS

✓ *The causes of perinatal mortality include maternal diseases, complications of pregnancy and congenital malformations.*

✓ *Intranatal causes include complications in labour such as obstructed labour and prolonged labour.*

✓ *Birth asphyxia, prematurity and low birth weight contribute to neonatal morbidity and mortality.*

Essay question
1. Define perinatal mortality rate and discuss the causes and factors that influence perinatal mortality.

Short answer questions
1. Define
   a) Stillbirth
   b) Neonatal mortality rate
2. What are the causes of stillbirth?
3. What is perinatal hypoxia?
4. Write a short note on birth injuries.

MCQs
1. Perinatal mortality rate is calculated as
   a) Stillbirth/1,000 live births
   b) Stillbirth + death in the first week of life/1,000 live births
   c) Stillbirth/1,000 total deliveries
   d) Stillbirth + death in the first week of life/1,000 total deliveries
2. The WHO definition for late fetal deaths has a cut-off of what weight?
   a) 500 g
   b) 1,000 g
   c) 1,200 g
   d) 1,500 g
3. Neonatal death refers to death till what day of life?
   a) Day 1
   b) Day 7
   c) Day 28
   d) Day 42
4. Which of these is not a cause of stillbirth?
   a) IUGR
   b) Abruption

c) Induction of labour
d) Diabetes mellitus

5. What is the most common cause of neonatal death?
   a) Prematurity
   b) Infection
   c) Hypoxia
   d) Congenital malformation

6. Which of these cannot increase the risk of hypoxia in a fetus?
   a) Postmaturity-related placental changes
   b) Cord prolapse
   c) Shoulder dystocia
   d) Cephalic presentation

7. What is the prevalence of fetal malformations?
   a) 1%
   b) 2–4%

c) 5%
d) 10%

Answers

1. (d), 2. (b), 3. (c), 4. (c), 5. (a), 6. (d), 7. (b)

Fill in the blanks

1. Neonatal death is defined as infant death occurring through _____ of age.
2. The prevalence of major congenital malformations among live-born infants is _____.

Answers

1. 28 days,   2. 2–4%

60 Coagulation Disorders

OG 10.2

Learning Objectives

» To understand the changes that occur in the coagulation system during pregnancy
» To know the causes and clinical manifestations of disseminated intravascular coagulation (DIC)
» To know the investigations and management of DIC

■ INTRODUCTION

In order to reduce the blood loss following any trauma, it is necessary for the blood vessels to be sealed off without affecting the circulation permanently. The same principle applies in pregnancy also, where following delivery, besides the myometrial contraction, the open vessels need to be sealed off to reduce the bleeding from the placental site. In order to achieve this hemostasis, the coagulation pathway gets activated after delivery. The activation of the coagulation cascade yields thrombin, which converts fibrinogen to fibrin. The stable fibrin clot is the final product of hemostasis. The activation of the fibrinolytic system generates plasmin, which breaks down fibrinogen and fibrin, thus resulting in the lysis of fibrin clots. The presence of plasmin is critical as it is necessary for the breakdown of clots. The breakdown of fibrinogen and fibrin results in polypeptides called fibrin degradation products (FDPs) (Fig. 60.1).

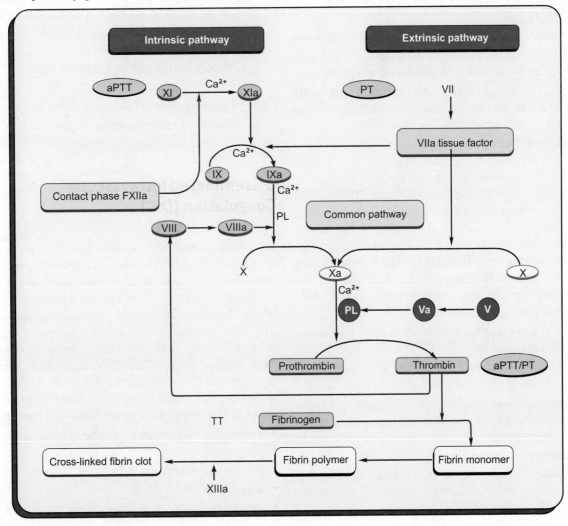

Fig. 60.1 Coagulation cascade

PHYSIOLOGICAL CHANGES IN THE COAGULATION SYSTEM DURING PREGNANCY

During pregnancy, there is an increase in the levels of the majority of clotting factors and a reduction in fibrinolytic activity. These changes lead to a hypercoagulable state, which is likely to be due to the hormonal changes of pregnancy. The increase in clotting activity is greatest at the time of delivery with placental expulsion and the subsequent release of thromboplastic substances. This is a physiological adaptive mechanism that promotes clot formation to reduce blood loss at delivery. These coagulation and fibrinolytic changes reverse and reach pre-pregnant levels 3–4 weeks postpartum.

The following changes occur during normal pregnancy:

- **Platelets:** The platelet count decreases in a normal pregnancy, possibly due to increased destruction and hemodilution, with the maximum decrease in the platelet count seen in the third trimester. On the other hand, the platelet width and volume increase.
- **Clotting factors:**
  — The levels of clotting factors VIII, von Willebrand factor (vWf), ristocetin cofactor (RCoA) and factors X and XII increase during pregnancy.
  — The levels of factor VII increase gradually during pregnancy and reach very high levels (up to 1,000%) by term.
- **Fibrinogen:** Levels of fibrinogen also increase during pregnancy. The concentration of plasma fibrinogen in normal, non-pregnant women is about 300 mg/dL and ranges from 200 to 400 mg/dL. During normal pregnancy, the fibrinogen concentration increases by about 50% to an average of about 450 mg/dL late in pregnancy with a range of 300–600 mg/dL (Table 60.1). The increase in the concentration of fibrinogen is the chief cause of the accelerated erythrocyte sedimentation rate (ESR) observed during pregnancy.
- **Factor V:** Concentrations increase in early pregnancy then decrease and stabilise.
- **Factor II (prothrombin):** Levels may increase or not change in early pregnancy but are normal by term.
- **Hemostatic functions:** Tests of hemostatic functions such as clotting time and bleeding time yield normal results in pregnancy.
- **Fibrinolytic activity:** Plasma fibrinolytic activity is decreased during pregnancy, remains low during labour and delivery and returns to normal within one hour of the delivery of the placenta.

Table 60.1 Coagulation factors in the non-pregnant state and in pregnancy

Factor	Non-pregnant state	Third trimester
Fibrinogen (mg/dL)	233–496	301–606
Prothrombin time—PT (seconds)	12.7–15.4	9.6–12.9
Partial thromboplastin time—aPTT (seconds)	26.3–39.4	22.6–35.0
INR	0.9–1.04	0.80–1.09
Platelets (X 109/L)	165–415	146–429

(*Source*: Modified from *Willam's Obstetrics*, 23rd Ed, P 1260)

COAGULATION DISORDERS ENCOUNTERED DURING PREGNANCY

- Disseminated intravascular coagulation (DIC)
- Thromboembolic manifestations during pregnancy and the puerperium
- Bleeding disorders due to medical conditions— certain medical conditions present with bleeding disorders during pregnancy, in the postpartum period and in the puerperium:
  — Idiopathic thrombocytopenic purpura
  — Von Willebrand disease
  — Disorders related to coagulation therapy
  — Drug-induced thrombocytopenia
  — Chronic renal and liver disease

Disseminated Intravascular Coagulation (DIC)

DIC, also known as consumptive coagulopathy, is a pathological process characterised by the activation of the clotting mechanism, and consequently, the formation of blood clots in the small blood vessels throughout the body. This leads to a reduction of tissue blood flow and ultimately, multiple organ damage. Since the intravascular coagulation process consumes clotting factors and platelets, bleeding can occur from various sites including venipuncture sites. DIC is a common contributor to maternal morbidity and mortality. Life-threatening coagulation disorders may occur during pregnancy in the following conditions:

- Premature separation of the placenta (abruptio placentae)
- Severe pre-eclampsia/eclampsia
- Intrauterine fetal death
- Septic abortion, chorioamnionitis

- Amniotic fluid embolism
- Acute fatty liver of pregnancy
- Massive blood transfusion

Abruptio placentae

This is the most frequent obstetric cause of coagulation failure. The risk of coagulopathy is high in severe abruptio placentae, when the placental abruption is severe enough to kill the fetus. Disseminated intravascular coagulation (DIC) occurs in 10% of all placental abruption, and the incidence is higher in cases of fetal death.

The placenta and decidua contain massive amounts of tissue thromboplastin which is pumped into the circulation following placental separation. This triggers the clotting system and also a secondary, and often excessive, fibrinolytic activity. Coagulation causes microcirculatory changes, especially in the kidneys, resulting in renal insufficiency. The increased fibrinolytic activity causes hemoglobinemia and hemoglobinuria. In addition, due to hypofibrinogenemia and increased levels of FDP, there is secondary uterine atony which can hinder effective labour and increase the bleeding from the abruption surface and aggravate the existing DIC.

All women diagnosed with abruption placenta should be investigated for coagulation failure. Early detection and timely correction of coagulation disorders can reduce maternal morbidity and mortality. As described in Chapter 22, *Antepartum hemorrhage—abruptio placentae*, clotting tests should be performed on admission and repeated every two hours or more frequently to diagnose the disorder. Hemostatic failure should be suspected if there is persistent oozing at the site of venipuncture or bleeding from the mucous membranes of the mouth or nose or hematuria or PPH not due to uterine atony or uterine trauma. Laboratory tests will show a low platelet count, low fibrinogen and greatly prolonged prothrombin time along with raised fibrin degradation products (FDPs) due to secondary fibrinolysis.

The mainstay of treatment is to restore the blood volume, fibrinogen and platelets. At the same time, steps should be taken to expedite delivery. Delivery should be completed within six to eight hours after the onset of placental abruption to avoid worsening of DIC and organ damage.

Pre-eclampsia/eclampsia

The majority of women with severe pre-eclampsia and eclampsia have subclinical consumptive coagulopathy. Frank manifestation of DIC occurs in association with complications such as placental abruption and HELLP syndrome. HELLP syndrome may progress to DIC in 15–30% of patients. The placenta is central to the pathophysiology of pre-eclampsia. Placental hypoperfusion produces oxidative stress leading to the activation of the vascular endothelium. This endothelial cell activation leads to the liberation of vasoactive substances and the activation of the clotting cascade.

In pre-eclampsia with laboratory reports suggesting DIC, immediate delivery is recommended to avoid clinically evident DIC. Management consists of early delivery with the adequate replacement of platelets and fibrinogen. In the setting of DIC, vaginal delivery is preferable with appropriate anti-DIC therapy. If vaginal delivery is difficult because of obstetric complications, then all measures should be taken to correct DIC before resorting to a cesarean section. The prothrombin time, activated partial thromboplastin time and serum fibrinogen levels remain normal in HELLP syndrome but will be prolonged in DIC. Aggressive treatment is indicated, and delivery should be expedited; at the same time, blood pressure and coagulation abnormality should be kept in control.

Intrauterine fetal death

Fetal death can occur at any time during pregnancy. The mechanism of coagulopathy is the activation of factor VII of the extrinsic pathway by the release of tissue thromboplastin from the fetoplacental unit. A coagulation disorder following IUFD is uncommon in modern obstetrics due to early aggressive treatment of intrauterine fetal demise (IUFD). The hemostatic derangements become evident after 4–5 weeks of IUFD. The coagulopathy may be subacute to chronic, with intravascular clotting and simultaneous lysis of the circulating fibrin. It is recommended that in all cases of IUFD, including missed miscarriages, a complete blood count and the estimation of PT, aPTT, D-dimers and fibrinogen should be done.

Septic abortion/chorioamnionitis

In cases of septic abortion and chorioamnionitis, due to the release of endotoxin due to gram-negative organisms, especially *E. coli*, patients may go into endotoxic shock and coagulation failure. Endotoxic shock is accompanied by circulatory changes, namely, slowing of the circulation in the arterioles and venules, increased capillary permeability, raised blood viscosity and hypovolemia. All these changes favour the development of DIC.

Uterine infection must be treated with broad-spectrum antibiotics. If the products of conception are present in the uterine cavity, they should be removed under antibiotic cover. DIC is managed as per the protocol.

Amniotic fluid embolism

In amniotic fluid embolism (AFE), amniotic fluid enters into the systemic maternal circulation. In this condition, maternal mortality is high. The particulate matter in the amniotic fluid causes mechanical obstruction of the pulmonary capillaries and elicits a vasoconstrictor response, resulting in pulmonary artery hypertension. This leads to right ventricular failure with secondary left ventricular failure. There is also an anaphylactic reaction due to the activation of complements and the release of immune mediators. The mechanism leading to DIC in AFE is the presence of a tissue factor in the amniotic fluid that activates factor VII in the extrinsic pathway.

This condition is often associated with strong uterine contractions following the rupture of the membranes, especially after oxytocin stimulation, cesarean section, rupture of the uterus, premature separation of the placenta and intrauterine fetal death. The immediate result of the embolism is right ventricular failure, followed by a drop in the left ventricular output and culminating in cardiogenic shock. If the patient survives this episode, in the ensuing hours, there is an increased risk of disseminated intravascular coagulation principally affecting the lungs, followed by increased fibrinolytic activity. The clinical presentation is unexplained sudden cardiovascular collapse, respiratory distress, cyanosis, altered mental status and bleeding due to DIC.

Management is mainly supportive with cardiorespiratory resuscitation and correction of coagulopathy with packed cells, FFP and platelet transfusion.

Acute fatty liver

Acute fatty liver is mostly reported in the third trimester and has a fulminant course. Genetic deficiencies in the beta oxidation of fatty acids play a role in the pathogenesis of acute fatty liver. Severe hepatic dysfunction and anti-thrombin III deficiency are hypothesised as the cause of DIC.

Major obstetric hemorrhage and massive blood transfusion

Women presenting with major obstetric hemorrhages require massive blood transfusions. In these women, if the blood loss is replaced only by stored blood, it will be deficient in the labile clotting factors V and VIII and platelets. Therefore, the circulation will be rapidly depleted of these essential clotting factors, which will manifest with DIC. This is called dilutional coagulopathy. The majority of healthy pregnant women can tolerate a massive transfusion without developing dilutional coagulopathy or dilutional thrombocytopenia.

Women receiving massive transfusion should have periodical screening with laboratory tests including platelet count, PT, APTT and serum fibrinogen. If the woman develops dilution coagulopathy, she should be treated with platelet transfusions and FFP.

Clinical features of DIC

Disseminated intravascular coagulation is an acquired thromboembolic disease in which the clinical findings usually depend on the underlying pathology.

- Bleeding is usually the most frequent clinical finding. It manifests as ecchymosis, petechia, mucosal oozing, prolonged bleeding at vein puncture sites and surgical incision sites, heavy vaginal bleeding and bleeds from various systems, especially the gastrointestinal system.
- It can also present with end-organ damage due to fibrin accumulation in the intravascular bed at the microvascular level.

Diagnosis of DIC

Bedside clinical test

Blood clotting and clot retraction time can be checked at the bedside if facilities for laboratory tests are not available. Normally, there is good clot formation in 10 minutes, which will remain stable for 30 minutes to 1 hour; this indicates adequate fibrinogen level. After 1 hour, the clot retracts and separates from the serum. In the presence of fibrinolysis, the clot does not retract, or it breaks easily due to the presence of FDP.

Laboratory investigations

- Coagulation tests (aPTT, PT, thrombin time [TT])
- Serum fibrinogen levels
- Markers of fibrin degradation product (FDP)—D-dimer
- Hemoglobin, PCV and platelet count
- Analysis of blood smear for evidence of fragmented RBCs

The tests should be repeated over a period of 6–8 hours because what begins as a mild abnormality can change dramatically into severe DIC. Common findings are prolongation of PT and/or aPTT; platelet counts <100,000/mm³ or rapid decline in platelet numbers and elevated level of FDP. The most sensitive test for DIC is the FDP level. The D-dimer test is more specific for the detection of fibrin degradation products.

Fibrinogen level <100 mg/dL is indicative of severe hypofibrinogenemia.

Prothrombin time, activated partial thromboplastin and platelet count reflect the consumption and activation of thrombocytes and clotting factors. The PT and its derived measure, the international normalised ratio (INR), are tests for factors II, V, VII and X and fibrinogen. Activated partial thromboplastin time is considered a good screening test for deficiencies of VIII, IX, XI and XII.

Management of DIC

The main goal of the treatment in DIC is to correct the underlying obstetrical cause. Supportive treatment should be implemented to correct the coagulation disorder.

- Delivery should be expedited, and the underlying cause should be corrected. Prolonging the exposure to the triggering factors will worsen DIC.
- Blood and blood products should be replaced based on the clinical presentation and the laboratory results.
  - Whole fresh blood may be the treatment of choice in coagulation failure associated with obstetric disorders. Stored blood is devoid of clotting factors and if used, it is advisable to transfuse 2 units of FFP for every 4–6 units of red cells administered.
  - Fresh frozen plasma (FFP) contains all the coagulation factors present in plasma. It is obtained from whole blood within 6 hours of donation, frozen rapidly and stored at −300°C. Clotting factors are well-preserved for at least one year. Fresh frozen plasma is a rich source of fibrinogen and is administered at a dose of 10–20 mL/Kg. However, caution must be exercised not to overtreat with fibrinogen in the presence of active DIC.
  - Although cryoprecipitate is richer in fibrinogen than FFP, it lacks antithrombin (AT) which is rapidly consumed in obstetric bleeding associated with DIC.
  - Platelet suspensions are administered to patients with platelet counts less than 50×109/L and who are actively bleeding. Blood group matching (ABO, RhD) is typically recommended before platelets are given. One unit of platelet transfusion increases the platelet count by 10,000 cells.

Pharmacological treatment

The use of pharmacological agents inhibiting the coagulation and fibrinolytic systems in disseminated intravascular coagulation is still controversial. Heparin will theoretically inhibit intravascular coagulation and subsequent fibrinolysis through the inhibition of the thrombin activity. It is especially recommended in DIC cases associated with thrombosis without bleeding. Tranexamic acid and ß-aminocaproic acid are in general contraindicated in DIC. There may be a place for recombinant factor VII. These medications may be effective when there is life-threatening bleeding.

▍ THROMBOEMBOLISM IN PREGNANCY

Women are at an increased risk of both venous and arterial thromboembolism during pregnancy. Thromboembolic events during pregnancy (discussed in detail in Chapter 49, *Puerperal infection and other postpartum complications*) occur in approximately 2 per 1,000 deliveries. Compared to women who are not pregnant, the risk of arterial thromboembolism (strokes and heart attacks) is increased three- to four-fold and the risk of venous thromboembolism (VTE) is increased four- to five-fold in pregnant women. The risk is 20-fold higher in the postpartum period. Approximately 80% of these events are venous and 20% are arterial (stroke and myocardial infarction). Approximately 80% of venous thromboembolic events during pregnancy are deep vein thrombosis (DVT) and 20% are pulmonary emboli. The majority of them occur in the postpartum period. When DVT occurs during pregnancy, it is more likely to be proximal, massive and in the left lower extremity. An increased risk of venous thromboembolism is seen in pregnant women and is due to:

- The hypercoagulable state of pregnancy due to increased clotting factors and decreased fibrinolytic activity
- Mechanical obstruction caused by the enlarged uterus on the venous system, which results in venous stasis
- Increased risk of trauma to the pelvic veins during delivery

Other conditions that could increase the risk of thromboembolism are as follows:

- Medical disorders such as hypertension, diabetes, heart disease and obesity
- Multiple gestation
- Acquired and congenital thrombophilia—Screening for inherited and acquired thrombophilia is recommended in women with a personal or strong family history of VTE, within or outside pregnancy
  - Thromboembolism is treated with unfractionated heparin/LMWH. Warfarin is rarely recommended

for use in pregnancy (exceptions include women with prosthetic heart valves) as it crosses the placenta and is teratogenic in the first trimester. Also, there is an increased risk of fetal intracerebral hemorrhage when warfarin is used in the third trimester.

— For postpartum contraception, estrogen-containing contraceptives should be avoided as they increase the risk of thromboembolism. Progestin-only contraceptives have not been found to increase the risk of thrombosis and hence can be recommended.

KEY POINTS

✓ *Physiological changes that occur during pregnancy affect the coagulation process. There is increased concentration of all coagulation factors and fibrinogen and a decrease in fibrinolytic activity.*

✓ *Coagulation disorders encountered in pregnancy are DIC and thromboembolic manifestations.*

✓ *The causes of DIC include abruptio placentae, severe pre-eclampsia, intrauterine fetal death, septic abortion, chorioamnionitis and amniotic fluid embolism.*

✓ *Clinical manifestations of DIC are ecchymosis, petechia, mucosal oozing, prolonged bleeding at vein puncture sites and surgical incision sites and heavy vaginal bleeding.*

✓ *In all patients who manifest with DIC or a risk of DIC, a coagulation profile should be undertaken without delay.*

✓ *In the management of DIC, delivery should be expedited, and the underlying cause should be corrected. Prolonging exposure to the triggering factors will worsen DIC. The required blood and blood products should be transfused without delay.*

✓ *Early recognition and prompt management can decrease maternal morbidity due to this disorder.*

Essay question

1. Discuss the pathophysiology, causes, diagnosis and management of disseminated intravascular coagulation in pregnancy.

Short answer question

1. Write a short note on thromboembolism in pregnancy.

MCQs

1. Which of these changes is not noted in pregnancy?
   a) Increased factors II, V, VII, VIII
   b) Increased fibrinogen
   c) Increased platelets
   d) Decreased fibrinolytic activity

2. Which of the following conditions is not associated with a coagulation disorder?
   a) Eclampsia
   b) Intrauterine fetal death
   c) Abruption
   d) Gestational diabetes

3. What is the most common obstetric cause of coagulation disorder?
   a) Abruption
   b) Amniotic fluid embolism
   c) Intrauterine fetal death
   d) Big baby

4. In amniotic fluid embolism, which factor is increased?
   a) Thromboplastin
   b) Fibrinogen
   c) Platelet
   d) Clotting factor

5. Changes that occur in the coagulation system during pregnancy include all EXCEPT:
   a) Decreased concentration of all clotting factors
   b) Decrease in fibrinolytic activity

c) Unchanged clotting and bleeding time
d) Increase in plasma fibrinogen level

6. Coagulation disorders may complicate all of the following conditions EXCEPT:
   a) Abruptio placentae
   b) Gestational diabetes mellitus
   c) Amniotic fluid embolism
   d) Septic abortion

Answers

1. (c), 2. (d), 3. (a), 4. (a), 5. (a), 6. (b)

Fill in the blanks

1. Platelets levels _____ during pregnancy.
2. Fibrinogen levels _____ during pregnancy.
3. Warfarin is rarely recommended for use in pregnancy except in women with _____.

Answers

1. decrease, 2. increase, 3. prosthetic heart valves

Case study-based discussion

1. A 32-year-old gravida 4, para 3 comes to the casualty with a history of 9 months of amenorrhea and painful bleeding per vaginum for the previous 4 hours and inability to feel fetal movements since then. On examination, she is pale, her pulse is 100/minute and BP is 90/70 mmHg. On abdominal examination, her uterus is 36 weeks in size, hard and tender; it is difficult to feel the fetal parts and the fetal heart is not heard. On vaginal examination, the cervix is 3 cm dilated, the membrane is absent, and the head is at the brim. There is bleeding per vaginum. The woman is started on crystalloids, and blood samples are taken for investigations. The intern notes bleeding from the puncture sites and reports it to the seniors.
   a) What is the condition we are dealing with?
   b) What investigations would you order?

c)   What are the other causes of DIC?
d)   How do you manage DIC?

Answers

a) The clinical findings are suggestive of abruptio placenta with possible DIC.

b) One should order coagulation tests (aPTT, PT, thrombin time [TT]), serum fibrinogen levels, D-dimer, hemoglobin and platelet count and analysis of blood smear for evidence of fragmented RBCs.

c) The other causes of DIC include severe pre-eclampsia, intrauterine fetal death, septic abortion, chorioamnionitis and amniotic fluid embolism.

d) The underlying obstetrical cause should be treated, and delivery should be expedited. Based on the clinical presentation and the laboratory results, blood and blood products such as FFP, cryoprecipitate and platelets should be replaced.

61

OG 10.2

Use of Blood and Blood Products in the Obstetric Practice

Learning Objectives

» To describe the indications for the use of blood and blood components in obstetrics
» To know the procedure of blood transfusion
» To discuss the monitoring of the transfused patient
» To know the complications of blood transfusion
» To know the management and reporting of adverse blood transfusion reaction

---

■ INTRODUCTION

In Africa and Asia, obstetric hemorrhage accounts for more than 30% of all maternal deaths. Blood transfusion has saved millions of mothers from death due to hemorrhage. Though blood transfusion is a life-saving measure, it is not without risks. Therefore, before ordering a blood transfusion, it is important to ensure that the benefits of transfusion outweigh the risks for the particular patient. It is also important to ensure that transfusion is given in a timely manner and in adequate amounts. Blood transfused too late or too little may not benefit the patient.

■ INDICATIONS FOR BLOOD TRANSFUSION

The clinical conditions that necessitate blood transfusion in obstetric practice are as follows:

- Severe anemia complicating pregnancy with hemoglobin <7 g
- Bleeding in early pregnancy due to miscarriages, ectopic pregnancy, molar pregnancy
- Bleeding in late pregnancy due to rupture of the uterus, abruption, placenta previa and abnormal placentation
- Bleeding after childbirth due to atonic and traumatic PPH, inversion of the uterus and retained placenta
- In HELLP syndrome, DIVC and idiopathic thrombocytopenic purpura (ITP)

■ BLOOD AND BLOOD COMPONENTS USED IN OBSTETRIC PRACTICE

The blood and blood products used in obstetric practice are as follows:

- Whole blood
- Packed red blood cells
- Fresh frozen plasma (FFP)
- Cryoprecipitate
- Platelet concentrate

Whole Blood Transfusion

Compatible whole blood is ideal for treating hypovolemia in acute hemorrhage. It increases hematocrit by 3–4% and also replaces coagulation factors, especially fibrinogen. It must be ABO- and RhD-compatible with the recipient.

Packed Cells

Packed cells are RBC concentrates derived from whole blood. The hematocrit of packed cells ranges from 65–80%. A single unit of packed cells increases the hematocrit level by 3–4%. Packed cells are useful in transfusing severely anemic patients in whom overload should be avoided.

Platelet Transfusion

Platelet transfusion would be indicated in ITP, HELLP syndrome and in DIVC. It is also indicated when the platelet count is <50,000 in an acutely bleeding patient. 6–10 units are generally transfused; one unit raises the platelet count by 10,000. When platelet transfusion is given, the following precautions should be taken:

- Preferably, a single-donor platelet transfusion should be given.
- It should be ABO-compatible.
- Rh-D negative women should receive Rh-D negative platelets.

- Occasionally, if the appropriate product is not available or would cause an unacceptable delay, it may be necessary to transfuse D-positive platelets. In these circumstances, prophylaxis against possible Rh-alloimmunisation with red cells contaminating the platelet product should be given. A dose of 300 µg of anti-D immunoglobulin should be sufficient to cover up to five adult therapeutic doses of D-positive platelets given within a 6-week period.

Fresh Frozen Plasma (FFP)

FFP is prepared by separating the plasma from the whole blood and freezing it. It contains stable clotting factors.

The indications for FFP are the following:
- When the fibrinogen concentration is <100 mg/dL
- When PT/aPTT are prolonged >1.5 times the normal
- In the event of massive transfusion, 4 units of FFP are given for every 6 units of red blood cells
- For the reversal of warfarin's effect

FFP is given in a dose of 12–15 mL/Kg. Before administration, FFP needs to be defrosted, which takes about 30 minutes. Subsequent use of FFP is guided by the PT/aPTT, which should be maintained at <1.5.

Cryoprecipitate

Cryoprecipitate is the precipitate obtained after centrifugation of FFP. It is an ideal source of fibrinogen and also contains factors VIII, IX and XIII and Vwf. Each unit contains 10–15 mL, which contains 150–250 mg of fibrinogen.

The indications for the use of cryoprecipitate are as follows:
- Fibrinogen <80–100 mg/dL
- Patient not responding to FFP
- In cases of massive obstetric hemorrhage, a standard dosage of 2–5 pools of cryoprecipitate is given in the early stages

FFP and cryoprecipitate, when administered, should be of the same group as that of the recipient. RhD-positive plasma products may be given to RhD-negative recipients. No anti-D prophylaxis is required if an Rh-negative woman receives RhD-positive FFP or cryoprecipitate. If the patient needs both FFP and platelets, the platelets should be given first, followed by FFP.

COLLECTION OF BLOOD FOR GROUPING AND CROSS-MATCHING

- A minimum of 3 mL of fresh clotted blood and an EDTA blood sample are required for grouping and cross-matching.

- After every third unit of blood, a fresh sample should be collected for cross-matching.
- Grouping and Rh typing should always be performed in the respective hospital's blood bank even if the patient's blood group and Rh type are known already.

BLOOD TRANSFUSION PROCEDURE

- There should be a clear indication for the blood transfusion.
- Consent for blood transfusion should be taken from the patient after explaining the indication.
- It should be ensured that the blood has been cross-matched and its compatibility checked. Before commencing transfusion, the blood bag and the patient details should be verified for accuracy (patient's name, age, hospital number, blood product, blood group and cross-matching details).
- Once the blood is released from the blood bank, it should be transfused within 15–30 minutes (delay will result in hemolysis).
- Once the blood is taken out of the blood bank, it cannot be returned to the blood bank under any circumstances.
- A new line with a wide-bore needle should be used for blood transfusion.
- No drug should be administered via the IV line through which blood is being transfused.
- There is no evidence to recommend the routine pre-transfusion of diuretics and steroids prophylactically as their use may mask minor reactions. However, if minor reactions do occur following blood transfusion, they can be used.
- Warming of blood is not required when the infusion is slow. However, blood should be warmed to prevent hypothermia in cases of massive blood transfusion wherein more than 6 units of blood are required. If necessary, blood should be warmed in a blood warmer. Blood should never be warmed in a bowl of hot water as doing so could lead to the hemolysis of the red blood cells and could be life-threatening.

In order to minimise the error of a wrong transfusion, as far as possible, vein-to-vein identity should be maintained (the person who draws the blood for cross-matching should be the person transfusing blood to the patient).

TIME FRAME FOR TRANSFUSION

It is important for blood and blood products to be transfused within a stipulated period of time (Table 61.1).

Table 61.1 The time frame for the infusion of blood products

Blood products	Starting infusion	Completing infusion
Whole blood/red cells	Within 30 minutes of removing the pack from the refrigerator	Within 4 hours or less in high temperature
Platelet concentrates	Immediately	Within 20 minutes
Fresh frozen plasma	As soon as thawing is complete (usually within 30 minutes)	Within 20 minutes
Cryoprecipitate	As soon as possible	Within 20 minutes

(Reproduced with permission from *The Clinical Use of Blood in General Medicine, Obstetrics, Pediatrics, Surgery and Anaesthesia, Trauma and Burns*, Geneva, World Trade Organization)

MONITORING THE TRANSFUSED WOMAN

A patient receiving blood transfusion should be closely monitored at the following stages:

- Before starting the transfusion, the patient's vitals should be checked, and the correct identity of the patient should be verified. It is also important to ensure the correct identify of the blood to be transfused. Emergency medications should be made available before starting the blood transfusion.
- After the transfusion is started, the patient should be monitored at the following stages:
  — 15 minutes after starting the transfusion
  — Every 15–30 minutes during transfusion
  — On completing the transfusion
  — Four hours after completing the transfusion
At each of these stages, the following information should be recorded in the patient's chart:
- General appearance
- Temperature
- Pulse
- Blood pressure
- Respiratory rate
- Urine output
- Fluid balance
  The following transfusion details should also be recorded:
- Time at which the transfusion was started

- Time at which the transfusion was completed
- Volume and type of all components transfused
- Unique numbers of all blood components transfused
- Any adverse reaction observed

The patient should be closely monitored during the first 15 minutes of the transfusion and regularly thereafter to detect early symptoms and signs of adverse effects.

ADVERSE REACTIONS TO BLOOD TRANSFUSION

- Blood transfusion reactions may range from minor skin reaction to anaphylactic reaction.
- The adverse symptoms include urticaria, rashes, chest pain, loin pain, headache, rigors, fever, restlessness, sweating, difficulty in breathing, vomiting, etc.
- The signs of adverse reactions include hypotension, tachycardia, hemoglobinuria and evidence of DIVC.

Management of Blood Transfusion Reaction

- When a transfusion reaction occurs, the transfusion should be stopped immediately and normal saline should be infused through another IV line.
- If a minor reaction is noted, it can be treated by administering an antihistamine such as chlorpheniramine by the intramuscular route.
- If a major anaphylactic reaction has occurred, shock is treated with appropriate measures.
- The airway is maintained, and high-flow oxygen is given by a mask. CPAP ventilation may also be required.
- Adrenaline (1:1,000 solution) 0.01 mg/Kg of body weight should be given by slow intramuscular injection.
- Hydrocortisone 4 mg/Kg (200–400 mg IV) should be considered.
- An H1-antihistamine, e.g., loratadine or cetirizine 10 mg per oral should be considered for itching or angioedema. Parenteral antihistamine may also be required.
- A diuretic such as frusemide 1 mg/Kg IV is given.
- A fresh urine specimen is checked visually for signs of hemoglobinuria.
- Renal, pulmonary and CVS functions should be monitored.
- Clotting failure should be looked for.

- The blood bank's medical officer should be informed of the incident and the superior or senior doctor attending the patient should be notified.
- In a case of hematuria/renal shut down a nephrologist's opinion should be sought for forced alkaline diuresis.
- An anesthetist's opinion should also be sought.
- The blood bag and the patient's identity should be checked for discrepancies.
- An immediate post-transfusion blood sample along with the blood bag and a urine sample should be sent to the blood bank for investigations for re-grouping and cross-matching and to look for evidence of hemolysis.
- If septic shock is suspected, blood samples should be sent for culture.

In all blood transfusion reactions, a hemovigilance notification should be sent to the blood bank.

MONITORING RESPONSE TO BLOOD TRANSFUSION

- Platelet count should be repeated after one hour and hemoglobin, after 48 hours of transfusion.
- Between two elective transfusions, there should be a gap of at least 48 hours.

BLOOD TRANSFUSION FOR MASSIVE BLOOD LOSS

Massive blood transfusion may be defined as the replacement of one blood volume (equivalent to 10 units of blood) in any 24-hour period or half of the blood volume (5 units of blood) in any 4-hour period in an adult. In the event of massive obstetric hemorrhage, the following blood and blood products should be ordered:

- Pre-warmed resuscitative fluids

- To enhance oxygen delivery to tissues, 4 units of packed cells should be transfused in 5–10 minutes
- During an emergency, for urgent use, the following blood can be used:
  — O group Rh-negative blood
  — Group-specific un-cross-matched blood
  — Fully matched blood
- Use of FFP
  — When PT and PTT are more than 1.5 times the control, 4 units of FFP should be transfused; if PT and PTT are not available, 4 units should be transfused after 1–1.5 litres of blood transfusion
- Use of cryoprecipitate
  — If bleeding is not corrected with FFP
  — If fibrinogen level is <100 mg/mL
- Use of platelets
  — If the platelet count is less than 50,000/mL, 6 units of platelets should be transfused
- Use of 10% injection calcium gluconate IV
  — 10 mL should be given for every litre of transfused blood

TRANSFUSION-RELATED COMPLICATIONS

The following complications can occur following blood transfusion:

- Risk of infection with HIV, syphilis, malaria, hepatitis B and C
- Anaphylaxis
- Fluid overload
- Septic shock
- Transfusion-associated acute lung injury (TRALI)
- Citrate toxicity
- Hypocalcemia, hyperkalemia
- Hypothermia

KEY POINTS

✓ *The blood and blood products used in obstetric practice are whole blood, packed red blood cells, fresh frozen plasma (FFP), cryoprecipitate and platelet concentrate.*

✓ *Patients receiving blood and blood products should be carefully monitored for blood transfusion reactions.*

✓ *In the event of a transfusion reaction, a hemovigilance notification should be sent to the blood bank and the respective authorities.*

Short answer questions

1. What are the indications for blood transfusion in obstetric practice?

2. What is a massive blood transfusion?
3. What are the indications for platelet transfusion?
4. What complications can occur following blood transfusion?

62 Prenatal Diagnosis

OG 8.8 and 20.3, AN 81.1, 81.2, 81.3, RD 1.13 and FM 3.21

Learning Objectives

» To know the indications for prenatal diagnosis
» To understand the various techniques used in prenatal diagnosis and their complications

■ INTRODUCTION

Prenatal diagnosis refers to the process of testing for diseases or conditions in a fetus in utero, before it is born. Diagnosing a problem in a fetus while in utero is important as it may enable timely medical and surgical interventions before or after birth in indicated cases. Also, in the event of a major birth defect or chromosomal abnormality, with timely identification and adequate counselling, parents may decide on the termination of pregnancy early or prepare physically, mentally and financially to care for such babies.

Prenatal testing includes screening tests and diagnostic tests. Screening tests are used to identify pregnancies that are at a high risk of a problem. If the test is screen-positive, diagnostic testing is offered to the pregnant woman to confirm or rule out a condition. Prenatal diagnostic procedures are used to identify the following conditions:

- Structural abnormalities such as congenital malformations
- Chromosomal abnormalities
- Genetic disorders
- Congenital infections

These procedures are also useful in planning therapeutic interventions.

■ STRUCTURAL ABNORMALITIES OF THE FETUS

Structural malformations may involve the internal or external parts of the fetus. With the widespread use of ultrasonography (USG), some anomalies such as anencephaly are identified in the first trimester itself and most others are identified in the second trimester during the targeted scan between 18 and 20 weeks of gestation. Anomalies such as cardiac anomalies may evolve later in the second trimester or in the third trimester. Therefore, repeat scanning is required in high-risk pregnancies. If an anomaly is identified, there should be a thorough search for anomalies involving other organs. Congenital anomalies may also be associated with chromosomal defects.

Craniofacial Abnormalities

Neural tube defects (NTD)

Between the 17th and 30th day after conception (or 4–6 weeks after the first day of the last menstrual period), the neural tube forms in the embryo and then closes. The neural tube later develops into the baby's spinal cord, spine, brain and skull. A neural tube defect (NTD) occurs when the neural tube fails to close properly, leaving the developing brain or spinal cord exposed to the amniotic fluid.

NTD include **anencephaly, encephalocele and spina bifida**. Women with diabetes, epilepsy and those on anticonvulsants are at a high risk of developing NTD. In these conditions, the alpha-fetoprotein levels are elevated and can be identified by testing the maternal serum at 16 weeks of gestation. With the advent of USG, anencephaly and encephalocele can be identified in the first trimester itself, whereas spina bifida is picked up during the anomaly scan at 18–20 weeks. In babies with encephalocele, there may be associated anomalies such as polycystic kidneys, polydactyly, cleft palate and congenital heart disease. This condition is diagnosed as **Meckel's syndrome**—an autosomal recessive condition with a 25% recurrence rate. In other types of NTD, the risk of recurrence is 5% with one affected child and 10% with two affected children. NTD can be prevented by starting tablet folic acid 0.4 mg/day before conception and continued through 12 weeks of pregnancy. In women who are epileptic and on anticonvulsant medications and those who have a previous history of NTD, the prophylactic dose should be 5 mg/day.

Anencephaly

In this condition, the cranial vault is absent, exposing the meninges. Along with the frontal, parietal and occipital bones, the cerebral hemispheres are absent.

The base of the skull, cerebellum and facial bones are unaffected. Such fetuses present with bulging eyes, a short neck and a large tongue (Fig. 62.1). Anencephaly is incompatible with life.

The condition can be diagnosed as early as 9–10 weeks by USG showing absent calvarium (Fig. 62.2) and a typical 'frog-eye' appearance (Fig. 62.3). If the condition goes undiagnosed and the pregnancy advances, problems such as postdated pregnancy, polyhydramnios and face presentation can occur. The pituitary and adrenal glands are observed to be small or atrophic in anencephaly.

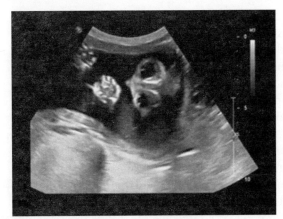

Fig. 62.3 'Frog-eye' appearance on USG

Encephalocele

It is the protrusion of the meninges and brain tissue through a bony defect in the cranial vault. Occipital meningomyelocele is the commonest type of encephalocele (Fig. 62.4 and 62.5).

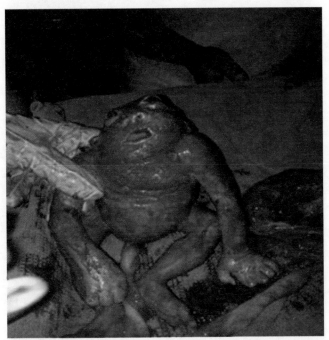

Fig. 62.1 An anencephalic fetus (*Source*: Dr Sravani Chithra, Assistant Professor, OBG, SMMCH & RI)

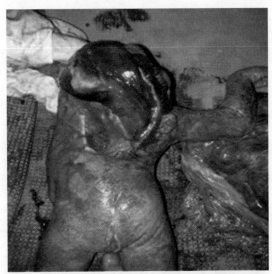

Fig. 62.4 Protrusion of the brain in the occipital region (*Source:* Dr Sravani Chithra, SMMCH & RI)

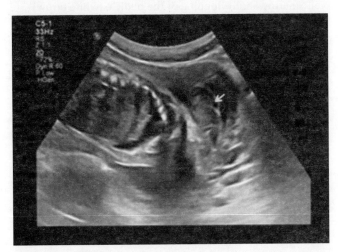

Fig. 62.2 Fetal brain with absent calvarium (yellow arrow) (*Source*: Dr Parameshwar Keerthi, Consultant Radiologist, BM Scans, Kancheepuram)

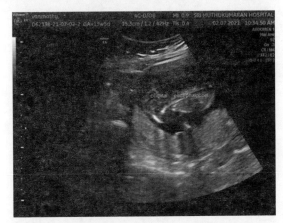

Fig. 62.5 Occipital encephalocele on USG (*Source*: Dr Parameshwar Keerthi, BM Scans, Kancheepuram)

Spina bifida

It is the non-closure of the spinal cord or a defect in the neural arch of the spine, which exposes the neural content. It is more common in the lumbosacral region. If only the meninges are exposed, the condition is called a meningocele; if the spinal cord is also prolapsed, it is called a meningomyelocele (Fig. 62.6, 62.7 and 62.8). Spina bifida is most often open.

In occult spina bifida, there is a defect in the bony arch but no protrusion of the neural content. It is identified by a dimple or a tuft of hair over the area. This form of spina bifida very rarely causes disabilities or symptoms and is often diagnosed only by accident on an X-ray. On USG, in a normal spine, in the transverse plane, two lateral processes and one midline vertical body of the spine can be seen. In spina bifida, the midline vertical body is absent, and the lateral processes are seen apart. There are also associated USG findings in the fetal brain.

In fetuses with open neural defects, there is a deformity in the frontal region of the brain and the anterior portion is elongated; this is called the 'lemon sign'. There is also flattening of the cerebellar surface, referred to as the 'banana sign'. Open neural defects are associated with elevated alpha-fetoprotein and acetylcholine esterase in the amniotic fluid.

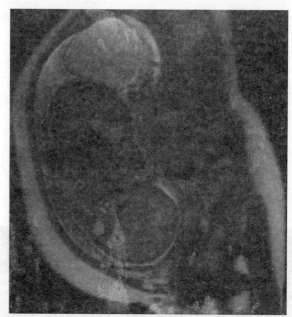

Fig. 62.7   Fetal MRI with T2 hyperintense myelomeningocele in the lumbosacral region (*Source:* Dr Parameshwar Keerthi, BM Scans, Kancheepuram)

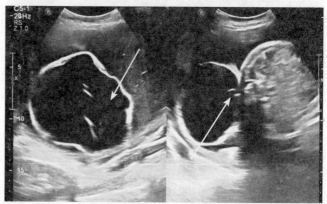

Fig. 62.8   Meningomyelocele in the lumbosacral region (yellow arrow) and widening of the pedicle (white arrow) (*Source:* Dr Parameshwar Keerthi, BM Scans, Kancheepuram)

Hydrocephalus

Hydrocephalus (Fig. 62.9 and 62.10) is the dilatation of the ventricular system of the brain. This may occur due to aqueductal stenosis, neural tube defects, infections such as CMV, rubella or toxoplasmosis or it may be associated with chromosomal abnormalities; hydrocephalus of unknown etiology may also develop. In hydrocephalus, the lateral ventricles are usually distended with fluid and the choroid plexus may be seen dangling in the CSF fluid.

If secondary to aqueductal stenosis, it may be X-inked with a 12% risk of recurrence in male infants. In other forms of hydrocephalus, the risk of recurrence is 2%. In Dandy–Walker syndrome, the fourth ventricle is distended with fluid.

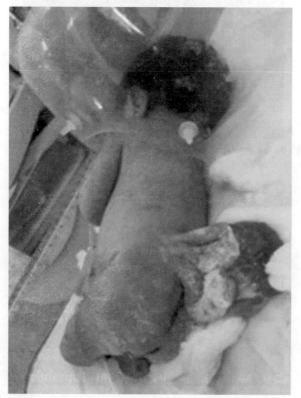

Fig. 62.6   Lumbosacral meningomyelocele (*Source:* Dr Parameshwar Keerthi, BM Scans, Kancheepuram)

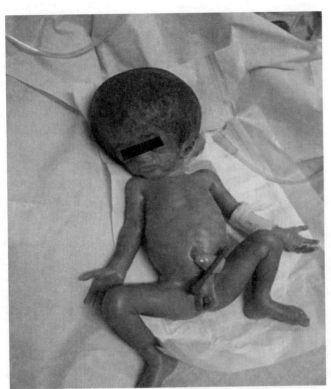

Fig. 62.9 Baby born with hydrocephalus (*Source:* Dr Sravani Chithra, SMMCH & RI)

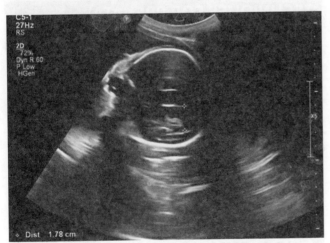

Fig. 62.10 USG image of dilated lateral ventricles in hydrocephalus (*Source:* Dr Parameshwar Keerthi, BM Scans, Kancheepuram)

Other craniofacial anomalies that are detected are microcephaly and cystic hygroma. In cystic hygroma, there is a fluid-filled space in the neck, usually associated with aneuploidy such as Turner's syndrome.

Cardiac Defects

Women suffering from diabetes and congenital heart disease are at an increased risk of having babies with cardiac defects. Cardiac anomalies account for nearly 10% of all fetal anomalies. Cardiac defects can also be associated with chromosomal anomalies such as trisomy 21. At the time of a targeted scan, cardiac evaluation is done using USG with a four-chamber view and visualising three vessels. Further evaluation with fetal echo is required in the third trimester of pregnancy if the mother has diabetes or an autoimmune disease or when there is a history of exposure to teratogens. IVF pregnancies, increased nuchal translucency and monochorionic twins are also indications for fetal echo. Commonly seen cardiac anomalies are ASD, VSD, Fallot's tetralogy and malposition of the great vessels.

Anterior Abdominal Wall Defects

Omphalocele

This condition is also known as exomphalos. It is a defect in the anterior abdominal wall in the midline. The defect is located at the base of the umbilical cord (Fig. 62.11). Through the defect, there is herniation of the abdominal contents. The herniated viscera are covered by the peritoneum and the amnion. When there is an isolated omphalocele, repair is possible with a good prognosis.

At 6 weeks of development, there is a rapid elongation of the gut, and the liver also increases in size; due to the reduced intra-abdominal space, the abdominal contents are pushed out of the abdominal cavity. Around the 10th week, the intestine returns to the abdominal cavity; the process is completed by the 12th week. The persistence of the intestine and other abdominal viscera (e.g., stomach, liver) in the umbilical cord results in an omphalocele.

Omphalocele occurs in 1 in 4,000 births and is associated with a high rate of mortality (25%) and severe malformations such as cardiac anomalies (50%), neural tube defect (40%) and exstrophy of the bladder. Associated chromosomal abnormalities are seen in 15% of live-born infants. 30% of live-born babies have other congenital abnormalities.

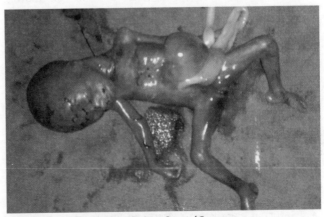

Fig. 62.11 Omphalocele in a fetus (*Source:* Dr Sravani Chithra, SMMCH & RI)

Gastroschisis

In gastroschisis, the umbilical cord is not involved, and the intestinal protrusion is usually to the right of the midline. There are free-floating loops of the bowel in the amniotic fluid without a covering membrane. Gastroschisis is less frequently associated with defects other than omphalocele. Exomphalos and gastroschisis need to be differentiated from each other and from other causes of an abdominal wall mass. Exomphalos is more centrally placed than gastroschisis, is covered with a membrane and is more likely to be associated with other congenital defects. In an omphalocele, the sac feels firm due to the presence of the liver and tightly packed bowel.

Gastrointestinal Defects

Common gastrointestinal defects are esophageal atresia and duodenal atresia.

Renal Tract Anomalies

Common renal tract abnormalities detected through prenatal diagnosis are polycystic kidneys, posterior urethral valves causing urinary tract obstruction and renal agenesis.

Skeletal Defects

Commonly encountered skeletal defects are talipes equinovarus, polydactyly, autoamputation of the limbs, multiple fractures and short limbs.

Hydrops Fetalis

Hydrops fetalis is an accumulation of fluid in the skin, scalp and in body cavities such as the pleural and pericardial cavities. The condition is often associated with polyhydramnios. Fetal hydrops can be classified into immune and non-immune types. Immune hydrops occurs in Rh-isoimmunisation due to circulating antibodies. Non-immune hydrops occurs due to various causes such as infections (CMV, toxoplasmosis), maternal diabetes, fetal conditions such as anemia, cardiac diseases and chromosomal abnormalities.

▌ INDICATIONS FOR PRENATAL TESTING

Prenatal screening and diagnostic tests are indicated in women who are at a high risk of having congenital anomalies and chromosomal aberrations. The indications include the following:

- Maternal age over 35 years
- History of congenital anomaly in a previous child
- History of chromosomal aberrations such as Down syndrome in the previous child
- History of consanguinity with previous pregnancy losses
- History of recurrent abortions
- Previous unexplained stillbirth/neonatal death
- Woman or partner a carrier of chromosomal inversion or translocation
- Family history of neural tube defects (NTD)
- Familial genetic disease
- Couples at risk of inborn errors of metabolism
- History of diabetes, epilepsy
- Exposure to certain drugs
- Exposure to environmental agents and infections
- Belonging to an ethnic group that is at high risk

Ethnic risk factors for genetic diseases
- South-East Asians: Thalassemia
- African/Afro-Caribbean: Sickle cell disease
- Jews: Tay–Sacks disease
- North European: Cystic fibrosis

TECHNIQUES FOR PRENATAL DIAGNOSIS

The techniques used for prenatal diagnosis include biochemical, non-invasive and invasive methods.

The Government of India, in the Prenatal, Preconception Diagnostic Tests (PCPNDT) Act, prohibits all tests performed with the intention of determining the sex of the unborn child. Before any prenatal diagnostic test is performed, it is imperative that the provisions of the Act are strictly followed.

▌ BIOCHEMICAL METHODS

Alpha-Fetoprotein (AFP)

It is the main **glycoprotein** in the fetus. Its concentration increases steadily in the fetal serum and amniotic fluid until week 13 and then decreases rapidly. AFP passes into the maternal circulation. **Maternal serum AFP (MSAFP)** screening is usually done between 15 and 20 weeks of gestation. The correct interpretation of AFP levels requires an accurate estimate of gestational age. Maternal serum values above 2.0 or 2.5 MOM (multiple of the median) are usually considered elevated. Women with abnormal levels of AFP are offered a targeted ultrasound and amniocentesis if indicated.

Conditions associated with abnormal maternal serum AFP levels

Elevated levels

- Open neural tube defects
- Esophageal or intestinal obstruction
- Cystic hygroma
- Gastroschisis and omphalocele
- Polycystic or absent kidneys
- Oligohydramnios
- Low-birth-weight babies
- Multiple pregnancy
- Underestimation of gestational age
- Abruptio placentae
- Rh-isoimmunisation and other conditions associated with fetal edema
- Fetal demise

Low levels

- Chromosomal trisomy such as trisomy 13, 18 and 21

DIAGNOSIS OF CHROMOSOMAL ABNORMALITIES

Prenatal screening tests are used for the diagnosis of aneuploidy, wherein the chromosomal number is abnormal (either more or less than normal).

- More number
  - Trisomy 21:   Down syndrome
  - Trisomy 18:   Edward syndrome
  - Trisomy 13:   Patau syndrome
  - XXY: Klinefelter syndrome
  - Triploidy: 69 chromosomes
- Less number
  - Monosomy: 45 XO

According to the Guidelines of the American College of Obstetricians and Gynecologists, all women should be offered aneuploidy screening before 20 weeks of gestation, regardless of maternal age.

Prenatal Diagnosis of Down Syndrome

Down syndrome is the most common aneuploidy. Here, there is an extra copy of chromosome 21. In >95% of cases, it occurs due to non-disjunction during meiosis, is sporadic and has a well-defined relationship to maternal age. The risk of trisomy increases with maternal age due to the ageing of oocytes (Table 62.1).

Table 62.1 Age-related risk of Down syndrome

Age in years	Frequency of risk
30	1 in 900
35	1 in 400
40	1 in 100
45	1 in 30

In <5% of cases, Down syndrome could be familial due to Robertsonian translocation or reciprocal translocation. In all affected babies, karyotyping should be carried out to know whether Down syndrome is due to non-disjunction or translocation. If karyotyping was not available for the affected baby, then parental chromosomal testing is mandatory to identify translocation.

Recurrence risk

The recurrence risk is 2–3% if Down syndrome is related to age-related non-disjunction. If it occurs due to translocation, the risk depends on the carrier status of the parents:

- If the parental chromosomes are normal, the recurrence risk is 1%
- If the mother is normal and the father is a carrier, the recurrence risk is 2–3%
- If the father is normal and mother is a carrier, the recurrence risk is 11%
- If both are carriers of balanced translocation, the recurrence rate is 100%

Morphological features of Down syndrome

Down syndrome is characterised by short stature, a flat face, wide epicanthic folds, slanting eyes, a flat nose, a small, open mouth, a protruding tongue with deep fissures, abnormal teeth and low-set, small ears that may be folded. Children with this chromosomal abnormality have a single palmar crease, short and stubby fingers with a fifth finger that curves inward (called clinodactyly) and extra-flexible joints; they also have a larger than normal space between the big and second toes (Sandal gap). These children also have cardiac and GI tract anomalies such as duodenal atresia, imperforate anus, and hearing defects and have low IQ and learning difficulties.

Aneuploidy screening

Screening for aneuploidy depends on finding soft markers on USG and on biochemical methods.

Ultrasound markers of Down syndrome

Only about 50% of fetuses with Down syndrome exhibit some markers on ultrasound, which may be non-specific. Therefore, USG cannot be used as a diagnostic test; i.e., if these soft markers are found on ultrasound, it may or may not indicate the need for further testing. If these findings are isolated and found in a young pregnant woman, further testing may not be required. However, if they are found in older women or in association with another anomaly or a positive biochemical marker, further testing is required.

Increased nuchal thickness

• Nuchal translucency >3.5 mm (between weeks 12 and 13) has been shown to predict Down syndrome (NT thickness is also increased in cardiac and renal anomalies and diaphragmatic hernia). NT is measured between 11 and 13+6 weeks of gestation. The detection rate for Down syndrome with NT is 75–80%.

Other markers suggesting Down syndrome in the first trimester are absent nasal bone, tricuspid regurgitation and increased impedance to flow in the ductus venosus (Table 62.2). USG markers of aneuploidy in the second trimester include ASD, VSD, exomphalos, duodenal atresia, echogenic bowel, choroid plexus cyst, echogenic focus in the heart, renal pyelectasis and shortening of the long bones.

Serum markers for Down syndrome (Tables 62.2, 62.3 and 62.4)

• **First trimester:** A double marker using pregnancy-associated plasma protein-A (PAPP-A) and free β-hCG is the most informative marker for Down syndrome. These two markers can detect 60–70% of cases of Down syndrome. PAPP-A is low and β-hCG is high in Down syndrome.

• **Second trimester (16–18 weeks):**
  — The triple screen uses the estimation of three hormones—MSAFP, hCG and unconjugated estriol (uE3)—to diagnose Down syndrome. In Down syndrome, hCG levels are high, while MSAFP and unconjugated estriol levels are low. The detection rate of this test is 65–70%.
  — Quadruple screen uses four serum markers—MSAFP, hCG, unconjugated estriol and inhibin-A (Table 62.3). In Down syndrome, MSAFP and unconjugated estriol levels are low and hCG and inhibin-A levels are high. The detection rate with this test is 80%.

Multiple marker screening

First-trimester combined test using nuchal translucency measurement as well as biochemical markers is an effective screening test for Down syndrome in the general population. It is performed between 11 and 13+6 weeks of gestation.

Table 62.2 Summary of screening and diagnostic tests for aneuploidy

Screening tests		
	First trimester	Second trimester
USG	Increased nuchal translucency	Increased nuchal fold thickness
	Absent nasal bone	Cardiac defects
		Duodenal atresia
Biochemical tests	Double marker test	Triple test
		Quadruple test

Diagnostic tests		
	Chorion villus sampling	Amniocentesis
		Cordocentesis

Table 62.3 Quadruple test—alterations in serum markers

Markers	AFP	uE3	hCG	Inhibin-A
NTD	↑	No change	No change	No change
Trisomy 21	Low	Low	↑	↑
Trisomy 18	Low	Low	↑	No change

First-trimester combined test with serum testing of beta-hCG and PAPP-A and USG measurement of NT can detect Down syndrome in 90–95% of cases.

Integrated tests

Integrated screening tests require the measurement of serum markers, with or without ultrasound in both first and second trimesters.

Full integrated test

This consists of ultrasound measurement of nuchal translucency at weeks 10–13, PAPP-A measured at weeks 10–13, and alpha-fetoprotein (AFP), unconjugated estriol (uE3), hCG and inhibin-A levels measured at weeks 15–18. The full integrated test has the highest detection rate for Down syndrome—>95%.

Serum integrated test

This test is the same as the full integrated test but without the ultrasound measurement of nuchal translucency. It may be used in areas where expertise in the measurement of nuchal translucency is not available. The serum integrated test also has the highest detection rates.

A disadvantage of integrated tests is that the patient has to wait until the second trimester to obtain her risk estimate. Sequential and contingent testing schemes have been developed to address this problem. In sequential testing, the first-trimester integrated test results are disclosed to the woman so that she can opt for invasive testing early if required. In the contingent test, following the first-trimester screening, those who are at low risk are reassured, those at high risk are offered invasive procedures and those in the intermediate risk group are counselled about invasive testing/second-trimester serum screening. The screening test results are reported as high-risk and low-risk; if the cut-off is 1 in 250 and above, it is considered screen-positive and necessitates further investigations to confirm or rule out trisomy.

Non-invasive prenatal testing in maternal blood (NIPT)

This test entails the isolation of fetal cells from maternal circulation. Pregnant women have been found to have a small number of fetal cells in their circulation. It is possible to isolate these cells by using a cell-sorting technique. This technique uses cell surface proteins to distinguish fetal from maternal cells. Isolated fetal cells may be evaluated for fetal red cell D antigen type, karyotype and some genetic diseases.

Table 62.4 Detection rates of various screening tests for aneuploidy

Screening test	Components	Gestational age	Detection rate
Double marker test	Free β-hCG and PAPP-A	10–13+6 weeks CRL: 33–84 mm (Cannot be done in multiple pregnancy)	60%
Nuchal scan	Nuchal translucency (NT)	CRL: 45–84 mm (Cost-effective)	75–80%
Combined screening test	NT, free β-hCG, PAPP-A	CRL: 45–84 mm	90%
Triple screening test	AFB, β-hCG, uE3	BPD: 32–52 mm	65–70%
Quadruple screening test	AFB, β-hCG, uE3, DIA	BPD: 32–52 mm	80%
Integrated test	Combined screening test in the first trimester and quadruple test in the second trimester	First and second trimesters	94%
NIPT	Cell-free fetal DNA from maternal blood	9–18 weeks	99%

Other non-invasive prenatal diagnostic tests:
- USG—3D, 4D
- Fetal MRI, echo

■ INVASIVE TECHNIQUES

In order to diagnose and confirm chromosomal abnormalities, genetic disorders single gene defects, infections (CMV, rubella, toxoplasmosis), amniotic fluid/blood samples are collected for karyotyping, biochemical investigations and tests for infections. In order to obtain samples, the following techniques are used:
- Amniocentesis
- Chorion villus sampling (CVS)
- Cordocentesis
- Fetoscopy

Amniocentesis

This is a technique for withdrawing amniotic fluid from the uterine cavity using a needle. Amniocentesis is the most commonly used invasive technique for prenatal diagnosis.

Procedure

The procedure is carried out under **ultrasound guidance** at 15–20 weeks. Amniocentesis should not be performed before 14 weeks of gestation because the procedure is difficult and is associated with a higher incidence of complications like membrane rupture, foot deformities and fetal loss. It is also associated with more cell culture failures.

A 20–22-gauge needle is introduced into the amniotic sac while avoiding the fetus, the placenta and the umbilical cord (Fig. 62.12). About 20 mL of amniotic fluid is withdrawn and used for genetic analysis.

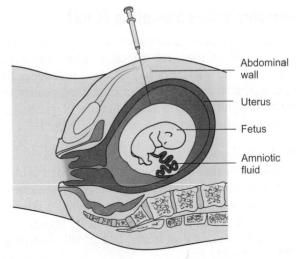

Fig. 62.12 Amniocentesis

Amniotic fluid contains desquamated fetal cells that can be:

- Cultured and karyotyped for the detection of aneuploidies (Fig. 62.13)
- Used for a variety of metabolic assays (for the detection of congenital adrenal hyperplasia [CAH], Tay–Sachs disease and Gaucher's disease)
- Used for DNA extraction (for the detection of cystic fibrosis, fragile X syndrome) and fluorescence in situ hybridisation (FISH) test
- Used to measure amniotic fluid—AFP to detect neural tube defects, duodenal atresia, omphalocele (exomphalos)

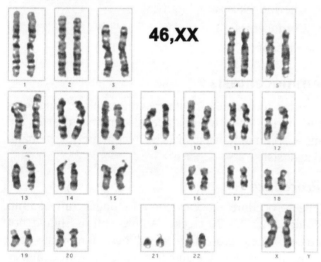

Fig. 62.13 Normal female karyotype

Complications of amniocentesis

- Vaginal spotting and amniotic fluid leakage
- Fetal loss: 0.5%
- Failed procedure: 1.0%
- Culture failure: <0.5%

Chorionic Villus Sampling (CVS)

CVS is a prenatal diagnostic technique that can be performed in the first trimester. It is performed between 10 and 13 weeks of gestation. It reduces the psychological stress of waiting until mid-pregnancy for a diagnosis and allows a safer method of pregnancy termination, should an abnormality be detected.

Techniques

1. **Transcervical:** The procedure is performed using a 1.5 mm diameter catheter (Fig. 62.14). The catheter is introduced under ultrasonographic guidance. Chorionic villi are aspirated with a syringe. An adequate sample is at least 5 mg of villi, but 10 to 25 mg is preferred.

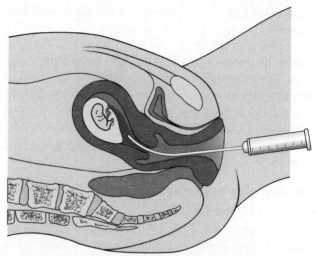

Fig. 62.14 Transcervical chorionic villus sampling

2. **Transabdominal:** This approach is advantageous when the placenta is located on the anterior uterine wall, near the fundus (Fig. 62.15).

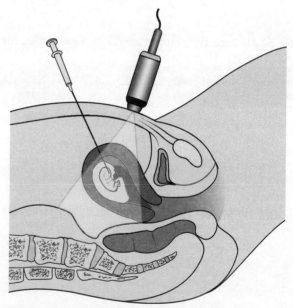

Fig. 62.15 Transabdominal chorionic villus

CVS is an alternative to mid-trimester genetic amniocentesis.

Complications of CVS

- Fetal loss of about 1%
- CVS at early gestation (<10 weeks) carries the risk of limb reduction defects
- Unsuccessful CVS in 1–5% (depends on operator experience and accessibility of placenta)
- Risk of placental mosaicism in 1–2% of cases
- Culture failure in 1–2%

Fetal Blood Sampling/Percutaneous Umbilical Blood Sampling (PUBS)

This technique, also known as **cordocentesis**, is used routinely after week 18 to evaluate fetuses with severe growth restriction, congenital infection, unexplained oligohydramnios, thrombocytopenia, hydrops and certain genetic diseases. Presently, it is most commonly used in the evaluation and management of fetal isoimmunisation.

Procedure

Blood is obtained from the umbilical vein under ultrasound guidance (Fig. 62.16) by puncturing it near the placental end. The procedure is indicated when fetal blood is needed for metabolic, hematological or immunological studies, acid–base analysis or viral cultures. It is also indicated for genetic analysis when the results of CVS and amniocentesis are equivocal and rapid diagnosis is necessary. Karyotyping of fetal blood can usually be done within 24–48 hours.

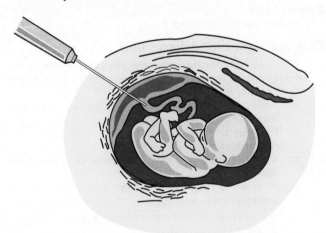

Fig. 62.16 Percutaneous umbilical blood sampling

Complications of PUBS

* Cord hematoma
* Transient fetal bradycardia
* Fetomaternal hemorrhage
* Fetal loss rate of <2%

Fetal Tissue Biopsy

Fetal tissue is obtained by ultrasound-guided skin or muscle biopsy. This has been used to identify fetuses with muscular dystrophy and epidermolysis bullosa.

■ UPCOMING TECHNIQUES

Pre-implantation Diagnosis

As the name suggests, this technique involves an **analysis of the embryo** before it is implanted. This may comprise **polar body analysis** or **blastomere biopsy**. It may be used to diagnose single gene disorders, sex determination in X-linked diseases and the identification of aneuploidy. This technique has the advantage that only healthy embryos can be allowed to be implanted, reducing the incidence of pregnancy termination.

■ FETAL THERAPY

Prenatal diagnostic techniques are also used for fetal therapy such as intrauterine fetal transfusion, management of acardiac twins and ablation of the posterior urethral valve. Medications such as antiarrhythmic drugs for fetal supraventricular tachycardia can also be administered.

KEY POINTS

✓ *Prenatal diagnosis is the detection of abnormalities in the fetus in utero.*

✓ *The methods of prenatal diagnosis include biochemical tests like the estimation of maternal serum AFP, β-hCG, PAPP-A and inhibin, non-invasive tests like ultrasound and invasive tests like amniocentesis, chorionic villus sampling, percutaneous umbilical blood sampling and fetal tissue biopsies.*

✓ *Pre-implantation diagnosis and evaluation of fetal cells from maternal circulation are the upcoming prenatal diagnostic techniques.*

Essay questions

1. What are the indications for prenatal screening and diagnostic tests?
2. Discuss the prenatal screening and diagnostic tests for Down syndrome.

Short answer questions

Write short notes on:
1. Alpha-fetoprotein
2. Amniocentesis
3. Chorionic villus sampling
4. Percutaneous umbilical blood sampling

MCQs

1. Which anomaly can be detected in the first trimester of pregnancy with USG?
   a) Microcephaly
   b) Anencephaly
   c) Meningocele
   d) Hydrocephalus

2. Maternal serum alpha-fetoprotein levels are raised in all except:
   a) Open spina bifida
   b) Omphalocele
   c) Cystic hygroma
   d) Down syndrome

3. At what gestational age is maternal serum AFP screening done?
   a) 5–10 weeks
   b) 11–15 weeks
   c) 16–20 weeks
   d) 21–25 weeks

4. All the following are associated with elevated levels of AFP except:
   a) Chromosomal trisomies
   b) Neural tube defects
   c) Esophageal atresia
   d) Omphalocele

5. Ultrasound markers for trisomies include all except:
   a) Thickened nuchal fold
   b) Echogenic bowel
   c) Hypoechoic long bones
   d) Choroid plexus cyst

6. Chorionic villus sampling is usually performed at:
   a) 6–8 weeks
   b) 8–10 weeks
   c) 10–13 weeks
   d) >14 weeks

7. Amniocentesis is carried out at:
   a) 15–20 weeks
   b) 10–12 weeks
   c) <10 weeks
   d) 14–16 weeks

8. Maternal serum alpha-fetoprotein levels are increased at 18 weeks in all the following conditions except:
   a) Down syndrome
   b) Multiple pregnancy
   c) Neural tube defects
   d) Gastroschisis

9. The most common presentation in anencephaly is:
   a) Brow
   b) Face
   c) Vertex
   d) Breech

10. The risk factors for anencephaly include the following except:
    a) Family history of NTD
    b) Previous history of NTD
    c) Antiepileptic drugs
    d) Pre-eclampsia

11. All the following biochemical markers are included in the triple test except:
    a) Human chorionic gonadotrophin
    b) Alpha-fetoprotein
    c) Acetylcholine esterase
    d) Unconjugated estriol

12. A 35-year-old gravida 2, para 1 with a previous history of delivering a baby with Down syndrome presents at 18 weeks of gestation. Which is the best investigation modality to diagnose Down syndrome in this case?
    a) Quadruple screening test
    b) Chorionic villus sampling
    c) Amniocentesis
    d) USG

Answers
1. (b), 2. (d), 3. (c), 4. (a), 5. (c), 6. (c), 7. (a), 8. (a), 9. (b), 10. (d), 11. (c), 12. (c)

Fill in the blanks

1. Pre-implantation genetic diagnosis is done by _____ or _____.

2. Nuchal translucency thickness as a screening test for Down syndrome is carried out at _____ weeks of gestation.

Answers
1. polar body analysis, blastomere biopsy,   2. 11–13+6

Case scenario-based discussion

1. A 30-year-old primigravida presents at 8 weeks of gestation for routine antenatal care. There is no significant medical or family history.
   a) Would you advise screening tests to this woman to diagnose Down syndrome?
   b) What are the screening tests that can be used in the first trimester?
   c) At what period of gestation will you carry out these investigations?
   d) What is the diagnosis if the first-trimester screening was reported as follows:
      • Increased NT for the gestational period
      • Nasal bone not visualised
      • PAPP-A is low and β-hCG is elevated

Answers
a) All women should undergo some screening to diagnose Down syndrome. At the age of 30, the risk of having a baby with Down syndrome is 1 in 900. Therefore, screening tests should be carried out.
b) The screening tests used in the first trimester are USG to look for increased nuchal translucency and biochemical tests using PAPP-A and serum β-hCG.
c) The best time to carry out the screening tests in the first trimester is between 11 and 13+6 weeks of gestation.
d) This woman is at a high risk of having a Down syndrome baby. Therefore, a definite diagnostic test should be carried out by CVS at 10–13 weeks, and chorionic tissue should be sent for karyotyping. The woman can also be offered non-invasive prenatal testing on maternal blood between 9 and 18 weeks.

63

Medical Termination of Pregnancy

Learning Objectives

» To describe the MTP act and its amendments
» To discuss the Preconception and Prenatal Diagnostic Techniques (PC & PNDT) Act, 1994, and its amendments
» To list out the indications for MTP
» To describe the pre-requisites for MTP
» To describe the various methods of first- and second-trimester termination of pregnancy
» To list out the complications of MTP

INTRODUCTION

Unsafe abortion has been recognised as one of the most significant causes of maternal mortality and morbidity in developing countries and is the third most common cause of maternal mortality in India. By preventing unsafe abortions, maternal mortality can be reduced significantly. In many countries, rigid laws regarding the induction of abortion have been liberalised to reduce maternal mortality resulting from illegal abortions.

THE MEDICAL TERMINATION OF PREGNANCY ACT (MTP ACT)

The Medical Termination of Pregnancy (MTP) Act, 1971, provides the legal background for making comprehensive abortion care services available in India. The MTP Act protects providers and empowers them with a tool to ensure that women do not approach unqualified providers for abortion services and put their health at risk.

This Act was passed by the Indian Parliament in 1971 and came into force on 1 April 1972 (except in Jammu and Kashmir, where it came into effect on 1 November 1976). The Act was further amended in December 2002 and the Rules, in June 2003. Under this Act, the termination of pregnancy can be performed up to 20 weeks of gestation. The revised Medical Termination of Pregnancy (Amendment) Bill, 2020 was introduced in Lok Sabha on 2 March 2020 and passed on 17 March 2020. This was officially notified in the Gazette of India as the Medical Termination of Pregnancy (Amendment) Act, 2021 ('Amendment Act'). This amendment increased the upper limit for the termination of pregnancy from 20 to 24 weeks for certain categories of women.

The Medical Termination of Pregnancy Act lays down the following guidelines:

- The conditions under which a pregnancy can be terminated
- The person or persons who can perform such terminations
- The place where such terminations can be performed
- Until what gestational age the pregnancy can be terminated

Conditions Under Which a Pregnancy Can Be Terminated

- **Medical:** Where continuation of pregnancy might endanger the mother's life or cause grave injury to her physical or mental health
- **Eugenic:** Where there is a substantial risk of the child being born with serious handicaps due to physical or mental abnormalities
- **Humanitarian:** Where the pregnancy is a result of rape
- **Failure of contraceptive devices:** Where the pregnancy resulted from a failure of a contraceptive method used by the woman or her partner

Persons Who Can Provide an Abortion

- In the case of a medical practitioner who was registered before the commencement of the MTP Act—should have experience in the practice of gynecology and obstetrics for a period not less than three years
- In the case of a medical practitioner who was registered after the commencement of the Act
  - Should have completed six months of house surgery in gynecology and obstetrics or

— Should have experience at any hospital for a period of not less than one year in the practice of obstetrics and gynecology or

— Should hold a postgraduate degree or diploma in gynecology and obstetrics or

— Should have assisted a Registered Medical Practitioner (RMP) in the performance of 25 cases of MTP, of which at least five have been performed independently in a hospital established or maintained by the government or a training institute approved for this purpose by the government

Where MTP Can Be Performed

A pregnancy can be legally terminated at one of the following two types of sites:

• Hospital established or maintained by the government
• Private site approved by the government or a district level committee constituted by the government for this purpose

Up to What Gestational Age Pregnancy Can Be Terminated

The MTP Act, 1971, allows termination of pregnancy only up to 20 weeks of gestation. In the revised Medical Termination of Pregnancy (Amendment) Act, 2021, the upper limit for termination was increased from 20 to 24 weeks for certain categories of women.

If the gestation is less than 12 weeks, a single medical practitioner can make the decision to terminate a pregnancy. However, where the pregnancy exceeds 12 weeks but is under 20 weeks, the opinion of two registered practitioners is required for the termination of pregnancy.

According to the Medical Termination of Pregnancy (Amendment) Act, 2021, the requirement of the opinion of one registered medical practitioner (instead of two or more) is enough for the termination of pregnancy up to 20 weeks of gestation. However, the opinion of two registered medical practitioners is required for the termination of pregnancy at 20–24 weeks of gestation. This extension allows the termination of pregnancy in cases where some anomaly in the fetus is reported after 20 weeks.

THE PRECONCEPTION AND PRENATAL DIAGNOSTIC TECHNIQUES (PCPNDT) ACT

The Preconception and Prenatal Diagnostic Techniques (Regulation and Prevention of Misuse) Amendment Act, 2002, prohibits sex selection before or after conception and regulates prenatal diagnostic techniques to prevent their misuse for sex determination leading to female feticide. Under this Act, sex determination tests and disclosure of the sex of the fetus are strictly prohibited. Hence, abortion solely for the purpose of sex selection constitutes an offence under this Act.

PREREQUISITES FOR TERMINATION OF PREGNANCY

When a pregnant woman approaches a doctor requesting an abortion, a decision regarding the termination of pregnancy can be taken only after counselling, clinical examination and the basic necessary investigations.

Pre-abortion Counselling

Pre-abortion counselling is essential for the following reasons:

1. It helps the woman to decide on a method of termination of pregnancy.
2. It ensures that the woman has consented to the procedure after receiving all the information about the procedure and the post-abortal complications.
3. It helps women to adopt a contraceptive method after abortion.
4. Some women may choose to continue with the pregnancy following counselling.

Whose Consent is Required for the Termination of Pregnancy

As per the provisions of the MTP Act, only the consent of the woman whose pregnancy is being terminated is required. However, in the case of a minor (below the age of 18 years) or a mentally ill woman, the consent of a guardian (the MTP Act defines a guardian as someone who is responsible for the care of the minor) is required for termination. The MTP Rules, 2003, prescribe that consent needs to be documented on Form C.

Mandatory Documentation for MTP Procedures Under The MTP Act

1. **Form C (consent form):** To be signed by the woman herself/her guardian
2. **Form I (opinion form):** To be certified by the RMP within three hours of the termination of pregnancy
3. **Form II:** To be sent by the head of the hospital or the owner of the establishment with a monthly statement of cases to the CMO of the district

4. **Form III (admission register):** An approved site will maintain case records in Form III

> This MTP register is maintained for a period of five years from the date of the last entry. It should be kept in safe custody and should not be opened for inspection by any person except under the authority of law.

The Amendment Act, 2021, also introduces a **new privacy clause** whereby registered medical practitioners are prohibited from revealing the name and other particulars of the woman whose pregnancy has been terminated except to authorised persons under any law.

Clinical Assessment

Clinical assessment for eligibility to undergo MTP is critical to avoid any complications. It also helps to identify women with complications who may have to be referred to higher centres for MTP or who may require additional care.

1. A detailed history regarding the following should be taken
   a. Menstrual history—LMP is important for gestational dating
   b. Obstetric history
   c. Previous history of MTP and the method used
   d. Prior attempts to terminate the current pregnancy
   e. Medical disorders
2. A detailed physical examination
   a. General examination is necessary to check for anemia, icterus, pulse and blood pressure
   b. Systemic examination should be performed to rule out cardiovascular and respiratory problems
   c. Bimanual pelvic examination usually gives a rough estimate of the gestational age
   d. Rule out pelvic infection and other abnormalities of the genital tract

Investigations

The fitness of the pregnant woman to undergo the procedure must be assessed by a few investigations. These include the following:

1. **Hemoglobin (Hb) estimation:** Anemia is quite prevalent among women in India. Hence, Hb estimation is mandatory before performing an abortion. MTP performed on an anemic woman will increase morbidity.
2. **Urine examination:** Urine is examined for the presence of albumin and sugar.
3. **Blood group and Rh typing:** MTP performed on an Rh-positive woman will not pose any problems, but in an Rh-negative mother, it may result in isoimmunisation, which will interfere with the outcome of a subsequent pregnancy. If the woman is Rh-negative, the administration of anti-D will reduce the risk of isoimmunisation.
4. **USG:** This is not mandatory if the woman has regular cycles and if the uterine size corresponds to the period of amenorrhea. However, ultrasound may be performed for dating a pregnancy in a woman with irregular cycles, in a woman who has conceived during lactational amenorrhea or when there is a clinical discrepancy between the dates and the size of the uterus to exclude ectopic gestation.

Medications

- All Rh-negative women undergoing MTP should be given 50 µg anti-D immunoglobulin if the gestational age is <12 weeks and 300 µg if the gestational age is >12 weeks.
- Antibiotic prophylaxis is not required for women undergoing a medical method of termination. In those undergoing surgery, in order to prevent post-abortal endometritis, injection ceftriaxone 1 g is given intravenously one hour prior to the procedure.

■ METHODS OF MTP

First-trimester methods
- Medical methods—Mifepristone+misoprostol
- Manual vacuum aspiration
- Suction evacuation
- Dilatation and curettage
- Menstrual regulation

Second-trimester methods
- Medical method—Mifepristone+misoprostol
- Extra-amniotic instillations
- Intra-amniotic instillations—these are not used anymore as a routine procedure
- Surgical method—hysterotomy

First-Trimester Termination of Pregnancy

1. Medical methods of terminating pregnancy

The medical method of abortion (MMA) is a non-invasive method of terminating pregnancy using drugs. Presently, the DCGI approves the use of RU-486 (mifepristone—an anti-progesterone) with misoprostol (prostaglandin E1) only up to 9 weeks or 63 days of amenorrhea. The termination of pregnancy with mifepristone (RU-486) followed by a synthetic prostaglandin E1 analogue (misoprostol) is an established and safe method for terminating early pregnancy. This combination has a success rate of 95–99% for pregnancies up to seven weeks.

Mechanism of action

RU-486 is a derivative of norethindrone with anti-progestin action. It binds to progesterone receptors at the endometrium and decidua, resulting in necrosis and detachment of the placenta. It also softens the cervix and causes mild uterine contractions. Mifepristone sensitises the uterus to the action of prostaglandin, which is given 1–2 days later. Misoprostol binds to myometrial cells, causing strong myometrial contractions and cervical softening and dilatation. This leads to the expulsion of the fetus from the uterus.

Pre-abortion counselling for medical methods of termination

Women who are given these medications must be willing to come to the hospital for a minimum of three visits and should have easy access to a healthcare facility. The abortion may be incomplete in 2–3% of women, necessitating a surgical procedure. Vaginal bleeding usually occurs for 8–13 days during the whole process and is similar to heavy menstrual bleeding. However, the amount and duration of bleeding differ from woman to woman.

Regimen of medical abortion

* Up to 49 days
    — Day 1: Mifepristone 200 mg orally; inj. anti-D to Rh-negative women
    — Day 3: Misoprostol 400 µg vaginally or orally
    — Day 14: Follow-up visit to assess completion of abortion
* From 49–63 days
    — Day 1: Mifepristone 200 mg orally; inj. anti-D to Rh-negative women
    — Day 3: Misoprostol 400 µg/800 µg vaginally or orally; the woman is observed for 4 hours in the hospital, during which time, expulsion may take place; after discharge from the hospital, if the woman has heavy bleeding at any time, she should be asked to return to the hospital immediately as surgical evacuation may be required in such cases
    — Day 14: Follow-up visit to assess completion of abortion by USG

Medical methods of abortion have been proven to be safe and effective. The reported success rate is >95%.

Side effects of medications

Side effects include nausea, vomiting, diarrhea, headache and uterine cramps.

Contraindications

The use of these drugs for abortion is contraindicated in anemic women (Hb <8 g%), those on long-term steroids (due to chronic adrenal suppression), those with cardiovascular and renal diseases or any seizure disorder and in those with uncontrolled hypertension.

2. Menstrual regulation/aspiration

Aspiration of the endometrial cavity using a flexible 5–6 mm Karman cannula and syringe within 6 weeks of amenorrhea is referred to as menstrual regulation (MR). Though this was one of the popular methods of terminating pregnancy in the past, this procedure is no longer preferred for the following reasons:

* It is an office procedure in which a woman who misses her period goes to the clinic to get the procedure done without checking whether she is pregnant or not.
* The implanted zygote may be missed by the cannula, resulting in the continuation of pregnancy.
* It is associated with a failure to recognise an ectopic pregnancy.

3. Manual vacuum aspiration (MVA)

This procedure provides for termination up to 12 weeks of gestation (up to eight weeks in PHCs). Other than MTP, MVA can also be used for evacuating a missed abortion and for removing retained products of conception.

Contraindications

* Acute vaginal, cervical or pelvic infection
* Suspicion of ectopic pregnancy

Procedure

* Before procedure
    — No need for overnight fasting or routine enema
    — No need to shave the perineum; pubic hair can be trimmed if required
    — Oral analgesia should be given one hour before the procedure '
    — A single dose of prophylactic antibiotic may be given
    — The woman is asked to empty her bladder
* Preparation for the procedure
    — Ensure that the required instruments are available

— Assemble the syringe and lock the valve buttons inside the syringe

— Connect the appropriate cannula; the syringe is now charged and ready for use

- Steps of the procedure

— The woman is placed in lithotomy position on the operation table

— The choice of anesthesia is determined by the surgeon and the acceptor and is a combination of oral analgesics and paracervical block; general anesthesia can even be used if the woman is very apprehensive

— The perineum is cleaned and draped. The cervix and vagina are cleaned with a povidone–iodine solution.

— A paracervical block is given.

— A speculum is inserted into the vagina and the cervix is visualised. The anterior lip of the cervix is caught with tenaculum forceps and gently pulled forward.

— The charged syringe is introduced into the cervical cavity and the valves are released.

— The contents of the uterine cavity can be seen flowing into the syringe and filling it.

— A gentle to-and-fro movement is applied with the cannula.

— The cannula SHOULD NOT be brought out of the external os.

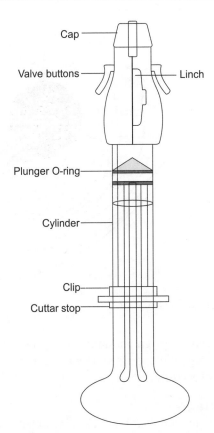

Fig. 63.1 MVA syringe

The MVA syringe is a 60 cc syringe with a plunger (Fig. 63.1). The cephalic end consists of a double valve which helps in producing negative pressure of 660 mmHg. It has different cannula ranging in size from 4–12 mm. Since it is made up of silicone, it can be chemically sterilised, boiled or autoclaved. The following are signs that the uterine cavity is empty:

- Red or pink frothy material passing through the cannula without tissue
- Gritty sensation
- Cervix gripping over the cannula
- Uterus contracting over the cannula

At the end of the procedure, the valve should be closed. The syringe and cannula should be removed, and the contents of the syringe should be emptied into a container.

4. Suction evacuation/vacuum aspiration

It is a quick and efficient method of emptying a pregnant uterus up to 12 weeks of gestation (Fig. 63.2).

Different vacuum aspiration pumps of various brands are available which may be manually or electrically operated. For aspiration, an electrical suction machine that produces at least 625 mmHg negative pressure is commonly used. It is important to ensure that the pump is constructed to suck and not blow air into the uterine cavity.

Procedure

After emptying the bladder, the woman is placed in the lithotomy position. A bimanual pelvic examination is performed to determine the size and position of the uterus. The cervix is then exposed using a Sims speculum, and sponge forceps are used to hold the anterior lip of the cervix. The cervical os is then dilated with Hegar's dilators to accommodate the cannula to be used for evacuation. Dilatation of up to 8 mm is recommended for seven weeks pregnancy (dilatation of 1 mm more than the period of gestation) and up to 11 mm for 10 weeks gestation. Plastic cannulae are used for the procedure. After the required dilatation is achieved, the cannula is introduced into the uterine cavity. When suction is applied, the cannula is systematically moved over the surface within the uterine cavity to cover the entire area. The operator will notice a characteristic grating when the uterus has been completely emptied.

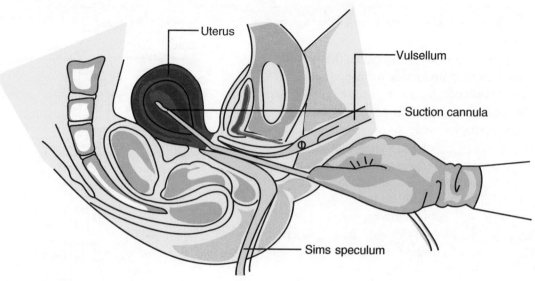

Fig. 63.2 Suction evacuation

Oxytocics can be given intramuscularly/intravenously if required. A gentle curettage may be performed at the end of the procedure.

Complications

The immediate complications are cervical tears, uterine perforation and hemorrhage.

Uterine perforation

This may occur at the time of dilatation, before the evacuation of the uterus or with a curette, when the evacuation is complete. Due to the high risk of perforation in a soft pregnant uterus, the introduction of uterine sound is usually avoided during evacuation. Depending on the instrument that causes perforation, there could be an intraperitoneal bleed necessitating laparotomy. If there is no clinical evidence of shock (hypotension, tachycardia), management will depend on the stage of the operation at which the perforation occurred.

- If the perforation occurred before evacuation, a laparoscopy can be done to visualise any bleeding, and suction evacuation can be completed vaginally under laparoscopic guidance. At the end of the procedure, if there is no significant bleeding from the perforation site, the woman may be kept under observation, There is no need for a laparotomy.

- If the perforation occurred at the end of the procedure and there is no evidence of an intraperitoneal bleed as assessed by the woman's general condition and ultrasound, conservative management is recommended.

- If there is evidence of bleeding, a laparotomy is required.

- If the perforation occurred while using a suction cannula, it is possible that it could have damaged the intraperitoneal structures, the omentum and the bowel. Therefore, it is mandatory to evaluate further with laparoscopy/laparotomy.

5. *Dilatation and curettage*

The method of dilatation and curettage is not preferred nowadays due to the availability of much safer and better alternative termination methods.

Cervical priming

Cervical priming agents are used before suction evacuation and dilatation and curettage to reduce the trauma to the cervix at the time of cervical dilatation. This is especially useful while evacuating a pregnancy in a nulliparous woman or in a woman who had a previous cesarean section.

- **Use of prostaglandins for cervical priming:** Misoprostol 200–400 µg is inserted intravaginally one hour prior to the MTP. Similarly, intracervical prostaglandin gel can also be used.

- **Use of hygroscopic dilators—laminaria tent:** This is made from seaweed that is dried and rounded into a stick-like shape. It is intensely hygroscopic. When placed in a moist environment, such as the cervical canal, it gradually swells to several times its original diameter over a 6–12-hour period, dilating the cervix in the process. In the dry state, laminaria tents come in 5.5–6 cm lengths and in three diameters—3–5 mm (small), 6–8 mm (medium), and 8–10 mm (large). A thread is placed at one end to facilitate removal.

Second-Trimester Termination of Pregnancy

Methods used in the second trimester include:
1. Mifepristone and misoprostol
2. Extra-amniotic instillations of drugs
3. Surgical method—hysterotomy

1. Mifepristone and misoprostol

Various regimens are used for the induction of abortion in the second trimester. The commonly used regimens are mifepristone 200 mg followed by misoprostol after 36–48 hours. Misoprostol is given orally/vaginally in doses of 400 µg every 4 hours for five doses or 800 µg vaginally followed by 400 µg orally for four doses.

There is enough evidence to show that these drugs can be safely used right up to 20 weeks of gestation. However, misoprostol is contraindicated in women with a scarred uterus such as in the case of previous cesarean section scars.

2. Extra-amniotic instillation of drugs

The various drugs used are as follows:
- Ethacridine lactate
- Prostaglandins
- Normal saline

Ethacridine lactate

Ethacridine lactate is a derivative of acridine, a yellow dye with antiseptic action, and is an inexpensive drug. It acts by releasing prostaglandins from the decidua. It is instilled extra-amniotically through a Foley's catheter introduced through the cervical canal at the rate of 10 mL for each week of pregnancy with a maximum limit of 150 mL. The inflated bulb of the catheter is pulled gently so that it blocks and lodges over the internal os. The catheter is removed after six hours. Successful complete abortion takes place in a high percentage of cases within 36 hours. Whenever there is a delay, oxytocic drugs can hasten the process. The use of extra-amniotic normal saline and prostaglandins is not widely practiced clinically.

3. Hysterotomy

Hysterotomy is the process of evacuating the uterine contents through the abdominal route. It is the last resort when all other methods of second-trimester abortion fail. In women who have undergone hysterotomy, the subsequent pregnancies should be delivered by cesarean section.

■ COMPLICATIONS OF ABORTIONS

- Anesthesia-related complications at the time of surgical procedures
- Uterine perforation during surgical evacuation (already discussed)
- Cervical laceration during the dilatation of the cervix
- Heavy bleeding during the procedure
- Incomplete abortion and retained products of conception, which can be managed medically with misoprostol or re-evacuation
- Post-abortal sepsis
- Failure to achieve abortion and continuation of pregnancy, which may occur rarely

■ POST-ABORTAL CONTRACEPTION

A women's fertility can return quickly after an abortion—as early as two weeks after an abortion. All modern contraceptive methods, both temporary and permanent, may be used at or immediately after surgical and medical abortions.

■ MEDICOLEGAL ISSUES RELATED TO MTP

Medicolegal issues can arise following the MTP in the following areas:
- Failure to obtain consent
- Failure of termination and continuation of pregnancy
- Retained products of conception
- Damage to the viscera
- Failure to administer anti-D immunoglobulin following MTP in an Rh-negative woman
- Sex determination tests and disclosure of the sex of the fetus prior to MTP, which are are punishable acts
- Death of the woman following MTP

KEY POINTS

✓ *The MTP Act, which was passed in 1971, was amended in 2021 to increase the upper limit for termination from 20 to 24 weeks.*

✓ *The Preconception and Prenatal Diagnostic Techniques (Regulation and Prevention of Misuse) Amendment Act (PCPNDT), 2002, prohibits sex selection.*

✓ The commonly used first-trimester abortion methods include mifepristone and misoprostol used in conjunction, MVA and suction evacuation.

✓ Second-trimester abortion methods are mifepristone and misoprostol used in conjunction and the extra-amniotic instillation of drugs.

✓ Cervical priming should be done prior to surgical evacuation.

✓ Pre-abortion counselling helps women to decide about the method of termination of pregnancy and adopt a contraceptive method after abortion.

Essay questions

1. Discuss in detail the MTP Act in India and its components.
2. Describe the steps of manual vacuum aspiration/suction evacuation and list the complications associated with this method.
3. A 25-year-old G2P1L1 comes to the clinic at 6 weeks of gestation for the termination of pregnancy due to contraceptive failure.
   a) Is she eligible for the termination of pregnancy?
   b) List the different termination methods available for this woman.
   c) What drugs can be used for termination?
   d) Mention two complications of suction evacuation.
4. A 32-year-old G2P1L1 diagnosed with anencephaly at 14 weeks of gestation wants an MTP.
   a) On what grounds can MTP be performed in this case?
   b) List two methods of termination for this patient.
   c) What is the upper gestational age limit for termination of pregnancy according to the MTP Amendment Bill, 2021?
   d) Which form should be signed by the patient prior to MTP?

Short answer questions

1. What are the different conditions under which termination of pregnancy can be performed legally?
2. What are the different methods of termination of pregnancy in the first trimester?
3. What are the different methods used for termination of pregnancy in the second trimester?
4. What are the complications of MTP?

MCQs

1. Which of these conditions for the termination of pregnancy is not permitted by the MTP Act?
   a) Following rape
   b) Anomalous baby
   c) Failure of contraceptive
   d) Gender-specific termination

2. What examination is not required prior to the termination of pregnancy?
   a) Hemoglobin
   b) Blood pressure
   c) Blood grouping and typing
   d) Renal function test

3. Which of these is not a first-trimester termination method?
   a) Hysterotomy
   b) Mifepristone and misoprostol
   c) Menstrual aspiration
   d) Manual vacuum aspiration

4. Which of these is not true of mifepristone?
   a) RU-486
   b) Progesterone agonist
   c) Softens the cervix
   d) Sensitises uterus to misoprostol

5. Menstrual regulation with a Karman cannula can be attempted until:
   a) 5 weeks
   b) 6 weeks
   c) 7 weeks
   d) 8 weeks

6. Manual vacuum aspiration cannot be used in a case of:
   a) 12 weeks pregnancy
   b) Missed abortion
   c) Retained products
   d) Active pelvic infection

Answers

1. (d), 2. (d), 3. (a), 4. (b), 5. (b), 6. (d)

Fill in the blanks

1. The Medical Termination of Pregnancy Act of India was passed by the Indian Parliament in _____.
2. The upper limit of termination of pregnancy according to the revised MTP act is _____ in certain categories of women.

Answers

1. 1971, 2. 24 weeks

64

AN 77.5, PH 1.39, FM 3.24,
OG 19.1, 19.2, 19.4, 21.1
and 21.2, PY 9.6 and CM 9.5

Contraception

Learning Objectives

» To enumerate the temporary methods of contraception
» To enumerate the permanent methods of contraception
» To know the selection of patients for temporary and permanent methods of contraception
» To know the eligibility criteria for temporary and permanent methods of contraception
» To know the counselling required for contraception
» To know the most common contraceptive methods and their use in the postpartum period
» To learn the different types of IUCDs, the techniques of insertion, contraindications and possible complications
» To know the indications, techniques, side effects, success and failure rates of temporary and permanent methods of contraception
» To know about male contraception
» To know about emergency contraception

■ INTRODUCTION

Contraception (fertility control) refers to methods or techniques used to prevent pregnancy as a consequence of sexual intercourse. This can be achieved either by preventing the fertilisation of an egg by a sperm (conception) or by preventing the implantation of the fertilised egg in the uterus. By using contraceptive methods, the number and timing of pregnancies can be controlled. Though birth control methods have been used since ancient times, effective and safe methods of birth control have been available only since the 20th century.

The Need for Fertility Control

Fertility control is required for various reasons; it may be for the benefit of the woman or for the benefit of the nation, from the standpoint of stabilising the population.

The woman's perspective

- Desire to limit childbearing
- To have an adequate birth interval between children
- In unmarried sexually active women who wish to prevent unwanted pregnancies
- In recently married women who wish to postpone pregnancy temporarily
- In women with medical conditions in whom pregnancy is contraindicated temporarily or permanently

To stabilise the population

India was the first country in the world to develop a population policy to stabilise the population and slow down population growth; the National Family Programme was introduced in 1952.

The population of India doubled to 1.2 billion between 1975 and 2010, reaching the billion mark in 1998. Currently, the population in India stands at 1,387,816,936 (1.38 billion), making it the second most populous country in the world after China, where the population stands at 1,446,312,871 (1.44 billion) people. India is set to become the world's most populous country by 2024, surpassing even China. With a population growth rate of 1.2%, India is predicted to have more than 1.53 billion people by the end of 2030 and to reach 1.7 billion by 2050. These figures show that India represents almost 17.85% of the world's population (living on 2.4% of the earth's land area), which means that one out of six people on this planet lives in India. 26 September marks World Contraception Day, which is devoted to raising awareness about contraception, education and sexual and reproductive health.

■ MEDICAL ELIGIBILITY CRITERIA

Medical eligibility criteria are a set of guidelines published by the WHO that help in making a decision about the suitability of a particular method for a client.

Eligibility Criteria for Reversible Contraceptives

Contraceptive methods are organised into four categories:

- **Category 1:** There is no restriction on the use of the contraceptive method. Therefore, it can be used under any circumstances.
- **Category 2:** The advantages of using the method generally outweigh the theoretical or proven risks. Therefore, it can be generally used.
- **Category 3:** The theoretical or proven risks usually outweigh the advantages of using the method. Hence, this method not generally recommended unless other, more appropriate methods are not available or acceptable.
- **Category 4:** An unacceptable health risk is associated with the use of this contraceptive method. Therefore, it should not be used.

Categories 1 and 4 are self-explanatory. While category 1 indicates that the method is suitable for all, category 4 indicates that the method is not suitable under particular conditions/circumstances. Categories 2 and 3 are relative contraindications. While category 2 indicates that the method can generally be used, but with careful follow-up, category 3 indicates that the method is best avoided unless no other method is available.

Criteria for Selecting Women for Sterilisation

- **Accept:** The procedure can be performed in a routine setting without delay.
- **Caution:** The procedure can be performed in a routine setting but with extra preparation and precautions, depending on the condition of the patient.
- **Delay:** The female sterilisation should be postponed. This applies to certain conditions (e.g., anemia and infection) that must be treated and resolved before female sterilisation can be performed. The client should be prescribed another method of contraception until the procedure can be performed.
- **Special:** This refers to special arrangements that need to be made before performing the procedure (such as heart disease, hypertension or any medical disorder) in a setting with an experienced surgeon

and staff, equipment to provide general anesthesia and other backup medical support.

GENERAL PRINCIPLES WHILE OFFERING CONTRACEPTIVE METHODS

- While using any contraceptive method, the cafeteria approach should be followed, whereby the woman should be informed about all the contraceptive choices available and their benefits and side effects and then she should be allowed to make a decision regarding what would be right for her.
- Before offering any contraceptive method to a woman, it is important to know the contraindications and complications related to that particular method. It is also important to provide adequate counselling to the woman, explaining the risks and benefits. The woman's consent should always be taken.
- At the time of counselling, the 'GATHER' approach should be used (**greet, ask, tell, help, explain and return**). It has been shown that the more the GATHER elements a counsellor uses, the more satisfied women are with their care and the more likely they are to use contraception.

Several methods are used for the control of fertility (Fig. 64.1 and Table 64.1). The success of a method depends on its acceptability by the user in particular and the community at large.

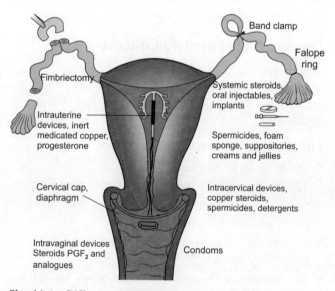

Fig. 64.1 Different methods of contraception

Table 64.1 Methods of fertility control

Temporary contraceptive methods	Permanent contraceptive methods
• Natural methods • Barrier methods • Intrauterine contraceptive devices • Oral contraceptives (hormonal and non-hormonal) • Injectable contraceptives • Hormonal implants • Vaginal rings • Transdermal patches • Emergency contraception	• Female sterilisation • Male sterilisation

 LONG-ACTING REVERSIBLE CONTRACEPTION

Long-acting reversible contraception (LARC) methods, which include copper-containing intrauterine devices, levonorgestrel-releasing intrauterine system (LNG-IUS) and contraceptive implants are the most effective reversible contraceptive methods available to women with failure rates less than 0.1–1%. They are convenient methods, especially for new mothers, and are also safe for use while breastfeeding. In addition to their ease of use, LARC methods are cost-effective and have the advantage of fertility being restored after removal. LARC devices can be placed immediately postpartum or at a later time. If IUDs are placed postpartum, the best practice is to place them within 10 minutes of placental delivery.

TEMPORARY CONTRACEPTIVE METHODS

Fertility Awareness Methods (Natural Family Planning Methods)

Fertility awareness methods involve determining the days when a woman is most likely to be fertile during her menstrual cycle and avoiding unprotected sexual intercourse during that period. In a woman who has a regular menstrual cycle, an ovum is released from one of the ovaries approximately 14 days before the start of the next menstrual cycle. The unfertilised egg survives for 12–24 hours, whereas the sperm survives in the genital tract for as long as five days. Therefore, fertilisation can occur from intercourse that occurred five days before ovulation as well as at ovulation.

There are several techniques to determine the most fertile period:
• Rhythm method or calendar method
• Cervical mucus method (based on the changes in the cervical mucus)
• Monitoring the basal body temperature
• Symptothermal method

These methods have typical first-year failure rates of 24%. However, with perfect use, the first-year failure rates range from 0.4–5% depending on the method used.

Calendar method (rhythm method):

It is based on the assumption (**Ogino–Knaus theory**) that in a woman with regular cycles, ovulation takes place 14 ± 2 days before the onset of the next period. The calendar method (also called the standard days method) can be used only by women who have regular menstrual periods. To calculate when to abstain from intercourse, a woman subtracts 18 days from the shortest and 11 days from the longest of her past 12 menstrual cycles. For example, if her cycles last from 26–29 days, she must abstain from intercourse from day 8 (26 minus 18) through day 18 (29 minus 11) of each cycle. The day that a menstrual period begins is considered day 1. In a woman with a regular 28-day cycle, abstinence is advised from 8–18th day of menstruation (this gives allowance for variation in ovulation timings even with regular cycles). Either sexual intercourse can be avoided or a barrier method of contraception such as a condom or a spermicide can be used during the above period. This method works well for women who have regular cycles. Cycle beads can be used to help women keep track of their fertile days. These beads are colour-coded, with each bead representing a day of the cycle.

Limitations
• This method is not suitable for women who have irregular cycles.
• This method does not protect against sexually transmitted diseases.
• These methods require training, discipline and effort by the clients.

Basal body temperature (BBT) method

This method is based on the fact that after ovulation, the progesterone level in the blood rises, increasing the basal metabolic rate (BMR) and causing a rise in temperature by 0.5–0.8°F (0.5°C) in the luteal phase of the menstrual cycle. In this method, the temperature has to be taken immediately after waking up, before doing any other chore. Moreover, the exact timing of ovulation cannot be predicted as the temperature rise occurs only after ovulation.

Billings ovulation method or the cervical mucus method

In this method, the woman determines her fertile period by observing the secretions (cervical mucus) from her vagina. Mucus usually has the following pattern during the menstrual cycle:

- There may be no mucus for a few days after the menstrual period stops. This is called the dry period.
- Then mucus appears and is cloudy, thick and inelastic. The wet period starts with the appearance of mucus.
- Due to the effect of estrogen, shortly before ovulation, more mucus is produced, which is thinner, elastic (can be stretched between the fingers—spinnbarkeit test), clearer and more watery (like raw egg white). These changes create an environment that helps sperm to travel through the cervix, uterus and fallopian tubes to the egg.
- Intercourse should be avoided from the time mucus first appears after a menstrual period until the mucus completely disappears. After the mucus disappears, intercourse is permitted without restrictions until the next period begins.

Limitations

- The woman may have trouble in interpreting the appearance of the cervical mucus.
- Vaginal or cervical infection alters the nature of the discharge.
- Women should not use douches or feminine hygiene sprays and creams when they follow the cervical mucus method for contraception as these can change the nature of mucus.

Symptothermal method

The symptothermal method combines the measurement of body temperature at rest (basal body temperature) with the mucus changes and calendar methods. Because it combines three methods, it is most reliable. The woman is instructed to note the cervical mucus changes as well as the date of temperature rise. She should abstain from intercourse from the first day requiring abstinence according to the calendar method until at least 72 hours after the day her basal body temperature increases and cervical mucus changes are noted.

Lactational amenorrhea method (LAM)

This method can be used by women who breastfeed their infants. Following delivery, the woman has natural postpartum infertility due to the elevated levels of prolactin, which inhibits the pulsatile release of GnRH, leading to anovulation. For this method to be effective, the following conditions have to be fulfilled:

- The mother should not have resumed her periods after delivery (in those who are exclusively breastfeeding, about 10% begin having periods before three months and 20% before six months. In those who are not breastfeeding, fertility may return four weeks after delivery).
- The baby should be exclusively breastfed, at least every four hours during the day and at least every six hours during the night. Breastfeeding should be the only source of food for the baby. Supplementing breast milk with formula or solid food or pumping breast milk makes this method less effective.
- The baby should be less than six months of age.

With exclusive breastfeeding, the failure rate of the LAM method is 2% in the six months following delivery. Failure rates increase to 4–7% at one year and 13% at two years. Feeding formula, pumping instead of nursing, using a pacifier for the baby and feeding solids all increase the failure rate of this method.

Coitus interruptus or withdrawal method

The withdrawal method (also known as coitus interruptus) is the practice of ending intercourse ('pulling out') before ejaculation. The main risk of the withdrawal method is that the man may not perform the manoeuvre correctly or in a timely manner. First-year failure rates vary from 4% with perfect usage to 22% with typical usage. Apart from the failure rate, there is significant stress and strain on both partners with this method.

Abstinence

Sexual abstinence may be used as a form of birth control. This means either not engaging in any type of sexual activity or specifically not engaging in vaginal intercourse. Complete sexual abstinence is 100% effective in preventing pregnancy.

Advantages of natural family planning methods

- No physical side effects
- Menstruation is not affected
- No financial cost is involved
- Culturally and socially acceptable
- Do not need follow-up

Disadvantages of natural family planning methods

- Need commitment, motivation, training and the cooperation of both partners
- They are less effective than other methods
- Do not protect against STDs and HIV
- Failure rate of natural methods could be as high as 25%

Barrier Method of Contraception

Barrier contraceptives physically block the sperm's access to a woman's uterus. In order to achieve this, direct insemination into the vagina/cervix during ejaculation must be prevented and any sperm deposited in the vagina must be immobilised before it can reach the cervix. This can be achieved by using mechanical barriers such as condoms, diaphragms, cervical caps or contraceptive sponges protecting the external os and using spermicides to destroy sperm.

The commonly used barrier methods include the following:

- Diaphragm
- Cervical cap
- Female condom
- Spermicides
- Male condom

Diaphragm

This is a soft latex cup that covers the cervix. Plastic and silicone diaphragms are also available. The silicone diaphragm is softer and more durable than diaphragms made of latex. The rim contains a firm, flexible spring that keeps the diaphragm in place. It comes in different sizes and requires training to be able to insert it properly. A diaphragm should cover the entire cervix without causing discomfort. After insertion, it should extend from the posterior fornix to the symphysis pubis. Neither the woman nor her partner should be able to notice its presence. The diaphragm is inserted before intercourse, but not earlier than 6 hours before. After the intercourse, it should be left in its place for at least 6–8 hours but no more than 24 hours. If intercourse is repeated while the diaphragm is in place, additional spermicidal cream or gel should be inserted into the vagina to continue protection. Diaphragms can be washed and reused multiple times. The diaphragm must be renewed every year. It must also be renewed in the event of a vaginal infection to prevent re-infection. A woman should inspect the diaphragm regularly for tears. This method of contraception is not completely reliable without the addition of a chemical spermicide.

The cap should be smeared both inside and outside with the spermicide before use. Side effects include an increase in the risk of bacterial vaginosis and urinary tract infections. If it is left in the vagina for more than 24 hours, toxic shock syndrome may occur. Though the diaphragm can reduce the incidence of STIs, it does not protect against HIV as the vagina is still exposed. During the first year of diaphragm use, the percentage of women who become pregnant is about 6% with perfect use and about 12% with typical use (the way most people use it) (Fig. 64.2).

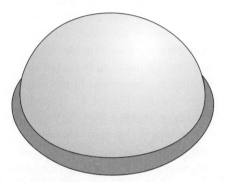

Fig. 64.2   A diaphragm

Cervical cap

The cervical cap, which is a hat-shaped silicone cup, is inserted into the vagina and positioned over the cervix. It prevents sperm from entering the cervix. Cervical caps resemble diaphragms but are smaller and more rigid (Fig. 64.3). It is shaped like a thimble with a raised rim and is made of rubber or plastic. It covers the cervix to its base. The circumference of the circular rim should fit that of the cervix tightly. The cervix must be long enough to protrude well into the bowl of the cap.

Cervical caps are available in different sizes—small, medium, large and extra large. A spermicidal cream or gel should always be used with a cervical cap. The cap

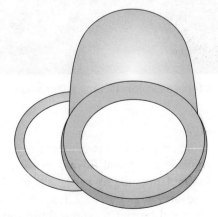

Fig. 64.3   A cervical cap

is inserted before sexual intercourse and left in place for at least 6 hours after intercourse but not more than 48 hours. A strap is attached to the cervical cap for easy removal. The cervical cap can be washed and reused for 1 year. During the first year, the pregnancy rate with typical use is about 8% in women who have not had a baby. In women who have delivered children, the failure rate is higher.

Female condom

The female condom is a pouch made of polyurethane and has an inner ring and an outer ring. The inner ring is inserted as far as it can go into the vagina, and the outer ring remains outside. The internal ring in the closed end of the pouch covers the cervix and the external ring remains outside the vagina, partially covering the perineum (Fig. 64.4). It works by forming a barrier that keeps sperm out of the vagina, preventing pregnancy. Spillage of semen should be prevented while removing the female condom.

The female condom should be inserted no more than 8 hours before sexual intercourse and should be removed soon after the intercourse. A new condom should be used each time a person has sexual intercourse, and the condom should be discarded if its integrity is in doubt. A spermicide, which may be included in the condom's lubricant or inserted separately into the vagina, may increase the effectiveness of condoms. Spermicide should be reapplied each time a condom is used.

A female condom also provides protection against STIs including HIV and HPV infections. The chance of pregnancy with female condoms during the first year is 5% with perfect use and 21% with typical use.

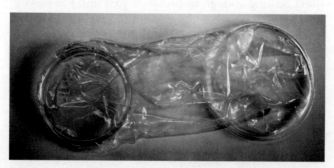

Fig. 64.4 A female condom (*Source*: Wikimedia Commons)

Spermicides

Spermicides are preparations that kill sperm on contact. They are available as vaginal foams, creams, gels and suppositories and are placed in the vagina before a couple has sexual intercourse. These contraceptives provide a chemical barrier to sperm by trapping and damaging sperm. Thus, they prevent sperm from fertilising an egg.

Even with the proper use of spermicides, about 19% of women become pregnant during the first year of use. Because their effectiveness is limited, spermicides are best used with another barrier contraceptive such as a condom or diaphragm. Spermicides should be placed in the vagina at least 10–30 minutes and no more than 1 hour before sexual intercourse. They should be reapplied each time a couple has intercourse. Modern spermicides contain surface-active agents that damage the sperm cell membranes.

The agents currently used are non-oxynol-9, octoxynol-9 and benzalkonium chloride. Most spermicides contain 60–100 mg of these agents. Chemical contraceptives are available in the following forms.

- **Foam tablets**: These dissolve in the presence of moisture with the formation of carbon dioxide foam and release the active spermicide into the vagina.
- **Creams, pastes, jellies**: These are contained in metal or plastic tubes with screw-on caps. Applicators are available for deposition in the vagina.
- **Aerosols**: These are pastes or creams compressed into strong containers with a gas. The foam is released by pressure on a release valve into an applicator from which it is injected into the vagina.

Side effects

Using spermicides several times a day may irritate the vagina and damage the tissues lining it. As a result, the microorganisms that cause sexually transmitted diseases (including HIV) can more easily enter the body and cause disease. Spermicides do not protect against sexually transmitted diseases.

Contraceptive sponge

A contraceptive sponge is a round, pillow-shaped polyurethane sponge about 4 cm in diameter. The sponge is made wet with water, folded and inserted deep into the vagina, where it blocks sperm from entering the uterus. The sponge also contains a spermicide. It is available over the counter and does not need to be fitted by a healthcare practitioner. The sponge can be inserted into the vagina by the woman up to 24 hours before sexual intercourse and provides protection through that period of time, regardless of how frequently intercourse is repeated. The sponge must be left in place for at least 6 hours after the last act of intercourse. It should not be left in place for more than 30 hours. Following the insertion, neither the female nor the male partner will be aware of its presence in the vagina. Pregnancy rates with typical use are 12% for women who have not had children and 24% for women who have.

Serious problems related to its use are uncommon. They include allergic reactions, vaginal dryness or irritation and difficulty removing the sponge. TODAY sponge is available in India and is incorporated with non-oxynol-9.

Its advantages are that it does not require a prescription and that it is a female control method and does not require a partner's cooperation. It cannot be used if the individual is sensitive or allergic to spermicide or polyurethane and has recently delivered or by women who have had a recent miscarriage. It can lead to frequent urinary tract infections; a forgotten sponge can result in toxic shock syndrome.

Male condom

Condoms are thin protective sheaths that cover the penis. The condom is an effective contraceptive method and is the only barrier method that can be used by men. The male condom is also effective against HIV infection and other sexually transmitted infections. Most condoms are made of latex, polyurethane or silicone rubber. These materials are thin and more likely to tear. Condoms must be used correctly to be effective.

A condom should be applied before penetration. A new condom of the correct size should be used for each act of sexual intercourse. It should be put on after the penis is erect and before any genital contact with the partner. After application, a 1/2 inch of the condom should be left at the tip of the condom to collect semen. With latex condoms, only water-based lubricants can be used, and oil-based lubricants should be avoided. Pre-lubricated and spermicide-containing condoms are also available. Incorrect use and breakage of condoms account for failures. Breakage rates vary from 1–8 per 100 episodes of vaginal intercourse.

Its advantages are that it is a safe non-hormonal method that almost every couple can use easily to prevent pregnancy and STIs including HIV. Disadvantages are that it requires a high degree of motivation for regular use; allergic reactions may occur in some couples with the use of spermicides, latex condoms, diaphragms and caps. Accidents like slippage and breakage during coitus necessitate a 'backup' use of emergency contraception. Some people are embarrassed to buy and ask their partner to use this method. It is a male-controlled method and can be used only after erection. During the first year that male condoms are used, the chance of pregnancy is about 2% with perfect use (when instructions are followed exactly) and about 18% with typical use (the way most people use them).

Intrauterine Contraceptive Devices (IUCDs)

Intrauterine devices are small, flexible, T-shaped plastic devices that are inserted into the uterus to prevent pregnancy. An IUCD can be left in place for 3, 5 or 10 years, depending on the type used. There are various types of intrauterine contraceptive devices (Table 64.2 and Fig. 64.5).

Table 64.2 Types of intrauterine devices

Type of IUCD	Examples
First-generation/ Unmedicated IUCDs	Lippe's loop, Saf-T-Coil, Chinese single coil ring, Chinese double-coiled ring (Mahua ring) and Ota ring
Second-generation/ Copper IUCDs	Copper-7, Copper-T 200, Multiload copper 250, Multiload copper 375, Copper T 380A, Copper T 380 Ag, Copper-T 380S, Nova T, and Copper T 220C
Third-generation/ Hormone-releasing IUCDs	Progesterone IUCD (Progestasert) and levonorgestrel IUCD (Mirena, LNG 20)
Fourth-generation IUCDs	Frameless IUCD (Gynefix) and frameless IUS (Fibroplant)

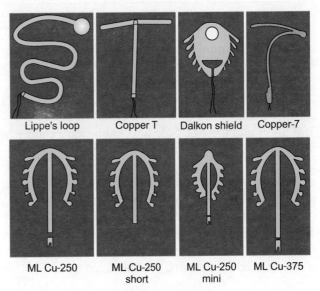

Fig. 64.5 Types of intrauterine devices

A specifically trained healthcare provider inserts an IUCD into a woman's uterus through her vagina and cervix. Almost all types of IUCDs have one or two strings or threads tied to them. The strings hang through the cervix into the vagina. An IUCD works primarily by causing a chemical change that damages the sperm and egg before they can meet.

Unmedicated IUCDs

The Lippe's loop is a polyethylene device in the shape of a double 'S' with a small polyethylene filament protruding through the cervix to facilitate identification. It is not used anymore.

Copper IUCDs

The copper-bearing intrauterine device is a small, flexible plastic frame with copper sleeves or a wire around it. Various types of devices varying in shape and size are available. The 'T' device of Tatum was originally introduced with a view to provide a design that could best adapt itself to the uterine cavity even when it is contracted maximally. The T-shaped device has lowered expulsion rate and bleeding complications when compared to others. Because of the lower incidence of side effects with the 'T' device and its anti-fertility properties, the idea of using the 'T' device as a carrier for copper emerged, and thus, the copper-T device emerged. Most of the T-shaped devices have a plastic T frame with a pure copper wire or copper sleeves wound around it.

All copper devices carry a number, which is the surface area of copper in mm² that the device has. These are the Cu-7, CuT-200, CuT-220C, Multiload-250 and the Nova-T. The Multiload-375 has 375 mm² of copper and the Copper T-380A contains 380 mm² of copper. The Nova-T is similar to the Copper-T 200, containing 200 mm² of copper. However, it has a silver core beneath the copper wire to prevent fragmentation of the copper, thereby increasing its lifespan.

Some copper-Ts have only copper in the stem. Examples are the Multiload Cu-375, Nova T-380, UT-380, UT3-380 Short and the Neo Safe-380. Some have copper in the sleeves as well. They are the most effective and long-lasting ones. Multiload devices are designed with flexible serrated arms, which facilitate placing the device in position without stretching the uterus.

The most popular copper IUCD is the Copper-T 380A, which is currently available all over India as part of the National Family Planning Programme (Fig. 64.6). It can be used for up to 10 years and can be considered a reversible alternative to sterilisation. Copper-T 380A has a surface area of 380 mm² of copper wire—314 mm² wound around the vertical stem and 33 mm² on each transverse arm of the device. The failure rate ranges from 0.6–0.8 per 100 women years.

The approved lifespan of Copper-T 380 A is 10 years, that of Copper-T 380 Ag is 4 years, that of Copper-T 380 S is 2.6 years and that of Mutiload Copper-375 is 5 years.

Mechanism of action

The copper IUD releases free copper and copper salts that cause biochemical and morphological changes in the endometrium. It also produces alterations in cervical mucus and endometrial secretions. Copper ions decrease sperm motility and function by altering the uterine and tubal fluid environment, thus preventing sperm from reaching the fallopian tubes and fertilising the egg. They prevent pregnancy by killing or immobilising sperms. The device also stimulates a sterile inflammatory reaction in the endometrium which is toxic to the sperm and prevents implantation.

Hormone-releasing IUDs

These intrauterine devices contain progesterone (Fig. 64.7a and b). Progestasert contains a reservoir of 38 mg of progesterone and releases it at a rate of 65 μg per day. However, Progestasert is not freely available. LNG-20 contains 52 mg of levonorgestrel, which is released at the rate of 20 μg per day. The lifespan of LNG-20 is 5 years. Besides its contraceptive use, it is being used successfully for dysfunctional uterine bleeding, simple hyperplasia, adenomyosis and fibroids.

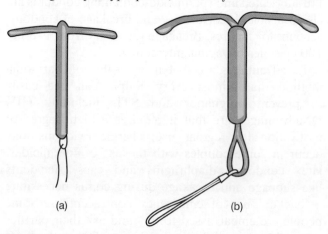

Fig. 64.7 Hormone-releasing IUDs: (a) Progestasert and (b) LNG-20

Mechanism of action

The progesterone in progesterone-releasing IUCDs causes endometrial decidualisation with atrophy of the

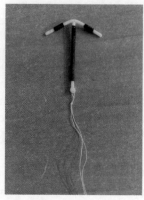

Fig. 64.6 Copper-T 380A

glands. The altered endometrial environment leads to the inhibition of implantation and sperm capacitation and survival. Progesterone also causes thickening of the cervical mucus, creating a barrier to sperm penetration.

Skyla and Kyleena are 'low-dose' levonorgestrel-releasing intrauterine systems (LNG-IUS) which have been researched and introduced to complement the currently available systems. Skyla LNG-IUS contains 13.5 mg and Kyleena LNG-IUS contains 19.5 mg of levonorgestrel. The major benefits of these low-dose devices are that they have a smaller frame and narrow inserter, have a lower rate of amenorrhea compared to LNG-IUS 20 and provide contraceptive protection for five years as in LNG-IUS 20.

Fourth-generation IUCDs

The frameless IUD (GYNEFIX)—made without the plastic T-shaped frame common to most other types of IUCDs—consists of several copper cylinders tied together on a string. It is anchored one centimetre deep into the fundus (top) of the uterus. This design is intended to cause less pain and bleeding than framed devices.

FibroPlant-LNG releases progestin levonorgestrel. Like the GyneFix IUCD, it also is anchored to the fundus of the uterus. FibroPlant-LNG delivers 14 μg of levonorgestrel daily and prevents pregnancy for at least three years.

Contraindications for IUCDs

- Active pelvic inflammatory disease (PID) or a sexually transmitted infection
- History of past PID/STI in the last 6 months
- Evidence of active cervical or vaginal infection
- Suspected pelvic tuberculosis
- In HIV-positive women
- Pregnancy
- Undiagnosed vaginal bleeding
- Distorted uterine cavity due to submucous fibroids
- A structural abnormality that distorts the uterus such as a septate uterus or a bicornuate uterus
- Cervical/uterine malignancy
- In breast cancer, LNG-IUCD is contraindicated
- Cu-T is contraindicated if there is an allergy to copper and in cases of Wilson disease
- Anemia is a relative contraindication and has to be corrected before IUCD insertion

Timing of IUCD insertion

The IUCD can be inserted in the postmenstrual, post-abortal or postpartum period or post-cesarean section. At times, postcoital insertion is also done.

- The most ideal time to insert an IUCD is the postmenstrual period.
- Postpartum IUCD insertion (PPIUCD):
  — Postplacental IUCD insertion (PPIUCD)—insertion is done within 10 minutes after the expulsion of the placenta following a vaginal delivery on the same delivery table (discussed later).
  — Intra-cesarean—insertion can be done during a cesarean delivery, after the removal of the placenta and before the closure of the uterine incision.
  — Within 48 hours after delivery—insertion is done within 48 hours of delivery and prior to discharge from the postpartum ward.
  — Extended postpartum/interval—insertion is done at any time after 6 weeks postpartum.
- Post-abortion: Insertion is done following an abortion if there is no infection, suspicion of retained products, bleeding or any other contraindication.

Technique of IUCD Insertion

Insertion of Copper-T differs from that of the Lippe's loop. The Lippe's loop is inserted by pushing it into the uterine cavity (Fig. 64.8a–d).

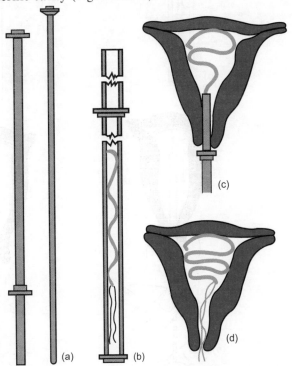

Fig. 64.8 Insertion of Lippe's loop: (a) Flexible plastic inserter with a plastic syringe, (b) the loop is negotiated into the bottom end of the inserter, (c) the loop is pushed into the uterine cavity and (d) the inserter is withdrawn, leaving Lippe's loop in the uterus

The IUCD should NOT be inserted from 48 hours to 6 weeks following delivery because there is an increased risk of infection and expulsion.

To insert a Copper-T, the introducer is placed in the fundus of the uterus and the plunger is withdrawn, leaving the device in the uterus (Fig. 64.9a–g). There are fewer chances of perforation in this technique, which is called the withdrawal technique.

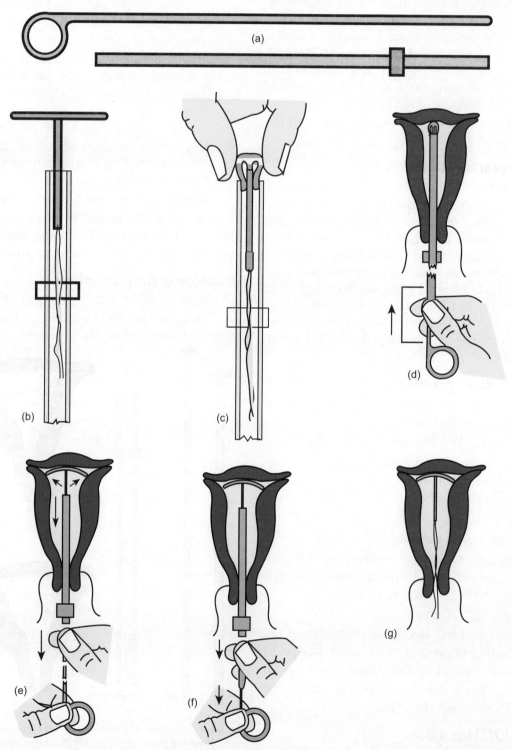

Fig. 64.9 Insertion of copper-T: (a) Flexible plastic inserter with a plastic plunger, (b–c) Copper-T is negotiated into the top end of the inserter, (d) Copper-T-loaded inserter with the plunger is introduced into the uterine cavity, (e) the inserter is retracted over the plunger, leaving Copper-T inside the uterus, (f) the plunger and inserter are withdrawn and (g) Copper-T in position

Before inserting an IUCD, the woman is placed in a dorsal position. Strict aseptic precautions should be followed. Speculum and bimanual examinations are done to rule out any contraindications. After introducing a bivalve speculum, the anterior lip of the cervix is held with Vulsellum forceps. The cervix is cleaned and painted with an antiseptic solution. A uterine sound is introduced to note the length and position of the uterus. The actual insertion varies with the type of IUCD. The currently used technique is the 'no touch technique' by which the arms of the Copper-T are inserted into the plunger before removing it from the pack.

- The adjustable collar is adjusted so that the size of the portion of the inserter above it corresponds to the size of the uterine cavity as determined by the uterine sound.
- The solid rod plunger is now introduced into the inserter tube up to the lower end of the vertical arm.
- The inserter loaded with the device is now negotiated into the uterine cavity until it touches the fundus and the collar touches the external os.
- The plunger is held firmly with the left arm, and the outer inserter tube is retracted over the plunger with the right hand for about 2 cm so that the Copper-T device is left high up in the fundus and lies transversely.
- The plunger is withdrawn.
- This is followed by the removal of the inserter tube.

This method of insertion is known as the withdrawal method; there are fewer chances of perforation if this method is used.

Post-insertion follow-up

- The woman should be asked to check her pad for three cycles to detect possible expulsion.
- The woman should be educated to feel the thread after each period and report if the thread is missing.
- Speculum examination should be performed in the subsequent menstrual cycle to look for the thread.
- The woman should be instructed to report if there is heavy bleeding, pain or abnormal vaginal discharge, if she cannot feel the thread or if she misses her period.
- Indications for removal include expiry of the device, pelvic inflammatory disease, pelvic pain, menopause and suspected malignancy. The Copper-T device can be removed by holding the thread with artery forceps and bringing it out by steady traction.

Complications

- **Expulsion:** Expulsion is more common following postpartum and post-abortal insertion and usually occurs during the first 4–6 months during menstruation. It is also more common in nulliparous women. Expulsion of the IUCD occurs in 2–8% of women in the first year. If the device is expelled and the loss is noticed only after a few days, backup contraception should be immediately adopted.
- **Menstrual disturbances:**
  - **Heavy menstrual bleeding/intermenstrual bleeding:** Soon after insertion and in the first two or three cycles, irregular spotting and heavy bleeding during periods are very common due to the aseptic endometritis caused by the IUCD. These side effects can be prevented/treated by prescribing NSAIDs/antifibrinolytic agents for the duration of menstruation for 2–3 cycles. These symptoms gradually reduce.
  - **Amenorrhea:** Women who have had an LNG-IUCD inserted may experience scanty periods/amenorrhea.
  - **Dysmenorrhea and pelvic pain:** These are more common in nulliparas. Such cases usually present with spasmodic dysmenorrhea in the first 3–6 months following insertion. The woman should be warned of these symptoms and treated with NSAIDs.
- **Vaginal discharge and infection:** Vaginal discharge is also common following IUCD insertion. However, pelvic infection and PID can also occur if aseptic precautions were not followed at the time of insertion.
- **Perforation:** This usually occurs at the time of insertion due to faulty technique and is reported in less than 1 per 1,000 insertions. It may manifest as lower abdominal pain. Perforation and migration into the peritoneal cavity lead to omental adhesions with copper-containing IUCDs; therefore, in such cases, the IUCD should be removed; this can be done laparoscopically. Uterine perforation may occur in 0.1 per cent of women during insertion.
- **Pregnancy:** Pregnancies can occur with the IUCD in situ. If the woman misses her period, it is important to rule out intrauterine and ectopic pregnancy. To do this, an immediate pregnancy test (urine/blood) and a USG of the pelvis should be carried out.
  - The overall risk of ectopic pregnancy is reduced in association with IUCD use versus using no contraception. However, if pregnancy does occur in a woman with an IUCD, then the risk of ectopic pregnancy is increased as the fallopian tubes are less protected.

— When there is an intrauterine pregnancy with an IUCD in situ, if the woman requests pregnancy termination, it can be carried out.

— In a woman who wishes to continue the pregnancy, if the thread is seen, the IUCD should be removed. If the thread is not seen, she can still continue with the pregnancy. However, complications such as infections, miscarriage, preterm labour and PPROM are higher in pregnancy with IUCD in situ. There is no evidence that the IUCD is teratogenic.

• **Missing IUCD thread**: If the IUCD thread is not seen, an ultrasound examination is carried out to see whether the device is within the uterine cavity or if it has migrated outside the uterus.

— If the IUCD is located within the uterus, an attempt can be made to retrieve the thread from the endocervical canal using artery forceps. If unsuccessful, hysteroscopic removal can be undertaken.

— If the IUCD cannot be located within the uterus, the possibilities are expulsion or migration into the peritoneal cavity. Due to the gas shadows caused by the bowel, USG may not be able to pick up the IUCD. Therefore, a plain X-ray should be carried out. IUCD found in the peritoneal cavity is removed through a laparoscope.

Advantages of IUCDs
• Involves less cost and minimal side effects
• Long-acting
• Can be used in the interval period or after an abortion or delivery
• Reversible—immediate return of fertility after removal

Disadvantages of IUCDs
• Needs high motivation to use
• Cannot be used by a woman who has irregular cycles, history of cervical surgery or an STI
• It doesn't offer any protection against sexually transmitted infections

Postpartum IUCD insertion (PPIUCD)
The CuT-380A is approved by the Government of India for immediate postpartum insertion as a method of contraception. The PPIUCD must only be inserted after the woman is counselled and her informed consent is recorded. Counselling should take place in the antenatal period, in early labour or immediately postpartum. Counselling for informed consent should not take place during the active phase of labour.

The PPIUCD can be performed immediately after the delivery of the placenta during a cesarean section or within 48 hours following childbirth. Insertions within 10 minutes of placental delivery are called 'post-placental insertions'. The IUCD must be inserted only by a person who has been trained in immediate PPIUCD according to national standards.

Specific advantages of an IUCD placed in the immediate postpartum period
• Convenience—saves time and additional visit
• Safe—because it is certain that the woman is not pregnant at the time of insertion
• High motivation (woman and family) for a reliable birth spacing method
• Has no risk of uterine perforation because of the thick wall of the uterus
• Reduced perception of initial side effects (bleeding and cramping)
• No effect on the amount or quality of breast milk
• The woman has an effective method for contraception before discharge from the hospital

Limitations of PPIUCD
• Increased risk of spontaneous expulsion—insertion by skilled clinicians with the right technique is associated with lower expulsion rates

Hormonal Contraception
Hormones that are used to prevent pregnancy include estrogens and progestogens. They act by preventing ovulation as well as by making the cervical mucus thick, which prevents the ascent of sperms through the cervical canal into the uterus. By the dual mechanism, hormonal methods prevent the fertilisation of the ova. All hormonal methods can have similar side effects and restrictions on use. There are different modes of administration of hormonal contraceptives (see box).

Routes of administration of hormonal contraceptives
• Oral contraceptives
• Injectable hormonal contraceptives
• Hormone-impregnated IUD (already discussed under intrauterine contraceptive devices)
• Vaginal rings
• Hormonal patches
• Hormonal implants

Oral contraceptives
Oral contraceptives, commonly known as birth control pills contain hormones—either a combination

of progestin and estrogen or progestin alone. The combined oral contraceptive pill was the first oral contraceptive method that was marketed in 1960. In the following decades, newer methods of oral contraception such as progestin-only pills and the non-hormonal pill—centchroman (ormeloxifene)—and emergency contraceptive pills have been popularised. Oral contraceptive methods are highly effective when taken correctly and consistently.

Types of oral contraceptives

There are two types of oral contraceptives—hormonal and non-hormonal.

- **Hormonal:**
  — Combined oral contraceptive (COC), which contains both an estrogen (usually ethinyl estradiol) and progestin
  — Progestin-only pill (POP), which contains only a synthetic analogue (progestin) of progesterone
  — Emergency contraception
- **Non-hormonal Centchroman (ormeloxifene):** This is non-steroidal, non-hormonal method, taken twice a week on fixed days for the first three months and once a week thereafter. It is safe for breastfeeding women.

Combined oral contraceptive pills

Combined oral contraceptive pills contain a highly potent, orally active, synthetic estrogen—ethinyl estradiol—combined with an orally active progestogen. They can be given in a continuous or a sequential fashion. Continuous combined oral pills are available in different formulations.

- Monophasic pill—each tablet contains a fixed amount of estrogen and progestin
- Biphasic pill—each tablet contains a fixed amount of estrogen, while the amount of progestin increases in the second half of the cycle
- Triphasic pill—the amount of estrogen may be fixed or variable, while the amount of progestin increases in three equal phases

In the sequential regimen, estrogen alone is taken for 15/16 days, beginning on the fifth day of the menstrual cycle, and is followed by estrogen plus progestogen in the last five days of the cycle.

The estrogen component of the OC pills

Low-dose pills have less than or equal to 35 µg of ethinyl estradiol (commonly used). High-dose pills contain 50 µg of ethinyl estradiol (not used commonly); ultra-low-dose pills contain 20 µg of ethinyl estradiol. Ultra-low-dose pills are as good at preventing pregnancy as

higher-dose options. They come with a lower risk of side effects such as headaches and fluid retention.

The progestogen component of OC pills

Progestogen compounds of varying potency are in use. Most progestational compounds used in oral contraceptives belong to the 19-norethisterone derivatives group. These include norethisterone, norethynodrel, lynoestrenol and ethynodiol diacetate (Table 64.3).

Table 64.3 Generations of COC pills based on the type of progestin

First-generation pills	• Norethynodrel, norethindrone, norethisterone and ethynodiol • These tablets contain high doses of both estrogen and progestogens
Second-generation pills	• Norgestrel and levonorgestrel (Mala-N, Mala-D) • These tablets have lower doses of hormones
Third-generation pills	• Desogestrel and norgestimate (Novelon, Femilon) • These are less androgenic, have a lesser effect on lipid profile and body weight but have a higher risk of venous thrombosis
Fourth-generation pills	• Drospirenone (Yasmin) • More anti-androgenic property

Mode of administration

When oral contraceptive pills are started for the first time, they are started on the first day of the menstrual cycle. In subsequent cycles, the new pack is started either from the fifth day of withdrawal bleeding or on the 7th day after stopping the pills. The pills should be taken continuously for 21 days without a break. Some preparations have inert tablets or tablets containing iron for 7 days so that the woman can take a pill continuously without a break.

Extended cycle regimen/short pill interval

In order to minimise the number of withdrawal bleeds, the COC is continued beyond 28 days. In this method, the number of bleeding episodes and the amount of bleeding are reduced. Seasonale (84/7), which contains 30 µg of ethinyl estradiol and 150 µg of levonorgestrel, is taken for 84 days with a 7-day drug-free interval.

Mechanism of action

- The mode of action of COC pills is mainly by suppressing ovulation by inhibiting gonadotropin secretion. The progestational agent in the pill primarily suppresses the luteinising hormone (LH), while the estrogenic component suppresses follicle stimulating hormone (FSH) secretion.

- COCs make the endometrium unsuitable for implantation.
- The cervical mucus also becomes scanty and viscous, which impairs sperm transport.

Prescribing oral contraceptives

- Before prescribing an oral contraceptive, detailed medical, social, medication and family history should be taken to determine whether there are any contraindications to the use of oral contraceptives. In those who have not had a pap smear, it should be taken.
- Blood pressure and weight should be measured at the first visit and a breast examination should also be performed. In obese women and those who have medical disorders, blood sugar and triglyceride levels should also be measured.

Contraindications for COC pill use

Combination oral contraceptives (tablets that contain estrogen and a progestin) should not be prescribed in any of the following conditions:

- They should not be prescribed within 21 days of delivery in the general population and within 42 days for women who have risk factors for thrombosis such as obesity and those who have had a cesarean section
- Women who smoke more than 15 cigarettes a day and are older than 35 or obese
- Women with untreated or poorly controlled high blood pressure
- Women who have had diabetes for more than 20 years or have diabetes with complications
- Women above the age of 35 suffering from migraines or women who have migraines with an aura
- Past or current history of deep vein thrombosis or pulmonary embolism
- Women who have coronary artery disease or valvular disease of the heart and those who have a history of peripartum cardiomyopathy in the previous pregnancy
- Active liver disease, cirrhosis or a liver tumour
- Breast/endometrial cancer
- Women who have a very high triglyceride level
- Those who have a gallbladder disorder and those who have had jaundice due to cholestasis
- Other risk factors for thrombosis such as systemic lupus erythematosus
- Family history of coagulation disorders
- Hereditary conditions such as Dubin–Johnson and Rotor syndromes

Relative contraindications include breastfeeding, family history of cardiovascular disease, obesity and hypertension without complications.

Drug interaction and OC pills

Taking certain drugs can make oral contraceptives less effective. These drugs include the following:

- Antiseizure drugs such as phenytoin, carbamazepine and primidone
- Drugs used in the treatment of HIV such as ritonavir
- Antibiotics such as rifampicin, ampicillin and doxycycline
- Antifungals such as griseofulvin and ketoconazole

These drugs induce the synthesis of liver enzymes, which reduce the level of ethinyl estradiol, and thereby, the efficacy of OC pills. If a woman taking oral contraceptives has to take one of these drugs, she should also be asked to use another contraceptive method for the duration for which she is taking the drug and resume the pill after her first period after stopping the drug.

When to start the pill

- Ideally, the OC pill should be started within five days from the start of the menstrual cycle.
- **If it is more than 5 days** after the start of monthly bleeding, combined oral contraceptives (COCs) can be started at any time as long as the woman is reasonably certain that she is not pregnant. However, she will need a **backup method** for the **first seven days** in addition to taking the oral contraceptive pill.
- If a woman is switching from an IUCD, she can start COCs immediately.
- The time for starting combination oral contraceptives after pregnancy varies:
  — After a miscarriage or an abortion during the first trimester of pregnancy, it can be started immediately.
  — Following a second-trimester miscarriage or preterm delivery up to 28 weeks, OC pills can be started within one week.
  — For any delivery after 28 weeks of gestation, OC pills can be started only after 21 days.
  — If a woman is breastfeeding or has risk factors for thrombosis such as obesity or cesarean delivery, it can be started after 42 days. However, COC pills can affect the quality and quantity of breast milk.

Efficacy of COC pills

It is a highly effective contraceptive method with a failure rate is 0.3% if taken as instructed. However, the failure rate increases to 9% if the pill is not taken properly.

Management of missed pills

It is easy to forget a pill or be late in taking it. Therefore, COC users should be instructed on what to do if they forget to take the pills (Table 64.4).

Table 64.4 Management of missed pills

Missed pill	What to do
Missed 1 or 2 pills/started new pack 1 or 2 days late	• Take one hormonal pill as soon as possible or two pills at the scheduled time
Missed 3 or more pills in the first or second week/ started a new pack 3 or more days late	• Take one hormonal pill as soon as possible and continue the scheduled pill • Use a backup method for the next 7 days • Can also consider taking emergency contraceptive pill in case of sex in the past 5 days
Missed 3 or more pills in the third week	• Take one hormonal pill as soon as possible and finish all hormonal pills in the pack as scheduled • Throw away the 7 non-hormonal pills in a 28-pill pack • Start a new pack the next day • Use a backup method for the next 7 days • Also consider using emergency contraception in case of sex in the past 5 days
Severe vomiting or diarrhea after taking the pill	• In case of vomiting within 2 hours after taking a pill, take another pill from the pack as soon as possible and continue taking the scheduled pills • If vomiting or diarrhea continues for more than 2 days, follow instructions for 1 or 2 missed pills above

(Reproduced with permission from Johns Hopkins Bloomberg School of Public Health, WHO and the United States Agency for International development [USAID]. Missed Pills, Family Planning: A Global Handbook for Providers. 2011. Global handbook. atendesigngroup.com/if-you-miss-pills)

Fertility following stopping the pills

Oral contraceptives do not have any long-term effects on fertility, and conception occurs in nearly 60% of women within three months of stopping the pill. In women who have had irregular periods prior to the use of OC pills, after stopping the pills, amenorrhea may continue; this is called 'post-pill amenorrhea'. These women should be investigated for other causes of secondary amenorrhea if it continues beyond six months.

Teratogenic effects

Oral contraceptives inadvertently taken early in pregnancy do not harm the fetus. No increase in fetal malformations or miscarriage is reported. However, the woman should stop using them as soon as she finds out that she is pregnant.

Effect on lactation

COC reduces the quantity of milk and also affects its composition. Therefore, COC should be avoided in lactating mothers, especially in the first six months. Progesterone-only pills are best suited for such women.

Follow-up after COC pills

• The woman should be reviewed after the first withdrawal period to assess the tolerability of the medication and to check whether there were any side effects. If the woman is able to tolerate the pill, the same preparation is continued. Her blood pressure and weight are checked.

• The woman may be reviewed one year later for compliance. At this juncture, besides weight and blood pressure, lipid profile and blood sugar levels are checked.

• If the woman is unable to tolerate the preparation or if there are considerable side effects, an alternate preparation should be considered.

Side effects of COCs

The use of COC may be associated with short-term and long-term side effects. Side effects may be related to the estrognic component or the progestogenic component of the pill (Table 64.5).

Table 64.5 Short-term side effects of combined oral contraceptive pills

Estrogenic side effects	Progestogenic side effects
• Breast tenderness/enlargement • Weight gain (fluid retention) • Nausea • Headache • Bloating • Chloasma • Non-infective vaginal discharge • Photosensitivity • Loss of libido	• Acne • Oily hair • Weight gain (increased appetite) • Hirsutism • Depression/mood swings • Loss of libido • Vaginal dryness

Breakthrough bleeding can occur when a woman forgets to take the tablet or if the estrogen content is low for the particular woman. In such a situation, the estrogen content should be increased. If the breakthrough bleeding persists, it should be evaluated for pathological causes such as endometrial polyps, cervical lesions, etc.

Long-term side effects

Taking oral contraceptives for a long time and in high doses increases the risk of developing various conditions.

- Venous and arterial thrombosis:
  - With long-term use, the risk of developing deep vein thrombosis (DVT) may be 2–4 times higher for women who are taking combination oral contraceptives than it was before they started taking the contraceptives. However, the risk of developing DVT is much lower in the general population using contraceptive pills than the risk of developing DVT during pregnancy. In those with a personal or family history of thromboembolic disease, combined oral contraceptives are absolutely contraindicated. Women who develop thromboembolic disease while on combined pills should be investigated for thrombophilias.
  - Obese women who have diabetes or hypertension and those who smoke are at an increased risk of myocardial infarction/stroke. For healthy women who do not smoke, taking low-dose combination tablets with a low dose of estrogen does not increase the risk of having a stroke or heart attack.
- Genital tract malignancy:
  - Women who have ever used oral contraceptives have a slightly increased relative risk of breast cancer compared to women who had never used oral contraceptives. This increase is seen especially with long-term oral contraceptive pill use.
- Women who have used oral contraceptives for five or more years have a higher risk of cervical cancer than women who have never used oral contraceptives. Pill users should have regular pap smear screening.
- Gall bladder and liver disease:
  - There may be a small increase in the incidence of gallstones in those on combined pills, but the risk is very less in women taking low-dose oral contraceptives.
  - Taking oral contraceptives for a long time and in high doses increases the risk of developing hepatocellular adenoma with the associated risk of rupture and bleeding. The tumour usually disappears after the pill is stopped.
- Effect on carbohydrate and lipid metabolism:
  - The progestogen content of combined pills may increase insulin resistance and LDL.
  - By increasing the angiotensinogen levels, estrogen may increase blood pressure; however, the effect is minimal with low-dose pills.

Non-contraceptive benefits of COCs

Other than for contraceptive purposes, OC pills are used in a number of gynecological conditions.

- Menstrual cycle regularity
- Treatment of dysmenorrhea
- In the management of abnormal uterine bleeding due to ovulatory dysfunction in adolescent girls, PCOS and in perimenopausal women
- To reduce blood loss and improve iron deficiency anemia
- Prevention of menstrual migraines
- Treatment of acne and hirsutism
- In the management of premenstrual syndrome
- In the management of benign breast disorders
- Treatment of pelvic pain due to endometriosis
- In the management of heavy bleeding due to leiomyoma
- OC pill use decreases the risk of endometrial, ovarian and colorectal cancers
- As prophylaxis in young women with a family history of hereditary ovarian cancer
- For improved bone mineral density in older women

Progesterone-only pill (POP)

It is also called the 'mini pill'. The progesterone-only pill does not contain estrogen. It contains a very low-dose of synthetic progestin—levonorgestrel or desogestrel. The available preparation is Cerazette, which contains 75 µg of desogestrel. The tablet is taken every day, without a pill-free interval. Effectiveness depends on the regular intake of POP at the same time every day (within a window of three hours). It is safe to use in breastfeeding women and can be started in <6 weeks after delivery. Progestin-only oral contraceptives may be taken immediately after the delivery of a baby.

Mechanism of action

- The POP makes the cervical mucus thick and prevents the entry of sperm.
- It also inhibits ovulation.
- By causing endometrial atrophy, it prevents implantation.
- It inhibits follicular development, leading to amenorrhea.

Failure rate

If taken every day at the same time and correctly used, the failure rate is less than 0.3%; with typical use, the failure rate is 9%.

Indications

- In lactating mothers, it can be safely used as it does not affect milk production and composition.

- It can also be used by women in whom estrogen is contraindicated (refer to the section on COC pills).

Disadvantages

- It has to be taken daily at the same time, and its efficacy depends largely upon the user's memory. The newer POP-containing desogestrel offers a margin of 12 hours in contrast to the three-hour grace period earlier available with conventional POPs.
- Menstrual abnormalities may occur such as a delay in the return of menstruation in breastfeeding women (lengthened postpartum amenorrhea), frequent, prolonged bleeding, infrequent, irregular bleeding and amenorrhea.
- The other side effects include nausea, headaches, dizziness and mood swings and enlarged ovarian follicles in those who are not breastfeeding.
- If more than 27 hours go by between tablets, the woman should be asked to take a backup contraceptive method for the next 7 days in addition to taking the progestin-only contraceptive each day.

Non-hormonal oral contraceptive (Centchroman)

Centchroman (ormeloxifene), also known as Chhaya or Saheli, is a non-steroidal, non-hormonal oral contraceptive that is taken once a week for spacing. It acts as a selective estrogen receptor modulator (SERM). In some tissues/organs of the body, it has weak estrogenic action (e.g., bones), while in others such as the uterus and breasts, it has strong anti-estrogenic action. It is available as a 30 mg tablet.

For initiation of the centchroman (ormeloxifene), the first pill should be taken on the first day of the period (as indicated by the first day of bleeding) and the second pill should be taken three days later. This pattern of days is repeated through the first three months. Starting from the fourth month, the pill is to be taken once a week on the first pill day and should be continued on the weekly schedule regardless of the woman's menstrual cycle. This OC is safe for lactating women.

Side effects

Centchroman causes delayed periods in a few women. However, this occurs in only around 8% of users and usually in the first three months. The periods tend to settle into a rhythm once the body gets used to the drug. Periods can get scanty over time in some women.

Emergency contraception

Emergency contraception or postcoital contraception refers to methods that can be used in the first few days after unprotected sexual intercourse to prevent an unwanted pregnancy. It is not a substitute for contraception and should not be used for that purpose. Women should be counselled that emergency contraception is for emergency use only and is not meant to use as an ongoing contraceptive method.

Indications

- For emergency use following unprotected sexual intercourse
- Sexual assault, when the woman was not protected by an effective contraceptive method
- When there is concern of possible contraceptive failure, from improper or incorrect use, such as:
  — Condom breakage, slippage or incorrect use
  — Three or more consecutively missed combined oral contraceptive pills
  — Delay for more than three hours in taking the progestogen-only pill (minipill)
  — More than 2 weeks late for the norethisterone enanthate (NET-EN) progestogen-only injection
  — More than 4 weeks late for the depot-medroxyprogesterone acetate (DMPA) progestogen-only injection
  — More than 7 days late for the combined injectable contraceptive (CIC)
  — Dislodgment, breakage, tearing, or early removal of a diaphragm or cervical cap
  — Expulsion of an intrauterine contraceptive device (IUD)

Methods of emergency contraception (Table 64.6)

The four methods of emergency contraception are as follows:

- Emergency contraceptive pills containing LNG
- Emergency contraceptive pills containing ulipristal acetate
- Combined oral contraceptive pills
- Copper-bearing intrauterine devices

Emergency contraceptive pill containing levonorgestrel (LNG)

- The emergency contraceptive pill with LNG is taken as a single dose of 1.5 mg; alternatively, LNG is taken in 2 doses of 0.75 mg each, 12 hours apart.
- It can be taken within up to 120 hours of unprotected sexual intercourse; however, it is most effective if taken within 72 hours.
- It acts by preventing or delaying ovulation. It can also act by making the cervical mucus hostile for the transportation of sperm.

- Caution should be exercised in women taking enzyme-inducing drugs such as phenytoin or rifampicin, as there is a risk of a higher failure rate.
- Contraindications include hypersensitivity to LNG, acute porphyria and severe liver disease.
- Emergency contraception containing LNG can be safely used during lactation.
- Side effects include nausea, vomiting, dizziness and delayed menstruation.

Emergency contraceptive pill containing ulipristal acetate

- Ulipristal acetate is a synthetic, orally active selective progesterone receptor modulator.
- It acts by inhibiting or delaying ovulation.
- It is used in a single dose of 30 mg within 5 days of the earliest episode of unprotected sexual intercourse, regardless of the number of coital acts within those 120 hours.
- Ulipristal is not recommended in women with severe hepatic impairment or asthma poorly controlled by oral glucocorticoids.
- Liver enzyme-inducing drugs may reduce plasma concentrations of ulipristal and thereby, efficacy.
- It cannot be used during breastfeeding. If inadvertently taken, breast milk should be expressed and discarded for 7 days.

Combined ethinyl estradiol and levonorgestrel (Yuzpe method)

- In situations where LNG or ulipristal are unavailable and the individual does not wish to use a copper-bearing intrauterine device, a combined oral contraceptive pill can be used within 72 hours of unprotected sexual intercourse.
- The dose of ethinyl estradiol should be 100 μg and that of LNG should be 0.5 mg. Two doses are given 12 hours apart. As separate packs are unavailable in these doses for emergency contraception purposes, four tablets of any contraceptive preparation containing levonorgestrel 150 μg and ethinyl estradiol 30 μg are given. 12 hours later, another four tablets are repeated. This regimen can be associated with severe nausea and vomiting and is not suitable for women in whom estrogen is contraindicated.

Emergency contraception using mifepristone

Mifepristone is a progesterone antagonist. It acts by preventing ovulation and implantation. Different dose regimens are recommended ranging from 10–600 mg given as a single dose within 72 hours of unprotected sexual intercourse. A low dose of mifepristone has been shown to be as effective as high doses with minimal side effects. The side effect of this treatment may be a delay in the onset of menstruation.

Copper-bearing intrauterine contraceptive devices (IUCDs)

- A copper IUCD can be inserted up to 5 days after the first episode of unprotected sexual intercourse.
- The mechanism of action is based on the direct toxicity of copper ions on sperms which inhibits fertilisation and the effect of the device on the endometrium which inhibits implantation.
- When used within 5 days of unprotected intercourse, the failure rate of the copper IUCD as a contraceptive is less than 1%.
- Once inserted, women can continue to use the IUCD as an ongoing method of contraception.
- Contraindications include PID, puerperal sepsis and unexplained vaginal bleeding.
- Copper-bearing IUCDs should not be inserted for emergency contraception following sexual assault as the woman may be at high risk of a sexually transmitted infection such as chlamydia and gonorrhea.

General points for women receiving emergency contraception

- The woman should be informed that her next period may be on time, early or late.
- She should be advised that if there is a delay of more than 7 days in the onset of menstrual bleeding, it would be appropriate to take a pregnancy test.
- She should be advised to see a doctor immediately if she develops lower abdominal pain (the possibility of ectopic pregnancy should be considered).
- The woman should be counselled about a more definitive method of contraception for the future.
- The woman should be forewarned that the method does not provide contraceptive protection for the remaining part of the cycle and that she should immediately use an alternative method.
- If she becomes pregnant following the use of emergency contraception, the woman should be assured that levonorgestrel or LNG+EE used for emergency contraception has no adverse effect on pregnancy and that teratogenicity has not been reported. Teratogenicity of ulipristal is not known.

Table 64.6 Emergency contraceptive methods

Method	Timing	Dose	Efficacy
LNG pill	Up to 120 hours after unprotected sexual intercourse (Efficacy is more if used within 72 hours)	Single dose of 1.5 mg can be used or 0.75 mg in 2 doses can be given 12 hours apart	98%
Ulipristal acetate	As soon as possible within 5 days of the earliest episode of unprotected sexual intercourse, regardless of the number of coital acts within those 120 hours	Single oral dose of 30 mg	99% if used within 5 days of unprotected sexual intercourse
Copper IUD	Up to 5 days after the first episode of unprotected sexual intercourse		99% if used within 72 hours of unprotected sexual intercourse

Injectable Contraceptives

Injectable contraceptives include:

1. Progestogen-only injectables (POI) containing only synthetic progesterone; these are of two types:
   - Depot medroxyprogesterone acetate (DMPA) given as three-monthly injections
   - Norethisterone enanthate (NET-EN) given as two-monthly injections
2. Combined injectable contraceptive (CIC)—contain estrogen (usually ethinylestradiol) and progesterone and are given as monthly injections

Depot medroxyprogesterone acetate (DMPA) injectable contraceptive

- DMPA injectable contraceptive (ANTARA) is included under the National Family Planning programme
- Depo-Provera (DMPA) comes as microcrystals suspended in an aqueous solution. The dosage for contraceptive purposes is 150 mg given intramuscularly (gluteal or deltoid) every three months. The injection must be given deeply by the **Z-track technique.**

Mechanism of action

- It acts by inhibiting ovulation by suppressing mid-cycle peaks of LH and FSH.
- It causes the thickening of the cervical mucus, thereby preventing sperm penetration into the upper reproductive tract.
- It causes the thinning of the endometrial lining, making it unfavourable for the implantation of the fertilised ovum.

When to start

- A DMPA injection can be started any day within 7 days of the beginning of the menstrual cycle with no need for a backup method.
- It can also be started any time later in the menstrual cycle (after 7 days) if it is reasonably certain that the woman is not pregnant (no history of unprotected sex since LMP). However, in such cases, the woman will need a backup method (e.g., condom) for the first 7 days after the injection.
- It can be started in the postpartum period in breastfeeding women.

Contraindications

It is absolutely contraindicated in the following scenarios:
- Women with unexplained genital bleeding
- Severe coagulation disorders
- Previous sex steroid-induced liver adenoma
  Relative contraindications include:
- Liver disease
- Severe cardiovascular disease

Efficacy

It is a highly effective contraceptive method. With a standard regimen, the first-year effectiveness is 99.7% when the drug is used correctly; however, the effectiveness decreases with typical use. The perfect use failure rate of 0.3% is lower in comparison to female sterilisation (0.5%), IUCD (0.8%) and combined oral contraceptives (0.3%) (WHO, Family Planning: A Global Handbook for Providers).

Advantages

- Injectable contraceptives are suitable for women who are breastfeeding.
- They are suitable for women who are not eligible to use estrogen-containing combined oral contraceptives.
- Unlike combination oral contraceptives, progestin injections do not increase the risk of high blood pressure.

- Interactions with other drugs are uncommon; therefore, these may be a good choice for women with seizure disorders.

Side effects of DMPA

The major problems are irregular menstrual bleeding. Up to 25% of patients discontinue usage in the first year due to menstrual problems.

- **Changes in bleeding patterns in the first three months**
  - Irregular bleeding
  - Prolonged bleeding
- **Changes at one year**
  - Amenorrhea
  - Infrequent bleeding
  - Irregular bleeding
- DMPA may cause a delay in the return of fertility, which may be delayed upto 7–10 months from the date of the last injection.
- Other side effects include breast tenderness, headache, weight gain, abdominal bloating, transient loss of bone density, loss of libido, mood changes and depression.

Non-contraceptive benefits of DMPA

- Improves anemia by reducing menstrual blood loss in AUB
- Reduces the symptoms of endometriosis
- Decreases benign breast disease
- Medroxyprogesterone acetate does not increase the risk of developing breast, ovarian or invasive cervical cancer
- Protects against endometrial cancer and possibly, ovarian cancer

Injectables containing a combination of estrogen and progesterone

This combination is given to overcome the problem of irregular menstrual bleeding. It is available as Cyclo-Provera or Cyclofem. This injectable consists of 25 mg DMPA and 5 mg of estradiol cypionate. It is administered monthly as a deep intramuscular injection. This method is as effective as Depo-Provera, but is not associated with menstrual irregularity. The method is rapidly reversible.

Contraceptive Implants

The subdermal implant system is a long-acting, low-dose, reversible, progestin-only method of contraception. Insertion and removal of these implants

have to be performed by the physician. Single-rod implants are easier to insert and remove as compared to the set of six capsules. The first progestin-only contraceptive implant was Norplant. Different types of implants have been in use over the years. These include:

- Norplant-containing: Six capsules or rods
- Jadelle and Norplant-2: Containing two rods
- Implanon: Containing one rod

Norplant

The Norplant system consists of six capsules containing a total of 216 mg of levonorgestrel (each capsule contains 36 mg levonorgestrel) (Fig. 64.10). Each capsule measures 34 mm in length with a 2.4 mm outer diameter. The capsules release approximately 85 µg of levonorgestrel every 24 hours during the first 6–12 months of use. The rate declines gradually to 50 µg by 9 months and 30 µg per day for the remaining duration of use. The system delivers a sustained level of levonorgestrel for a long time (up to 7 years), though its use is approved for only five years.

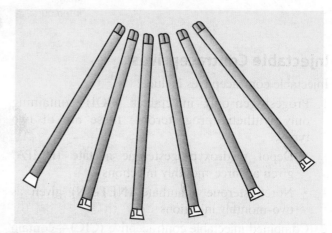

Fig. 64.10 Norplant

Norplant-2

This implant consists of two levonorgestrel rods. Each rod measures 43 mm in length and 2.5 mm in diameter; it contains 75 mg of the drug and releases the drug at the same dosage as the six capsules.

Implanon

This is a long-acting, single-rod subdermal implant (Fig. 64.11). The rod measures 4 cm in length and 2 mm in diameter. The core of the implant contains 68 mg of crystalline etonogestrel, dispersed in a matrix of ethylene vinyl acetate copolymer. The initial release rate is 60–70 µg per day and declines to 25–30 µg at the end of the third year. Its use is recommended for 3 years.

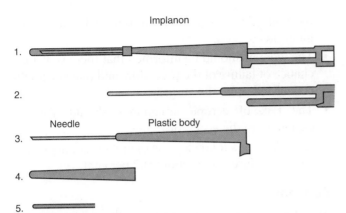

Fig. 64.11 Implanon

Mechanism of action of implants

Implants like Depo-Provera produce a sustained release of progestin, which inhibits ovulation and thickens the cervical mucus. An implant can also be inserted immediately after a miscarriage, an abortion or the delivery of a baby.

Side effects

The side effects include menstrual disturbance and weight gain, headaches, nausea, breast tenderness, mood swings and irregular bleeding. These are temporary and are seen during the first few months. For immediate protection, another mode of effective contraception must be used for at least seven days following insertion.

Advantage

High effectiveness of up to 99% within seven days of implant insertion provides long-term continuous contraception independent of user memory and sexual intercourse.

Transdermal Contraceptive Patch

A contraceptive transdermal patch releases estrogen and progesterone directly into the skin. Each patch contains a 1-week supply of hormones, both norelgestromin and ethinyl estradiol. It releases a sustained low daily dose of steroids—150 µg norelgestromin and 20 µg ethinyl estradiol—equivalent to the lowest-dose oral contraceptive. The patch is removed and replaced with a new patch every week and is used consecutively for three weeks; no patch is used during the fourth week, allowing time for withdrawal.

The advantages of this method include greater compliance and fewer adverse effects such as nausea and vomiting due to the avoidance of the first-pass effect. However, the patch may cause skin irritation, and if removal goes unnoticed, it may compromise efficacy. The patch may be less effective in overweight women. If more than two days go without using the patch, the woman should use a backup contraceptive method for seven days in addition to the patch. If two days go by and the woman has had unprotected intercourse in the five days before those two days, the woman should consider emergency contraception.

Vaginal Rings

A vaginal ring is a small, flexible, soft, transparent device that is placed in the vagina.

Two types of rings are available:

- One that must be replaced each month
- One that must be replaced only once a year

Both types are left in place for three weeks and then not used for one week to allow the menstrual period to occur. A woman can place and remove the vaginal ring herself. Usually, the vaginal ring is not felt by the woman's partner during intercourse. The ring does not dissolve and cannot be pushed too far up.

A flexible vaginal ring (NUVARING) is available that releases 120 µg of etonogestrel (a progestin) and 15 µg of ethinyl estradiol (an estrogen) each day of use. The ring is inserted into the vagina for a three-week period, then removed for one week, during which time, the woman has a menstrual period.

Annovera (segesterone acetate and ethinyl estradiol) vaginal system is the first vaginal ring contraceptive that can be used for an entire year. Annovera is a reusable donut-shaped (ring), non-biodegradable, flexible vaginal system that is placed in the vagina for three weeks followed by one week out of the vagina, at which time women may experience a period (a withdrawal bleed). This schedule is repeated every four weeks for one year.

Usually, there are no side effects. If women use a patch or a ring for 3 weeks (replacing it each week), followed by 1 week when no patch or ring is used, they typically have a regular menstrual period. Spotting or bleeding between periods (breakthrough bleeding) is uncommon.

▌ PERMANENT CONTRACEPTIVE METHODS

Permanent contraception includes vasectomy for men and tubal procedures for women, which are highly effective.

Female Sterilisation

For women who have decided not to have any more children, tubal sterilisation is one of the best and most effective methods. Sterilisation of the woman can be carried out at any time and also as a postpartum procedure.

Case selection

- Clients should be married (including ever-married).
- Female clients should be below the age of 45 years and above the age of 22 years.
- The couple should have at least one healthy child whose age is above one year unless the sterilisation is medically indicated.
- Clients or their spouses/partners must not have undergone sterilisation in the past (not applicable in cases of failure of previous sterilisation).
- Clients must be in a normal state of mind so as to understand the full implications of sterilisation.
- Mentally ill clients must be certified by a psychiatrist, and consent should be given by a legal guardian/ spouse.

Timing of the surgical procedure

- Interval sterilisation should be performed within seven days of the menstrual period (in the follicular phase of the menstrual cycle).
- Postpartum sterilisation should be done after 48 hours up to seven days of delivery.
- Concurrent sterilisation can be done during a cesarean section, medical termination of pregnancy (MTP) or other surgeries like ovarian cystectomy.

Postpartum sterilisation

- It is customary to perform the operation within the first 72–96 hours of delivery. The uterus during this period is well above the symphysis and the chances of infection are less. Another advantage of postpartum sterilisation is that, if performed within the first 72 hours of delivery, it does not prolong hospital stay unnecessarily.
- Prior to the surgery, medical history, menstrual and obstetric history should be taken and physical examination and laboratory investigations should be performed as needed to ensure the eligibility of the client for surgery.

Counselling

- Counselling before surgery is important but is often missed. It should be emphasised to the acceptor that for all practical purposes, tubal sterilisation is a permanent procedure. The success rate of

recanalisation procedures (if required) cannot be guaranteed.
- The woman should be informed that there is a small chance of failure of the procedure and that she might conceive despite the surgery.
- The risk of ectopic pregnancy should also be explained to the acceptor.
- Complications following the operation are negligible and the failure rate is about 0.2 per cent.

Consent

After the woman fully understands the implications of permanent methods of sterilisation, consent is taken from the woman while she is mentally stable; the husband's signature is not required.

Routes of performing tubal sterilisation

- Female sterilisation can be carried out through a mini-laparotomy, laparotomy, laparoscopy or hysteroscopy. Occasionally, it is carried out by the vaginal route concurrently along with a vaginal procedure such as prolapse repair.
- In the postpartum period, tubectomy is carried out through a mini-laparotomy incision.

Technique of tubal sterilisation

- While the modified Pomeroy's technique is the preferred method, any standard method of tubal sterilisation is permitted.
- The laparoscopic methods include the use of Fallope rings, Filshie clips and diathermy. However, the Fallope ring is the preferred method of ligation during laparoscopic tubal ligation in India.

Modified Pomeroy's technique

The modified Pomeroy technique is the most commonly used method for occluding the fallopian tubes. The basic concept of the technique is to pick up a loop of fallopian tube in an avascular area, tie a knot at the base of the loop and excise the loop of the tube above the ligature. Care should be taken to minimise tissue destruction. Absorbable suture material should be used.

Steps of the procedure for postpartum sterilisation:

- The woman is prepared as for any major abdominal surgery.
- The operation can be carried out under local, spinal or general anesthesia. The best practice is to sedate the patient with good pre-medication and operate under local infiltration anesthesia using 0.5–1% novocaine or lignocaine.

- The fundus of the uterus is identified. As the tubal take-off is below the level of the fundus, a small, transverse skin incision is made 2–2.5 cm below the level of the fundus of the uterus. After opening the peritoneal cavity, the tubes are identified under direct vision and brought out of the peritoneal cavity by holding them with **Babcock's forceps** or other suitable **atraumatic tissue forceps** as needed

- The operating surgeon should identify each fallopian tube clearly, following it right up to the fimbria. It is essential to **identify the tubes** by visualising the fimbrial end, as otherwise, the round ligaments which are anterior to the tubes may be mistaken for the latter and resected.

- The site of the occlusion of the fallopian tube must always be within 2–3 cm from the uterine cornu in the isthmal portion, so that after resection, a fair length of the tube with its fimbria remains (should the couple desire another pregnancy, there will then be a sufficient length of tube for **re-anastomosis** or **recanalisation**).

- After identifying the tube, it is picked up to form a loop. The base of the loop is tied with 1–0 chromic catgut suture passed through the mesosalpinx, avoiding the blood vessels. The knuckle of the tube so isolated is then cut off.

- 1 cm of the tube is removed, and the ends are ligated. The suture material should be absorbable; 1-0 chromic catgut is commonly used. Delayed absorbable sutures should be avoided. The use of cautery and crushing of the tube should be avoided as they can cause extensive tubal damage.

- The process is repeated on the other side and the abdomen is closed.

- The overall **failure rate** in tubal sterilisation using various techniques is 0.5%; with Pomeroy's technique, it is about 0.2%.

Vaginal tubal ligation

Tubal sterilisation can also be performed **per vaginum**, but never as a postpartum procedure. This procedure is not commonly performed as the risk of pelvic inflammatory disease is higher. However, vaginal tubal ligation is performed with other vaginal operations like the Manchester operation for uterine prolapse.

Laparoscopic sterilisation

Tubal sterilisation through a laparoscope is popular all over the world. In India, it is widely used as a routine procedure and also in mass programmes. A ring or band is applied over a knuckle of the tube by an applicator through a laparoscope and under vision (Fig. 64.12a and b). In many cases, this can be done in a short time. Only one stitch is required over the wound, following which, the woman can go home the same day or the next day.

General anesthesia is usually used for laparoscopic sterilisation. Although unipolar electrosurgical techniques were popular in the early days of laparoscopic sterilisation, this method was abandoned due to an increased risk of surgical complications. The most common techniques used today include bipolar cautery, the Filshie clip, and the silastic band (Fallope ring). Laparoscopic sterilisation should not be done in the postpartum period and following second-trimester abortions due to surrounding edema. The Government of India does not approve cautery for tubal sterilisation at the time of laparoscopy.

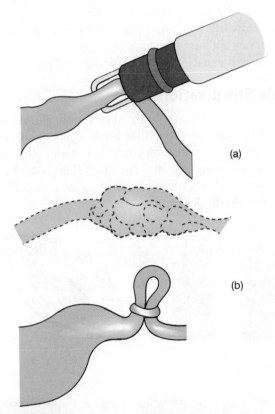

(a)

(b)

Fig. 64.12 Laparoscopic sterilisation by silastic band (Fallope ring): (a) The tube is picked up with an operating laparoscope so as to push the silastic band into the loop of the tube and (b) a silastic band is placed on the tube

Mini-lap sterilisation

In interval cases and in patients undergoing MTP, the same Pomeroy's technique of tubal ligation can be employed. Even though the uterus is not palpable, as in puerperal cases, the operation can be done easily with some training. A pre-op packing of the vagina or elevation of the uterus using a uterine elevator can help in pushing the uterus out of the pelvis. Then, the tubes can be easily identified. The only difference is that a small incision is made just above the pubic hair line. Precautions like emptying the bladder are important.

Failure of operation leading to pregnancy

This may be due to either a technical deficiency in the surgical procedure such as a round ligament being mistaken for a fallopian tube or due to spontaneous recanalisation.

Hysteroscopy

Sterilisation using the Essure device involves the introduction of a microinsert device transcervically through a hysteroscope. The device is placed in the proximal portion of the fallopian tube. Over time, the device causes tissue ingrowth and permanent tubal occlusion. As with vasectomy, another method of birth control must be used to prevent pregnancy until occlusion is confirmed.

Male Sterilisation

A vasectomy (male sterilisation) is a surgical procedure to cut or seal the tubes that carry a man's sperm to permanently prevent pregnancy. It is easier than tubal sterilisation and equally effective (Fig. 64.13a–d). Vasectomy is less expensive and has a lower failure rate than female sterilisation.

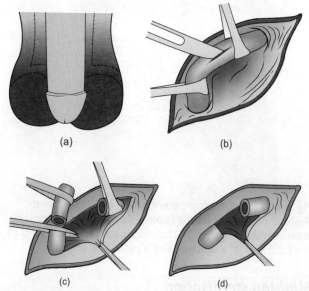

(a) (b)

(c) (d)

Fig. 64.13 Steps of vasectomy: (a) Incisions are made on the skin (b) the sheath of the vas is cut open, (c) a portion of the vas is removed and (d) the vas is ligated at the cut ends

No-scalpel vasectomy

No-scalpel vasectomy is a simple method of performing vasectomy; it is now being advocated by the Government of India to promote male sterilisation. In this procedure, after local anesthesia, instead of making an incision, the skin of the scrotum is pierced with specially designed dissection forceps at the level of the junction of the middle and upper thirds of the median raphe. The puncture is enlarged with dissecting forceps; the vas deferens is held in position and lifted out of the skin opening with a 'fixing clamp'. Each vas can be occluded through the same skin opening by ligation, heat or by using a clamp.

Advantages

- Male sterilisation is intended to provide lifelong, permanent and very effective protection against pregnancy.
- It involves a safe, simple surgical procedure.
- It does not affect male sexual performance.

Disadvantages

- The contraceptive efficacy starts only after 3 months.
- The couple must use condoms or another contraceptive method for three or more months until semen analysis shows azoospermia after the vasectomy.

▌CONTRACEPTION IN MEDICAL DISORDERS

Seizure Disorder

- The concurrent use of COCs and hepatic enzyme-inducing anti-convulsants can affect the contraceptive's efficacy. There may also be increased seizure risk (for example, with lamotrigine). Depo-Provera can be used in such cases since it does not undergo first-pass metabolism.
- LNG-IUCDs, copper IUCDs and barrier methods are safe.
- Women with migraines and facial neurological symptoms or other risk factors for stroke (smoker, >35 years) should be counselled to use IUCDs, barriers or POP.

Obesity

COCs when used in cases of obesity, increase the risk of venous thromboembolism. LNG-IUCDs provide protection against pregnancy and endometrial hyperplasia associated with obesity.

Diabetes Mellitus

Combined oral contraceptives are safe for use in women with type I and II diabetes mellitus without nephropathy, retinopathy, hypertension or other cardiovascular risk factors. IUCDs and POPs are safe in women with diabetes.

Human Immunodeficiency Virus Infection

Caution should be exercised while prescribing COCs to women on antiretroviral therapy (ART), which increase or decrease the efficacy of contraceptive steroids. IUCDs are efficacious and do not increase the risk to women with HIV and their partners. However, the risk of infection should be kept in mind. DMPA can also be prescribed.

Systemic Lupus Erythematosus

COCs are safe for women who have systemic lupus erythematosus if the disease is mild and there is no antiphospholipid syndrome. IUCDs are also safe.

Sickle Cell Disease

DMPA use is associated with the inhibition of sickling and improvement of anemia. Low-dose OCPs can also be given.

▌EFFICACY OF VARIOUS CONTRACEPTIVES (Table 64.7)

The pearl index is used for measuring the effectiveness of a contraceptive method. It is defined as the number of contraception failures (pregnancies) per 100 woman years (HWY) of exposure. It is calculated by the formula:

$$\text{Pearl index} = \frac{\text{Number of pregnancies} \times 1{,}200}{(\text{Patients observed} \times \text{Months of exposure})}$$

- The efficacy of a contraceptive method is high if the pearl index is less than 10.
- The efficacy of a contraceptive method is low if the pearl index is more than 10.

▌NATIONAL FAMILY PLANNING PROGRAMMES

- India was the first country in the world to have launched a National Programme for Family Planning in 1952.
- For improved access to contraceptives and family planning services in high-fertility districts spreading

Table 64.7 Percentage of women with an unintended pregnancy within the first year of contraception use (modified from Trussell et al.)

Method	Perfect use (%) (theoretical effectiveness)	Typical use (%) ('real-world' effectiveness)
Vasectomy	0.10	0.10
Tubal sterilisation	0.50	0.50
Progestogen subdermal implant	0.05	0.05
LNG-IUS	0.20	0.20
Cu-IUCD	0.60	0.80
DMPA injection	0.20	6.00
Progestogen-only pill	0.30	9.00
Combined hormonal contraception pill/ring/patch	0.30	9.00
Condom	2.00	18.00
Diaphragm	6.00	12.00
Fertility awareness	0.40–5.00	24.00
No contraception	85.00	85.00

(*Cu-IUCD*, copper intrauterine contraceptive device; *DMPA*, depot-medroxyprogesterone acetate; *LNG-IUS*, levonorgestrel-containing intrauterine system)

over seven high-focus states, the Ministry of Health and Family Welfare launched '**Mission Pariwar Vikas**' in 2016.

- Special attention has been given to 146 high-fertility districts of **Bihar, Uttar Pradesh, Assam, Chhattisgarh, Madhya Pradesh, Rajasthan and Jharkhand** with an aim to ensure the availability of contraceptive methods at all the levels of healthcare systems.
- The overall goal of this programme is to reduce India's fertility rate to 2.1 by the year 2025.
- **Postpartum Sterilisation Programmes:**
  — Postpartum IUCDs, including postplacental insertion
  — Injectable contraceptives, MPA (medroxy-progesterone acetate) under the Antara programme
  — The government has initiated efforts to expand oral contraceptive options by including progestin-only pills and centchroman (ormeloxifene) in the national programme and providing them through the public health delivery system

KEY POINTS

✓ *Temporary methods of contraception include natural methods, barrier methods, oral contraceptives, intrauterine contraceptive devices, injectables and implants. Male and female sterilisation are permanent methods.*

✓ *Diaphragm, cervical cap, female condom and spermicides are barrier methods used by women; the condom is the barrier method used by men. The male condom provides protection against STIs including HIV.*

✓ *IUCDs containing copper and low-dose oral contraceptives are provided free by the National Family Welfare Programme in India.*

✓ *Progesterone-containing injectables and implants are associated with menstrual irregularity.*

✓ *Female sterilisation can be performed in the postpartum period or following MTP. Laparoscopic sterilisation is performed in the non-pregnant state or after first-trimester MTP.*

✓ *Male sterilisation has been made easier with non-scalpel vasectomy (NSV).*

✓ *Emergency contraception can be used as a backup method after unprotected coitus and is effective if used within 72 hours.*

Essay questions

1. Discuss in detail the natural methods of contraception.
2. What is a copper-T? What is its mechanism of action? List the various copper-containing contraceptive devices.
3. What are the different types of oral contraceptives available? Describe their mechanism of action and non-contraceptive benefits.

Short answer questions

1. List the temporary and permanent methods of contraception.
2. Discuss the various types of injectable contraceptives and implants that are available.
3. List the various methods of female sterilisation.
4. Describe postpartum sterilisation.
5. What is emergency contraception? Describe the various methods available.
6. Describe the contraceptive choices for a woman who has:
   a) Diabetes mellitus
   b) Seizure disorder
   c) HIV infection
7. Describe the non-contraceptive benefits of COCs and LNG-IUCDs.
8. Discuss non-scalpel vasectomy.
9. Describe the contraceptive choices for a newly married woman.

MCQs

1. Which of the following is not a barrier method of contraception?
   a) Today sponge
   b) Female condom
   c) Diaphragm
   d) Implanon
2. Non-oxynol-9 is a:
   a) Barrier contraceptive
   b) Emergency contraceptive
   c) Hormonal contraceptive
   d) IUCD
3. In a woman with a regular 28-day menstrual cycle, what is the safe period?
   a) First 14 days of a menstrual cycle
   b) Last 14 days of a menstrual cycle
   c) First seven days of a menstrual cycle
   d) First and last 7 days of a menstrual cycle
4. The best contraceptive choice in lactating women is:
   a) Barrier method
   b) Lactational amenorrhea method
   c) Progesterone-only pill
   d) Continuous combined oral contraceptive pill
5. What is the minimum effective dose of ethinyl estradiol required for contraception in oral contraceptive pills?
   a) 20 µg
   b) 30 µg
   c) 35 µg
   d) 50 µg
6. Regarding the use of oral contraceptives, all the following are true except:
   a) Increases the risk of myocardial infarction in smoking and obese women
   b) Increases the risk of endometrial carcinoma
   c) Decreases the risk of ovarian carcinoma
   d) Increases the risk of venous thromboembolism
7. The following are the absolute contraindications for oral contraceptive pills except:
   a) Past history of deep vein thrombosis
   b) Past history of cerebrovascular accident
   c) Active viral hepatitis
   d) Diabetes mellitus
8. Regarding DMPA, all the following are true except:
   a) Safe in lactating women
   b) Safe to use in seizure disorders
   c) Acts by inhibiting ovulation
   d) There is a quick return of fertility after discontinuing DMPA
9. All the following are used for emergency contraception except:
   a) Levonorgestrel pill
   b) LNG–IUS
   c) Copper T
   d) Ulipristal
10. The life span of Copper-380A is:
    a) 1 year
    b) 3 years
    c) 5 years
    d) 10 years

11. The site of ligation of the tube in female sterilisation is the:
    a) Fimbrial end
    b) Cornual end
    c) Isthmus
    d) Ampullary region
12. The contraceptive choice for a woman with a past history of ectopic pregnancy is:
    a) Oral contraceptive pills
    b) IUCD
    c) Barrier methods
    d) Progesterone-only pill
13. Barrier methods of contraception used by the woman include all the following EXCEPT
    a) Diaphragm
    b) Cervical cap
    c) Female condom
    d) Intrauterine device
14. The amount of ethinyl estradiol in the first-generation oral contraceptives is:
    a) 50 µg
    b) 40 µg
    c) 30 µg
    d) 20 µg

Answers

1. (d), 2. (a), 3. (d), 4. (c), 5. (a), 6. (b), 7. (d), 8. (d), 9. (b), 10. (d), 11. (c), 12. (a), 13. (d), 14. (a)

Fill in the blanks

1. In India, the National Family Planning Programme was launched in _____.
2. The set of guidelines published by the WHO which help in decision-making as to the suitability of a particular contraceptive method to the client are called the _____.

Answers

1. 1952, 2. medical eligibility criteria

Case scenario-based discussion

1. A 24-year-old unmarried woman presents with a history of having had unprotected sexual intercourse the previous night. What is the emergency contraceptive method you would advise?

Answer

She should be advised to take tablet levonorgestrel 0.75 mg one tablet immediately and a second tablet 12 hours later. The second option is to prescribe a single dose of 30 mg ulipristal orally. If tablet levonorgestrel and ulipristal are unavailable, she may be prescribed a combined oral contraceptive pill 4 tablets immediately, followed by another 4 tablets 12 hours later. However, contraindications to the use of high doses of estrogen should be ruled out. The side effects would include nausea and vomiting.

2. A 36-year-old woman with two children of 10 years and 7 years presents with a history of unprotected sexual intercourse 4 days before and is requesting an emergency contraceptive method.
   a) Which is the most suitable method for this woman?
   b) The woman has agreed to have the Cu-T IUCD inserted. What advice you would give her?

Answers

a) A copper T 380-A intrauterine contraceptive device would be most suitable for this woman. The efficacy of the emergency contraceptive pill levonorgestrel is greater if it is used within 72 hours of sexual intercourse. Cu-IUD gives effective protection if used within 5 days of sexual intercourse. Moreover, it can be used as an ongoing, long-term contraception for up to 10 years.

b) The woman should be informed that there may be some amount of bleeding for a few days and that her periods may be heavier than usual for 3–4 cycles. During menstruation, she should be asked to check for the thread and report for follow-up after one month and then a year after. In the meantime, if she misses her periods, develops severe abdominal pain or is unable to feel the thread, she should be asked to report immediately.

65

FM 3.19

Ethics and Medicolegal Issues in Obstetrics

Learning Objectives

» To understand the principles of ethical practice and human values
» To know the application of ethical principles in day-to-day practice
» To know the medicolegal issues related to intrapartum care and cesarean section
» To know how to avoid medicolegal issues in obstetrics

■ DEVELOPING ETHICAL PRACTICE

Medical ethics is a branch of knowledge that deals with moral principles (what we should and should not do) applied to clinical practice to protect and promote the interest of the patient. The importance of medical ethics was emphasised nearly 2,500 years ago by Hippocrates.

Establishing Integrity of the Profession

Ethical standards should not be based solely on individual assessments of what is and what is not morally acceptable. Rather, the adoption of a set of core values that reflect a consensus among members of a discipline enhances public confidence in individuals who have been trained to meet the profession's ethical standards.

Public Trust

As pregnancy and labour are normal physiological phenomena, only favourable outcomes are expected and accepted by the general public. This perception combined with the easy availability and accessibility of medical information to patients (although beneficial in many ways), inadvertently exposes obstetricians to undue persecution by the public.

■ APPLICATION OF ETHICAL PRINCIPLES IN OBSTETRIC PRACTICE

Medical ethics is an important aspect of medical professionalism and should serve as a guide for decision-making and interaction with patients. Ethics provide a moral compass, especially in situations that are not straightforward. On the other hand, violations of ethical principles can result in inappropriate medical care of the patient that may be considered medical negligence or malpractice. The major principles that

should be followed by medical professionals as guides to professional action or resolution of conflicting situations in the healthcare setting are autonomy, beneficence, non-maleficence and justice.

Autonomy

- Patient autonomy refers to patients' right to make decisions for themselves according to their systems of morals and beliefs.
- Respect for a patient's autonomy acknowledges an individual's right to hold views, to make choices and to take actions based on her own personal values and beliefs.
- Respect for autonomy also provides a strong moral foundation for informed consent, wherein the patient is adequately informed about her medical condition, the available therapies and the associated benefits and risks. After ensuring that the patient has understood what has been explained to her, she should be allowed to freely choose a specific treatment or non-treatment.

Paternalism

- Broadly defined, paternalism is an action performed with good intention by the doctor but against the patient's will or without the patient's consent. Historically, medical practices have predominantly adopted this approach, as doctors assumed the responsibility for their patients' health in good faith in the context of poor medical literacy, understanding and decision-making ability of patients.
- However, in recent times, with easily available medical information, higher levels of education and awareness among the public, there has been an evolution in the medical practice wherein a collaborative and partnering approach with the

patient in all decision-making is recommended and must be emphasised.

- Unilateral decisions excluding patient and family's wishes may result in mistrust and lead to violations of the basic ethical principles. Patient education and counselling and allowing patients an opportunity for a second counsel or opinion may provide solutions to resolving situations of disagreement and protect the interests of the patient.

Beneficence

- Here the provider acts or recommends courses that are in the patient's best interests. It is not done through coercion or manipulation but through education, support and counselling.
- When patient autonomy is compromised (e.g., incapacity), beneficence must be the guiding ethical principle for decisions.

Non-maleficence

- This ethical principle is closely related to beneficence. It means abstaining from any action that may bring harm to the patient—best known as '*Primum non nocere*' or 'First, do no harm'.
- Simply remembering and self-enforcing this rule while making decisions or offering therapies to patients should uphold this ethical principle.

Distributive Justice

- This refers to the proper allocation of resources in a manner that is fair and just. It does not necessarily mean equal allocation of resources. An example would be triaging of patients—the first patient who presents to labour and delivery is not necessarily attended to first (routine labour versus abruption).

In addition to these four principles, **veracity** (truthfulness/honesty) is an important attribute of the medical profession. A crucial part of this is revealing all the pertinent details of the patient's condition and prognosis to them and explaining the risks and benefits of treatments offered. It also includes informing patients of any mistakes that have been made under the medical practitioner's care. Other critical aspects within the reach of ethical principles include informed consent, confidentiality and privacy, which are also important aspects to be considered during the care of patients. Using the core principles of medical ethics, clinical scenarios such as assisted reproduction, medical termination of pregnancy or similar scenarios that have ethical and legal implications should be carefully approached and managed.

Generally, in obstetrics, it is prudent to value the well-being of the mother and potential offspring as paramount. Apart from this, all patients have a right to a standard of healthcare, transparency and treatment with respect and dignity. There should be no discrimination.

There should be training on medical ethics and areas where problems can arise, which includes the following:

- Malpractice and negligence—it is important to provide the right treatment to the best of the practitioner's knowledge and without negligence; it amounts to negligence if the doctor fails to carry out his professional duties with competence and integrity due to insufficient knowledge or skills or an incorrect approach
- Incompetence
- Breach of confidentiality
- Irrational drug use
- Unlawful activities such as issuing fake certificates, advertisements and performing unwanted surgeries
- Not taking informed consent from the patient
- Right-to-issues arising in ART, MTP, sex selection, female feticide and the birth of a disabled child

MEDICOLEGAL ISSUES IN OBSTETRIC PRACTICE

Cases related to medical litigations are increasing throughout the world, both in developed and developing countries. The claims arising from obstetrics and gynecology account for >30% of these cases. Litigation in obstetrics and gynecology is far more common than in any other specialty. Obstetricians are especially vulnerable to medical negligence cases because they are responsible for the well-being of two lives—those of the mother and the baby. The higher number of litigations against obstetricians is also attributable to the fact that pregnancy and childbirth are natural physiological phenomena that are expected to culminate in a healthy mother and a healthy baby. However, emergencies are very common in obstetrics; occasionally, they are life-threatening and can result in damage to both mother and the baby. Despite excellent professional care and infrastructure, complications can occur in a small number of cases. Therefore, medicolegal problems cannot be totally avoided, only minimised. This being the case, practitioners should be aware of the potential areas where they may face legal problems and should be equipped to find solutions to minimise medical litigation.

The reasons for the claims could be due to the negligence of the physician, incompetence, malpractice, medication errors and inadequate logistics support such as inadequate personnel, operating room malfunctions, etc. Examples of potential scenarios leading to medicolegal issues during the different stages of pregnancy are mentioned in this section. Medicolegal issues in obstetrics are mostly related to cesarean section, MTP, maternal and perinatal deaths and failure of sterilisation.

The common causes of litigations in obstetrics are as follows:

A) Claims related to antenatal care:
— Lack of privacy, failure to treat patients with courtesy and respect
— Failure to elicit a comprehensive medical history, resulting in valuable information being missed and leading to inappropriate antenatal care
— Failure to identify risk factors such as HIV status, Rh-isoimmunisation, previous h/o deep vein thrombosis (DVT)
— Drug-induced teratogenicity
— Failure in detecting congenital anomalies during obstetric scans—most litigations are due to this
— Failure to make necessary referrals where indicated

B) Claims related to intrapartum care:
— Intrapartum hypoxia
— Perinatal deaths
— Perioperative injuries to mother and baby
— Retained swabs and instruments
— Issues related to intrapartum monitoring, either failure to perform CTG, failure in the interpretation of CTG or delay in taking action following an abnormal CTG resulting in an adverse outcome
— Failure to document and maintain labour records appropriately—documents such as partographs should be correctly dated and signed; all recordings should be continuous
— Sympathetic explanation to patients
— Issues related to VBAC—malpractice claims arise due to failure to warn women about the risk of scar rupture in VBAC, scar rupture with induction/augmentation, failure to institute effective continuous electronic fetal monitoring or violation of protocols

C) Issues related to operative procedures:
— Failure to warn patients of recognised complications like the risk of anesthesia, bowel and bladder injury, broad ligament hematoma, etc., during cesarean section
— Failure to take precautionary measures like catheterisation prior to surgery
— Failure to seek a senior's help when indicated
— Failure to recognise complications intraoperatively like retained placental bits, bladder injury or bowel injury during cesarean section
— Retention of swabs or instruments in the peritoneal cavity
— Injury to the fetal scalp is considered to be an act of negligence
— Failure to administer anti-D immunoglobulin when indicated
— Instrumental delivery is another potential area fraught with the danger of lawsuits—injuries arising out of the application of instruments, wrong choice of instruments, double instrumentation, fetal injury, etc.

D) Issues related to postnatal care:
— Failure to arrange rubella immunisation for seronegative mothers
— Failure to administer anti-D immunoglobulin when appropriate

E) Causes of litigation in relation to the termination of pregnancy:
— Failure to abort
— Retained products of conception
— Missed ectopic
— Damage to viscera
— Death from any cause
— Failure to administer anti-D prophylaxis when indicated

F) Causes of litigation in relation to sterilisation
— Not recognising pregnancy at the time of sterilisation
— Failure to obtain proper informed consent
— Failure of sterilisation (pregnancy following sterilisation procedures)

Avoiding Medicolegal Issues in Obstetrics

In order to avoid unpleasant medicolegal issues, it is important to focus on preventive measures as follows:

1. **Good communication:** A good patient–doctor relationship is essential right from the beginning. The rapport thus created ensures a positive impact

throughout the treatment. While taking history, it is essential to maintain eye contact with the patient. The doctor should listen patiently and attentively to whatever the patient has to say. The details of her health conditions and the treatment should be discussed with her in clear and simple language. Her comprehension of what has been discussed should be ensured. There should not be any communication gap. While the patient is consulting, the doctor should avoid using cell phones. Discussing cases in public places like a lift or corridor should also be avoided. Significant consequences can result from inappropriate electronic communication. Communication through personal e-mail must be avoided. Social media poses confidentiality risks. Inappropriate and unprofessional commentary on patients or medical cases with peers or co-workers in non-educational settings could amount to a breach of confidentiality and privacy and should be avoided. To gain the patient's confidence, the clinician should exhibit empathy and good behaviour, and should take an interest in the patient's apprehension and complaints.

2. **Documentation and record keeping:** Documentation is the cornerstone that protects the doctor and acts like a lifeline when he/she faces medicolegal issues. It is important to document every discussion with the patient along with the time and date. A management plan with its associated risks and benefits and any alternate mode of treatment available must be explained. If the patient is unwilling to opt for the treatment plan after the discussion, the fact should be documented and duly signed by the patient. For documentation, records should be written legibly, with the date and time of each entry and should not include unknown abbreviations. There should be no attempt to alter or disguise an entry in the records or computer. Each entry should be signed.

3. **Informed consent:** Failure to obtain consent to perform any procedure can lead to criminal prosecution for assault and civil claim for damages. Informed consent protects the individual's autonomy to freely choose whether or not to abide by the doctor's prescription/suggestions/mode of treatment. The process involves three components:

a) Providing relevant medical information (nature of treatment, risks and benefits, alternative methods available), preferably in the patient's vernacular language

b) Ensuring the information relayed by the doctor has been comprehended by the patient

c) Voluntary participation without coercion with an opportunity for questioning.

— Failure to obtain informed consent amounts to medical negligence. The consent form should be signed by the patient and the doctor who has explained the procedure.

— Any individual who is >18 years, in sound mind and not under the effect of alcohol, drugs or pre-medication is eligible to give their consent; this is mandatory. The consent form should be in a language the patient understands.

— Since a minor is not considered competent to give legal consent, a parent or guardian can give consent on behalf of the minor.

— In the case of a mentally disabled person, the validity of consent depends on the severity of the mental handicap. In a severely handicapped individual, either a parent or guardian can give their consent. However, one may have to seek a psychiatric opinion and legal advise, and if necessary, permission from a court of law.

— In an emergency situation, where it is impossible to get consent from the patient, in order to protect the patient's life, consent may be taken from the next of kin.

— Third-party consent—taking consent from the relatives like husbands, parents, brother, etc., has no legal validity.

— Consent for research—it is necessary to obtain valid written consent from the participants after explaining the nature of research, its benefits and risks.

4. **Risk management:** Near-miss cases and cases of untoward mishaps must be reported to the concerned authorities. After identifying the error, the situation should be assessed and evaluated, and remedial measures should be recommended and implemented. This should be monitored periodically.

5. **Training and education:** Periodical training and updating of knowledge and skills are very important. Medical practitioners should stay abreast of the newest and latest updates in their field.

— All medical practitioners should strive to provide quality service by ordering the right investigation at the right time, carrying out the appropriate treatment and ensuring adequate supervision of patients and timely referral if necessary.

— Appropriate training—adequate training is the basic requirement for any profession.

It is dangerous to venture beyond one's capability and qualification. Important areas of training and retraining are USG, CTG and drills for obstetric emergencies like PPH and shoulder dystocia. For the purpose of training, instructional videos, simulations and supervised labour ward training for instrumental delivery, cesarean section and safe obstetric practice can be employed.

6. **Asset protection:** In order to protect doctors, patients and infrastructure from mob-frenzy and vandalism in the event of an untoward mishap, a good security system is essential. Professional protection laws have been amended in favour of doctors.

The medical profession has got ethical, moral and legal obligations to the community and patients. The responsibilities of medical professionals are as follows:

- All the decisions and actions should be rational and scientific.
- Doctors should be kind, humble and show empathy.

- Doctors should keep themselves abreast with the recent advances.
- They should make no distinctions between the rich and the poor and between private and public hospital patients.
- Inadvertent damage should be explained to patients and their relatives.
- Once he has taken the responsibility for a case, the doctor should be available until the treatment is no longer required.
- The patient should not be neglected during critical stages.
- Negligence and rashness should be avoided at all costs.

All doctors should know the potential areas of litigation and follow the recommended guidelines in these areas. They should get themselves insured in order to avoid a heavy financial burden in the event of litigation.

KEY POINTS

✓ *Medical ethics is a branch of knowledge that deals with moral principles (what should and should not be done) that is applied to clinical practice to protect and promote the interests of the patient.*

✓ *The major principles of ethics in healthcare are autonomy, beneficence, non-maleficence and justice.*

✓ *Litigation in obstetrics and gynecology is far more common than in any other specialty.*

✓ *Medicolegal issues in obstetrics are mostly related to cesarean section, MTP, maternal and perinatal deaths and failure of sterilisation.*

✓ *In order to avoid unpleasant medicolegal issues, it is important to focus on preventive measures. Medical practitioners should be aware of the potential areas of litigation and follow recommended guidelines in these areas.*

✓ *The medical profession has got ethical, moral and legal obligations to the community and patients.*

Essay questions

1. Discuss in detail how medicolegal problems can be avoided in obstetrics.
2. Discuss the potential areas where medicolegal problems can arise in the antenatal, intrapartum and postnatal care of the patient.

Short answer questions

1. What is medical ethics?
2. What are the major principles of ethics?
3. What are the causes of litigation in relation to the termination of pregnancy?
4. Write a short note on documentation and record-keeping.
5. Define informed consent.

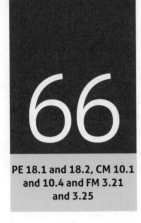

66

PE 18.1 and 18.2, CM 10.1 and 10.4 and FM 3.21 and 3.25

Maternal and Newborn Health: Initiatives and Programmes by the Government of India

---

Learning Objectives

» To know the various govt. initiatives and programmes to reduce MMR and PNMR
» To discuss the major results of the National Family Health Survey

---

▌ INTRODUCTION

The Government of India has launched a number of initiatives and introduced a number of programmes to reduce the maternal mortality ratio (MMR), perinatal mortality (PNM) and infant mortality rate (IMR). India's MMR has seen a decline from 130 per 1 lakh live births in 2014–2016 to 122 per 1 lakh live births in 2015–2017. From 2015–2017, the north-eastern state of Assam had the highest maternal mortality ratio at 229 deaths per 100,000 women, whereas Kerala had the lowest mortality ratio with 42 fatalities during pregnancy. The maternal mortality ratio in India for the period 2016–2018 as per the latest report in the National Sample Registration system (SRS) data is 113/100,000 live births.

Infant mortality rate (IMR) is defined as the number of infant deaths (less than one year) per thousand live births. At the national level, the IMR in India is reported to be 33; in 2017, it ranged from 37 in rural areas to 23 in urban areas. Among the larger states and UTs, it varies from 10 in Kerala to 47 in Madhya Pradesh. The IMR was higher among female infants than male infants in all states except Chhattisgarh, Delhi, Madhya Pradesh, Tamil Nadu and Uttarakhand.

The remarkable pace of decline in MMR and INR can be attributed to the schemes launched by the Government of India that are aimed at improving maternal and child health through various programmes. Apart from the initiatives launched by the central government, individual states have also introduced their own maternity and neonatal benefit schemes and insurance programmes for the weaker sections of society so that no woman or child dies for want of timely medical services.

▌ THE NATIONAL FAMILY HEALTH SURVEY

Since 1992, the International Institute for Population Sciences, Mumbai, has conducted the National Family Health Survey (NFHS) for the Government of India's Ministry of Health and Family Welfare. The survey provides detailed information on population, health and nutrition in each state and union territory of India. The 2019–20 (NFHS-5) survey was published on **24 November 2021**. The survey, which was conducted from 2 January 2020 to 30 April 2021, sampled 636,699 households, covering 724,115 women and 101,839 men. The report contains data on 131 socio-economic and health indicators like education, fertility, family planning, infant and child mortality and maternal and child health. It also gathered information on reproductive health, sexual behaviour, marriage, domestic violence and attitudes towards gender roles. The survey has shown the following important key facts that can help in planning future programmes:

- India's total fertility rate decreased from 2.2 children per woman in 2015–16 to two children per woman in 2019–21.

- There has been an increase in the use of family planning measures from 53.5% in 2015–16 to 66.7% in 2019–2021. At 37.9 per cent, female sterilisation remains the most popular method of family planning in the country, followed by condoms (9.5%) and contraceptive pills (5.1%).

- The sex ratio in India increased from 991 to 1,020 females per 1,000 males between 2015–16 and 2019–21. The number stands at 1,037 and 985 females per 1,000 males in rural and urban areas respectively.

- The percentage of institutional births increased from 78.9% in 2015–16 to 88.6% in 2019–21.
- About 57% of women in the age group of 15–49 years are anemic—58.5% of women in rural India and 53.8% in urban areas.

(National Family Health Survey [NFHS-5], 2019–21, Compendium of Fact Sheets: Key Indicators – India and 14 States/UTs [Phase-II])

MATERNAL AND NEWBORN HEALTH—INITIATIVES BY THE GOVERNMENT OF INDIA

Essential Obstetric Care

Provision of quality antenatal care is essential for improving maternal and newborn care. The components of essential obstetric care include treatment of anemia, institutional/safe delivery services and postnatal care. These have been facilitated by the round-the-clock services available from primary health centres (PHCs) onwards and by training the staff nurses, lady health visitors/auxiliary nurse midwives (SNs/LHVs/ANMs) in skilled attendance at birth.

Quality Antenatal Care

Quality antenatal care (ANC) includes a minimum of four antenatal visits, including early registration (before 12 weeks of gestation). In addition to physical and abdominal examinations, Hb estimation and urine investigations are also performed at these visits. The pregnant woman is also given two doses of tetanus toxoid immunisation and 100 mg of iron and folic acid (IFA) tablets for 100 days.

Skilled Attendants at Birth

Every birth should be attended by a skilled birth attendant (SBA). According to the WHO, a skilled attendant is an accredited health professional such as a midwife, doctor or nurse who has been educated and trained in the skills required to manage normal (uncomplicated) pregnancies, childbirth and the immediate postnatal period and in the identification, management or referral of complications in women and newborns (WHO, 2005). To achieve this goal, staff nurses and ANMs are being trained in emergency and essential obstetric and newborn care and being posted to community and institutional centres for round-the-clock skilled birth attendance for every birth. To manage and handle common obstetric emergencies at the time of birth, a policy decision has been taken permitting staff nurses and ANMs to administer certain injections and to perform certain interventions in specific emergency situations to save the life of the mother.

Postnatal Care for the Mother and the Newborn

It is essential that every birth is managed in a healthcare facility with a skilled birth attendant. Newly delivered mothers should also be advised to stay in the facility for 48 hours after normal delivery. Subsequently, the woman should be reviewed either through home visits or in the hospital facilities on the third, seventh and forty-second day for the identification and management of emergencies occurring during the postnatal period. ANMs, LHVs and staff nurses are being oriented and trained to tackle emergencies identified during these visits.

Provision of Emergency Obstetric and Neonatal Care at First Referral Units (FRUs)

The provision of emergency obstetric and neonatal care at FRUs is being ensured by making all FRUs functional in the country. The thrust is on critical components such as manpower, blood storage units, referral linkages and so on. The availability of trained manpower (skill-based training for MBBS doctors) is linked with the functioning of FRUs. The following initiatives are being taken in this regard.

Augmentation of skilled human resources for maternal health

To overcome the shortage of skilled manpower, particularly anaesthetists and obstetricians, the following key skill-based training programmes have been undertaken:

- An 18-week training programme for doctors (MBBS) in life-saving anesthesia skills for emergency obstetric care (24 weeks in Tamil Nadu)
- A 16-week training programme for doctors (MBBS) in obstetric management skills including C-section in collaboration with the Federation of Obstetric and Gynaecological Society of India (24 weeks in Tamil Nadu)
- A ten-day training programme in basic emergency obstetric care for medical officers (BEmOC)
- A three-week training programme for ANMs/staff nurses/LHVs to act as skilled birth attendants (SBA)

Referral services at the community and the institutional levels

The national ambulance service is functional in all states to ensure basic patient care. Transportation ambulances will reach the beneficiary in rural areas within 30 minutes of a call for quick service delivery.

Safe abortion services/medical termination of pregnancy (MTP)

This ensures the provision of comprehensive and safe abortion services at public health facilities—PHCs, hospitals and community health centres (CHCs)—with a focus on delivery points.

Capacity building of medical officers in safe MTP techniques

In order to ensure safe abortions, doctors are trained in safe abortion techniques. Along with this, the ANMs, SNs and other field functionaries are also being trained to provide confidential counselling for MTP and to promote post-abortion care, including contraception.

Supply of Nischay pregnancy detection kits

Subcentres are provided with kits for early detection of pregnancy so that safe abortion services can be provided for unwanted pregnancies.

Provision of RTI/STI Services

Under NRHM, the provision of reproductive tract infections/sexually transmitted infections (RTI/ STI) care services is a very important strategy to prevent HIV transmission and other infections. There are also services to promote sexual and reproductive health under the National AIDS Control Programme (NACP-III) and Reproductive and Child Health (RCH-II). Enhanced syndromic case management (ESCM) with minimal laboratory tests is the cornerstone of (RTI/ STI) management under NACP-III. These services are being provided at all FRUs, CHCs and at block PHCs.

■ GENERAL MEASURES

Setting up of Blood Storage Centres (BSC)

Blood storage centres are being set up at FRUs to overcome delays in starting blood transfusions.

Village Health and Nutrition Day

This is a unique programme under which village health and nutrition day (VHNDs) is organised at *anganwadi* centres at least once every month to provide antenatal/postpartum care for pregnant women, promote institutional delivery, immunisation, family planning and nutrition counselling.

Delivery Points (DPs)

All states and union territories have identified DPs above a certain minimum benchmark of performance to prioritise and direct resources in a focused manner to these facilities for filling the gaps like trained and skilled human resources, infrastructure, equipment, drugs and supplies, referral transport and so on for providing quality and comprehensive RMNCH (reproductive, maternal, neonatal and child health) services.

Web-Enabled Mother and Child Tracking By STEM

Name-based tracking of pregnant women and children has been initiated by the Government of India as a policy decision to track every pregnant woman, infant and child by name up to three years for the provision of timely ANC, institutional delivery and postnatal care along with immunisation and other related services.

Maternal Death Review

The process of maternal death review (MDR) has been implemented and institutionalised by all states as a policy since 2010. Guidelines and tools for conducting community-based MDR and facility-based MDR have been provided to the states. States are required to report deaths along with an analysis of the cause of death in each case.

Joint MCP Card

This card, which was jointly launched by the Ministry of Health and Family Welfare (MOHFW) and the Ministry of Women and Child Development (MOWCD), is a tool for documenting and monitoring antenatal, intranatal and postnatal services for pregnant women and immunisation and growth monitoring of infants.

Tracking of Severe Anemia During Pregnancy and Childbirth by PHCs

Severe anemia is a major cause for pregnancy-related complications that may lead to maternal deaths. Effective monitoring of these cases by the ANM as well as the medical officer in charge of a PHC has resulted in the necessary treatment being given to these women.

GOVERNMENT OF INDIA PROGRAMMES

Government programmes related to maternal and child health are discussed in Chapter 58, *Maternal mortality*. A few programmes are discussed in detail in this chapter.

Child Survival and Safe Motherhood Programme (CSSM)

The programme was launched in August 1992. Its objectives were to improve the health status of infants and improve child and maternal mortality and morbidity rates. The programme includes oral rehydration therapy, universalising prophylaxis schemes for the control of anemia in pregnant women, control of blindness in children and control of acute respiratory tract infection, training of traditional birth attendants, provision of aseptic delivery kits and strengthening of first referral units.

Reproductive and Child Healthcare (RCH) Programme Phase-I

It was launched by the Govt. of India in October 1997. It provides services under the CSSM and family welfare programme along with management of RTIs, STIs and adolescent reproductive health.

RCH Phase-II

It was launched in April 2005. The additional features of this programme are the promotion of state ownership of the programme and its decentralisation.

Reproductive, Maternal, Newborn, Child + Adolescent Health (RMNCH)

Under this programme, efforts were made to tailor programmes to the needs of underserved and vulnerable sections of the Indian population.

- The package for mothers includes:
  — Early registration
  — Antenatal care—four or more visits
  — Anemia prophylaxis and treatment
  — Two doses of tetanus toxoid or a booster
  — Institutional deliveries and deliveries by skilled birth attendants
  — Referrals to first referral units for obstetric emergencies
  — Home-based postnatal care
  — Counselling for birth spacing and limiting
  — Increased facilities for MTP

- The package for newborn and child health includes:
  — Skilled care at birth by establishment of newborn facilities
  — Early initiation of breastfeeding, promotion of exclusive breastfeeding, timely and appropriate complementary feeding
  — Integrated management of neonatal and childhood illnesses for common illnesses
  — Immunisation
  — Management of children with malnutrition
  — Vitamin A, iron and folic acid prophylaxis
  — Child health screening and early interventions services

- The package for adolescents includes:
  — Adolescent nutrition, iron and folic acid supplementation
  — Care for mental health, substance abuse, injuries, violence, non-communicable diseases
  — Facility-based adolescent reproductive and sexual health services (adolescent health clinics)
  — Information and counselling on adolescent sexual and reproductive health and other health issues
  — Menstrual hygiene
  — Preventive health screening and check-ups

The long-term goal of RMNCH is to establish and operationalise the following:

- BEmOC—Basic emergency obstetric care (Fig. 66.1)
- CEmOC—Comprehensive emergency obstetric care centres as per the expected delivery load in the state and district

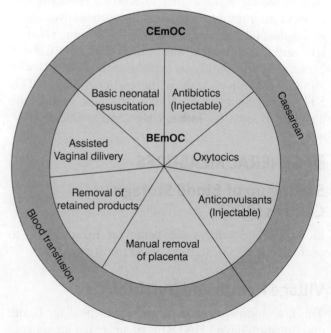

Fig. 66.1 Facilities provided by BEmOC and CEmOC centres

Janani Suraksha Yojana (JSY)

Janani Suraksha Yojana is a safe motherhood initiative under the National Rural Health Mission (NRHM), which was launched in 2005 with the aim to reduce maternal and infant mortality by focusing on increasing institutional deliveries. This scheme includes urban mothers too. Under the JSY, an amount of Rs 700 is paid to resident rural mothers and Rs 600 is paid to resident urban mothers who deliver at accredited institutions. Women who deliver at home are entitled to an amount of Rs 500. All BPL/ SC/ST mothers delivering at public health centres and accredited private institutions are eligible to receive this benefit, irrespective of age and parity.

Janani Shishu Suraksha Karyakram (JSSK)

The Government of India launched the Janani Shishu Suraksha Karyakaram (JSSK) on 1 June 2011.

Free entitlements for pregnant women under the JSSK
- Free and cashless delivery
- Free cesarean section
- Free drugs and consumables
- Free diagnostics
- Free food during stay in the institution
- Free provision of blood
- Exemption from user charges
- Free transport from home to the institution
- Free transport facilities in case of referral
- Free drop from institution to home after a 48-hour stay

Free entitlements for sick newborns and infants upto 30 days after birth (now extended to cover sick infants)
- Free treatment
- Free drugs and consumables
- Free diagnostics
- Free provision of blood
- Exemption from user charges
- Free transport from home to the institution
- Free transport in case of referrals
- Free drop from the institution to home

Pradhan Mantri Matritva Vandana Yojana (PMMVY) – 2017

It promotes appropriate practice, care and institutional service utilisation during pregnancy, delivery and lactation. Under this programme, women are counselled about optimal nutrition and feeding practices, including early and exclusive breastfeeding for the first 6 months. The scheme makes provision for cash incentives for improved health and nutrition to pregnant and lactating mothers. Under the PMMVY, a cash incentive of Rs 5,000 is deposited in three instalments directly in the bank/post office account of pregnant women and lactating mothers (PW&LM) for the first living child of the family, subject to fulfilling specific conditions relating to maternal and child health.

Pradhan Mantri Surakshit Matritva Abhiyan (PMSMA) – 2016

The programme aims to provide assured, comprehensive and quality antenatal care, free of cost and universally to all pregnant women on the 9th day of every month.

Dr Muthulakshmi Reddy Maternity Benefit Scheme

This maternity scheme was launched in 1987. Under this useful scheme, the Tamil Nadu state government provides financial help to poor pregnant women during maternity. Financial help is provided for pregnant women over 19 years of age and only for the first two pregnancies. The Muthulakshmi Reddy Maternity Benefit Scheme provides a total of Rs 18,000 in a total of five instalments and two nutrition kits. The final instalment is allotted when the child has received all the essential vaccines between 9 and 12 months of age.

Criteria
- The pregnant woman must have completed 19 years of age.
- Eligible pregnant women may receive all five instalments for the first two deliveries only.
- The pregnant woman must register the application form of her pregnancy before 12 weeks of pregnancy with the village health nurse/urban health nurse (VHN/UHN).

Laqshya

It is labour room quality improvement initiative that was launched by Ministry and Family Welfare on 11 December 2017. The goal is to reduce preventable maternal and newborn mortality, morbidity and stillbirths associated with the care and delivery in the labour room and maternity OT and ensure respectful maternal care. The components of this initiative are as follows:

- Reorganising the labour room and maternity operation theatre layout and workflow as per 'Labour Room Standardisation Guidelines'

- Ensuring that at least all government medical college hospitals and high-case-load district hospitals have dedicated obstetric HDUs for managing complicated pregnancies
- Ensuring strict adherence to clinical protocols for the management and stabilisation of the complications before referral to higher centres
- Ensuring the availability of optimal and skilled human resources as per case load
- Ensuring skill assessment of all staff of LR and OT through OSCE testing
- Application of skills-lab training, simulations and drills
- Ensuring dedicated staff working in the labour room and maternity OT
- Sensitising care providers for the delivery of respectful maternity care and close monitoring of language, behaviour and conduct of the labour room, OT and HDU staff
- Creating an enabling environment for the natural birthing process
- Operationalisation of C-section audits and corrective and preventive actions for ensuring that C-sections are undertaken judiciously
- Instituting an ongoing system of capturing of beneficiaries' independent feedback and taking action to address concerns
- Ensuring the availability of essential support services
- Use of digital technology for record keeping and monitoring for maternity wing (MIS), including use of E-partograph
- Piloting technology for managing care, such as computerised physician order entry

Pregnancy and Infant Cohort Monitoring and Evaluation (PICME)

PICME is an initiative of the Govt. of Tamil Nadu that was instituted on 1 April 2008. It is an online registration system to ensure that pregnant women receive proper medical care and assistance. Upon registration, the pregnant woman receives a unique 12-digit RCH identification number that is used for surveillance by the local nurses and *anganwadi* workers. This number is mandatory for obtaining a birth certificate for the child.

Manyata Programme

The FOGSI launched 'Manyata'—a nationwide initiative to improve the quality of maternal and neonatal care in the private sector in India.

Under this programme, there are 16 parameters to quality maternal care:

1. Screen for clinical conditions and for complications like HIV, anemia, etc.
2. Prepare for safe care during delivery
3. Assess all pregnant women at admission
4. Conduct PV examination, follow infection prevention practices, and record findings
5. Ensure respectful and supportive care
6. Monitor the progress of labour
7. Assist the pregnant woman to have a safe and clean birth
8. Assess and perform immediate newborn care
9. Perform active management of the third stage labour and examine the placenta thoroughly
10. Identify and manage postpartum hemorrhage
11. Identify and manage severe pre-eclampsia/eclampsia
12. Perform newborn resuscitation if the baby does not cry immediately
13. Ensure care of newborns that are small for gestational age at birth
14. Adhere to universal infection prevention protocols
15. Offer postpartum care package to the mother and baby at discharge
16. Review clinical practices related to C-section at regular intervals

Navjaat Shishu Suraksha Karyakram (NSSK)

The infant mortality in India is high. According to the latest government data released by the Sample Registration System, India's infant mortality rate (IMR) has reduced by 42% over 11 years—from 57 per 1,000 live births in 2006 to 33 in 2017. Despite the reduction, India's IMR in 2017 is higher than the global average of 29.4.

Neonatal mortality accounts for two-thirds of all infant mortality. Birth asphyxia and serious infections account for nearly 50% of all neonatal deaths. If these two factors are addressed, it would have a telling effect on the infant mortality rate.

The Government of India, keeping this in mind, has developed a programme on basic newborn care and resuscitation to address these causes in a large way. This programme trains all health professionals in basic newborn care and simple resuscitation techniques. This programme is timely and will certainly contribute significantly to bringing down neonatal mortality and other serious long-term morbidities such as neurodevelopmental sequelae in survivors of asphyxiated newborn babies.

Rashtriya Bal Swasthya Karyakram (RBSK)

Rashtriya Bal Swasthya Karyakram (RBSK) is a new initiative aimed at early identification and early intervention for children from birth to 18 years to cover the 4 'D's.

1. Defects at birth
2. Deficiencies
3. Diseases
4. Development delays, including disability

Besides focussing on maternal mortality, it is important to evaluate 'near-miss' cases as well. A near miss case is one in which the woman survives a life-threatening complication during pregnancy, following an abortion or childbirth or within 42 days of the termination of pregnancy. The Ministry of Health and Family Welfare has introduced guidelines for reviewing near-miss cases in 2014.

Health Programmes for Adolescents (Table 66.1)

Rashtriya Kishor Swasthya Karyakram (RKSK)

The Ministry of Health and Family Welfare has launched this health programme (also called the National Adolescent Health Programme) for adolescents. The Rashtriya Kishor Swasthya Karyakram was launched on 7 January 2014 to comprehensively address the health needs of about 243 million adolescents. It introduces community-based interventions through peer educators and is underpinned by collaborations with other ministries and state governments. The objectives of the programme are to improve nutrition, improve sexual and reproductive health, enhance mental health, prevent injuries and violence and prevent substance misuse.

The key principles of this programme are adolescent participation and leadership, equity and inclusion gender equity and help adolescents in India to realise their full potential by making informed and responsible decisions related to their health and well-being and access the services and support they need in order to do so.

Table 66.1 Health programmes for adolescents

Programme	Year	Goals
National Iron Plus Initiative	2013	Iron and folic acid supplementation for adolescents and women in the reproductive age group, children between the ages of 6 and 60 months and pregnant and lactating women
Weekly Iron and Folic Acid Supplementation Scheme (WIFS)	2000	Weekly supplementation of iron (100 mg) and folic acid (500 μg) for all adolescents b/w 8th and 12th standards in govt. schools
12/12 Initiative for Anemia Control	2007	Every child to have hemoglobin of 12 g% by the age of 12
National Nutritional Anemia Control Programme	1970	Promotion of regular consumption of iron-rich foods
	1989 (renamed)	Provision of iron and folate supplements for 100 days to high-risk groups
		Identification and treatment of severe anemia
Anemia Mukt Bharat	2018	Designed to reduce prevalence of anemia by 3% points per year among children, adolescents and women in the reproductive age group (15–49 years), between 2018 and 2022
Promotion of menstrual hygiene	2011	Sanitary napkins 'free days' distributed by ASHAs under NRHMs
Rastriya Kishor Swastiya Karyakram	2014	Age group 10–19 years—improve nutrition and sexual, mental, reproductive health
SABLA	2011	Provision of supplementary nutrition
		IFA supplementation, health check-up, referral services, nutrition and health education
UJJAWALA	2007, 2016	Comprehensive scheme for prevention of trafficking and rescue, rehabilitation and re-integration of victims of trafficking for commercial sexual exploitation
ARSH Strategy (RCH II–Adolescent, reproductive and sexual health strategy)	2013	Reduction of IMR, MMR, TFR and reducing incidence of STD and HIV

Weekly Iron and Folic Acid Supplementation (WIFS) Programme

Adolescents are at a high risk of iron deficiency anemia; this is due to accelerated growth, poor dietary intake of iron and a high rate of worm infestation. The problem is more acute in girls due to menstruation and the problem of adolescent pregnancy and conception. Clinical evidence indicates that weekly supplementation of 100 mg elemental iron and 500 µg folic acid (IFA) is effective in decreasing the incidence and prevalence of anemia in adolescents. Hence, the Ministry of Health and Family Welfare (MOHFW) launched the Weekly Iron and Folic Acid Supplementation (WIFS) Programme for school-going adolescent girls and boys and for out-of-school adolescent girls. The programme envisages the administration of supervised weekly IFA supplementation and biannual deworming tablets to approximately 13 crore rural and urban adolescents through schools and *anganwadi* workers. To guide the implementation of this programme, the Ministry of Health and Family Welfare (MOHFW), in collaboration with the United Nations Population Fund (UNFPA), has developed a National Adolescent Health Strategy.

Sabla—Rajiv Gandhi Scheme for the Empowerment of Adolescent Girls

This programme involves providing nutritional support to out-of-school girls who are 11–14 years old and all girls aged 14–18 years. This scheme makes provision for supplementary nutrition containing 600 calories, 18–20 g of protein and micronutrients per day for 300 days in a year. Girls aged 11–18 years are also provided with IFA supplementation, health check-ups and referral services, nutrition and health education, guidance on family welfare, life skills education, guidance on accessing public services and vocational training.

Ujjwala

In effect since 1 April 2016, Ujjwala is a comprehensive scheme for the prevention of trafficking and the rescue, rehabilitation and re-integration of victims of trafficking for commercial sexual exploitation.

Contraceptives under National Programmes

Currently, the following contraceptive methods are available under various national programmes:

- Spacing methods
- Injectable contraceptive DMPA under ANTARA programme
- Oral contraceptives Mala N and centrochroman 'CHHAYA'
- Condoms
- IUCDs—Cu T-380A (10 years) and Cu T-375 (5 years)
- Permanent methods
- Emergency contraceptive pills for unplanned/unprotected intercourse

National AIDS Control Programme

This programme was launched in 1987, aimed at the prevention of parent-to-child transmission of HIV/AIDS (PPTCT). The programme was launched in India in 2002. Under this national programme, it is recommended to provide lifelong ART for all pregnant and breastfeeding women living with HIV, whereby all pregnant women living with HIV receive a 'single-pill' triple-drug ART regimen (TDF +3TC + EFV) regardless of their CD4 count or clinical stage both for their own health and to prevent vertical HIV transmission and for additional HIV prevention benefits.

The PCPNDT Act

The Preconception and Prenatal Diagnostic Techniques (Prohibition of Sex Selection) Act (PCPNDT) is a statute enacted to stop the female feticide which has resulted in a decline in the female sex ratio in India. In 1994, the Prenatal Diagnostic Techniques (Regulation and Prevention of Misuse) Act (PNDT) was passed by the Indian government and came into effect on 1 January 1996. Amendments were made in 2003, at which time the Act was renamed the PCPNDT Act. The main purpose of the Act is to prohibit the use of sex selection techniques before or after conception and prevent the misuse of prenatal diagnostic techniques for sex-selective abortion. It regulates prenatal diagnostic techniques for detecting genetic, metabolic disorders, chromosomal abnormalities, congenital malformations and sex-linked disorders.

Prenatal diagnostic techniques include ultrasonography, fetoscopy and collecting samples of amniotic fluid, chorionic villi, blood or any tissue or fluid from a man or woman before or after conception. The Act prohibits sex determination/selection absolutely. All techniques must be conducted by qualified persons only (holding any medical qualification recognised by the MCI, whose name is entered in a State Medical Register and who have six months' ultrasound training). Every centre/institute conducting these tests must be registered under the Act. Approved applicants receive form B as a certificate that must be displayed in the centre. The certificate is valid for five years. Before conducting a test, form F must be filled (patient details, indication for the test, patient's declaration that she does not want to know the sex of fetus, doctor's declaration that he/she has not determined/conveyed the sex of fetus, etc.). Every centre/institute must display a notice delineating that sex determination/selection is prohibited under law.

Offences and penalties

- Any medical geneticist, gynecologist or registered medical practitioner or any person who owns a genetic counselling centre, a genetic laboratory or a genetic clinic who contravenes any of the provisions of this Act or rules laid down thereunder shall be punishable with imprisonment for a term which may extend to three years and with a fine which may extend to ten thousand rupees and on any subsequent conviction, with imprisonment which may extend to five years and with a fine which may extend to fifty thousand rupees.

- Any medical geneticist, gynecologist or registered medical practitioner or any person who owns a genetic counselling centre, a genetic laboratory or a genetic clinic who contravenes any of the provisions of this Act or rules laid down thereunder shall have his/her name removed from the medical council register for a period of five years for the first offence and permanently for the subsequent offence.

The Preconception and Prenatal Diagnostic Techniques (Prohibition of Sex Selection) (Six Months Training) Rules 2014, were amended in 2020. As per the amendment, existing registered medical practitioners who are conducting ultrasound procedures in a genetic clinic or ultrasound clinic or imaging centre on the basis of one-year experience or six-month training are exempt from undertaking the said training provided they are able to qualify the competency-based assessment.

KEY POINTS

✓ The Government of India has launched a number of initiatives to reduce the maternal mortality ratio (MMR), perinatal mortality (PNM) and infant mortality rate (IMR).

✓ Quality antenatal care is essential for optimum outcomes for the mother and the newborn. A skilled birth attendant should be present to conduct deliveries.

✓ First referral units (FRUs) should be well-equipped with manpower and facilities. RTI/STI and abortion services should also be provided.

✓ Various programmes of the government aim to improve maternal and fetal outcomes. These include JSY, JSSK, NSSK, RBSK, RKSK and WIFS.

✓ LAQSHYA is labour room quality improvement initiative launched by the Ministry and Family Welfare on 11 December 2017.

Essay question

1. Discuss the various government programmes to improve adolescent health.

Short answer question

1. Write short notes on the following:
   a) LAQSHYA
   b) PICME
   c) Dr Muthulakshmi Reddy Maternity Benefit Scheme
   d) Pradhan Mantri Surakshit Matritva Abhiyan

2. Who is a skilled birth attendant?

Annexure 1
Normal Blood Values

Tests	SI units	Traditional units
Albumin (serum)	35–50 g/L	3.5–5.0 g/dL
Bicarbonate (HCO3B) (serum)	23–29 mmol/L	23–29 mEq/L
Bilirubin (serum)*—Adults conjugated	0–5 mmol/L	0–0.3 mg/dL
Bilirubin (serum)*—Total	3–22 mmol/L	0.2–1.3 mg/dL
Bleeding time (Ivy)	<5 min	<5 min
Chloride (serum)	96–106 mmol/L	96–106 mmol/L
Cholesterol (serum)**	<5.2 mmol/L	<200 mg/dL
Creatinine (serum)	50–110 µmol/L	0.6–1.2 mg/dL
Creatinine (urine)—females	7.0–15.8 mmol/d	0.8–1.8 g/24 h
Erythrocytes (RBCs)—females	$4.2–5.4 \times 10^{12}$/L	4.2–5.4 million/mm³
Ferritin (serum)	20–200 µg/L	20–200 ng/mL
Glucose—Fasting (plasma or serum)	3.9–6.1 mmol/L	70–110 mg/dL
Hematocrit—Females	0.37–0.47	37–47%
Hemoglobin (Hb)—Females	120–160 g/L	12.0–16.0 g/dl
High density lipoproteins (HDL) (recommended range)	>0.91 mmol/L	>35 mg/dL
International normalized ratio	0.9–1.1	0.9–1.1
Iron (serum)—Females	5–29 µmol/L	28–162 µg/dL
Lactate dehydrogenase (LDH) (serum)—Adult	45–90 IU/L	45–90 U/L
Leukocytes – Total	$3.5–12.0 \times 10^9$/L	3,500–12,000/mm³
Differential—Neutrophils	$3,000–5,800 \times 10^6$/L	3,000–5,800/mm³
Differential—Lymphocytes	$1,500–3,000 \times 10^6$/L	1,500–3,000/mm³
Differential—Monocytes	$300–500 \times 10^6$/L	300–500/mm³
Differential—Basophils	$50–250 \times 10^6$/L	50–250/mm³
Basophils	$15–50 \times 10^6$/L	15–50/mm³
Low density lipoproteins (LDL) (recommended range)	<3.4 mmol/L	<130 mg/dL
Magnesium (serum)	0.65–1.05 mmol/L	1.3–2.1 mg/dL
Mean corpuscular volume (MCV)	76–100 fL	76–100 mm³
Oxygen (arterial saturation)	94–99%	94–99%
Partial thromboplastin time (PTT)	22–37 sec	22–37 sec
pCO$_2$	35–45 mmHg	35–45 mmHg
pH	7.35–7.45	7.35–7.45
Phosphatase, alkaline (serum)	40–160 IU/L	40–160 U/L
Platelet count	$150–400 \times 10^9$/L	150,000–400,000/mm³
pO$_2$ (arterial)	80–100 mmHg	80–100 mmHg

Potassium (serum)—Adult	3.5–5.1 mmol/L	3.5-5.1 mEq/L
Protein (serum)—Total	60–80 g/L	6.0–8.0 g/dL
Albumin	35–55 g/L	3.5–5.5 g/dL
Protein (urine)	10–150 mg/d	10–150 mg/24h
Prothrombin time (PT)	9–12 sec	9–12 sec
Reticulocytes	25–75 × 109/L	25,000–75,000/mm³
Erythrocyte sedimentation rate (ESR)	0–15 mm/h	0–15 mm/h
Sodium (serum or plasma)	135–145 mmol/L	135–145 mEq/L
Thrombin time (plasma)	<17 sec	<17 sec
Thyroid-stimulating hormone (TSH) (serum)—Adults	0.4–4.8 mIU/L	0.4–4.8 mIU/L
Thyroxine (T4) (serum)**	66–155 nmol/L	5–12 µg/dL
Thyroxine, free (FT4) (serum)**	13–27 pmol/L	1.0–2.1 ng/dL
Transaminase (serum)—AST	7–40 IU/L	7–40 mU/mL
(SGOT) ALT (SGPT)	5–35 IU/L	5–35 mU/mL
Triiodothyronine (T3) (serum)	1.1–2.9 mmol/L	70–190 ng/dL
Triglycerides	0.45–1.71 mmol/L	40–150 mg/dL
Urea (plasma or serum)	4.0–8.2 mmol/L	24–49 ng/dL
Urea nitrogen (BUN) (plasma or serum)	8.0–16.4 mmol/L	22–46 mg/dL
Uric acid—enzymatic (serum)	2.0–7.0 mg/dL	120–420 µmol/L

*Test values are method dependent
**Test values vary with age
***Test values are diet dependent
Modified from Clinical Laboratory Tests, Normal Values, Royal College
www.royalcollege.ca/common/documents/exams/normal_values_e.pdf

Annexure 2
Obstetric Instruments

SPONGE-HOLDING FORCEPS

Sponge-holding forceps (Fig. 1) are long forceps with ring-like ends. These rings have serrations for better grip. The handles are provided with a ratchet for locking.

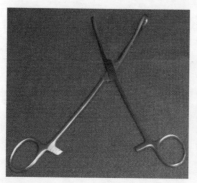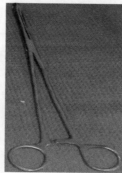

Fig. 1   Sponge-holding forceps

Sponge-holding forceps are used for:
- Cleaning the abdomen and vagina with a gauze soaked in antiseptic solution.
- Used with gauze, can be used for pushing the bladder down in abdominal hysterectomy or cesarean section.
- Can be used as a means to ensure that there is no cervical tear by going around the cervix after forceps delivery. This procedure is known as 'walking the cervix'.
- Also used in cervical cerclage procedure.

OVUM FORCEPS

Ovum forceps (Fig. 2) resemble sponge-holding forceps. Unlike the sponge forceps, they have two fenestrated or non-fenestrated blunts ends which come close together. There is no locking mechanism in this instrument.

Ovum forceps are used for:
- To remove products of conception (POC) following first trimester abortion (induced or spontaneous).
- To remove adherent placental bits or POC.

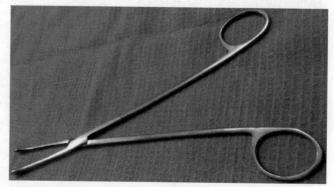

Fig. 2   Ovum forceps

PINARD'S FETOSCOPE

Pinard's fetoscope (Fig. 3) is made of aluminium, though earlier, it used to be made of wood. It is used for listening to the fetal heart. The broad end should be placed over the mother's abdomen. The narrow end is meant for listening to the heart sounds of the fetus by placing the ear to it. The fetoscope should not be held by the hand as this may muffle the heart sounds. Nowadays, with the easy availability of the hand-held Doppler, the fetoscope is being used less frequently.

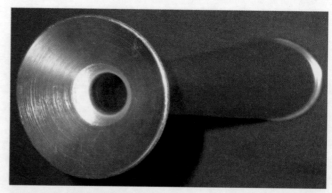

Fig. 3   Pinard's fetoscope

STRAIGHT SCISSORS

Straight scissors (Fig. 4) are used for cutting suture material. Since both the blades are straight and the tips are sharp, it is not advisable to use them for cutting tissues.

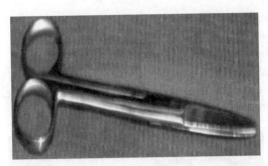

Fig. 4 Straight scissors

CURVED SCISSORS

Curved scissors (Fig. 5) are used for cutting tissues. The curve should always face upwards so that the surgeon has a clear view of the structure being cut.

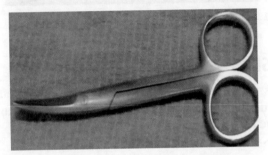

Fig. 5 Curved scissors

- They are used for cutting tissues, including the uterus, during cesarean section.
- When episiotomy scissors are not available, a pair of curved scissors may be used.

EPISIOTOMY SCISSORS

Episiotomy scissors (Fig. 6) have an angled blade and the end of the lower blade is blunt. They are used for episiotomy. The angling makes it convenient for entering the vagina while performing an episiotomy.

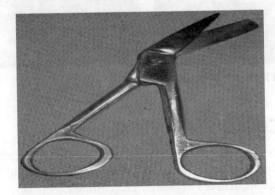

Fig. 6 Episiotomy scissors

OUTLET FORCEPS

Outlet forceps (Fig. 7) are otherwise known as low forceps and also as short forceps. These forceps have two blades which can be articulated and fixed by an English lock. The blades are fenestrated. Both the cephalic and pelvic curves are on the blades.

- As the name suggests, they are used only when the head is at the outlet.
- The only permissible movement while using these forceps is the extension of the head.
- There is no need for anesthesia, except local infiltration anesthesia, for episiotomy.
- They are used to prevent the mother from straining during labour, in cases of maternal exhaustion, heart disease, anemia in pregnancy, vaginal birth after cesarean section (VBAC).

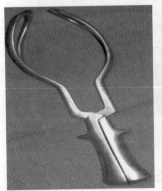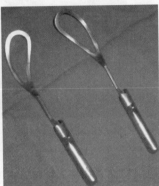

Fig. 7 Outlet forceps

SILASTIC CUPS FOR VACUUM EXTRACTION

Silastic cups for vacuum extraction (Fig. 8) have slowly replaced the metallic Malmström's cups for vacuum extraction. These cups are flexible, and therefore, less traumatic. They are available in different sizes, the most common ones being the 50 mm and 60 mm sizes.

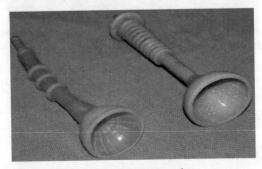

Fig. 8 Silastic cups for vacuum extraction

The chignon formed is also bigger than with the metallic cup and the chances of slipping are less. The cup is fixed either to a vacuum bottle which is connected to either a hand-held vacuum pump or a mechanical pump.

■ MUCUS SUCKER-BULB

With the liberal availability of disposable mucus suckers like De Lee's, bulb suckers (Fig. 9) are being slowly phased out.

The bulb is pressed down and the nozzle is gently lead into the throat of the newborn, and the pressure on the bulb released. This sucks out the mucus.

The bulb sucker can be reused after sterilising it. However, it should be washed thoroughly before being sterilised.

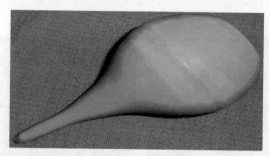

Fig. 9   Mucus sucker bulb

■ DE LEE'S MUCUS SUCKER

De Lee's mucus suckers (Fig. 10) are disposable, single-use mucus suckers. There are two tubes attached to a plastic trap. One tube is introduced into the baby's mouth or nostrils and the other tube is used for sucking out the secretions.

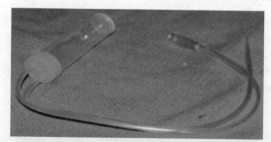

Fig. 10   De Lee's mucus sucker

The operator is protected from accidentally swallowing the secretions by the plastic trap wherein all the secretions are collected.

■ CORD CLAMP

Cord clamps (Fig. 11) made of plastic have largely replaced cord ties and strings. They are supplied as sterile packs. There are two serrated arms which fit into one another with a lock.

- The clamps are left *in situ* till the cord falls off.
- Caution should be exercised when the cord is thick or more gelatinous, when there is a risk of the clamp slipping.

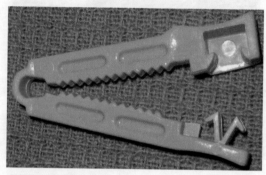

Fig. 11   Cord clamp

■ SIMS SPECULUM

Sims speculum (Fig. 12) is the most commonly used speculum in obstetrics and gynecology. It is also known as the duck-bill speculum.

Its role in obstetrics is limited. It is used:

- To visualise the vagina and cervix following instrumental vaginal delivery.
- To rule out any vaginal or cervical tear when traumatic postpartum hemorrhage is suspected.
- For the evacuation of the uterus in missed abortion or inevitable abortion and also in medical termination of pregnancy.

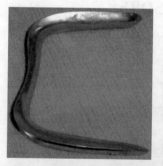 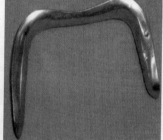

Fig. 12   Sims speculum

■ CUSCO'S SPECULUM

Cusco's speculum (Fig. 13) is a self-retaining speculum and hence there is no need for an assistant to hold the speculum. Its role in obstetrics is limited.

- It can be used in the evacuation of products of conception as in abortion.

- This speculum is useful in cases where antenatal pap smear needs to be done routinely.

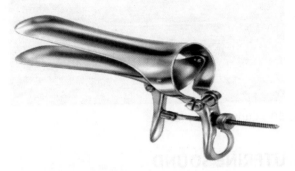

Fig. 13 Cusco's speculum

■ HEGAR'S DILATOR

Hegar's dilator (Fig. 14) is used more commonly in obstetric practice as it is less traumatic. It has a round body with tapering ends. Each end is of two different sizes.

It can be used:

- For dilating the cervix prior to first trimester evacuation of the uterus.
- In the evacuation of vesicular mole.
- As a method to diagnose an incompetent cevical os.

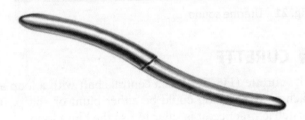

Fig. 14 Hegar's dilator

■ MATHEW DUNCAN DILATOR

The Mathew Duncan dilator (Fig. 15) is used more commonly in gynecological procedures. Each dilator is long and unlike the Hegar's dilator, is only of one size. The indications are as for the Hegar's dilator.

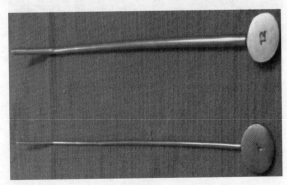

Fig. 15 Mathew Duncan dilator

■ TOOTHED FORCEPS

The toothed forceps (Fig. 16) come in various sizes. The tip of the instrument has a single tooth-like projection which fits into the corresponding hollow on the opposite end.

- They are used for holding the skin during episiotomy suture or for skin suture following cesarean section.
- Since the tooth is sharp and can be very painful, they should not be used without local anesthesia during episiotomy suturing.

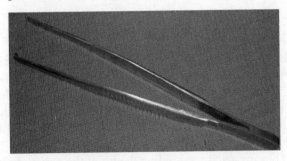

Fig. 16 Toothed forceps

■ ALLIS TISSUE FORCEPS

The Allis tissue forceps (Fig. 17) are available in two sizes. The end of the blade has three to four teeth-like projections. A lock is also provided in the handle.

They are used for:

- Holding the rectus sheath both during cutting and also during its suturing.
- For holding the cut edges of the uterus in cesarean section.

Since the teeth could be traumatic, they should be used with caution in obstetric practice.

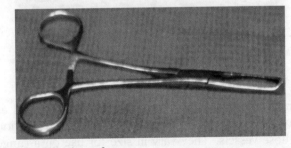

Fig. 17 Allis tissue forceps

■ BABCOCK'S FORCEPS

Babcock's forceps (Fig. 18) are used extensively:

- In female sterilisation to hold the fallopian tube
- To hold the vas in vasectomy
- To hold the appendix
- To hold any tissue with minimal trauma

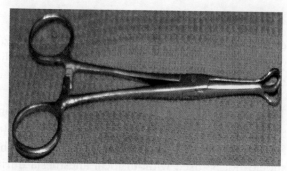

Fig. 18   Babcock's forceps

■ VOLSELLUM FORCEPS

Volsellum forceps (Fig. 19) are a long instrument with minimal curvature of the blades. The tip of the blade has three teeth-like projections which fit into the hollow in between two teeth-like projections on the other blade. This gives a good grip on the structure held by the forceps.

They are used for holding the lip of the cervix. Since they can traumatise a pregnant cervix, their use in obstetrics is restricted to early first trimester for the evacuation of the uterus.

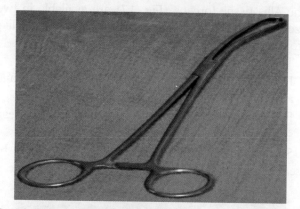

Fig. 19   Volsellum forceps

■ CURVED ARTERY FORCEPS

Curved artery forceps (Fig. 20) are primarily used as hemostatic forceps to grasp vessels and allow ligation of those vessels. They vary in size for use on a range of vessels, from fine, delicate vessels to large vascular pedicles. Artery forceps can also be used to grasp tissues, sutures and other prosthetic materials.

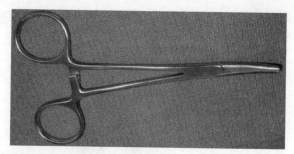

Fig. 20   Curved artery forceps

■ UTERINE SOUND

Uterine sound (Fig. 21) is used for measuring the cervical length. It has a handle with a long portion which is graduated in inches or centimeters to measure the length of the cervix. It not only measures the uterine length but also the direction of the uterus—anteversion or retroversion.

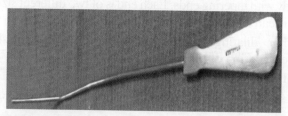

Fig. 21   Uterine sound

■ CURETTE

The curette (Fig. 22) has a central shaft with a loop at each end. The loop could be either blunt or sharp. In obstetric practice, it is safer to use the blunt loop.

It can be used for the following purposes:

- To check curettage following evacuation of uterus.
- After evacuation of a vesicular mole.
- To remove any retained placental bits in postpartum hemorrhage.
- To confirm the completeness of the procedure of termination of pregnancy.

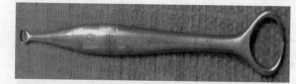

Fig. 22   Curette

Index